HANDBOOK OF

Institutional Pharmacy Practice

HANDBOOK OF

Institutional Pharmacy Practice

Edited by

Thomas R. Brown, M.S., Pharm. D.

Professor of Health Care Administration
and Clinical Pharmacy Practice
School of Pharmacy
University of Mississippi

Mickey C. Smith, Ph.D.

Professor
Department of Health Care Administration
School of Pharmacy
University of Mississippi

SECOND EDITION

WILLIAMS & WILKINS

Baltimore • London • Los Angeles • Sydney

Editor: John Butler
Associate Editor: Victoria M. Vaughn
Production: Anne G. Seitz

Accurate indications, adverse reactions, and dosage schedules for drugs are provided
in this book, but it is possible that they may change. The reader is urged to review
the package information data of the manufacturers of the medications mentioned.

Made in the United States of America

First edition published 1979

Library of Congress Cataloging in Publication Data

Main entry under title:

Handbook of institutional pharmacy practice.

    Includes bibliographies and index.
    1. Hospital pharmacies. I. Brown, Thomas R.
II. Smith, Mickey C. [DNLM: 1. Pharmacy
Administration. 2. Pharmacy Service, Hospital
WX 179 H236]
RA975.5.P5H28 1986   362.1'782   85-12091
ISBN 0-683-01090-5

86 87 88 89 90   10 9 8 7 6 5 4 3 2 1

DEDICATION

To

George and Lottie Lester

and

Bonnie, Dennis, and Jeffrey

TRB

To

Franklin W. Dixon (all of them), who introduced me to the glory
of the printed word, and to my family

MCS

Preface

More frequently than not, a second edition of a book is indicative of at least reasonable success with a first edition. Since the first edition "was designed for both student and practitioner" with the hope of providing the former "with a thorough grounding in institutional pharmacy" and the latter "with a ready reference to use in addressing any problem in practice," there seems little need to modify the logic but rather to improve on the substance.

The adopted framework for organization of this edition is the competency statement of the American Society of Hospital Pharmacists. We urge careful reading of this statement since it provides considerable insight into the nature of practice as well as the expected talents required to be a competent pharmacist. As editors, we endeavored to identify talented people to further define and explore the elements of competency in a given subject area. As in the first edition, we attempted to use practitioners as authors to the extent possible.

The extent of success of the book relies on the ability of each author to distill a large volume of material into a single contribution that hopefully will provide an appreciation for the nature and scope of the subject. As a supplement to these contributions, we urge the reader to purchase the *Practice Standards of the American Society of Hospital Pharmacists*. These extremely important standards and guidelines were included as appendices in the first edition, but in keeping with current cost-containment concepts in practice, it was decided to strongly encourage the reader to purchase them as a separate reference. Their importance to this book as well as to the development of practice and competencies to practice cannot be overemphasized.

In a reference text to which so many have contributed, it is difficult to retain consistency in form and content. In fact, it is probably not totally desirable to do so from an editorial point of view. It may be helpful for the reader to remember that texts are references which, in general, seem never complete, perhaps because the topics they cover are themselves incomplete. The prudent student or practitioner will continue to update this reference through knowledge of current practice as well as current literature.

As was the case with the first edition, this text is intended as a practical guide, but it does not ignore the underlying theory important to the practice. It further attempts to provide material of value to pharmacists in any institutional setting. It should not be construed as "all things to all institutional practitioners," but rather as a framework from which a healthy understanding of the required competencies can be obtained.

Thomas R. Brown
Mickey C. Smith

Acknowledgments

The editors appreciate the assistance of everyone who contributed to this and the first edition, for without individual contributions the collective work would not be possible. Special appreciation is due the American Society of Hospital Pharmacists for their development of acknowledged standards for hospital pharmacy practice, including the competencies required for practice on which this book is based.

At the University of Mississippi, graduate students Pat Condon and Li-Yin Yang were especially helpful. To Karen Mifflin and Pat Henderson, for their typing and understanding, a grateful thanks.

To those contributors who agreed to contribute and further met their deadlines, we owe a special debt of gratitude.

Bonnie Brown and Mary Smith, who agreed to "love" and "honor," if not "obey," gave us their long-standing support, which provided an opportunity to complete this work.

Contributors

Ann B. Amerson, Pharm.D.
Associate Professor and Director, Drug Information Center, College of Pharmacy, University of Kentucky, Lexington, Kentucky

David M. Arrington, M.S.
Department of Pharmacy Services, Carnegie 180, The Johns Hopkins Hospital, Baltimore, Maryland

Kenneth N. Barker, Ph.D.
Professor and Head, Pharmacy Care Systems, School of Pharmacy, Auburn University, Auburn University, Alabama

Thomas R. Brown, M.S., Pharm.D.
Associate Professor, Health Care Administration and Clinical Pharmacy Practice, School of Pharmacy, University of Mississippi, University, Mississippi

G. Edward Collins, M.S.
Research Triangle Park, North Carolina

James W. Cooper, Jr., Ph.D., F.C.P.
Professor and Head, Department of Pharmacy Practice, College of Pharmacy, University of Georgia, Athens, Georgia

Timothy R. Covington, Pharm.D.
Professor and Chairman, Department of Clinical Pharmacy, School of Pharmacy, West Virginia University Medical Center, and Associate Director of Pharmaceutical Services for Academic Affairs, West Virginia University Hospitals, Inc., Morgantown, West Virginia

Frederic R. Curtiss, Ph.D., R.Ph.
Vice President, Reimbursement Services, HPI Health Care Services, Inc., Los Angeles, California

William J. Dana, Pharm.D.
Director, Drug Information and Clinical Services, Department of Pharmacy, M.D. Anderson Hospital and Tumor Institute, Houston, Texas

Charles E. Daniels, Ph.D.
Assistant Director, Pharmaceutical Services, University of Minnesota Hospitals, Minneapolis, Minnesota

Mary Lou Ebbert, Pharm.D.
Berwyn, Illinois

W. Gary Erwin, Pharm.D.
Assistant Professor, Clinical Pharmacy, The Philadelphia College of Pharmacy and Sciences, Philadelphia, Pennsylvania

Ronald P. Evens, Pharm.D.
Assistant Director, Clinical Research, Medical Department, Bristol Laboratories, Syracuse, New York

Joseph L. Fink III, J.D.
Assistant Dean and Professor, College of Pharmacy, and Professor of Health Administration, College of Allied Health Professions, Albert B. Chandler Medical Center, University of Kentucky, Lexington, Kentucky

Robert A. Freeman, Ph.D.
The Upjohn Company, Kalamazoo, Michigan

Joseph F. Gallelli, Ph.D.
Chief, Pharmacy Department, The Clinical Center, Department of Health and Human Services, Public Health Service, National Institutes of Health, Bethesda, Maryland

James B. Gantenberg
Staff Assistant to the President, American College of Hospital Administrators, Chicago, Illinois

Dewey D. Garner, Ph.D.
Professor, Health Care Administration, School of Pharmacy, University of Mississippi, University, Mississippi

Ms. Jacqueline P. Gary, RN, BS
Vice President for Professional Services, Dallas–Fort Worth Hospital Council, Dallas, Texas

William K. Ginnow
Director, Health Services, Group Health Plan of Greater St. Louis, St. Louis, Missouri

Jeanette Bousquet Goudreau, M.S.
Department of Pharmacy, Brockton Hospital, Brockton, Massachusetts

Dick R. Gourley, Pharm.D.
Dean, Southern School of Pharmacy, Mercer University, Atlanta, Georgia

William A. Gouveia
Director, Pharmacy, New England Medical Center, Boston, Massachusetts

George J. Grimes, Jr., B.S.
Supervisory Pharmacist, Pharmaceutical Development Service Section, Pharmacy Department, The Clinical Center, National Institutes of Health, Department of Health and Human Services, Bethesda, Maryland

Zachary I. Hanan
Assistant Director, Department of Pharmacy, Cabrini Medical Center, New York, New York

Philip D. Hansten, Pharm.D.
Associate Professor, Clinical Pharmacy, College of Pharmacy, Washington State University, Spokane, Washington

Joseph A. Harris, M.B.A.
Director, Department of Pharmaceutical Services, Sinai Hospital of Detroit, Detroit, Michigan

Charles D. Hepler, Ph.D.
Associate Professor, Pharmacy and Pharmaceutics, Virginia Commonwealth University, Richmond, Virginia

James M. Hethcox
Director, Pharmacy, Presbyterian Hospital, Oklahoma City, Oklahoma

Paul K. Hiranaka, B.S.
Pharmacist Review Officer, Office of Biologics Research and Review, Center for Drugs and Biologics, Food and Drug Administration, Bethesda, Maryland

William B. Hladik III, M.S.
Associate Professor, College of Pharmacy, University of New Mexico, Albuquerque, New Mexico

Clifford E. Hynniman, M.S.
Director, Pharmacy/Central Supply, University Hospital, Albert B. Chandler Medical Center, University of Kentucky, Lexington, Kentucky

Rodney D. Ice, Ph.D.
President, Triar Enterprises, Edmond, Oklahoma

Louis P. Jeffrey, Sc.D.
Director, Pharmacy Services, Rhode Island Hospital, Providence, Rhode Island

Ralph Kalies, Ph.D.
President, Konsult, Oskosh, Wisconsin

Ingo S. Kampa, Ph.D.
Head, Clinical Chemistry, Department of Pathology, Valley Hospital, Ridgewood, New Jersey

Charles M. King, Jr.
Assistant Vice President, HCA Management Company, Nashville, Tennessee

James C. King, Ph.D.
Professor, Clinical Pharmacy, School of Pharmacy, University of the Pacific, Stockton, California

Duane M. Kirking, Ph.D.
Assistant Professor, Pharmacy Administration, College of Pharmacy, The University of Michigan, Ann Arbor, Michigan

Michael L. Kleinberg, M.S.
Director, Pharmacy, Memorial Sloan-Kettering Care Center, New York, New York

David A. Knapp, Ph.D.
Professor, School of Pharmacy, University of Maryland, Baltimore, Maryland

Herman Lazarus, M.S.
Director, Pharmacy Services, University of Alabama Medical Center, Birmingham, Alabama

Dennis W. Mackewicz, Pharm.D.
Senior Associate Director, Pharmacy Services, Memorial Medical Center of Long Beach, Long Beach, California

Leslie Reuss Mackowiak, B.S.
Pharmacy Supervisor, Duke University Medical Center, Durham, North Carolina

John I. Mackowiak, Ph.D.
Assistant Professor, Pharmacy Administration, School of Pharmacy, University of North Carolina, Chapel Hill, North Carolina

Ray R. Maddox, Pharm.D.
Associate Director for Clinical and Educational Programs, Department of Pharmaceutical Services, Emory University Hospital, Atlanta, Georgia

Charles D. Mahoney, M.S.
Associate Director, Pharmacy Services, Rhode Island Hospital, Providence, Rhode Island

James C. McAllister, M.S.
Associate Director, Pharmacy, Duke University Medical Center, Durham, North Carolina

Alan B. McKay, Ph.D.
Assistant Professor, Pharmacy Practice, School of Pharmacy, University of Maryland, Baltimore, Maryland

Robert F. Miller, M.S.
Director, Pharmacy Services, Stanford University Hospital, Palo Alto, California

Jay M. Mirtallo, M.S.
Clinical Pharmacist, Nutrition Support Service, Department of Pharmacy, The Ohio State Hospital, Columbus, Ohio

Joseph M. Morrissey, M.S.
Department of Pharmacy, Brockton Hospital, Brockton, Massachusetts

Charles E. Myers
Associate Director, Pharmacy Services, Medical College of Virginia Hospitals, and Assistant Professor, School of Pharmacy, Virginia Commonwealth University, Richmond, Virginia

Arthur A. Nelson, Jr., Ph.D.
Dean, College of Pharmacy, University of Nebraska, Omaha, Nebraska

Paul W. Niemiec, Jr., Pharm.D.
Clinical Pharmacy Coordinator, Surgery—Critical Care Division, The Johns Hopkins Hospital, Baltimore, Maryland

Michael Norvell, Pharm.D.
Assistant Professor, Clinical Pharmacy, Department of Pharmacy Practice, College of Pharmacy, University of Nebraska, Omaha, Nebraska

Welton O'Neal, Jr., Pharm.D.
Assistant Professor and Clinical Pharmacist in Pediatrics, Department of Pharmacy Services, Medical University of South Carolina and Medical University of South Carolina Hospital, Charleston, South Carolina

Jayant A. Patel, Pharm.D.
Director, Drug Analysis and Toxicology Laboratory, University of Michigan Hospitals, Ann Arbor, Michigan

Robert E. Pearson, M.S.
Associate Professor, Hospital Pharmacy, Pharmacy Care Systems, School of Pharmacy, Auburn University, Auburn University, Alabama

John J. Piecoro, Jr., Pharm.D.
Professor, Division of Clinical Practice, College of Pharmacy, University of Kentucky, Lexington, Kentucky

James A. Ponto, M.S.
Nuclear Pharmacist, University of Iowa Hospitals & Clinics, and Associate Clinical Professor, College of Pharmacy, The University of Iowa, Iowa City, Iowa

Michael F. Powell, M.S.
Associate Director, Pharmacy Services, Detroit Receiving Hospital and University Health Center, and Adjunct Assistant Professor, Hospital Pharmacy, Wayne State University College of Pharmacy and Allied Health, Detroit, Michigan

George Provost, M.S. (Deceased)

Stephen L. Priest
Director, Information Resources, Brockton Hospital, Brockton, Massachusetts

C. Eugene Reeder, Ph.D.
Assistant Professor, Pharmacy Administration, College of Pharmacy, University of South Carolina, Columbia, South Carolina

Thomas P. Reinders, Pharm.D.
Associate Professor of Pharmacy and Associate Director of Pharmacy Services, Medical College of Virginia, Virginia Commonwealth University, Richmond, Virginia

M. J. Roberts, M.S.
Assistant Director of Pharmacy for Patient Service, Hermann Hospital, Houston, Texas

Jack M. Rosenberg, Ph.D.
Associate Professor and Director, Clinical Pharmacy, Arnold and Marie Schwartz College of Pharmacy and Health Sciences, Long Island University, Brooklyn, New York

Bruce E. Scott, M.S.
Assistant Professor and Assistant Director, Pharmacy, University of Kansas Medical Center, Kansas City, Kansas

Neal W. Schwartau
Director, Pharmacy and Central Supply, Rochester Methodist Hospital, Rochester, Minnesota

Hazel H. Seaba, M.S.
Clinical Associate Professor and Director, Iowa Drug Information Service, The University of Iowa, Iowa City, Iowa

Thomas R. Sharpe, Ph.D.
Acting Director, Research Institute of Pharmaceutical Sciences, University of Mississippi, University, Mississippi

Harold M. Silverman, Pharm.D.
Rye, New York

F. Mauriece Smith, M.S.
Supervisor, Pharmaceutical Production, University of Kansas Medical Center, Department of Pharmacy, Kansas City, Kansas

Mickey C. Smith, Ph.D.
Professor, Health Care Administration, University of Mississippi, University, Mississippi

William E. Smith, Pharm.D., M.P.H.
Director, Pharmacy Services, Memorial Medical Center of Long Beach, Long Beach, California

Glen L. Stimmel, Pharm.D.
Associate Professor, Clinical Pharmacy, Clinical Psychiatry and The Behavioral Sciences, School of Pharmacy, University of Southern California, Los Angeles, California

Ronald B. Stewart, M.S.
Professor and Chairman, Department of Pharmacy Practice, College of Pharmacy, University of Florida, Gainesville, Florida

Marc Summerfield, M.S.
Director, Pharmacy, Arkansas Children's Hospital, Little Rock, Arkansas

Bonnie L. Svarstad, Ph.D.
Associate Professor, Social Studies of Pharmacy, School of Pharmacy, University of Wisconsin, Madison, Wisconsin

Carmencita Tranquilino, B.S.
Director, Pharmacy, TLC Advanced Home Therapies Inc., New Hyde Park, New York

Timothy W. Vanderveen, M.S., Pharm.D.
Clinical Affairs Department, IMED Corporation, San Diego, California

Albert I. Wertheimer, Ph.D.
Professor and Chairman, Department of Graduate Studies in Social and Administrative Pharmacy, University of Minnesota, Minneapolis, Minnesota

Henry F. Wedemeyer, M.S.
Director of Pharmacy, Saint Luke's Hospital, Denver, Colorado

Stuart A. Wesbury, Jr., Ph.D., F.A.C.H.A.
President, American College of Hospital Administrators, Chicago, Illinois

Sara J. White, M.S.
Associate Director, Pharmacy Services, University of Kansas Medical Center, Kansas City, Kansas

Robert B. Williams, M.S.P.
Clinical Professor and Assistant Dean, College of Pharmacy, and Director, Department of Pharmacy, Shands Hospital, University of Florida, J. Hillis Miller Health Center, Gainesville, Florida

Michael Z. Wincor, Pharm.D.
School of Pharmacy, University of Southern California, Los Angeles, California

W. Allan Woodward
Department of Pharmacy Services, Rochester Methodist Hospital, Rochester, Minnesota

David Zilz, M.S.
Director, Pharmacy, Respiratory Care and Materials Services, and Clinical Professor, University of Wisconsin–Madison, Madison, Wisconsin

ASHP Guidelines on the Competencies Required in Institutional Pharmacy Practice

Preface

The practice of pharmacy in health care institutions continues to undergo evolutionary and even radical changes. It has changed to a personal health service charged with assuring pharmaceutic and therapeutic appropriateness of all its functions in the care of patients. Professional, societal, governmental and economic factors will continue to force further changes and the pharmacist practicing in an institution must be ready not only to adapt to these changes but to take the lead in introducing them. In all cases, the basis for the institutional pharmacist's contribution to health care is a thorough knowledge of drugs and their actions. To bring this expertise to bear in the most effective manner, the institutional pharmacist must interact and cooperate closely with all other health professionals practicing in the institution and he must assist the patient and the patient's family to cope with the problems of illness.

It is recognized that a large and diverse body of expertise is required in the operation of a pharmacy department. No one pharmacist may possess or have opportunity to demonstrate this breadth of expertise. For a variety of reasons, some institutions offer greater opportunity than others for the pharmacist to use his unique skills. All institutional pharmacists should, however, develop minimal competencies in each area and be capable of becoming expert in any one or several of them. This requires more than casual acquaintance with a broad area of knowledge and emphasizes the need for a sound professional education grounded on a firm base of physical, biological and social sciences.

This statement addresses itself to the various competencies which must be demonstrated collectively by the professional staff of an institutional pharmacy department. The statement recognizes not only the need for but the responsibility of a department to make pharmaceutical services available to both inpatients and ambulatory patients as well as to promote the rational use of drugs by health professionals and the public. The department must participate in all programs and functions of the institution where pharmaceutical expertise is needed. The professional staff of the pharmacy department must have the ability to carry out collectively the following service functions.

I. Effective Administration and Management of a Pharmacy Department in an Institution

The successful delivery of any pharmacy service offered will be based on expert management and administrative procedures. The director of pharmacy services or personnel specializing in departmental administration must be familiar with the health care system in general and the specific function of the institution in particular so that the pharmacy's goals can be achieved in cooperation with all other departments in the institution and with other programs that insure continuity of care for the patient.

Broad areas of administrative and management responsibilities include planning and integrating professional services, budgeting, inventory control, cost review, cost effectiveness, audit, maintenance of records and preparation of reports. As a basis for this responsibility, pharmacy personnel must be thoroughly familiar with the organization of a hospital, with staff and line relationships and with appropriate lines of communication.

Pharmacy activities must be coordinated with medical, nursing and other services and with the administrative elements of the hospital. Pharmacy administrative personnel must be able to prepare suitable written communications to the hospital staff concerning pertinent pharmacy matters.

The director of pharmacy services, or his designee, is responsible for the justification and accountability of all pharmaceutical services in terms of patient care and the expenditure of funds. He must be able to analyze and interpret prescribing trends and the economic impact of new drug developments, which for budgeting purposes are translated to his forecast of future drug expenditures. He must maintain an adequate system of stock and inventory control. He must have the ability to control operational costs without compromising services.

The director of pharmacy services is responsible for records on all pharmacy operations which may be legally or administratively required. The data collected should be translated into periodic or special reports. These may include, but usually are not limited to, data on prescriptions dispensed, controlled drugs dispensed, drug purchases, inspections and improvements in operations. The use of au-

xv

tomated data processing systems may allow more effective and efficient handling of pharmacy records and data. A basic knowledge and understanding of the applications of such systems to pharmacy operations is important to the department.

II. Assimilation and Provision of Comprehensive Information on Drugs and Their Actions

Fundamental to the pharmacist's contribution to health care is his knowledge of drugs and their actions. The pharmacy department is the primary source of information concerning drugs. The pharmacy must maintain the appropriate information sources and develop mechanisms for evaluating information and transmitting it to the institution's professional staff and to patients.

The pharmacist must have the ability to use his basic science knowledge and his knowledge of the effects of drugs on biological systems in assessing such determinants of drug action as absorption, distribution, metabolism and excretion of a drug; drug interactions with other drugs, foods or diagnostic agents; effects of a disease state on the drug's action; and miscellaneous patient and drug variables. Thus, the pharmacist practicing in an institution must be knowledgeable in chemistry, pharmacology, toxicology, pathophysiology, pharmaceutics, therapeutics, and patient care techniques, and he should have some background in the social sciences.

III. Development and Conduct of a Product Formulation and Packaging Program

Frequently, the institutional pharmacist must respond to the need for special dosage forms and formulations not available commercially. Not infrequently, this also involves a knowledge of appropriate packaging. An adequate understanding of the principles involved in the formulation and preparation of pharmaceutical dosage forms is needed. This involves the concepts of biopharmaceutics, bioavailability, pharmacokinetics, pharmaceutics, stability, physicochemical, kinetics, microbiology, quality assurance and techniques of medication administration. In some instances, as in the case of intravenous admixtures and total parenteral nutrition, the pharmacist must also be familiar with patient variables such as electrolyte and fluid balance, and such factors as personal hygiene, environmental control and equipment performance. Similar concepts hold true in radiopharmacy. Furthermore, the pharmacist must be able to evaluate the economic factors involved, including the cost of labor, raw materials, space, equipment depreciation and other items of fixed overhead.

IV. Conduct of and Participation in Research

The institutional pharmacist must be prepared to participate in clinical research originated by the medical staff and to conduct pharmaceutical research or initiate research himself. In doing so, he may act as the principal or coprincipal investigator or he may use the resources of the department to support a particular research study. The pharmacist must be able to establish a data base, either for the drugs being used or the patients participating in the study. Equally important, he must have the ability to collect appropriate data, interpret them, apply the conclusions drawn from the data and transmit the results in an adequate manner.

An educational background with appropriate orientation and training in research methodology, including criteria for and structure of a research report, is mandatory.

V. Development and Conduct of Patient-oriented Services

Pharmacy, as practiced in health care institutions, is developing a wide spectrum of clinical services which have become part of overall pharmaceutical service but may not be directly associated with drug distribution. Fundamental to these clinical services is the pharmacist's knowledge of drugs, diseases and patient and drug variables, and his ability to interact closely on a personal basis with other health professionals. Academic training in such areas as toxicology, pathophysiology and therapeutics, as well as extensive clinical experience, provide the background for a pharmacist to function in this clinical role.

These services include (1) drug information, which encompasses the collection, organization, retrieval, interpretation and evaluation of the applicable literature and the ability to present the excerpted data in an appropriate fashion; (2) collection of the pharmacy patient data base; (3) patient education; (4) the monitoring (either subjectively or objectively) and auditing of therapeutic regimens; (5) drug use review; (6) the monitoring of specific adverse drug reactions to decrease their incidence; and (7) other similar functions designed to improve patient care by optimizing drug use. Further, clinical functions may extend to the pharmacist's role in primary care as well as in the management of chronic care patients.

VI. Conduct of and Participation in Educational Activities

A wide range of educational activities is performed routinely in the institution and involves all health practitioners and students of the various health professions. The director of pharmacy services, or his designee, is responsible for coordinating the department's contribution to these educational activities. Further, he is responsible for training new personnel and for carrying on a continuous educational program for pharmacists and pharmacy supportive personnel. In institutions having a pharmacy residency program, the pharmacist must develop a well planned and coordinated program so that the residency is a meaningful educational experience in the development of future practitioners. In institutions offering a pharmacy residency program in conjunction with an academic program, the pharmacist must have a thorough understanding of his own program and the course material and objectives of the academic phase to assist in coordinating one with the other.

VII. Development and Conduct of a Quality Assurance Program for Pharmaceutical Services

A major responsibility of the department must be the assurance of the quality of its services and of products dispensed, coupled with a control program for the distribution of drugs throughout the institution.

The pharmacist must conduct service audits, either by process or outcome, or both, to assure the quality of patient care services rendered and to assure the appropriate patient benefit of all pharmaceutical services offered.

Contents

SECTION III/Drug Information and Drug Actions **247**

SECTION IV/Product Formulation, Packaging, and Distribution **323**

SECTION V/Research **423**

SECTION VI/Patient-Oriented Services **507**

SECTION VII/Educational Activities **591**

Overview

As noted in the Preface, the materials in this *Handbook* are built around the Guidelines on the Competencies Required in Institutional Pharmacy Practice of the American Society of Hospital Pharmacists. Relevant excerpts from those Guidelines appear at the beginning of each section of this *Handbook*. The intact Guidelines appear just before Section I. The Preface to the Guidelines follows.

The practice of pharmacy in health care institutions continues to undergo evolutionary and even radical changes. It has changed to a personal health service charged with assuring pharmaceutic and therapeutic appropriateness of all its functions in the care of patients. Professional, societal, governmental and economic factors will continue to force further changes and the pharmacist practicing in an institution must be ready not only to adapt to these changes but to take the lead in introducing them. In all cases, the basis for the institutional pharmacist's contribution to health care is a thorough knowledge of drugs and their actions. To bring this expertise to bear in the most effective manner, the institutional pharmacist must interact and cooperate closely with all other health professionals practicing in the institution and he must assist the patient and the patient's family to cope with the problems of illness.

It is recognized that a large and diverse body of expertise is required in the operation of a pharmacy department. No one pharmacist may possess or have opportunity to demonstrate this breadth of expertise. For a variety of reasons, some institutions offer greater opportunity than others for the pharmacist to use his unique skills. All institutional pharmacists should, however, develop minimal competencies in each area and be capable of becoming expert in any one or several of them. This requires more than casual acquaintance with a broad area of knowledge and emphasizes the need for a sound professional education grounded on a firm base of physical, biological and social sciences.

This statement addresses itself to the various competencies which must be demonstrated collectively by the professional staff of an institutional pharmacy department. The statement recognizes not only the need for but the responsibility of a department to make pharmaceutical services available to both inpatients and ambulatory patients as well as to promote the rational use of drugs by health professionals and the public. The department must participate in all programs and functions of the institution where pharmaceutical expertise is needed. The professional staff of the pharmacy department must have the ability to carry out collectively the following service functions.

CHAPTER 1

Health Care Institutions and the Health Care System

ALBERT I. WERTHEIMER and FREDERIC R. CURTISS

"If you are not part of the solution, then you must be part of the problem."
ELDRIDGE CLEAVER
Soul on Ice

It is essential for the pharmacist as well as any helping professional to understand the environment or universe in which we function. The health care delivery system is the second largest industry in the United States, and it is important for us to know who does what and the means for reaching them. Moreover, by understanding the area of activity and the capabilities and limitations for each of the nearly 400 professions and subprofessional groups identified within that system, we are better able to make informed decisions. The conscientious pharmacist will know where patients may be served and how they may be referred, the differences in costs and prices for various types of care and the legal, organizational, political, and, most important, economic considerations involved in the delivery of health care services. We owe patients no less than this.

Pharmacists in patient care settings will be called upon to answer questions and provide explanations to patients and to their families and friends. Taking time to explain the details of a particular diagnostic test or to discuss the advantages and safeguards of transferring a patient to a given facility may be more valuable, and surely less harmful, than simply dispensing drugs intended to deal with problems such as anxiety arising from the uncertainty surrounding these events.

The first step to take in becoming a problem solver for patients is to gain a perspective on the U.S. health care delivery system. This perspective then should help us to serve patients seeking referral and information, as well as to be a reliable and trusted source of drugs and related products.

PERSPECTIVE ON THE HEALTH CARE SYSTEM

Health has to do with well-being and the ability to engage in the activities that we want to be able to do. As such, "health" is a personal and emotional matter. Small wonder, then, that the availability, quality, and cost of health care services are as important as social/political issues. This prominence in the social political arena guarantees political debate and legislation intended to improve the quality of the health care system or access to it or to moderate its cost. In the 1980s and beyond, the focus is on the cost of health care services and ways to moderate these costs. This focus on *costs* contrasts with the greater attention paid to *access* to health care services during the 1950s and 1960s and to the *quality* of health care in the 1970s.

Concern regarding the cost of health care has lead to significant legislative changes by federal and state legislators and regulatory changes by federal and state agencies. The legislative and regulatory changes are affecting the financing of health care services. As the method of payment for services and the financial incentives change, significant effects are being seen in the organizational structure of the health care system. Proprietary companies, once insignificant in the health care delivery system, now are becoming increasingly important determinants of the shape of this system. Financial incentives are causing a change in focus away from the acute care hospital as the center of the health care system to alternative care delivery sites, including emergency and surgical care centers, and home health care. While the direction of future changes may be difficult to predict, what is not speculative is that change in the structure of the health care delivery system will be commonplace through the 1980s and probably into the 1990s. The pharmacist will be better prepared to serve patients in this changing environment through understanding the current health care delivery system, including its shortcomings, and how this system evolved.

In our study of the health care delivery system, the first thing that strikes us is that it is not really a "system" at all, but rather a quasisystem of health care delivery that often lacks organization and a rational distribution of services. Gaps and overlaps, undercare and overcare result in many patients not receiving the care they need and others receiving perhaps too much care (1). Moreover, virtually all care commands high prices. Throughout this and any examination of the health care delivery system, it is particularly helpful to think of the major issues, problems, and solutions in terms of three evaluative parameters: *cost, quality,* and *access.*

In your analysis of the health care system, it will become clear that the problems associated with the delivery of health care have not gone unanswered. Indeed, the number of proposed solutions probably exceeds the number of problems. Remember that the generation and choice of solutions probably is directed as much by politics and emotion as by rationality. Appropriate balance often is not achieved among the parameters of access, quality, and cost. Our analysis here will involve a review of the major shortcomings in current "systems" of health care delivery in the hope of obtaining insight to help us in our task of providing efficient, optimal care.

MALDISTRIBUTION OF PERSONNEL

The U.S. health care delivery system probably has sufficient resources to meet all patient needs, but proper distribution of these resources is still problematic. Geographic distribution of manpower, particularly physicians, is a major concern of experts and planners in health care. Some states have over 1000 persons for each practicing physician, while others have just over 400 (2). Many communities are completely without physician services, while some urban and suburban areas of the country report physician-to-population ratios two and three times that of rural and economically depressed urban areas (3,4). Furthermore, the percentage of physicians reporting patient care as their major activity has declined to about 85% (5).

Efforts intended to encourage physicians to establish practice in "physician shortage areas" have been attempted by federal, state, and local governments and by many private institutions (6). And despite significant spending in these programs, population size continues to influence practice location for many categories of physicians; the best predictors of distribution of physicians are median area income (7) and factors unrelated to the health care needs of the population (8).

Maldistribution of the total number practicing physicians also is coupled with an inadequate distribution by type of practice. The "specialty" of general practice has a particularly acute physician shortage. The proportion of physicians in general practice has declined steadily over the years to less than 15% in 1981, and this figure includes more than 7000 physicians in family practice (5). The specialties, particularly surgery, continue to attract an increasing proportion of physicians, and American specialty boards now number 23. The fastest growing physician specialities over the 10-year period from 1971 to 1981 were radiology, neurology, and gastroenterology.

Adequate distribution of physicians is a concern extending even beyond maldistribution by geography and type of practice. As we have seen, the proportion of physicians engaged in direct patient care has decreased to the point

where only four out of five physicians are treating patients directly (9). Further, specialization has decreased patient access to general practitioners. Access to the health care delivery system for the poor and for minorities is even less than for whites, with the portal of entry being the hospital emergency room or outpatient department or the community clinic rather than private practitioners (10). In addition, women physicians still accounted for less than 10% of the total number of physicians in 1982 (11).

While other providers such as dentists, pharmacists, and nurses may not be quite as maldistributed as physicians, their distribution usually parallels that of physicians, contributing to the problem of difficult access to care for many persons.

MALDISTRIBUTION OF FACILITIES

Hospitals and other health care institutions may be defined by several characteristics, such as ownership, types of service rendered, size, average length of patient stay, etc. General acute care hospitals have become the center for the delivery of health care services in the United States over the last 50 years. The average length of patient stay in these short-term hospitals is less than 30 days. These are the most numerous of health care facilities, with approximately 4.4 beds/1000 population throughout the United States (12). In contrast to health care systems in other developed countries, the majority of hospitals in the United States are nongovernmental facilities. Acute care hospitals also are classified as to whether they are teaching institutions and, often, according to specialization and intensity of care. For example, some categories of specialty hospitals are those for children, mental diseases, women, tuberculosis, cancer, alcohol rehabilitation, and drug rehabilitation. Some hospitals, particularly small, rural hospitals, are equipped to handle only primary care patients and refer patients requiring more intensive or sophisticated services to other hospitals that possess intensive care units (ICUs), coronary care units (CCUs), burn units, etc. Hospitals providing sophisticated services, usually teaching hospitals, often are referred to as tertiary care facilities and are equipped to handle the most severely ill patients and those with rare diseases or other special needs.

Hospitals with the average length of stay of 30 days or more are referred to as long-term hospitals. Examples include hospitals focusing their care on mental disease, tuberculosis, rehabilitation, and some cancers. Long-term care services of a less acute nature also are provided by long-term care (LTC) facilities, generally referred to as "nursing homes." The two largest categories of nursing homes are intermediate care facilities (ICFs) and skilled nursing facilities (SNFs), differentiated largely by accreditation criteria, including the requirement that skilled nursing services be available 24 hours a day in a SNF.

While there was an average of 4.4 short-term hospital beds per 1000 population throughout the United States in 1982, there was not an even distribution of hospitals and other health care facilities according to geographic area and urban vs rural setting. Because of this maldistribution of health care facilities and services, care is not accessible to many population groups. National studies of medical care utilization indicate that persons who need health care are not necessarily those most likely to receive it (14). In particular, nonwhites, rural farm people, the poor, and those who do not have a regular source of care have been found to have less access than they "should," based on medical evaluation of severity of reported symptoms.

Various health plans have advocated a 30-minute travel time to general hospitals as a criterion of accessibility. Using this standard, 10% of the entire population (extrapolated from one state under study) and nearly 20% of rural residents live in areas of inaccessibility to health care services (15).

Accessibility to care is a function of more than the availability of services, however. Utilization of services also is impacted by economic and cultural barriers. Perceived symptoms and ability to pay are the major predictors of utilization of health services, and cultural barriers (e.g., cultural differences, expectations, and differential ordering of values) still exist when economics is no longer a barrier (16). Further, organizational barriers to entry, such as long queues to obtain services and long travel time to care in some areas, still exist (17). These organizational barriers contribute to problems of differential access and perpetuation of two levels of health care in this country, i.e., a level of care for the poor and a separate level of care for the nonpoor (18-20). Furthermore, while distribution statistics directly address the issues of patient access and efficiency in the delivery of services, variations in individual community requirements for health care are disregarded. Patterns of utilization of services (demand), as well as local health care needs, also should be considered. The supply of care, in terms of both health manpower and health facilities, is of principal interest as it relates availability of care to the needs of the local population.

REGIONALIZATION

The concept of regionalization of health care providers represents one approach to combating the maldistribution of personnel and facilities. The concept is based on tiered levels of care and adequate referral relationships. Primary ambulatory care is provided in small towns and rural areas. Secondary level care is provided by community hospitals in larger towns, such as the county seat. These community hospitals are linked to medical centers that provide tertiary care. Very specialized procedures may be performed by experts in tertiary care centers located in university teaching facilities. This tiered system of regionalized care requires local responsibility for medical care for specific population groups and formal and informal referral mechanisms to allow access to the proper level of care for all persons.

ORGANIZATIONAL CHANGES IN DELIVERY OF CARE

The social goal of making necessary and proper health care readily available to everybody has spawned major changes in the organization of health care services in the United States. Not many years ago, medical care was delivered from black bags toted by "family docs" who traveled from house to house, generally treating patients in their homes. Most of these practitioners worked alone, out of their own houses or possibly small, rented offices. Indeed, all of health care was organized as a "cottage industry," each individual practitioner working independently of other practitioners and facilities.

Today, physician solo practices are much less common. Solo physicians are more likely to practice in urban locations and in counties where per capita incomes are relatively high (21). Solo physicians are more highly concentrated in the older portions of the United States, such as New England and the mid-Atlantic areas, while the number of physicians in organized group practice is significantly greater in the Pacific Coast states. The Council on Medical Services of the American Medical Association (AMA) defines medical group practice as the delivery of medical services "by three or more physicians formally organized to provide medical care, consultation, diagnosis and/or treatment through the joint use of equipment and personnel, and with income from medical practice distributed in accordance with methods previously determined by members of the group."

Group practice has become increasingly popular as an organizational form and may be defined by the following three categories: single-specialty groups, composed of physicians restricting their practice to one specialty; general practice groups, composed only of general practitioners (or family medicine practitioners); and multispecialty groups, consisting of physicians in at least two major specialities. General practice groups possess characteristics that overlap with the other two groups, composed only of general practitioners (or family medicine practitioners); and multispecialty groups, consisting of physicians in at least two major specialities. General practice groups possess characteristics that overlap with the other two groups, resembling single-specialty groups in the provision of more diversified medical care services.

Pharmacy, like medicine, shows less resemblance to a "cottage industry" today. More and more health care is being delivered through institutions. Hospitals and chain pharmacies* have recorded steady, substantial increases in prescription dispensing. In the early 1900s, independent community pharmacies dispensed virtually all prescriptions filled in this country. Today, hospitals dispense prescriptions to outpatients as well as deliver drugs and intravenous solutions to inpatients, and chain pharmacies now dispense 27% of all retail prescriptions in the United States (22). Many medical clinics also have incorporated pharmacy services in their delivery of care. This trend toward institutional pharmacy practice is in sharp contrast to the one-man drugstores and apothecaries that were so characteristic at the turn of the century. Small pharmacies continue to be replaced by large pharmacies having several millions of dollars of sales each year. Fifteen percent of all prescriptions dispensed in 1982 were in supermarkets, discount, variety, and department stores (23).

In general, the changes in the organization of health care services might be described as centralization and institutionalization. A related, but perhaps parallel, shift in the organizational structure has been coined "corporatization," referring to corporate-oriented health care delivery (24).

---

*A chain pharmacy is defined by the National Association of Chain Drugstores (NACDS) as common ownership of four or more retail pharmacies.

Many of these corporate-oriented delivery systems involve proprietary providers such as investor-owned chains of hospitals, nursing homes, home health agencies, medical equipment suppliers, and dialysis centers that sell patient services for a profit. For example, for-profit companies owned 1118 hospitals with 131,109 beds in 1983 and managed another 282 hospitals with 35,499 beds (25). Hospitals also are investigating shared services and other forms of horizontal integration, such as multihospital systems, in order to optimize management efficiencies and increase access to capital. It is estimated that by 1990, 80% or more of all hospitals will be part of some multihospital arrangement, either investor owned or not for profit.

ALTERNATE DELIVERY MODES

At the same time that corporatization is taking place in the delivery of health care services in the United States, there is a seemingly dichotomous trend developing in which the hospital is no longer the principal and central source of care. "Alternate care" services now are being touted as substitutes for more expensive hospital care. While some of these alternate care modes involve centralized delivery structures, such as health maintenance organizations (HMOs), restructured hospital outpatient departments (OPDs), neighborhood health centers, and prepaid group practices (PGPs), often these alternate care services are provided in freestanding centers. Particularly popular in the 1980s are freestanding primary care clinics, freestanding emergency care units (referred to as "emergicenters"), ambulatory "surgicenters," birthing centers, retail dentistry outlets, and freestanding urgent care units (referred to as "urgicenters") (26). These alternate care services tend to be more consumer oriented in that patients can stop in without appointments and receive care after only a short time. Most alternate care facilities feature longer hours than physicians offices, usually ranging from 16-24 hours a day.

The number of alternate care service sites is expected to increase greatly, particularly as the predicted surplus of physicians in the United States begins to materialize during the late 1980s. The growth of alternate care facilities increases access to primary health care services for much of the population. However, many alternate care centers will handle only certain patient cases, often based on an ability to pay, and these centers may not be integral parts of referral networks that provide continuity of care.

The HMO is an alternate care organizational structure that has become an important part of the U.S. health care delivery system. HMOs provide comprehensive health care services in exchange for a fixed monthly premium amount, negotiated and paid in advance. The number of HMOs in the United States grew from 72 in 1973 to an estimated 280 in 1983, serving more than 12.5 million people, or approximately 5.5% of the entire population (27). Accelerated growth for HMOs is expected as the capitation payment method becomes increasingly popular among insurance companies, employers, and federal and state governments. However, HMOs have shown disappointingly slow growth in low-income communities and, because of the large amount of capital required, may not be feasible for serving nonurban populations (28). Also, despite evidence that prop-

erly structured ambulatory care service can reduce higher cost hospitalization (29), HMOs and PGPs have been criticized for achieving savings by making it more difficult for patients to obtain appointments and requiring long waiting times for care (30). What *is* clear is that HMOs have significantly lower hospitalization rates than traditional health insurance programs (31).

The competitive struggle for patients has spawned another alternate care delivery structure, referred to as a preferred provider organization (PPO). PPOs generally offer comprehensive health care services to insurance companies, employers, and other payers at a discounted rate in exchange for being designated as the "preferred provider" for the given population of patients (32). Many of the PPOs have been formed by hospitals in an effort to compete with HMOs and other hospitals (33).

Home health care is expected to show perhaps the most dramatic growth in the next 10 years. Home care can be a less expensive substitute for institutional care, and many fairly acute and intensive services are now being provided in the home environment (34). Also, many patients have been shown to prefer the comfort and familiarity of the home as the site of care (35). Yet the growth of home health care services will depend on both the generation of evidence that these are indeed substitutes for institutional care rather than additions to it and the development of payment mechanisms that recognize home care products and services as covered benefits.

THE PRICE OF HEALTH CARE

Health care spending has become one of the major social/political issues of the 1980s. An estimated $322 billion was spent for health care in the United States in 1982, or approximately $1400 per person. This amount was equal to 10.5% of the total output of all goods and services and grew 12.5% over the previous year, during a time when the economy as a whole was in recession. As a country, we spend more of our gross national product on health care services than any other country in the world, and in just 20 years we have doubled the percentage of the gross national product that is spent on health care. Part of this tremendous spending of course is due to greater access to care, resulting in higher utilization of services. However, a larger part of this increase in health care spending is due to higher prices and inflationary increases in those prices. Politicians are increasingly inclined to claim that too much is being spent on government-financed health programs. Economists and others suggest that we would be just as healthy a population if we spent half what we do today on health care services and addressed ourselves more to those factors that have a significant effect on health status: smoking, drinking, overeating, stress, and insufficient exercise.

MEDICARE/MEDICAID AND HEALTH INSURANCE

Economists attribute much of health care spending and the spiraling costs to the Medicare and Medicaid entitlement programs and to private health insurance. Because health care services are financed through these programs, the users (patients) are effectively insulated from the price of these services. Most of the reforms being proposed today for the financing of health care services include features that reintroduce the factor of price to the patient at the point when health care services are purchased.

The greatest impact on the U.S. health care system in the last two decades has perhaps been enactment of Medicare/Medicaid legislation. When Medicaid (P.L. 89-97) was initiated on July 30, 1965, the predominant view was that an infusion of money into the system would correct many of the deficiencies (37). Now it seems difficult to understand how Congress could have been persuaded to appropriate funds for health care without attention to the organization of services. Medicare/Medicaid enactment fueled rising health care expenditures by paying hospitals their actual costs. This caused hospitals to be largely unconcerned about their operating costs. Reimbursing physicians at prices set by physicians also contributed to spiraling health care prices and spending. With Medicaid patients being totally insulated from the price of health care services and Medicare patients having only a small degree of price sensitivity, and with no effective means to control utilization, health care spending in these government programs grew from less than 2 billion in 1966 (38) to over $80 billion in 1984 (39).

Proposals for reform of Medicare and Medicaid include restrictions on eligibility, greater cost sharing by Medicare beneficiaries and Medicaid recipients, and new reimbursement systems with altered financial incentives for hospitals, physicians, and other providers. These reforms directly affect the delivery of health care services to approximately 20% of the U.S. population, i.e., the elderly, disabled, and those with severe kidney disease through the Medicare program and the poor through the Medicaid program. However, changes in Medicare and Medicaid reimbursement methods also tend to have a major influence on the structure and delivery of health care services to the entire population. After 15 years of relatively little change in government reimbursement methods and with the government share of total health care spending increasing from 20% to over 40%, the first major reform occurred with P.L. 97-35, the Omnibus Budget Reconciliation Act of 1981. This legislation significantly affected Medicaid programs in several ways, primarily by allowing state Medicaid agencies greater flexibility in setting eligibility criteria for recipients, requiring copayments of patients at the time when they use services, and establishing limits and fixed rates of payments to hospitals and physicians (40). Even more dramatic changes were prescribed by Congress the following year when a prospective pricing system was adopted for Medicare payments to hospitals (41). The new payment method established fixed prices for specific patient cases, categorized according to the admission diagnosis of the patient in one of 470 diagnosis related groups (DRGs).

As revolutionary as these changes were, they still were not perceived as sufficient to bring government spending for health care services into control. As the solvency of the Medicare Hospital Insurance Trust Fund was called into question in the early 1980s, a 13-member Advisory Council on Social Security was commissioned. Their recommendations included new sources of revenue, such as increased taxes on alcohol and tobacco, and new limits on eligibility

and coverage, as well as ways to reduce the use of health care services and payments to health care providers (42). A parallel but separate report on the Medicaid program was released by the Center For The Study of Social Policy in early 1984. The study recommended the use of prepaid capitated financing by the federal government and called for reform of long-term care for the elderly and mentally retarded (43). Long-term care services account for approximately 50% of the entire Medicaid budget in most states.

Private health insurance, including Blue Cross and Blue Shield and commercial companies such as Aetna, Metropolitan, and Prudential, account for approximately 30% of health care financing. The role of private health insurance in financing of services grew most dramatically after World War II, when the U.S. Supreme Court ruled that fringe benefits, including health insurance, were a legitimate part of the bargaining process in labor contract negotiations with management. Since that time the number of persons insured has increased greatly, and health insurance coverages have broadened significantly. In a chicken vs egg manner, health insurance became necessary to protect people from personal bankruptcy resulting from the use of costly medical care services, and simultaneously fueled inflationary increases in health care spending by insulating users for these services from their cost.

Blue Cross and Blue Shield plans are tax-exempt organizations, tied by membership to the national Blue Cross/Blue Shield Association (BCA), but otherwise are independent corporations. The "Blues" and the commercial insurers historically have had less influence then Medicare and Medicaid in the structure of the U.S. health care delivery system. However, these companies are making increased efforts to control health care prices and spending, as they have watched their payments to providers balloon and subsequently have had to increase their premiums to employers and individual subscribers. Prepaid capitated financing of health care in the United States would help control health care prices and the use of services, as well as promote further centralization and institutionalization in the structure of the health care delivery system. If prepaid capitation financing does not bring health care spending under control, the obvious alternative is a nationalized health care system in which the government is the provider as well as the payer for health care services to the entire population.

QUALITY OF CARE

There is more than price at issue, and the impact of Medicare/Medicaid legislation has been felt in more than economic terms. Federal legislation has influenced the quality of health services provided to beneficiaries, and to the entire U.S. population, by tying Medicare payments to accreditation standards for facilities, licensure, and other certification requirements for personnel and by mandating the establishment of watchdogs, such as pharmacy and therapeutics and (P&T) committees in hospitals and utilization review mechanisms for hospitals and ambulatory care facilities. The utilization of services, quality of program administration, and relationships of providers of health services to fiscal intermediaries all have come under scrutiny as government has increased its role in health care delivery (44).

Superior quality of health care services in the United States often is cited as the reason for the high cost of these services. Certainly, there is some direct and proportional relationship between quality and cost. Yet we still are unable to measure quality precisely and therefore also are unable to determine the "price" of quality. Quality assurance (QA) has become commonplace in hospitals, and QA programs are mandated by the conditions of participation for the Medicare program. Most QA programs attempt to define standards and measure performance according to the parameters of structure, process, and outcome of hospital services. Proposed changes in the Medicare conditions of participation would give hospitals greater flexibility in designing these QA programs and monitoring the quality of hospital services (45). These new Medicare conditions signal clearly that the issue of quality of health care services will take a back seat to concerns regarding the costs of these services during the 1980s.

Quality of health care services in the United States is protected by more than accreditation of health care facilities, educational institutions and teaching programs, and the licensure of personnel. Peer review also is performed in an attempt to protect quality. Peer review is both formal and informal and may be either retrospective, current, or prospective in nature. Retrospective peer review involves examination of patient chart information in a case-by-case medical audit or employs a computerized review of this information, sometimes referred to as patient care monitor (PCM) (46). Hospital charts usually are the basis for evaluation, but physician office records also may be used in the retrospective peer review process (47).

Concurrent review is becoming a more common means of health care evaluation, and may be more effective because it involves evaluation of care as it is rendered. Major aspects of concurrent review are hospital admission certification, continued stay review, and discharge planning. Admission certification is concerned with appropriateness of institutionalization. Continued stay review monitors the length of stay of patients according to their diagnosis, severity of illness, and major complications. Discharge planning involves weighing alternate courses of action regarding discharge, such as extended care vs hospitalization, home care vs extended care, and the need for specific health care services after discharge. Prospective review involves the establishment of standards of care and the design and implementation of provider education programs to meet these standards.

Efforts to protect the quality of health care services also include some indirect methods, such as voluntary and compulsory continuing education for practitioners and relicensure of personnel via reexamination. These methods probably will become more important in the future, particularly as health care technology and the amount of health care information continue to grow. Continuing education and reexamination for licensure are only indirect methods of quality protection, however, since they tell us what the practitioner has learned or should be doing, not what is actually being done or the consequent health care outcome.

Utilization review (UR) is a more direct, but not necessarily more effective, means of protecting the quality of health care services. UR first was formalized in 1972 with the establishment of professional standard review organizations (PSROs) by the 1972 Amendment to the Social Security Act (P.L. 92-603). The purpose of the PSRO program was to assure that health care services and items for which payment was made by the government through Medicare and Medicaid and other programs are medically necessary, conform to certain professional standards, and are delivered effectively and efficiently. Overall, PSROs had only limited success in achieving these goals, largely as a result of the obstacles that plague all UR activities, i.e., the use of incomplete and inaccurate medical record information as the basis for monitoring and evaluating health care services and outcomes, and a reluctance on the part of organized medicine to control those practitioners who deviate from ethical and professional norms (48). PSROs were replaced by peer review organizations (PROs) in 1984 in an attempt to better control hospital utilization under the Medicare Prospective Payment System by examining the medical necessity and appropriateness of hospital admissions and hospital services to Medicare patients (49). We will be better able to measure the performance of PROs as opposed to other quality protection efforts because PROs will focus primarily on the costs associated with medically unnecessary or inappropriate services.

LONG-TERM SERVICES

Long-term care is the fastest-growing segment of the U.S. health care industry. In terms of revenues and spending, nursing homes dominate the long-term care sector (50). The other institutional components of long-term care include chronic disease hospitals, domiciliary care facilities, and retirement homes, sometimes referred to as "lifecare" centers. Many personal and supportive care services also are provided in the home and in noninstitutional environments to the elderly, chronically infirm, and mentally retarded. Therefore, counting the long-term care population is difficult. Moreover, many long-term care services, particularly supportive and personal care, are delivered by friends and relatives.

Nursing homes are so designated on the basis of scope and organization of services and the level of care required by the patient. Chronic disease facilities include institutions for mental retardation, tuberculosis, and the mentally ill, among others. Domiciliary care institutions essentially are living accommodations without health-related services. Personal care institutions, which provide services related to activities of daily living, such as dressing, eating, walking, etc, and sheltered care institutions, which provide a protective environment and occasional personal service, complete this category of health care–related institutions.

Long-term care institutions, particularly nursing homes, have been found to suffer from major deficiencies such as unsatisfactory compliance with various codes and regulations and inappropriate patient placements (51,52). Nursing homes seem chronically prone to fail to meet federal requirements for Medicaid and Medicare programs (53). Required medical and nursing attention were not being rendered to patients in these facilities, and noncompliance with prevailing safety codes was widespread. A comprehensive report by the U.S. General Accounting Office (GAO) in 1983 highlighted several problems and challenges for the nursing home industry: (1) the availability of nursing home services varies widely from state to state, (2) some elderly persons are unable to gain access to nursing homes, (3) unavailability of nursing home beds may be due in part of unnecessary use of nursing homes by some persons, (4) the new Medicare Prospective Payment System for hospital reimbursement may unintentionally increase the demand for nursing home beds and thereby further reduce the availability of nursing home services to some persons, and (5) efforts by states to keep their Medicaid costs down by limiting reimbursement or the supply of beds, or both, is expected to continue to restrict the availability of beds for the elderly at a time when the demand for these beds is growing significantly (54).

Remedial efforts in the provision of long-term care services are hampered by inadequate participation by consumers, community advisory groups, and even physicians. Physician services are in short supply in long-term care because such care is a neglected aspect of the medical student's socialization process; when combined with the very nature of long-term care (i.e., little hope for real improvement in patients' health status), this often results in provider apathy and apparent indifference. Some claim that too few physicians are involved in nursing home care in the community, and of those involved even fewer devote much attention to such patients on a regular basis (55).

Major reform in long-term care services appears unavoidable. The increasing proportion of elderly persons in the population will come into direct conflict with further legislative efforts to cut spending at the federal and state level. One alternative in the financing of long-term care may involve a greater role for the private health insurance industry (56).

PATIENT MANAGEMENT

Patient misplacement is a major problem in health care delivery, with many thousands of patients placed in facilities inappropriate to their needs. Misplacement contributes to great inefficiencies in economic terms, as well as to inappropriate personal care of the patient. The factors contributing to misplacement of patients are many, including the lack of suitable alternatives to institutionalization, reimbursement based on factors other than patient needs, and the insensitivity of utilization review to detect much care that is inappropriate or unnecessary.

In order to place patients where they could receive all of the services they need, the concept of progressive patient care was developed and promoted by the U.S. Public Health Service in the early 1960s. Six levels of care were delineated, and judgments could be made to transfer patients so that a person would not occupy a bed associated with unnecessary services and concomitant costs. The six levels are:

1. *Intensive care*. For critically and seriously ill patients.

All necessary lifesaving emergency equipment, drugs, and supplies are immediately available.

2. *Intermediate care*. For patients requiring a moderate amount of nursing care. Emergency care and frequent observation rarely are needed.

3. *Self-care*. For ambulatory and physically self-sufficient patients requiring tests or convalescence.

4. *Long-term care*. For patients requiring skilled, prolonged medical and nursing care.

4. *Home care*. For patients who can be cared for adequately in the home with the addition of specific services delivered to them by visiting nurses or others.

6. *Outpatient care*. For ambulatory patients requiring specific diagnostic or treatment services on a scheduled basis, primarily through clinics.

A general preference for analyzing structure and process components of health care rather than health outcomes inhibits improvements in the patient misplacement problem.

COORDINATION OF SERVICES AND CONTINUITY OF CARE

Specialization of medical practice and the independence of providers at various levels in delivery of health care services contribute to a lack of continuity of care; better coordination of care is needed and may be achieved through more comprehensive and sophisticated information systems and more communication among practitioners. The practice of medicine and the delivery of health care services demand verbal and written communications among other providers as well as patients. However, the quality and quantity of communication are concerns voiced by experts, planners, and providers. Interprofessional communication often is strained, causing inadequate coordination of services and threatening the quality of care (58-60).

Referral networks are illustrative of interpersonal relationships among providers, both intraprofessionally and interprofessionally. The failure of physicians to use the referral process adequately and to effectively use the information available to primary care physicians leads to inefficiencies in the provision of health care services (61,62). The referral process also may be viewed as a means for the medical profession to exert control over the health care delivery system and its own members (63).

Provider-patient interaction also is plagued by an inadequate exchange of information. Social distance and status differentials impair physician-patient communication (64,65), and pharmacist-patient communication is compromised because of physical barriers such as the prescription counter and a time commitment to the technical tasks involved in dispensing prescriptions. Furthermore, evidence suggests that even when support personnel are used in pharmacies, presumably to free pharmacist time for greater patient interaction, patient contact actually may decrease rather than increase (66).

EXPANSION OF PROVIDER ROLES

Physicians are the captains in the health care delivery system. Physicians admit and discharge patients from hospitals, write prescriptions for drugs and diagnostic tests, refer patients to other providers, etc. These functions are restricted to physicians through state medical practice act and physician licensure requirements. However, many nonphysician providers are assuming expanded roles in specialty areas as a means to increase productivity in the health care system. Productivity can be increased through the use of paramedical or support personnel (67-70). Most studies have shown that nonphysician practitioners in these expanded roles deliver primary care of quality comparable to that delivered by physicians (71-75). Yet despite this evidence and the need for greater productivity, several factors augur limited expansion of nonphysician roles. Patient acceptance of support personnel in surrogate physician roles is an important factor (76-78). Physician resistance to expanded roles for nonphysician providers is a significant limiting factor (79).

Greater interprofessional cooperation and a more appropriate division of labor in health care would lead to a more efficient delivery system. However, state legislation will be necessary to bring about change in statute and regulation to permit overlap in responsibility and authority in patient care among health professionals.

CONSUMER PARTICIPATION

Delivery of health care services in the United States involves more than a simple provider-patient relationship. Many third parties are important in the delivery of care. As we have seen, government is playing a greater role in all aspects of health care; employers are having greater influence in the delivery of health care services through business coalitions (80). Consumer participation in planning and management of health care programs was mandated by federal legislation in 1972 (P.L. 92-603) and in 1974 (P.L. 93-641) and has continued to be included in all subsequent health care legislation (81).

At the same time, several forces have been at work to limit greater consumer participation in planning and regulation of the health care industry. The role of the consumer sometimes is unclear in federal legislation. Health practitioners may be reluctant to consider their work in terms of a service industry responsive to consumer input (82), and providers dominate the accreditation process, licensure boards, and total health care management (83). Also, consumers need to be better organized and more informed.

MALPRACTICE

Medical malpractice suits by patients precipitated a near crisis in the middle 1970s (84). Malpractice insurance premiums had increased to the point where some U.S. physicians were paying as much for malpractice insurance as the entire annual income of physicians in other countries (85). Nearly every state responded by approving legislation oriented toward either arbitration and other quasilegal approaches to resolving medical disputes, setting limits on malpractice awards, or establishing malpractice insurance pools (86). Nevertheless, medical malpractice problems persist, and medical malpractice insurance rates increased an average of 20-30% in 1983 (87). For example, a neurosur-

geon in Long Island, New York, may pay $66,500 a year in premiums or as much as $199,400 with a poor loss experience record. Some physicians have gone "bare," dropping medical malpractice insurance altogether, as a result of these high insurance premiums.

The sources of the malpractice problem, apparently unique to the U.S. health care system, are unclear. The U.S. health care system may be partly responsible because of its commercial nature, creating a demanding patient who is inclined to rush off to the courts if things go wrong; an impersonal provider-patient relationship in the delivery of health care also has been cited (88). Medical incompetence appears to be a factor in many of the malpractice cases (89). The growth of medical malpractice law as a specialty predicts further increases in the number of malpractice suits and concomitant expense in the health care delivery system (90).

SUMMARY

The U.S. health care delivery system is a complex mix of mostly independent facilities and practitioners, financed via a myriad of payment mechanisms. Increasing centralization and institutionalization may bring providers together but not necessarily result in better coordination of care and patient management. The delivery of health care in the United States will continue to be the subject of much sociopolitical debate until health care spending is contained. Inevitably, society will be faced with making increasingly difficult decisions regarding the structure and financing of the health care delivery system. "Access" may have to be more restricted and perhaps "quality" compromised in some manner in order to contain "cost."

REFERENCES

1. McLaughlin CP, Sheldon A: *The Future and Medical Care*. Cambridge, MA, Ballinger, 1974.
2. U.S. Department of Health, Education and Welfare: Press release. January 8, 1976.
3. Fahs I, Peterson O: Towns without physicians and towns with only one: A study of four states in the Upper Midwest. *Am J Public Health* 58:1200, 1968.
4. Elesh D, Shollaert PT: Race and urban medicine: Factors affecting the distribution of physicians in Chicago. *J Health Soc Behav* 13:236-250, 1972.
5. Bidese CM, Danais DG: *Physician Characteristics and Distribution in the U.S.* Chicago, American Medical Association, 1982.
6. Eisenberg BS, Cantwell JR: Policies to influence the spatial distribution of physicians: A conceptual review of selected programs and empirical evidence. *Med Care* 14:455-468, 1976.
7. Guzick DS, Jahiel RI: Distribution of private practice offices of physicians with specified characteristics among urban neighborhoods. *Med Care* 14:469-488, 1976.
8. Fuchs VR, Kramer MJ: *Determinants of Expenditures for Physicians' Services in the United States, 1948-1968*. National Bureau of Economic Research, Paper No. 17, DHEW Publication No. (HSM) 73-3013. Washington, DC, U. S. Government Printing Office, December 1972.
9. Anon: *Health—United States 1982*. DHHS Publication No. (PHS) 83-1232. Hyattsville, MD, U.S. Department of Health and Human Services, December 1982.
10. Ginzberg E: A new physician supply policy is needed. *JAMA* 250:2621-2622, 1983.
11. Anon: *Physician Characteristics and Distribution in the U.S., 1982*. Chicago, American Medical Association, 1983.

12. Roemer MI: *An Introduction to the U.S. Health Care System*. New York, Springer, 1982.
13. United States National Center for Health Statistics. Series 10, Nos. 9, 64, 74, 75, 87, Series 3, No. 7, Series 11, No. 125.
14. Taylor DG, Aday LA, Anderson R: A social indicator of access to medical care. *J Health Soc Behav* 15:39-49, 1975.
15. Bosanac EM, Parkinson RC, Hall DS: Geographical access to hospital care: A 30-minute travel time standard. *Med Care* 14:616-624, 1976.
16. Berkanovic E, Reeder LG: Can money buy the appropriate use of services? Some notes on the meaning of utilization data. *J Health Soc Behav* 15:93-99, 1974.
17. Aday LA: Economic and noneconomic barriers to the use of needed medical services. *Med Care* 13:447-456, 1975.
18. U.S. National Center for Health Statistics: Health Characteristics of Low Income Persons. Public Health Service Publication No. 73-500, Series 10, No. 74, 1972.
19. Leo PA, Rosen G: A bookshelf on poverty and health. *Am J Public Health* 59:591, 1969.
20. Smith DB, Kaluzny AD: Inequality in health care programs: A note on some structural factors affecting health care behavior. *Med Care* 12:860-870, 1974.
21. Lorant JH: *Characteristics of Group and Solo Physicians, Practices, and Populations Served. Profile of Medical Practice*. Chicago, Center for Health Services, Research and Development, American Medical Association, 1974.
22. Anon: American Druggist annual pharmacy survey. *Am Druggist* 187(5):12, 16, 1983.
23. Glaser M, Chi J: Drug Topics' 35th annual report on consumer spending. *Drug Top* 126(13):2-4, 7, 8, 1983.
24. Anon: The corporatization of American health care. *Wash Report Med Health* November 14, 1983.
25. Anon: Management companies' progress enables industry to maintain growth pattern. In *1984 Directory of Investor-Owned Hospitals and Hospital Management Companies*, Little Rock, Federation of American Hospitals, 1983.
26. Anon: Doctor surplus breeds new practice forms. *Wash Report Med Health* April 25, 1983.
27. Punch L, Johnson DEL: HMO's predict rapid employee growth as consumers' cost concerns mount. *Mod Healthcare* 14(1):54-56, 1984.
28. Blendon RJ: The reform of ambulatory care: A financial paradox. *Med Care* 14:526-534, 1976.
29. Bellin SS, Geiger HJ, Gibson CD: The impact of ambulatory health care services on the demand for hospital beds. *N Engl J Med* 280:808, 1969.
30. Tessler R, Mechanic D: Consumer satisfaction with PGP: A comparative study. *J Health Soc Behav* 16:95-113, 1975.
31. Greenlick MR, Lamb SJ, Carpenter TM, Fischer TS, Marks SD, Cooper WJ: Kaiser-Permanente's Medicare plus project: A successful Medicare prospective payment demonstration. *Health Care Fin Rev* 13(4): 85-97, 1983.
32. Lundy RW, Blacker RA: Preferred provider organizations: The latest response to healthcare competition. *Healthcare Fin Mgt* 13(7):14-18, 1983.
33. Kuntz EF: Hospitals forming PPO's to fend off HMO rivals. *Mod Healthcare* 13(2):22-24, 1983.
34. Curtiss FR: Third party reimbursement for home parenteral nutrition and IV therapy. *NITA J* 6:193-197, May/June, 1983.
35. Anon: *The Elderly Should Benefit from Expanded Home Health Care but Increasing These Services Will Not Insure Cost Reductions*. Report No. IPE-83-1, Gaithersburg, MD, U.S. General Accounting Office, December 7, 1982.
36. Gibson RM, Waldo DR, Levit KR: National health expenditures. *Health Care Fin Rev* 5(1):1-31, 1983.
37. Breslow L: The organization of personal health services. *Millbank Mem Fund* 50(4):365, 1972.
38. Muse DN, Sawyer D: *The Medicare and Medicaid Data Book, 1981*. Office of Research and Demonstrations, Healthcare Financing Administration, April 1982.
39. Anon: Reagan budget: What's new? *Wash Rep Med Health* February 6, 1984.
40. Anon: Medicaid program; miscellaneous Medicaid provisions—increased state flexibility. *Fed Reg* 46(190):48524-48561, 1981.
41. Anon: Medicare program; final rules: Prospective payment for Medicare inpatient hospital services. *Fed Reg* 49(1):233-340, 1984.
42. Anon: Advisory Council on Social Security recommends major Medicare reforms. *Hotline* November 15, 1983.
43. Anon: Report recommends drastic Medicaid program reform. *Hosp Week* 20(6):1, 1984.
44. Costanzo GA, Vertinsky I: Measuring the quality of health care: A decision oriented typology. *Med Care* 13:417-431, 1975.
45. Anon: Medicare and Medicaid programs; conditions of participation for hospitals: Proposed rule. *Fed Reg* 48(2):299-315, 1983.
46. Novick LF, Dickinson K, Asnes R, Maylan SP, Lowenstein R: Assessment of ambulatory care: Application of the tracer methodology. *Med Care* 14:1-12, 1976.
47. Wirtschafer DD, Mesel E: A strategy for redesigning the medical record for quality assurance. *Med Care* 14:68-76, 1976.
48. Bellin LE: PSRO—quality control? Or gimmickry? *Med Care* 12:1012-1018, 1974.
49. Anon: Medicare: Utilization and quality control peer review organization (PRO) area designations and definitions of eligible organizations; final rule and notice. *Fed Reg* 49(39):7201-7210, 1984.
50. Scanlon WJ, Feder J: The long-term care marketplace: An overview. *Healthcare Fin Mgt* 14(1):18, 19, 24-26, 28, 30, 34, 36, 1984.
51. Comptroller General of the United States: *Problems in Providing Proper Care to Medicaid and Medicare Patients in Skilled Nursing Homes*. Report B-16403 (13), Washington, DC, U.S. Government Printing Office, 1970.
52. Zimmer JG: Characteristics of patients and care provided in health-related and skilled nursing facilities. *Med Care* 13:992-1010, 1975.
53. Ruchlin HS, Levey S, Miller C: The long-term care marketplace: An analysis of deficiencies and potential reform by means of incentive reimbursement. *Med Care* 13:979-991, 1975.
54. Anon: *Medicaid and Nursing Home Care: Cost Increases and the Need for Services Are Creating Problems for the States and the Elderly*. Publication No. GAO-IPE-84-1, Washington, DC, U.S. General Accounting Office, October 21, 1983.
55. Solon JA, Greenwalt LF: Physicians' participation in nursing homes. *Med Care* 12:486, 1974.
56. Lifson A: Financing long-term care: HIAA's evaluation. *Healthcare Fin Mgt* 14(3):64-65, 1984.
57. Starfeld DH, Simborg DW, Horn SD, Yourte SA: Continuity and coordination in primary care: Their achievement and utility. *Med Care* 14:626-636, 1976.
58. Banta HD: Role strains of a health care team in a poverty community. *Soc Sci Med* 6:697-722, 1972.
59. Nathansan CA, Becker NH: Physicians, nurses and clinical records. *Med Care* 11:213-233, 1973.
60. Brown CA: The division of laborers: Allied health professions. *Int J Health Serv* 3:435-444, 1973.
61. Clute KF: *The General Practitioner: A Study of Medical Education and Practice in Ontario and Nova Scotia*. Toronto, University of Toronto Press, 1963.
62. Johnson AC et al: The office practice of internists: III. Characteristics of patients. *JAMA* 193:916-921, 1965.
63. Shortell SN: *A Model of Physician Referral Behavior: A Test of Exchange Theory in Medical Practice*. Chicago, University of Chicago. Center for Health Administration Studies, Reserve Series, 1972.
64. Freidson E: *Professional Dominance*. Chicago, Atherton, 1970.
65. McKinley JB: Who is really ignorant—physician or patient? *J Health Soc Behav* 16:3-11, 1975.
66. Dickson WM, Rodowskas CA: Verbal communication of community pharmacists. *Med Care* 13:486-498, 1975.
67. Lees REM: Physician time-saving by employment of expanded-role nurses in family practice. *Can Med Assoc J* 108:871-875, 1973.
68. Rafferty J: *Health Manpower and Productivity*. Lexington, MD, 1974.
69. Hepler CD: A primer on productivity. *Top Hosp Pharm Mgt* 1:55, 1981.
70. McGhan WF, Smith WE, Adams DW: A randomized trial comparing pharmacists and technicians as dispensers of prescriptions for ambulatory patients. *Med Care* 21:445-453, 1983.
71. Lewis CG, Resnick BA: Nurse clinics and progressive ambulatory patient care. *N Engl J Med* 277:1236-1245, 1967.
72. Charney E, Kitzman H: The child-health nurse (pediatric nurse practitioner) in private practice: A controlled trial. *N Engl J Med* 285:1353-1358, 1971.
73. Sackett DL, Spitzer WO, Gent M, Roberts RS: The Burlington Randomized Trial of the nurse practitioner: Health outcomes of patients. *Ann Intern Med* 80:137-145, 1974.

74. Levine DM, Morlock LL, Mushlin AI, Shapiro S, Malitz FE: The role of new health practitioners in a prepaid group practice: Provider differences in process and outcomes of medical care. *Med Care* 14:326-347, 1976.

75. McCloud BC: Clinical pharmacy: The past, present and future. *Am J Hosp Pharm* 33:29-38, 1976.

76. Litman T: Public perception of the physician's assistant—a survey of attitudes and opinions of rural Iowa and Minnesota residents. *Am J Public Health* 62:343-346, 1972.

77. Weinstein P, Demers JL: Rural nurse practitioner clinic: The public's response. *Am J Nurs* 74:2022-2026, 1974.

78. Lawrence LS: Patient acceptance of the family nurse practitioner. *Med Care* 14:356-364, 1976.

79. Wriston S: Nurse practitioner reimbursement. *J Health Politics Policy Law* 6:444-462, 1981.

80. Anon: *Managing Health Costs: Strategies for Coalitions and Business.* Washington, DC, Clearinghouse on Business Coalitions for Health Action, Chamber of Commerce of the United States, 1982.

81. Metsch JM, Veney JG: Consumer participation and social accountability. *Med Care* 14:283-293, 1976.

82. Wingate MB, Silver T, McMillen M, Zeccardi J: Obstetric care in a family health oriented university associated neighborhood health center. *Med Care* 14:315-325, 1976.

83. Stein GH: The use of a nurse practitioner in the management of patients with diabetes mellitus. *Med Care* 12:885-890, 1974.

84. Anon: Survey shows liability law gains in '75. *Am Med News* 19:1, 1976.

85. Klein R: Few suits in British medicine. *Washington Post* May 23, 1976.

86. Congressional Record Proceedings: Medical Malpractice Reinsurance Program. *Congr Rec* 121:5302, 1975.

87. Taravella S: Physicians faced with ballooning malpractice rates. *Lauer Rep* 1(5):2-3, 1983.

88. Mechanic D: *Public Expectations and Health Care.* New York, Wiley-Interscience, 1972.

89. Klaw S: Bad medicine: When practice makes imperfect. *Washington Post* December 21, 1975.

90. Holder AR: *Medical Malpractice Law.* New York, John Wiley & Sons, 1975.

CHAPTER 2

The Organizational Structure of the Hospital

STUART A. WESBURY, Jr., and JAMES B. GANTENBERG

HISTORICAL DEVELOPMENT

During the 17th century, the primary role of the hospital was that of community servant. This role consisted of ridding the community of the sick, dying, and insane. Not until 1840, with the advent of the voluntary hospital and the philanthropic movement, did hospitals alter their goals to serve individual patients rather than the community. In the 19th and early 20th centuries, profound social and technologic change (anesthesia, sterilization, surgery, etc) further altered the goals of hospitals. At this point, hospitals clearly established "curing" patients as their primary goal.

In the mid- to late 20th century, the U.S. hospital industry expanded as a result of the Hill-Burton program (a federally sponsored program begun in 1946 to provide communities with funds for building hospitals). Furthermore, Blue Cross and insurance programs grew rapidly and improved the financial base for hospitals. The year 1965 ushered in the age of health care services entitlement with Medicare (over 65 years of age) and Medicaid (welfare) programs. The technologic boom also continued unabated.

As hospitals moved into the 1970s, concerns developed about the high cost of providing health care services to the citizens of our nation. The federal government made significant attempts to control the construction of new hospital beds and the creation of new hospital services. National health planning programs were implemented. Yet in spite of these efforts, costs continued to climb at a rate higher than the cost of living, creating even greater pressure on the federal government to find ways to slow down cost escalation.

The latest federal response to this problem was the implementation, on October 1, 1983, of the Medicare prospective payment system. This new system pays for hospital stays of Medicare patients based on the use of diagnosis related groups (DRGs). It provides for a specific payment to the hospital for the cost of providing hospital care to a Medicare patient without regard to specific services provided. In other words, the diagnosis of the patient determines the payment made to the hospital. Those hospitals whose costs are below the DRG payment will earn a surplus for treating a particular patient. The reverse is also true: the hospital potentially can suffer a loss if its costs are higher than its payment. Thus, the federal government now has reached a point where the individual hospital is at risk concerning the care provided to Medicare patients. Previous hospital reimbursement mechanisms, which essentially paid hospitals for the cost of services rendered, are now rapidly disappearing from the industry.

ORGANIZATIONAL STRUCTURE

Hospital organizational structures have been altered over time not only to accommodate changes in the way health care services are delivered, but also to reflect the changing environment and external pressures. Until the 20th century, hospitals were simple organizations, with nursing as the primary function and service. The lack of diagnostic and treatment services put few management demands on the institution. Frequently, a physician or nurse was "in charge," and often the role was part time or reserved for someone at or near retirement. The burden on management was slight. Communication was direct and followed the professional to nonprofessional chain of command (physician–nurse–aide–other nonprofessional).

As time moved on, technologic advances, medical specialization, and complicated financing programs forced hospitals to adopt increasingly complex organizational structures. New departments within hospitals were created (respiratory therapy, medical records, electrodiagnosis, etc). These new departments and services required higher levels of integration to assure the effective delivery of patient care. The profession of hospital administration was created in the early 1930s in response to the hospitals' need to employ professionally educated individuals to manage complex institutions. Specialization had reached even the ranks of management.

Today, the organization of a modern hospital demonstrates the integration of many elements not even present in hospitals 75 years ago. Committees of the governing body, a highly organized medical staff and its committees, growing numbers of specialized departments, and numerous special functions (public relations, fund-raising, planning, etc) must now be linked together in a highly coordinated way. Thus, the organizational structure of a modern hospital includes a complex of formal and informal structures. These are designed to provide for direct management of specific patient services and support activities while reflecting the influence of many committees created to serve specific purposes. Figure 2.1 is a prototype of today's modern hospital (1). It indicates that the board of trustees (governing body) is the central authority for the institution, responsible for the care rendered by the hospital. Through a president/chief executive officer, the policies of the board are implemented on a day-to-day basis, with the president taking responsibility for the management of the institution's activities and programs. Supporting the president is a staff of executives managing activities involved with delivery or support of patient care services. In addition, functions such as planning, public relations, industrial engineering, and fund raising are carried out under the supervision of the president.

The medical staff is organized as a separate body with its own bylaws, which must be approved by the hospital's governing body. Its linkage with the governing body and the president is through a joint conference committee. This committee coordinates medical staff appointments and responsibilities in addition to integrating medical staff activities with the long-range planning and management of the hospital. The medical staff is supported by its own committee structure as indicated in Figure 2.1. The pharmacy and therapeutics committee is responsible for creating a hospital formulary and providing necessary and appropriate controls on drug utilization in the hospital. All these medical staff committees then influence the activities of hospital departments that are directly involved with providing patient services. This is indicated by the dotted line box linking the medical staff with the departments that report to the vice-president of nursing and the vice-president for professional services.

Legally, the governing body is responsible for the quality of care rendered to patients. Medical staff appointments, reviewed and recommended by the medical staff, ultimately must be approved by the governing body. From the oper-

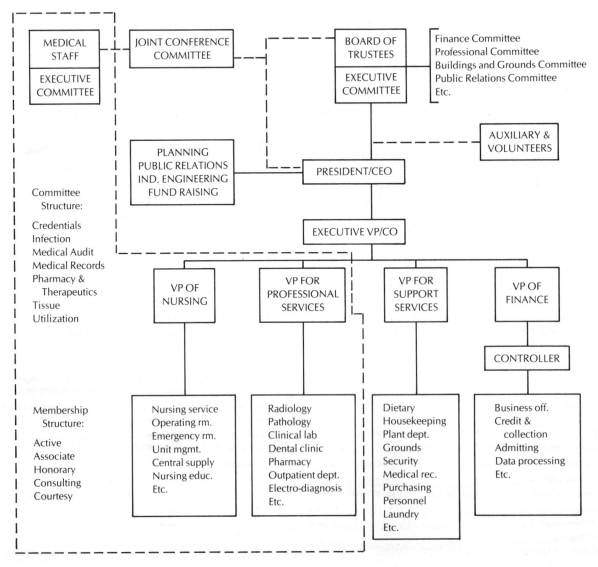

FIGURE 2.1 Organizational structure of a modern hospital.[1]

ational perspective, all hospital activities report directly to the president/CEO and through the president to the governing body. Thus, the board has the opportunity to monitor, control, and evaluate the quality of care rendered and the operation of the entire institution. The hospital structure, therefore, focuses the total responsibility on the governing body (2).

EVOLVING HEALTH CARE ORGANIZATIONS

As hospitals move into the mid-1980s and beyond, significant trends will affect hospital organizations. These movements are related directly to concerns over cost and the changing methods by which hospitals are paid, partic-

ularly by government and other third-party payers. Reduced income, greater difficulty in obtaining funds for capital expansion, modernization, and new treatment modalities, plus the need to create greater operational economies, have combined to encourage massive restructuring of hospital organizations and a large number of mergers and corporate consolidations. In addition, medicine now stresses "wellness" care as well as traditional "illness" care. This movement will likely alter organizations also, as the supplemental readings indicate.

For-profit corporations now own or lease more than 10% of the nation's hospitals. Close to 30% of all hospitals belong to some multihospital system (not for profit or for profit). It is estimated that, by 1995, 95% of all hospitals

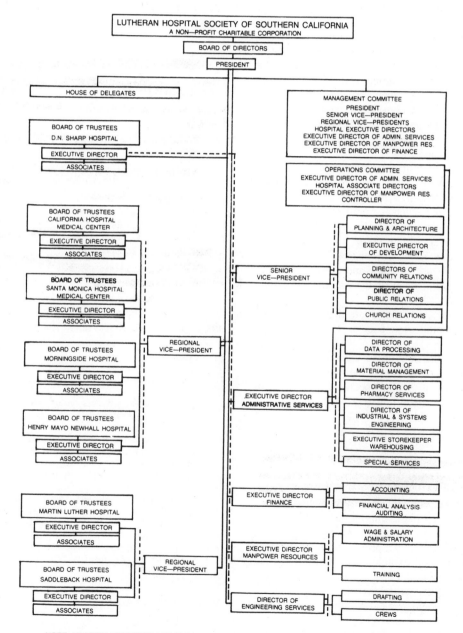

NOTE: HILLSIDE COMMUNITY HOSPITALS, SAUGUS, CALIFORNIA, HAS BEEN ADDED RECENTLY.

FIGURE 2.2   Organizational chart of large not-for-profit multihospital system.[4]

will be part of a multihospital system (3). These developments offer the hospital an opportunity to be part of a system and draw on the knowledge and skill of management/technical experts at the corporate level. Increased access to capital and cost savings through economies of scale also add to the list of advantages.

For health care professionals, such as pharmacists, this multi-institutional movement brings additional opportunities. For example, transfers/promotions can occur as an individual is moved from one hospital to another within a multihospital system. Also, consultant pharmacist roles may be available at corporate headquarters. Thus, upward mobility may be enhanced for a variety of professionals.

Contract management of a department's services is still another alternative. A single firm may contract with many hospitals to provide pharmacy or other services to a hospital. The hospital benefits through backup support available from a central organization and elimination of some day-to-day operational problems. Unfortunately, these methodologies fail to offer entirely positive outcomes. Hospitals must be prepared to accept some loss of autonomy as they join larger systems or contract out some of their services. Each merger or contract decision must be considered carefully in light of the individual hospital's objectives and current and future needs. These are major decisions that affect both patient services and employee careers.

Part of the decision to join with other organizations is related to whether a hospital wishes to join with other hospitals (horizontal integration), with other kinds of health care delivery organizations, such as ambulatory care clinics, nursing homes and hospices (vertical integration), or both. Some multi-institutional organizations are nationwide; others are restricted to a single city or town. Again, these organizational decisions are complex and must be made at the highest policy-making level of the organization (i.e., the governing body).

As a reference, the organizational chart of a large not-for-profit multihospital system is presented in Figure 2.2 (4).

For the pharmacist, the new organizational structure offers new and exciting opportunities. Pharmacists should examine carefully the extent of a prospective employer's involvement in such multi-institutional systems.

NEW STRUCTURES FOR THE FUTURE

The single most predominant trend in the health care system is the linking of complex health care organizations into multi-institutional systems. These organizational linkages potentially will improve health care quality while reducing costs. Already, an increasing number are occurring between hospitals and group practices, nursing homes, health care agencies, and other providers of health care services. Successful models exhibit leadership, innovation, growth, and vertical/horizontal integration. Each system or model contains a group of institutions with common sets of goals, shared services, management resources, and clearly defined ''markets''(5).

Examples of such systems include:

1. Sisters of Mercy Health Corporation in Farmington Hill, Michigan, owns, leases, sponsors, or contract manages 20 hospitals in four different states with a total bed com-

plement of 5713 beds. On a smaller scale, the Sisters of Charity Health Care Systems of Cincinnati, Ohio, owns, leases or sponsors seven hospitals in four different states with a total bed complement of 3014 beds.

2. In the for-profit sector, Hospital Corporation of America, Nashville, Tennessee, owns, leases, or sponsors 195 hospitals and contract manages another 145 hospitals in 41 states with a bed complement of 45,386 beds. Humana, Inc., of Louisville, Kentucky, owns, leases, or sponsors 87 hospitals in 23 states with a bed complement of 15,294 beds (6).

All of these systems exhibit important characteristics of growth and synergistic operations between member institutions. Other systems in the United States also are successful models. In the years ahead, many variations of these systems will be organized.

CONCLUSION

Whether a hospital is freestanding or part of a large for-profit or not-for-profit multihospital system, the organizational structure begins at the top with the governing body. Three primary functions must be fulfilled by the governing body (7):

1. Accepting legal responsibility for organizational effectiveness
2. Gaining support from the community for the hospital
3. Being accountable to the community for services rendered by the hospital

Governing bodies set policy to assure that institutional objectives are met using the management expertise of the CEO and the management team. The CEO, in turn, organizes, plans, controls, and directs operations and services through the executive staff, divisional and departmental directors, and employees.

Futuristic views of the health care system point to growing complexity and changing roles of institutions, organizations, and highly qualified specialists such as pharmacists.

REFERENCES

1. Schulz R, Johnson AC: *Management of Hospitals*. New York, McGraw-Hill, 1976, p 55.
2. Dornblaser BM: The social responsibility of general hospitals. In *Foundations for Excellence*. Chicago, American College of Hospital Administrators, Pluribus Press, 1982, pp 178-187.
3. McManis Associates, Inc: *American College of Hospital Administrators Strategic Planning Committee. An Environmental Assessment*. Chicago, American College of Hospital Administrators, 1984, p 15.
4. Tibbitts SJ: Multiple hospital systems. *Hosp Health Serv Admin* 18(2):15, 1973.
5. Ross A: Organizational linkages: Management issues and implications. In *Foundations for Excellence*. Chicago, American College of Hospital Administrators, Pluribus Press, 1982, pp 1-10.
6. American Hospital Association: *Directory of Multi Hospital Systems*. Chicago, American Hospital Association, 1982, pp 18-40.
7. Schulz R, Johnson AC: *Management of Hospitals*. New York, McGraw-Hill, 1976, p 47.

ADDITIONAL READING

McCormick TR, Frado RL: Corporate reorganization—a case study. *Hosp Health Serv Admin* 28(6):21-29, 1983.
Anon: Comprehensive report of the Cooperative Commission on Wellness, 2030. In *Health Care: Three Reports from 2030 A.D.* Washington, DC, American Council of Life Insurance, 1980.

CHAPTER 3

The Institutionalized Patient

BONNIE L. SVARSTAD

Why is it important to understand the patient's feelings, attitudes, and behavior? Does it simply enable the practitioner to provide more compassionate or humane care, as some believe? Or does it enable the practitioner to make better clinical judgments and decisions, as others believe (1)? In this chapter we will suggest that becoming more informed about the processes that govern patient perceptions and behavior can help the practitioner to provide more humane service and that it can aid practitioners in other ways, too. For example, we may be able to elicit more complete and accurate information when interviewing patients if we have a better understanding of the social and psychologic factors that influence patients' willingness and ability to report symptomology, what drugs they have been taking, noncompliance, adverse drug reactions, and other data that may be useful in assessing patients' pharmacy-related needs. If we are aware of the psychosocial factors affecting the patient's response to surgery and other stressful aspects of illness and treatment, then we may be able to devise more effective techniques of helping them to cope with such experiences and hence reduce the reliance on antianxiety agents, hypnotics, and other drugs commonly used to manage institutionalized patients. Moreover, improved understanding and communication can have a significant impact on patient satisfaction (2), the patient's ability to cooperate during painful or noxious procedures (3), postoperative complications and recovery time (4,5), demand for narcotic analgesics (4,5), and the length of hospitalization (4,5).

The purpose of this chapter is to review some of the social and psychologic factors that can influence the perceptions and behavior of institutionalized patients. In the first section, we will provide a brief overview of two different approaches to the understanding of patients and their problems—the purely physiologic or biomedical approach and the biopsychosocial approach. It will be suggested that the traditional biomedical approach is limited and that contemporary practitioners should consider a broader approach that includes social, psychologic, and cultural considerations. In the second and third sections, we will review some of the studies that have examined the role of social and psychologic factors in illness and treatment. Emphasis will be placed on the stresses of physical illness and treatment and the social and psychologic factors affecting the patient's response to illness and treatment. Readers who have an interest in mental illness or specific health conditions should consult the additional reading list, as there is a vast literature of potential interest to specialists.

THE BIOMEDICAL AND BIOPSYCHOSOCIAL APPROACHES

Although there has been increased interest in the social and psychologic dimensions of illness, many practitioners still rely on a purely physiologic or biomedical approach when thinking about patients and their problems (1,6,7). This approach has its base in the biologic sciences and does not explicitly consider the social and psychologic dimensions of disease and its treatment. Instead, it assumes that physical symptoms and disease can be understood in purely physiologic terms. The basic assumptions are that bodily sensations and symptoms result from physical causes, that variations in symptomology reflect variations of physiologic functioning, and that differential response to therapy reflects a change that occurs at the physiologic level. In other words, there is believed to be a one-to-one correlation between the actual bodily state and the way in which this bodily state is perceived, evaluated, and acted on by different people and in different situations.

Although variations in symptomology and illness-related behaviors often reflect true variations in physical functioning, there can be problems if practitioners rely on a purely physiologic model when assessing patient needs and monitoring their response to therapy. For example, they may overestimate or underestimate the effectiveness of certain drug regimens if they assume that perceptions and reports of pain are always correlated with the true extent of injury or trauma. In fact, there is considerable evidence to the contrary. As noted by Skelton and Pennebaker (7) in their recent review, perceptions of pain are not always correlated with the extent of injury, and there often is a low correlation between objective measures and an individual's perception or report of physiologic events having known concomitants in bodily sensations (e.g., perceived and actual heart rates, breathing rates, and nasal congestion). This means that the patient's perceptions and illness-related behaviors cannot be fully explained in physiologic terms. As a result, practitioners and researchers are devoting more serious attention to alternative approaches or models. These newer models are referred to as "sociomedical" or "biopsychosocial" models because they explicitly consider the physiologic as

17

well as the social, psychologic, and cultural dimensions of illness and treatment.

The proponents of the biopsychosocial approach suggest that there is a hierarchy or continuum of natural systems, including molecules, organelles, cells, tissues, organ/organ systems, the person, the dyad or two-person system, the family and other social groups and institutions, the community, the culture-subculture, the society-nation, and the biosphere (1). It is argued further that each system has distinctive properties that can and should be studied with scientific methods and that each system can be influenced by the larger system(s) of which it is a part. This means that we cannot fully understand or interpret patient symptomology and response to therapy unless we become more informed about patients as persons, doctor-patient and nurse-patient relationships, and the power of families and other social groups and institutions. In short, the biopsychosocial approach encourages us to take a broader view of the patient and provides us with a framework for considering the biologic and psychosocial determinants of disease as well as the full range of factors that can influence how physical symptoms and disease are perceived, evaluated, reported, and acted on by different kinds of people in different situations. To illustrate the potential importance of social and psychologic factors in the care of institutionalized patients, let us review some of the studies that have been conducted in this area.

THE STRESSES OF ILLNESS AND TREATMENT

Common sense tells us that a person who has to enter a hospital or long-term care facility probably will experience a certain amount of stress at some point during the diagnostic and treatment process. But what is meant by "stress"? What are its key features and how does it develop? What types of stress are experienced by institutionalized patients? How do they attempt to cope with the potentially stressful and dehumanizing aspects of illness and treatment, and what are the outcomes of these efforts?

Since there are several excellent reviews of the vast literature on stress and coping in illness and treatment (8-11), we will not attempt a thorough review here. However, it might be useful to highlight some of the major conclusions that have been reached by authorities in this area. First, it is clear that people have very different ways of appraising internal and external events and that these cognitive appraisals influence whether or not the event will be viewed as stressful, how the individual will cope with the event, and the emotional, behavioral and physiologic reactions to the event (9). Mechanic (8) suggests that the key is not in the event itself but in the interaction between an event and a person's capacity to deal with it. In other words, patients will experience a stress response (i.e., physiologic changes, feelings of discomfort, and concern) only when there is a discrepancy between the demands of a situation and their capacity to deal with it comfortably. Second, patients experience and attempt to cope with a wide variety of threats when they have a serious illness and must enter an institution. Of course, these threats include the threat to life and the fear of death. In addition, there is evidence that patients

experience many other threats. For example, individuals who experience a myocardial infarction or other serious acute illness may perceive threats to their self-concept and future plans, threats to their emotional equilibrium, threats to their social roles and relationships, and/or other threats associated with the intensive care unit or hospital environment (9). Third, it has been shown that the patient's mode of coping can positively or negatively affect the course of illness in a variety of ways. It can influence the patient's emotional response or level of anxiety, thereby influencing the severity of pain or other symptomology. It can facilitate or interfere with the patient's ability to perform certain tasks that are necessary for proper diagnosis, treatment, or rehabilitation. The patient's coping style also can affect the way in which complaints are presented to the physician, which, in turn, affects the physician's diagnostic and treatment decisions. Furthermore, the patient's mode of coping can have direct physiologic effects. Although there have been some attempts to determine how the patient's mode of coping influences the nature and outcome of drug therapy, there is an urgent need for more systematic work in this area, as will be suggested in the following sections. Fourth, patients adopt many different modes of coping with the same event. These general modes include information-seeking, taking direct action (e.g., requesting medication), avoiding certain actions (e.g., withdrawing), seeking attention or support from others, and using intrapsychic techniques or defenses (e.g., minimizing pain) (9). Given the different modes of coping, it is logical that many factors can affect the degree of threat and the person's ability to cope successfully with it. These factors include the importance of the situation, the degree of discrepancy that is anticipated or experienced, the availability of material resources and social supports, the individual's problem-solving and communication skills, the adequacy of psychologic defenses, and whether the individual maintains a continuing commitment to social relationships and activities (8). Theoretically, this means that there are many potentially effective ways of helping patients to cope with the stresses of illness and treatment. A few of these strategies will be described in a later section. Finally, the processes that govern an individual's perception of physical symptoms, disease, and treatment effects appear to be the same as the processes that govern the perception of other phenomena (7). Similarly, there is a parallel between the processes that determine how an individual will cope with illness and treatment and the processes that govern other types of behavior. Thus, health practitioners and researchers might find it useful to become more knowledgeable and skillful in applying the research that has been conducted by perceptual and cognitive psychologists, learning theorists, and behavioral scientists with other theoretical orientations that might enable us to better predict and explain variations in patient perception and behavior. The potential utility of these perspectives will be illustrated in the next section, in which we discuss some of the specific social and psychologic factors known to affect patient reactions to illness and treatment.

FACTORS AFFECTING PATIENT RESPONSE TO ILLNESS AND TREATMENT

The Patient's Social and Cultural Background

Although health professionals have long noted striking differences in their patients' reactions to pain, scientific interest in the role of social and cultural factors did not fully emerge until the 1950s, when Zborowski (12) published his now classic study of the cultural components in response to pain. His investigation was unique because it focused on patients from four ethnocultural backgrounds—Italians, Jews, Irish, and a group of ''Old Americans'' who were native-born and did not identify themselves with a particular nationality. One of the main findings was that these groups had very different attitudes toward pain and reactions to it, even though they were suffering from similar medical problems (mainly herniated discs, spinal lesions, and other neurologic diseases). The Jewish and Italian patients tended to have a more emotional response to pain, i.e., they felt free to discuss their pain, complain about it, groan, cry, and ask for help. In contrast, the Irish and Old American patients tried to deny their pain and appear more stoic. The meaning of pain and attitudes toward pain medications also varied considerably. For instance, the Italian patients tended to call for pain relievers and easily forgot their suffering after pain relief was achieved. On the other hand, Jewish patients were apprehensive about the effects of analgesics and continued to express concern after being relieved of pain. Unlike the Italian patients, they were worried about the source or meaning of pain and sometimes seemed as if they would prefer to suffer. Using observational and interview data, Zborowski traced the different reactive patterns back to the patients' social and cultural backgrounds, concluding that the patients had learned different ways of reacting to pain and that they had behaved in a manner that was ''expected, accepted, and approved'' by their families and others in their social environment.

Since the publication of this work, there have been other experimental and nonexperimental studies confirming Zborowski's basic hypotheses regarding the role of cultural patterns in the perception and presentation of other symptoms and complaints (13,15). For example, it is well known that an individual's educational, socioeconomic, and religious backgrounds can affect the willingness to recognize and express psychologic distress and to seek help for emotional problems. Because medical diagnosis and treatment depend partly on the patient's report of symptomology, these social factors can then have a significant impact on the physician's diagnosis and treatment plan. A good illustration of this point can be found in Bart's study of women entering the neurology and psychiatry services of a hospital (16). In this case, the investigator compared women who entered the neurology service but were discharged with a psychiatric diagnosis with women who had come directly to the psychiatry service. As expected, she found that the first group was less educated and more likely to have come from low socioeconomic, rural, and non-Jewish backgrounds. In addition, she found that these women were more likely to have had a hysterectomy. Her hypothesis is that certain social groups feel less comfortable than others about expressing their psychologic distress. Consequently, they tend to focus on their physical complaints and to express their emotional problems in physiologic terms, thereby increasing their exposure to unnecessary tests and surgical intervention.

Similar hypotheses have been used to explain why women consistently report more physical and mental health symptoms than men and why women are more likely to use physicians, hospital services, and prescription and nonprescription drugs (17-18). Researchers in this area have suggested that men and women develop different attitudes or orientations toward illness, medical care, and drugs. It is believed that these attitudes are learned or acquired through the process of socialization and are linked to traditional male and female roles in society. In other words, girls are encouraged to seek care for their complaints, whereas boys are encouraged to deny their pain and to avoid ''feminine'' or ''sissy-like'' behaviors (19). As a result, women may have a higher sensitivity to symptoms, a greater willingness to talk about their symptoms, a higher tendency to request help or relief, a higher tendency to express their fears and concerns, and more confidence in health professionals and medications. In addition, men may be less willing to report that they have used certain types of medication, especially if there is some stigma associated with these medications. In one study, for example, men were significantly more likely than women to underreport their actual use of psychotropic medications but were no less likely to report their use of antibiotics (20). If the investigators had inquired about the use of alcohol, they would probably have obtained the opposite result. In other words, men may be more willing to give accurate reports about the extent of their alcohol use because alcohol is viewed as a more socially acceptable coping mechanism for men in our society (21).

In summary, there are many ways in which the patient's social and cultural background can affect his or her response to illness and treatment. Unfortunately, most of the available work has been conducted by researchers who have little familiarity with prescription drugs and pharmacy. As a result, there is a need for more research in these areas.

The Patient's Emotional Status and Coping Style

One of the first studies to examine the role of psychologic factors in the course of illness was Janis' study of emotional disturbance among surgical patients (22). This study stimulated considerable interest because it showed that there was a relationship between preoperative anxiety levels and postoperative emotional disturbance. Since the publication of this study in 1958, there have been many studies on the psychologic factors affecting recovery from illness and surgery. Because these studies have involved diverse patient populations and the use of different measures, they have produced some contradictory findings (9). On the other hand, there have been some consistent results. One of the recurring themes in the literature is that there is a large psychologic component in postoperative or illness-related pain (9,13). This conclusion is based on a number of interesting studies. One of the most well-known studies was reported by Beecher (23). In this study of drug effects and surgery, he found than civilian patients reported more severe pain that wounded soldiers even though the soldiers had more severe tissue damage, suggesting that the two groups of patients attached different meaning to their pain and that the psychic element must be considered when managing pain. Similar findings have been obtained in studies that compare the amount of pain medication sought by patients having different types of surgery. For example, one study found that patients having general surgery sought less pain medication than patients having relatively painless but threatening eye surgery, suggesting the importance of emotional factors in determining the patterns of postoperative drug utilization (24). Other studies consistently have shown that anxiety reduction and pain relief are associated and that about one third of all patients achieve significant pain relief when given a placebo. On the other hand, placebos are not particularly effective in relieving pain if the pain is experimentally induced, if anxiety is not present, of if anxiety remains high because of other factors (13,23,25). These findings are consistent with results of intervention studies aimed at alleviating the stresses associated with surgery (discussed below).

Another interesting set of studies has been reported by physicians and behavioral scientists who are interested in the treatment of asthma (26-27). These researchers acknowledge the role of psychologic factors in the etiology or development of the illness and its characteristics, but remind us that it is also important to consider how psychologic factors can influence the patient's *response* to asthma attacks and the course of drug therapy. Using the Asthma Symptom Checklist (ASC), they were able to show that patients have very different ways of responding to an asthma attack. For example, patients with high panic-fear scores were more likely to report feeling scared, panicky, and afraid of dying or being left alone when they experienced asthma attacks. In a subsequent analysis, they found a weak correlation between the patient's panic-fear scores and pulmonary function levels, suggesting that the patient's coping or response style is not solely related to the patient's actual medical condition, but that it may be a function of personality and behavioral factors (26). To test this hypothesis, they examined the correlation between the patient's scores on the panic-fear scale derived from the Asthma Symptom Checklist and their scores on a 15-item panic-fear scale derived from the Minnesota Multiphasic Personality Inventory (MMPI) (27). As predicted, there was a strong correlation. The patients who reported feeling panicky or frightened during asthma attacks also described themselves as highly emotional and inclined to give up when faced with other difficulties, whereas the patients who reported low fear during asthmatic attacks generally described themselves as calm, stable, and self-controlled in other situations.

These investigators also found a close relationship between the patient's coping or response style and the patient's request for medications (28). Low-scoring panic-fear patients were least likely to request prn medications, regardless of their objectively measured pulmonary function levels. Similarly, the high-scoring panic-fear patients frequently requested prn medications, regardless of their pulmonary functioning. The patients with moderate panic-fear scores were the only patients who requested medication according to their medical condition as measured by their pulmonary

functioning levels. This led the researchers to conclude that the patient's request for medication cannot be used as an accurate index of the effectiveness of therapy unless one explicitly considers the patient's response style. They also suggest that the patient's response style should be considered when evaluating the patient's need for discharge medications and counseling, because there is evidence that the patient's behavior can have a direct influence on medical decisions and the course of treatment. For example, there is evidence that patients with high panic-fear scores receive more intensive oral corticosteroid regimens at discharge, thereby becoming exposed to the potential risks of side effects or overuse (26). How these patients influence their physicians' prescribing decisions is not clear, but it is believed that panicky patients receive more intensive regimens because their subjective reports make them appear worse. On the other hand, low-scoring panic-fear patients may present a ''serene picture of well-being,'' which, in turn, leads to earlier discharge, less intensive drug regimens, and possibly less counseling by the physician and other health care providers. As a result, these patients may continue to minimize or disregard their asthmatic distress and fail to follow their scheduled drug regimens, thereby becoming exposed to other potentially serious consequences (28).

In summary, there are a number of different problems that can arise if the practitioner is not cognizant of the psychologic factors that can influence the patient's subjective symptomology and his or her ''style'' of coping or responding to illness and treatment. It is clear that we need to have a better understanding of these different ''coping styles,'' whether these coping styles are adopted by patients who have other types of illness, and how these coping styles actually influence drug-related decisions and therapeutic outcomes.

The Provider's Characteristics and Behavior

How patients respond to their illness and treatment also is influenced by the characteristics and behavior of their physicians and other health care providers. Some of the major considerations are listed below.

Prescriber Expectations and Suggestion

It is well known that an individual's physiologic and psychologic responses to a placebo depend in part on what that individual has been led to expect by the person who prescribed or administered the placebo (25). A good illustration can be found in Brodeur's study of pharmacy students (29). In order to determine the effects of suggestion, the investigator divided the students into three groups. The first group was told that they had been given a meprobamate-like tranquilizer, the second group was told that they were to take an amphetamine-like stimulant, and the third group was led to believe that they had been given the placebo. Actually, everyone was given cornstarch. When the students' responses were compared, it was found that their pulse rates were in the expected direction and that 60% of the students felt that they had experienced the suggested drug effect.

Other studies have shown a correlation between the patient's response to an active drug and the physician's personality, attitudes toward a drug, and general level of optimism about drug therapy. One of the earliest studies to examine the role of physician attitudes was conducted by Uhlenruth et al (30). They selected two psychiatrists who were known to have very different views about the use of drugs in the treatment of neurotic patients. The first doctor was noncommittal in his views about drug therapy, whereas the second doctor expected significant differences to occur. These psychiatrists then were asked to treat two matched groups of psychoneurotic patients who would be given meprobamate, phenobarbital, or a placebo. A double-blind design was used, and the patient's responses to drug therapy were evaluated using a variety of techniques, including the patient's overall judgment, the physician's judgment, and a 45-symptom checklist. One of the main findings was that there was no difference among the drug groups if the patient was treated by the first doctor but that there was an improvement among the meprobamate and phenobarbital groups if the patient was treated by the second doctor. These findings led the authors to conclude that the physician's expectations are an important influence even though double-blind procedures are used. How physician expectations actually affect the patient's reaction to drug therapy is unknown. However, there are a number of interesting hypotheses that have been advanced recently by cognitively oriented psychologists. For example, Skelton and Pennebaker (7) suggest that the physician's behavior may lead patients to adopt a certain hypothesis about how the drug will affect them. These patients then engage in a "selective monitoring" of bodily sensations. In other words, they actively search for signs that are consistent with the suggestion-induced hypothesis and ignore sensations that are inconsistent, thereby increasing the probability that the expected effect will be perceived and reported to the physician.

Although there has not been much research on the factors affecting the patient's perception and reporting of adverse drug reactions, some interesting hypotheses have been advanced. To test some of these hypotheses, Schachter and Singer (31) asked healthy volunteers to participate in a study testing the effects of a vitamin on vision. Although all subjects were told that they would receive an injection of the vitamin, they actually were given an injection of epinephrine or an injection of saline solution. The subjects then received varied communication about the potential side effects. One group was correctly informed about what to expect (warm and flushed face, hand tremors, heart pounding, etc); one group was misinformed about what to expect (numb feet, itching, headache, etc); and one group received no information about the potential side effects. Finally, the subject was told to wait with another person while the drug took effect. In fact, the other person was a confederate who had been instructed to behave in one of two specified ways. This research design enabled the researchers to assess the effect of the drug, the communication about side effects, and the environmental cues provided by the confederate. Basically, they found that the subjects were more susceptible to social influence and mislabeling of side effects if they had received the epinephrine and had no appropriate explanation for their sensations.

To our knowledge, this study has never been replicated in a clinical setting. But it does suggest another approach to the study of communication effects as well as some interesting hypotheses about the conditions that might lead to patient error and bias in the reporting of adverse drug reactions. Controlled studies of this kind are especially important as pharmacists become more involved in clinical trials, discharge counseling, and the design and evaluation of package information leaflets and other educational materials. Moreover, there is some evidence that some package-information leaflets are more likely than others to cause patient bias or error in naming potential side effects and other problems associated with the use of a drug (32). Why these differences occur and how such errors can be prevented are issues that need to be explored in future studies.

Provider Communication Before Surgery and Other Stressful Events

We now turn to a series of studies that are primarily concerned with the effects of information or emotional support on the patient's reactions to diagnostic procedures, surgery, and heart attacks. These studies are of interest here because they often include a systematic assessment of drug utilization before and after patients have been exposed to varying kinds and amounts of information and support. In their recent review of this literature, Mumford et al (5) found 34 experimental studies testing the effects of various "psychologic interventions" on recovery from surgery and heart attacks. While the kind and amount of information and support varied from study to study, the findings generally showed that the patients who receive high amounts of information and support from their providers have significantly shorter hospital stays and fewer postoperative complications. Of the 34 studies they reviewed, 13 also included measures of postoperative drug use. The majority of these studies showed that the patients who receive high amounts of information or emotional support use a significantly lower number of narcotic analgesics, tranquilizers, and sleep medications. One of the most widely quoted studies of this kind involved an examination of 97 patients receiving elective intra-abdominal operations (33). The patients who were assigned to the experimental group received detailed instruction and encouragement from an anesthetist the night before the operation. They were told the nature of the pain to be experienced, what would be done at various times, how to relax, how to turn, and how to use the trapeze. The surgical residents ordered the narcotic analgesics and the nurses administered the medications, but both groups were blinded or unaware of which patients had been assigned to the experimental and control groups. As predicted, there was a considerable reduction in the use of narcotic analgesics and the length of hospitalization. The experimental patients required one half the narcotic analgesics required by the other patients and were able to leave the hospital an average of 2.7 days earlier.

Other investigators have examined the effects of special instruction on the patient's reactions during a painful or noxious medical examination. One of the best examples of this work is a study examining 48 hospitalized patients who received an endoscopic examination (3). This study was designed to test several hypotheses derived from social psychologic theory about negative affect and behavior during threatening situations. The first hypothesis was that people are less likely to experience negative affect or emotional reactions if they can accurately anticipate what they will feel during the threatening event. Therefore, it was expected that patients would experience less emotional distress if they received accurate information about what would be done and the specific sensations that would be experienced during each step of the endoscopic examination (e.g., how the drug would affect them, the size of the tube, how it feels to have air pumped into the stomach). A second hypothesis was that people are better able to perform danger-controlling behaviors if they have received detailed instructions or behavioral preparation. Thus, it was expected that patients would be better able to perform certain required tasks (e.g., controlled breathing and swallowing) if they received prior instruction and rehearsal about how and when to act during the diagnostic procedure. To test these hypotheses, the authors divided the patients into four groups: a group receiving detailed sensory information, a group receiving specific behavioral instructions, a group receiving both types of information, and a control group. To control the nature and extent of information given, all instructions were provided by tape-recorded messages and booklets that had been prepared by a participating nurse. The clinic staff and observer were blind to the group assignment, permitting an objective evaluation during the endoscopic examination. As predicted, the group receiving sensory information experienced fewer emotional reactions during the procedure. They required significantly less diazepam during the procedure, showed more stable heart rates, and had a lower frequency of gagging. The behavioral instruction group also used fewer milligrams of tranquilizers and showed a stabilization of heart rate and less gagging, but these differences were not significant. Another major finding was that both sensory information and behavioral instructions were needed to help the patient achieve better control over tube swallowing. This led the authors to conclude that the patient's ability to cope with threatening events is affected by two key processes—emotion and competency to deal with danger. In summary, there is abundant evidence that the provision of information and support can significantly alter patterns of recovery and drug utilization. Therefore, we would agree with Mumford et al (5) when they conclude that more attention needs to be given to the education and counseling of institutionalized patients and their families.

It is often argued that the medical care system cannot afford to take on the emotional status of the patient as its responsibility. Time is short and costs are high. However, it may be that medicine cannot afford to ignore the patient's emotional status, assuming that it will take care of itself. Anxiety and depression do not go away by being ignored.

The Provider's Style of Medication Counseling

Another factor that can affect the patient's perceptions and behavior is the physician's style of medication counseling. Since it is extremely difficult to conduct scientific research in this area, there are only a few studies available. However, the existing data suggest that physicians adopt different styles of interviewing and counseling their patients about drugs and that these varied styles are correlated with different outcomes. These data were collected as part of a sociologic study that included systematic observation and analysis of physician-patient interaction in an outpatient clinic, review of medical and pharmacy records, follow-up interviews, and unannounced "bottle checks" conducted in the patient's homes about a week after their clinic visit (34-35). When we examined the physicians' methods of interviewing and counseling about drugs, we found that they used a wide variety of interpersonal techniques and that some of these techniques were more effective than others in terms of gaining the patient's understanding and acceptance of the treatment plan. We also found that the physicians could be divided into two groups based on their general style of relating to patients. The first style can be called the "participative style," because the physicians in this group made a rather consistent effort to increase their patients' understanding and acceptance of the treatment plan and to solicit patient feedback and participation in drug-related decisions. A quantitative analysis of the transcripts indicated that these physicians gave more specific and complete medication instructions, a higher number of verbal and nonverbal cues of approachability or friendliness toward the patient, and a higher number of statements indicating the purpose or rationale for drug therapy. They also used more effective interviewing techniques and reacted in a nonjudgmental and flexible manner when their patients complained about their medications or admitted noncompliance. Although they were firm when the circumstances warranted it, they rarely exerted their authority when trying to gain their patients' cooperation. Instead, they tried to identify and resolve the patient's concerns and drug-taking problems, ultimately enhancing the patient's faith in and acceptance of the physician and the drug regimen. The second group of physicians adopted one of several autocratic styles. A few gave the impression that the patient could "take-it-or-leave-it," whereas others were more authoritarian in their approach. Unlike the participative physicians, the autocratic physicians prescribed medications without much instruction or explanation. They also tended to ignore their patients when they complained or mentioned side effects and often became angry or upset if the patient admitted noncompliance.

To determine how these varied styles might influence the course of drug therapy, we conducted an in-depth analysis of a subsample of patients being treated for the same condition (hypertension). As predicted, there was a close correlation between the physician-patient relationship and different outcome measures. The patients who were being treated by a participative or nonautocratic physician had a more accurate understanding of how to take their medications, a more positive evaluation of the prescribed drugs, higher compliance after the visit, and fewer broken appointments. We also observed that the patients of the autocratic physicians were less likely to trust the physician, in the sense that they asked fewer questions, were less likely to express their concerns about side effects, and were more likely to conceal or deny their noncompliance when visiting the physician. In effect, the autocratic physicians received inaccurate information and feedback and, as a result, we observed a number of cases where they made errors in clinical judgment. For example, they tended to overestimate the patient's compliance and underestimate the efficacy of the drug regimen when the patient's condition did not stabilize or improve. Rather than question the accuracy of the patient's report, they simply assumed treatment failure and proceeded to change the drug regimen, thereby creating further confusion and problems for the patient. This may explain why they were given a larger number of prescriptions even though their medical records indicated no major difference in the severity of their condition. The following excerpt of a research interview illustrates the sequence of events and potential problems from the patient's perspective.

PATIENT: The doctor said, "Well, the 25 mg pills must not be enough so we'll try the 50 mg." I couldn't tell him at that point that I wasn't taking it regularly before. I was worried though, so I began by taking those 50 mg pills. I got so sick that I couldn't even walk to the bathroom . . . was in bed and after a short while the whole bed seemed to be moving around. My heart felt like it was going to come out, pounding. I had to crawl to the bathroom to vomit . . . thought I was going to die. I flushed them down the toilet.

AUTHOR: Does the doctor know you're not taking them now?

PATIENT: No. He thinks I'm taking them.

AUTHOR: Did you tell him what happened when you took the 50 mg pills after not taking any medicine at all?

PATIENT: No. I couldn't tell him that. I told him that they gave me headaches.

AUTHOR: Why couldn't you tell him the truth?

PATIENT: He would fuss and fuss. I don't want to go through all those "changes."

Whether this patient would have revealed her true feelings and experiences to an inquiring pharmacist can only be speculated. But our experience leads us to believe that it is difficult to evaluate the patient's report of drug use without considering the patient's relationship with his or her physician. We also suspect that pharmacy practitioners are like other practitioners in that they adopt various "styles" or approaches to the interviewing and counseling of patients. As a result, there may be considerable differences among pharmacists in terms of their ability to achieve patient trust and participation during an interview or counseling session. This hypothesis was supported in a recent study of 588 pharmacist-patient transactions that took place in a hospital pharmacy (36). In this study, we found that the pharmacist's age and interviewing style had a significant effect on the degree to which the patient asked questions and made statements about the drugs being dispensed. Patients were more expressive with younger pharmacists and pharmacists who used certain techniques for eliciting patient questions and feedback.

It is known that community pharmacists have different attitudes about medication counseling and that these attitudes are highly correlated with their interviewing and counseling behaviors (37), but relatively little is known about how institutional pharmacists actually conduct medication histories and discharge counseling sessions. Do they also adopt different styles or approaches? What factors lead them to adopt these styles? Are certain styles more effective than others? Under what circumstances and with what types of patients are these techniques more effective? Can these styles be taught and/or modified? These are just a few ques-

tions that deserve more attention if we are to do a more effective job of preparing pharmacy students for institutional practice.

Nurse Attitudes and Practices

Although institutionalized patients often receive pain and sleep medications that are to be administered by nurses on a prn or "as needed" basis, there are only a few studies that have examined the nurse-patient relationship and its potential impact on the course of drug therapy. One of these studies was conducted by a pharmacist who was interested in the administration of hypnotics (38). To gain a better understanding of the patient's role in drug administration, he interviewed and reviewed the records of 100 adult admissions to the general medicine ward of a university hospital. He found that 87 patients received a prn hypnotic order and that seven nurses were involved in the administration of 310 prn hypnotic doses. When he examined nurse differences in drug administration, several interesting findings emerged. First, there was considerable variation in the degree to which patients were involved in the nurse's decision to administer a prn hypnotic dose. One half of the doses were initially requested by the patient; 30% were given after the nurse offered the medication; and 20% were given without any patient discussion. Of the latter group, one half were unaware that they had received a sleep medication and did not think they needed it. Interestingly enough, the majority of these "routine" prn doses were administered by the same nurse. This raises the possibility that there are significant differences in nurse knowledge of therapeutics, nurse attitudes toward sleep and sleep medications, and/or nurse perception of various roles and responsibilities. Whether and how these differences actually influence the nurse's performance of drug-related tasks are issues that need to be explored.

Nurse-patient interaction regarding pain medication is a second area that deserves more careful attention, because there is some evidence that nurses have variable pain philosophies and that these varied philosophies affect nurse interpretation of drug orders and performance of other drug-related tasks. Most of the work in this area is anecdotal and exploratory in nature, making it difficult to draw definitive conclusions about the role of nurse attitudes. However, the available data are provocative. For example, Fagerhaugh and Strauss (37) studied nurse-patient interaction in nine California hospitals and found wide variation in nurse attitudes about pain management. They found varied opinions about who should give information about pain medications, how much information should be given about the pain and pain medications, how much pain the patient should endure before calling the nurse, the amount of control that patients should have, when the nurse should consult a physician for changes in the drug order, and other issues. They also observed that physicians varied in the amount of discretion they allowed nurses and that nurses varied in their interpretation of these orders. Some nurses consistently gave the lowest amounts permitted; other nurses consistently gave the highest amounts permitted. Given these opposing views and practices, the researchers were not surprised to find considerable patient confusion, patient dissatisfaction and mistrust, and conflict in patient-staff and staff-staff interactions. Why these varied philosophies exist, how they can be managed, and how they ultimately affect the quality of patient care are questions that are virtually unexplored.

Institutional Differences

A close examination of the literature reveals that there are considerable differences in drug use from one institution to another. For instance, specialists in oncology have reported wide variation in the extent to which psychotropic drugs are used by cancer patients in five major centers (40). They noted that 22% of all antianxiety agents were given for "medical procedures" but that this was due entirely to the prescribing practices at two of the five participating institutions. They speculated that these differences may be due to staff attitudes, not the incidence of psychologic disorder.

. . . different staffs hold distinct postures concerning the prescription of pychotropic drugs, and these attitudes determine in large measure the utilization rates of these drugs.

Others have observed that there is extraordinary variation in the use of antipsychotic drugs among nursing homes. In their study of 173 Tennessee nursing homes, Ray et al (41) found 43 homes in which none of the continuous patients received antipsychotic medication on a chronic or daily basis. On the other hand, they found 15 homes in which 20-46% of the patients received these drugs on a chronic basis. Because there was a positive correlation between home size and chronic drug usage and because none of the high-volume facilities were devoted to psychiatric care, it is possible that social or economic factors were at work. However, more information is needed if we are to gain a better understanding of these trends and why they occur.

My colleagues and I also observed considerable institutional differences in a study that is not yet published (42). This study examined the prescribing and administration of hypnotic drugs among 372 newly admitted residents in six proprietary and three nonprofit church-related nursing homes. As expected, the prescribing rate did not vary from one facility to another; the patients who resided in proprietary facilities received about the same number of hypnotic drug orders as did the patients residing in nonprofit facilities. However, there was wide variation in the amount of medication that was actually administered by the nurses in these facilities. The patients who had a hypnotic drug order and resided in a proprietary facility received four times the amount of sleep medication that was administered to their counterparts in nonprofit facilities (12.5 vs 3.0 doses per patient month). Of course, there are many possible explanations. The "biomedical" model would suggest that these differences are due merely to differences in patient mix or the incidence of physical and psychologic problems that are disruptive of sleep. The "biopsychosocial" model would suggest a broader approach. It would acknowledge that admissions and referral policies ultimately can affect patient mix, thereby influencing patient demand and patterns of drug administration. However, it would add other factors to the equation. These factors would include possible differences in the social and cultural background of the patients,

the nurses' training and attitudes, staff-patient ratios and the availability of other resources, and other social and economic factors that must be explored. Robers and I now are examining some of these issues in a more comprehensive study that involves an examination of pharmacy and nursing records, a survey of nurses responsible for administering sleep medications, and a survey of nursing home administrators. It is hoped that this kind of behavioral research will increase our understanding of the full range of factors that influence patterns of drug utilization, thereby aiding practitioners in their attempts to control the quality and cost of drug therapy in long-term care facilities. Whether this type of approach will prove to be useful remains unseen.

CONCLUSION

There are a wide variety of factors affecting the patient's reactions to illness and treatment. These factors include the patient's medical condition as well as the patient's social and cultural background, the patient's emotional status and coping style, the physician-patient relationship, the nurse-patient relationship, and the institution in which these transactions occur. This means that the institutional pharmacist may find it helpful to explicitly consider these factors when conducting medication histories, monitoring the patient's response to drug therapy, providing discharge counseling, and/or conducting drug utilization reviews. We believe that pharmacists who become more informed and skillful in applying behavioral science principles will be in a better position to care for their patients, but a detailed blueprint cannot be provided at this time. We only can urge pharmacy practitioners and researchers to accept the challenge of learning more about the social and psychologic dimensions of illness and drug therapy.

REFERENCES

1. Engel GL: The clinical application of the biopsychosocial model. *Am J Psychiatry* 137:534-544, 1980.
2. Ley P, Bradshaw PW, Kincey JA, et al: Increasing patients' satisfaction with communications. *Br J Soc Clin Psychol* 15:403-413, 1976.
3. Johnson JE, Leventhal H: Effects of accurate expectations and behavioral instructions on reactions during a noxious medical examination. *J Soc Psychol* 29:710-718, 1974.
4. Ley P: Psychological studies of doctor-patient communication. In Rachman S (ed): *Contributions to Medical Psychology*, vol 1. Oxford, Pergamon Press, 1977.
5. Mumford E, Schlesinger H, Glass G: The effects of psychological intervention on recovery from surgery and heart attacks: An analysis of the literature. *Am J Public Health* 72:141-151, 1982.
6. Engel GL: The need for a new medical model: A challenge for biomedicine. *Science* 196:129-136, 1977.
7. Skelton JA, Pennebaker JW: The psychology of physical symptoms and sensations. In Sanders GS, Suls J (eds): *Social Psychology of Health and Illness*. Hillsdale, NJ, Lawrence Erlbaum Associates, 1982, pp 99-128.
8. Mechanic D: *Medical Sociology*, ed. 2. New York, Free Press, 1978.
9. Cohen F, Lazarus RS: Coping with the stresses of illness. In Stone GC, Cohen F, Adler NE, et al (eds): *Health Psychology—A Handbook*. San Francisco, Jossey-Bass, 1979, pp 217-254.
10. Cohen F, Lazarus RS: Coping and adaptation in health and illness. In Mechanic D (ed): *Handbook of Health, Health Care, and the Health Professions*. New York, Free Press, 1983, pp 608-635.
11. Dimond M: Social adaptation of the chronically ill. In Mechanic D (ed): *Handbook of Health, Health Care, and the Health Professions*. New York, Free Press, 1983, pp 636-654.

12. Zborowski M: Cultural components in response to pain. *J Soc Issues* 8:16-30, 1952.
13. Sternbach RA (ed): *The Psychology of Pain*. New York, Raven Press, 1978.
14. Kotarba JA: *Chronic Pain: Its Social Dimensions*. Beverly Hills, Sage Publications, 1983.
15. Mechanic D: Social psychologic factors affecting the presentation of bodily complaints. *N Engl J Med* 286:1132-1139, 1972.
16. Bart PB: Social structure and vocabularies of discomfort: What happened to female hysteria. J Health Soc Behav 9:188-193, 1968.
17. Nathanson CA: Sex, illness, and medical care: A review of data, theory, and method. *Soc Sci Med* 11:13-25, 1977.
18. Verbrugge LM: Sex differences in legal drug use. *J Soc Issues* 38:59-76, 1982.
19. Lewis CE, Lewis MA: The potential impact of sexual inequality on health. *N Engl J Med* 297:863-869, 1977.
20. Parry HJ, Balter MB, Cisin IH: Primary levels of underreporting psychotropic drug use. *Pub Opin Q* 34:582-592, 1970-71.
21. Svarstad BL: The sociology of drugs. In Wertheimer AI, Smith MC (eds): *Pharmacy Practice: Social and Behavioral Aspects*. Baltimore, University Park Press, 1981, pp 261-277.
22. Janis IL: *Psychological stress: Psychoanalytic and Behavioral Studies of Surgical Patients*. New York, John Wiley & Sons, 1958.
23. Beecher HK: *Measurement of Subjective Responses: Quantitative Effects of Drugs*. New York, Oxford University Press, 1959.
24. Drew FL, Moriarty RW, Shapiro AP: An approach to the measurement of the pain and anxiety responses of surgical patients. *Psychosom Med* 30:826-836, 1968.
25. Jospe M: *The Placebo Effect in Healing*. Lexington, Lexington Books, 1978.
26. Konsman RA, Dahlem NW, Spector S, et al: Observations on subjective symptomatology, coping behavior, and medical decisions in asthma. *Psychosom Med* 39:102-119, 1977.
27. Dirks JF, Jones NF, Kinsman RA: Panic-fear: A personality dimension related to intractability in asthma. *Psychosom Med* 39:120-126, 1977.
28. Dahlem NW, Kinsman RA, Horton DJ: Panic-fear in asthma: Requests for as-needed medications in relation to pulmonary function measurements. *J Allergy Clin Immunol* 60:295-300, 1977.
29. Brodeur DW: The effects of stimulant and tranquilizer placebos on healthy subjects in a real-life situation. *Psychopharmacologia* 7:444-452, 1965.
30. Uhlenhuth E, Canter A, Neustadt J, et al: The symptomatic relief of anxiety with meprobamate, phenobarbital and placebo. *Am J Psychiatry* 134:659-662, 1977.
31. Schachter S, Singer JE: Cognitive, social and physiological determinants of emotional state. *Psychol Rev* 69:379-399, 1962.
32. Berry SH, Kanouse DE, Hayes-Roth B, et al: *Informing Patients about Drugs: Analysis of Alternative Designs for Flurazepam Leaflets*. Santa Monica, Rand Corp, 1981.
33. Egbert LD, Battit GE. Welch CE, et al: Reduction of postoperative pain by encouragement and instruction of patients. *N Engl J Med* 270:825-827, 1964.
34. Svarstad BL: Physician-patient communication and patient conformity with medical advice. In Mechanic D: *The Growth of Bureaucratic Medicine*. New York, John Wiley & Sons, 1976, pp 220-238.
35. Svarstad BL: Doctor-patient communication. In Currie B (ed): *Patient Education in the Primary Care Setting*. Proceedings of the Conference on Patient Education in Primary Care Setting, Madison, WI, April 11-12, 1978, pp 17-29.
36. Svarstad BL, Mason HL, Schuna AA. Factors affecting pharmacist-patient communications: A multivariate analysis. Paper presented at the American Association of Colleges of Pharmacy Annual Meeting, Denver, July 1979.
37. Mason HL, Svarstad BL: Medication counseling behaviors and attitudes of rural community pharmacists. *Drug Intell Clin Pharm* 18:409-414, 1984.
38. Parker WA: Effect of hospitalization on patient use of hypnotics. *Am J Hosp Pharm* 40:446-447, 1983.
39. Fagerhaugh SY, Strauss A: *Politics of Pain Management: Staff-Patient Interaction*. Menlo Park, Addison-Wesley, 1977.
40. Derogatis LR, Feldstein M, Morrow G, et al: A survey of psychotropic drug prescriptions in an oncology population. *Cancer* 44:1919-1929, 1979.
41. Ray WA, Federspiel CF, Schaffner W: A study of antipsychotic drug use in nursing homes: Epidemiologic evidence suggesting misuse. *Am J Public Health* 70:485-491, 1980.
42. Svarstad BL, Bond CA, Peterson RP. *The Use of Hypnotics in Proprietary and Non-Profit Church-Related Nursing Homes*. (Mimeographed)

ADDITIONAL READING

Howard J, Strauss A (eds): *Humanizing Health Care*. New York, John Wiley & Sons, 1975.
Jospe M: *The Placebo Effect in Healing*. Lexington, Lexington Books, 1978.
Ley P: Practical methods of improving communication. In Morris LA, Mazis MB, Barofsky I (eds): *The Banbury Report No. 6: Product Labeling and Health Risks*. Cold Spring Harbor Laboratory, 1980, pp 135-146.
Mechanic D. *Medical Sociology,* ed 2. New York, Free Press, 1978.
Mechanic D. *Mental Health and Social Policy,* ed 2. Englewood Cliffs, NJ, Prentice-Hall, 1980.
Mechanic D (ed): *Handbook of Health, Health Care, and the Health Professions*. New York, Free Press, 1983.
Pennebaker JW. *The Psychology of Physical Symptoms*. New York, Springer-Verlag, 1982.
Sanders GS, Suls J (eds): *Social Psychology of Health and Illness*. Hillsdale, NJ, Lawrence Erlbaum Associates, 1982.
Stone GC, Cohen F, Adler NE et al (eds): *Health Psychology—A Handbook*. San Francisco, Jossey-Bass, 1980.
Svarstad BL: The sociology of drugs. In Wertheimer AI, Smith MC (eds): *Pharmacy Practice: Social and Behavioral Aspects*. Baltimore, University Park Press, 1981, pp 261-277.

Administration and Management

EFFECTIVE ADMINISTRATION AND MANAGEMENT OF A PHARMACY DEPARTMENT IN AN INSTITUTION

The successful delivery of any pharmacy service offered will be based on expert management and administrative procedures. The director of pharmacy services of personnel specializing in departmental administration must be familiar with the health care system in general and the specific function of the institution in particular so that the pharmacy's goals can be achieved in cooperation with all other departments in the institution and with other programs that ensure continuity of care for the patient.

Broad areas of administrative and management responsibilities include planning and integrating professional services, budgeting, inventory control, cost review, cost effectiveness, audit, maintenance of records, and preparation of reports. As a basis for the responsibility, pharmacy personnel must be thoroughly familiar with the organization of a hospital, with staff and line relationships, and with appropriate lines of communication.

Pharmacy activities must be coordinated with medical, nursing, and other services and with the administrative elements of the hospital. Pharmacy administrative personnel must be able to prepare suitable written communications to the hospital staff concerning pertinent pharmacy matters.

The director of pharmacy services, or his designee, is responsible for the justification and accountability of all pharmaceutical services in terms of patient care and the expenditure of funds. He must be able to analyze and interpret prescribing trends and the economic impact of new drug developments, which for budgeting purposes are translated to his forecast of future drug expenditures. He must maintain an adequate system of stock and inventory control. He must have the ability to control operational costs without compromising services.

The director of pharmacy services is responsible for records on all pharmacy operations that may be legally or administratively required. The data collected should be translated into periodic or special reports. These may include, but usually are not limited to, data on prescriptions dispensed, controlled drugs dispensed, drug purchases, inspections and improvements in operations. The use of automated data processing systems may allow more effective and efficient handling of pharmacy records and data. A basic knowledge and understanding of the applications of such systems to pharmacy operations is important to the department.

CHAPTER 4

JCAH Accreditation Standards*

JACQUELINE P. GARY

The Joint Commission on the Accreditation of Hospitals (JCAH) is an offshoot of the Hospital Standardization Program begun by the American College of Surgeons (ACS) in 1918. At that time the ACS came to the realization that surgeons are a product not only of their medical schools and instructors but of the institutions in which they train. Members of the ACS devised a five-part standard, four parts of which were related to the functioning of the medical staff and their review of care; the fifth included a requirement for adequate laboratory and radiology facilities. Hospitals participated in the program at their request; representatives were sent to those hospitals to evaluate their compliance with the standard. In the 1918 survey, the first, the results were so poor and the findings so onerous that all information concerning the hospitals was destroyed and not made public. From that low point the Hospital Standardization Program thrived as hospitals throughout the country accepted the standard and attempted to comply. Although the five-part standard stayed basically the same, explanations of the standard eventually occupied over 100 pages of small print.

By 1950, the program was in trouble because of its own success; it was too expensive for the ACS to fund alone, despite the contributions of individual members to its upkeep. The ACS was forced to ask for assistance in maintaining such a program. After considerable infighting for control among the prospective members, the JCAH was formed and incorporated in 1951. It was composed of seven members from the American Medical Association, seven members from the American Hospital Association, three members of the College of Physicians, and three members of the College of Surgeons. A representative of the Canadian Medical Association also was a member. In 1957, the Canadians withdrew to form their own program, but in 1979 the American Dental Association was added as a member with one representative, and in 1980 a consumer was added. The JCAH has two primary charges. The first is to develop standards for hospitals and other health care–related facilities, and the second is to evaluate the facilities against those standards. If they are in compliance, they are issued a certificate and are said to be accredited. The JCAH maintains that compliance with their standard represents optimal achievable care. This is in contrast with state and federal regulations, which represent minimal standards.

To understand the JCAH in relation to the accreditation process, it is important to realize that it is, in reality, a dichotomy. The standards are the first part of the dichotomy—the survey process is the second. The standards are developed with input from experts in their respective fields, are sent to various health care professionals and institutions for review and comment, and finally are approved by the JCAH Board of Commissioners before they become effective. Every effort is made to develop standards that reflect current thinking in medicine and related fields. The standards also show the influence of landmark legal decisions. The standards are as valid as they can be made. Contrary to the opinion of some, the JCAH tries very hard not to dictate how hospitals should be managed or to dictate the practice of medicine. The standards tell what should be done, and the individual health care facilities and medical staffs decide how to do it.

Despite continuing efforts, the survey process to date does not reflect the same validity as the standards. Perhaps this is because the surveys are done by individuals, and individuals are bound to be variable. Much of the criticism leveled against the JCAH is actually the result of the survey process. The survey process, by its very nature, may never be perfect, but those who think to solve problems by eliminating or diminishing the standards may be "throwing the baby out with the bath water." Without definite standards, health care facilities would have little direction and nothing to live up to.

Accreditation is entirely voluntary; no health care facility will find it necessary to be accredited in order to be reimbursed by third-party payers. The JCAH, in reality, reflects the efforts of the health care industry to police itself.

The Pharmacist in an Accredited Hospital

The pharmacist in an accredited hospital occupies a unique position. Knowledgable and an expert in his field, he may be virtually powerless in the hospital structure and seldom called on to share his expertise. JCAH standards require the director of pharmacy services to develop policies and procedures for the pharmacy and for drug use throughout the hospital; yet, by that same mandate, those same policies and procedures can be carried out only with the approval of the medical staff. Although practitioners and nurses may ask for his advice, they are under no obligation to follow it. Administration expects the pharmacy services to show a

---

*Portions of this chapter are adapted by permission from publications of the Dallas–Ft. Worth Hospital Council.

profit, but the medical staff dictates which drugs he must stock, even if those drugs are neither medically nor cost effective. He must coax a reluctant medical staff to participate in the pharmacy and therapeutics function, a function delegated by the JCAH standards to the organized medical staff, not to the pharmacist. He, more often than not, finds himself assigned to review antibiotic usage, a JCAH medical staff requirement that physicians feel interferes with the individual practice of medicine and that they therefore resent. He incurs the animosity of nursing service by participating in the review of medication errors. In small hospitals where he is the only pharmacist, he is on call 24 hours a day, 7 days a week.

As if contending with the administration, medical staff, and nursing service were not enough, the pharmacist also must contend with JCAH requirements and prepare for a JCAH survey. At least a portion of those responsibilities can be eased through the elimination of misunderstandings about JCAH standards and the acquisition of an expertise concerning the survey process.

THE SURVEY PROCESS

Preparing for Survey

The first principle of survey preparation is to know the standards. You may not be held to anything that is not in the standards. Because people are variable and come from differing backgrounds, the wording of the standards may not mean the same thing to everybody. This is particularly true of the JCAH surveyor because the person responsible for the pharmacy section of the standards is the administrative member of the team. He often has no background in pharmacy and was trained to survey pharmacy not by a pharmacist but by another administrative surveyor. He may do an adequate evaluation of the pharmacy, but it is easy to see how he and a pharmacist might interpret standards differently.

You should also understand certain key words in the standards. If the words "shall" or "must" are used, they mean just that. However, "should" allows more latitude. "Should" means that you must meet the intent of the standard in an equivalent or better way. The surveyor will not be allowed to judge if your method of meeting the standard is equivalent. He must document his findings and forward the report to the central office of the JCAH for final judgment. Other phrases used are "it is desirable" or "it is recommended" or similar terminology. Failure to comply with standards worded like this does not generally affect your accreditation status, but the words are meant to encourage compliance.

Obtain a copy of the recommendations from the previous survey. Make certain that they are implemented to the best of your ability. Recommendations not implemented carry more weight each time they are made. If you have any questions regarding their implementation, call the JCAH hotline. Since the number changes occasionally, call 1-800-555-1212 to obtain the correct number.

The Hospital Survey Profile (HSP) developed by the JCAH will be given to you to complete about 3 months prior to most surveys. Use it as a guide in preparing for

survey because it includes the same questions the surveyor will ask. You may be certain that if the HSP asks a question with a yes or no answer, not only is the correct answer generally a "yes," but the surveyor will ask to see a policy or procedure relating to the question.

Organize the policy and procedure manual according to the standards and the HSP; use key words from the standards and the HSP to title policies and procedures. Surveyors are pressed for time; they must answer well over 1000 questions in the course of a hospital visit. It is much easier for them to find familiar key words than it is to make the translation from different terminology. Prior to survey, use the HSP to go through your manual and mark the questions so that you will be able to locate them easily. Otherwise, on survey you will thumb frantically through your manual, knowing that the policy or procedure is there but being unable to locate it. You will find that with a little preparation surveys are not so bad.

The Survey

The JCAH administrative surveyor will come to your department, usually the second day of a 2-day survey, or in the afternoon of a 1-day survey. He will stay between half an hour and an hour. You will need the following documentation:

1. Licenses for the pharmacy and pharmacists and Drug Enforcement Administration (DEA) registration
2. Policies and procedures as discussed in the following pages
3. Your copy of the minutes of the Pharmacy and Therapeutics (P&T) Committee (Not all administrative surveyors look at these.)
4. Records pertaining to the use of control drugs
5. Reports of monthly inspection of all medication centers and drug storage areas throughout the hospital
6. The continuing education program for the pharmacy, including attendance records
7. Information about the antibiotic review program if the pharmacy is involved (Not all administrative surveyors will check this.)
8. Quality assurance records

The surveyor will review the policies and procedures to make certain you have everything that is asked for in the JCAH standards and will ascertain as he tours the hospital that you are following your own policies and procedures. He will check the pharmacy records you are required to keep to make certain that you are complying with the law.

Whether the physicians or the administrative surveyor read the P&T minutes, the following items must be included:

1. Quarterly meetings
2. Minutes of meetings that reflect that the P&T Committee is functioning as required in the medical staff bylaws
3. Attendance at meetings (Representation is required from the medical staff, nursing service, pharmacy service, and administration.)
4. Topics covered and reported to the medical staff through the Executive Committee of the medical staff. These must include:

a. Choice of drugs available for patient care and diagnostic testing

b. Addition or deletion of drugs in the hospital formulary or drug list

c. Review of formulary or drug list for currentness at stated intervals

d. Review of all drug reactions

e. Evaluation and approval of protocols concerned with use in investigational or experimental drugs

f. Discussion of policies and procedures related to the pharmacy, particularly those related to the scope and safety of administration

g. Any problems that have been noted or discovered in the use of drugs

h. Identification of problems arising during the meeting and any plans made to solve them

The administrative or physician surveyor will also check the antibiotic usage review, if the medical staff has assigned the pharmacist that responsibility. Whoever is responsible will look to see that:

1. The medical staff bylaws determine how and by whom the function is to be implemented

2. The review is based on preestablished criteria, and ''ongoing,'' meaning no fewer than quarterly reports of this function

3. The review includes all types of patients and services, including emergency service and ambulatory care

4. Criteria are established for the prophylactic use of antibiotics

   The prophylactic use of antibiotics is monitored and studied if necessary

5. Criteria are established for the therapeutic use of antibiotics

6. The therapeutic use of antibiotics is monitored and studied if necessary

7. Effective corrective action is taken when problems are discovered

8. The use of antibiotics has improved as a result of the antibiotic review program

If the pharmacist has been assigned the responsibility of antibiotic review in conjunction with the medical staff and keeps the documentation of this activity, be sure that the physician surveyor knows this and has access to the documentation. Otherwise, he may assume that antibiotic review is not done and wrongly cite the hospital.

The surveyor will look at patient drug profiles. He wants to know whether they are being done, if they contain all the required information, if they are current and complete, and if they are being utilized.

The surveyor will examine physicians' orders. He wants to know whether they are complete, legible, properly signed, and only approved abbreviations used. He will report this information to the physician surveyor.

He will look at the documentation of the pharmacy quality assurance (QA) activities to make certain that there is an organized system to identify problems that impact on patient care and that, once identified, they are addressed, resolved, and monitored or referred on for assistance in resolution and are not lost or ignored. There must be evidence that not only are problems looked at individually, but an effort is made to identify overall trends. He will look for reports to the Quality Assurance Committee as required by the hospital QA plan. *He will not look for drug studies as such.*

He will read the minutes of pharmacy departmental meetings. If problems relating to patient care are identified there, he will look to see whether they are being addressed in some way or have been solved.

He will look at the monthly checks of drug storage locations throughout the hospital to make certain that all areas are covered and that any problems identified during these checks are corrected and remain corrected.

The surveyor should review with the director of pharmacy any recommendations concerning the pharmacy service made during the last survey to ensure that they have been implemented. By the time the surveyor leaves the department, you should have a good idea of the recommendations he plans to make and the reasons for making them.

Summation Conference

When all the surveyors have completed their observations of the hospital, they will hold a summation conference. Present at this conference must be representatives of the medical staff, administration, governing body, nursing service, and anyone else invited to attend by the hospital. This almost always includes department heads. At the summation conference the survey team will present verbally all the recommendations they plan to make in writing. The conference will be taped by the survey team and, generally, by the hospital. Listen carefully to make certain that the recommendations made concerning pharmacy services and any other areas in which you are involved are accurate and that you understand them. If, as far as you are concerned, there is a problem with accuracy or you do not understand the reason for the recommendation, ask appropriate questions. The survey findings must be justified. The conference is taped as the first step in the appeals process. Should there be problems with the results of the survey, the tape will be evaluated in the JCAH central office. The questions you have asked and the objections you have raised will be considered. In general, no recommendations may be made in the final report that were not made at the summation conference. Participation in the summation conference is just as important as participation in the survey.†

DIRECTION

Director

Whether the hospital has a licensed pharmacy or a drug room, all pharmacy services must be directed by a currently licensed pharmacist who is responsible for the proper storage, preparation, dispensing, and administration of drugs. This pharmacist should be knowledgable concerning the operation of hospital pharmacies and clinical pharmacy. The knowledge may be gained either by several years of experience working in hospital pharmacies or by serving a residency in hospital pharmacy approved by the American So-

---

†NOTE: The following pages are arranged according to the JCAH standards. If occasionally there appears to be repetition and duplication, it is because the standards are organized in that manner.

ciety of Hospital Pharmacists (ASHP) (AMH84, page 133, lines 16-25). Ideally, the pharmacist should maintain a current active membership in the ASHP. The director of pharmacy services must report to the hospital administrator or the designated associate or assistant director of the hospital (AMH84, page 133, lines 16-17).

Availability of Pharmacist

The JCAH does not require that the pharmacist be a full-time employee. However, it does recommend that a pharmacist be available at all times. (The standard does not define "available.") According to the JCAH, the workload is to determine whether the hospital requires a full-time, part-time, or consultant pharmacist. However, the service must meet the needs of the patients "as determined by the medical staff" (AMH84, page 133, lines 25-29).

If the pharmacy is decentralized, then each satellite pharmacy must be supervised by a licensed pharmacist who reports to the director of pharmacy (AMH84, page 133, lines 30-34).

Administration

The JCAH has few administrative standards that apply to the pharmacy. One is a requirement for departmental budgeting. The other concerns personnel requirements including, orientation to the hospital and the pharmacy, verification of current licensure, and periodic performance evlauations, based on the job description (AMH84, page 78, lines 25-31).

In order to be effective, the director of pharmacy services must be familiar with current trends in the provision of institutional pharmacy practice and in professional practice. The director should be responsible for hiring and training pharmacy personnel. He should develop job descriptions and should ensure that all pharmacy employees are evaluated periodically based on those job descriptions. Ultimately, he is responsible for making certain that all pharmacist employees possess valid, current licenses.

Personnel

Once the scope of pharmacy services to be provided has been determined, there must then be an adequate number of trained personnel to provide that service. One point made in the Accreditation Manual for Hospitals (AMH) is so important that it must be quoted. "Non-pharmacist personnel shall work under the direct supervision of a licensed pharmacist and in such a relationship that the supervising pharmacist is fully aware of all activities involved in the preparation and dispensing of medications. . . . The duties and responsibilities of non-pharmacist personnel must be consistent with this training and experience, and they shall not be assigned duties that by law or regulation, must be performed only by a licensed pharmacist" (AMH84, page 133, lines 35-40; page 135, lines 1-5). The interpretation of this standard is perplexing, and, because of state pharmacy laws, not the same everywhere. The surveyors are guided by the state laws. It would be well to have a copy of the state pharmacy act available, since the issue arises in several instances in the standards.

Drug Rooms

If the hospital does not have an organized pharmacy service (generally taken to mean that there is no license to operate a pharmacy), the pharmaceutical services must be obtained from a community pharmacy or from another hospital that does provide pharmacy services. In that case, only prepackaged drugs may be stored in the drug room, and only prepackaged drugs may be distributed from the drug room. The drug room must be under the supervision of a licensed pharmacist. The prepackaged drugs obtained from outside pharmacies are required to be labeled appropriately with name, strength, lot number or control number, and expiration date. This is necessary in case of any recall and to implement a system of control. The procedure for obtaining these drugs on both an emergency and routine basis must be documented (AMH84, page 134, lines 9-17).

Infection Control

At few places in the hospital are infection control measures more important than in the pharmacy. The pharmacy is generally a central area from which drugs are dispensed throughout the hospital. A single break in techniques here can affect many patients. If the pharmacy has the responsibility for the admixture program, special care must be taken. Policies and procedures should be developed and implemented to minimize any possible problems that could arise concerning admixtures, drug reconstitutions, or hyperalimentary solutions (AMH84, page 73, lines 36-39). If laminar airflow hoods are used, quality control measures should include cleaning of equipment on each shift during which hood is in use, checks for operational efficiency at least annually, microbiologic monitoring as required by the hospital infection control committee (AMH84m page 135, lines 19-24), and biologicals and thermolabile medications stored in their own refrigerator or in a separate compartment within a refrigerator (AMH84, page 134, lines 48-51).

Although it is not required by the JCAH, you might want to develop a policy concerning the use of multiple-dose vials.

Infection control policies developed for the pharmacy itself should relate to physical environment and might cover such items as the pharmacy layout, separation of clean and soiled areas, handwashing facilities and procedures, traffic control, and cleaning schedules. They also might relate to equipment and supplies, both clean and dirty, and to proper disposal of outdated drugs, trash, needles, and syringes. Policies regarding pharmacy personnel themselves are especially important (in a sense, they are like food handlers) and might relate to immunizations, clothing, restricted assignments in the event of communicable disease, and appropriate inservices relating to infection control in the provision of pharmaceutical services.

Although the JCAH does not require it, the pharmacist makes a good member of the Infection Control Committee (ICC). He frequently is involved in the admixture program.

He knows about the prevalence of infections because he dispenses antibiotics. He is knowledgeable about antibiotics and their usage. Sometimes the medical staff delegates to the ICC its responsibility for monitoring antibiotic usage. In this instance, the representation of the pharmacist on the ICC is absolutely necessary.

Space

The JCAH says that the pharmacy department must have ". . . the necessary space, equipment, and supplies for the storage, preparation, and dispensing of drugs" (AMH84, page 134, lines 28-30). Supplies and most equipment almost always are available, but the pharmacy appears to be one of those areas that is chronically short of space, both storage areas and work space for the pharmacist. A few pharmacies are absolutely unsafe because of an overcrowded working area. Some state laws specify the amount of work space required. New Mexico, for example, requires that the compounding counter must provide a minimum of 16 square feet of unobstructed compounding and dispensing space for one pharmacist and a minimum of 24 feet when two or more pharmacists are on duty (Regulation No. 6, Board of Pharmacy, Section 302B, 11-13-80). Even this space is lacking in many hospital pharmacies. However, space cannot be allocated according to rigid numbers. One state, Texas, specifies that allotment of space in the pharmacy should be based on:
1. Basic functions and the extent to which each function is to be carried on in the pharmacy
2. Methods used in performing each function
3. Types and needs of patients to be served
4. Establishment of a viable and effective formulary system to reduce the amount of storage space necessary

Bulk Storage

The director of pharmacy services is responsible for drug storage and preparation areas, not only in the pharmacy itself, but throughout the hospital. Drugs must be stored properly. This takes into consideration sanitation, temperature, light, moisture, ventilation, and segregation (AMH84, page 134, lines 5-37). Problems frequently occur in bulk storage areas, particularly when drugs are warehoused. Some bulk storage areas have no heating or cooling systems. Obviously, drugs are then subjected to temperature extremes beyond those which ensure stability, generally agreed to range from 59° to 89°F. Drugs may be left on loading docks for long periods of time and be exposed to the same temperature extremes. IV solutions present storage problems too. As the use of IV solutions increases, it becomes apparent that hospitals were not built to accommodate the bulk of IV solutions necessary for the practice of today's medicine. IV solutions are placed wherever a spot can be found for them, however unsuitable. One hospital stored them in a closet in the back of the soiled linen collection room. The director of pharmacy must make certain that he knows where, and under what conditions, drugs are stored prior to the time they are delivered to the pharmacy.

Frequently the pharmacist is responsible for the storage of flammables, such as alcohol, ether, and acetone. Flammable liquids must be stored in rooms or enclosures with a 1-hour fire-resistant rating. Combustibles may not be stored with flammable liquids. If alcohol is stored in a large drum, then the drum must be kept in an upright position and the alcohol withdrawn by the use of a hand pump (AMH84, page 39, lines 49-53; page 40, lines 7-8).

Drug Storage for Dispensing and Administration

All areas where drugs are prepared must have good lighting and be located where personnel working to prepare drugs for dispensing or administration will not be disturbed (AMH84, page 134, lines 37-41). This includes the pharmacy and any other place where drugs are prepared for administration. To avoid interruptions, dispensing areas should be located in the rear, not by the service area. Nursing units must be designed so that drugs can be stored and administered safely. Locked drug storage or locked medication carts must be provided.

Routine Inspections

The director of pharmacy or his "qualified designee" is required to inspect monthly all areas of the hospital where "medications are dispensed, administered, or stored" (AMH84, page 134, lines 41-44). A qualified designee need not be a pharmacist, but a person the pharmacist has delegated to perform the task. That person must be qualified by previous training.

Documented checks are to be made monthly to make certain that:
1. External drugs are stored separately from internal drugs.
2. Drugs are stored under the proper conditions.
3. Outdated and other unusable drugs are removed from locations where they could be administered in error.
4. The use of control drugs is correctly documented and in compliance with state and federal laws.
5. The use of investigational drugs conforms with the pharmacy policies and procedures.
6. Emergency drug supplies are in order and adequate.
7. The metric system is used for all medications. Metric-apothecary conversion charts should be available where medications are given or medication orders written (AMH84, page 134, lines 39-54; page 135, lines 1-18).

Drug storage locations include all crash carts, anesthesia carts and supplies, operating rooms, recovery room, labor and delivery rooms, nurseries, emergency rooms, radiology, nuclear medicine, respiratory care, ambulatory clinics, special procedure rooms, all nurses stations, special care units, and the pharmacy itself.

When outdated stock is removed, it must be put somewhere out of the way until it can be picked up for refund or destroyed. Label the storage area prominently with a warning. Others who come into the pharmacy when it is closed should run no risk of using outdated drugs in error.

Emergency Drugs

The pharmacist, medical staff, and other departments, as appropriate, decide what is to be stocked on the crash cart and emergency trays. It then becomes the responsibility of the director of pharmacy to establish procedures for the inspection of emergency carts and trays throughout the hospital to make certain that the contents are intact and the supplies are not outdated (AMH84, page 135, lines 11-15). The JCAH has several standards applying to the routine checks for crash carts. The checks are required so frequently that the responsibility generally is delegated to the appropriate department, usually to the nursing service or whatever department in which the cart happens to be located. In the ambulatory care service, which includes day surgery, emergency carts and emergency drug storage areas must be checked each day and immediately after each use (AMH84, page 65, lines 43-48). The emergency carts in all special care units are to be checked during every shift and after each use by "an appropriate, designated member of the hospital staff to assure that all items required for immediate patient care are actually in place . . . and in usable condition" (AMH84, page 185, lines 37-44). In radiology, an emergency drug tray is required "where parenteral administration of diagnostic agents is performed." There is to be a system in use to ensure that the emergency tray will not have "missing or outdated items." Also required is "ready access" to oxygen and airways and "the capacity to administer IV support" (AMH84, page 154, lines 9-12). The emergency service calls for "standard drugs, antivenin, common poison antidotes, syringes and needles, parenteral fluids and infusion sets, plasma substitutes and blood administration sets, and surgical supplies. . . ." Here emergency carts and emergency drug storage areas are to be checked at least every shift and following each use. In all cases, a sealed cart or medication kit is acceptable, provided that the seal is checked as required to make sure it is intact. Carts and supplies should be arranged uniformly (AMH84, page 30, lines 1-11). Many nursing units, physical therapy departments, operating rooms, stress-testing laboratories, and other areas throughout the hospital also are equipped with crash carts and emergency drugs. The JCAH standards do not specifically refer to them, but the contents and a method of ensuring their integrity fall under the responsibility of the director of pharmacy. Generally, nurse surveyors expect crash carts on nursing units to be checked every shift. *Each check of emergency supplies and crash carts in all areas throughout the hospital must be documented. Checks to verify the integrity of the seals also must be documented.*

Parenteral Medications

If your pharmacy service has the responsibility for parenteral medications, the JCAH requires that you also have appropriate space, location, and equipment. Preferably, this would include a separate room for the purpose. If laminar airflow hoods are used, the equipment must be cleaned on each shift. The ICC, taking into consideration the Centers for Disease Control guidelines, should determine what type of bacteriologic monitoring will be done, and their advice should be followed. At least annually the equipment must be checked for operational efficiency by a qualified person. Documentation must be kept concerning the performance, maintenance, and all checks of the hood (AMH84, page 135, lines 19-24).

Delivery Service

If necessary, the pharmacy service should provide for the delivery of drugs (AMH84, page 135, lines 26-27). The surveyor probably will not even check for this, yet it can cause the pharmacy and hospital personnel more grief and more hard feelings than almost any item in the JCAH standard for pharmacy services. Problems in this area might be a good topic for the QA Committee, since many of the issues are interdisciplinary. One problem seems to be based on the interpretation of stat orders. What is "stat?" How fast should "stat" orders be filled? Are there any medications for which stat orders would not be appropriate? A detailed study of this problem with input from all sides might lead to an amiable solution.

References

The JCAH requires current reference material to be available to the pharmacy. The purpose, according the JCAH, is to furnish not only the pharmacy staff, but also the medical and nursing staffs, with drug information. No specific books are required; types of references are suggested, such as official pharmaceutical compendia, textbooks concerning toxicology, pharmacology, chemistry, therapeutics, bacteriology, sterilization and disinfection, compatability and drug interactions, and other topics related to pharmacy. Current antidote information is required, as well as the posting of the poison control number. This also is a requirement for the emergency service. Federal and state drug acts and information are also needed (AMH84, page 135, lines 28-40). It is only a courtesy to the pharmacist to make certain that he has copies of the minutes of the P&T and Antibiotic Usage Review Committees. Since he generally is expected to implement any recommendations made there, most surveyors look at the minutes of the P&T Committee in their review of pharmacy service. Physician surveyors also check these minutes during their review of medical staff functions.

THE SCOPE OF PHARMACEUTICAL SERVICES

"As Determined by the Medical Staff"

According to the JCAH, the scope of pharmaceutical services must be decided by the hospital medical staff, taking into consideration the medication needs of the patients (AMH84, page 135, lines 44-45). Leaving the determination of the scope of pharmaceutical services to the medical staff alone seems a particularly archaic attitude and does not take into consideration the great strides that have been made in the practice of hospital pharmacy in recent years. Indeed, many physicians are unaware of the variety of services a modern hospital pharmacy has to offer.

"All drugs should be obtained and used in accordance with written policies and procedures that have been approved by the medical staff." At the very least, this means that the pharmacist must get the P&T Committee together and request that the chairman or the chief of staff approve and sign the pharmacy policy and procedure manuals. Actually, committees of the medical staff only recommend. Their work is submitted to the Executive Committee of the medical staff, which is charged with ''. . . receiving and acting upon reports and recommendations from medical staff committees. . .'' (AMH84, page 97, lines 19-20). The JCAH surveyor will be looking for appropriate medical staff signatures. Policies and procedures are to relate to ''. . . the selection, the distribution, and the safe and effective use of drugs in the hospital'' (AMH84, page 102, lines 15-17).

Actually, policies and procedures are an important part of a good pharmacy service. They help to ensure uniformity and consistency. Policies, carefully developed and adhered to, can be your best defense in the event of litigation. Once developed, policies should be followed, and the occasional exception carefully documented, giving a reason for the exception. Never throw away all copies of old policies and procedures. When they are changed or updated, retain one copy of the old policy for your files. In the event of legal action against you or the hospital, the policies and procedures in effect at the time of the incident will be important. It is not necessary to date each policy and procedure individually every time they are reviewed, but they should be dated when they are developed and each time they are changed. The manual itself should be dated at the time of each review, which is required annually.

The Pharmacy and Therapeutics Committee

The P&T function of the medical staff (it need not be a committee) is held responsible for ''. . . the development and surveillance of pharmacy and therapeutics policies and practices, particularly drug utilization within the hospital.'' The function must be performed at least quarterly and minutes documented. Not only the medical staff, but nursing service, administration, and pharmacy must participate (AMH84, page 102, lines 32-35).

Those performing the P&T function are responsible for advising on the use of all the drugs in the hospital. The duties of the committee are considerable; yet it is often difficult to persuade medical staff members to participate in this important role. Furthermore, many medical staff members and pharmacists lack the expertise to make the P&T function the vital activity that it should be. Some influential directors of pharmacy services have developed job descriptions for the chairman of the P&T Committee and refuse to accept as chairman anyone who does not fit the description. Generally, they ask that the physician chairman be an internist, willing to attend meetings and devote time to the committee. Once a good chairman has been found, it is desirable that he serve as long as he is willing and effective in the position. Changing medical staff committee chairmen annually is not always in the best interest of the medical staff functions. It takes some time to learn what the committee should be doing and how to go about it. At about the time the chairman learns his task, it would be time for a new chairman.

By custom, the pharmacist is secretary of the P&T Committee. However, this is not always a good idea. It is not easy to take notes and participate in a meeting at the same time. A better system is to have the medical staff or administrative secretary keep minutes, after first giving her an agenda and some instructions on pertinent points that must be documented. Many times the pharmacist is responsible for preparing the committee agenda. If that pharmacist is knowledgable and enthusiastic and prepares the agendas accordingly, the committee can be very effective.

The JCAH standards require that the P&T function:

- Advise the medical staff and pharmacy service on matters pertaining to the choice of drugs available for patient care and diagnostic testing
- Concern itself with the addition and deletion of drugs in the hospital formulary or drug list and continually review it for currency
- Review all drug reactions occurring in the hospital
- Evaluate and approve the protocols for the use of investigational and experimental drugs

In addition, the P&T function should focus on the safe use of drugs within the hospital and consider problems such as drug interactions, medication errors, and the misuse of drugs (AMH84, page 102, lines 20-35).

Antibiotic Review

The review of the clinical use of antibiotics throughout the hospital, including inpatients, ambulatory care patients, and emergency patients is the responsibility of the medical staff. Many P&T committees are assigned this function. This is often a thankless task, since many physicians see antibiotic review as an effort to interfere with their personal practice of medicine. As a result, it has not been effective, or even attempted, in some hospitals. Antibiotic review is not merely a statistical accounting of the numbers and types of antibiotics used. Criteria must be set for the prophylactic and therapeutic use of antibiotics, and actual usage must be monitored using these criteria (AMH84, page 103, lines 14-35). The criteria can be very simple. One example might be, ''The antibiotic used must be effective against the identified organism as demonstrated in culture and sensitivity testing.'' This could be monitored on a concurrent basis in the pharmacy if the lab would furnish the pharmacy a copy of the culture and sensitivity report. This information could then be compared with the patient profile, and the prescribing practitioner could be notified if the antibiotic that the patient is receiving is not appropriate. Other simple criteria may be developed and used. From these, patterns of antibiotic usage can be established and any problem areas identified. Then, if necessary, a full-blown study may be initiated.

Both the P&T function and antibiotic usage review are considered to be part of the overall hospital quality assurance program, since they serve to identify real or potential problems.

Responsibilities of the Director of Pharmaceutical Services

The standard explaining the scope of pharmaceutical services gives a sort of a job description for the director of pharmaceutical services by defining the responsibilities of the position. The director of pharmaceutical services:

1. *Maintains an adequate drug supply* (AMH84, page 136, line 7). However, the problem in many hospitals is not maintaining an adequate drug supply (what is adequate?) but in preventing overstocking. Extensive drug inventories are expensive and can be reduced considerably by developing an adequate formulary or drug list and allowing generic substitutions. However, it is worthy of note that the JCAH says that unless the medical staff rules and regulations or legal requirements say differently, prescribing practitioners may refuse to accept generic substitutions. Any problems should be worked out by the P&T Committee (AMH84, page 141, lines 9-13).

2. *Participates, through the P&T function, in the development and updating of a current hospital formulary or drug list* to present to the medical staff for approval. A good formulary serves as a guide for the practice of good medicine. It lists drugs that represent the best and latest treatments available and it eliminates obsolete drugs. It also prevents duplication in stocking of drugs and allows the deletion of medications no longer used. It does not mean that unlisted drugs cannot be used, only that they will not be stocked routinely. In fact, a written policy and procedure concerning obtaining unlisted drugs must be developed. The JCAH surveyors will accept formularies developed outside the hospital, such as the *American Hospital Formulary Service,* but only if it is indicated, preferably by each entry, which drugs are stocked. The notations must be current, and the entire system and drugs utilized must be approved by the medical staff (AMH84, page 102, lines 27-30; page 136, lines 50-52; page 137, lines 1-7). It is perhaps worthy of note that the ACS said in 1946 in its *Manual of Hospital Standardization* that "the most efficient means of securing efficiency and economy . . . is the adoption of a well-compiled hospital pharmacopeia that will facilitate uniform prescribing of drugs and limit them to the official pharmaceutical preparations."

3. *Establishes "specifications for the procurement of . . . drugs"* (AMH84, page 136, lines 8-9). Most pharmacists use the specifications found in the *United States Pharmacopeia* and *National Formulary.* However, procurement also refers to purchasing. In making generic substitutions, specifications for drugs, chemicals, and biologicals become especially important because the substitute must be of the same high quality as the original. A trend in hospital economics is group purchasing. The pharmacist must be assertive with regard to the purchasing practices related to the pharmacy to make certain that the drugs meet specifications. In purchasing generic, repackaged drugs for use in unit dose, the pharmacist must make certain of the quality of generic drugs used and the validity of the expiration date. In the case of repackaging, he might also want to develop specifications regarding the packaging materials and procedures.

4. *Participates in orientation and the continuing education of all persons responsible for the preparation or administration of sterile parenteral medications and fluids.* He furnishes literature and instructions about incompatibilities (AMH84, page 136, lines 30-33). This means that the pharmacist must see to the education of his own personnel if the pharmacy is involved in an admixture program. He also must provide in-service training to nursing personnel and other concerned individuals in the correct use of admixtures. These in-service programs must be documented.

5. *Assumes responsibility for the preparation, sterilizing, and labeling of parenteral medications and solutions manufactured in the hospital* (AMH84, page 136, lines 11-12). Not many hospitals manufacture their own solutions to any great extent. The exception may be those large institutions that provide tertiary care. When the hospital has a hyperalimentation program, overall direction must be provided by a physician to ensure safety in preparation and administration and proper nutritional content (AMH84, page 136, lines 26-29).

6. *Assumes responsibility for the compounding and admixture of large volume parenterals (LVP), both medications and solutions.* He makes certain that persons who prepare and administer LVPs have appropriate training. If anyone other than the pharmacy is responsible for the preparation and administration of LVPs, he provides written guidelines and gives his approval to the procedure (AMH84, page 136, lines 17-26).

7. *Assumes responsibility for any pharmaceuticals manufactured within the hospital* (AMH84, page 136, lines 34-35).

8. *Assumes responsibility for emergency drugs and antidotes throughout the hospital.* Both must be readily available throughout the hospital in patient care areas and in the pharmacy. In all areas where these drugs are stored, current antidote information should be available, as should the phone number of the regional poison control information center (AMH84, page 136, lines 36-41).

9. *Assumes responsibility for the dispensing of drugs throughout the hospital* (AMH84, page 136, lines 42-43).

10. *Keeps detailed records of controlled drugs within the hospital* to comply with federal, state, and local laws (AMH84, page 136, lines 44-46). An in-depth understanding of the drug laws is necessary. For example, in hospitals with full-time pharmacists, only Schedule I drugs are required to be securely locked at all times. Most hospital pharmacies will not have any Schedule I drugs, since by definition they are not considered suitable for use in the treatment of disease. According to the DEA, Schedule II, III, IV, and V drugs may be disbursed throughout the stock unless the pharmacist is a part-time employee or a consultant. One problem that occurs frequently is how to dispose of controlled drugs. What is the procedure on the nursing units when only part of an ampule of a Schedule II drug is used? Schedule IV? The pharmacy also has problems with the disposal of controlled drugs. Is someone from the state responsible for picking them up? May the pharmacist destroy them in front of witnesses? Should they be returned to someone? Specific procedures should be developed concerning all aspects of controlled substances, stating how things are done in *your* hospital. General references to the drug laws are not enough. The ASHP has excellent guidelines for controlled substance record keeping.

Not only should the director of pharmacy be responsible for controlled substances, but he must be accountable for the use of all drugs in the hospital. Therefore, he must know where and how the drugs are being used. To accomplish this, he must make certain that good records are kept for the requisitioning and dispensing of all pharmaceutical supplies (AMH84, page 136, lines 46-48). In keeping with this, he should develop and implement effective procedures for obtaining drugs when the pharmacy is closed.

11. *Ensures that personnel working in the pharmacy on all levels have an appropriate orientation to the hospital and the pharmacy.* He develops training programs to teach personnel new procedures. He provides relevant in-service programs. He sends persons of supervisory level to outside educational programs. The participation of each person must be documented. The director of pharmacy determines the type and frequency of educational programs based on the scope of services offered. This is subject to the approval of the administrator (AMH84, page 137, lines 8-13). Administrative approval for educational programs is required nowhere else in the JCAH standards except in pharmacy services.

12. *Attends all meetings of the P&T Committee and implements their decisions "throughout the hospital"* (AMH84, page 137, lines 24-35).

13. *Reviews pharmaceutical policies and procedures annually to make certain that they reflect hospital practices* (AMH84, page 137, lines 26-28). This requirement does not refer to the pharmacy department only. All policies and procedures relating to pharmaceutical practices throughout the hospital should be developed in conjunction with the pharmacy service to make certain that they are acceptable pharmaceutically and not in conflict with any pharmacy policies. The pharmacist is an expert in his field and should be consulted when policies and procedures need to be developed relating to medication orders and administration (AMH84, page 116, lines 16-18). Anesthesia, the operating suite, the recovery room, labor and delivery, respiratory care services, nuclear medicine, radiology, and the emergency service may also have policies and procedures relating to pharmacy services.

14. *Maintains confidentiality of information relating to patients and medical staff* (AMH84, page 137, line 29).

15. *Devises a method of identifying the signatures of all practitioners* allowed to prescribe for ambulatory care patients. He also must have a list of their DEA numbers and assume that they are correct (AMH84, page 137, lines 30-34).

16. *Cooperates in any hospital teaching or research programs* (AMH84, page 137, line 84).

17. *Participates in "those aspects of the overall hospital QA program that relate to drug utilization and effectiveness* (AMH84, page 137, lines 16-21).

18. *Assumes responsibility for monitoring the drugs each patient is receiving* "in keeping with each patient's needs." To accomplish this, a drug profile or medication record should be kept for each patient. The profile must include name, age, weight, current diagnosis, allergies and sensitivities, responsible physician, and current drug therapy. The best profiles also include current lab work, and some pharmacists are working with dieticians in coordinating diets and drugs. To be effective, the profile must be current and must be reviewed frequently, especially as medications are changed, for any drug-related problems that could arise, such as interactions, incompatibilities, and interferences. If any problems or potential problems are noted, the pharmacist must notify the prescribing practitioner immediately.

If the problem or potential problem is serious and the practitioner is unresponsive, administration and nursing service should be informed (AMH84, page 137, lines 35-48). Document when practitioners are notified about problems in relation to drug therapy and their responses. When physicians are uncooperative, it might be well to forward copies of all documentation to the P&T Committee or to the appropriate medical staff department.

Much, if not all, of the background information required to begin the drug profiles can be obtained through nursing service. If the pharmacy is not decentralized, this may be the only practical way of obtaining such information. Teach the nursing personnel about drug profiles and their benefits for the patients. The cooperation you receive will be much better if the reason that such information is needed is clearly understood.

Frequently, all parenteral medications and fluids are not recorded on the same drug profiles. This is true most often in hospitals in which the pharmacy is not responsible for the admixture program. Obviously, a profile that does not include *all* the medications that a patient is receiving is almost useless. Rarely seen on profiles are tests that the patients have undergone that involve the use of chemicals and drugs, e.g., intravenous pyelograms. Medications given during the course of surgery and recovery also are not customarily noted on the profile. How detailed the individual profile will be in your hospital is a decision for the director of pharmacy services and ultimately, through the P&T Committee, the medical staff.

19. *Assists in the current education of the nursing, medical, and other appropriate hospital staff* concerning such topics as new drugs and biologicals stocked in the pharmacy—their appropriate use and possible hazards; incompatibilities and sensitivities; signs and symptoms of toxicity; and other topics of importance in drug therapy. Persons who administer drugs or who are responsible for drug storage should be taught to recognize the signs of drug deterioration (AMH84, page 138, lines 5-11).

20. *Makes certain that patients are receiving correct instruction concerning take-home medication given at discharge,* either by giving the instruction himself, designating another pharmacist, or teaching members of nursing service how to instruct about the use of drugs and what to teach about the individual medications (AHM84, page 137, lines 49-51; page 138, lines 1-3). Pharmacists and nurses frequently do not cooperate in the provision of drug therapy for patients. An example is teaching patients about their medications. It is rare to find handouts concerning take-home drugs that have even been reviewed by a pharmacist. They are, however, almost universally approved by the medical staff.

21. *It is highly desirable that the director of pharmacy establish a drug information service* (AMH84, page 138, lines 11-13). However, it is not universally agreed on as to exactly what constitutes a drug information service. The JCAH surveyors differ as to what they look for and tend to be too lenient. "If they have current references, they have a drug information service," said one surveyor.

From the scope of services that JCAH requires of the pharmacy, it should be apparent that more hospital pharmacies are understaffed than overstaffed, especially because of the increasing emphasis on clinical pharmacology. The clinical functions of pharmacists are just beginning to be recognized in many parts of the country. Yet a hospital that allows the clinical aspects of pharmacy to be neglected is delivering less than optimal patient care. To ask a pharmacist to be responsible for clinical duties, administrative duties, and dispensing in any but the smallest hospitals places an impossible burden on the pharmacist. Hospitals must examine the pharmacy services they provide to make certain that such services enhance, rather than inhibit, patient care.

INTRAHOSPITAL DRUG DISTRIBUTION

The JCAH says that the medical staff makes the decision concerning the scope of pharmacy services. However, policies and procedures having to do with intrahospital drug distribution are to be developed by the director of pharmacy service "in concert" with the medical staff and other appropriate disciplines (AMH84, page 138, lines 16-20).

Drug Preparation and Dispensing

The JCAH says that "drug preparation and dispensing shall be restricted to a licensed pharmacist or his designee under the direct supervision of a pharmacist" (AMH84, page 138, lines 24-25). The JCAH does not require that the designee be a pharmacist. The surveyor will look for a policy concerning this. Direct supervision, in JCAH language, generally is taken to mean that the supervisor is on the premises and immediately available. This requirement causes problems for hospitals with a part-time pharmacist and full-time pharmacy employees. What are they to do when the pharmacist is not there? The situation is a puzzle for the surveyor too. He never is quite certain whether to make a recommendation or not. In this case, the JCAH surveyor has an escape. He describes the individual situation to the JCAH central office on the Surveyors Report Form (SRF) and asks central office to make the decision.

Pharmacist Review of the Prescriber's Orders

The prescriber's order or a direct copy of it should be reviewed by a pharmacist before the medication is dispensed. When the pharmacist is not available, the order should be reviewed by a pharmacist within 24 hours or earlier (AMH84, page 135, lines 25-31). This requirement is much more important than the question of who performs the actual mechanics of dispensing, since this requires some clinical expertise. The standard is a good one and deserves to be taken seriously by all hospitals. However, at least two problems arise:

The first is that the pharmacist simply is not available. The pharmacy department is small, employing only one pharmacist, who has weekends off. In this event, the surveyor is within his rights to write a recommendation. However, the recommendation does not carry much weight with regard to accreditation or nonaccreditation. More important is the harm that could result to the patient. When the hospital pharmacist is not available, another pharmacist should arrange to take the call and should review all drug orders at least daily.

A second, more serious problem exists when the hospital medical staff does not choose to insist that a pharmacist review orders prior to dispensing. In fact, the system of obtaining medication often makes this impossible. Perhaps there is an automated dispenser on each nursing unit, perhaps floor stock is still in use, or perhaps a unit clerk transcribes the order to a computer and the medication magically appears from the pharmacy. These systems have tremendous potential for errors. A pharmacist who values his license would be unwise to work in such a situation, because in the event of litigation, the pharmacist can be sued, too. In court, it would be difficult to support such antiquated methods of dispensing medication. Fortunately, they are no longer in common use.

It is worth noting here that the ACS in the "Eighteenth Annual Hospital Standardization Report" made in 1935 observed that, "a legal requirement which is not sufficiently observed is the keeping on file of the original of all prescriptions. Physician's order forms can be provided in duplicate, the original being sent to the pharmacy and the duplicate retained on the floor." Even today, 50 years later, some hospitals have not met the intent of this standard.

For safe patient care, and to be in compliance with the JCAH, floor stock medications should be used minimally. If floor stock is to be used, some system of accountability should be developed for control. One method would be to include a list of the amount and kind of drugs that would be supplied to each unit. However, the unit dose distribution system is encouraged and recommended (AMH84, page 138, lines 32-24). The hospital will get a recommendation if the unit dose system is not in use, but again, the recommendation does not tend to affect the accreditation status of the hospital. The unit dose system does not mean only that patients receive their medication in individual little packages; it implies a pharmacy-coordinated method of dispensing and controlling medication in which each patient has his own medication tray, identified and checked by a pharmacist. Medications are contained in single-unit packages, and the supply of doses is limited, preferably to 24 hours.

The following documented policies and procedures relating to the intrahospital drug distribution system are required and must be implemented. You must have evidence that these and all pharmacy policies and procedures are reviewed annually.

- *Labeling:* All drugs must be labeled appropriately. Labels must include any accessory or cautionary statements and the expiration date (AMH84, page 138, lines 39-41). A policy should be developed that states what constitutes correct labeling.
- *Return of unusable drugs to the pharmacy:* Discontinued, outdated drugs, or drugs in containers with damaged, unreadable, or missing labels must be returned to the pharmacy, where they can be disposed of properly (AMH84, page 138, lines 42-43). The procedure should state the method of returning drugs to the pharmacy, whose responsibility it is to dispose of them, and what constitutes proper disposal.
- *Obtaining drugs in the absence of a pharmacist:* If a pharmacist is not available, then only a designated *registered* nurse or physician may remove drugs from the

pharmacy. These drugs must be prepackaged and only enough needed for the immediate therapeutic needs of the patient may be taken. These drugs should be stored separately and be appropriately labeled. The person taking the drug should record the name and quantity of the drug taken. Ask the person removing the drug to leave the container from which the drug was taken near the signout book with a copy of the prescriber's order. When the pharmacist returns, he will verify the use of any drugs removed in his absence (AMH84, page 138, lines 47-53). For the best control, persons who are not pharmacy personnel should not be allowed in the pharmacy. A locked night cabinet in a convenient location for the nursing supervisor, who usually is the "designated registered nurse," can be employed. A pharmacist should be on call for questions and any problems that might arise.

- *Recalls:* There must be a recall procedure both for inpatient and outpatient medications. The procedure must be easy to implement, and the results of any recall must documented (AMH84, page 139, lines 1-3).
- *Drug defects:* If a drug is found to have a product defect, it should be reported according to the ASFP-USP-FDA Drug Product Problem Reporting Program (AMH84, page 139, lines 4-5). The pharmacist should provide information to the medical staff and nursing service as to what constitutes a drug defect, and the correct action to take if problems arise should be noted.
- *Dispensing to discharged inpatients:* When medications are dispensed to inpatients at the time of their discharge, the labeling must be the same as the labels for ambulatory care patients. These labels must include:
  1. Name, address, and phone number of the hospital pharmacy
  2. Date and pharmacy's prescription number
  3. Full name of the patient
  4. Name of the drug, strength, and amount dispensed
  5. Directions for use
  6. Name of the prescribing practitioner
  7. Identification of individual dispensing
  8. Any required DEA cautionary label and any other pertinent cautionary labels (AMH84, page 139, lines 12-22).
- *Identification of outpatients:* There must be an effective system to identify ambulatory care patients when they pick up their prescribed medications (AMH84, page 139, lines 8-10). Large outpatient services issue clinic cards to patients. Some pharmacists check driver's licenses or other identification.
- *Samples:* Drug samples brought into the hospital must be controlled by the director of pharmacy services. Drug samples should not be distributed in the hospital (AMH84, page 139, lines 23-25). It is good practice to eliminate drug samples in the hospital completely. However, if they are available, one good policy is that no charge will ever be made if they must be given to patients. There are tales of hospital Medicare audits in which years of retroactive denials were made for drugs because it was discovered that patients had been charged for samples. If sample drugs do happen to be administered to patients, the pharmacy should be no-

tified so that appropriate information can be included on the patient's drug profile.

SAFE ADMINISTRATION

Policies and procedures having to do with the safe administration of drugs and biologicals are to be developed by the medical staff in cooperation with the director of pharmacy, nursing service representatives, and other appropriate disciplines (AMH84, page 139, lines 29-32). As everywhere, these policies and procedures must be reviewed annually, reflect actual practices, and be enforced. Policies and procedures must include the following.

Medication Orders. Only members of the medical or house staff or other persons granted clinical privileges to write such orders may order the administration of drugs to patients. Medical staff rules and regulations must state what personnel are designated to accept verbal orders and require that the verbal orders must be signed within 24 hours (AMH84, page 139, lines 39-44; page 81, lines 37-45; page 100, lines 46-48). To enforce policies concerning medication orders, the pharmacist should know positively who is authorized to order medication in his hospital and should have a current list of such persons by name. The pharmacist should know who may accept verbal orders and should have access to the medical staff bylaws, rules, and regulations.

Who May Administer Medications? "All medications shall be administered by, or under the supervision of, appropriately licensed personnel in accordance with laws and governmental rules and regulations governing such acts and in accordance with the approved medical staff rules and regulations" (AMH84, page 139, lines 45-48). This required policy deserves comment because of the current discrepancies between Medicare and JCAH regulations. Medicare says that, except for physicians and dentists, only RNs and LVNs/LPNs may administer medications in hospitals. The JCAH is more flexible and realistic. Certainly, respiratory therapists administer medications. In many hospitals, radiology technologists administer diagnostic agents such as radioopaque dyes. This also is the case with nuclear medicine technologists. Some pharmacy technicians prepare medications and administer them to patients. In the military, nonlicensed persons administer medications under the supervision of RNs. Perhaps a more important point to be considered is who may administer certain categories of drugs. For example, may any RN or LVN/LPN administer chemotherapeutic agents? Another consideration is the route of administration. Who may give IV medications? Who may administer oral medication? Any policies you develop must reflect what is actually happening in your hospital. Once the issue is resolved, rules and regulations reflecting any decisions should be added to the medical staff bylaws.

Automatic Stop Orders. All standing drug orders must stop automatically when a patient goes to surgery (AMH84, page 139, lines 49-50). This is the only automatic stop order required by the JCAH. The problem with this policy is what happens after surgery. Physicians want to write, "Resume all orders." Pharmacists and nurses want them to completely rewrite all orders to prevent errors. Actually it is a matter of common sense and depends on how long and how complicated the patient's stay was before surgery. It also has to do with how many physicians wrote orders for the patient preoperatively. Charts can get very confused. It is almost as if a fresh start is made following surgery. The JCAH standards do not say that orders must be rewritten. This is a matter for the P&T Committee to take under consideration.

• • •

The medical staff, through the P&T function, should determine whether any other automatic stop orders will be required and add them to their rules and regulations. There must be some way to notify the prescribing practitioner that an order is about to expire so that he can decide to reorder, change the order, or allow the order to expire (AMH84, page 139, line 52; page 140, lines 1-2). Automatic stop orders really are an extension of the use of the patient profile. They will be most effective when monitored by the pharmacy service, although enforcement will require the cooperation of nursing service. Automatic stop orders contribute to patient safety and economy of care. Perhaps in some instances, stop orders should not be dependent on time limits, but on certain mandatory laboratory tests, such as prothrombin time. The P&T Committee is the appropriate vehicle for developing good, effective automatic stop orders and a method of enforcing them.

Parenteral Drugs. "Cautionary measures for the safe use of parenteral products shall be developed." Your policy may want to include any requirements about the use of filters when administering IV solutions or blood, routine changes of IV sites and tubing, length of time that bottles can hang, a uniform keep vein open rate, and any of the myriad details involved in the administration of parenteral products. The JCAH says that if drugs are added to IV solutions, then a label must be attached to the container. The label must include patient name, location, name and amount of drug added, date and time of addition, name of the basic parenteral solution, rate of administration, identity of person who prepared the admixture, supplemental instructions, and the expiration date of the compounded solution (AMH84, page 140, lines 3-10).

Correct Medication Administration. Before drugs are administered they must be checked against the original orders and prepared correctly. The person administering the drug must identify the patient prior to administration. Once the medication is given, it must be charted correctly (and promptly) in the patient's medical record (AMH84, page 140, lines 11-14). Individual doses of drugs should be administered as soon as possible after preparation, especially parenteral drugs, and, if possible, by the person who prepared the medication, except where unit dose is in use (AMH84, page 141, lines 4-8).

Most policies and procedures concerning correct administration of medication will be developed by the nursing service. However, since the JCAH standards make the pharmacist responsible for pharmacy policies and procedures throughout the hospital, he will want those policies and procedures in his manual to the extent of being practical. Actually, policies and procedures concerning drug administration should be developed jointly by the nursing and pharmacy services. Policies and procedures should discuss whose responsibility it is to check the prescribers' orders and how and when this will be done, especially from the

nursing point of view. How does the nurse verify that the drug has been prepared correctly, especially in the case of unit dose? How will the patient's identity be verified prior to administration of medication? What is nursing's role in the admixture program? These are only a suggested few of the policies and procedures concerned with the correct administration of medications.

Medication Errors. Medication errors must be reported immediately, according to hospital procedure. The procedure must include notification of the prescribing practitioner, and prompt entry of the medication given must be made in the patient's medical record (AMH84, page 140, lines 15-17). To discuss medication errors with any meaning they must first be defined for medical staff, pharmacy, nursing service, and appropriate others. Good reporting of medication errors is necessary, openly and without fear of retribution. It is not necessary to state in the medical record that the medication was given in error, only that it was given and the prescriber notified. If serious consequences are anticipated, prompt, corrective measures must be taken. One of the most important aspects of medication errors is an effort to learn from experience and make certain that they will not happen again. Therefore, they should be reviewed as a group, and the lessons learned should be publicized to appropriate persons or groups within the hospital. They must be reviewed by the Safety Committee or the P&T Committee or some other appropriate forum. It is not desirable to have only one discipline involved in the review. Different disciplines have different points of view and can contribute much to what may be a perplexing problem for one group. Each discipline must be careful not to be critical of the other, or there can be no open discussion. The object is to learn from each other and not to condemn.

Any study of medication errors will be enhanced by reducing them to statistics. The number of medication errors that occur in the hospital each month is, by itself, meaningless. A better method of reporting is to use a formula similar to calculating the attack rate for nosocomial infections:

$$\frac{\text{No. of medication errors}}{\text{No. of doses administered}} \times 100$$
$$= \% \text{ errors per dose administered}$$

Adverse Reactions. Adverse drug reactions must be reported immediately as they are identified and according to hospital procedure. The procedure must include notification of the prescribing practitioner and pharmacist, and prompt entry of the reaction must be made in the patient's medical record. Unexpected or significant reactions should be reported to the Food and Drug Administration and the manufacturer (AMH84, page 140, lines 15-21). Better reporting of adverse drug reactions might occur if some information describing what constitutes a drug reaction and what should be reported were provided. Establishing hospital-wide criteria for the recognition of drug reactions will help. For example, respiratory therapy has a requirement to develop policies and procedures concerning "the steps to be taken in the event of adverse reactions, based on established criteria for the identification of undesirable side effects" (AMH84, page 172, lines 34-35). When was the last time an adverse reaction was reported to pharmacy from respiratory therapy? On reviewing drug profiles, if instances can be identified when medications were stopped and a stat dose of Benadryl was administered, this is a good indication of a drug reaction. Drug reactions, even minor ones, should be examined by the P&T Committee. Perhaps an unexpected number of patients complain of headache after receiving a certain drug. It is possible that a given lot has an undetected defect. But if reports are not made, the pattern will never be identified.

Drugs Brought into the Hospital by Patients. If patients bring their own drugs into the hospital, they may not be administered unless they have been properly identified and there is a written order from the responsible practitioner that the drugs may be given. If they will not be used, they are to be packaged and sealed and returned to the family of the patient or given to the patient on discharge, with the permission of the responsible practitioner (AMH84, page 140, lines 22-30).

Patients often bring their medications to the hospital. Sometimes their physicians ask them to so that it can be determined what medications the patients have been taking. It is not a good policy to administer medications that do not come from the hospital pharmacy at the time of the current admission. To allow a physician to "identify" the drug and write an order for its administration is foolhardy. Physicians have neither access to really dependable information about drug identification nor the time to pursue it adequately. The pharmacist is the appropriate person to identify drugs. Identity is not the only concern. The drug might be expired or deteriorated or not what it appears to be. If the pharmacist determines that the drugs are acceptable and may be given to the patient, he relabels them appropriately. One exception to this procedure might be the patient who is receiving investigational drugs through another hospital or drug program and must receive them without interruption. A check with the research institution usually will resolve any problems. The P&T Committee should recommmend the exact policies and procedures concerning drugs brought into the hospital by patients.

Self-Administration. Self-administration of drugs by patients may not be allowed except on written order by the responsible practitioner (AMH84, page 140, lines 31-33). The P&T Committee should recommend appropriate policies and procedures concerning this subject too. On psychiatric and rehabilitation units partcularly, part of the therapy may be assuming the responsibility for one's own medications. This also is a part of the program of some self-care units.

Investigational Drugs. The use of investigational drugs in the hospital is definitely a matter for the P&T Committee, and they are so charged in the standards (AMH84, page 102, lines 27-32). They must decide whether investigational drugs are to be permitted at all, and, if so, by whom. They must require that the drugs be properly labeled and stored and that they be used only under the direction of the authorized principal investigator. A protocol for the administration of investigational drugs must be developed. It must include requirements for appropriate informed consent from the patient or family. Nurses may administer these drugs only with the approval of the principal investigator and only

after they have been taught basic facts about these drugs, including possible problems and other pharmacologic effects. The pharmacy service is responsible for maintaining essential information about these drugs (AMH84, page 140, lines 34-44).

Written Orders. The medical staff must approve a list of symbols and abbreviations. Orders may be carried out only if the approved symbols and abbreviations are used. The use of abbreviations in prescribing should be discouraged to prevent error. The leading decimal point should never be used. The prescriber must state the administration times or the time intervals between doses. If "prn" or "on call" are used, they must be qualified, i.e., "prn for pain." The order must be legible (AMH84, page 140, lines 45-51). The JCAH standards have much to say about abbreviations. They are mentioned in two other places besides "Pharmacy Services." A rule about them is required in the medical staff rules and regulations (AMH84, page 100, lines 44-45), and their use is explained further in Medical Records Services (AMH84, page 84, lines 48-52). The pertinent facts for the pharmacy service are that there must be an explanatory legend available, and each abbreviation and symbol may have only one meaning.

Discharge Drugs. If a drug is to be released to a patient on discharge, the responsible practitioner must write such an order. It must then be appropriately labeled as for ambulatory care patients and recorded in the medical record. Instruction regarding the use of the drug should be given to the patient by the physician, pharmacist, or nurse responsible, and appropriately documented (AMH84, page 140, lines 52-53; page 141, lines 1-3).

QUALITY ASSURANCE

Most pharmacists have a deep commitment to quality assurance whether they are aware of it or not. They make certain that medication orders are filled accurately. They remove outdated drugs from stock, and they head off problems in the pharmacy before they have a chance to happen. They serve on the infection control, safety, pharmacy and therapeutics, and other committees concerned with patient care. They assist the medical staff in performing antibiotic usage reviews. They enforce automatic stop orders. They help the nursing service to review medication errors. They note and solve problems in carrying out medication orders. They, probably more than anybody in the hospital, are aware of how medications really are being used. They know which physicians overmedicate or prescribe drugs without good indications. They are aware of the popularity trends in drugs, perhaps because of the new and personable detail representative assigned to the area. The pharmacist is aware of many problems in the hospital. Those that concern himself and his department, he solves. Those that concern other services or practitioners, he may assist in solving, or he may learn to live with them.

Now, we have *quality assurance* as mandated by the JCAH. Basically, QA calls for an organized approach to finding and solving problems pertaining to patient care, if possible at a departmental level, and then monitoring them to make certain that they are solved and stay solved. If any problem is to be solved within the department, the problem may be referred to the hospital-wide QA function. This is most often a QA Committee. It is obligated to respond to the problem in some way. Since the QA Committee receives periodic reports from all the QA activities in the hospital, it may learn of some problems involving the pharmacy service of which the director of pharmacy service is unaware. These may be referred to him for investigation and solution, or he and other concerned individuals may be asked to study the problem and to suggest solutions. The point is that problems adversely affecting patient care must not be allowed to persist. The pharmacy service must report on an ongoing basis to the QA Committee, at least as often as specified in the hospital QA plan. These reports consist of the problems you have noted in the reporting period, how they were found, what caused them, what you did or are doing about them, and a follow-up to make certain the corrective action was effective.

It is not necessary that each problem be solved at the time of reporting. Some situations are much too involved to be resolved in one reporting period, but you must report at what stage of the solution you are to ensure that a problem is not "lost." You may note problems over which you have no control for the benefit of the QA Committee. Since most of the problems identified through the pharmacy are concerned with drug utilization in one form or another, you should take any practitioner-related problems to the P&T Committee for discussion and possible solution. If the P&T Committee cannot resolve a problem, it must refer it to the appropriate committee of the medical staff.

There is no JCAH mandate to do studies on a regular basis unless, in your judgment, they seem absolutely necessary. For example, you may have to prove to a skeptical medical staff that a problem really exists before you can persuade them to take corrective action. That will take a study. You may have to undertake a study to prove that a proposed solution is the correct one. *You are not required to do a study just to do a study.* What you must do is to develop an organized procedure to identify problems and apply it constantly. As a part of the overall QA program you may be asked to determine usage patterns for various drugs or categories of drugs, specific clinical services, or individual practitioners (AMH84, page 137, lines 17-21). Remember that usage patterns are not an end in themselves but are only a tool in determining the presence or absence of problems. It is not required that this be done on a regular basis.

The pharmacy QA program must be reviewed at least annually to make certain that problems pertaining to patient care are indeed being identified by the procedure in use and that, once identified, they are tracked to solution. If this is not happening as a result of the QA program, then the program is not effective and should be revised. But the pharmacist can hardly avoid finding problems. Now, at least, there is hope that most of them will find a solution.

CONCLUSION

Actually, dealing with the JCAH is not difficult. It just involves knowing how to prepare. The JCAH pharmacy standards were developed in cooperation with ASHP and, as such, provide a basis that the director of pharmacy service can use to provide the best professional pharmaceutical services to the hospital's patients and staff.

REFERENCES

Pharmacy Services from Accreditation Manual for Hospitals, 1984 Edition, Joint Commission on the Accreditation of Hospitals

Anesthesia Services
   Standard IV; page 5; lines 5-7
Dietetic Services
   Standard III; page 15; lines 48-50
Emergency Services
   Standard V; page 26; lines 13-14, 50-51
   Standard V; page 28; lines 18-21
Functional Safety and Sanitation
   Standard II; page 39; lines 5-10, 18-28, 36-40
                  page 40; lines 7-10
                  page 41; lines 12-15; 33-34
                  page 42; lines 37-38
Home Care Services
   Standard V; page 57; lines 14-20, 37-40
Hospital-Sponsored Ambulatory Care Services
   Standard III; page 64; lines 3-7, 14
   Standard IV; page 65; lines 43-49
   Standard VI; page 67; lines 9-10, 11-12
Infection Control
   Standard I; page 70; lines 6-8
   Standard II; page 71; lines 14-17
   Standard III; page 73; lines 11-18, 36-38
Management and Administrative Services
   Standard I; page 78; lines 29-31
Medical Record Services
   Standard II; page 81; lines 37-45
Medical Staff
   Standard III; page 100; lines 2-8, 33-35, 44-45, 46-48
   Standard IV; page 102; lines 10-35; page 103; lines 14-36
Nuclear Medicine Services
   Standard I; page 105; lines 30-32
   Standard IV; page 108; lines 14-16, 19-23
Nursing Services
   Standard I; page 112; lines 5-10
   Standard IV; page 115, lines 10-13
   Standard VI; page 116, lines 16-18
Radiology Services
   Standard III; page 154, lines 9-12
Respiratory Care Services
   Standard III; page 174; lines 34-35, 43-44
Special Care Units
   Standard IV; page 184; line 19
   Standard V; page 186; lines 6-8

If you wish to order the *Accreditaion Manual for Hospitals,* check with JCAH for the price, since it is subject to change. All orders must be prepaid. Send your orders with payment in U.S. dollars to:

Cashier
Joint Commission on the Accreditation of Hospitals
875 North Michigan Ave.
Chicago, IL 60611

ADDITIONAL READING

Accreditation Manual for Hospitals, Chicago, Joint Commission on the Accreditation of Hospitals, 1984.
American College of Surgeons *Bulletin,* vol 66, No. 2, February 1981.
American College of Surgeons *Bulletin,* vol 20, p 113, September 1935.
Gary J: *Coping with the Joint Commission,* Pharmacy Services, Dallas, Dallas–Fort Worth Hospital Council, 1983.
Manual of Hospital Standardization, Chicago, American College of Surgeons, 1946.

The Policy and Procedure Manual

CHARLES M. KING, Jr., WILLIAM K. GINNOW, and JAMES M. HETHCOX

The policy and procedure manual is simply a compilation of written policy and procedural statements. As such, the policy and procedure manual serves as a guide containing specific information regarding administrative and professional policy decisions as well as the accepted methods of implementing those decisions. Thus, for an institutional pharmacy staff, a policy and procedure manual serves as a guide to effective and efficient provision of pharmaceutical services. For that institution's administration, medical and dental staff, and, perhaps most important, pharmacy department's management, the manual serves to promote the safe, efficient, and uniform performance of departmental functions by all pharmacy personnel.

NEED FOR POLICIES AND PROCEDURES

The need to develop policies and procedures to govern the functions of the pharmacy department has been clearly stated in recognized standards relative to the delivery of pharmaceutical services in institutional settings. In adopting the *Minimum Standard for Pharmacies in Hospitals* (1) in 1950, the American Society of Hospital Pharmacists (ASHP) charged the pharmacy director with responsibility for initiating and developing rules and regulations regarding the operation of the pharmacy department in the hospital:

The director of pharmacy service, with approval and cooperation of the director of the hospital, shall initiate and develop rules and regulations pertaining to the administrative policies of the department . . . [and] with the approval and cooperation of the Pharmacy and Therapeutics Committee, shall initiate and develop rules and regulations pertaining to the professional policies of the department.

In the *Minimum Standard for Pharmacies in Institutions* (2), as adopted by the Board of Directors of the ASHP in August 1977, the need for written policies and procedures was emphasized. Standard I of this document states:

An operations manual governing all pharmacy functions should be prepared. It should be continually revised to reflect changes in procedures, organization, etc. All pharmacy personnel should be familiar with the contents of the manual.

Standard III of this document further states that policies and procedures should be "developed by the pharmacist with input from other involved hospital staff . . . and com-

mittees" to govern "procurement, distribution and control of all drugs used within the institution."

Finally, the *Minimum Standard for Pharmacies in Institutions,* in Standard V, charges "the pharmacist, in concert with the medical staff," to develop "policies and procedures for assuring the quality of drug therapy."

In summary, the following points relative to the development of policies and procedures are to be found in the *Minimum Standard for Pharmacies in Institutions:*

A comprehensive operations manual should be prepared.
Lines of authority and areas of responsibility should be clearly defined.
Written job descriptions should be developed and revised as necessary.
Revisions in the operations manual should be continually made to reflect procedural and/or organizational changes.
All personnel should be familiar with the contents of the manual.
Input from other disciplines should be obtained; and for the necessary familiarity with the medical and nursing procedures relative to the use of drugs, a rapport with these disciplines must be established.

The Joint Commission on Accreditation of Hospitals (JCAH) has also established standards for delivery of pharmaceutical services within the hospital (see Chapter 4). These standards also require the pharmacist's active participation in the development of policies and procedures specific to the operation of the pharmacy department. The interpretation of Standard III of JCAH's standards for pharmaceutical services states (3):

. . . policies and procedures should relate to the selection, the distribution, and the safe and effective use of drugs in the hospital, and should be established by the combined effort of the director of the pharmaceutical department/service, the medical staff, the nursing service, and the administration.

When any part of . . . [preparing, sterilizing, and labeling parenteral medications and solutions] is performed within the hospital but not under direct pharmacy supervision, the director of the pharmaceutical department/service shall be responsible for providing written guidelines and for approving the procedure to assure that all pharmaceutical requirements are met.

[The director of the pharmaceutical service should be responsible for] . . . a written policy and procedure for the procurement [of non-formulary drugs].

[The director of the pharmaceutical service should be responsible for] performing an annual review of all pharmaceutical pol-

43

icies and procedures for the purpose of establishing their consistency with current practices within the hospital.

Standard IV of the JCAH standards further states:

Written policies and procedures that pertain to the intrahospital drug distribution system shall be developed by the director of the pharmaceutical department/service in concert with the medical staff and, as appropriate, with representatives of other disciplines.

The interpretation of this standard states that "written policies and procedures that are essential for patient safety and for the control, accountability, and intrahospital distribution of drugs shall be reviewed annually, revised as necessary, and enforced." Such policies and procedures include, but are not limited to, those relative to:

Labeling, including accessory or cautionary labeling
Disposition of discontinued, outdated, or improperly labeled drugs
Dispensing of drugs by pharmacy personnel
Removal of drugs from the pharmacy when a pharmacist is not available
Recall of drugs
Reporting of drug product defects
Dispensing to inpatients at the time of discharge
Identification of ambulatory care patients
Labeling of ambulatory care patient prescriptions
Distribution of drug samples

In addition, Standard V of these JCAH standards states:

Written policies and procedures governing the safe administration of drugs and biologicals shall be developed by the medical staff in cooperation with the pharmaceutical department/service, the nursing service, and, as necessary, representatives of other disciplines.

The interpretation of this standard requires:

Written policies and procedures governing the safe administration of drugs shall be reviewed at least annually, revised as necessary, and enforced.
Such policies and procedures shall include, but not necessarily be limited to, the following:
• Delineation of authority to write medication orders and to receive verbal medication orders
• Delineation of authority to order and administer medications
• Establishment of automatic drug stop orders
• Establishment of cautionary measures for the safe admixture of parenteral products
• Verification of prescriber's orders at time of drug administration
• Reporting of medication errors and adverse drug reactions
• Use/handling of medications brought into the institution
• Self-administration of medications
• Control and use of investigational drugs
• Use of abbreviations and symbols in writing drug orders
• Dispensing of drugs prescribed for ambulatory care patient use
• Preparation and administration of drugs

In a comparative analysis of the standards for pharmaceutical services of the JCAH and the *Minimum Standard for Pharmacies in Institutions,* many similarities are quickly identified. In regard to the subject of the need for policies and procedures, JCAH standards similarly stress:

The pharmacist's participation in the development of policies and procedures regarding:

• Selection of drugs
• Distribution of drugs
• Safe administration of drugs
• Safe and effective use of drugs
An annual review by the pharmacist of all pharmaceutical policies and procedures
The revision, as necessary, of pharmaceutical policies and procedures
The enforcement of pharmaceutical policies and procedures
Cooperation with the medical staff, nursing service, administration, and other disciplines as necessary

BENEFITS FROM A POLICY AND PROCEDURE MANUAL

Although various standards relative to the delivery of institutional pharmacy services have clearly emphasized a need for written policies and procedures, sufficient incentive to develop a policy and procedure manual should be provided through a recognition of the many benefits potentially derived from the development and proper utilization of such a manual. Among these is a more effective management of the department, a benefit which can result from:

Creation of a foundation from which the department's administrative and professional activities can evolve
Coordination of the department's resources (i.e., personnel, supplies, and equipment) for the production of an efficient, economical service with a reduction in or an elimination of waste of time and/or materials that otherwise results from error, inexperience, and/or need for direct supervision
Improvement of intradepartmental communications through (1) reduction of those errors otherwise resulting from the verbal transmission of policy and/or procedural information among personnel and (2) provision of information which is current, reliable, and readily retrievable
Improvement of employees' security, job satisfaction, and productivity as the result of management's statement of expectations relative to the performance of departmental functions
Rapid detection of inefficient or inferior performance of personnel through evaluation against a written standard
Establishment of a means by which the quality of service provided by the department can be evaluated.

Consistency in the orientation and training of new personnel can be achieved better if a current, comprehensive policy and procedure manual is utilized as an orientation and training guide. Therefore, with consistency in the orientation and training of new personnel and the provision of a ready reference that is both current and comprehensive for the other personnel as well, uniformity in the actions of the entire personnel of the department is promoted. Ultimately these factors contribute toward realization of yet another benefit, uniformity in the provision of the services of the department.

Interdepartmental relations can also be improved through the development of departmental policies and procedures. Specifically, if departmental policies and procedures are established with proper input from other disciplines and services, interdepartmental communication will be improved and the other services or departments will be familiarized with the policies and procedures of the department. Perhaps more important, interdepartmental conflicts will be reduced as many potential interdepartmental problems or conflicts will be identified in advance, and departmental policies and procedures will be written so as to avoid those conflicts.

A benefit to which reference has already been made in this chapter is the compliance with the requirements of various accrediting bodies that is afforded by the proper development of a policy and procedure manual. This compliance might also be advantageous with regard to third-party reimbursements (e.g., Medicare).

Finally, the policy and procedure manual can serve as evidence of standards of practice. With evidence of compliance with and periodic review of the written policies and procedures, a manual can serve as verification that the department has taken due precaution to protect patient safety and can serve as an important element in the institution's defense in a negligence suit arising from a departmental error. However, it is imperative that the written policies and procedures be continually reviewed, revised as necessary, and enforced.

The pharmacy department manager should discover that written policies and procedures, when properly developed and utilized, are effective administrative tools that are useful in planning, developing, improving, and extending pharmaceutical services. When effectively utilized, these tools can aid the department in obtaining resources necessary for fulfillment of departmental responsibilities and accomplishment of administrative and professional objectives.

DIFFICULTIES IN THE DEVELOPMENT OF POLICY AND PROCEDURE MANUALS

Despite the well-established value of written policies and procedures and the compilation of these statements as a policy and procedure manual, many pharmacy departments have not developed such a manual.

In a 1957 survey of pharmaceutical services in this nation's hospitals reported in *Mirror to Hospital Pharmacy* (4), only approximately one of three pharmacy departments had written procedures regarding administrative practices, and even fewer had written policies and procedures regarding professional practices. However, a significant majority of the departments did have established, but unwritten, policies and procedures concerning both administrative and professional functions. Reasons cited for the failure of the pharmacist to have developed written policies and procedures include:

Failure of the administrator to be insistent in encouraging the pharmacist to develop written policies and procedures
Pharmacist's lack of knowledge regarding the preparation of such statements
Lack of time to devote to this activity

Some believe that the current status in regard to the development of written policy and procedural statements by pharmacists is little changed from that of the 1957 survey. Furthermore, established policy and procedure manuals are not being utilized maximally; frequently their contents are ambiguous or outdated, and too often such manuals serve only as "handsome ornaments for the management book-case" (5) to lend an aura of organization and well-ordered communication to the department.

With a recognition of such deficiencies, the remainder of this chapter will be devoted to material relevant to the de-

velopment of a useful policy and procedure manual, or operations manual, which when properly maintained and utilized, will produce those desired benefits discussed previously. However, affirmation is first made that the principal motivation for developing any departmental policy and procedure manual should come from the department manager himself, in this case the pharmacist, and not from an insistent administrator. A manual developed through a motivation from the latter would surely seem doomed to failure.

DEVELOPMENT OF A POLICY AND PROCEDURE MANUAL

Definitions

In beginning a discussion of the development of a policy and procedure manual, it is appropriate to attempt to provide workable definitions of the two key terms, "policy" and "procedure." Formally defined, a policy is "a definite course or method of action . . . to guide and determine present and future decisions" (6). More simply stated, a policy is a broad, general plan that provides a framework for action. A policy statement addresses specifically what must be done and sometimes addresses the questions of: *Why? When? By whom?*

A procedure is formally defined as "a particular way of accomplishing something or of acting" or "a series of steps followed in a regular definite order" (6). More practically stated, however, a procedure is a "how-to" statement, i.e., it addresses the question of how the thing that must be done is to be done. It provides an explanation of the means or method by which a policy is carried out and, in so doing, starts at the beginning of the task and, in a step-by-step process, outlines that task through a complete cycle. In the procedure statement, responsibility for each specific function should be assigned to specific personnel.

Therefore, in combination, the policy and procedural statements answer the questions:

What must be done?
What is its purpose?
When should it be done?
Where should it be done?
Who should do it?
How should it be done?

Administrative vs Professional Statements

As indicated in the earlier reference to the *Minimum Standard for Pharmacies in Hospitals,* policies and procedures are characteristically either administrative or professional. Administrative statements, i.e., administrative policies and procedures, relate primarily to:

Control of resources (i.e., personnel, supplies, and equipment)
Departmental relationships
1. Relationships to administration
2. Relationships with other departments

Such administrative policies and procedures should be developed primarily with the advice and consent of the institution's administration (1).

Policies and procedures of a professional nature pertain primarily to the care of the patient, whether that care be direct or indirect. Professional policies and procedures relate to areas such as:

Drug procurement
Drug preparation
Dispensing of drugs
Handling and control of drugs
1. Within the department
2. Within the institution
Clinical services

Although subject to the approval of the institution's administration, professional policy and procedural statements are developed primarily through cooperation with the institution's medical and dental staff through its Pharmacy and Therapeutics Committee (1).

Writing Policies and Procedures

A primary objective in developing written policy and procedural statements should be to present information in a concise, easily understood form. To accomplish this objective, language should be simple and direct, i.e., words should be short and familiar. Sentences should be short, simple, and declarative, with each expressing only a single idea. Finally, the format, whether outline, narrative, or dialogue, should be uniform.

Various suggestions have been offered with regard to the individual or individuals most qualified or best suited to write policy and procedural statements. Some have recommended that the department manager and/or the supervisory staff of the department prepare such statements. Others have suggested that policies and procedures are best prepared by a staff member who regularly performs the activity himself or who immediately supervises it. Still others have recommended that policies and procedures be written by a committee of the department. Regardless, the following concepts seem to be valid:

It is desirable for the person(s) writing the policy and procedural statements to have an analytical mind and to avoid creative writing because of the relatively fixed pattern of writing desired for policy and procedural statements.

It is desirable to have input from the staff when writing policy and procedural statements. Acceptance of and understanding of the statements are improved with the involvement of the staff in the preparation of the statements. The comprehensiveness of such statements is generally increased with input from those persons actually performing the associated tasks.

When practical, it might be desirable to develop within the department a procedure analyst or specialist (7). This person could be given responsibility for:

Proofing, standardizing, and editing all rough and final drafts
Preparing illustrations and figures
Circulating drafts for comment and/or approval
Preventing unnecessary duplication of material
Coordinating periodic review

The pharmacy manager should investigate the availability of a word processing system in the hospital for the purpose of entering and maintaining the department's policy and procedure manual. Drafting, revising, and reviewing policies and procedures can be performed much more efficiently with the use of this equipment. The word processing function may also be added to the pharmacy computer system, if available, through the installation of additional software.

Contents of a Policy and Procedure Manual

It is important that one begin to develop a policy and procedure manual only after much thought and planning regarding the contents of the manual. One should carefully analyze the mission, goals, and purposes of both the department and the institution it serves and also determine the needs and purposes the manual is to satisfy. The latter will be affected by:

Organizational structure
Size of physical facilities
Scope of services
Complexity of operations
Maturity of department
Nature of staff (e.g., size, caliber, and turnover)

The contents of manuals therefore will vary considerably among institutional pharmacy departments, and one should develop a manual following an outline designed to accommodate the specific needs identified for a particular department.

Although reviewing manuals from other institutions may be helpful in stimulating content ideas as one plans the development of a manual, it cannot be overemphasized that each institutional pharmacy department is unique and that, for effectiveness, each policy and procedure manual must be designed to meet that department's specific needs. Furthermore, severe legal consequences could occur should one simply duplicate the contents of another's manual without effectively implementing all policies and procedures specifically included therein.

Organization of Contents

The contents of most policy and procedure manuals could generally be divided into several primary divisions. A very basic scheme could consist of only three primary divisions:
1. General information: Included within this division would be information regarding both the institution's and the department's:
   a. Description
   b. Development
   c. Philosophy
   d. Objectives
   e. Goals
2. Administrative information: This division would include, but not be limited to, information regarding:
   a. Personnel policies and procedures
   b. Organizational relationships
   c. Job descriptions
   d. Control procedures for use of departmental resources
3. Professional policies and procedures: Using this basic scheme of content organization, professional policies and procedures, i.e., those which either directly or indirectly relate to patient care, should represent the major portion of the manual. For example, statements relative to the following would be included:

a. Drug distribution, including unit dose drug distribution and other inpatient drug distribution
b. Compounding and manufacturing (including IV admixture preparation and other special formulation)
c. Dispensing for ambulatory care patients
d. Control and distribution of investigational drugs
e. Control and distribution of controlled substances
f. Drug information services
g. Other clinical services

Another approach to content organization is a scheme based on the delineation of management responsibilities within the department (Fig. 5.1). Other organizational schemes of varying complexity are provided for illustration purposes in Figure 5.2 (8-11).

In addition, various specialized manuals may be utilized. These may include master formula and compounding manual, computer procedures manual, and pricing manual.

DIVISION 01 General

CHAPTER 05 Introduction

SECTION 05 Anytown Hospital

    PART 05 General Statement
       10 Statement of Mission and Goals
       15 Maps

SECTION 10 Department of Pharmaceutical Services

    PART 05 General Statement
       10 Statement of Mission and Goals
       15 Division Purposes
       20 Objectives for the Current Fiscal Year
       25 Floor Plan and Location Guide
       30 Departmental Appearance

CHAPTER 10 Department of Pharmaceutical Services Organization

SECTION 05 Organization Chart
       10 Acting Authority
       15 Position Descriptions

    PART 05 Drug Distribution Division

SUBPART 05 Assistant Director
       10 Inpatient Supervisor
       15 Outpatient Supervisor
       20 Staff Pharmacist
       25 Senior Data Entry Operator
       30 Pharmacy Technician
       35 Pharmacy Intern

SECTION 20 Committees

CHAPTER 15 Standards

SECTION 05 American Pharmaceutical Association Code of Ethics
       10 Joint Commission on Accreditation of Hospitals—Pharmaceutical Services
       15 American Society of Hospital Pharmacists—Minimum Standard for Pharmacies in Institutions
       20 State Board of Health—Pharmacy Department of Standards
       25 American Society of Hospital Pharmacists—Accreditation Standard for Pharmacy Residency in a Hospital
       30 American Society of Hospital Pharmacists—Guidelines on the Competencies Required in Institutional Pharmacy Practice
       35 Minimum Expectations of a Pharmacist
       40 Hospital Code of Ethics
       45 Patient's Bill of Rights

CHAPTER 20 Policy and Procedure Manual

SECTION 05 Format
       10 Writing Style
       15 Distribution
       20 Responsibility
       25 Revisions and Additions
       30 Review

CHAPTER 25 Personnel Policies
       30 Staffing and Scheduling
       35 Security
       40 Interdepartmental Relationships
       45 Communications
       50 Safety Program—Accident Prevention
       55 Fire Emergency Plan
       60 Disaster Plan
       62 Bomb Threat
       65 Public Relations

DIVISION 02 Drug Distribution

CHAPTER 05 General
       10 Central Inpatient Pharmacy Service
       15 Outpatient Pharmacy Service
       20 Satellite Pharmacies

DIVISION 03 Administration and Technology

CHAPTER 05 Administration
       10 Purchasing and Inventory
       15 Quality Assurance
       20 Technology
       25 Transportation

DIVISION 04 Drug Information

CHAPTER 05 Drug Information Requests
       10 Pharmacy and Therapeutics Committee
       15 Publications
       20 Investigational Drugs
       25 Library
       30 Adverse Drug Reaction Reporting Program
       35 Drug Allergy Reporting Program
       40 Drug Interaction Reporting Program

DIVISION 05 Clinical Services, Education, and Research

CHAPTER 05 Clinical Services
       10 Education
       15 Research

FIGURE 5.1 Portion of table of contents.

ILLUSTRATION A

- Organization
- Facilities
- Personnel
- Services and activities

ILLUSTRATION B

- Philosophy
- General
- Administrative
- Dispensing
- Interdepartmental
- Bulk compounding and sterile solutions

ILLUSTRATION C

- General
- Pharmacy standards
- Preparation, handling, and dispensing of pharmaceuticals
- Narcotics, hypnotics, amphetamines, alcoholic liquors, and other controlled drugs
- Pharmacy stores and inventory management
- Records and reports

ILLUSTRATION D

- Administrative services
- Education and training
- Pharmaceutical research
- Assay and quality control
- Manufacturing and packaging
- Sterile products
- Inpatient services
- Outpatient services
- Drug information services
- Departmental services
- Purchasing and inventory control
- Central supply services
- Radiopharmaceutical services
- Intravenous admixtures

FIGURE 5.2 Schemes of content organization.

Regardless of the organizational scheme chosen for the contents of the policy and procedure manual, it is recommended that the manual contain a preface (Fig. 5.3) that states:

Purpose(s) of the manual
Major headings within the manual
Authority of the manual
How other published instructions affect the use of manual
Explanation of the classification system, i.e., the organization of the manual, and how to locate material
Method for handling new material and revisions
What is expected of users

Furthermore, to enhance the value of the manual as an orientation and training guide, as well as for completeness, the manual should contain:

Statement of mission and goals (1) of institution and (2) of department
Current fiscal year objectives (1) of institution and (2) of department
Purposes of specific areas of the department
Organization charts (1) of institution and (2) of department (Fig. 5.4)
Job descriptions (Fig. 5.5)
Floor plans and location guides
Description of interdepartmental relationships

Before proceeding, it must be noted that organization charts should clearly reflect the department's relationship to the institution's administration and to other departments. The organization charts should accurately and clearly depict the department's internal organization including the relationships among the department's staff. All direct and indirect lines of authority affecting the department should be readily identified from these charts (Fig. 5.4).

Stepwise Approach to Preparing a Policy and Procedure Manual

Before presenting a summary of a suggested stepwise approach to the preparation of a policy and procedure manual, several comments are appropriate. Although one should begin a manual only after much thought and planning, this should not deter one nor provide an excuse for not developing a manual. Rather, one should find encouragement in the fact that a manual has indeed been established with the writing of the first policy and procedure statement and that success can be had through a "divide and conquer" approach in which existing policies and procedures are dealt with first before new ones are developed and easier statements are approached first. One must also realize that a manual should never be "completed," for pharmacy is a dynamic practice in which that which is suited for today may be archaic tomorrow.

Considering the above points, the following stepwise approach is presented as a suggested method for developing an effective policy and procedure manual:

PREFACE

I. PURPOSE

The purpose of a policy and procedure manual is to provide an authoritative source of official organizational policies, procedures, and practices, as well as to define operational responsibilities and the line of authority in the various areas within a department.
The department Policy and Procedure Manual will serve:
A. As a means of standardizing and coordinating procedures
B. As a reference and guide for daily operations
C. As a means of orientation for new pharmacy personnel
D. As a central record of the department policies

II. MATERIALS INCLUDED IN THE MANUAL

The Policy and Procedure Manual is divided into five main divisions as follows:
DIVISION 01 General
DIVISION 02 Drug Distribution Division
DIVISION 03 Administration and Technology Division
DIVISION 04 Drug Information Division
DIVISION 05 Clinical Services, Education, and Research Division
The Divisions are subdivided into various chapters as listed in the Table of Contents to cover the topics included in each Division.

III. AUTHORITY OF THIS MANUAL

A. The instructions contained in this manual are official and shall be relied upon as the basis for the performance of work. It is the responsibility of each employee to be thoroughly familiar with each policy and procedure covered in the manual which affects the scope of responsibility of that employee. Questions about any specific policy or procedure should be referred to the employee's supervisor for clarification. Since all conceivable work situations cannot be anticipated by an instruction, the policies and procedures set forth in this manual shall be regarded as guides to performance under related or analogous conditions.
B. Situations may arise where conformance with the instructions in this manual may not be possible. This may be because the original instructions may not have anticipated additional factors, which may be present in a given situation. Whenever such a situation arises, the supervisor is expected to exercise judgment as to whether the instruction shall be suspended pending review by the Director of Pharmacy or in emergency situations whether other action is required, provided there is no violation of law or fixed Anytown Hospital policy. This does not mean that supervisor may, at will, suspend the effect of instruction with which he may not be in agreement. This shall be regarded as an emergency authority only, and in every case of the exercise of this authority, a full written report shall be made to the Director of Pharmacy. This report shall justify why emergency exception to the rules was taken without prior authorization.

IV. OTHER GENERAL PUBLISHED INSTRUCTIONS

A. Other general published instructions of the Pharmacy Department shall be within the framework of the policies and procedures of this manual or shall be supplementary to it. In the event of conflict between other published instructions and this manual, the manual shall take precedence, unless otherwise specified.
B. Occasionally, it may be necessary to issue temporary instructions which will take precedence over materials in the manual. When this is done, the temporary instruction shall clearly state the exception and shall include a time limit for the temporary instructions.
C. If a supervisor should issue verbal or written instructions in conflict with this manual, such superseding instructions shall be followed, but it is the responsibility of the person receiving them to point out the conflict with the manual. This shall be regarded as an emergency authority only, and in every case of the exercise of this authority, a full report shall be made to the Director of Pharmacy. This report shall justify why emergency exception to the rules was taken without prior authorization.

V. HOW TO FIND MATERIAL

The material covered by this manual has been organized into divisions, chapters, sections, parts, and subparts. All subdivisions are numbered with Arabic numerals. A typical section designation, therefore, would be 01-20-15:
DIVISION 01 General
CHAPTER 20 Policy and Procedure Manual
SECTION 15 Distribution
When more than one page is required for a particular part or subpart, a dash and the letter "A" shall follow the page number. The second page would be "B" and so on as necessary. Through reference to the Table of Contents, one may ordinarily find all related material together. Sample forms will appear at the end of each division and will be numbered consecutively within each division.

VI. NEW MATERIAL AND REVISIONS

Chapters, sections, parts, and subparts are numbered so that additional information may be inserted without altering the numbering system; that is, originally every fifth digit was used.
In most cases, a draft of proposed new material will be sent to all concerned individuals so that suggestions and recommendations can be made.
All new material, as well as revisions of old material, will be placed in each volume of the manual by the secretarial staff, at which time a copy, under cover of a transmittal memo, where necessary, will be sent to each employee concerned, stating that the enclosed policy and procedure has been placed in the manuals.
A copy of the Policy and Procedure Manual will be located in each area of the Pharmacy Department and will be available to any departmental employee.

FIGURE 5.3 Preface.

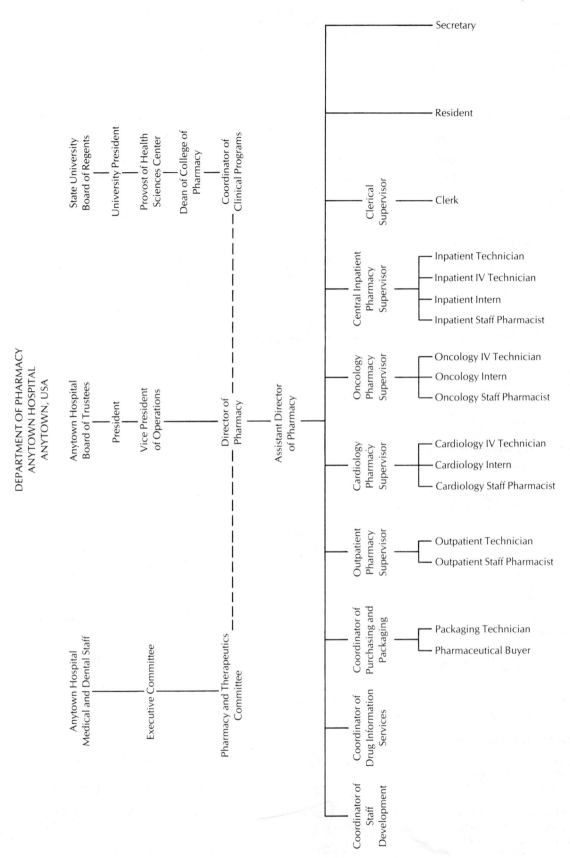

FIGURE 5.4   Organizational chart.

Step 1. Analyze the mission, goals, and purposes of the institution and the department. Then define the purpose(s) of the manual.

Step 2. Determine the method of (a) content organization and (b) presentation.

In addition to the table of contents, an alphabetical index should also be included for cross-referencing purposes.

Step 3. Determine the specific subjects requiring policy and procedural statements. Helpful information can be obtained from (a) old policies and procedures, (b) minutes of staff meetings, Pharmacy and Therapeutics Committee meetings, interdepartmental meetings, and other meetings, (c) departmental memoranda, (d) departmental reports, (e) instructions on forms, (f) instructions on equipment, (g) job descriptions, (h) input from staff and other departments, (i) interviews, (j) manuals of other departments of the institution, and (k) manuals of other pharmacy departments.

Step 4. Compile a table of contents and circulate a draft to the staff to ensure that the material will meet the needs of the department.

Step 5. Develop a suitable referencing system. Options include (a) open numbering (Figs. 5.6 and 5.7), (b) closed numbering, e.g., Dewey decimal system (Fig. 5.8), and (c) alphabetical.

The system selected must be flexible so as to permit additions or deletions without the disruption of the previous sequence of material in the manual.

Step 6. Develop policies and procedures regarding (a) format (Fig. 5.6), (b) writing style (Fig. 5.7), (c) placement of illustrations or figures, (d) distribution, (e) responsibility, (f) revisions and additions, and (g) review.

Step 7. Develop other policies and procedures in accordance with the previously developed policies and procedures.

Distribution of the Policy and Procedure Manual

Specific policy and procedural statements regarding the location, i.e., distribution, of all manuals as well as who

---

JOB TITLE: Inpatient Staff Pharmacist

POSITION NUMBER: _____

DATE: _____

SUPERVISOR: Central Inpatient Pharmacy Supervisor

DEPARTMENT: Pharmacy

UNIT: Central Inpatient Pharmacy

SHIFT: To Be Arranged

JOB SUMMARY:

Under the indirect supervision of the central inpatient pharmacy supervisor, maintains and dispenses pharmaceuticals and other pharmacy-supplied items utilizing a unit dose drug distribution system and an intravenous admixture service; assists in the provision of drug information services; provides direct supervision of pharmacy interns, other supportive personnel, and students in the performance of their respective duties; participates in educational programs provided by the department and the hospital for patients, staff, and other health care personnel; and functions periodically in other pharmacy units under the job description for the staff pharmacist of the respective unit.

DAILY JOB DUTIES:

1. Enters pertinent patient information and medication orders into computerized patient files and monitors these files for undesirable pharmacologic implications.

2. Receives, interprets, and fills medication orders including those for intravenous solutions and admixtures.

3. Receives and fills requisitions for personal care items as well as requisitions for supplies for other departments and nursing divisions.

4. Directly supervises pharmacy interns, other supportive personnel, and students in the performance of their respective duties.

5. Verifies contents of patient cassettes after filling of cassettes by pharmacy interns, other supportive personnel, or students.

6. Provides drug information upon request.

7. Assists in drug procurement by reporting needed items to the unit's pharmaceutical buyer or by initiating purchase orders in accordance with established departmental procedures as necessary in the absence of the buyer.

8. Maintains statistics and unit records as prescribed.

9. Verifies perpetual inventory records of controlled substances as prescribed.

10. Serves as liaison pharmacist to assigned nursing division(s).

11. Maintains work areas in neat and orderly condition.

FIGURE 5.5 Job description.   *Continued.*

JOB TITLE: Inpatient Staff
Pharmacist

PERIODIC JOB DUTIES:	HOW OFTEN?
1. Inspects nursing division(s) to which assigned as liaison pharmacist for deteriorated drugs, drugs stocked without approval, and general compliance with standards.	Not less than monthly
2. Participates in patient education programs.	As assigned
3. Participates in orientation and staff development programs of the Department of Pharmacy.	As programs are offered
4. Participates in orientation and inservice programs of other departments.	As assigned
5. Conducts or assists in research.	As assigned
6. Initiates the established recall procedures.	Upon recall notification
7. Participates in the inventory process.	Annually or as required
8. Performs other duties.	As necessary

EQUIPMENT USED:	HOW OFTEN?
Cathode Ray Tube (CRT)	Daily
Electric Typewriter	Daily
Compounding Equipment Including LAF Hood	Daily
Packaging Equipment	Occasionally

Personnel	Job Incumbent	Supervisor	Dept. Head
Date	Date	Date	Date

FIGURE 5.5, cont'd   Job description.

should receive copies of new and revised policies and procedures should be developed early. Such accomplishment serves to control the number of manuals issued and ensure that the right persons get material when it is needed.

Manuals should be distributed only to individuals or areas having a continuing and frequent requirement for such. However, a change in interdepartmental relationships may warrent a modification of an established distribution. Should a copy of a manual be used less than once daily, the distribution of that copy would probably be unwarranted (5). By limiting distribution, one reduces costs as well as the difficulty encountered in maintaining and updating manuals.

All departmental employees should be responsible for reading, understanding, and complying with the written policies and procedures. As previously suggested, the preface to the manual should clearly state this obligation.

Review/Revision of a Policy and Procedure Manual

If the policy and procedure manual is indeed to clarify rather than confuse, information contained therein must be

ANYTOWN HOSPITAL
HOSPITAL PHARMACY
POLICY AND PROCEDURE MANUAL

CLASSIFICATION NUMBER

01-20-05-A

DIVISION 01 General

CHAPTER 20 Policy and Procedure Manual

SECTION 05 Format

<u>**POLICY**</u>

A standard format shall be used in the preparation of all pages for the Policy and Procedure Manual.

<u>**PROCEDURE**</u>

1. All policies and procedures shall be typed on Hospital Pharmacy Policy and Procedure Manual letterhead paper. The top margin shall be 1½″ from the edge of the paper; the right, left, and bottom margins shall be 1″ from the edge of the paper. The words ''Policy'' and ''Procedure'' shall be underlined and centered appropriately. All paragraphs shall be single-spaced. Double-space between the subject heading and the body, between paragraphs, and below the words ''Policy'' and ''Procedure.'' Information published in an acceptable format may be inserted into the manual provided numbers 2, 3, and 4 of this procedure are adhered to.

2. Each page that begins a new division, chapter, section, part, or subpart shall have a subject heading on the upper left-hand side. The words ''DIVISION,'' ''CHAPTER,'' ''SECTION,'' ''PART,'' and ''SUBPART'' shall be in all capitals. The specific subject titles shall be in initial capitals. The subject heading shall be double-spaced.

3. Every page shall have a classification number in the upper right-hand corner. When more than one page is required for the same classification number, the number shall be followed by an ''A.'' The second page shall be ''B'' and so on. Each classification number shall be on the fourth line from the top and end exactly at the 1″ margin.

4. Each policy and procedure shall be followed by the word ''New:'' or ''Revised:'' and the effective date. This shall begin at the left margin 2 spaces above the bottom margin. The words ''Approved by:'' and the signature of the Director of Pharmacy shall be on the same line beginning in the center of the page. The word ''Reviewed:'' shall begin at the bottom left margin and shall be followed by a 3″ underscore line.

5. Capitalization rules for subject headings shall apply to the Table of Contents. All lines in the Table of Contents shall be double-spaced. Division and chapter headings shall begin at the left-hand margin. Section, part, and subpart headings shall begin under the chapter, section, and part numerals, respectively.

ANYTOWN HOSPITAL
HOSPITAL PHARMACY
POLICY AND PROCEDURE MANUAL

CLASSIFICATION NUMBER

01-20-05-B

The information stated in number 4 of this procedure shall follow the Table of Contents for each division.

6. Figures for purposes of clarification or exemplification shall be placed serially at the end of each division. The classification number shall consist of the division number followed by the word ''Figure'' and the appropriate figure number. Figure classification numbers shall be on the fourth line from the top and end exactly at the 1″ margin.

New: (Date)_____ Approved by: (Director of Pharmacy Signature)

Reviewed: _____ (Dates)_____

FIGURE 5.6   Format statement.

ANYTOWN HOSPITAL
HOSPITAL PHARMACY
POLICY AND PROCEDURE MANUAL

CLASSIFICATION NUMBER

01-20-10-A

DIVISION 01 General

CHAPTER 20 Policy and Procedure Manual

SECTION 10 Writing Style

POLICY

A standard writing style shall be used in the preparation of policy and procedural statements for the Policy and Procedure Manual.

PROCEDURE

1. Give essential information only. Begin with important information; omit unnecessary and tiresome preliminaries.

2. Use third person nouns, more specifically position titles (e.g., "the pharmacist shall initial the form").

3. Use the verb "shall" in the preparation of all policy and procedural statements where practical.

4. Use an outline style as in this statement where practical; where this is not possible, a 1, 2, 3, stepwise order is preferred.

5. Clarity is achieved when the reader understands the meaning of the instructions precisely in the way intended by the writer. The following is an aid in achieving clarity:
   a. Present ideas and facts in a logically ordered sequence.
   b. Give complete information.
   c. Qualify or amplify general rules or statements with specific subrules or substatements.
   d. Define unfamiliar terms or those which have a special or unique meaning.
   e. Be specific as to quantity, time, and place.
   f. Write sentences in direct, straight order as subject, predicate, and object (e.g., "the pharmacist shall fill the bottle," rather than "the bottle is filled by the pharmacist").

6. Brevity is an aid to clarity provided it is sought through economy of language, not economy of thought or detail.
   a. Statements shall be in sufficient detail to allow an individual who is unfamiliar with procedure to carry it out.

ANYTOWN HOSPITAL
HOSPITAL PHARMACY
POLICY AND PROCEDURE MANUAL

CLASSIFICATION NUMBER

01-20-10-B

   b. All repetitious and nonessential words shall be eliminated.

7. Paragraph structure
   a. A paragraph shall contain only one central thought.
   b. The central thought is usually expressed in the first sentence.

8. Sentence structure
   a. In the sentence, the single thought is important.
   b. Compound sentences shall be avoided.
   c. Use short, simple sentences.

9. Vocabulary
   a. The words used to convey instructions shall be as definite, specific, precise, and concrete as possible.
   b. Action words should be used wherever possible (e.g., "the pharmacist shall type a label," rather than, "the pharmacist shall prepare a label").

10. Numerical figures shall be written in Arabic numerals rather than words.

New: (Date) _____ Approved by: (Director of Pharmacy Signature)

Reviewed: _____ (Dates) _____

FIGURE 5.7 Style statement.

ANYTOWN HOSPITAL
POLICY AND PROCEDURE

QUALITY ASSURANCE/UTILIZATION REVIEW   (New or Revision Date)

19.21 Antibiotic Usage Review Program

I. Policy

There shall be an ongoing review of the clinical use of antibiotics in the hospital and long-term care facilities. This program shall be a component of the Drug Usage Review Program.

II. Procedures

A. Physician's Antibiotic Order Form

All inpatient orders for antibiotics shall be ordered on the preprinted "Antibiotic Order Form" PHARM 20 12/83 (Exhibit I). When writing antibiotic orders, physicians shall categorize the use of antibiotics as prophylactic, empirical, or therapeutic and write the prescription in the corresponding section of the form. The prescription categories shall be defined as follows:

Prophylaxis refers to antibiotic therapy given with the intent of preventing infection at a non-infected site.
Empiric therapy refers to the treatment of suspected or known infections for which bacteriologic confirmation is not available at the time antibiotic therapy is initiated.
Therapeutic refers to the use of antibiotics when the site and microorganism of an infection are known.

Changes in antibiotic therapy shall require a new order written in the appropriate section of the form.

Automatic stop orders are not in effect if the length of therapy or number of doses to be administered is specifically ordered.

All order forms shall be complete and contain the following information before the pharmacy will begin preparation:
1. Patient identification plate
2. Date and time of order
3. Depending on the category of antibiotic therapy, basic clinical information such as the planned surgical procedure, the suspected site of infection, and the culture results shall be recorded.
4. Name of drug, route, strength, and frequency of administration.
5. Physician's signature. Note: Chief resident's or attending physician's signature is also required if antibiotic is a nonformulary agent.

QUALITY ASSURANCE/UTILIZATION REVIEW   Page 2

19.21 Antibiotic Usage Review Program

B. Pharmacy Responsibilities

1. The pharmacy will monitor all Automatic Stop Orders. A "Medication Stop Order Reminder" PHARM 54 (Exhibit II) shall be sent to the nursing station 24 hours in advance of the time at which the medication will no longer be supplied, unless the length of therapy or number of doses to be administered has been specifically ordered.
2. The pharmacy will compile statistical/prevalence information to serve as a data base from which more specific assessment may be performed.

C. Pharmacy and Therapeutics Committee

The Pharmacy and Therapeutics Committee shall:
1. Review all statistical/prevalence information, susceptibility/resistance trend studies, all adverse drug reaction reports, and other appropriate hospital reports to identify problem areas associated with antibiotic use.
2. Establish clinically valid criteria for the assessment of potential problem areas.
3. Review the assessment results and make recommendations to the Quality Assurance Committee for problem resolution.
4. Document Antibiotic Usage Review activities by quarterly written reports of the findings and action taken.
5. Evaluate the Antibiotic Use Review Program annually to assure that the program is ongoing, comprehensive, effective in improving patient care and clinical performance, and conducted with cost efficiency.

FIGURE 5.8   Revision example.

current and *reliable*. Because the pharmacy department is a dynamic rather than static entity, it is imperative that the manual be flexible and readily revisable. A manual that fails to satisfy these two characteristics will become static and thus will not be utilized to its fullest. As previously indicated, the entire contents of a manual should be reviewed or revised frequently, at least annually, "to ensure currency and conformity with new laws, rules, and regulations of government agencies . . . and with the standards of the joint Commission on Accreditation of Hospitals" (12).

For continued revision, and also for expansion when necessary, it is recommended that the manual be maintained as a loose-leaf volume(s) rather than as a permanently bound book. This obviously facilitates immediate entry of new materials and removal of that which has been superseded. A regular three-ring binder is recommended over a post binder to permit easier insertion and deletion of materials (13).

Policies and procedures should be established that clearly identify the method of handling revisions in the manual. In these policies and procedures, attention should be directed toward:

Who can initiate change
How change is accomplished
Who reviews and comments on change
Processing of revised material that is no longer in effect

Copies of all old policy and procedures that have been revised should be maintained on file for reference purposes.

Maintaining control of policies and procedures that are issued, revised, and/or reviewed can be accomplished through (1) individual signatures and dates of issuance, revision, and/or review on each document (Figs. 5.6 and 5.7) or (2) a policy indicating that all policies and procedures must be approved by the pharmacy director before insertion into the manual. The original date of issuance or revision can be indicated on the document (Fig. 5.8). A policy requiring annual review and a central file of review dates will provide assurance of current information and necessary documentation.

CONCLUSION

In this chapter, the need for written policies and procedures, the benefits afforded a department by the establishment and maintenance of a policy and procedure manual, and the actual development and maintenance of a useful manual have been reviewed. In closing, a final note of caution: a policy and procedure manual should inform and guide, not suppress professional judgment, personal initiative, or creativity.

REFERENCES

1. *Minimum Standard for Pharmacies in Hospitals.* Washington, DC, American Society of Hospital Pharmacists, 1950.
2. *Minimum Standard for Pharmacies in Institutions.* Washington, DC, American Society of Hospital Pharmacists, 1977.
3. *Accreditation Manual for Hospitals, 1984.* Chicago, Joint Commission on Accreditation of Hospitals, 1983, pp 135-141.
4. Francke DE, Latiolais CJ, Francke GN, Ho NFH: *Mirror to Hospital Pharmacy.* Washington, DC, American Society of Hospital Pharmacists, 1964, pp 88-91.
5. McNairn WN: Three ways to wake up procedure manuals. *Mgt Advisor* 10:26-33, 1973.
6. *Webster's New Collegiate Dictionary.* Springfield, MA, GC Merriam, 1976, pp 890, 917.
7. Coughlin CW: The need for good procedures. *J Systems Mgt* 24:30-33, 1973.
8. Latiolais CJ: Pharmacy procedure manual: Policy guide and evaluation tool. *Hospitals* 33:77-78, 1959.
9. Gonzales, Sr M, Reilly MJ: The preparation of a procedure for a hospital pharmacy. *Am J Hosp Pharm* 21:458-463, 1964.
10. Eckel FM: Developing a policy and procedure manual. *Drug Intell Clin Pharm* 1:128-131, 1967.
11. *Remington's Pharmaceutical Sciences,* ed 14. Easton, PA, 1970, pp 1784-1785.
12. *Reference Manual on Hospital Pharmacy.* Chicago, American Hospital Association, 1970, p 16.
13. Ginnow WK, King CM, Jr.: Revision and reorganization of a hospital pharmacy policies and procedures manual. *Am J Hosp Pharm* 35:698-704, 1978.

CHAPTER 6

Marketing

MICKEY C. SMITH

While marketing is certainly not a new subject in pharmacy circles, its introduction as a subject of serious study and activity in the institution, especially the hospital, is a relatively recent phenomenon. This is true at least insofar as we are speaking of marketing *qua* "Marketing." The functions of marketing have always been performed by hospitals and other health care institutions. Their identification as *marketing* functions may be what is in fact recent.

In any case, in this chapter we will present a bit of marketing background and vocabulary for those who have not already been forced to absorb them. We will also provide a brief framework for market and marketing analysis for pharmacists who practice in the institutional environment. First, a definition or two.

One possible definition of marketing is the process of planning and managing all transactions between an organization and its constituents. Surely that is a relevant field of study for any institutional pharmacist.

A bit broader definition was composed more than 20 years ago by the marketing faculty of The Ohio State University (1):

Marketing is the process in a society by which the demand structure for economic goods and services is anticipated or enlarged and satisfied through the conception, promotion, exchange, and physical distribution of such goods and services.

Are we talking about the same thing here? That second definition sounds like something from a Fourth of July speech. The truth is that "marketing" is viewed by some as a cornerstone of the American economy and by others as an insidious plot to make people buy things they don't want—and obvious hazard when some of those "things" are actually dangerous.

Because marketing *has* been rather cruelly criticized and because the idea of marketing, e.g., *hospital* services, seems to discomfort some patients and professionals alike, we will take the time to offer some defenses of marketing that have been provided by its defenders.

MARKETING AND SOCIAL GOALS

Because marketing is a social process, its goals should be consistent with and contribute to the broader social goals. The number of societal goals is doubtless as great as the variety of areas of social concern. Statements of such goals are therefore as diverse as the varied viewpoints that exist in a world of social conflict and high dynamics. Within a democratic society, however, such as exists in the United States, certain goals are widely accepted. Among those that are closely related to or affected by marketing may be the following:

1. All institutions of the society must enhance the dignity of the individual citizen, contribute to the maximal development of his capabilities, stimulate individual responsibility, and continually widen the range and effectiveness of opportunities for individual choice.

2. There should be an opportunity for all members of the society to enjoy a reasonable and rising standard of living.

3. The centers or sources of economic power should be as diffused and as balanced as possible to preserve the productive results of fair competition and to foster maximal freedom for individuals in their choice of occupation, location, goods, services, and style of life.

4. The economy should grow at the maximal rate consistent with the primary dependence on private enterprise and the avoidance of marked inflation. Such growth is essential to achieve and maintain reasonably full employment, to raise living standards, and to assure competitive strength in international affairs.

5. Technologic change and managerial progress should be stimulated and encouraged as a means for advancing the economy and opening new opportunities for satisfying human needs and wants.

Within the context of these goals, marketing is practiced and, as with other fields of endeavor (such as pharmacy), there are certain normative criteria that serve as ideals, perhaps never completely reached but always in sight. For marketing these would include:

1. Goods and services wanted by society are produced and offered in the right quantities and qualities.

2. Desired goods and services are made available at the time and place that they are wanted.

3. A fair price is charged for goods and services marketed. This is a price that in the long run covers the cost of making the goods and providing for their effective distribution. (The same principle, of course, applies to services.)

4. Adequate and reliable market information is provided for all market participants, both producers (including marketing agencies) and consumers, as well as other final buyers.

5. Institutions performing marketing functions are dynamic, modifying their character and offerings in response to changes in customers' wants and needs.

6. The market is regulated by law to the extent necessary to prevent abuse and for the ultimate welfare of society.

With expected continuing increases in population, productive capacity, and living standards, marketing will become increasingly important by developing better means of enlarging and servicing markets, thereby enabling the economy to produce more and better goods and services. The ends served by the marketing process are, it is hoped, the more complete satisfaction of human, business, and public wants, and at the same time provision for the highest attainable degrees of utilization of technologic and human resources.

As an economy reaches an advanced stage of development, the variety as well as the quantity of goods and services is multiplied. The choices available to consumer and business buyers become much more numerous, and each one has an enlarged opportunity to select those that are more closely related to his specific wants or needs. This condition places a heavy premium on marketing, first, in more accurately ascertaining the magnitude and the qualitative characteristics of demand and, second, in providing the necessary information to prospective buyers. Of course, all of this is complicated by two characteristics of the health care market: First, demand and need may be appreciably mismatched, in either direction and, second, the actual payment for the good or service rendered may come from the consumer only indirectly, or not at all.

Grauer (2) has recognized these problems and provided some advice to the profession:

Pharmacy should implement this marketing concept by first recognizing "unmet" health care needs and then by developing cost-efficient services to meet those needs. However, caution must be exercised, so that fictitious wants and needs are not created during this process. The ability of pharmacy to accomplish this

facet of consumer satisfaction will contribute greatly to the value society will place on the profession as a contributor to health care in the future.

The last evolutionary era and pinnacle of marketing is called the societal area. Few, if any, firms or professions are marketing themselves in this manner. The orientation is toward societal satisfaction. For pharmaceutical services, this means a total dedication toward such societal trends as cost containment, instant gratification, life simplification, and self-actualization. Pharmaceutical services should not be implemented purely on the basis that someone will use the service. Instead, implementation should be done on the basis that society as a whole will benefit from that service.

Grauer's mention of the "marketing concept" deserves special attention. The marketing concept, widely discussed in the literature of the discipline, suggested that "good" marketing consists of determining customer wants and needs and then attempting to satisfy them. The difference between this approach and earlier practices is shown in Table 6.1. A bit of reflection will certainly furnish pharmacists with examples of pharmacy services that the customer was "too stupid to appreciate." An honest determination of client needs might very well have found those same customers very intelligent with regard to another service.

THE FOUR P'S OF MARKETING*

In health care terms, the *product* or good is presented in terms of service offered. Some organizations basically provide inpatient care; others offer outpatient care; still others specialize in rehabilitation services. These offerings are determined by two factors: the demands of the patients or consumers of health care service in the target market and the resources that the organization has available for providing these particular services.

---

*Most expositions on marketing will finally get around to the "four P's." This one is no different. Kubica (see additional reading list) has done a thorough job on this aspect of marketing.

TABLE 6.1 Some Differences in Outlook between Adopters of the Marketing Concept and Typical Production-Oriented Businessmen[a]

Marketing Orientation	Attitudes and Procedures	Production Orientation
Customer needs determine company plans	Attitudes toward customers	They should be glad we exist, trying to cut costs and bring out better products
Company makes what it can sell	Product offering	Company sells what it can make
To determine customer needs and how well company is satisfying them	Role of marketing research	To determine customer reactin, if used at all
Focus on locating new opportunities	Interest in innovation	Focus is on technology and cost cutting
A critical objective	Importance of profit	A residual, what's left after all costs are covered
Seen as a customer service	Role of customer credit	Seen as a necessary evil
Designed for customer convenience and as a selling tool	Role of packaging	Seen merely as protection for the product
Set with customer requirements and costs in mind	Inventory levels	Set with production requirements in mind
Seen as a customer service	Transportation arrangements	Seen as an extension of production and storage activities, with emphasis on cost minimization
Need-satisfying benefits of products and services	Focus of advertising	Product features and quality, maybe how products are made
Help the customer to buy if the product fits his needs, while coordinating with rest of firm—including production, inventory control, advertising, etc	Role of sales force	Sell the customer, don't worry about coordination with other promotion efforts or rest of firm

[a]Modified from Vizza RF, Chambers TE, and Cook EJ: *Adoption of the Marketing Concept—Fact or Fiction?* New York, Sales Executives Club of New York, Inc, 1967, pp 13-15.

Price is sometimes determined by the government, as in the case of Medicare or Medicaid, where there are limits beyond which reimbursement will not be made. At other times price is determined by insurance companies, which set maximal rates for particular services. At still other times, price is determined by competitive organizations, in which case the hospital or health care facility structures its prices according to the general market. Finally, sometimes price is determined by "what the traffic will bear" in that, for sophisticated or complex lifesaving surgery, some people are willing to supplement their insurance by paying whatever is necessary for the operation or for the use of the equipment.

Place refers to where the services are offered. For surgery, people are accustomed to coming to the hospital. For minor procedures, they often are content to visit a satellite unit located near their home. Today it is becoming evident that many people do not need to remain in the hospital for extended periods of time; most of them can profit from outpatient visits. So, health care now is becoming mobile in the sense that hospitals are setting up units around town where people can come for minor maintenance service.

Promotion refers to how the organization lets people know about its services. Typical examples include newspaper stories, radio and television reporting, letters and brochures mailed to local organizations and former patients, and word-of-mouth advertising by volunteers and satisfied patients. The "right" kind of promotion is going to be determined by the targeted customer/patient market that will be interested in the service, the health care organization itself, and the promotion efforts currently being used by the competition.

MARKETING IN HOSPITAL PHARMACY

Many people believe that marketing techniques are rarely used by modern hospitals and even fewer expect to find them in hospital pharmacies. For the most part, they are wrong.

Marketing techniques are widely employed, although the specific applications do vary greatly. For example, it has been reported that attitude surveys among current or discharged patients were used by 70% of their respondents. Other common marketing techniques uncovered by the researchers included studies of services offered by nearby hospitals (64%), formal definition of the institution's target market (59%), development of a demographic profile of the patient population (47%), use of marketing research techniques to assist in feasibility studies (34%), and patient-oriented advertising (24%) (3).

However, it should be noted that less than 10% of the respondents reported that their organization had a formal marketing plan, and only 4% said that they had a staff member with the word "marketing" in his/her title. So, a variety of marketing functions are being practices by hospitals, but little recognition currently is being given to marketing through either staff titles or the preparation of a formal, integrated, marketing plan.

Despite reports to the contrary, hospital administrators believe that marketing is a legitimate function of their institution. However, their perceptions of the appropriateness of specific marketing techniques vary widely. Whittington

and Dillon (3) report that only 6% of the administrators in their study disagreed with the statement, "marketing is a legitimate function of hospitals." However, when asked whether specific techniques should be included in the hospital's program, there was a diverse set of responses. Over 90% of the administrators said that an attitude survey of current or discharged patients "probably" or "certainly" should be included in the hospital's program. The same was true for such areas as patient demographic profiles, definitions of target market, formal marketing plans, and studies of service of medical professionals. However, about one in three of the respondents said that patient-oriented advertising should not be included, and 25% thought the same for direct-mail promotion to physicians. In summary, activities related to knowledge of patients were viewed as appropriate for hospital marketing, but those associated with the creation of demand were regarded with a more critical eye.

We are fortunate to have, in addition to the study just quoted, the results of a survey of hospital *pharmacy* directors (4). They showed that hospital pharmacy directors generally were familiar with marketing concepts, although they did not always identify them as such. By whatever name they knew marketing concepts, the directors had clear perceptions of pharmacy goals, target segments among relevant publics, and the need for adaptation to changes in the health care marketplace.

The researchers in this study expressed surprise at the finding that directors did not emphasize third parties as one of their relevant publics, in spite of their role in the financing of health care institutions. However, they were gratified by the finding that most directors recognized that different patient types had different pharmacy service needs and that a market segmentation policy might offer some promise.

It may be well to point out here that it *is* service that is being marketed and that service marketing can be different in some ways from product marketing. Some of these differences are identified in Table 6.2.

MARKETING TO WHOM?

A hospital has three broad options in defining its target population. First is a community orientation. In this option, the hospital defines its target market as all people in the local community who have health care needs. Second is a special public orientation. With this option, the hospital serves special groups that are not often defined by the surrounding community. Examples include hospitals that serve psychiatric patients, veterans, terminally ill patients, and other special groups. These hospitals have a narrower target market than those that cater to all ill people in the local area. Third is the referral orientation option. In this case, the hospital specializes in the skilled treatment of certain types of medical problems and attempts to build a national/international name for these specialties.

Of course, not all hospitals opt for just one of these options. Some try to straddle two or three orientations. When a hospital decides to add a referral orientation to its community orientation, this happens. In other cases, an institution may have trouble making up its mind as to just what target patient population it should pursue.

The identification of a target patient population helps to

TABLE 6.2 Service Marketing

Special considerations of marketers of service

1. Services cannot be stockpiled.
2. The entire service mix is usually not visible to the consumer.
3. The intangibility of services makes pricing difficult.
4. The intangibility of services makes promotion difficult.
5. The existence of a direct service organization-consumer relationship makes employee public relations skills important.
6. Services often have high costs and low reliability.
7. Peripheral services are frequently needed to supplement the basic service offering.

Basic differences between services and products

Services	*Products*
1. Services are often intangible. Services are acts, deeds, performances, efforts. Most services cannot be physically possessed. The value of a service is based on an experience; there is no transfer of title.	1. Products are tangible. Products are objects, things, materials. The value of a product is based on ownership; transfer of title takes place.
2. Services are usually perishable. Unused capacity cannot be stored or shifted from one time to another.	2. Products can be stored; product surpluses in one period can be applied against product shortages in another period.
3. Services are frequently inseparable. One cannot separate the quality of many services from the service provider.	3. Products can be graded or built to specifications. The quality of a product can be differentiated from a channel member's quality.
4. Services may vary in quality over time. It is difficult to standardize some services because of their labor intensiveness and the involvement of the service user in diagnosing his or her service needs.	4. Products can be standardized through mass production and quality control.

define the organization's objectives and provide inputs for the planning process. For example, a community hospital in a poor neighborhood is likely to develop specialties in areas such as trauma, communicable diseases, and maternity. Meanwhile, a Veterans Administration hospital will develop specialties in orthopedics, rehabilitation, and substance-abuse programs. From these specialties come guidelines for the type of "doctor mix" that will be needed.

Keep in mind, of course, that hospitals tend to be much more doctor oriented than patient oriented. Patients choose the doctor, and the latter has a great deal of authority in determining which hospital to use in case of admission. So it is to the hospital's benefit to be very concerned with physician marketing, a topic that will be addressed in the next section. Meanwhile, how can the hospital ensure that it is sensitive to the patients' needs and expectations? The answer is by concentrating attention on the three key phases of a person's experience in a hospital, i.e., admission, patient care, and exit.

Marketing during the admission phase is important because this is the time when the incoming patients get their first impression of the hospital. An individual who has to wait in a long line, is asked a large number of questions (many of which relate to financial responsibility), and is treated "like a number" will develop a poor mental image of the hospital. Patients want to feel from the very beginning that the hospital staff is concerned primarily with their comfort and well-being and that everything else is secondary.

Then comes the patient's bed-care experience. Several factors are important here. One is the overall environment of the hospital. Does it smell like a hospital? It is clean and bright? Does it look like a place where people come to die? Are there enough nurses and are they responsive? What is the quality of the food? With what degree of efficiency does the hospital provide such services as medications, diagnostic tests, telephone, and television.

Some hospitals find that even if they have handled things well thus far, they can lose all of this goodwill by bungling the exit phase of the individual's stay. For example, the person who arrives at the cashier's office and finds an extraordinarily high bill containing many items that were unanticipated is going to be very angry. At this point, the exit staff members must make a concerted effort to explain these costs and smooth the exit procedure. This can be quite difficult if the hospital has a rule that patients cannot leave until payment of all outstanding obligations has been made or a plan of action for resolving the bills is worked out. Money discussions can be particularly painful at this point in time. That is why many hospitals are now estimating the patient's bill on arrival and asking for some payment up front. Then, when the individual leaves and the insurance claims are made, the remainder of the bill is sent to the person for payment. This makes the entry phase a little less pleasant but helps to preserve the goodwill that has been built up during the individual's stay.

Physician Marketing. Hospitals and other health care agencies cannot afford to overlook physician marketing. They know that many of the people in their institution have been referred by their doctor. Furthermore, if the hospital has built a reputation in a particular specialty, such as cardiac surgery, it often will be looking for outstanding doctors in this area who will help to maintain the name of the institution. Therefore, there are a number of important aspects to physician marketing.

In trying to market itself to physicians, a health care organization must understand a doctor's requirements and desires. What is the physician seeking, and what is the hospital capable of offering? Physician motivation will vary by specialty.

Physicians will want to know aspects such as the amount of time they will have to be at the hospital, the research orientation of the institution, and the overall social environment in the hospital. The medical staff recruitment committee charged with bringing in new doctors has to be sensitive to these desires while determining whether or not they can be met. One of the poorest marketing strategies of all is to hire physicians with false promises, for not only will the physician leave but will let other doctors know that the hospital is not a very good place for a top-flight physician. This negative image could be carried around the country and could result in a severe backlash on the hospital.

Community Marketing. Hospitals and other large health care institutions often affect the local community. Ambulance noise, litter, parking problems brought about by hospital traffic, and the impact of the institution on real estate

TABLE 6.3   The Market and Market Segments[a]

- How large is the territory covered by your market? How have you determined this?
- How is your market grouped?
  —Is it scattered?
  —How many important segments are there?
  —How are these segments determined (demographics, service usage, attitudinally)?
- Is the market entirely urban, or is a fair proportion of it rural?
- What percentage of your market uses third-party payment?
  —What are the attitudes and operations of third parties?
  —Are they all equally profitable?
- What are the effects of the following factors on your market?
  —Age
  —Income
  —Occupation
  —Increasing population
  —Decreasing birthrate } demographic shifting
- What proportion of potential customers are familiar with your organization, services, programs?
  —What is your image in the marketplace?
  —What are the important components of your image?

The Organization

- Short history of your organization:
  —When and how was it organized?
  —What has been the nature of its growth?
  —How fast and far have its markets expanded? Where do your patients come from geographically?
  —What is the basic policy of the organization? Is it on "health care," "profit"?
  —What has been the financial history of the organization?
    —How has it been capitalized?
    —Have there been any account receivable problems?
    —What is inventory investment?
  —What has been the organization's success with the various services promoted?
- How does your organization compare with the industry?
  —Is the total volume (gross revenue, utilization) increasing, decreasing?
  —Have there been any fluctuations in revenue? If so, what were they due to?
- What are the objectives and goals of the organization? How can they be expressed beyond the provision of "good health care"?
- What are the organization's present strengths and weaknesses in:
  —Medical facilities
  —Management capabilities
  —Medical staff
  —Technical facilities
  —Reputation
  —Financial capabilities
  —Image
- What is the labor environment for your organization?
  —For medical staff (nurses, physicians, etc)?
  —For support personnel?
- How dependent is your organization upon conditions of other industries (third-party payers)?
- Are weaknesses being compensated for and strengths being used? How?
- How are the following areas of your marketing function organized?
  —Structure
  —Manpower
  —Reporting relationships
  —Decision-making power
- What kinds of external controls affect your organization?
  —Local?
  —State?
  —Federal?
  —Self-regulatory?
- What are the trends in recent regulatory rulings?

Competitors

- How many competitors are in your industry?
  —How do you define your competitors?
  —Has this number increased or decreased in the last 4 years?
- Is competition on a price or nonprice basis?
- What are the choices afforded patients?
  —In services?
  —In payment?
- What is your position in the market—size and strength—relative to competitors?

Products and Services

- Complete a list of your organization's products and services, both present and proposed.
- What are the general outstanding characteristics of each product or service?
- What superiority or distinctiveness of products or services do you have, as compared with competing organizations?
- What is the total cost per service (in-use)? Is service over/under utilized?
- What services are most heavily used? Why?
  —What is the profile of patients/physicians who use the services?
  —Are there distinct groups of users?
- What are your organization's policies regarding:
  —Number and types of services to offer?
  —Assessing needs for service addition/deletion?
- History of products and services (complete for major products and services):
  —How many did the organization originally have?
  —How many have been added or dropped?
  —What important changes have taken place in services during the last 10 years?
  —Has demand for the services increased or decreased?
  —What are the most common complaints against the service?
  —What services could be added to your organization that would make it more attractive to patients, medical staff, nonmedical personnel?
  —What are the strongest points of your services to patients, medical staff, nonmedical personnel?
  —Have you any other features that individualize your service or give you an advantage over competitors?

Price

- What is the pricing strategy of the organization?
  —Cost-plus
  —Return on investment
  —Stabilization
- How are prices for services determined?
  —How often are prices reviewed?
  —What factors contribute to price increase/decrease?
- What have been the price trends for the past 5 years?
- How are your pricing policies viewed by:
  —Patients
  —Physicians
  —Third-party payers
  —Competitors
  —Regulators

Promotion

- What is the purpose of the organization's present promotional activities (including advertising)?
  —Protective
  —Educational
  —Search out new markets
  —Develop all markets
  —Establish a new service
- Has this purpose undergone any change in recent years?

[a]Reprinted by permission from Berkowitz EN, Flexner WA: The marketing audit: A tool for health service organizations. *Health Care Mgt Rev* 3:51-57, 1978.

Continued.

TABLE 6.3 The Market and Market Segments—cont'd

- To whom has advertising appeal been largely directed?
  - —Donors
  - —Patients
    - —Former or current
    - —Prospective
  - —Physicians
    - —On staff
    - —Potential
- What media have been used?
- Are the media still effective in reaching the intended audience?
- What copy appeals have been notable in terms of response?
- What methods have been used for measuring advertising effectiveness?
- What is the role of public relations?
  - —Is it a separate function/department?
  - —What is the scope of responsibilities?

Channels of Distribution

- What are the trends in distribution in the industry?
  - —What services are being performed on an outpatient basis?
  - —What services are being provided on an at-home basis?
  - —Are satellite facilities being used?
- What factors are considered in location decisions? When did you last evaluate present location?
- What distributors do you deal with (e.g., medical supply houses, etc)?
- How large an inventory must you carry?

values are all examples of this. Additionally, the local residents will want to know whether the hospital is open to all patients in the community, how efficient and responsive its emergency room services are, and what its specialties are.

In answering these kinds of queries, many hospitals have appointed a director of community relations. This person is responsible for such functions as developing a close relationship with important organizations in the local areas, including business firms, women's clubs, and community groups; gathering information on the community's health needs and its perception of the hospital; preparing and sending out news and information about the hospital using annual reports, the news media, and public appearances before local groups as vehicles; offering community education programs that will help to improve the health of local residents; and helping to establish outreach programs through the formation of drug, alcohol, and cigarette smoking withdrawal clinics. In this way, the individuals help the hospital to build positive goodwill in the local community.

Employer Marketing. The employer has not been a major concern for most hospitals or administrators. The health care facility has received reimbursement for services performed through health insurance coverage purchased by the employer, but there has been little, if any, employer-hospital contact. Today this is beginning to change as employers express concern about the high costs of health care and the need for greater accessibility, less waiting time, and more services for their people. Interest is also beginning to grow in health maintenance organizations (HMOs), freestanding health centers designed to provide timely, low-cost health services, and surgical centers that can provide one-day outpatient surgery. Businesses are becoming more aware of the large sums that they are expending for employee health premiums, and in many cases the result is a customer who is becoming dissatisfied with the status quo.

There are a number of important steps that hospitals can take in marketing to businesses. The first is to identify the local employers. The second is to develop a strong education program for relating services and health care benefits provided by the hospital. These can be explained by inviting key members of industry or employer groups to industrial dinner meetings.

Marketing to Governments

One of the best ways to market a health care institution to government and regulatory agencies is to present an image of an organization that keeps health costs under tight control. Of course, these agencies are the ones that ultimately decide whether or not a program is effective. However, the health care facility must take the initiative and present its programs as those that should be accepted. The hospital has to lead rather than follow!

The importance of this last statement becomes clearer when we realize that, in the eyes of regulatory agencies,

TABLE 6.4 Questions Regarding Innovative Services[a]

1. Are there market segments (such as the aged) for which you could develop a new service program (e.g., day care, nutrition services, speech and hearing)?
2. Do you now have the basic capability of providing those services or would you have to start from scratch?
3. What is your present competition and what does it offer in terms of product, price, and place to that segment?
4. What other organizations have a better basic capacity to provide such services (personnel, equipment, facilities, location) and might decide to do so?
5. What can you do that is better than existing and potential competition?
6. What would be the impact on your organization if you succeeded in implementing such a program? At what levels of utilization?
7. What internal groups must be won over to the idea for it to succeed?
8. What external groups?
9. How might the program be developed so as to improve the probability that internal groups will support it?
10. Can you involve potential consumers or referral agencies in developing the program?
11. What groups or individuals might oppose the development and for what reasons?
12. Can they be won over or is it necessary to defeat them?
13. What strategies can you use for either?
14. What benefits can you promise to interested groups as a result of implementing the program and at what costs?
15. How can you communicate most effectively to the precise segments of the market most likely to use the program?
16. What message will be most likely to stir their interest?

[a]Modified from MacStravic REF: *Marketing by Objectives for Hospitals,* Germantown, MD, Aspen Systems, 1980, p 263.

the image of many hospitals is a negative one. Hospitals have opposed regulation and claimed that the government simply does not understand their problems. This has merely served to infuriate the regulators, who then have proceeded to view the situation as "us against them."

Regulatory health care strategies have been some of the most difficult to understand in light of the fact that these agencies have tremendous potential for creating major change in the health care system.

THE MARKETING AUDIT

The marketing audit, a sequential process, consists of:
- Goal specification
- Operational objectives
- Strategy development
- Implementation
- Evaluation

It is usually offered as an early and ongoing marketing process, and pharmacy should be prepared both to understand the audit of the overall hospital operation and to conduct its own audit. Table 6.3 shows the kind of elements in a good marketing audit.

The detailed marketing audit shown in Table 6.3 is a useful exercise, but pharmacists may find it desirable to start from a more general perspective. Such a perspective, applicable to decisions such as offering an outpatient counseling service, is provided in Table 6.4.

CONCLUSION

The intention, in this brief chapter, was not to teach techniques of marketing, but rather to introduce the subject. Institutional pharmacy has experienced a period of rapid growth and diversification. It has done so through the application of marketing principles, though perhaps not consciously so.

In the era that lies at the end of the 20th century, apparently one of limited expansion, growth in institutional pharmacy probably will require more clever and conscious application of marketing concepts. The "institutional outreach programs" described by Oddis (5), among others, are precisely the kinds of initiations that marketing is designed to augment. Successful pharmacists of the future will bring a firm grasp of marketing to their workplace.

REFERENCES

1. Marketing Staff of Ohio State University: A statement of marketing philosophy. *J Marketing* 29:43-44, 1965.
2. Grauer DW: Marketing concepts for pharmaceutical service development. *Am J Hosp Pharm* 38:233-236, 1981.
3. Whittington FB, Dillon R: Marketing by hospitals. *Health Care Mgt Rev* 4:33-37, 1979.
4. Grauer DW, Pathak DS: Marketing perspectives of hospital pharmacy directors. *Am J Hosp Pharm* 40:984-988, 1983.
5. Oddis JA: Current and future pharmacy initiatives in institutional and corporate practice. *Am J Hosp Pharm* 41:279-281, 1984.

ADDITIONAL READING

Cooper PD, Robinson LM: *Health Care Marketing Management.* Rockville, MD, Aspen Systems, 1982.
Kotler P: *Marketing for Non-Profit Organizations,* ed 2. Englewood Cliffs, NJ, Prentice-Hall, 1983.
Kubica AJ: Marketing management concepts for contemporary pharmacy practice. *Top Hosp Pharm Mgt* 2:55-65, 1982.
MacStravic RE: *Marketing Health Care.* Rockville, MD, Aspen Systems, 1977.
McMillan NH: *Marketing Your Hospital.* Chicago, American Hospital Association, 1981.

CHAPTER 7

Pricing and Reimbursement

ROBERT F. MILLER

Not so many decades ago hospitals were a place in which to die. They were supported almost totally by charitable contributions and staffed largely by volunteers. Today, hospitals utilize expensive technology to prolong life beyond most expectations. They collectively compose a multibillion dollar industry and are staffed by competitively paid professionals and specialists. Today, like any businesses, hospitals are quite concerned about being adequately reimbursed for their products and services.

This chapter will review the methods by which hospitals and their pharmacies are paid for products and services; some of the significant changes under way in reimbursement procedures; and various methods used by hospital pharmacies for pricing.

REIMBURSEMENT

Reimbursement is simply another name for the payment that hospitals receive for the care of patients. As we continue, it will become clear that this payment often is not equivalent to the charges that appear on the hospital bill. The methods used to determine how much the hospital is reimbursed for services have become quite complex and vary significantly, depending on the source of the payment.

This review deals only with reimbursement for inpatient hospital services. Additionally, ''reimbursement'' is used in the broad sense to mean general payment for hospital services, rather than specific payment for pharmacy services. Hospital pharmacies usually do not bill directly for their products and services. Rather, pharmacy is one of the several types of charges included on the hospital bill.

Historical Perspective

A brief look back may help to put into perspective the current state of hospital reimbursement and the changes that are under way. Our ''health care system,'' as we call it, is not very old. Only within the last 50 years has there been a ''system'' at all. Prior to that time, most care was rendered by the family and individual medical practitioners. Medical knowledge was limited, and a significant portion of the practitioner's role was to comfort the dying. Payment for services was as likely to be by the barter system (e.g., a chicken or some produce) as it was to be by cash. In the early 1930s, the ''system'' began to evolve with advances

in medical science and development of a structure of infirmaries, clinics, and hospitals in industrial areas. Prepaid health insurance also came into being at this time.

Blue Cross is said to have had its beginning in 1929 (1). A prepayment plan for hospital care was developed under which schoolteachers who joined the plan could pay $6.00 a year and be assured of up to 21 days of hospital care in a semiprivate room at Baylor University Hospital in Dallas. The prepayment plan relieved the problem of cash shortage facing the hospital and the pressure of hospital bills for the teachers. These plans became popular rather quickly, and commercial insurance companies also began to offer health insurance. By 1947, there were 27 million members of Blue Cross plans, equal to 19% of the U.S. population.

At about this time, the second stage in the evolution of the health care system began with the inception of the Hill-Burton program. This was an enormous, ongoing federal commitment to hospital construction and aid to schools, colleges, and individuals entering the health professions. This period witnessed a growth in technology and resources and an immense expansion of health insurance coverage for the general population. A peak was reached in 1965 with the establishment of Medicare and Medicaid. The philosophy of health care as a public utility and health care benefits as a human right was evolving. By the mid-1970s, the federal government was becoming increasingly concerned about the cost and the quality of health care. Professional standards review organizations, health systems agencies, health maintenance organizations, as well as hospital cost-containment legislation were established to control costs and assure quality. Regulation and bureaucracy were the tools.

In 1981, ''Reaganomics'' hit the health care system (2). The Reagan administration's goals for the health care system were to (1) develop alternatives to regulation to promote cost containment and quality control through competition and (2) increase the roles of state and local governments and the private sector to increase competition. The Omnibus Reconciliation Budget Act of 1981 initiated this process. This legislation called for major federal health spending reductions over the next 3 years, primarily in the Medicare and Medicaid programs. It also provided state Medicaid programs more flexibility in determining reimbursement rates to providers. Next came The Tax Equity and Fiscal Responsibility Act of 1982 (TEFRA) (3). This very significant legislation:

1. Placed a per case limit on total reimbursement to hospitals for Medicare patients

2. Set a "target amount" of costs for each hospital and made provisions for the hospital to retain 50% of the amount by which actual costs fall below the target

3. For the first time, brought ancillary services, such as pharmacy, under the total reimbursement limit

4. Required that the Secretary of Health and Human Services present a plan for a "prospective payment system" to Congress by the end of 1982.

This latter provision of TEFRA laid the groundwork for conversion to the diagnosis related group (DRG) method of Medicare reimbursement, which will be discussed in more detail later in this chapter.

Sources of Hospital Reimbursement

Hospitals receive payment for their services from several different sources, depending on which type of health care "insurance" covers each patient. The major sources of payment are "third parties." These are sources (other than the hospital or the patient, who are the first two parties) such as Blue Cross, Medicare, Medicaid, commercial insurance companies, or any agent other than the patient who contracts to pay all or part of the patient's hospital bill. Not all third parties pay the hospital under the same set of rules or at the same rate or price. The mix and relative proportion of reimbursement sources vary from one hospital to the next. Reimbursement usually is provided by one of the following sources. The percentages are an estimate of the "mix" in the average hospital (4).

Medicare. Also known as Title XVIII of the Social Security Act, this program helps to pay for two kinds of health services for persons 65 years of age or older and for certain disabled persons. Part A pays for hospital care and related services, and Part B pays doctors' bills for services in and out of the hospital. Both parts require some "copayment" by the patient. Medicare reimbursement has been based on reasonable costs as detailed in a Medicare cost report that the hospital must file annually.

Medicaid. Also known as Title XIX of the Social Security Act, or as "state welfare," this program helps to pay for medical care for the indigent. Medicaid also generally pays hospitals on a reasonable cost basis. However, because Medicaid is administered at the state level, the specific provisions of the program may vary from state to state. Medicare and Medicaid account for a combined 50% of reimbursement in the average hospital.

Blue Cross. This is a nongovernmental prepayment program for hospital expenses that originally was founded to save hospitals from financial ruin. In 1980, there were 69 autonomous Blue Cross plans in the United States. These plans generally provide more comprehensive coverage than commercial insurance. The majority of Blue Cross plans reimburse hospitals on the basis of cost; the rest pay a percentage of charges. Blue Cross payments provide about 18% of reimbursement in the average hospital.

Commercial Insurance. These health insurance plans pay hospitals on a charge basis for the specific benefits allowed under the insurance contract with the subscriber. An initial "deductible" amount, as well as the charges for services not covered, are the responsibility of the patient. Commercial insurance payments provide about 24% of reimbursement in the average hospital.

Self-pay. Patients who pay all or part of their hospital bills provide the remaining 8% of reimbursement to the average hospital. They pay at the full hospital charge rate.

Charge vs Cost

In the reimbursement vocabulary, "charge" means the charges that appear on the hospital bill. In the same vocabulary, the meaning of "cost" is not as clear. Logically, "cost" would seem to refer to the cost of providing hospital services. This cost would include all of the costs of operating the hospital: the direct and indirect costs of producing a service; education and community service costs; the cost of providing new equipment and facilities; and the cost of bad debts and free services. The "costs" that some third-party payers pay do not include all of these operation costs.

In actuality, Medicare, Medicaid, and Blue Cross pay less than the full cost of providing service to patients. In their agreements with hospitals, these payers "disallow" or exclude certain real costs. In effect, because of their bargaining power and the precarious financial positions of most hospitals, these third parties can manage to pay less than their "fair share" of hospital costs. This practice results in "cost shifting." Hospitals must recover their costs by setting the charges paid by commercial insurance companies and self-pay patients considerably above the actual cost of providing services.

This practice of cost shifting makes published hospital charges appear much higher than the income they actually produce. Cost shifting also causes commercial insurance premiums (and the resulting costs to the employers, who pay most of the premiums) to be much higher than would be necessary if Medicare and Medicaid, in particular, paid a "fair share" of costs.

Retrospective vs Prospective Payment

Retrospective payment refers to the practice of paying hospitals for services after their provision. This type of payment may be based on hospital costs or charges. However, the amount of payment is determined on the basis of the services actually provided during the patient's stay. Under retrospective payment, there is little incentive for the hospital to contain costs because payments increase as more costs are incurred. All third parties traditionally have paid hospitals on a retrospective basis.

Under prospective payment, also known as incentive reimbursement, the amount of payment is set prior to the provision of services. The rates of prospective payment can be based on per day costs, per episode of illness, per hospital admission, on a capitation basis, on services rendered, etc. This type of payment puts the hospital at risk to provide services within the costs covered by the predetermined rates. Under prospective payment, the hospital also usually shares in any savings that accure when service is provided at less cost than that covered by the payment rate. Thus, there is an incentive to provide services at less cost.

State-Legislated Hospital Cost-Containment Programs

Since 1969, 18 states have enacted legislation that requires the disclosure, review, or regulation of hospital rates or budgets by some type of commission (5). The requirements of such legislation has ranged from public disclosure of budgets and rates in some states (e.g., California) to full hospital budget approval authority down to the departmental level in other states (e.g., Connecticut). Although the objective of these programs was to reduce hospital expenditures, it is not clear that this objective has been achieved in most of the affected states. These legislated programs have, however, had an impact on hospital budgeting and financial management in these states and have increased the scrutiny of the budgets of hospital departments.

Prospective Payment Systems

The prospective payment system (PPS), developed to fulfill a requirement of the TEFRA legislation of 1982, became effective in October 1983 for hospitals whose fiscal years began on or after that date. The PPS regulations implement the Social Security Amendments of 1983, which change the method of Medicare payment for inpatient hospital services from a cost-based, retrospective reimbursement system to a diagnosis-specific prospective payment system (6,7). This payment system, which uses the DRG as the service unit for which payment is made, promises to have far-reaching impact on hospital reimbursement systems.

The DRG reimbursement unit is a positive incentive to hospitals to provide services more efficiently. Under this system, the hospital is paid a predetermined amount specific to the DRG into which the patient is classified. The single payment covers the entire episode of care, regardless of how many days the patient remains in the hospital, regardless of how many tests are performed, and regardless of how many drugs are used. This system is to be phased in over a 3-year period that began October 1, 1983. By 1987, 100% of a hospital's Medicare reimbursement is to be based on the DRG-PPS system that uses a single national payment rate for each of the 470 DRGs.

The calculation of the specific reimbursement for the care of an individual patient under this system is currently somewhat complex. However, there are several general factors involved:

- There are two national DRG rates (specific regional rates are used during the 3-year phase-in period) composed of a labor and nonlabor component. One rate applies to urban hospitals and the other applies to rural hosptials. The rates in 1984 were urban, $2837.91; and rural, $2264.00.
- National rates for a specific DRG are derived by multiplying by a weighted factor intended to reflect the relative cost, across all hospitals, for treating patients classified in that DRG. For example, the national urban rate in 1984 for DRG 126, Acute & Subacute Endocarditis, was $2.6645 \times \$2837.91 = \$7561.61$.
- During the 3-year phase-in period, regional rates are used that take into account regional differences in personnel costs. Also during this period, a portion of the payment is based on hospital-specific base year costs and individual hospital case mix.

- Additional payment amounts, above the prospective payment rates, are made to cover some specific costs, including:
  1. Outliers—cases that have an extremely long length of stay in comparison to most discharges classified in the same DRG
  2. Capital costs—equipment and construction costs
  3. Direct and indirect medical education costs—to ease the adverse impact of PPS on teaching hospitals
- Special provisions or exemptions are made for certain specialty hospitals and hospitals that are the only hospital in a community.

Although the government's PPS currently applies only to inpatient hospital reimbursement from Medicare, it is believed that similar payment systems eventually will be extended to other payment categories. In addition, the conversion of Medicare to this system has increased the anxiety of other third-party payers and employers who pay the insurance premiums with regard to "cost shifting" by hospitals. This concern has stimulated the development of innovative payment systems by nongovernmental payers.

Medicaid Reimbursement System Changes

The state-administered Medicaid programs are also attempting to reduce health care costs. In 1983, 56% of all state Medicaid reimbursement systems used prospective payment, and another 32% were pursuing conversion to prospective payment (8).

Preferred Provider Organizations

One of the innovative payment systems developed in the private sector is the preferred provider organization (PPO). These are groups of hospitals and physicians that contract on a fee-for-service basis with employers, insurance carriers, or other third parties to provide comprehensive medical services to subscribers (9,10). These arrangements are characterized by:

1. A negotiated, discounted schedule of fees
2. A provider panel that includes a limited number of hospitals and physicians
3. Utilization control mechanisms
4. Flexibility for the consumer to choose non-PPO providers, although financial incentives to use PPO providers usually are present

The discounted fees, which may be paid on a per diem or per case basis, create pressure to provide care at reduced cost. However, these programs provide more rapid payment to providers and can enlarge the provider's patient population base.

Exclusive Provider Organizations

A more restrictive modification of the PPO removes the subscriber option of receiving partial coverage for use of a provider not covered by the program. Under the exclusive provider organization (EPO) model, the insurer makes payments only for services rendered by providers with EPO contracts. The Medi-Cal (Medicaid) program in California, for example, negotiates contracts with hospitals at significantly reduced per diem rates. Medi-Cal patients may use only contracted hospitals for service.

Other Health Care Incentives Reform Proposals

A number of other mechanisms to limit health care spending have been proposed and are in various stages of development. These include limitations on the amount of annual tax-exempt employee health benefits, increased cost sharing by Medicare beneficiaries and Medicaid recipients, and an optional voucher plan for Medicare beneficiaries to purchase private health insurance. All of these mechanisms are designed to encourage less frequent use of health care services or use of the least costly alternatives.

Effect of the New Reimbursement Systems on Hospitals and Hospital Pharmacies

The changes described in this section represent current developments in the methods of payment for inpatient hospital services. All of these changes are directed toward reducing the utilization and cost of these services. During the next few years, terminology and specific methodologies may change. However, the trend toward reduced inpatient reimbursements from all payers is very likely to continue.

In order to remain financially viable, hospitals must also change. Among the effects already evident are:

- Increased attention to analyzing the costs of providing the various components of care
- Increased emphasis on cost containment at all levels
- Increased competition among hospital services and departments for limited resources
- An emphasis on discharging patients are early as possible
- Limitation of new programs and services to those that reduce overall costs
- Increased competition between hospitals for PPO and EPO contracts
- Increased tension between hospitals and their medical staffs as administrators take increased interest in the cost effectiveness of the resource use by individual physicians
- A trend toward diversification into the provision of non-inpatient services (e.g., home care) and into nonhealth for-profit business ventures (e.g., real estate)
- Services that previously were revenue centers (i.e., produced extra income for the hospital), such as pharmacy and laboratories, are becoming cost centers as all-inclusive per diem and per case PPSs replace separate ancillary charges

More time is needed to determine what impact these changes will have on the overall cost and quality of health care.

PRICING

Although hospital reimbursement is being moved toward prospective payment systems, charging for specific products and services continues to be important. A number of Blue Cross plans, most commercial insurance plans, and, of course, self-pay patients still pay hospitals based on what the hospital charges. Charge-based payment may account for 50% or more of the average hosptial's reimbursement.

This section will review some of the theoretical, as well as the practical, determinants of hospital pharmacy prices (or charges); the usual sources of charge documentation; the common methods used to price hospital pharmacy products and services; and several factors to be considered in designing the pharmacy pricing system.

The Basis for Prices

The price for a pharmacy product or service should be set to cover the following components:

1. *Direct personnel costs:* Salaries for the man-hours required; a percentage for vacation and absences; a percentage to account for an average productivity of less than 100%; and a percentage for fringe benefits

2. *Drug costs:* Actual acquisition costs for the drugs included in the product or unit of service being priced

3. *Other direct supply costs:* Labels, vials, syringes, needles, etc used in preparing or distributing the product

4. *Fixed overhead costs:* A percentage of fixed departmental management, supervision and clerical costs, office supplies, subscriptions, equipment depreciation, etc

5. *Indirect costs:* A percentage of utility costs and other costs allocated to pharmacy for operation of nonrevenue-producing departments, which support the functioning of the pharmacy and the hospital

6. *Revenue deductions:* A percentage of third-party disallowances, contractual allowances, bad debts, etc, which reduce the actual revenue received from charges

7. *Profit margin:* An amount that is above the break-even cost of providing a product or service and that is necessary to provide for replacement and upgrading of hospital equipment and facilities

Each pharmacy charge should contribute to covering a share of each of these cost components as well as a share of the profit-margin requirement. Although initially set on this theoretical basis, as time goes on prices are often changed on the basis of financial expediency. Pharmacy prices may be increased to support cost increases in non-revenue-producing departments. Pharmacy prices may be increased to avoid increases in the more visible daily room rates, increases which would affect the hospital's competitive position relative to neighboring institutions. Selected pharmacy prices may be increased without relation to cost because the standard prices in neighboring institutions allow increases for these items. In an effort to remain competitive, hospital pricing decisions are often influenced by what neighboring institutions are charging for similar products and services. The prices resulting from these somewhat arbitrary adjustments may have a less logical relation to actual costs than did the original pricing. As will be discussed subsequently, it is important that the pricing structure retain a logical relationship to the actual cost of providing associated products and services.

Sources of Charge Documentation

Pharmacy revenue is derived primarily from charges for discrete drug product units, e.g., a single-dose or multidose container. In most cases, the charging transaction also generates necessary data on the cost of drugs dispensed by the pharmacy. These cost data then are used to reduce "book inventory" and to record the "cost of goods sold."

Reliable systems must be established for collecting data on the dispensing and/or administration of drugs. Unless pharmacy charges are based entirely on a per diem rate, this system must record the use of specific quantities of specific drugs for individual patients. The documents most commonly used as charge sources are the pharmacy medication profile and the nursing medication administration record (MAR).

The patient-specific pharmacy medication profile is an integral part of the drug distribution system. The profile indicates the quantities of drugs dispensed for administration to the patient. The profile also usually indicates the quantities of drugs returned unused, allowing determination of the net quantity used. The profile may be computerized, in which case the pricing is usually done automatically. When the profile is maintained manually, the quantities used must be either priced manually or entered separately into a computer for computation of price and summation of charges.

The MAR is maintained by the nurse as drugs are administered to patients. The MAR indicates the doses actually administered and is a permanent part of the medical record. Like the profile, the MAR may also be computerized, with pricing and charge summation done automatically. If a manually maintained MAR is used as a charge document, it usually must be routed to the pharmacy for pricing or data entry.

Both the medication profile and the MAR have advantages and disadvantages as charge documents. The quality of the profile is under the control of a relatively limited number of pharmacy personnel and may present an accurate record of drugs dispensed from the pharmacy. However, it does not necessarily reflect the doses of drugs actually administered, or recorded as administered, in the medical record. The medical record is the legal record of drug use. It is the record used to substantiate charges when these are questioned by third-party payers. Thus, charges that are accounted for on the profile may de disallowed if not accounted for by medical record. The MARs are maintained by a relatively large number of nurses and may not account for all doses dispensed by the pharmacy. Also, problems with consistent, timely delivery of manually maintained MARs to the pharmacy for charge processing are common, resulting in lost or late (unpostable) charges. However, the MAR is the legal medical record documentation of drug use. Charges based on the MAR are likely to be substantiated more easily if questioned.

Other charge documents, such as controlled substance disposition records, copies of the physician's orders, IV admixture records, and operating-room charge sheets may be used to supplement the medication profile and MAR.

Pharmacy Pricing Methods

The methods and formulas used to price pharmacy products and services vary considerably among hospitals. The more common methods will be described here.

The Percentage Markup Method

Pricing based on a percentage markup of the product cost is one of the oldest pricing methods. A common method used in retail businesses, the percentage markup method is based on the assumption that the inventory holding cost of a higher cost product is proportionally higher. Although this assumption also applies to pharmaceutical products, this method, used exclusively, is one of the most inequitable for hospital pharmacy pricing. It ignores the professional service component and the fact that the cost of this component of pharmacy services has no relationship to the cost of the drug product. Under this method, the patient receiving a more costly drug pays for a proportionately larger part of overall pharmacy service costs regardless of the amount of service received. Fortunately, this method rarely is used alone for hospital pharmacy pricing.

The Dispensing Fee Method

The most commonly used pricing method is the dispensing fee. The price is calculated by adding a fixed fee to the acquisition cost of the unit of product dispense. The fee is established to cover the direct, indirect, and fixed costs of providing pharmacy services as well as the profit margin required by the hospital. This method allocates the charge for pharmacy services evenly without any relationship to the cost of the product dispensed.

In practice, more than a single dispensing fee is used. For example, separate fees are often added to the acquisition cost of oral doses and parenteral doses because of the usually higher cost of preparing and administering parenteral doses.

A similarly derived "professional" fee may be used to charge for clinical pharmacy services (e.g., pharmacokinetic dosing consultation or patient teaching) when such services are charged separately from the product (11,12).

The Per Diem Charge Method

Making a single, per diem charge for drugs and pharmacy services has been promoted on the premise that pharmacy costs do not vary sufficiently among patients to warrant the clerical and logistical costs of processing charges for individual units or doses of drugs (13,14). Under the per diem charge method, the average drug cost per patient day, the average pharmacy service cost per patient day, and the desired profit margin are computed to arrive at a single pharmacy charge for each day that a patient is in the hospital. Separate per diem rates may be established for the various clinical service areas. This method takes into account the differences in pharmacy resource use between, for example, a patient in an intensive care unit and a patient in an obstetric unit.

Combinations and Modifications of the Standard Methods

Several pricing procedures that modify and/or combine the percentage markup, the dispensing (or professional) fee, and the per diem charge have been described by pharmacy managers (15-17). The combined approach can take advantage of the beneficial characteristics of the separate methods, while avoiding some of the disadvantages that may exist with exclusive use of a single method.

An example of this synergistic effect is the charging system described by Smith and Weiblen (15). This system consists of four parts:

1. *Drug product costs:* The actual acquisition cost of each

specific drug administered appears on the patient's bill. This clearly shows what portion of pharmacy charges is for the drug product.

2. *Per diem charge:* This charge covers basic pharmacy services, including drug information and general drug therapy monitoring. Three different per diem rates were established initially: cirtical care, general care, and minimal care. This categorization allows differentiation among the pharmacy personnel resource use by different types of patients. A per diem charge is made to any patient who receives medication.

3. *Intravenous drug admixtures:* A separate, all-inclusive charge is made for IV admixtures for each unit received by a patient.

4. *Special clinical service charge:* This charge covers the time required for pharmacists to perform specific physician-prescribed clinical services, such as patient drug histories and implementation of a heparin infusion protocol.

According to the authors, this charging system allows for a more equitable distribution of charges based on actual services received; makes it clear to patients and third parties what they are paying for; and allows logical adjustment in service charges as services and costs change. The reader is referred to the specifically cited references for further details on the implementation of individual pricing methods.

Judicious combination and modification of the basic pharmacy charging methods is likely to result in the most workable and logical system for pricing pharmacy products and services.

Considerations in Designing a Pharmacy Pricing System

Each of the basic pharmacy pricing methods has advantages and disadvantages. As already noted, a combination of methods probably works best. The following considerations should be kept in mind as the components of a pricing system are selected:

1. *Collection of charge data:* Regardless of the pricing method used, data on the number and type of product or service units provided must be collected in order to make charges. A reliable process for collecting these data must be established to avoid problems. For example, if the MAR is to be used as the charge source for the dispensing fee method, consideration should be given to the consistency of nurse charting and the logistics of collecting the MARs on a timely basis. Deficiencies in these areas can result in "lost" charges and charges received too late to process within the limited billing period following patient discharge. Computerization can make a major contribution here.

2. *Clerical and administrative time requirements:* The personnel time required to collect, calculate, and process charges and to administer the charging system should be considered. This should also include time required outside the pharmacy, e.g., in the data processing and patient accounting departments. Per diem charging probably requires the least time, whereas manually accounted, individual dose-dispensing fee methods probably are the most time consuming.

3. *Generation of adequate charge detail:* Hospital bills, including pharmacy charges, are often questioned and challenged by patients and third-party payers. Most recently, employers, who ultimately pay most health care insurance premiums, are contracting with organizations specifically set up to challenge hospital bills. The pharmacy charging system must generate adequate detail on the charges in order to answer such inquires. If charges cannot be substantiated adequately, the hospital may not be able to collect on the charge. Per diem charges that include drug products may be most vulnerable to such problems.

4. *Assurance of adequate revenue:* Many hospital and pharmacy costs are relatively fixed. They cannot be adjusted easily on the basis of fluctuations in patient census or drug prescribing volume. Pricing methods must assure adequate revenue to cover these fixed costs when the volume or type of product or service consumption fluctuates. A percentage markup alone may not assure adequate revenue if prescribing patterns shift to lower cost drugs. A per dose dispensing fee may not assure adequate revenue if the number of doses administered decreases, e.g., because of a shift to drugs that require less frequent dosing. A per diem fee may not produce adequate revenue if patient census declines because of fewer admissions or a shortened length of stay. Many of our clinical pharmacy services are directed at producing these types of changes in order to contain costs. Thus, the pharmacy charging system should ideally produce an amount of revenue that is not dependent on drug product use or patient days of service. A per admission or per discharge pharmacy charge that is similar to the DRG rate may be effective. Alternatively, a charging system that incorporates a combination of dispensing fees and per diem charges may help to buffer against the revenue impact of product or patient-day volume fluctuations.

5. *Ease of logical revision:* Pharmacy charges require periodic revision as operating costs and services change. Usually, revision is required at least annually. The pricing methods should allow easy and logical revision as frequently as necessary. The system should allow specific change in the drug-cost component when drug costs change; and in the personnel component when personnel costs or requirements change. When a new service is initiated or a current service is discontinued, the system should allow specific changes in the charges to those patients affected by the service change.

6. *Explainability:* Increasingly, patients, third-party payers, employers, and physicians are insisting on an explantion of specific hospital charges. Pharmacists should be prepared to explain how their charges are derived and how the charges relate to the cost of supplies and services. The pharmacy pricing system must be logical and should be based on real costs. Basing charges on fictitious "costs," such as the average wholesale price of drugs, or saying that "hospital administration tells us what to charge" is not adequate. A logical pricing system that reasonably relates charges to actual costs is desirable.

7. *Acceptance by third-party payers:* Deviations from traditional pricing methods, even though logical and innovative, may not be acceptable to third-party payers. As already noted, the system should be clearly explainable and based on real costs. Additionally, pharmacists should ask the advice of the hospital finance department with regard to the advisability of seeking specific approval from the principal third-party payers.

CONCLUSION

Adequate reimbursement for the products and services used in caring for patients is critical to the financial viability of hospitals. Health care, and especially hospital reimbursement regulations, procedures, and practices are undergoing significant change. Most of this change, which is directed at lowering the overall cost of health care, has broad support from government agencies, Congress, employers, insurers, and consumers. Much of it is also supported by hospitals.

For the next several years, hospitals will be dealing with a mixture of dissimilar, sometimes contradictory, reimbursement systems. Cost reduction, decrease in ancillary service use, and shortened length of stay are important to survival under the Medicare prospective reimbursement system. Yet an adequate volume and level of daily room charges and ancillary service charges are important to survival under the charge- and cost-based reimbursement systems of Blue Cross and private insurers. For the foreseeable future, pharmacy charges and pricing methodologies will be important for reimbursement from these latter payers.

Hospital pharmacists must understand the basic hospital reimbursement systems; how they are changing; and how the design of the pharmacy pricing and charging system contributes to hospital reimbursement so that they can adequately adapt and plan for the future.

REFERENCES

1. Berman HJ, Weeks LE: Blue Cross. In *The Financial Management of Hospitals* Ann Arbor, Health Administration Press, 1982.
2. Enright SM: Effect of Reaganomics on the U.S. health-care system. *Am J Hosp Pharm* 39:1169-75, 1982.
3. Curtiss FR: Current concepts in hospital reimbursment. *Am J Hosp Pharm* 40:586-91, 1983.
4. Anon: Reaction of providers. In *Prospective Payment: What It Is/How to Cope*. Concord, MA; International Health Services, Ltd, 1983.
5. Berman HJ, Weeks LE: Charges and rate setting. In *The Financial Management of Hospitals*. Ann Arbor, Health Administration Press, 1982.
6. Health Care Financing Administration: *Fed Reg* 48:39752-39890, 1983.
7. Enright SM: *Prospective Payment Regulations*. Bethesda, American Society of Hospital Pharmacists, 1983.
8. Anon: Reaction of insurers to prospective payment. In *Prospective Payment: What It Is/How to Cope*. Concord, MA; International Health Services, 1983.
9. Enright SM: Preferred provider organizations. *Am J Hosp Pharm* 40:551, 1983.
10. Schroer K, Elsworth T: A survey of preferred provider organizations, *Hospitals* 85-88, 1984.
11. Nold EG, Pathak DS: Third party reimbursement for clinical pharmacy services: philosophy and practice. *Am J Hosp Pharm* 34:823-26, 1977.
12. Schad R, Schneider P, Nold E: Reimburseable pharmacy teaching program for adrenalectomy patients. *Am J Hosp Pharm* 36:1212-1214, 1979.
13. Bower RM, Helper CD: A statistical approach to per diem pharmacy pricing. *Am J Hosp Pharm* 31:1179-1188, 1974.
14. Dirks I, Pang FJ: Charging for hospital pharmaceutical services: Combined product-service per diem fees. *Am J Hosp Pharm* 36:363-365, 1979.
15. Smith WE, Weiblen JW: Charging for pharmaceutical services: Product cost, per diem fees and fees for special clinical services. *Am J Hosp Pharm* 36:355-359, 1979.
16. Fish KH: Charging for hospital pharmaceutical services: Computerized system using a markup and a dose fee. *Am J Hosp Pharm* 36:360-363, 1979.
17. Wyatt BK: Charging for hospital pharmaceutical services: Flat fee based on the medication record. *Am J Hosp Pharm* 36:365-367, 1979.

CHAPTER 8

Work Analysis and Time Study

CHARLES D. HEPLER

PURPOSE OF WORK ANALYSIS

The purpose of work analysis is expressed succinctly in the motto, "work smarter, not harder." Work analysts attempt, through the application of logic and knowledge of how the human body functions in performing physical tasks, to devise methods for task performance that are easier to learn, less fatiguing, quicker, safer, and more reliable than those methods which may first occur to the worker or to management. A classic example is F. B. Gilbreth's improvement of methods used in laying brick. By changing the method used by the mason and the layout of the mason's work area, Gilbreth was able to obtain average productivity per man-hour almost three times that of the very best masons using the standard methods of the time. Another of the pioneers in work analysis, F. W. Taylor, was able to reduce the labor requirement for ore or coal handling by his methods to 25-35% of the labor requirement of earlier methods. Neither of these improvements involved introduction of machinery (1).

Hospital pharmacy, especially in medium- and small-sized hospitals, includes many labor-intensive activities. Because of the scale of most hospital pharmacy operations, major replacement of human activity with capital equipment for performing physical tasks appears unlikely in the forseeable future. Therefore, methods improvement can be important to many hospital pharmacy managers.

PLACING RESPONSIBILITY FOR WORK ANALYSIS

Work analysis is frequently assumed, perhaps unconsciously, to be the sole province of "methods engineers." This assumption is implicit in some of the older methods engineering literature and may have had some basis in reality in the age of Taylor and the Gilbreths. Today, however, the assumption must be examined critically, for the worker frequently is able to improve his own methods and is willing to do so if management will support his efforts and if the net effect of the improvement includes benefits to him. Managers also can frequently devise methods improvements merely by critical examination. Management can promote continual methods improvement by (1) encouraging all workers to think critically about their work, (2) consulting the workers involved when considering new methods or equipment, (3) supporting methods improvement suggestions, and (4) increasing the chance that improved methods will be seen by the worker as bringing personal benefits of some kind.

Mankind's understanding of the psychology and sociology of work has undergone drastic change since the early days of work analysis. The assumption that man works reluctantly, only under close supervision, and only for wages is no longer considered to be universally valid, as it once was. Ironically, the beginnings of modern theories of human behavior at work may be found in a study done at the Hawthorne Works of Western Electric. The study was initiated as a straightforward work analysis project that ignored the psychologic aspects of work. Significant amounts of variation were found that could be explained only by psychological factors. Today, the work analyst must recognize the possibility, for example, that people working in a system that is "suboptimal" (according to objective work analysis criteria) may be more productive than they would be in an "optimal" system. Part of the work analyst's and the manager's challenge today is to develop systems that best permit workers to satisfy their own needs by satisfying the needs of the organization and to avoid whenever possible methods improvements that degrade the motivational content of a job (2).

Authority for the final acceptance or rejection of a work analyst's recommendations, therefore, must reside in the person responsible for the work itself. In a hospital pharmacy service, this person is the pharmacy director or the professional worker who takes personal responsibility for his work and the work of the technicians he supervises. Consequently, pharmacy managers should be acquainted with at least the major concepts and techniques of work analysis. Occasionally, a methods engineer's recommendations may carry considerable weight because of the engineer's superior knowledge of the field. The pharmacy director may be able to balance such weight more confidently if equipped with the fundamentals presented in this chapter.

EMPHASES IN HOSPITAL PHARMACY WORK ANALYSIS

The principal setting of work analysis traditionally has been industry. Application of work analysis to the hospital pharmacy setting requires a shift of emphasis but not a shift of basic approach. For example, hospital pharmacy equipment tends to be less expensive and less elaborate than in manufacturing industries, so the work analyst's concern with the relationship between men and machines is different in the two settings. An individual worker in a hospital pharmacy may perform a wider variety of tasks and have a wider variety of outputs than an industrial worker, so the hospital pharmacy work analyst may be relatively unconcerned with such traditional topics as detailed standardization of methods, time standards, and productivity incentives. The scale of operations is different, so the expected return per unit of methods improvement expense may be lower in hospital pharmacy than in industry. Finally, the issue of quality of output may be dealt with differently in hospital pharmacy settings than in industrial settings, because hospital pharmacy outputs include many services in addition to goods. Quality is frequently much harder to define and to measure

in hospital pharmacy than in industry, and in-process quality control may have more general importance.

The aspects of work analysis that are of prime importance to hospital pharmacists are discussed in three categories: process analysis, operation analysis, and workplace design.

DEFINITIONS

In this chapter, the term "work analysis" denotes the systematic decomposition, modification, and reorganization of tasks (operation analysis) or relatively small collections of tasks (process analysis) for the purpose of improving the tasks or process according to given criteria. Although no sharp distinction between process analysis and systems analysis can be made, process analysis is more specifically oriented toward the tasks or operations themselves and, in general usage, connotes a relatively more qualitative approach than systems analysis.

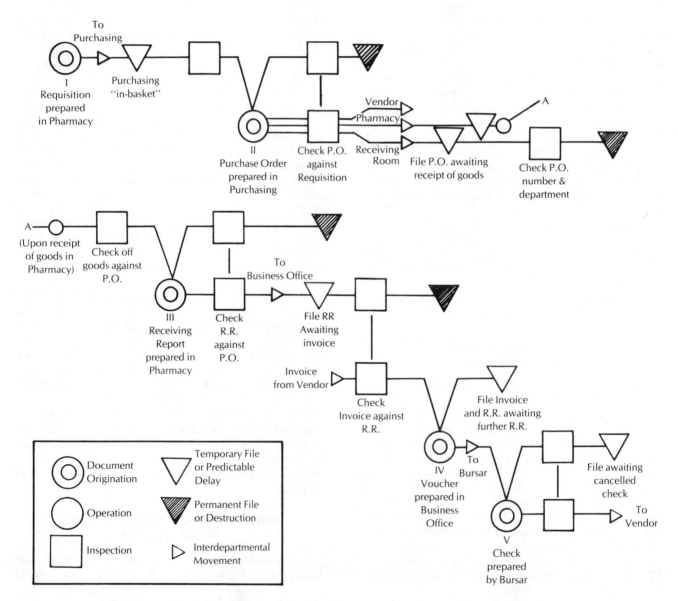

FIGURE 8.1 Process flow diagram—pharmaceutical procurement system in a large university hospital.

"Workplace layout" denotes the arrangement of the immediate area in which a specific task is carried out. "Facility design" denotes the geometric arrangement of workplace modules into systems in a given area.

"Time study" denotes the estimation of time actually spent by a properly trained person, working at a normal pace, doing certain tasks or small collections of tasks, primarily for the purpose of comparing alternative methods or establishing time requirements.

PROCESS ANALYSIS

Process analysis is work analysis applied to groups of tasks; it usually should be performed before detailed analysis of the individual operations. Process analysis techniques can be applied to materials flow (e.g., prescription filling) or to information flow (e.g., procurement) aspects of systems.

Process Charts

A process chart is a type of flow chart used to abstract relevant aspects of a process into graphic form. It is frequently possible to see major improvements in a system merely by observing and flow charting it. Figure 8.1 is an example of a process chart.

Example: Procurement System

The procurement procedure flow charted in Figure 8.1 was used at an Eastern medical center for many years. The procedure had evolved over a number of years. Although it had become inconvenient and consumed inordinate amounts of time, it was accepted by those using it. Merely flow charting this system, so that its essential elements are compactly and graphically displayed, suggests significant improvements. For example, five documents are initiated in the original procedure: the requisition, the purchase order, the receiving report, the voucher, and the check. A few moments spent thinking about the information contained in these documents (Table 8.1) suggests that the purchase order can be made to contain all the information needed for the receiving report and voucher. The voucher need only contain a small fraction of the information on the purchase order (e.g., department, account number, vendor, purchase order number). If departments check in their own merchandise, then the copy of the purchase order for the receiving room need only include purchase order number, vendor, and department. These two documents can be stubs, i.e., partial copies, of the purchase order. Initiation of the requisition from pharmacy to purchasing can also be eliminated for standard items if a "traveling requisition" is used.*

These changes are rather obvious, the products of common sense. The need and possibilities for change, however, were not fully apparent during the many years that the original system was in use. The necessary modifications were not obvious until the system was flow charted.

---

*A traveling requisition is one which contains all the information needed to identify a drug product. The pharmacy need only write in the number of units to be purchased. Purchasing then returns the traveling requisition to pharmacy for reuse.

OPERATION ANALYSIS

Operation analysis is work analysis applied to individual tasks (e.g., prescription filling, prepackaging, patient profile maintenance, drug information storage/retrieval) or to even more elementary operations (e.g., tablet counting, liquid measurement, label printing). The purpose of operation analysis is to eliminate unnecessary steps in the execution of a task and to arrange the necessary steps in the most efficient sequence. Although operation analysis can be applied to any physical task performed by people, it provides the greatest benefit when applied to tasks which are repeated frequently. For example, suppose that operation analysis were performed on the procedure used by a pharmacy technician to load a delivery cart, or on the procedure used by a pharmacy technician in prepackaging liquids into screw-capped bottles. The analyses presumably can reduce the time and effort required to complete either task. If cart loading occurs relatively infrequently, e.g., once each day, while liquid prepackaging occurs much more frequently, e.g., continuously for 4 hours each day, the packaging analysis is likely to produce the larger total time savings. If the costs of performing either analysis are about the same, the prepackaging analysis would obviously be the better choice.

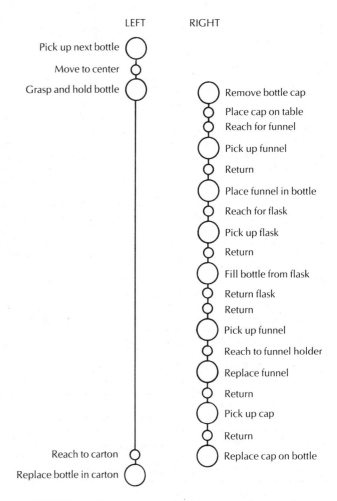

FIGURE 8.2 Operation chart of fluid prepackaging procedure.

TABLE 8.1 Paper Work Simplification Checklist

Form Name				Form No.
Analysis by		Date		
No.	Consider These Principles of Paperwork Simplification	Present Method No	Present Method Yes	Remarks and Suggestions
1	Does the form make someone's job **easier?**			
2	Does the form provide information essential to the running of our business?			
3	Is the form properly designed so it is **easy** to process?			
4	Is the source of information being worked with in the same order as on the form?			
5	Are all items or columns on form being used?			
6	Is the form of standard size which permits easy processing and filing?			
7	Is the form being processed in multiples?			
8	Are the forms being furnished in unit sets with carbons inserted?			
9	Are the forms being furnished in continuous forms?			
10	Does the form contain complete and adequate information?			
11	Are all items on the form clearly understood by all?			
12	Is part of the information preprinted on the form?			
13	Is a rubber stamp(s) being used to add information to the form?			
14	Is a checklist system being utilized?			
15	Is the form being filled out by machine?			
16	Are all the copies *really* needed to accomplish the purpose?			
17	Does the form flow smoothly through the house without backtracking?			
18	Are the principles of motion economy being adhered to at all stations?			
19	Are all signatures necessary and made by the lowest classification echelon?			
20	Is there a punched card with this information on it?			
21	Is the information microfilmed?			
22	Is the form presorted before filling?			
23	Is it necessary to file the forms in all cases? WHY?			
24	Will the information be referred to frequently after filing?			
25	Is this the only place where the information is filed?			
26	Are the files located near the people who use them?			
27	Is noncurrent information removed from active files periodically?			

Methods and Principles

Flow charting is as useful in operation analysis as it is in process analysis, but a different type of flow chart may be used. An "operation chart" is a flow chart that shows the movements of the two hands simultaneously. Figure 8.2 is an operation chart of a procedure used to prepackage liquids into screw-capped bottles using a flask and a funnel. It shows how the two hands are used in the procedure, and it is complete except that refilling the flask is not shown. This chart greatly facilitates analysis of the procedure.

Guidelines for Operational Analysis and Design

Operations analysts have developed a number of guidelines that are useful for the analysis and design of tasks much as that depicted in Figure 8.2. Barnes (3) offers a rather complete list of such guidelines, which are summarized in Table 8.2. As Barnes points out, not all of his "principles" are applicable to every operation, but they do provide a useful checklist to prompt consideration of whichever principles may be applicable to a given operation.

Example: Liquid Prepackaging

A review of Table 8.2 suggests a number of improvements that can be made in the liquid prepackaging operation. First, principles 1-3 and 18 call attention to the use of the left hand: it is idle throughout most of the operation, since it is used to support the bottle. This suggests the use of some mechanical means of supporting the bottle so that the left hand is freed for more useful effort. According to the principles, this will reduce the time required to perform the operation not only because both hands are available, but also because speed can be improved (or fatigue reduced) by introducing more symmetry of motion. The bottles could be left in the original carton, which would hold them in position and save the time required to remove and replace them. If this were not practical, the bottles could be slid against a rail. Principle 4 suggests that simpler and coarser motions are preferred to complex and finer motions. Positioning of the bottle, funnel, and flask requires fairly fine and complex motions which it would be desirable to simplify. Principles 19 and 20 suggest that the "tools," i.e., funnel and flask, should be prepositioned and combined whenever possible. If we preposition the funnel and flask, we have improved our compliance with principle 4 as well as principles 19 and 20. The idea of combining the flask and funnel suggests a number of approaches, e.g., an Erlenmeyer flask with a small orifice such as an old-fashioned schoolroom ink bottle.

Since we want to position our combination flask/funnel permanently, we might think of a large separatory funnel with a stopcock. These are expensive and easily broken, and we might finally decide to have one made out of stainless steel with an automatic closure (Fig. 8.3).

TABLE 8.2   Principles of Motion Economy[a]

A Check Sheet for Motion Economy and Fatigue Reduction		
These 22 rules or principles of motion economy may be profitably applied to shop and office work alike. Although not all are applicable to every operation, they do form a basis or a code for improving the efficiency and reducing fatigue in manual work.		
Use of the Human Body	*Arrangement of the Workplace*	*Design of Tools and Equipment*
1. The two hands should begin as well as complete their motions at the same time.	10. There should be a definite and fixed place for all tools and materials.	18. The hands should be relieved of all work that can be done more advantageously by a jig, a fixture, or a foot-operated device.
2. The two hands should not be idle at the same time except during rest periods.	11. Tools, materials, and controls should be located close to the point of use.	19. Two or more tools should be combined wherever possible.
3. Motions of the arms should be made in opposite and symmetric directions and should be made simultaneously.	12. Gravity feed bins and containers should be used to deliver material close to the point of use.	20. Tools and materials should be prepositioned whenever possible.
4. Hand and body motions should be confined to the lowest classification with which it is possible to perform the work satisfactorily.	13. Drop deliveries should be used wherever possible.	21. Where each finger performs some specific movement, such as in typewriting, the load should be distributed in accordance with the inherent capacities of the fingers.
5. Momentum should be employed to assist the worker wherever possible, and it should be reduced to a minumum if it must be overcome by muscular effort.	14. Materials and tools should be located to permit the best sequence of motions.	22. Levers and wheels should be located in such positions that the operator can manipulate them with the least change in body position and with the greatest mechanical advantage.
6. Smooth continuous curved motions of the hands are preferable to straight-line motions involving sudden and sharp changes in direction.	15. Provisions should be made for adequate conditions for seeing. Good illumination is the first requirement for satisfactory visual perception.	
7. Ballistic movements are faster, easier, and more accurate than restricted (fixation) or "controlled" movements.	16. The height of the workplace and the chair should preferably be arranged so that alternate sitting and standing at work are easily possible.	
8. Work should be arranged to permit easy and natural rhythm wherever possible.	17. A chair of the type and height to permit good posture should be provided for every worker.	
9. Eye fixations should be as few and as close together as possible.		

[a]Reprinted by permission from Barnes RM: *Motion and Time Study: Design and Measurement of Work.* Copyright © 1968, John Wiley & Sons.

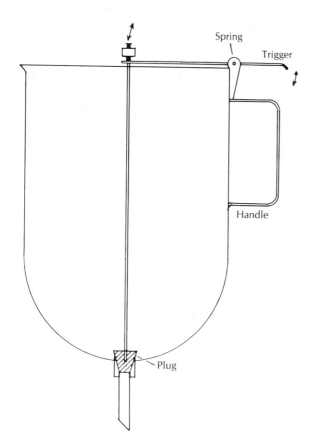

FIGURE 8.3 Stainless steel liquid filling can.

We can now arrange a holder which will position the filler can and leave enough room for the carton of bottles to slide underneath it. Figure 8.4 shows the operation chart for the modified procedure. We have drastically reduced the number of movements in the bottle-filling procedure and have introduced more symmetry of hand motion. Operation analysis can simplify procedures considerably with a minimum of capital investment. The modified procedure is not presented as optimal. Further modification or a different procedure may be needed because of various actual circumstances.

Our analysis has not yet considered the arrangement of the operator. Principles 15-17 move the focus of our concern

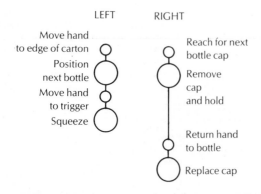

FIGURE 8.4 Revised liquid prepackaging operation chart.

from the *procedure* used to perform a task to the *environment* in which the task is performed, i.e., workplace design.

WORKPLACE DESIGN

Workplace design, or workplace layout, is concerned with the physical environment within which a specific task is performed. Obviously, the physical arrangement of the workplace may be as important as the procedures used, since either set of factors can be rate limiting. As suggested by the sequence of this chapter, process analysis ordinarily precedes operation analysis, which ordinarily precedes workplace design. The full benefit of the first two analyses may not be manifested in improved productivity unless the work area is designed appropriately.

Workplace design logically begins with recognition of the geometry and mechanics of human movement and the adaptation of the workplace to a human. Since building materials and buildings are based on the rectangle, the notion of work areas based on the circle does not seem very congenial at first. The natural boundaries for human movement, however, are circular, e.g., the small arc described by the hand rotating around a stationary wrist, the arc described by the forearm rotating around a stationary elbow, the larger arc described by the extended arm rotating around the shoulder, the still larger arc described by the extended arm and trunk rotating around the waist (Figs. 8.5 and 8.6). Each of the larger circles requires more effort. A work area based on rectangles does not fit the human body very efficiently: each rectangular plane must include areas which are harder to reach than other areas. It is not mandatory, of course, that equipment such as worktables be circular in their outside dimensions, but it is necessary that the work area be so constructed. A somewhat greater problem may be expected in obtaining a three-dimensional circular arrangement, e.g., for cabinets and shelves, because a horizontal shelf protruding into easily reached space would be a barrier. In some applications this challenge can be met with gravity feed bins. Construction of pharmacy equipment such as that described here may (or may not) be within the capability of a hospital cabinet shop, but is commercially available (Fig. 8.7) (4).

In operations that require the worker to remain in one place for a long time, special attention should be given to posture and positional fatigue. A workbench of suitable height for standing workers (36-40 inches) and a chair of adjustable height (26-35 inches) which permits the operator to remain at the same height while seated or standing can be quite important in reducing monotony and fatigue. The chair should be designed with a proper backrest to encourage proper posture (5,6). Illumination should be provided at the appropriate levels (70-100 footcandles, more for visually demanding work) and positioned so that direct or reflected light does not glare into the operator's eyes (7,8). Proper noise, humidity, and temperature control is also important in delaying operator fatigue (9,10).

FACILITY DESIGN

In this chapter the term "facility design" is used to denote the planned arrangement of the functional modules devel-

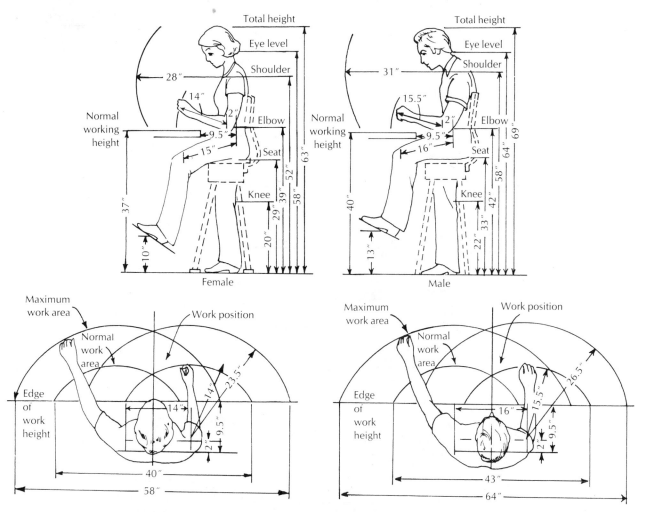

FIGURE 8.5 Dimensions of normal and maximum working areas in the horizontal and vertical planes as developed and used by the Process Development Section of the General Motors manufacturing staff. (Reprinted by permission from Farley RR: Some principles of methods and motion study as used in development work. *General Motors Engineering J* 2(6):20-25.)

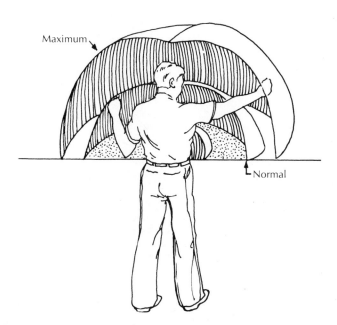

FIGURE 8.6 Normal and maximum dimensions of working space. (Reprinted by permission from Barnes RM: *Motion and Time Study: Design and Measurement of Work,* New York, John Wiley & Sons, 1968.)

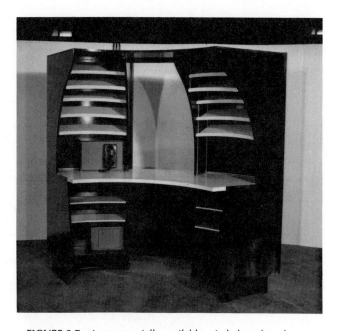

FIGURE 8.7 A commercially available, circle-based work area.

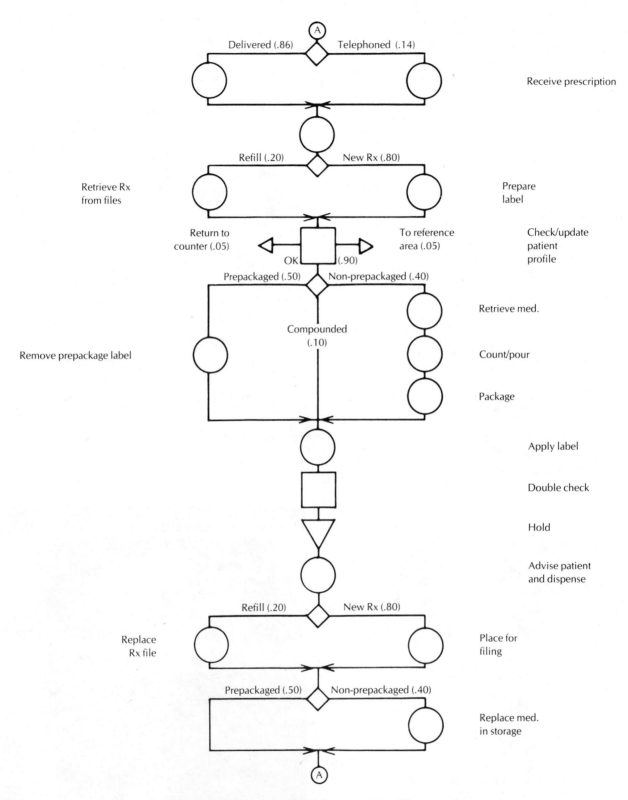

FIGURE 8.8 Flow chart of outpatient prescription-filling procedure.

TABLE 8.3 Relative Frequency Data for Outpatient Prescription-Filling Operation

New		0.80
Presented by patient	0.76	
Telephoned	0.04	
Refill		0.20
Presented by patient	0.10	
Telephoned	0.10	
Noncompounded		0.90
Prepackaged	0.50	
Nonprepackaged	0.40	
Compounded (nonprepackaged)		0.10
Acceptable as received or after clarification		0.95
Require pharm. reference		0.05

oped through operation analysis and workplace design. For example, the bottle-filling procedure may be viewed as one discrete functional module in a larger liquid prepackaging process. The actual packaging of a prescription may be considered as a module of the larger prescription-filling process which begins with receipt or retrieval of the prescription order and ends with advising the patient. Facility design is concerned with the physical organization of the modules comprising an overall system.

Like other aspects of work analysis, facility design employs a flow chart which depicts the system. Figure 8.8 is an example of such a flow chart. In this application, the relative frequencies of each module are the characteristics of primary interest (Table 8.3).

Unlike other aspects of work analysis, the objective of facility design can be expressed in a concise mathematical statement. We wish to minimize the sum of the products of each distance and each frequency of travel:

$$E = \sum_{ij} D_{ij}F_{ij} \qquad (1)$$

where D_{ij} is the distance and F_{ij} is the frequency of travel between points i and j. To facilitate the use of equation 1, a traffic summary table, which shows frequency of trips between locations, can be constructed. The frequencies are constant for a given system, while distances vary with a particular design. Table 8.4 is a traffic summary for the outpatient dispensing system flow charted in Figure 8.8.

(The numbers in parentheses are the proportions of prescriptions represented by each alternative, as shown in Table 8.3.) If the system is in operation, the traffic summary table should be constructed from direct observation. Otherwise, the traffic summary must be constructed from direct observation and simulation, or from simulation alone. The construction of the traffic summary itself usually provides considerable insight into the layout problem. Table 8.4 shows that the prescription bench is the center of activity in this system: the four most frequent trips involve this location. Chief among these are trips to or from the prescription bench and service counter (93) and profiles (90). Sometimes a "proximity diagram" or "string diagram" is drawn at this point to graphically represent an initial design (11,12). In this example, however, we assume that the system is already operating in a room measuring 40 × 50 feet, designed according to Figure 8.9A. Table 8.5A gives the traffic summary, distances, and products ($P_{ij} = F_{ij}D_{ij}$) for the existing design. The value of E has dimensions of feet per 100 prescriptions, and represents an estimate of the average distance that would be traveled in filling 100 prescriptions with the given assumptions, system, and design. There are four outstandingly large P_{ij} values in Table 8.5A, suggesting that any major improvements probably must be made by reducing the distances between the prescription benches and the patient profiles, service counter, drug storage area, and incoming prescription stack. Figure 8.9B shows the first alternative design, and Table 8.5B summarizes this design. E has dropped to 7662 feet, a substantial improvement. The largest distance-frequency product now involves the prescription bench–drug storage area distance. The third design (Figure 8.9C, Table 8.5C) was made to reduce this distance without increasing the other important distances. It shows minor improvement (499 feet per 100 prescriptions) over the second alternative.

This method, unfortunately, does not provide any indication of best layout, but merely allows alternatives to be compared. There may be other designs that would give even lower E values. The relatively small improvement achieved in the third design, however, suggests that this particular line of redesign is reaching its limit, and we may be willing to accept the third design as final. We have reduced the distance per 100 prescriptions by about 28% under the original design and probably have increased the speed of the system and reduced the amount of effort required.

TABLE 8.4 Traffic Summary, Outpatient Dispensing System (Trips per 100 Prescriptions)[a]

Locations	Incoming Stack	Prescription Bench	Prescription Files	Compounding Area	Reference Area	Drug Storage	Profiles
Service counter	43	93[b]	0	0	0	0	5
Incoming stack		64[b]	10	0	0	0	40
Prescription bench			10	20	0	80[b]	90[b]
Prescription files				0	0	0	10
Compounding area					5	5	0
Reference area						0	5
Drug storage							0
Profiles							

[a]Assumptions: Mean number of prescriptions per patient = 2; telephones are located at counter, profile area, and compounding area.
[b]The most frequently occurring trips.

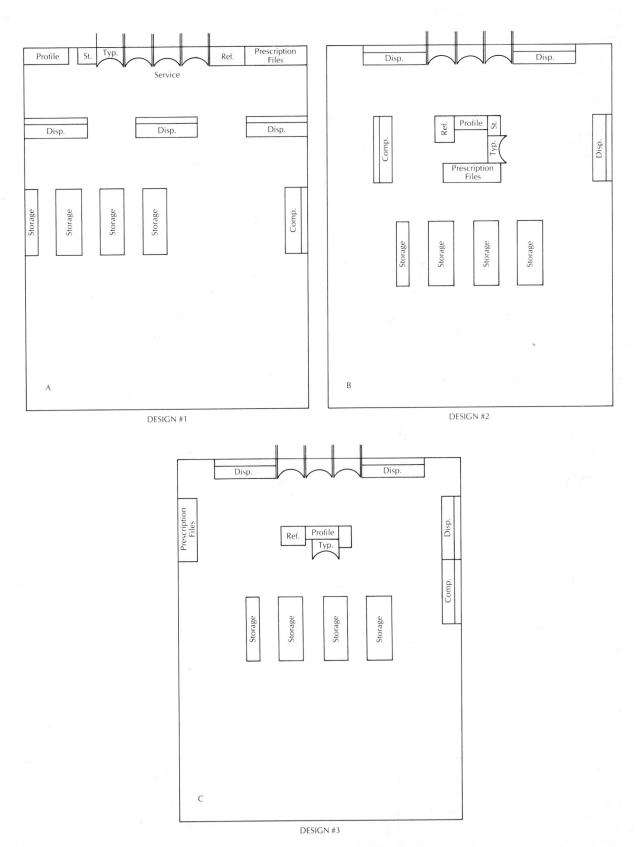

FIGURE 8.9 Three alternative facility layouts for the outpatient prescription-filling procedure. *A,* Design 1. *B,* Design 2. *C,* Design 3.

TABLE 8.5A   Traffic-Distance Summary for Outpatient Prescription Facility, Design 1

		Incoming Stack	Prescription Bench	Prescription Files	Compounding Area	Reference Area	Drug Storage	Patient Profiles
Service counter	F	43	93	0	0	0	0	5
	D	12	20.5	—	—	—	—	17
	P	516	1906.5	—	—	—	—	85
Incoming stack	F		64	10	0	0	0	40
	D		22.3	26	—	—	—	6
	P		1427.2	260	—	—	—	240
Prescription bench	F			10	20	0	80	90
	D			24.5	22.3	—	20	27.1
	P			245	446	—	1600	2439
Prescription files	F				0	0	0	10
	D				—	—	—	32
	P				—	—	—	320
Compounding area	F					5	5	0
						23	33	—
	F					115	165	—
Reference area	F						0	5
	D						—	25
	P						—	125
Drug storage	F							0
	D							—
	P							—

E = 9889.7.

TABLE 8.5B   Traffic-Distance Summary for Outpatient Prescription Facility, Design 2

		Incoming Stack	Prescription Bench	Prescription Files	Compounding Area	Reference Area	Drug Storage	Patient Profiles
Service counter	F	43	93	0	0	0	0	5
	D	7.5	14	—	—	—	—	6
	P	322.5	1302	—	—	—	—	30
Incoming stack	F		64	10	0	0	0	40
	D		12.5	23	—	—	—	5
	P		800	230	—	0	—	200
Prescription bench	F			10	20	0	80	90
	D			27	24.5	—	27.3	14.7
	P			270	490	—	2184	1323
Prescription files	F				0	0	0	10
	D				—	—	—	28
	P				—	—	—	280
Compounding area	F					5	5	0
	D					7	22	—
	F					35	110	—
Reference area	F						0	5
	D						—	17
	P						—	17
Drug storage	F							0
	D							—
	P							—

E = 7661.5; ΔE = 2228.2.

TIME STUDY

Time study is complementary to work analysis. Work analysis primarily involves design of procedures, while time study primarily involves measurement. Although the term "time study" usually invokes an image of a stopwatch on a clipboard, there are two basic approaches to the estimation of time requirements for certain tasks. Direct time study is the straightforward timing of specified activities. Work sampling is an indirect method of estimating time requirements that does not involve actual timing of individual activities. Work sampling is widely used in hospital pharmacy.

Time study has a number of purposes in industry that are seldom important in hosptial pharmacy applications and that will not be considered here. They are estimating labor costs before pricing a product or submitting bids, determining time standards for piecework incentive payments, and evaluating productivity of individual workers. The purposes of time study in common between hospital pharmacy appli-

TABLE 8.5C　Traffic-Distance Summary for Outpatient Prescription Facility, Design 3

		Incoming Stack	Prescription Bench	Prescription Files	Compounding Area	Reference Area	Drug Storage	Patient Profiles
Service counter	F	43	93	0	0	0	0	5
	D	8	13.3	—	—	—	—	6.5
	P	344	1236.9	—	—	—	—	32.5
Incoming stack	F		64	10	0	0	0	40
	D		11.3	22	—	—	—	5
	P		723.2	220	—	—	—	200
Prescription bench	F			10	20	0	80	90
	D			23.3	21.7	—	24.7	13.7
	P			233	434	—	1976	1233
Prescription files	F				0	0	0	10
	D				—	—	—	19
	P				—	—	—	190
Compounding area	F					5	5	0
	D					35	28	—
	P					175	140	—
Reference area	F						0	5
	D						—	5
	P						—	25
Drug storage	F							0
	D							—
	P							—

$E = 7163$; $\Delta E = 499$.

cations and industrial applications include comparing of alternative procedures or systems and estimating labor requirements for budgeting purposes. For example, the revised liquid prepackaging procedure described above could be evaluated in part by comparing its time requirement to the existing procedure's requirement. The times required for all prepackaging operations can be used to estimate budgetary labor requirements for prepackaging.

Direct Time Study

The equipment required for most direct time studies in hospital pharmacy is as simple as a stopwatch and clipboard. Usually, the stopwatch is calibrated in decimal minutes (or decimal hours) rather than in seconds. A preprinted form is mandatory for systematic recording of observed times.

Standardization

More important, but less obvious, prerequisites for direct time study are standardization of the procedure and specification of the procedure's component elements with unequivocal starting and ending points. Precise results are unlikely if an entire procedure is timed, especially if exact starting and ending points are left to the observer. Usually, the elements should be logical parts of the sequence (e.g., "positions bottle"), should be as short as can be accurately timed, and should have physically observable starting and ending points, e.g., "operator touches bottle" and "operator releases bottle." Active elements, e.g., "applies label," should be separated from passive elements such as waiting. The resulting elemental times can be added to estimate process times for the existing procedure or various modifications of the procedure. Furthermore, if a well-standardized procedure is decomposed into well-standardized elements, the observer can repeatedly time a given element,

using the time occupied by the other elements to read the stopwatch and record the time. This is likely to be more accurate and precise, especially for nonexpert observers, than attempting to read the watch and record the time while simultaneously timing the next element.

Poorly standardized procedures are frequently found in hospital pharmacy systems. Such procedures are seldom acceptable in industrial settings and may offend industrially oriented work analysts; nevertheless, suitability for direct time study is not a major criterion for the acceptability of a procedure. Deciding to standardize a procedure only to make it easier to time is putting the cart before the horse.

Some poorly standardized procedures may benefit from standardization, and increased suitability for direct timing is a nice fringe benefit. Other procedures may benefit little or may even suffer from standardization. Deciding whether to standardize a procedure is the responsibility of management, as discussed earlier. The average time required for a poorly standardized procedure can be estimated with work sampling or by timing the entire procedure if the relatively low precision can be tolerated.

When two or more observers are used in direct time study, their agreement with each other (or with the analyst in charge of the study) should be checked by comparing each observer's simultaneous timings of the same operations. Since some variability is to be expected, an appropriate statistical test, e.g., analysis of variance, is frequently employed.

Statistical Aspects of Direct Time Study

Three parameters are usually of interest in direct time study: the mean element time τ, the standard deviation of element times σ_t, and the standard error of the mean element σ_τ. These are estimated with equations 2-4.

$$\tau \simeq \bar{t} = \frac{1}{N} \sum_{i=1}^{N} t_i \qquad (2)$$

$$\tilde{\sigma}_t = \sqrt{\frac{N}{N-1} \frac{\Sigma t_i^2}{N} - \bar{t}^2} \qquad (3)$$

$$\tilde{\sigma}_\tau = \tilde{\sigma}_t / \sqrt{N} \qquad (4)$$

where the t_is are the individual time observations.

When N is large, $(N/N - 1)$ in equation 3 is approximately equal to 1 and can be ignored. Estimation of σ_t can be greatly simplified by the use of tables that relate range, sample size, and standard deviation for normally distributed variables (13,14).

The standard error statistic σ_τ is related to the amount of variability in $\bar{t}$ values between sets of N observations. If N is moderately large, the mean values $\bar{t}$ are well approximated by a normal (Gaussian) distribution, and one can predict the probable precision of time estimates. For example, suppose that 30 observations of some element yield a mean time $\bar{t}_1 = 5.25$ minutes and $\sigma_t = 2.00$ minutes. $\tilde{\sigma}_\tau$ therefore equals $2/\sqrt{30} = 0.365$.

Recognizing that the 30 observations are merely a sample from a vary large universe of times for that element, one may wonder how close one's estimate may be to the true mean τ of the universe of times, i.e., how *precise* the estimate is. It is customary in time study to express precision of observation in terms of relative error. The relative error of a time estimate may be conveniently defined as

$$\epsilon = \pm \frac{(\bar{t} - \tau)}{\bar{t}} \qquad (5)$$

For example, if the true mean $\tau = 5.55$ minutes, relative error $\epsilon = \pm(5.25\text{-}5.55)/5.25 = 0.054$, or 5.4% relative error. Of course, we do not know the value of τ and are trying to estimate it with $\bar{t}$.

Statistically speaking, we can never be absolutely certain of the precision of any observation and must specify a minimum acceptable degree of certainty. For example, we can specify that we want to be 90% certain that our estimate $\bar{t}$ is no more than $100\epsilon\%$ in error. Since we have 30 observations, we can use normal sampling theory to evaluate the precision of our example. It can be shown that the upper bound ϵ_b of relative error ϵ is related to our mean $\bar{t}$ and standard error $\tilde{\sigma}_t$ by

$$\epsilon_b = \frac{Z\tilde{\sigma}_t}{\bar{t}} \qquad (6)$$

where Z is obtained from Table 8.6 for the desired confidence level.

$$\epsilon_b = (1.65)0.365/5.25$$
$$= 0.115$$

This result says that we are 90% confident that the true mean τ is within 11.5% of the observed mean $\bar{t}$. For most work, this relative error is somewhat high: ordinarily 5-10% relative error is desired. There are two possible ways to reduce the relative error. First, we should be satisfied that random measurement error is as small as possible, i.e., that there is little variation being introduced by the manner in which the timing is done. This reinforces the importance of unequivocal starting and stopping points for the element being

TABLE 8.6 Z Values Corresponding to Various Confidence Levels, Assuming a Normal Distribution of Random Measurement Error

Confidence Level	Z
0.80	1.28
0.85	1.44
0.90	1.65
0.95	1.96
0.99	2.58

timed. In addition, we should check for distractions present during timing that prevent the observer from correctly reading and recording times. Second, we should determine whether the element being timed as well standardized. If it is not, we must either decide to standardize it or to accept the low precision. If we accept the times as they are, the only way to improve the precision of our estimate of τ is to increase sample size. Combining equations 4 and 6, we get

$$\epsilon_b = \frac{Z\tilde{\sigma}_t}{\bar{t}\sqrt{N}} \qquad (7)$$

and, rearranging,

$$\sqrt{N} = \frac{Z\tilde{\sigma}_t}{\epsilon_{b_i}} \qquad (8)$$

If we desire a relative error of 5%, we can calculate the necessary sample size for our example.

$$\sqrt{N} = \frac{1.65 \cdot 2.00}{0.05 \cdot 5.25} = 12.57$$

$$N \simeq 158$$

We conclude that unless we can standardize the element or improve the timing procedure (reduce $\tilde{\sigma}_t$), we will require about 160 observations to estimate τ within 5% relative precision at 90% confidence.

Work Sampling

Work sampling permits the estimation, without direct time study, of the proportion of a worker's time spent in various activities. While direct time study is more continuous and short term, work sampling is more intermittent and long term.

Work sampling rests upon the idea that a random sample tends to have the same "composition" as the universe from which it is drawn. Therefore, a series of instantaneous qualitative observations at random times tends to have the same proportion of observations in each class as the entire segment. For example, suppose that a nurse is engaged in medication-related activity for some proportion ϕ of the time she is working. For example, she spends an average of 2 hours on medication-related activity in each 8-hour shift, so $\phi = 2/8 = 0.25$. Now suppose that we observe this nurse's activity at random times, making N observations, of which n_1 observations find her engaged in medication-related activities. Obviously, the proportion $p = n_1/N$ will depend on ϕ. As the total number of observations is increased, p will get closer and closer to ϕ. To put it another way, p is the sample probability that an observation will find the nurse engaged in medication-related activity and is directly related to the true proportion of time she spends in such activity. To estimate the time T, in hours spent in medication-related activity, we need only multiply the total length of the time period observed by p. To estimate the average time required for some unit of activity, we can divide T by the number of units.

Advantages and Disadvantages of Work Sampling

Work sampling is most applicable in the study of multiple operators, when the events of interest are not closely clustered in time, or when direct time study is likely to interfere with the operations being observed. For example, the time spent in medication-related activity by a large number of nurses is easier to estimate by work sampling all nurses during the same period than by direct time study of individuals. If it is difficult or impossible to predict just when the medication-related activity will occur, direct time study is inefficient because the observer must wait for such activity during prolonged periods when it is not occurring. Many people are made to feel uncomfortable by prolonged periods of continuous observation, but work sampling involves only intermittent "instantaneous" observation. In some instances, workers who are being directly timed may alter their behavior for the relatively short duration of timing. In work sampling, the period of intermittent observation is usually prolonged, making representative behavior more likely and decreasing the likelihood of bias from other transient causes. Work sampling often requires less training for observers and is less fatiguing for them.

Work sampling is usually not advantageous for studying single operators or when the operators are widely scattered. Direct time study usually is better for estimating relatively short times and for obtaining detailed time breakdowns. Work sampling is usually not advantageous if the observer cannot easily classify the activity observed. Although in some instances the operator can be asked to state what he is doing or to classify his work for the observer, this is likely to interfere with the normal work, so that the observations become artificial to an unknown extent. The observer's ability to classify activities accurately and rapidly is an extremely important consideration in work sampling studies.

Statistical Aspect of Work Sampling

Most work sampling applications are based on the binomial probability distribution

$$P[n_j] = \frac{N!}{n_j!(N - n_j)!}\phi_j^{n_j}(1 - \phi_j)^{N - n_j} \qquad (9)$$

where n_j denotes the number of times that some activity (activity j) was observed in a total of N independent observations and ϕ_j denotes the "true" fraction of a very large number of observations in which activity j would be observed; ϕ_j is estimated by p_j:

$$\phi_j \simeq p_j = \frac{n_j}{N} \qquad (10)$$

The standard deviation of ϕ, σ_ϕ, is estimated by σ_p:

$$\sigma_\phi \simeq \sigma_p = \sqrt{\frac{p(1 - p)}{N}} \qquad (11)$$

For example, if a nurse is observed in medication-related activities 25 times in 500 observations,

$$\phi \simeq 25/500 = 0.0500$$

$$\sigma_\phi \simeq \sqrt{\frac{(0.05)(0.95)}{500}} = 0.00975$$

As with direct time study data, we must recognize that our observations are from a *sample*, and that another sample might yield a different estimate of ϕ. As before, we need to specify a desired level of precision for estimating ϕ and an acceptable level of confidence. The situation is different with work sampling than with direct time study in three ways. First, the standard deviation of the mean σ_ϕ depends both on sample size N and the value of the mean ϕ, whereas in our earlier example, $\tilde{\sigma}_\tau$ did not depend on τ. Second, relative error may have different implications, since p and ϕ are always less than 1. For example, suppose that $\phi = 0.004$ and $p = 0.010$. The absolute error of our estimate of ϕ is only 0.006, but the relative error is 60%. Finally, the binomial distribution is approximated well by the normal distribution only when p is close to 0.5 and N is large.†

We can, as with direct time study, define relative error ϵ as

$$\epsilon = \pm \frac{\phi - p}{p} \qquad (12)$$

If we can assume that the normal distribution provides a reasonable approximation to the distribution of ϕ, then the maximum relative error in estimating ϕ is given by

$$\epsilon_b = \frac{Z\sigma_p}{p} \qquad (13)$$

where Z is as defined earlier (Table 8.6). In our example, at the 95% confidence level,

$$\epsilon_b = \frac{(1.96)(0.00975)}{0.05}$$
$$= 0.382$$

We are 95% sure that our random error in estimating ϕ is 38.2% or less.

To estimate the number of observations required for a desired relative error, we can substitute equation 11 into equation 13 and rearrange it as follows:

$$\epsilon_b = \frac{Z\sqrt{\dfrac{p(1 - p)}{N}}}{p}$$

---

†As a rule of thumb, if either pN or $(1 - p)$N is greater than 5, we can approximate the binomial with the normal distribution (15).

$$\sqrt{N} = \frac{Z \sqrt{p(1-p)}}{\epsilon_b \cdot p} \quad (14)$$

In our example, the number of observations required to obtain maximum relative error of 5% at the 95% confidence level is

$$\sqrt{N} = \frac{(1.96)(0.218)}{(0.05)(0.05)} = 170.9$$
$$= 29,196$$

This example emphasizes an important aspect of work sampling. The P value is always less than 1, and as examination of equation 11 shows, small P values are associated with large N values for a given relative error, frequently to the dismay of the persons conducting the study. Compare this result to the number of observations required for an activity for which $P = 0.20$:

$$\sqrt{N} = \frac{(1.96)(0.4)}{(0.05)(0.2)} = 78.4$$
$$N = 6,147$$

Because of the large number of observations that may be required to estimate small ϕ values within desired relative error, careful consideration should be given to the amount of detail needed in a work sampling study. If various activities can be combined, the ϕ value of the grouped activity will be larger. Second, the uses intended for the results should also be considered. There is nothing magical about a relative error below 5-10%, and some applications may permit less precise measurement. Finally, in some cases, relative error is not really appropriate, and absolute error can be used instead. For example, we may be satisfied with a statement like, "Nurses spent from 4-6% of their time in medication-related activities." Absolute error E may be conveniently defined as

$$E = \phi - p \quad (15)$$

Using this definition, equation 13 becomes

$$E_b = Z\sigma_p \quad (16)$$

and equation 14 becomes

$$\sqrt{N} = \frac{Z \sqrt{p(1-p)}}{E_b} \quad (17)$$

To demonstrate the difference in sample size between a relative error criterion of $\pm 5\%$ and an absolute error criterion of ± 0.01, the sample size required for the latter criterion is calculated (compare to $N = 29,196$).

$$\sqrt{N} = \frac{(1.96)(0.218)}{0.01} = 42.7$$
$$N = 1826$$

Unfortunately, if we will be interested in relative precision of the values finally calculated, we should confine ourselves to relative precision criteria for ϕ. For example, suppose the purpose of the work sampling is to estimate the total time per day spent by nurses in medication-related activities

and that there are 480 man-hours of nursing per day in the wards of interest. We calculate

$$t_{mra} = (0.05)(480) = 24 \text{ hours/day}$$

If 29,000 observations were made, so that $\epsilon_b = 0.05$, then we are 95% confident that the true value of t_{mra} is 24 hours/day $\pm$ 5% (22.8-25.2 hours/day). If 1826 observations were made, so that $E_b = 0.01$, then we are 95% confident that t_{mra} is 24 hours/day $\pm$ 4.8 hours. Two final comments on statistical aspects are pertinent. First, tables and "alignment charts" are available (16) that can save the trouble of calculating equations 13 and 14 or 16 and 17. Second, if small sample sizes or small ϕ values are involved, alternative methods should be used for estimating the confidence interval for ϕ (17-19).

Temporal Variation and Validity

The primary criterion in evaluating a work sampling study is the validity (i.e., accuracy or representativeness) of the sample. A sample can be invalid for a particular purpose from two principal causes: if it includes too many atypical observations and if the sampling scheme itself were biased.

The operations observed may themselves be atypical for a number of reasons, e.g., operators working in an unfamiliar procedure, especially high or low workload volume, unusually complicated work being done, and poorly trained observer. In work sampling, many such atypical operations can be detected by watching the change in p_j with time. Of course, as a sample statistic, ρ_j will vary randomly around the true ϕ_j value. A method is needed for deciding whether a transient, large change is ρ_j is due to random sampling error or to an actual change in ϕ_j. An example will serve to illustrate such a method. Suppose that medication-related activity is being observed in a group of nurses and that the P values in Table 8.7 are obtained from 11 days of observation. Our best estimate of ϕ is

$$\phi \simeq p = \frac{\sum_{i=1}^{11} n_i}{\sum_{i=1}^{11} N_i}$$

TABLE 8.7 Work Sampling Results for Medication-Related Activity

i	Date	n_j	N_i	P_u	σ_p
1	10/20	6	120	0.050	0.020
2	10/21	7	119	0.059	0.022
3	10/22	7	120	0.058	0.021
4	10/23	6	120	0.050	0.020
5	10/24	6	121	0.050	0.020
6	10/25	3	120	0.025	0.014
7	10/26	6	120	0.050	0.020
8	10/27	7	121	0.058	0.021
9	10/28	7	120	0.058	0.021
10	10/29	7	120	0.058	0.021
11	10/30	7	110	0.058	0.021
Totals		67	1321		

$\phi \simeq p = 67/1321 = 0.051$.

$$= \frac{67}{1321}$$

$$= 0.051$$

We are interested in the result for day No. 6. The P value for that day, 0.25, is much smaller than the P values for the other days, and a decision should be made either to accept the result as a normal sampling error or to investigate its validity. A rational and commonly employed decision rule is to accept the result if the probability that it could arise due to sampling error alone is greater than 1% (or 5%) and to investigate further (or reject it) otherwise.

The most exact way to determine the probability of three observations out of 120 when $\phi = 0.051$ is to use equation 9.‡

$$P\,(3) = \frac{120!}{3!(117)!}\,(0.051)^3(0.949)^{117}$$

$$= \frac{(210)(119)(118)}{6}\,(0.051)^3(0.949)^{117}$$

$$= 0.0815$$

We find that there is an 8.15% chance of getting 3 out of 120 observations when $\phi = 0.051$, so our "odd" observation is probably due to sampling error and should be retained unless other evidence can establish that it is atypical.

Alternatively, 95-99% confidence intervals for ϕ are available in tables (20,21). The 99% confidence interval for $\phi = 0.500$ is 0.00116-0.1243. Since this includes 0.025, we draw the same conclusion as before. When N is large and P is fairly close to 0.50, a normal distribution approximation may be used (22,23).

More than one sample p value may be evaluated with respect to the confidence interval. A 95% confidence interval implies that, on the average, five of each 100 observations will lie outside the interval limits even if they actually came from the same population as the others, so all outliers cannot automatically be rejected. It is helpful to plot each p value on a control chart in which the date or cardinal number of the observation is on the abscissa and the p values are on the ordinate. The appropriate confidence limits can also be drawn on the chart. This greatly facilitates detection of cyclic or other time-related changes in p values. For example, if work sampling is begun too soon after the institution of a new procedure, before the operators have become familiar with it, we may find that daily p values tend to decline with time while the new procedure is being learned, and then level off. This violates the requirement of the binomial distribution that ϕ be a constant value, invalidates our estimates of precision, and biases our estimate of ϕ. It can, of course, result in rejection of a new procedure that would have been accepted if measurement had been done after ϕ had stabilized.

Sampling Schemes

The second major source of invalidity in work sampling is the appropriateness of the sampling scheme itself. There are two major issues involved in choice of sampling scheme: random vs systematic sampling and stratified vs homogeneous sampling.

Randomness is an elusive and troublesome concept. For this purpose a random sample is one in which the probability of selecting any instant of time to make an observation is equal to the probability of choosing any other instant. The purpose of random sampling is to increase the likelihood that the sample will be representative of the entire time period from which the sample is drawn. "Random" does *not* mean "accidental." To achieve randomness, a formal randomization procedure must be followed. Use of a random numbers table (24,25) is usually most convenient. A random numbers table is a list of digits, each of which has an equal probability of being found. For example, each 1 million random digits would contain very close to 100,000 zeros, 100,000 ones, 100,000 twos, etc. If two digits were drawn at a time, there would be very nearly 10,000 of each combination, "00" through "99." To set up a random sampling scheme, we must first choose the minimum acceptable sampling interval a and the desired mean sampling interval m. For example, suppose we wish to sample, on the average, 10 times an hour, but not less than 1 minute from the preceding observation. Then $m = \frac{60}{10} = 6$ and a = 1. The maximum sampling interval b is given by

$$b = 2m - a \tag{18}$$

In this case b = 12 − 1 = 11. We enter a random number table at any point, and, since b has two digits, we select digits two at a time, rejecting all digit pairs less than a or greater than b. In this case we would reject "00" and "12" through "99." The digits selected will range between "01" and "11" and represent our random sampling intervals. These intervals can readily be converted to actual observation times.

Selection of random digits is greatly facilitated by use of a computer or programmable calculator with a random number generator. Computers usually generate random digits with values between zero and one. Digits on the (0,1) scale can readily be converted to the desired (a,b) scale:

$$I = a + bd \tag{19}$$

where I is a sampling interval between a and b, rounded off to the desired amount, e.g., nearest minute, and d is a digit on the (0,1) scale. Of course, equation 19 can be used with a random number table, but the rejection method is easier to use without a computer.

To fully employ random sampling, a different sequence of random numbers is drawn for every observation period. It is possible that any one sequence may bias observations in some way, and the use of different sequences further reduces the chance of bias.

Systematic sampling often seems much simpler to use than random sampling but is conceptually more difficult to use correctly. In systematic sampling, an observation is made at equal time intervals throughout an observation period, e.g., every 6 minutes. (Sometimes the same series of unequal observation intervals is used for every observation period.) The risk of systematic sampling is that it may be "in phase" with some periodic occurrence in the work. A

---

‡Since 120! is an unwieldy number, the calculation is simplified if we note that 120!/117! = [(120) (119) (118) (116) . . . (3) (2) (1)] divided by [(117) (116) . . . (3) (2) (1)] = (120) (119) (118).

WORK SAMPLING OBSERVATION FORM

Set _____ of _____
Page _____ of _____

Study and phase:_____

Observer:_____ Date:_____ BOP_____ EOP_____

Route: _____

| Operator level codes: | Professional (P) | Clerical (C) | Technical (T) |

Activity Codes

1. Transcribing orders to Kardex
2. Preparing medications for adm.
3. Preparing pharmacy requis.
4. Ward stock inventory checking

5. Passing medications
6. Charting administrations
7. Personal
8. Out of area

TIME	AC	1	2	3	4	5	6	7	8	TIME	AC	1	2	3	4	5	6	7	8
	P										P								
	C										C								
	T										T								
	P										P								
	C										C								
	T										T								
	P										P								
	C										C								
	T										T								
	AC	1	2	3	4	5	6	7	8		AC	1	2	3	4	5	6	7	8
	P										P								
	C										C								
	T										T								
	P										P								
	C										C								
	T										T								
	P										P								
	C										C								
	T										T								
	AC	1	2	3	4	5	6	7	8		AC	1	2	3	4	5	6	7	8
	P										P								
	C										C								
	T										T								
	P										P								
	C										C								
	T										T								
	P										P								
	C										C								
	T										T								
	AC	1	2	3	4	5	6	7	8		AC	1	2	3	4	5	6	7	8
	P										P								
	C										C								
	T										T								
TALLY	P									TALLY	P								
	C										C								
	T										T								

FIGURE 8.10 Sample work sampling observation form.

systematic sampling scheme may tend to miss (or include) this activity to an unrepresentative extent, and to give misleading results. The analyst must be satisfied that he has accounted for all important periodic activities. This is sometimes difficult. Many jobs contain important periodic elements. For example, most workers begin work, take coffee and lunch breaks, and end work on the hour or half-hour. They may operate machinery that is inherently periodic or may work according to a schedule. For example, a nurse may check her medication records every hour on the hour. Repetitive tasks that all require approximately equal lengths of time may introduce periodicities into work.

If an analyst chooses a constant sampling interval longer than the duration of the longest activity being observed, so that each activity is observed at most once in each occurrence, he can use binomial sampling theory (equations 9-11, 14 and 17) but may bias his observations by missing some periodic activity. If the interval is set equal to or less than the duration of the shortest activity, periodic activity will not be missed, but binomial sampling theory cannot be used (26).

The second major issue in sampling is whether to consider the total observation period as homogeneous or broken up into separate sections (strata). The statistical question involved here is whether the probability ϕ_j is constant throughout the observation period or not. For example, it may be that medication-related activity by nurses is more likely during the day shift than during the night shift. In such cases, the precision of an estimate of the overall ϕ_j can be increased (i.e., required sample size decreased) by dividing the observation period into strata in which the individual ϕ_j values are constant (27).

If wide variations in ϕ_j are discovered, or if the observation period is subdivided anyway, e.g., for administrative convenience, then stratified sampling procedures should be considered.

Designing and Conducting a Work Sampling Study

Work sampling can be performed for a variety of purposes. It can be used to satisfy informal managerial information needs or to support informal process evaluations. It can be used to support formal proposals for procedural change or to provide research data for publication. Regardless of the application, the project manager must be unequivocal about the study's purpose, especially with regard to which activities are most important and how precisely their times must be estimated. Such clarity will reduce the project's requirements of time and other valuable resources.

Planning a work sampling project is seldom a linear, stepwise process. The analyst usually wishes to achieve the greatest possible precision for as many activities as possible. Frequently, a project will initially include more activities than ultimately can be included with acceptable precision and cost.

Consequently, it is normal for a project to include a preliminary or pilot study for the purpose of obtaining the information needed to plan the main study.

The first steps in designing a work sampling study are defining the activity categories and specifying the ways in which each activity can be recognized by the observer. The categories must be mutually exclusive and should include at least one category for "personal" or "nonproductive" time and one category for "out of area." When this is accomplished, the observation form should be designed. Usually, the observation form is adapted to the particular study (28). The only general requirements for the form are that it (1) indicate the times at which each observation is to be made, (2) permit the recording of the activity classifications found in every observation, (3) include the number of personnel on duty during the observation period, and (4) include the beginning and ending times of each observation period. If times are to be estimated per unit of activity, the *total* number of *occurrences* (not observations) of each activity unit should be recorded for each observation period. Figure 8.10 shows one example of an observation form. This example is very specific, in that it is intended for exactly eight activity classifications and three of fewer personnel classifications, but is not intended to show the identity of the operators, to distinguish between individual operators within a personnel classification, e.g., by ward, or to establish time required per activity. Randomly selected times would be written into the "Time" column before observations begin.

Ordinarily, the next step is selection, training, and testing of observers. After the observer's performance is judged to be satisfactory, a pilot study should be done for preliminary estimation of ϕ_j for each activity. During the pilot study, it is usually wise to subdivide the observation period into strata to investigate the possibility that ϕ_j is not the same at different times of day. Usually, 100-200 observations are enough to find large differences in ρ_j values between strata and to estimate sample size.

Following the pilot study, estimated ϕ_j values for an activity from different strata should be compared. The strata can be combined if they do not appear sufficiently different. After the strata (if any) have been established, sample size can be estimated by means of equation 14. After sample size is estimated, the average sampling rate m can be chosen and the number of days or strata required for the study can be estimated. If too large a sample is required for one or more activities, either the precision criteria should be relaxed or activities combined, as described earlier. These decisions influence the uses to which the study can be put and, therefore, require the clear conception of purpose described at the beginning of this section.

After the observation form is revised and additional observers are hired, as needed, the main study can commence. As the study progresses, stratified observations (if any) can be rechecked. Sample size should be reestimated, and checking for temporal changes in *P* should be carried out intermittently.

CONCLUSION

This chapter has presented a brief summary of those aspects of "methods engineering" that seem most pertinent to hospital pharmacy administration. The reader is directed to the references at the end of the chapter for further information. As in most human endeavor, work analysis and time study include multitudes of details that seem important to the expert and confusing to the novice. The material in this chapter should, at minimum, acquaint the hospital pharmacist with the essentials of the subject and demystify the methods and jargon of the engineer. At maximum, it should permit the reader to undertake some methods improvement and time study projects on his own or with the advice of a methods engineer.

REFERENCES

1. Barnes RM: *Motion and Time Study: Design and Measurement of Work*. New York, John Wiley & Sons, 1963, Chap 2.
2. McGregor DE: *The Human Side of Enterprise*. New York, McGraw-Hill, 1960.
3. Barnes RM: *op. cit.*, Chap 10-15.
4. Swensson ES: An innovative design in hospital pharmacy facilities. *Am J Hosp Pharm* 28:442-446, 1971.
5. Barnes RM: *op. cit.*, pp 283-286.
6. Ayoub MM: Work place design and posture. *Hum Fact* 15:265-268, 1973.
7. Buffa ES: *Models for Production and Operations Management*. New York, John Wiley & Sons, 1963, pp 106-110.
8. Staley K: Research points to new lighting levels. *Mod Hosp* 93:160, 1959.
9. Buffa ES: *op. cit.*, pp 96-106.
10. Greenberg A: Hospital air conditioning must be flexible. *Mod Hosp* 100:103, 1963.
11. Craig RJ: Tools for facility layout. *Hospitals* 46:60-64, 1972.
12. Buffa ES: *op. cit.*, pp 44-64.
13. Grant EL: *Statistical Quality Control*. New York, McGraw-Hill, 1946.
14. Snedecor GW, Cochran WG: *Statistical Methods*, ed 6. Ames, Iowa State University Press, 1967, p 40.
15. Ferguson GA: *Statistical Analysis in Psychology and Education*, ed 2. New York, McGraw-Hill, 1966, p 158.
16. Barnes RM: *op. cit.*, Chap 33.
17. Miller L, Freund J: *Probability and Statistics for Engineers*. Englewood Cliffs, NJ, Prentice-Hall, 1956.
18. Hald A: *Statistical Theory with Engineering Applications*. New York, John Wiley & Sons, 1952.
19. Pieruschka E: *Principles of Reliability*. Englewood Cliffs, NJ, Prentice-Hall, 1963, Chap 11.
20. Diem L, Lentner C (eds): *Documenta Geigy Scientific Tables*, ed 7. Basle, Switzerland, Geigy, 1970, p 99.
21. Arkin H, Colton RR: *Tables for Statisticians*, ed 2. New York, Barnes and Noble, 1963.
22. Barnes RM: *op. cit.*, Chap 33.
23. Miller I, Fruend J: *loc. cit.*
24. Diem K, Lentner C (eds): *op. cit.*, p 131.
25. Rand Corp: *A Million Random Digits with 100,000 Normal Deviates*, Glencoe, IL, Free Press, 1955.
26. Davidson HO, Hines WW, Newberry TL: The error of the estimate in systematic activity sampling. *J Industr Engineer* 11:290-292, 1960.
27. Conway RW: Some statistical considerations in work sampling. *J Industr Engineer* 8:107-111, 1957.
28. Johnston LJ: Using a work sampling study. *Hosp Pharm* 7:313-316, 1972.

CHAPTER 9

Work Measurement*

M. J. ROBERTS

The possibility of using management engineering concepts in the hospital pharmacy has been neglected for many years. The motto "working smarter, not harder" has recently captured the interest of the hospital pharmacy manager because of the expansion of labor-intensive services such as unit dose, IV additives, packaging, and drug monitoring during a time of cost constraints.

This chapter will familiarize you with work measurement—the assessment of work in terms of time to determine realistic and justifiable levels of man-hour input to handle varying levels of workload. Work measurement is concerned with identifying and minimizing the under- and overutilization of personnel resources. It can be used to (1,2):
- Compare the efficiency of alternative methods
- Determine labor and equipment requirements
- Divide work equitably among workers
- Set realistic labor standards
- Provide information for the planning and scheduling of personnel resources
- Ascertain output unit cost
- Ascertain machine utilization
- Assist in comparing performance with respect to workload and resource usage

Work measurement can enable pharmacy managers to perform effectively in the tasks of scheduling, job analysis, personnel budgeting, cost containment, productivity measurement, and expansion of services.

WORK MEASUREMENT TECHNIQUES

Seven techniques used for work measurement are subjective evaluation, statistical data, self-reporting, stopwatch time study, work sampling, standard data, and predetermined motion-time systems (3,4).

---

*This chapter is adapted in part from Roberts MJ, Kvalseth TO, Jermstad RL: Work measurement in hospital pharmacy. *Top Hosp Pharm Mgt* 2(2):1, 1982, with permission.

Subjective Evaluation

Labor standards determined by subjective evaluation are based on judgment, observation, past experience, and tradition (3). These standards are estimates and usually deviate from measured standards by about 25% on the average (4). The establishment of consistent and fair standards cannot be established simply by observing the work and judging the time to perform it. Therefore, subjective evaluation is not a desirable method for obtaining labor standards.

Statistical Data

Statistical data are a tabulation of completed work units obtained either through manual recording or data processing. Standards are established by mathematically relating the completed work units to personnel time. No detailed methods description or real work measurement is performed.

To establish standards from statistical data, the number of completed work units or outputs are obtained from manual recording or data processing. Such data in hospital pharmacy may be the number of IV admixtures prepared, unit dose drawers filled (census), prescriptions filled, new orders, discontinued orders, doses administered, items prepackaged, admissions, and discharges. The work time may be taken from past payroll or attendance records or gathered simultaneously with output data. Gross standards are obtained by mathematical relating of labor to output. Standards from statistical data are usually expressed as "output per manhour" or "output per full-time equivalent."

Standards from statistical data are used in work situations where detailed time measurement is not justifiable because of job variation or lack of cost benefit. Such standards are not exact, but are useful in providing rough measurement of the work being performed. Standards derived from statistical data are more reliable than those established through subjective evaluation, but do not provide sufficiently valid results to assure the efficient use of human resources (4). Discretion must be used by management when using standards from statistical data because standards derived this way do not represent all factors that affect a work force (1).

Self-Reporting

Self-reporting is a method of establishing time standards in which workers document their use of time and the work they complete. The study should be restricted to a base period of sufficient length to provide a representative sample of the work under study (2). This methodology involves recording all identifiable work units on a continuous log or a machine-readable data form. Attempts at maintaining a continuous reporting system of both time and work performed often fail. Personnel biases and data collection inaccuracy can result in extremely imprecise standards. These biases can be minimized by clearly informing workers of the purpose and importance of the study. The more professional the status of the workers, the more emphasis needs to be placed on the importance of study results (3).

Stopwatch Time Study

Work is measured through stopwatch time study by directly timing a task as it is performed. A sufficient number of work cycles must be timed in order to obtain a representative sample with a minimal variance. In developing the standard time, delay allowances and performance ratings (pace setting) must be considered. The use of performance rating may introduce error into the study because of its subjective nature (2,4).

Before a stopwatch time study can be conducted, the work to be measured must be divided into elements for timing. The elements should have a logical sequence, be as short as possible, and have physically observable beginning and ending points. For example, well-defined elements could be (1) taking a drug from a shelf, (2) opening the container, (3) counting the tablets, and (4) returning the drug to the shelf.

Stopwatch study is most frequently used when the work being measured is highly repetitive in nature. The technique may be used when the task has a single repeated cycle, subcycles, or a limited variety of cycles. It is of limited value when a variety of cycles exist that are not repeated in a short period of time (2).

Work Sampling

Work sampling is an indirect method of work measurement not requiring the actual timing of individual activities. A work sampling study consists of a large number of instantaneous observations taken at random intervals. The ratio of the number of observations of a given activity to the total number of observations taken will approximate the percentage of time spent on that activity. The accuracy of a work sampling study is dependent on the number of observations and the observer's ability to correctly interpret and classify the activities under study (5,6).

Work sampling is based on the laws of probability. The probability (p) exists that some category will be observed at a given instant. The probability $(1 - p)$ that it will not

be observed is equal to the summation of the probabilities of all other activities occurring (4). These probabilities are distributed through the binomial distribution. Therefore, each given activity is either occurring or not occurring, with all other activities being considered a nonoccurrence of the specified activity. Work sampling studies conducted on multiple activity work are defined so that the occurrence of a defined activity is dependent on the occurrence or nonoccurrence of other activities. This phenomenon is best described by multinomial probability distribution (7).

Work sampling is particulary useful in the analysis of nonrepetitive or irregularly occurring activities in which a difference in work content exists from cycle to cycle (4). This method can be used not only to establish standards, but also to obtain important managerial information concerning job analysis, personnel utilization, and possible areas of work simplification.

Work sampling can be used to measure any kind of work, does not require trained observers, can be done easily and economically (usually as a collateral duty of supervision), does not interrupt work flow, can be conducted over a long period of time, may be interrupted without affecting the results, and is usually the technique preferred by workers being studied (5,6,8).

Standard Data

Standard data are tabulated results of previous time studies (stopwatch time study, work sampling, or any other applicable work measurement approach) used to derive time standards by mathematical manipulation (2). The advantages of synthetic times over times compiled by individual studies (1,2,9) are that the former:

- Are based on data from large number of studies and thus are more reliable than times derived from a single study
- Are valuable in estimating time for planning and budgeting
- Allow an almost infinite range of times to be available
- Reduce number of individual studies that must be conducted
- Can be based on data from outside sources

The final accuracy of time standards set from synthetic times is a function of the accuracy of the compiled data from previous studies.

Time studies used to establish synthetic times must distinguish constant elements from variable elements. A constant element is one in which required performance time will stay approximately the same. A variable element is one in which performance time will vary within a specified range (4). Standards for constant elements are established by obtaining the average time required to complete those elements, as determined in previous time studies. One example of a constant element would be the typing of a prescription label. The time it takes to type one prescription label is relatively constant and depends on the quantity of medication dispensed. Standards for variable elements are determined by plotting the time required, as measured by the study, against the variable or variables, and fitting a curve through the plotted points. For example, the time required to prepare an IV admixture is a function of the number of additives that must be added. In this case, only one variable is involved, so that the equation takes the following form (10):

$$Y = MX + B$$

where Y = time required to prepare IV admixture, B = Y intercept, M = slope, and X = number of additives.

When the parameters B and M are known or have been estimated by means of least squares regression, the time required to prepare an admixture with any number of additives can be calculated from this equation by substituting the appropriate values for X. Therefore, the time required to prepare an admixture with four additives could be calculated by knowing the time it takes to prepare admixtures with one, three, and ten additives.

When the required time is a function of many variables, the equation takes the form of:

$$Y = B + M_1 + M_2X_2 + M_3X_3 \ldots$$

in which the values of the parameters B, M_1, M_2 . . . may again be determined by least squares regression.

Standard data allow for consistent work standards to be established rapidly and inexpensively, without the need for separate performance ratings. However, standard data require skilled personnel to perform complex calculations and may not accommodate small variations in methods (4).

Predetermined Motion-Time Systems

Predetermined motion-time systems (PMTS) provide the times required to perform fundamental human motion or groups of motions. Examples of such basic movements are reach, move, grasp, position, turn, disengage, and release. These times have been established by analyzing, frame by frame, films of many persons performing a given motion while doing diversified operations (10). Standards are derived by observing or mentally visualizing the work, dividing work tasks into basic movements (therbligs), assigning time values, and adding the assigned time values for each basic movement or groups of movements together. The time to perform these basic movements has shown to be a function of (2):

1. Distance
2. Complexity of action
3. Amount of body involved
4. Whether use of feet accompanies the action
5. Eye-hand coordination
6. Sensory requirements
7. Weight of resistance involved
8. Context and pattern of task
9. Direction of movement
10. Place of motion in performing task
11. Number of motions in performing task (4)

There are many types of PMTS. Examples are work factor, methods time measurements, basic motion time study, dimensional motion times, and motion-time analysis. These systems differ from each other by (3,4):

1. The number of variables that must be taken into account

2. Assumptions concerning independence of individual motion times
3. Level of performance on which time values are based
4. Manner of classifying motions, groups of motion, or body movements

PMTS have broad applications. However, these are complex techniques requiring a highly skilled individual who must be trained in the use of one of the PMTS and must be able to perform a detailed and accurate method analysis.

CHOOSING A WORK MEASUREMENT TECHNIQUE

The selection of an appropriate work measurement technique depends on the nature of the work being measured, purpose of the study, available resources, desired accuracy, and worker receptiveness (2).

The nature of the work being measured is a major determinant in the technique to be chosen. A given task may be more suitable for measurement through the use of one or several techniques. The purpose of the study will aid in determining the desired accuracy. When work measurement results are used for personnel resource determination, the accuracy and reliability of the time standards are not critical. Increased accuracy is required when the measurement is being used to establish expectations of a worker's output (11). Two types of costs are associated with the setting of time standards: the costs related to obtaining measurements and the incurred cost of using erroneous standards (12). In order to obtain a balance between these expenditures, a cost-benefit analysis should be conducted in the planning stages of any time study. The acceptability of the measurement technique to the workers under study is extremely important. Any work measurement system will fail without the cooperation of the workers concerned.

Work Measurement in Hospital Pharmacy

Self-reporting can be used to gather information regarding job content and establishment of estimated standards. It is helpful for measuring work performed in scattered locations and where observations are not feasible. Self-reporting also can be used for establishing preliminary information for work where the time required to perform tasks has never been quantified. It requires neither a large number of analysts nor observers to identify and classify the work. Self-reporting does not allow for any unreported idle time to be extracted from the data or for the performance rate to be established. Data are accepted as reported by the workers. Standards established through self-reporting, although better than estimates or historical data, lead to inefficient use of personnel resources. Self-reporting is useful only in cases in which labor costs are minor and no special desire for methods improvement exists (3).

The use of subjective evaluation, statistical data, and self-reporting is very common in hospital pharmacy. These techniques, although better than none, may result in poor standards and inefficient use of personnel resources. Scheduling, job analysis, personnel budgeting, and productivity measurement may not be accurately estimated by these techniques. In this era of inflation and cost containment, the cost of using these techniques is greater than the cost of obtaining more precise results. Standard time data, predetermined human work times, stopwatch time study, and work sampling represent better ways to establish equitable staffing needs.

The applicability of standard time data in hospital pharmacy is limited. Because work measurement in hospital pharmacy is at an evolutionary stage, time standards with well-defined variables are nonexistent. Hospital pharmacies vary in complexity of operation, facility design, and intensity of service, factors which represent variables in the time required to perform many tasks. Therefore, the development of standard time data applicable from hospital to hospital is highly unlikely in the near future.

The complexities and expenses involved in using predetermined human work times in hospital pharmacy are overwhelming and impractical. This technique requires a very detailed methods analysis, which is limited to manual labor and should be used only by individuals who have been properly trained.

Much of the work performed in the hospital pharmacy is nonrepetitive, has a long work cycle, and does not have a clear daily pattern. Work sampling (1) allows for the simultaneous study of several workers, (2) yields complete information about the total operation, and (3) is the technique most acceptable to professional workers. Therefore, it is postulated that the measurement technique most applicable to hospital pharmacy is work sampling.

In cases in which refined standards are desirable, and the work is highly repetitive and of too short a duration to be practically measured by work sampling, the stopwatch time study method would be more practical. Stopwatch time study can be used in hospital pharmacy for measuring monotonous technical tasks, such as preparing IV solutions prepackaging, and filling unit dose carts, but not for the more professional functions, for which judgment or clinical expertise is required.

Initial work measurement studies should be used to review the operation for possible changes. Subsequent studies should increase in complexity and specificity. Work sampling will suffice for initial studies, with stopwatch time study being required later to give a more detailed evaluation.

ESTABLISHING STANDARD TIMES

Work Sampling

Define the Objectives

Defining the objectives of the study is the initial step needed to plan a work sampling study. The objectives should identify the resources required to obtain reliable information. Work sampling studies can be used for appraising operational problems, analyzing personnel and equipment utilization, analyzing facility design, planning and budgeting, analyzing observance of policy and procedures, assessing the operation and efficiency of a given department, establishing job descriptions, and establishing time standards and allowances (5,6). Once the objectives of the study

have been defined, an estimate of the resources and the cost involved can be made.

Obtain Background Information

Obtain background information about the work to be studied. Time should be spent with supervisors and workers until the purpose and functions of the work to be studied are completely understood.

Defining the Activities

The work under study must be broken down into classifications compatible with the objectives of the study. The activities should be defined clearly in writing and should be easily recognizable by visual observation. Careful definition of categories will help to avoid observer bias or misinterpretation of activities (3). An example of categories applicable to hospital pharmacy is presented in Table 9.1.

There is no optimal number of categories. A gross analysis requires only a few categories, whereas a detailed analysis will require several categories. Limiting the number of categories increases the reliability of the results and decreases the cost and difficulty of conducting the study. This is because each category will have a greater number of observations, thus decreasing the variance and the required total number of observations.

It is advisable to have several narrow categories, particularly if well-defined objectives do not exist or performance and time standards are to be established. Categories can always be combined but can never be broken down after the completion of the study.

Identifying Measurable Output and Input Values

In order to establish standards, all inputs and outputs must be identified and a means of data collection devised. Inputs are the resources required to complete work (e.g., manhours worked by the employees). Such data can be collected through the use of time cards, observation, or a continuous log. Employee hours should be tabulated by job classification (i.e., pharmacists, technicians, interns, clerks) in order to calculate personnel costs accurately. Outputs are

TABLE 9.1 Work Sampling Categories Applicable to Hospital Pharmacy Work

Admission histories	IV admixture preparation
Breaks	Inventory ordering, stocking
Checking (chemotherapy, IV admixtures prepacking, profiling, unit dose cassettes)	Nonproductive time
	Omitted doses
Chemotherapy preparation	Parenteral nutrition monitoring
Clerical (charging, credits, profiling, recopying profiles, typing)	Patient discharge counseling
Controlled substances	Pharmacokinetic monitoring
Communication (interprofessional, intraprofessional)	Prepackaging
	Rounds
Drug information	Technician delivery
Exchanging unit dose cassettes	Walking
Medication administration	Verifying orders
Filling (orders unit dose cassettes)	Other

the tasks performed or completed by the employees undergoing study. Data can be collected through self-reporting (a less desirable method), computer output, or observer tabulation. All outputs that can be feasibly measured should be tallied.

Performing a Preliminary Study

A preliminary study can test the selected categories and study procedures, obtain a preliminary estimate of percentages of time developed to each activity, give the observers practice, and decrease the anxiety of the workers under study. Useful preliminary studies usually consist of 100-200 observations (5).

An estimate of the activity percentage is required to estimate the needed sample size. This estimate may be obtained by a preliminary study, previous time studies, or historical data. The activity of particular interest is the one in which an estimated percentage is used to calculate the needed sample size.

Selecting the Confidence Level

Before the required number of observations can be determined, the desired confidence level interval must be selected. A 95% confidence level is most commonly used. In some cases, too high a confidence level may be unrealistic, costly, and incompatible with the objectives of the study. Likewise, too low a confidence level may result in unreliable results for an activity of special interest.

Determining the Number of Observations

The required number of observations is dependent on the desired precision, as defined by the study objectives. Guidelines for the selection of the required sample size are presented in Table 9.2. Equations, tables, graphs, and nomograms represent alternative ways of estimating the needed sample size (Table 9.3, Figs. 9.1 to 9.3). Appropriate sample size can also be determined through the use of a computer (13).

The following equation can be used for multiple-activity work sampling studies (7):

$$N = \left[\frac{BP_1 (1 - P_1)}{A} \right]^2$$

where N = number of observations; B = upper (α/K) × 100 percentile of the chi-square distribution with one degree of freedom, K is the number of defined activities, and α is the level of significance; P_1 = estimated proportion of time of event closest to 0.5; and A = absolute accuracy expressed as a proportion (e.g., ±0.05). Approximate values of B can be determined from Figure 9.4. Divide the selected significance level (α) by the number of defined activities (K). Locate the quotient on the horizontal axis and move up to the curve and left to the vertical axis, where the resultant value of B is read.

For example, the formula would indicate a sample size of 3149 when P_1 is 0.35, A is 0.03, and B is 7.4 from Figure 9.4.

TABLE 9.2 A Guide for Selecting the Required Number of Work Sampling Observations[a]

Objectives of the Study	Suggested No. of Observations
Obtain general picture of the operation	100-200
Pinpoint specific condition	1000-2000
Appraise personnel and machine utilization	4000
Set allowances and time standards	Maximum of 10,000 (fewer is often sufficient)

[a]Modified from Barnes RM: *Work Sampling.* New York, John Wiley & Sons, 1957, and Krick EV: *Methods Engineering.* New York, John Wiley & Sons, 1962.

$$N = \left[\frac{7.4 \, (0.35) \, (1 - 0.35)}{0.03} \right]^2 = 3149$$

The equation given above ensures that the required steady criteria are met, but yields a sample size estimation. A more traditional method of estimating sample size is (10).

$$N = \frac{4a^2 \, P \, (1 - P)}{I^2}$$

where N = number of observations; a = 1.96 or 1.645 for 95% or 90% confidence limits, respectively, I = the designated confidence interval, and P = percent occurrence for a given activity.

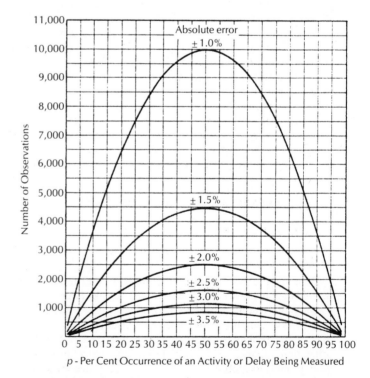

FIGURE 9.1 Curves for determining the number of observations for a given absolute error and value of p, 95% confidence level. (Reprinted by permission from Barnes RM: *Work Sampling.* New York, John Wiley & Sons, 1957.)

TABLE 9.3   Table for Determining the Number of Observations for a Given Absolute Error or Absolute Degree of Accuracy and Value of p, 95% Confidence Level[a]

% Total Time Occupied by Activity or Delay, p	Absolute Error						% Total Time Occupied by Activity of Delay, p	Absolute Error					
	±1.0%	±1.5%	±2.0%	±2.5%	±3.0%	±3.5%		±1.0%	±1.5%	±2.0%	±2.5%	±3.0%	±3.5%
1	396	176	99	63	44	32	51	9996	4442	2499	1599	1110	816
2	784	348	196	125	87	64	52	9984	4437	2496	1597	1109	815
3	1164	517	291	186	129	95	53	9964	4428	2491	1594	1107	813
4	1536	683	384	246	171	125	54	9936	4416	2484	1590	1104	811
5	1900	844	475	304	211	155	55	9900	4400	2475	1584	1099	808
6	2256	1003	564	361	251	184	56	9856	4380	2464	1577	1095	804
7	2604	1157	651	417	289	213	57	9804	4357	2451	1569	1089	800
8	2944	1308	736	471	327	240	58	9744	4330	2436	1559	1083	795
9	3276	1456	819	524	364	267	59	9676	4300	2419	1548	1075	790
10	3600	1600	900	576	400	294	60	9600	4266	2400	1536	1067	784
11	3916	1740	979	627	435	320	61	9516	4229	2379	1523	1057	777
12	4224	1877	1056	676	469	344	62	9424	4188	2356	1508	1047	769
13	4524	2011	1131	724	503	369	63	9324	4144	2331	1492	1036	761
14	4816	2140	1204	771	535	393	64	9216	4096	2304	1475	1024	753
15	5100	2267	1275	816	567	416	65	9100	4044	2275	1456	1011	743
16	5376	2389	1344	860	597	439	66	8976	3989	2244	1436	997	733
17	5644	2508	1411	903	627	461	67	8844	3931	2211	1415	983	722
18	5904	2624	1476	945	656	482	68	8704	3868	2176	1393	967	710
19	6156	2736	1539	985	684	502	69	8556	3803	2139	1369	951	698
20	6400	2844	1600	1024	711	522	70	8400	3733	2100	1344	933	686
21	6636	2949	1656	1062	737	542	71	8236	3660	2059	1318	915	672
22	6864	3050	1716	1098	763	560	72	8064	3584	2016	1290	896	658
23	7084	3148	1771	1133	787	578	73	7884	3504	1971	1261	876	644
24	7296	3243	1824	1167	811	596	74	7696	3420	1924	1231	855	628
25	7500	3333	1875	1200	833	612	75	7500	3333	1875	1200	833	612
26	7696	3420	1924	1231	855	628	76	7296	3243	1824	1167	811	596
27	7884	3504	1971	1261	876	644	77	7084	3148	1771	1133	787	578
28	8064	3584	2016	1290	896	658	78	6864	3050	1716	1098	763	560
29	8236	3660	2059	1318	915	672	79	6636	2949	1659	1062	737	542
30	8400	3733	2100	1344	933	686	80	6400	2844	1600	1024	711	522
31	8556	3803	2139	1369	951	698	81	6156	2736	1539	985	684	502
32	8704	3868	2176	1393	967	710	82	5904	2624	1476	945	656	482
33	8844	3931	2211	1415	983	722	83	5644	2508	1411	903	627	461
34	8976	3989	2244	1436	997	733	84	5376	2389	1344	860	597	439
35	9100	4044	2275	1456	1011	743	85	5100	2267	1275	816	567	416
36	9216	4096	2304	1475	1024	753	86	4816	2140	1204	771	535	393
37	9324	4144	2331	1492	1036	761	87	4524	2011	1131	724	503	369
38	9424	4188	2356	1508	1047	769	88	4224	1877	1056	676	469	344
39	9516	4229	2379	1523	1057	777	89	3916	1740	979	627	435	320
40	9600	4266	2400	1536	1067	784	90	3600	1600	900	576	400	294
41	9676	4300	2419	1548	1075	790	91	3276	1456	819	524	364	267
42	9744	4330	2436	1559	1083	795	92	2944	1308	736	471	327	240
43	9804	4357	2451	1569	1089	800	93	2604	1157	651	417	289	213
44	9856	4380	2464	1577	1095	804	94	2256	1003	564	361	251	184
45	9900	4400	2475	1584	1099	808	95	1900	844	475	304	211	155
46	9936	4416	2484	1590	1104	811	96	1536	683	384	246	171	125
47	9964	4428	2491	1594	1107	813	97	1164	517	291	186	129	95
48	9984	4437	2496	1597	1109	815	98	784	348	196	125	87	64
49	9996	4442	2499	1599	1110	816	99	396	176	99	63	44	32
50	10000	4444	2500	1600	1111	816							

[a]Reprinted by permission from Barnes RM: *Work Sampling,* New York, John Wiley & Sons, 1957.

For example, the formula would indicate a sample size of 3585 when P is 30% and the confidence level is 95%.

$$N = \frac{4(1.96)^2 \, 0.3 \, (1 \, - \, 0.3)}{(0.025)^2} = 3585$$

Setting the Study Duration and Frequency of Observations

The study duration and frequency of observations are dependent on work variations by day, week, or season, as well as the objectives of the study, availability of the observers, the time needed to make an observation, and the number of workers observed per observation. The time involved in conducting one observation is a function of the number of workers to be observed and the dimension of the work area.

The number of workers to be observed per observation influences the length of the study and the frequency of observations. If multiple workers are to be observed, then

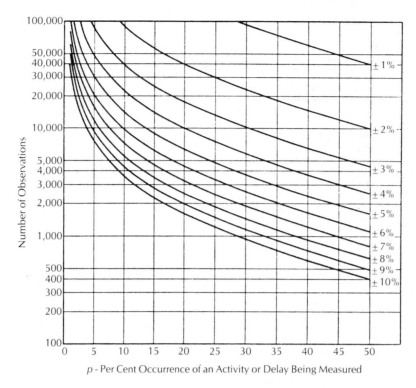

FIGURE 9.2 Curves for determining the number of observations for a given degree of accuracy and value of p, 95% confidence level. (Reprinted by permission from Barnes RM: *Work Sampling.* New York, John Wiley & Sons, 1957.)

the number of required observations should be divided by the number of workers observed per observation.

Rarely can the study duration be too long. A study extending over a long period of time, with a few observations per day (e.g., eight observations per day extended over several months of time) is relatively simple and inexpensive to perform and usually has a decreased variance because the sample will be more representative of a "typical day." Too short a study duration can result in a sample's reflecting bias because of seasonal or cyclic differences. Observations made too frequently (e.g., two or three per minute) become overwhelming for the observer as well as the workers and limit the advantages that work sampling has over stopwatch time study.

Choosing the Sampling Technique

Sampling is the process of making inference concerning the characteristics of population by examining closely the characteristics of a smaller number of items drawn from the population. Three different types of work sampling techniques can be used: randomized, systematic, or stratified. In random sampling, a sample is drawn from the population in such a way that each member of the population has an equal chance of being included. Observations are randomized to minimize systematic error that may otherwise occur. In systematic sampling, members of the population are selected on an equal interval basis. Systematic sampling is used when the work under study is felt to be random in nature and not subject to bias. A disadvantage of systematic

sampling is that workers have a greater tendency to anticipate observations when they are made at equal intervals. Stratified sampling is the selection of a sample randomly or systematically from a portion (stratum) of the population. Strata may be segmented by day, week, month, or worker type. Stratified sampling is used to minimize any known or suspected significant variance. The use of stratified sampling can result in an overestimate of both the required sample size and the final true variance, which in most cases is ignored in work sampling (5,12).

Developing Observation Times

The method used to develop observation times depends on the chosen sampling technique. If stratified or unstratified random sampling is selected, observation times are established in essentially the same manner. The only difference is that in stratified sampling the selection probability for a given time is the same within each stratum, but differs among strata (5).

Observation times are developed by (1) defining time limits for the study period, (2) determining the average frequency of observations, and (3) establishing random times (3). Random times can be established through the use of a computer (14), programmable calculator, or random number table. A random number table can be used to generate random times by the first two digits to represent the hour and the next two digits to represent the minutes (6).

The selection of observation times in systematic sampling is done by using random or nonrandom starting times. Ran-

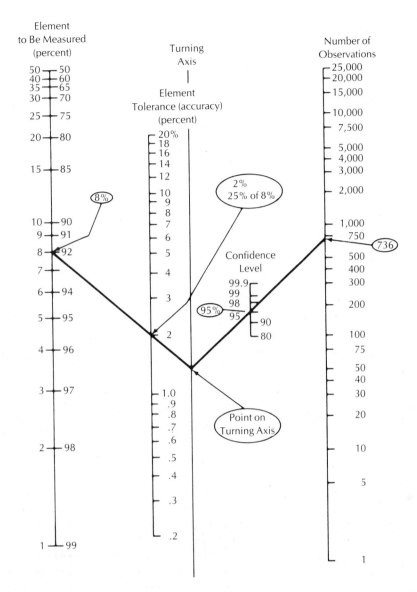

FIGURE 9.3 Nomogram to determine the number of random observations for various confidence levels (Reprinted by permission from Niebel BW: *Motion and Time Study.* Homewood, IL, Richard D Irwin, 1956.)

domized starting times eliminate biases that could occur with a nonrandom starting time. Starting times can be randomized by assigning a number for each interval minute, putting the numbers "into a hat," and then adding the corresponding interval time to the selected starting time. For example, when the interval time equals 10 minutes, slips of paper numbered 1-10 are placed in a hat, and one is picked at random. The number picked establishes the first observation, with subsequent observations made by adding 10 minutes to each successive observation (5).

Designing Necessary Forms

Since each work sampling study is unique (number of required observations, number of activities, number of workers to be observed, random times, etc), no standard forms exist. Forms are fairly similar, with modifications made to meet the objectives of each particular study.

Necessary forms include observer instructions, category definitions, data collection forms, and summary sheets. The observer instructions should be distributed to all observers and include all necessary procedures to be followed during the study. Clearly written category definitions should be distributed to all observers to minimize differences in observer judgments. The data collection form should allow for easy and accurate data collection. Computer-generated or computer-readable data collection forms can be used to reduce the time and cost involved in conducting the study. Computer-readable data forms facilitate data processing and subsequent analysis. If computer-readable forms are not utilized, summary forms will be needed to save time, especially considering the inordinate amount of paperwork

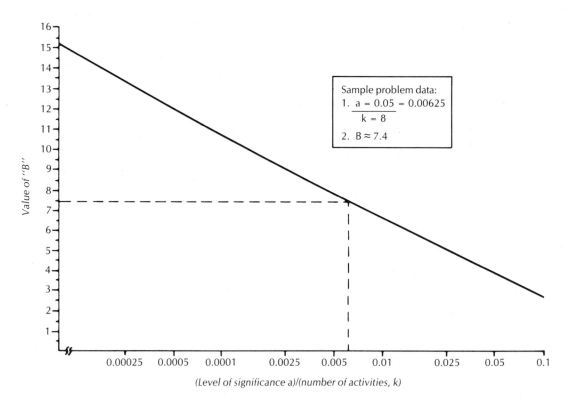

FIGURE 9.4 Determination of item B when level of significance and number of activities are known. (Reprinted by permission from Allen DS: Multiple activity work study needs and samples. *J Indust Engineer* 30:79, December 1979.)

WORK SAMPLING DATA   TIMES

FUNCTIONS
1. Receiving prescriptions
2. Coding prescriptions
3. Computer entry
4. Sorting labels
5. Filling prescriptions
6. Checking prescriptions
7. Counseling patients
8. Inventory ordering
9. Inventory stocking
10. Problem solving
11. Telephone
12. Idle time
13. Meals and breaks
14. Multiple dose prepackaging
15. CFS—clinic stock
16. Controlled substances count
17. Education—staff mtgs., etc.
18. Other

Observation day #   OUTPUT DATA
Day of Week   # of prescriptions: _____
                                 # of CFS _____
                                 # of patients: _____

FIGURE 9.5 Observation form for outpatient pharmacy study.

involved in manual analysis. For an example of a work sampling data collection form, see Figure 9.5.

Selecting and Orienting Observers

The results of the study will be inaccurate without observers who are conscientious, impartial, familiar with the work to be observed, and conversant with the methodology and objectives of work sampling (3,6). Observer orientation should cover work sampling theory, uses of work sampling, activity definitions, objectives of the study, uses of necessary forms, biasing effects, and observation procedures (5). Practice observations are highly recommended. The time involved in orienting observers should not require more than 4 or 5 hours (3).

Three types of observers who can be selected for work sampling studies are measurement personnel, trained workers, and first-line supervisors (5). The selection of the person(s) to do the observing depends on the objectives of the study and on available resources.

Measurement personnel or trained industrial engineers are essential when performance rating is desired. In most cases, the industrial engineer will be unfamiliar with the work and considered an outsider by the observed workers (3). Trained workers are staff personnel trained to conduct studies when many observers are required or the classification of the work activities is difficult. The fact that the worker may bias the results is offset by the fact that the worker is familiar with the work.

The use of first-line supervisors for observing or assisting in observing is preferred whenever possible. Benefits that may result include greater awareness of personnel utilization, methods improvement, and work simplification (5).

Orienting Workers under Study

It is common for workers to anticipate observations and to "act busy" when they are being observed. These biases can be minimized through proper orientation before the study is conducted. The orientation should cover how the study will be performed, what the purpose of the study is, and how the results are going to be used. Misunderstanding and suspicion can be avoided by presenting the information as frankly and informally as possible and allowing for questions as necessary.

Performing the Study

Observations are made by observing the work visually and recording what is seen at a designated instant. The observation schedule should be adhered to as strictly as possible. When an observation has been missed, or adherence to the observation schedule is not feasible, the missed observation should be made as soon as possible.

The observer's preconceived judgments should not bias the results. Observers should accurately observe, classify, and record the instantaneous activity that was seen, not what has happened or will happen (3,6). If any doubt exists concerning which classification the observed work belongs to, the observer should document this observation in an "other" category and explicitly define what was observed for subsequent review.

The use of a random activity analysis camera can help to minimize biases caused by worker apprehension and observer anticipation. Photographic work sampling enables a large number of observations to be obtained at minimal expense but may limit the number of activities that can be studied accurately.

There is a limit to the number of subjects that can be observed and the area that can be feasibly covered by an observer. These situations can be resolved by increasing the number of observers or randomly selecting observation sites and/or workers to be observed. In the case in which it is desirable to observe a large area, the observers should vary their travel routes whenever possible. This randomization can be accomplished by designating numbers to the work areas or observation routes and using the "pick out of the hat" technique.

If it is desired to have time standards include performance rating (pace settings), a performance rating will have to be recorded as the observations are being made. Performance rating is used to adjust measured work so that standards represent the time required by an average worker to complete a task at a normal pace. Standards can be established with or without performance rating (15). If performance rating is used, it should be done with caution. Performance rating is subject to error and must be done by a highly skilled individual. Also, work sampling was not designed to be used with performance rating. Barnes and Andrew (16) have proposed a method of using performance rating with work sampling. Work sampling studies done in hospital pharmacy usually are done by observing many different workers with varying skills and under various working conditions. The results already may represent the average worker performing at a normal pace. Therefore, pace setting in hospital pharmacy work sampling studies may be superfluous and lead to error.

Analyzing the Data

All inputs, outputs, and observation data must be compiled. This can be accomplished manually or through computerization. The data can be entered into a computer either through machine-readable observation forms or through key punching on line or on cards.

The data can be analyzed graphically on a periodic (daily, weekly, etc) basis during the study. A simple progress chart can be constructed by plotting the accumulated percent occurrence along the Y axis and accumulated number of observations along the X axis. An example of such a chart is illustrated in Figure 9.6. A stabilization of the accumulative percent occurrence indicates the approximate end of the study. Such a graph can be used as a basis for deciding when a sufficient number of observations have been accumulated (3,6,10). Another graphic method is control charting. An example of such a chart is illustrated in Figure 9.7. The graph consists of subsample percentages found in a single category or group of categories plotted along the Y axis, with time or subsample number along the X axis. The initial center line is established using the estimated percent

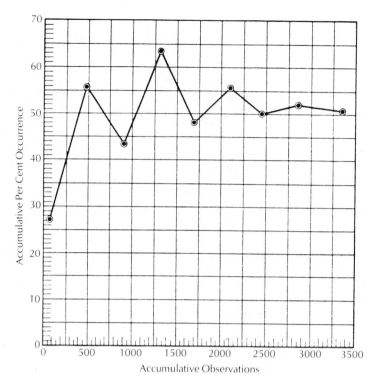

FIGURE 9.6 Work sampling progress chart. (Reprinted by permission from Barnes RM: *Work Sampling*. New York, John Wiley & Sons, New York, 1957.)

occurrence from the preliminary study or historical data. The control limits are established using the following formula for three sigmas (4):

$$\text{Control limit} = p \pm 3 \sqrt{\frac{p(1-p)}{n}}$$

where n = sample size of subsample and p = percent occurrence of an activity being measured.

The observed percentage of each subsample is routinely plotted on the graph. Appearance of stabilization is indicated by all points falling within the limit lines, falling outside, and by points clustering around the center line. If the graph does not follow these guidelines and no explanation exists for the deviation, the chart is out of control. An out-of-control chart requires a recalculation of the estimated percentage, control limits, and required sample size. This technique can be used to determine whether a representative sample has been acquired, whether the work is cyclic in predictable intervals, and whether trends indicate changes in the work or working conditions (3).

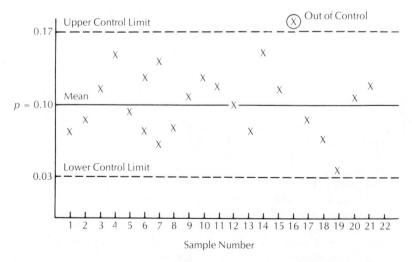

FIGURE 9.7 Work sampling control chart. (Reprinted by permission from Niebel BW: *Motion and Time Study*. Homewood, IL, Richard D Irwin, 1976.)

The probability of occurrences for each category, standard error, and confidence limits are derived using the following formulas (3,6,10):

Probability of occurrence for a given activity (p) =

$$\frac{\text{Total No. of observations for a given activity}}{\text{Total No. of study observations}}$$

$$\text{Standard error} = S_p = \sqrt{\frac{p(1-p)}{n}}$$

where p = probability of occurrence of activity concerned and n = total number of study observations.

$$\text{Confidence limits at 95\% level} = \pm 1.96\, S_p.$$

The combination of categories should be considered for categories with a small percentage of occurrence.

Standards can be calculated using the following formula (6):

Standard time for a given activity =

$$\frac{\text{Total input hours} \times \text{Proportion of occurrence for activity}}{\text{Total output of activity}}$$

When allowances and performance ratings are included, the following formula is used:

Standard time for a given activity =

$$\frac{\text{Total input hours} \times \text{Proportion of occurrence for activity} \times \text{Average performance rating}}{\text{Total output of activity}} + \text{\% allowance time}$$

Allowances are taken into account to represent personal delay, fatigue, and unavoidable delays. Allowances can either be calculated into each category or incorported into the calculation of productivity.

For categories with immeasurable outputs or outputs that would be difficult to obtain, the standard is equal to the percent occurrence multiplied by the man-hours worked. Work sampling results can be summarized on charts and graphs by worker type and day of the week, patient census, patient intensity, day of the week, work area, time of the year, and dollars spent to complete a given acitvity.

STOPWATCH TIME STUDY

Planning, execution, and analysis are three phases of any work measurement study. The planning phase should include all information gathering, job analysis, and decision-making processes to ensure that the results are accurate and reproducible. The execution phase consists of the actual observation of the work being performed, during which data on elapsed time and worker performance are gathered. In the analysis phase, the results are analyzed with basic times, and standard times, including allowances, are calculated.

Check the Method

The method being used by the worker to be studied must be checked before the study is performed. First, a methods study should be performed to ensure that all steps are necessary and that all principles of motion economy are being maximized. If changes should be made, the worker(s) should be given adequate training and practice time in the new method before the study proceeds. Second, it must be assured that the worker(s) perform the work as specified by carrying out all steps as outlined in the preferred methodology.

Planning

Establish Standard of Practice

Establishment of a written standard of practice is essential. All general information pertinent to the task to be measured must be documented so that the job and surrounding conditions may be examined or reproduced in the future. Recorded information should include description of work measured, output, work conditions, supplies, worker(s), workplace, layout, machine(s), forms, actual manual details of the job, and the purpose and duration of the study. Incomplete information makes subsequent evaluation of systems changes very difficult, if not impossible, and decreases the usefulness of results obtained from the study.

Perform Job Analysis

A complete job analysis must be performed in order to divide the job into elements. A detailed breakdown of elements is necessary to (1):
1. Ensure that productive work is separated from unproductive work
2. Permit ease of performance rating
3. Permit the checking of time standards and later deletions or insertions of elements
4. Establish future standard data
5. Facilitate a detailed and accurate description of the job

General rules for dividing a task into elements are that the elements should be easily identifiable, with definite beginnings and endpoints, be of as short a duration as can be accurately measured, consist of group-unified basic motions, and be separated by element type (1,2,17).

The five types of elements observed are repetitive, constant, variable, occasional, and foreign. Repetitive elements are those which occur in every cycle of a given activity or task. Constant elements are identical in time and specifications, whereas variable elements vary in some characteristic of the product, equipment, or process. Occasional elements do not occur in every cycle, but at regular or irregular intervals. Foreign elements are not a necessary part of the task under study (1).

The degree of detail with which the elements are divided depends on the type of work being measured, the results desired, and the future use of the results as standard data.

Select Worker(s)

The results of a work measurement study should represent the average time it takes an average worker to perform the job under normal conditions. Ideally, the individual(s) selected should be experienced and well trained, like their work, show interest in doing a good job, be cooperative, and work at a normal pace. The analyst conducting the study must inform the worker(s) of the purpose of the study, the timing techniques to be utilized, and the method of rating and allowances.

In cases in which the analyst performing the work measurement is not trained in performance rating, it will be necessary (if possible) to observe more than one worker performing the job under study. This will help to ensure that the results are representative of an "average" worker.

Choosing the Equipment

The most common equipment used for conducting a stopwatch time study includes a stopwatch, a clipboard, and a series of forms on which to record information. The stopwatch can be either spring loaded or electronic. For hospital pharmacy work, a timing device with decimal minutes (0.01 minute) is sufficient. The device should enable the user to record "split times" when necessary. The time study form should facilitate the gathering of all required data. The form should be designed so that the analyst can correctly and quickly record information regarding the method being studied, the condition of the study, watch readings, elemental times, foreign elements, and rating factors. The use of relatively inaccurate time devices, such as a wristwatch or wall clock, is acceptable when elements are exceptionally long and the output is of low volume. Alternative equipment includes electronic time-recording machines and videotape/motion picture devices for analysis.

Execution of Study

Observe and Record

The observer should be in a position so as not to distract or interfere with the worker being measured. The position taken should enable the analyst to visualize the operator, timepiece, and data sheet easily. The observer should be able clearly to observe all elemental breakpoints. During the study, the observer should avoid doing anything that may change the routine of the worker. For an example of a data reporting form, see Figure 9.8.

All elemental times should be recorded consecutively as performed by the worker. All missed readings should be indicated as missed, and no attempt should be made to approximate the missed value. When an element is missed, it should be indicated and not time recorded. When elements are performed out of order, this should also be recorded, and time values should be placed with appropriate elements. If elements are routinely omitted or performed out of order, the study should be stopped and the methods analysis reperformed or the worker retrained. All interruptions and delays should be recorded as foreign elements. When the work to be measured is performed by two or more workers, each worker should be studied separately.

Three methods used for timing are continuous, repetitive, and accumulative timing. In the continuous method (most commonly used), the time is measured during the entire duration of the study. The breakpoint of each element is measured by reading the stopped hand on a double-action

watch. Elemental times are obtained by successive subtractions after the study is completed. In the repetitive method, the watch is read at the termination of each element and at virtually the same time that the watch is reset to zero. This procedure is performed for each element until the study is completed. The accumulative method utilizes multiple stopwatches. In this method, one watch is stopped and another started at each elemental breakpoint.

Determine Number of Cycles to Be Studied

Stopwatch time study is a sampling technique. Therefore, the accuracy of the measured value with respect to the true value is a function of the size of the sample. Variations in measured times are caused by differences in worker pace and movements, positions of supplies, and slight measurement errors (4).

The number of cycles to be studied is a function of the observed time variances, the degree of accuracy desired, and the length of the cycle. The analyst should perform the study until a representative sample has been measured. A large number of samples will be required when elemental times have a large variance or very short cycles.

The sample size can be calculated using the equation (4)

$$N = \left(\frac{St}{K\bar{x}}\right)^2$$

where N = sample size, S = sample standard deviation, t = student "t" distribution, $\bar{x}$ = estimated mean of population, K = an acceptable percentage of $\bar{x}$.

The following shortcut formula can be used to determine the number of readings (2):

$$N = 205\frac{R}{\bar{x}} - 42$$

where N = number of observations required, R = range of cycle time, and $\bar{x}$ = mean cycle time.

Another shortcut method to estimate sample size to achieve ±5% or ±10% precision at the 95% confidence level is (2,18)

$$\frac{H - L}{H + L} = \text{Ratio}$$

where H = highest value in sample readings and L = lowest value in sample readings.

This ratio is then matched to the appropriate answers under the columns for 5 and 10 sample size in Figure 9.9. For example, element readings are 0.4, 0.4, 0.3, 0.4, 0.4, 0.4, 0.4, 0.5, 0.4, 0.4 (sample size = 10). Using the first equation, estimated sample size is 60.

$$N = 205\frac{R}{\bar{x}} - 42 = 205\frac{0.2}{0.4} - 42 = 60$$

In the second method,

$$\frac{H - L}{H + L} = \frac{0.5 - 0.2}{0.5 + 0.3} = \frac{0.2}{0.8} = 0.25$$

Look up 0.25 for 10 samples. The estimated sample size is 42. The element with the greatest variance should be used

TIME STUDY OBSERVATION SHEET   Page _____ of _____

Activity: _____   Date:_____

Operator:_____   Time Start:_____

Observer:_____   Time End:_____

                                                            Time Elapsed:_____

No.	Item Description	Clock Time	Element Time	Category	Comments
1					
2					
3					
4					
5					
6					
7					
8					
9					
10					
11					
12					
13					
14					
15					
16					
17					
18					
19					
20					
21					
22					
23					
24					
25					

FIGURE 9.8 Example of data reporting form.

when calculating the number of cycles to be observed. After the study is complete, the confidence interval should be calculated using the equation (4)

$$\bar{x} \pm t \frac{s}{\sqrt{N}}$$

where $\bar{x}$ = population mean, t = student's "t" distribution, s = standard deviation, and N = sample size.

In calculating the confidence interval, the analyst is ensuring that a representative mean time has been obtained. If the accuracy is deemed unsatisfactory after the confidence interval has been calculated, the analyst should obtain more readings.

It is optimal if samples can be taken at random times. Stopwatch time readings can be randomized by time of the day, day of the week, and workers observed. As the randomization occurs, so does the reliability of the measured time.

Performance Rating

Performance rating is an attempt to normalize the observed time so that it is representative of the average worker. Worker performance rating is a function of skill, aptitude, and execution. By definition, rating is a comparison between the level of performance observed and the analyst's subjective reference of normal pace. Observed times are normalized by adding time performed by better-than-average workers and subtracting time performed by poor workers.

On short-cycle, repetitive work, the analyst usually assigns one rating for the entire study. When the elements are

of long duration, each element is rated as it occurs during the study. The rating is documented simultaneously with elapsed time for each particular element.

Performance ratings should be done by a trained person. Therefore, it is beyond the scope of this chapter. The observation and measurement of multiple workers can be used

No. of Readings Required
for ± 5%; 95/100 Probability*

$\dfrac{H - L}{H + L}$	Data from sample of		$\dfrac{H - L}{H + L}$	Data from sample of		$\dfrac{H - L}{H + L}$	Data from sample of	
	5	10		5	10		5	10
0.05	3	1	0.21	52	30	0.36	154	88
0.06	4	2	0.22	57	33	0.37	162	93
0.07	6	3	0.23	63	36	0.38	171	98
0.08	8	4	0.24	68	39	0.39	180	103
0.09	10	5	0.25	74	42	0.40	190	108
0.10	12	7	0.26	80	46	0.41	200	114
0.11	14	8	0.27	86	49	0.42	210	120
0.12	17	10	0.28	93	53	0.43	220	126
0.13	20	11	0.29	100	57	0.44	230	132
0.14	23	13	0.30	107	61	0.45	240	138
0.15	27	15	0.31	114	65	0.46	250	144
0.16	30	17	0.32	121	69	0.47	262	150
0.17	34	20	0.33	129	74	0.48	273	156
0.18	38	22	0.34	137	78	0.49	285	163
0.19	43	24	0.35	145	83	0.50	296	170
0.20	47	27						

Example: Suppose you took a time study
in which the ten elapsed time values
for each of three elements were as follows:

	el 1	el 2	el 3	
	0.07	0.12	0.50	
	0.09	0.13	0.55	
	0.06	0.15	0.53	
	0.07	0.16	0.51	
	0.08	0.1	0.54	
	0.08	0.14	0.49	
	0.07	0.12	0.52	
	0.08	0.15	0.51	
	0.09	0.11	0.55	
	0.07	0.12	0.52	
H to L	0.09 – 0.06	0.16 – 0.11	0.55 – 0.49	
H – L	0.03	0.05	0.06	
H + L	0.15	0.27	1.04	
$\dfrac{H - L}{H + L}$	0.20	0.185	0.077	
Total readings	27	23	4	No. cycles obtained from above chart

For ± 10%, 95/100 probability, divide above required readings by four.
H = high value   L = low value

FIGURE 9.9 Short cut to calculating sample size.

to attain normality for work measured in the hospital pharmacy.

Analysis

Check Quality

All work measured should yield results that meet acceptable quality standards. Standards should be set and arrangements should be made to have all results checked against them. Quality that is too high or substandard is unacceptable. Normal fluctuations in quality are acceptable, and observed differences in time as a result of these fluctuations should be considered routine.

Allowance Time

Allowance time is time for which the elemental time must be adjusted, such as personal time and delay time. Personal time is the time required by workers because of fatigue or for meeting personal needs, such as trips to the restroom and the water cooler. The actual time required for personal needs is a function of the working environment, the nature of the work, the workload, and the general health of the worker. Two kinds of delay time exist: avoidable and unavoidable. Unavoidable delay times are frequently called "management" delays. These include talks with the supervisor, material problems, machine malfunctions, set-up time, clean-up time, etc. Avoidable delays consist of time used for social visits between workers and idleness other than resting to overcome fatigue. Usually allowance is not given for avoidable delays.

The allowance time is obtained through one of three methods: regular time study, all-day time study, or work sampling (19). Allowance time measured by a regular time study is observed foreign time for personal and unavoidable delays. The problem with this approach is that the probability exists that some occurrences will not be observed. All-day time studies conducted for a few days can also be used for allowance time. Gross activities are used for recording times; again, the items of interest are occurrences of other than productive activities. Work sampling is the preferred procedure for determining allowances. The categories are classified appropriately for measuring the desired allowances.

Allowance time is usually expressed as a percentage of that work time. Allowances must be realistically set to allow the average worker to complete his or her work at a normal pace. Allowances set too high will lead to inefficient use of personnel resources, while setting them too low may cause poor labor relations and the eventual failure of the performance measurement system.

Determine Time Standard

The standard time is calculated by the following equation (4):

Standard time = (Mean elapsed elemental time ×
Performance rating) + (Mean elapsed elemental
time × Allowance factor)

The performance rating and allowance factors are expressed as percentages. For example:

Mean elapsed elemental time = 28 seconds
Performance factor = 0.90
Allowance = 0.18
Standard time = (28 × 0.90) + (28 × 0.18) = 30.2

The mean elemental time is obtained by adding all observed times for each element, subtracting the total foreign time observed, and dividing by the number of times that element was observed. The performance factor is obtained by averaging either overall rating times or ratings collected simultaneously with elemental times. The allowance time is obtained as previously mentioned. The standard cycle time is obtained by adding up the standard elemental times for all elements in a cycle.

SELF-REPORTING

Develop Work Units

All work performed must be identified and classified into distinct, clearly defined, and documented work units. No task should be classified into more than one work unit. As many work units as possible should be related to measurable output, although some work units do not have output frequency, e.g., communicating, walking, problem solving, idleness, and taking personal time. All related functions should be defined in a given work unit. Definitions of the work units should be tested by the workers to be measured for understanding, clarity, and inclusiveness.

Devise Codes

A coding system for work units should be devised to facilitate data collection and analysis. An open number system such as 1.0, 1.1, 2.0, 2.1 can be used. Work units should be classified to allow the workers to record their data efficiently. Codes should be classified by work area, job description, and related tasks.

Example: Pharmacy Technician
1.0 Inpatient
    1.1 Drug distribution
        1.1.1   Filling unit dose carts
        1.1.2   Checking unit dose carts
        1.1.3   Exchanging unit dose carts
    1.2 Intravenous admixtures
        1.2.1   Preparing antibiotic syringes
        1.2.2   Preparing total parenteral nutrition
        1.2.3   Preparing antibiotic piggybacks

If data are to be machine analyzed, the coding system should facilitate data entry.

Develop Data Collection Form(s)

Data forms for output and worker reporting must be devised. For an example of a self-reporting data form, see Figure 9.10. If output data are to be gathered simultaneously by the workers, a column for output counts should be included on the workers' time report form.

DATE:_____					
NAME:_____					
AM SHIFT		JOB TITLE:_____			

TIME	CODE	TIME	CODE	TIME	CODE
0630		0940		1225	
0635		0945		1230	
0640		0950		1235	
0645		0955		1240	
0650		1000		1245	
0655		1005		1250	
0700		1010		1255	
0705		1015		1300	
0710		1020		1305	
0735		1025		1310	
0740		1030		1315	
0745		1035		1320	
0750		1040		1325	
0755		1045		1330	
0800		1050		1335	
0805		1155		1340	
0810		1100		1345	
0820		1105		1350	
0825		1110		1355	
0830		1115		1400	
0835		1120		1405	
0840		1125		1410	
0845		1130		1415	
0850		1135		1420	
0855		1140		1425	
0900		1145		1430	
0905		1150		1435	
0910		1155		1440	
0915		1200		1445	
0920		1205		1450	
0925		1210		1455	
0930		1215		1500	
0935		1220		1505	

FIGURE 9.10 Self-reporting data form.

Orient Workers

The orientation of the workers is the most crucial step in conducting a self-reporting study. Workers should be informed as to the purpose of the study, its duration, the methods of reporting data and interpreting the work unit definitions, and the fact that idle and personal time are acceptable and expected. Without total cooperation and proper training, workers will report their use of time haphazardly, and inaccurate data will result.

Data Collection

The study should be conducted over a period of time so that it yields representative results. A period of 1 or 2 weeks is most common for hospital pharmacy work. All workers should receive copies of both the data collection form and the work code list. They should be given a practice period for collecting data and the name of a contact person who will answer their questions. To record data, workers can record the beginning and end of each work unit by writing the code beside the start and stop times listed on the time log.

Checks should be made during the study period both during and immediately after each shift to ensure that the workers are recording data correctly and thoroughly. All time during each shift period should be accounted for during the study period.

Data Analysis

Time for each work unit is calculated by adding up all time assigned to that particular work unit. Some work units may need to be combined because of low frequency. The percentage of time spent by a work unit can be calculated by dividing the time spent in each given work unit by total time. Standard time can be obtained by dividing the time recorded for a work unit by its number output.

WORKLOAD MONITORING

Once standards are established, they can be applied to future or past output frequency data. All outputs are evaluated separately. The standard time taken to perform an output is multiplied by the standard time required to perform the work. Each output type is weighted in this fashion and added to all the others to yield total variable time for a given period. All allowances for constant time (allowances) are added to the variable time to yield resulting personnel time required.

A labor utilization ratio can be established by dividing the total personnel time required by staffing time worked. A percentage of 100 represents adequate staffing for a given workload with employees working at a normal pace. A percentage of greater than 100 represents inadequate staffing, which causes employees to work at a faster than normal pace, possibly omitting breaks and lunches or taking inadequate personal fatigue time. A percentage of less than 100 represents excessive staffing, which results in excessive time being utilized to complete work assignments, to partake in extended breaks or lunches, or to recover from fatigue.

Control limits for utilization percentages should be established to define acceptable and unacceptable variance. For example, labor utilization ratios within 95-105 could be defined as acceptable, while any labor utilization ratios

above or below these limits would be unacceptable and should result in some investigation or staffing changes. Control limits can be established arbitrarily by means of trial and error or statistical techniques.

The utilization ratio can be plotted on a daily basis (Figure 9.11) and can be analyzed weekly, monthly, or quarterly. This ratio can be plotted against man-minutes scheduled and percent utilization by day of the week (Figs. 9.12 and 9.13). These plots help to indicate whether personnel are being scheduled optimally. Other plots of the percent utilization ratio vs patient census, intensity indicators, census, admission, and number of prescription orders can be obtained and analyzed for correlations for predicting pharmacy workload.

REVIEW OF LITERATURE

Many different work measurement techniques have been used to determine time spent performing hospital pharmacy tasks. Examples of studies utilizing self-reporting (20,21), work sampling (22-36), stopwatch time study (36-51), and predetermined data (40,53,54) can be found in the hospital pharmacy literature. Self-reporting has been used to establish measurable and nonmeasurable workloads (20) and to develop a workload monitoring system (21). Work sampling has been used for the following purposes: establish less than optimal utilization of pharmacist time (22-23); establish the use of technicians; compare nursing time for medication-related activities in centralized and decentralized pharmacy systems (24); examine system changes in an IV additive area (25); establish the impact of computer system implementation (26,27); establish time spent in clinical pharmacy activities (28); compare staffing patterns (29); analyze an

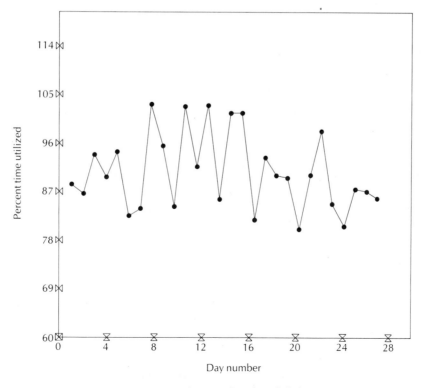

FIGURE 9.11 Utilization plotted on daily basis.

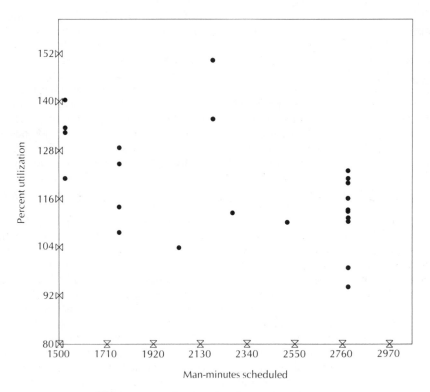

FIGURE 9.12 Utilization plotted against man-minutes.

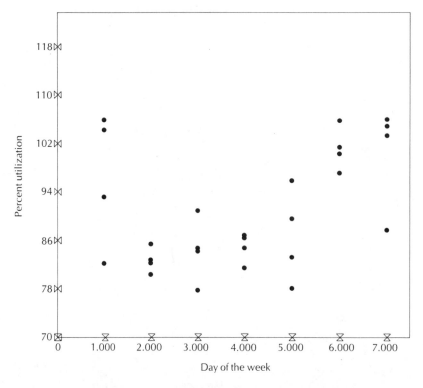

FIGURE 9.13 Utilization plotted against day of week.

outpatient pharmacy operation (30); document the usefulness of technicians (31); ascertain personnel activities and costs associated with decentralized and centralized unit dose distribution systems (32); establish relationship between staffing patterns and variations in the mix of professional and nonprofessional functions by pharmacists and technicians (33); compare the activities of decentralized pharmacists engaged in medication administration as well as in medication order transcription, rounding with physicians, and unit dose cart upkeep (34); and establish technician manpower requirements for a unit dose distribution system (35). Stopwatch time study has been used for the following: measure time differences in the handling of medications between unit dose and non–unit dose packaging (37); project staffing patterns for a centralized IV admixture program (38); ascertain the time required for unit dose packaging of respiratory therapy solutions (39); measure time used to prepare IV additives (40-43); establish the costs involved in distribution of controlled substances (44); compare the time spent filling unit dose carts among various workplace designs (45); measure the time involved in production and distributive tasks (46); establish differences in medication delivery times for centralized and decentralized unit dose systems (47); ascertain the costs associated with different IV infusion systems (48); evaluate differences in workload activities between centralized and mobile decentralized unit dose systems (49); and establish workload measurement and monitoring systems (46,50,51).

Workload monitoring systems have been developed using standards established by estimates and supervisory observation (52); stopwatch time studies and estimates (46); self-reporting (20,21); predetermined data (53,54); and self-reported work sampling (55).

A controversy exists regarding the use of fixed and variable work sampling observations. In a community pharmacy, Dickson (56) found no differences between the two methodologies. However, the study was conducted in an outpatient setting, where the work is more cyclical than in an inpatient hospital pharmacy.

CONCLUSION

Work measurement can be a valuable tool for pharmacy managers, facilitating the equitable allocation of personnel resources. This tool, although valuable, is imprecise, and therefore should not be abused. At all times, managers must be aware of the human approach to management.

REFERENCES

1. International Labor Office: *Introduction to Work Study.* Geneva, Switzerland, Atar, 1967.
2. Mundel ME: *Motion and Time Study.* Englewood Cliffs, NJ, Prentice-Hall, 1978.
3. Heiland RE, Richardson, WJ: *Work Sampling.* New York, McGraw-Hill, 1957.
4. Niebel BW: *Motion and Time Study.* Homewood, IL, Irwin, 1982.
5. Hansen BL: *Work Sampling.* Englewood Cliffs, NJ, Prentice-Hall, 1960.
6. Barnes RM: *Work Sampling.* New York, John Wiley & Sons, 1957.
7. Allen DS: Multiple activity work study needs x samples. *J Indust Engineer* 30:79, December 1979.

8. Conway RW: Some statistical considerations in work sampling, *J Indust Engineer* 8:107, March/April 1957.
9. Whitmore DA: *Measurement and Control of Indirect Work.* New York, American Elsevier, 1971.
10. Krick EV: *Methods Engineering.* New York, John Wiley & Sons, 1962.
11. Fein M: How "Reliability," "precision," and "accuracy" refer to use of work measurement data." *J Indust Engineer* 32:26, July 1981.
12. Moder JJ: Activity sampling with applications to time standards estimation. *J Indust Engineer* 18:24, January 1967.
13. Whithouse GE, Washburn DA: Work sampling analyzer. *J Industr Engineer* 32:22, April 1981.
14. Whitehouse GE, Washburn DA: Work sampling observation generator. *J Industr Engineer* 32:16, March 1981.
15. Haines IL: Work sampling by fixed interval study. *J Indust Engineer* 9:266, July/August 1958.
16. Barnes RM, Andrew RB: Performance sampling in work measurement, *J Indust Engineer* 6:8, November/December 1955.
17. Kargar DW, Bayha FH: *Engineered Work Measurement.* New York, Industrial Press, 1977.
18. Brisley CL, Fiedler WF: Balancing cost and accuracy in setting up standards for work measurement. *J Indust Engineer* 33:82, May 1982.
19. Nadler G: *Motion and Time Study.* New York, McGraw-Hill, 1955.
20. Rothenbuhler EF, Archambault GF: A preliminary study based on total departmental measurable and non-measurable workloads. *Am J Hosp Pharm* 19:163, 1962.
21. Mackewicz DW: Developing a workload measurement system for a decentralized hospital pharmacy service. *Top Hosp Pharm Mgt* 2(4):22, 1983.
22. Summerfield MR, Go HT, Lamy PP, Derewicz HJ: Determining staffing requirements in institutional pharmacy. *Am J Hosp Pharm* 35:1487, 1978.
23. Dipiro JT, Grovsse GC, Kubica AJ: Work sampling to evaluate staff pharmacist productivity. *Am J Hosp Pharm* 36:201, 1979.
24. Wodd WB, Blissenbach TJ: Medication-related nursing time in centralized and decentralized drug distribution. *Am J Hosp Pharm* 41:477, 1984.
25. Sebastian G, Thielke TS: Work analysis of an admixture service. *Am J Hosp Pharm* 40:2149, 1983.
26. Sikoria RG, Kotazan JA: Analysis of the change in work patterns following installation of an inpatient pharmacy computer. *Contemp Pharm Pract* 4:160, 1981.
27. Kohout TW, Broekemeier RL, Daniels CE: Work-sampling evaluation of an upgraded outpatient pharmacy computer system. *Am J Hosp Pharm* 40:606, 1983.
28. Nelson AN, Gourley DR, Tindall WN, Anderson RJ: Task analysis of a pharmacist's activities in a 45-bed rural hospital with comprehensive pharmaceutical services. *Am J Hosp Pharm* 33:38, 1976.
29. Strandberg LR, Smith MC, Sanger JM: A method for comparing hospital pharmacy staffing patterns. *Top Hosp Pharm Mgt* 2(3):27, 1982.
30. Roberts MJ, Kvalseth TO, Jermstad RL: Work measurement in hospital pharmacy. *Top Hosp Pharm Mgt* 2(2):1, 1982.
31. Barker KN, Smith MC, Winter ER: The work of the hospital pharmacist and the potential use of auxiliaries. *Am J Hosp Pharm* 29:35, 1972.
32. John GW, Burchart VD, Lamy PP: Pharmacy personnel activities and costs in decentralized and centralized unit dose drug distribution systems. *Am J Hosp Pharm* 33:38, 1976.
33. Dostal MM, Daniels CE, Roberts MJ, Giese RM: Pharmacist activities under alternative staffing arrangements. *Am J Hosp Pharm* 39:2098, 1982.
34. Thielke TS: Activity analysis of clinical pharmacist. *Am J Hosp Pharm* 28:704, 1971.
35. Johnston LJ: Using a work sampling study. *Hosp Pharm* 7:313, 1972.
36. Segall EL, Kotzan JA: Comparison of two methods of observing work areas in a hospital pharmacy. *Am J Hosp Pharm* 36:59, 1979.
37. Blasingame WG, Drevno H, Godley LF, et al: Some time and motion consideration with single-unit packaged drugs in five hospitals. *Am J Hosp Pharm* 26:310, 1969.
38. Sherrin PT, Miller WA, Latiolais CJ: Projecting staffing patterns from time study data in centralized intravenous admixture programs. *Am J Hosp Pharm* 29:1013, 1972.

39. Read OK: Unit dose packaging of respiratory therapy solutions. *Am J Hosp Pharm* 32:49, 1975.

40. Alligson RR, Stach PE, Sherrin TP, Latiolais CJ: Compounding times and contamination rates associated with the preparation of intravenous admixtures in three types of plastic containers. *Am J Hosp Pharm* 36:513, 1979.

41. Pohorylo EM, Lewis EM, Anderson ER: Time and cost comparison of four methods of filling piggyback bottles. *Am J Hosp Pharm* 40:87, 1983.

42. Gordon AY, Willcox GS, Jeffrey LP: Effectiveness of a volumetric pump for preparing sterile products. *Am J Hosp Pharm* 40:821, 1983.

43. Markowsky SJ, Kitrenos JG: Comparison of six methods for preparing cefazolin sodium for intermittent injection. *Am J Hosp Pharm* 40:1653, 1983.

44. Norwell MJ, McAllister JC, Bailey E: Cost analysis of drug distribution for controlled substances. *Am J Hosp Pharm* 40:801, 1983.

45. MacPherson DR, Brown TR, Nothern RE: Function-structure relationship and unit dose dispensing: a time study. *Am J Hosp Pharm* 30:1034, 1973.

46. Toohey JB, Herrick JD, Trautman RT: Adaptation of a workload measurement system. *Am J Hosp Pharm* 39:999, 1982.

47. Reynolds DM, Johnson MH, Longe RL: Medication delivery time requirements in centralized and decentralized unit dose drug distribution systems. *Am J Hosp Pharm* 35:941, 1978.

48. Paxinos J, Hammel RJ, Fritz WL: Contamination rates and costs associated with the use of four intermittent intravenous infusion systems. *Am J Hosp Pharm* 36:1497, 1979.

49. Kvancz DA, Cummins BA, Bennett DL, Fontana LC: Evaluating pharmacist workload activities: Centralized versus mobile decentralized pharmacy service. *Top Hosp Pharm Mgt* 2(2):50, 1982.

50. Trudeau T: A simple work measurement system that can aid ineffective production planning. *Hosp Pharm* 15:229, 1980.

51. Hunt ML, Tuck BA, Adams CT: System to measure the use of pharmacy personnel. *Am J Hosp Pharm* 39:82, 1982.

52. Levin RH, Letcher KI, DeLeon RF, McCart GM: Patient-care unit system for measuring clinical and distributive pharmacy workload. *Am J Hosp Pharm* 34:969, 1980.

53. Hammel RJ, King CM, Jones TF: Administrative case study: Analysis of hospital pharmacy's manpower requirements. *Am J Hosp Pharm* 34:969, 1977.

54. Bartscht KG, Estrella MA, Rothenbahler EF: Pharmacy staffing methodology—a management tool. *Am J Hosp Pharm* 22:564, 1965.

55. Hudsall RS, Gourley DR, Anderson RJ, et al: Work sampling in contemporary pharmacy practice: A multidimensional approach. *Top Hosp Pharm Mgt* 2(3):15, 1982.

56. Dickson WM: Measuring pharmacist time use: A note on the use of fixed-interval work sampling. *Am J Hosp Pharm* 35:1241, 1978.

ADDITIONAL READING

Barnes RM: *Work Sampling.* New York, John Wiley & Sons, 1957.

Heiland RE, Richardson, WJ: *Work Sampling.* New York, McGraw-Hill, 1957.

Kargar DW, Bayha FH: *Engineered Work Measurement.* New York, Industrial Press, 1977.

Krick EV: *Methods Engineering.* New York, John Wiley & Sons, 1962.

Mundel ME: *Motion and Time Study.* Englewood Cliffs, NJ, Prentice-Hall, 1978.

Nadler G: *Motion and Time Study.* New York, McGraw-Hill, 1955.

Niebel BW: *Motion and Time Study.* Homewood, IL, Richard D Irwin, 1982.

CHAPTER 10

Employee Compensation

CHARLES E. MYERS

Employee compensation may be defined as anything of value given to an employee in exchange for his labor. The thing of value most often given, of course, is money in the form of wages, salaries, and bonuses. In hospital pharmacy practice, the principal monetary compensations offered are wages (money earned proportionate to the number of hours worked) or salaries (monetary compensations at predetermined, fixed amounts regardless of the number of hours worked). In general, managerial and professional employees receive salaries. Technical, clerical, and courier employees receive salaries, as well, but in some organizations may receive wages.

Some portions of wages and salaries may be paid to employees as overtime compensation. These represent payments for sustained labor in excess of certain predetermined hours per period. Because it is important for directors of pharmacy services to understand the legal constraints involving overtime compensation, this topic will be further examined later in the chapter.

Bonuses are monetary rewards for especially valuable and exceptionally good employee performance. Bonuses, while fairly common in profit-oriented, non–health care businesses, have not been utilized much in hospitals until recently. An increasing number of hospitals, however, now operate as investor-owned, profit-oriented enterprises and utilize bonuses as incentive rewards for managerial employees.

While money is the most common medium for employee compensation, numerous other compensations exist and are frequently used in hospitals. These compensations typically fall into ten broad categories: (1) relocation, (2) leave, (3) insurance, (4) education, (5) subsistence, (6) profit/ownership sharing, (7) discounts, (8) fitness/recreation, (9) transportation, and (10) pensions (1,2). These compensations will be described more fully later but are mentioned early to emphasize their relative importance in the overall compensations offered to employees. Once termed "fringe benefits" because of their relatively small proportion of overall employee compensations, such compensations may now represent 15-41% of the total cost of compensations paid by hospitals (2). They require substantial amounts of managerial attention.

Compensation management may be viewed as those managerial efforts devoted to the establishment and promulgation of goals, objectives, policies, and operating procedures relating to employee compensation. In hospitals, the overall responsibility for compensation management is generally centralized in a personnel or payroll department head or in a corporate-level executive who authorizes department heads such as the director of pharmacy services to execute various aspects of the overall compensation program within prescribed limits of freedom. Wage and salary boundaries for pharmacy technicians in a given hospital, for example, most likely would be established by an upper level compensation manager. The director of pharmacy services might be consulted regarding industry norms for technician compensation as those boundaries are initially defined. However, once established, the boundaries would function as constraints on the pharmacy director, although he might be offered some latitude within the boundaries for determining appropriate starting salaries or compensation advancement rates for specific employees. Non wage and salary benefits are generally established at hospital administrative or corporate levels without the input or control of directors of pharmacy services. Benefit programs are generally administered centrally, without the granting of discretionary freedoms to the pharmacy director.

Fundamental to the successful management of compensation is the understanding of the term "employee." The understanding is important, because those persons legally entitled to the designation will be due compensation from their employers. In hospital pharmacy practice, the determination of who is or is not an employee is seldom an issue. Generally, the determination would actually be made by the hospital's administration, corporate management, or legal counsel. The legal definition of an individual as an employee, however, may not always be as clear as one would expect, and it is therefore important to know the general legal views. In practical terms, most members of a hospital pharmacy staff will be readily identifiable as employees, since they receive wages or salaries from the hospital. Less clear, however, is the case of unpaid students present for clerkship experiences or the case of volunteer workers. Such questions, if they arise and are not answerable through the hospital's local U.S. Department of Labor office, may have to be determined by the courts according to the specific facts and circumstances in each case.

The general legal definitions, which will suffice for most routine determinations, include the following (3):

Employee. [a] A person in the service of another under any contract of hire, express or implied, oral or written, where the employer has the power or right to control and direct the employee in the material details of how the work is to be performed. . . . [b] Generally, when person for whom services are performed has right to control and direct individual and performs services not only as to result to be accomplished by work but also as to details and means by which result is accomplished, individual subject to direction is an "employee". . . . [c] "Servant" is synonymous with "employee". . . .

Executive employees. [a] Persons whose duties include some form of managerial authority, actually directing the work of others. . . . [b] persons whose duties relate to active participation in control, supervision and management of business, or who administer affairs, or who direct, manage, execute, or dispense. . . . [c] the term executive employee carries the idea of supervision of or control over ordinary employees. . . ."

Personnel expenses in hospital pharmacy practice are generally substantial, usually occupy the second position in overall department expense category rankings, and therefore demand much of a pharmacy director's control efforts. Unlike most other hospital departments, in which labor represents the single most expensive element in departmental expenses, hospital pharmacy departments must devote primary management attention to drug and supply expenses (4,5). Compensation management requires considerable attention, as pharmacy directors must seek to balance budgetary constraints with complex legal requirements, employee wishes, and issues of equity.

LEGAL REQUIREMENTS

The Civil Rights Acts and the Fair Labor Standards Act of 1938 (FLSA), its 1963 amendment involving equal pay on the basis of sex, and related regulations create the primary body of regulatory controls over compensation practices (6,7). In most hospitals, internal hospital policies will be established with a conscious aim toward conformity with these acts. The provisions of these acts are complex, however, and abundant opportunities exist for violations by unknowledgeable department heads. It is therefore important that directors of pharmacy services understand the acts and their requirements. The reader is cautioned that changes in the acts and labor regulations stemming from them may occur periodically. The Labor Department offices in the hospital's locale should be contacted for up-to-date copies of the acts and regulations, when the need arises.

Title VII of the Civil Rights Act of 1964, also known as the Equal Employment Opportunity Act of 1964, and subsequent amendments prohibit employment practices (including, e.g., compensation) that have the *effect* of discriminating among employees on the basis of race, color, religion, sex, or national origin. Predating those laws, are the Civil Rights Acts of 1866, 1870, and 1871, which prohibit discrimination in employment practices on the basis of race (6,8).

The amended FLSA addresses five broad topics: equal pay requirements regardless of sex, the employment of workers less than 18 years of age, minimum wages, overtime pay eligibility, and record-keeping requirements (2,9). The equal pay provisions apply to all executives, professionals, administrators, and other employees. The provisions require that men and women be compensated equally for equal work. Equal work is defined as work requiring equal skill, effort, and responsibility under similar working conditions. Men and women may be compensated unequally if the unequalness is based on a seniority system, a merit reward system, a pay system in which earnings are proportionate to the quantity or quality of production, or a differential based on some factor other than sex (e.g., a night-shift differential). These conditions constitute what are known as the "four affirmative defenses" of the equal pay provision. All of the exemptions, if used, must be applied equally to men and women (7).

The FLSA prohibits the hiring of individuals less than 18 years of age if the work they are to perform is hazardous. The hiring of individuals who are 14 and 15 years of age is permitted, but only outside of normal school hours. With the exception of child actors, persons who are 12 and 13 years of age may be hired only by parents for agricultural work outside of normal school hours. Although hospitals often utilize minors for volunteer activities, most do not actually hire them, despite freedom to do so under the FLSA. Hospitals generally have been reluctant to hire minors, since the responsibilities inherent in the care of patients, the potential for harm, and the relative unaccountability of minors might increase legal liabilities.

Under the FLSA, all employees not specifically exempted must be paid at least a minimum wage. The minimum wage rate is revised periodically according to a schedule specified in the statute. The current minimum wage level may be determined through the hospital's local Labor Department office. In some states, state minimum wage rates may exceed the federal rate, in which case the higher rate must be paid. If the hospital supplies room, board, or lodging, their value may be computed, and corresponding adjustments may be made in the minimum pay provided to employees. Student assistants may be paid at less than the minimum wage rate via a special exemption through the Wage and Hour Division of the Department of Labor (2,6,7).

Under the FLSA, a normal workweek is defined as a period of 168 hours during seven consecutive 24-hour periods. All employees not specifically exempted must be paid at 150% of regular pay for all hours worked in excess of 40 hours during each workweek. Hospitals are permitted an exception to this rule. If they choose, they may establish 14-day pay periods instead of "workweeks" and must then pay overtime to nonexempt employees at 150% of regular pay for all hours worked in excess of 80 hours during the period. This option, if chosen, is permanent and carries with it the added requirement that the 150% overtime rate will apply to any hours worked in excess of 8 hours per day, whether or not 80 hours are exceeded for the overall period (2,9). The option may be applied to some departments at the same time that it is not applied to others.

There is no requirement that an employee's normal workweek be 40 hours in length or that overtime (at 150%) be paid for hours worked beyond the normal workweek but less than 40. If, for example, a nonexempt employee's normally scheduled workweek is 38 hours long, and if on some occasion the employee is required to work 42 hours within a workweek, the hospital will be expected to compensate the employee at a regular pay rate for the thirty-ninth and fortieth hours and at a 150% rate for the forty-first and forty-second hours.

Compensation practices may be used as evidence regarding the wage vs salary designation of an employee. If an organization normally pays what it regards as a salaried, exempt employee for hours worked beyond some normal workweek, the employee may, in legal fact, be found to be a nonexempt, wage-earning ("hourly") employee and therefore eligible for the 150% overtime rate (6).

The calculation of overtime pay is relatively simple for wage-earning ("hourly") employees. Their wage rates per hour should be a matter of record in the hospital's payroll and personnel files. For salaried, nonexempt personnel, however, the salary per hour in overtime calculations must be derived by a specific procedure in order to account for the fact that all months are not of the same length. To derive the rate per hour, multiply the employee's monthly salary by 12. Divide the answer by 52. Divide that answer by the number of hours normally worked per week by the employee (2). This arithmetic procedure presumes employment year-round. If faced with seasonal employment, such as for summer interns or "9-month" faculty members or teachers, the "52" in the procedure must be altered to reflect the normal number of weeks of employment per year.

Certain employees are exempted from the minimum wage and overtime requirements of the FLSA. Exempt employees fall into three categories and must meet certain criteria in order for employers to include them in the categories. Exempt are executives, administrative employees, and professionals. In order to be defined as an executive, an individual must meet six tests: (1) Fifty percent or more of the employee's time must be devoted to management of the organization or one of its major subdivisions, such as a department. This is known as the "primary duty" test. It is possible for an individual's primary duty to be management or his attention to be devoted so significantly to management that he meets the first test even if he devotes less than 50% of his time to the activity. The distinction can become unclear, however, if the individual occasionally performs nonexecutive work—e.g., a director of pharmacy services who performs in an executive capacity Monday through Friday during the day but who occasionally works a night or weekend shift in his own pharmacy department as a dispensing staff member.

The "wage" rate of the director relative to other dispensing staff members then becomes important to the Department of Labor in deciding whether the pharmacist is, in fact, an executive who occasionally dispenses or a staff pharmacist who earns slightly more than others in exchange for some managerial responsibility. In the former case, he would be exempt; in the latter, he would not. (2) No more than 40% of the employee's work can be of the "nonexempt" nature. (3) The employee must supervise at least two full-time employees. (4) The employee must possess the authority to hire and dismiss or effectively to recommend

hirings or dismissals. The recommendation power of the individual must be substantial and carry (or very nearly carry) the weight of decision. (5) The employee must customarily and regularly exercise discretionary power in his decisions. (6) The employee must be paid at least $155 per week on a salaried basis by the employer. Grant-supported employees may actually be seen as employees of the grantor and thus may be ineligible for exempt status in the hospital (6,7).

Five tests must be met for an employee to be exempted as administrative: (1) The employee's primary duties must be either responsible office or nonmanual work directly related to management or business operation or responsible work directly related to academic instruction or training carried on in administering the educational effort—e.g., pharmacy school faculty members working in a hospital. (2) The employee must customarily and regularly exercise discretionary power in his decisions. (3) The employee must regularly assist a bona fide executive or administrative employee, perform work only under general supervision, and execute special assignments only under general supervision. (4) No more than 40% of the employee's work can be of the "nonexempt" nature. (5) The employee must be paid at least $155 per week on a salaried basis by the employer. A slightly different rule applies to academic administrative employees. The salary must be at least $155 or a salary equivalent to the prevailing entrance for similar work in that academic institution (6,7).

A professional employee may be exempt if he meets the following tests: (1) The employer must be paid at least $170 per week. (2) The employer must meet the primary duty test relating to the proportion of his time devoted to professional activities. (3) The employee must meet the discretionary power test related to professional decisions. (4) No more than 20% of the employee's work can be of the "nonexempt" nature. Generally, to qualify for a professional exemption, the individual would need to possess a license or certificate and would have to be a graduate of an advanced study program in a field of science. A short test of $250 per week plus the discretionary power and primary duty requirements may also be used to determine professional employees (6,7). For staff pharmacists, the distinction between an exempt vs nonexempt designation is not generally difficult, since most of them earn in excess of $250 per week and meet the primary duty and discretionary power tests.

In most hospitals, staff pharmacists are exempt, as are hospital pharmacy residents. Department heads and assistant and associate-level employees in hospital pharmacy departments are generally exempt. Less certain and more dependent on the individual circumstances and tests is the exempt status of pharmacist supervisors, purchasing agents, or administrative assistants. Technicians, secretaries, receptionists, clerks, and couriers are not exempt (6). There is no FLSA requirement that overtime be paid (at any rate) to exempt professional, administrative, or executive employees. However, in many hospitals, staff pharmacists and supervisors are—by internal institutional policy—paid overtime at a regular (100%) rate (or some other rate) for hours worked beyond the normal workweek.

Compensation records required under the FLSA will, in most hospitals, be maintained by a payroll department. The following records must be maintained (2):

1. Employee name, address, occupation, and sex
2. Hour and day when workweek begins
3. Total hours worked each workday and workweek
4. Total basic pay on daily or weekly basis
5. Regular hourly pay rate for any week when the employee works overtime
6. Total overtime pay for the workweek
7. Deductions from or additions to wages
8. Total wages paid during the pay period
9. Date of payment and pay period covered
10. Special information when uncommon pay arrangements exist, or when board, lodging, or other facilities are counted as part of pay

In addition to the federal statutes discussed, state laws and regulations may affect compensation procedures. Some states, for example, stipulate the frequency of pay for both salaried and wage-earning employees. Some states stipulate the maximal number of consecutive workdays permitted for employees and allow employees to choose particular days of the week to have off as rest days. Local Labor Department rules should be investigated to determine such requirements.

NONMONETARY COMPENSATIONS

Nonmonetary compensations vary widely by institution. Most institutions offer several nonmonetary compensations and expand them from time to time, depending on economic circumstances and perceptions of recruitment and retention competition from other employers. Once established as benefits, these compensations are seldom reduced or discontinued except in the severest of economic circumstances. Alterations in the mix of benefits may occur, however, if economic pressures or employee preferences change. In cases in which the hospital forms formal contracts with collective bargaining groups, benefit packages are more likely to become topics of extensive negotiation.

A flexible benefit approach is utilized by many hospitals. Central to the approach is the concept that not all employees may prefer the same mix of benefits and that, as long as the dollar value of benefits given to employees is equivalent, then employees may be permitted some personal choice in the benefits to be received. Three flexible benefit plans typically are seen: core cafeteria, buffet, and alternative dinners (10).

A core cafeteria plan provides a consistent set of specific benefits to all employees. In addition, it offers employees the freedom to supplement those core elements with expansions of those elements (10). Within the core, for example, an employee might be offered 2 weeks of annual vacation time and $10,000 in life insurance. If the employee wishes, he might choose to keep his insurance at the $10,000 level and to expand his annual vacation allowance to 3 weeks. As an alternative, he might keep his vacation allowance at 2 weeks and expand his life insurance to $12,000.

A buffet plan is more flexible than the core cafeteria plan. In the core cafeteria plan, there is a certain minimal level of each benefit that each employee will receive. In the buffet plan, employees are permitted to reduce the levels of some of the benefits offered in exchange for increases in others (10). In the extreme, an employee could choose to have zero life insurance benefits in exchange for higher benefits of other kinds.

An alternative dinners plan resembles the core cafeteria plan except that the employer offers the employee several alternative mixes within the core and then allows the employee to add to the chosen mix with expansion options (10). One mix, for example, might be made up of life insurance, vacation time, and educational leave. Another might consist of health insurance, child care, and sick leave. Employees are allowed to choose only one of the mixes.

Common to most of the flexible plans in hospitals is the permission for employees to alter their choices from time to time. The pricing of the various benefit components is difficult, however, and prices would vary with market conditions. Frequent changes therefore are usually not permitted, as these would be expensive to administer.

The first non wage and salary benefit an employee may receive from a hospital employer may be relocation assistance. This may take the form of paid moving expenses, real estate searches, and paid reestablishment expenses (e.g., moves of licenses, real estate closing costs, startup deposits for utility services, or school enrollment fees). The degree of relocation assistance varies widely by institution. In some hospitals, the benefit is not available at all. In some, relocation benefits may be limited to moves within corporate operations; e.g., a move from one hospital in an investor-owned chain of hospitals to another hospital within the same chain. In most hospitals, relocation benefits are offered to executive, administrative, and some professional personnel.

A major category of benefits is leave. Leave is paid time away from work. Leave may occur for many reasons, including vacation, personal illness, family illness, education, childbearing, family bereavement, holidays, court attendance, public affairs, and professional office. Leave is an attractive benefit to most employees and poses both opportunities and hazards to pharmacy directors. For those employees to whom leave is desirable, the benefit can be an opportunity for the manager. Leave, in addition to being a routine benefit, can be expanded as a reward for good performance. Leave can also be problematic. It is a particularly visible benefit and one especially sensitive to employee perceptions of inequity. If not administered in a manner that employees perceive to be fair and evenhanded, leave policies can become morale destructive and major topics for disagreement.

Insurance is a common type of benefit. Four types are seen most often: (1) health, (2) dental, (3) life, and (4) indemnity. Health insurance typically pays for medical expenses associated with hospitalization and often ambulatory medical care. The degree of insurance coverage varies widely among institutions and underwriters. In some hospitals, health-insurance plans include coverage for dental expenses. In others, separate dental insurance plans exist, often underwritten by different insurance firms. Life insurance may be of the whole or term type. In the case of whole-life policies, the insured accumulates and permanently owns some of the assets invested. In term policies, the insured does not accumulate retrievable assets. Most hospital-purchased life insurance offered as an employee benefit is of the term type. Some hospitals offer other indemnity insurance, which is intended to recompense a "victim" for some loss. Insurance may be provided for an incurred disability that interferes with an employee's ability to perform his work, for example. Such insurance might pay the insured for wages lost because of extended work absence secondary to major illness or an accident.

Educational benefits may be temporary or ongoing. For example, employees may be provided extensive, one-time blocks of full-time, paid leave to pursue specific education or training expected to be especially valuable to the organization. A hospital pharmacy initiating a major computer system, for instance, might wish to enroll its intended system manager in a tuition-paid, full-time program of study to prepare for implementing or managing the system. More commonly, staff members who might benefit from continuing education or refresher education are allowed leave or hospital-paid registration at seminars or courses. In some hospitals, educational leave serves less as a benefit than as a reward for good performance and is made available only to those who "earn" it. When used in its broadest form as a benefit or reward, the nature of education benefits need not be organization related. A pharmacy technician might be allowed to enroll in a course at a local community college at hospital expense to study real estate sales or automobile repairs, for example. Such benefits may be ongoing in the sense that within prescribed limits, employees may be allowed to enroll repeatedly in courses or seminars over time.

Subsistence benefits are generally of two types: allowances for meals on the job and allowances for meals, travel, and lodging when an employee must travel to perform work for the hospital. A pharmacist on educational leave to attend an out-of-town national professional seminar will often receive a subsistence allowance for expenses associated with his attendance. Although less common than it used to be, some hospitals provide a meal per day to working employees at no out-of-pocket charge to the employee.

Profit sharing or ownership sharing is a benefit that may be made available to employees of corporate, for-profit hospitals. The benefit is generally made available in the form of the privilege to purchase shares of stock in the corporation or options to purchase shares in the future at guaranteed discounts.

Discounts are price reductions offered to employees for services or products available through the employing organization. Hospitals may offer discounts to employees for things such as medical-surgical supplies or equipment, prescription drugs, or other inpatient or outpatient services.

Hospitals may directly offer employees fitness and recreation facilities such as gymnasiums, swimming pools, aerobic exercise centers, muscle development centers, or racquet game courts. These are sometimes associated with fitness-monitoring services such as stress-testing laboratories.

Transportation benefits usually take the form of free or discounted parking privileges and are more commonly offered by hospitals in suburban sites than in urban areas. The benefits are usually extended to all employees but for selected employees may have "VIP" features such as reserved parking spaces associated with them.

Pensions, or retirement plans, are designed to provide income to employees after their retirement. They also delay the receipt of income and, presuming continual escalations in tax rates over time and tax allowances for retirees, they shelter income from taxation. Pension benefits are sometimes offered in the form of profit sharing and stock options, described earlier. Pension plans vary in their sources of funds. In some, the contributions are provided exclusively by the hospital. In others, both the employee and the employer contribute. The right of an employee to take with him the investments in his pension account on his leaving the hospital *before* retirement is termed "vesting." In some pension plans, all of the employee's pension account is vested dating from his initial hiring. In other plans, vesting begins only after a certain period of employment, or the proportion vested grows with the employee's length of employment.

EQUITY AND COMPRESSION

Two compensation problems that inevitably require attention from pharmacy directors and others responsible for compensation management are issues of perceived inequity and pay compression. The equity issues are of three types. These, along with pay compression problems, often require rather different management activities and efforts. Sometimes, irreconcilable objectives relating to these problems must be blended to create less than optimal overall solutions.

The three types of equity issues with which compensation managers must content are external, internal, and individual. External equity is the perception by employees that, relative to others outside the hospital in similar jobs or jobs requiring similar skills or knowledge, they are being paid at comparable levels (2). The most common external equity issue faced by a hospital pharmacy director is a perception by his staff pharmacists that they could work in staff positions in many community pharmacies (particularly chains) or possibly at other area hospitals at higher salaries. If the perception of inequity becomes severe enough, the hospital may lose pharmacists or be unable to recruit new ones. Salary adjustments may have to be made eventually.

Internal equity is the perception that, relative to others inside the hospital (particularly in other departments), one is being compensated comparably (2). This issue is common among pharmacy technicians. Technicians may compare their work hours, job duties, and pay levels with those in other groups, including laboratory technicians, radiology technicians, licensed practical nurses, clerical personnel, orderlies, and various other "assistant" classifications. Perceptions of inequity will create pressures on the pharmacy director to seek salary revisions and, if unaddressed, may lead to various secondary expressions of discontent such as deterioration in work volumes or work quality or increased absence.

Individual equity can be the most managerially troublesome and time-consuming of all the equity issues. Individual equity is the perception by an individual employee that his compensation is appropriate for his absolute worth and relative contribution to the organization (2). Inevitably, the individual measures the adequacy and "rightness" of his compensation relative to that of fellow workers doing essentially identical work. The opportunity for perception of inequity is particularly high in organizations that utilize performance-based compensation systems. Among staff pharmacists, perceptions of individual inequity are easily aroused if positions involving certain duties are compensated differently compared to others. In some hospitals, for example, pharmacists whose practices are related primarily to drug distribution systems may not be paid at the same level as those practicing in more clinical roles. The comparable worth of such duties is not easy to determine, and the conflicting temptation to base individual compensation differences strictly on the education and training credentials of employees poses inevitable problems. Over the next 15-20 years, as hospital pharmacy practice is infused with more and more pharmacists with nonbaccalaureate degrees and residency experience, it is highly likely that individuals with very different education and training credentials and experience backgrounds will be expected to perform similar duties (and vice versa). A compensation policy assigning salaries purely on the basis of either duties alone or credentials alone ultimately might be problematic.

As may be readily seen, an adjustment of one individual's salary to resolve a specific individual equity problem may lead to the creation of an inequity perception by a different worker. A change in salary levels for laboratory technicians, for example, might lead to the development of internal inequity perceptions by pharmacy technicians. An improvement in pharmacist salaries at hospital *A* might lead to an external inequity perception by pharmacists at hospital *B*.

An additional factor that may aggravate and increase the incidence of equity issues is pay compression. Hospitals in remote locations and hospitals with highly specialized pharmacy services may have to pay premium salaries to attract pharmacists, particularly during inflationary periods when relocation expenses are substantial. Often, the necessary starting salaries match or exceed the salaries to which existing staff members have advanced only after years of dedicated service. If discovered by existing staff, the salaries of the new staff members may stimulate perceptions of individual inequities. The phenomenon of the newer employees' salaries rapidly approaching that of employees in higher grades or that of employees with greater seniority is termed "pay compression" (11). It is common in most businesses during inflationary periods and in organizations inattentive to external developments in salary levels among comparable groups.

Issues of equity and pay compression appear to be somewhat inevitable. In some institutions, as a mechanism intended to minimize the necessity to deal with the issues, a policy of pay secrecy exists. The premise behind the policy is that if employees lack the evidence of inequities, inequity perceptions will not be created, and management will not have to respond to the related problems. The premise may be flawed. There is no assurance that employees will assume that equity exists, even in the absence of contrary evidence. A policy toward openness regarding compensation infor-

mation is intuitively attractive, but managers must be prepared for the fact that revealing one set of facts generally leads to requests for others. With each release of information, the potential exists for various types of inequity perceptions. Even more troublesome, a return to secrecy following a previous policy of openness would likely be interpreted with suspicion and distrust. In deciding on a policy of openness, managers must balance, on the one hand, the benefits to be derived from such a policy, and on the other, the expense and hazards associated with it. Managers who choose a policy of openness must be prepared to devote substantial amounts of time to conferences with individual employees and must possess good interpersonal skills to deal tactfully and honestly with questions of equity. Hospital compensation managers are especially sensitive to the harmful potential of inequitable treatment of employees and therefore strive to create systems that ensure equitable and objectively defensible decisions.

JOB ANALYSIS, EVALUATION, AND PRICING

Given sufficient time in most organizations, problems of pay compression and equity will eventually stimulate a general reassessment of the entire wage and salary structure and hierarchy. A systematic means of accomplishing this is needed. Similarly, if one were the first director of pharmacy services charged with the responsibility of establishing a salary and wage structure for pharmacy personnel in a new hospital, some organized means would be needed to do it. The new pharmacy director could, of course, simply duplicate the structure used in some other hospital, but he would have no assurance that that structure was free from internal or external equity flaws. Therefore, the need for some structured analysis would still exist.

A comprehensive analysis would generally consist of three parts: a job analysis, a job evaluation, and pricing. Job analysis is a process by which the content of jobs is defined. The outcome of the analysis is a set of job descriptions. Job evaluation is a process by which the relative worth of various work assignments is determined. Pricing is the actual selection of wages and salaries to be assigned to the various jobs (2,7).

A full description of the analysis, evaluation, and pricing process is beyond the scope of this chapter, but some broad elements will be discussed. The reader is referred to any up-to-date textbook on compensation management for further details (2,7).

The creation or revision of job descriptions for existing personnel may proceed by any of several different methods, including interviews with workers and supervisors, observation of the work performed, questionnaires, logs or diaries completed by workers, checklists, or combinations of these. The analysis, once completed, should specify why the job is performed; what tasks are performed in the job; which tasks are the most critical; what knowledge and skills are needed to perform the tasks; what results are expected and will be used as criteria for performance appraisal; what the job's physical, emotional, and intellectual demands are; and what the health and safety risks are for the employee. Numerous standardized questionnaire and data interpretation tools have been developed to assist in job analysis, including the Job Analysis Questionnaire, the Position Analysis Questionnaire, the Department of Labor Methodology, the Functional Job Analysis, and the Critical Incident Technique (2,7).

With job descriptions in hand, job evaluation can proceed. Four approaches are commonly used: ranking, classification, factor comparison, and the point factor method. The ranking method is the simplest, but is vulnerable to great subjectivity. Some group, usually an upper management group, simply arranges all the job descriptions in a rank order from most valuable to least valuable. The classification method creates an arbitrary number of groupings of jobs (15, for example) and broadly defines them relative to several elements thought to be important, e.g., complexity, degree of supervisory responsibility, or degree of public contact. The individual job descriptions are then sorted into the various classes on the basis of those elements (2,7). Wages and salaries are later assigned, not to the particular jobs, but to the classes. All jobs in a particular class would be allocated the same wage or salary scale.

In the factor comparison method, certain aspects of jobs are compared among jobs and, relative to those aspects, the jobs are ranked. Five job aspects typically are used as ranking factors: working conditions, responsibility, skills required, physical requirements, and mental requirements. The method is complex and requires that the jobs be weighted in some manner (usually by the average market wage for such a job) in order to arrive at an overall ranking (2,7). The use of market rates as weighting factors may appear to involve circuitous logic. Job evaluation is expected to be an enabling step leading to objective pricing of jobs. Starting from a premise that current or past market prices for the same jobs should determine or influence future prices tends to perpetuate existing rankings of the jobs. On the other hand, there may be no practical alternative, as the hospital will, in the end, have to compete against other hospitals to fill its positions. To do so, the hospital's wage and salary structure will have to be somewhat comparable to that of competitors.

The point factor method is the most common. Factors of value in each job are listed. The list of factors may be quite lengthy and may include a wide variety of elements. An arbitrary number of maximal points is specified for the list overall, and then points are assigned to the individual factors, totaling to the maximum (2,7). To minimize the influence of individual subjectivity, point allocations can be obtained from numerous employees, supervisors, employers, or "customers" (e.g., patients) to determine collective norms for the perceived importance and compensable worth of the various factors. Jobs with overall high point scores would be ranked higher in a compensation schedule than others. Several commercial job evaluation systems are available, including the Hay system, the National Position Evaluation Plan, EVALUCOMP, and the Position Analysis Questionnaire. The systems differ somewhat in the factors evaluated and the degree to which they ensure internal and external equity (2,7).

Following the ranking of jobs, pricing can occur with some confidence that the relative worth of the jobs will be reflected in the wages and salaries assigned. Prevailing market prices will therefore influence the assignments markedly. It is common to establish for each job a predecided range, i.e., a minimum starting salary and a maximum salary. The prevailing rate of competitors should fall somewhere within the range. Whether the competing rate falls near the bottom, in the middle, or near the top of the range depends on how competitive the institution is willing to be in providing attractive monetary and nonmonetary benefits. The breadth of the range and the size and number of the progressive increments through which employees may advance by raises will depend on the institution's strategic wishes relative to employee retention, development, and loyalty. An institution wishing to develop its employees, to create high employee loyalty, and to generate long-term employee retention will establish broader ranges, leaving employees considerable room for future pay advancement. The ranges for various jobs may overlap, so that, for example, a staff pharmacist with many years of seniority in a hospital might earn the same wage or salary as a new, inexperienced supervisor. Caution must be exercised in establishing the ranges to minimize such occurrences, as they pose particular opportunities for perceptions of individual inequity.

Information regarding prevailing wage and salary levels for various jobs is usually obtained through commercially available survey data, published survey data, or hospital-conducted surveys. To be most useful, data should be obtained from competing employers. Identifying the competing employers may not be easy, but it is essential for meaningful interpretation of survey data. For pharmacists, a hospital's competitors may be local community pharmacies, pharmaceutical research and production industries, industry sales forces, other local hospitals, regional medical centers and teaching-research hospitals, colleges of pharmacy, or some combination of these. For supportive pharmacy personnel, a hospital's competitors may be almost any businesses or service organizations that offer comparable wages, salaries, and benefits. These competitors are generally local.

Commercial surveys seldom include information regarding hospital pharmacists and, because of the wide diversity of specific recruitment markets for individual hospitals, such surveys are often of limited benefit. Similarly, unless elaborate in their regionalization and characterization of institutions surveyed and unless conducted over a large number of hospitals, published surveys are also usually less than ideal. The relative lack of specific data on pharmacy positions generally leads to some estimation based on the three survey sources described and on the relative ranking of pharmacy positions in job evaluation findings. The wages and salaries of other jobs specifically reported in surveys, plus the ranking of pharmacy jobs relative to them, yield estimated prices for the pharmacy positions. Two commercial surveys that *do* include data on hospital pharmacists are *Hospital Salary Survey Report* (published by John R. Zabka Associates, Hawthorne, N.J.) and *Hospital and Health Care Report* (published by Executive Compensation Service, Inc., Fort Lee, N.J.). The former lists data for the pharmacy directorship and is available to any health care practitioner. The latter lists data for the pharmacy directorship and for staff pharmacists. The report is available only to institutional purchasers. Each is published annually.

Published literature on hospital pharmacy wages and salaries is meager. Even less literature exists regarding nonmonetary benefits (12). The U.S. Bureau of Labor Statistics periodically publishes geographic area surveys, industry surveys, and national surveys of professional, administrative, technical, and clerical pay. At this writing (early 1984), the most recent of these that included data on hospital pharmacists was the *Industry Wage Survey: Hospitals and Nursing Homes, September 1978* (published in November 1980). The geographic area surveys do not list data regarding pharmacists. A separate Bureau of Labor Statistics report, based on 1981 data, ranked 247 occupations by their average weekly earnings. Hospital pharmacists were not listed separately; pharmacists in general were. They ranked twentieth on the list at $464 per week. Physicians ranked fourteenth at $501 per week (13).

In September 1981, 657 hospitals reported data showing that the annual salaries of hospital pharmacy directors varied considerably, depending on geographic location, hospital bed size, staff size, hospital ownership, size of city of location, and educational affiliation. By geographic region, the salaries ranged from $30,000-$40,000. By hospital bed size, the range was $30,000-$35,000. Governmental, nonfederal hospitals offered the lowest median salaries, at $30,000. Federal governmental hospitals offered the highest, at $36,000. In cities with populations of less than 20,000, the median salary of pharmacy directors was $29,062. In cities with more than 500,000, the median was $35,000. Nonteaching hospital pharmacy directors had the lowest median salaries at $30,000. Teaching hospitals instructing both medical and pharmacy students had the highest median directors' salaries of $36,000 (14).

A November 1982 survey of Michigan hospital pharmacists revealed average annual salaries of $28,792 for staff pharmacists, $31,712 for ''clinical'' pharmacists, and $32,023 for supervisory-level pharmacists (15). Medinger, Inc., reported a July 1982 national survey on 22 hospital positions, including directors of pharmacy services. The annual salaries of the directors varied by hospital bed size. In hospitals of 450 or more beds, they ranged from $33,000-$40,100. In hospitals of 350-500 beds, they ranged from $31,100-$36,300. In hospitals of 250 to 400 beds, they ranged from $32,500-$36,500. In hospitals with fewer than 300 beds, they ranged from $28,600-$35,700. The median salary of a pharmacy director was 49% of that of the median salary of hospital administrators (16). Cole Surveys, Inc., reported, in a June 30, 1982, survey that the director of pharmacy's annual salary varied by hospital revenue and ranged from a median of $26,000 in hospitals generating up to $7 million in annual revenue to $40,400 in hospitals generating over $80 million in revenue (17).

Hospital-conducted surveys are common and generally involve hospitals within a given competitive market. Surveys may be conducted by mail or by telephone. Surveys are usually more successful if they are easy to answer, are brief, and promise either absolute confidentiality or confidentiality among the respondents.

PERFORMANCE-BASED COMPENSATION

A performance-based compensation system is one in which employees individually receive compensation proportionate to the quality of their performance. The concept of compensation determined by employee performance is intuitively attractive. It appeals to the popular American cultural values of justice and earned rewards. Unfortunately, objective appraisal of employee performance is extremely difficult. When performance is judged subjectively or inconsistently and when the results then affect pay, the potential for perceptions of internal or individual inequity is substantial. Some cautions follow for pharmacy directors considering performance-based compensation policies.

A thorough discussion of performance appraisal in this chapter is not possible but, briefly stated, performance appraisal is an assessment or audit of what individual employees do and how well they do it. Appraisals most often are conducted by immediate supervisors, but can be conducted by peers or through self-appraisal by employees, or through some combination of these methods (18).

In some organizations, performance appraisal is designed to serve as a feedback tool to assist managers in coaching employees and to (hopefully) help employees to develop their knowledge and skills to their maximal potential. That objective may be achievable if certain procedural precautions are observed (18). However, when the results of performance appraisals conducted for coaching and development purposes are also used as the basis for pay decisions, problems occur. A major premise underlying a performance-based compensation plan is that all employees do not function at equivalent levels. If they *do,* then a performance-based plan is not needed. Thus, in the allocation of limited funds for monetary compensation, some employees will have to receive greater rewards than others. If the feedback, both formal and informal, provided to employees during performance appraisals does not correlate well with the monetary rewards received, perceptions of internal or individual inequity may be stimulated. There is evidence, as well, that negative feedback does not stimulate better performance (18). Additionally, employees who receive monetary rewards that are disappointingly small—even if small for the most uncontrollable reasons, such as general recessionary constraints, and even if employees lack specific knowledge of the monetary rewards given to fellow workers—may make mental connections between the rewards received and criticisms remembered from appraisal feedback. The eventual result is an erosion of trust in the appraisal process for coaching and developmental purposes and a regard of the process as being inextricably directed toward reward decisions. Moreover, if the appraisal occurs at a time considerably in advance of reward announcements, there is ample time for apprehension and anxiety to be generated in response to negative feedback received in the appraisal.

The burden of responding to inquiries or disputes regarding appraisal decisions and their ties to monetary rewards rests most heavily upon employees' immediate supervisors. Evidence exists that supervisors who know that appraisals will (or must) be shared with employees tend to avoid confrontations by inflating their ratings (18). Supervisors who know that appraisal results will be used in making compensation decisions may be even more reluctant to offer appraisals that would have adverse effects. Too often, appraisal results will then evolve to exhibit a flatness, except to identify employees whose performance is markedly substandard. What originally started out to be a system to reward excellence then *(presto!)* becomes a demerit system. Everyone receives an equivalent reward unless they perform poorly.

These problems may be reduced somewhat by utilizing two separate appraisals, one for development purposes, and another for compensation purposes. The potential exists, however, for employees to suspect that the two are not truly separated. In some organizations, compensation appraisals are not shared with employees (18). Another approach to performance-based compensation is to make reward differentations among employees nonmonetary in nature. In such an approach, employees would receive monetary compensation changes based on factors other than performance, e.g., seniority, or length of service. In addition, the extent of certain nonmonetary benefits would be flexible, depending on performance. This approach may also be the only practical way to continually reward excellent performance by employees who have risen to the ceiling wage or salary in their job class or pay grade.

SUMMARY

Employee compensation may take the form of monetary or nonmonetary rewards. Directors of pharmacy services in hospitals bear certain regulation-adherence and discretionary responsibilities for managing monetary and nonmonetary reward programs relating to their staff members. Overtime and minimum wage exemptions, under the FLSA, must be given particular attention. Nonmonetary benefit compensations vary widely among hospitals and are offered in varying degrees of flexibility. Pay compression and issues of external, internal, and individual equity create special, and to some extent inevitable, problems for pharmacy directors. These can be minimized or corrected somewhat by the careful use of job analysis, job evaluation, and job pricing methods. Job pricing may be assisted through the use of wage, salary, and benefit surveys. Performance-based compensation is associated with some special risks and must be managed carefully if these are to be minimized.

REFERENCES

1. Cunningham M: *Non-wage Benefits*. London, Pluto Press, 1981.
2. Wallace MJ, Fay CH: *Compensation Theory and Practice*. Boston, Kent, 1983.
3. Black HC: *Black's Law Dictionary*. St. Paul, MN, West, 1979.
4. Anon: Labor costs seen as culprit in rising hospital costs. *Trustee* 35:39-44, October 1982.
5. Deiner CH (ed): *Lilly Hospital Pharmacy Survey 1983*. Indianapolis, IN, Eli Lilly and Company, 1983.
6. Costello BG: A primer on regulations and controls affecting employee compensation. *Health Care Mgt Rev* 7:59-69, Fall, 1982.
7. Henderson RI: *Compensation Management: Rewarding Performance*, ed 3. Reston, VA, Reston, 1979.
8. Title 42, Ch 21 USC S1981-1983.
9. Title 29, USC S201-219 (1938), 29 CFR S500-889.
10. Cole A: Flexible benefits are a key to better employee relations. *Personnel J* 62:49-53, January 1983.
11. Bergmann TJ, Hills FS, Priefert L: Pay compression: causes, results, and possible solutions. *Compensation Rev* 15:17-26, 1983.
12. Herbert WJ, Mergener MA, DeMuth JE: Continuing education support as a fringe benefit. *Am J Hosp Pharm* 39:852-3, 1982.
13. Ward P: Occupational earnings from top to bottom. *Occupational Outlook Q* 26:21-5, Winter, 1982.
14. Oakley RS, Bradham DD: Factors affecting the salaries of pharmacy directors in large hospitals. *Am J Hosp Pharm* 40:591-7, 1983.
15. Anon: Pharmacists salaries in Michigan. *Parenterals* 1:5, 1983.
16. Collins LI: Survey of hospital salaries. *Hospitals* 56:59-66, December 1982.
17. Cole BS: Top hospital managers win 11.4% salary increase. *Mod Health Care* 12:67-90, December 1982.
18. Miner JB: Management appraisal: A review of procedures and practices. In Hamner WC, Schmidt FL (eds): *Contemporary Problems in Personnel*. New York, John Wiley & Sons, 1977, pp 228-239.

CHAPTER 11

Unions and Collective Bargaining

DEWEY D. GARNER

It has been suggested that the professions are currently undergoing an industrial revolution similar to the one experienced centuries ago by the crafts (1). Large-scale organizations are emerging to accomplish societal goals. They, in turn, challenge the individualistic nature of our free enterprise system as professional work roles become more standardized and mechanized and more bureaucratically structured. Perhaps the single most important goal that emerges as one studies unions and the motivation of professionals is power, followed by parity with peers and other professionals. Those who have held power, such as physicians, want to maintain or improve their position; those who have not had power want to gain their share (2).

A major effect of this revolution is that professionals at all levels are increasingly turning to the collective bargaining process and unionized assistance as a means of "protecting" their interests.

There are almost 3 million members of unions and employee associations in the United States who are classified as professional and technical workers (3). About 30,000 pharmacists belong to union-oriented organizations (4). Bearing in mind that about half of all practicing pharmacists are employees, the figure of 30,000 unionized pharmacists means that perhaps as many as 40% of all employed pharmacists are unionized to some degree. The Retail Clerks International Association (AFL-CIO) has claimed a membership of over 20,000 pharmacists enrolled in various locals (5).

Many and varied reasons may be presented for an increase of interest in unions and union-like activities. One of the most striking reasons is that there has been a complete change in the character of employment, resulting in the dramatic transition of pharmacists from private fee-for-service practitioners to paid employees within organizational settings.

Pharmacists have become employees of chain drugstores, individually owned stores, and hospitals. Corporate diversification has placed retail drug chain management in such diverse hands as A & P, Kroger, Penney's, and other nonpharmacist groups. The pharmacist, who 50 years ago owned his own pharmacy, today may find himself standing next to the meat counter in supermarkets dispensing drugs to shoppers. Denzin and Mettlin's conclusion is 1968 that pharmacy had achieved a state of incomplete profession-

alization seems equally true today (6). The pharmacist may be disillusioned as full professional recognition is difficult to achieve because of his employer's attitude that there is nothing "unique" about his occupational role requirements.

A second and most vital factor is purely economic. As a salaried employee, the pharmacist is faced with the necessity of gaining greater job control and greater economic security. In many instances, the employee pharmacist is far removed from the decision- and policy-making level of management. He is forced to recognize that his overall interests are tied to group interests and that, as an isolated professional, he is virtually powerless to influence his economic destiny.

A third factor to consider is a change in the attitude of the employee pharmacist. This, in part, relates to the first reason given, the complete change in the character of employment. Many pharmacists do not have the inclination to enter the profession at the management level, whether as entrepreneurs or as managers in institutional pharmacy. However, many of these young pharmacists feel that they are entitled to a "piece of the action" regardless of the level on which they find themselves.

PHARMACISTS' ATTITUDES

What is the attitude of the hospital pharmacists toward unions and collective bargaining? Hidde and Covington (7) conducted a study to determine the attitudes of hospital pharmacists regarding professionalization and labor organization. A questionnaire was mailed to a national random sample of 403 active members of the American Society of Hospital Pharmacists (ASHP). The questionnaire was designed to determine (1) professional orientation, (2) attitudes toward labor organization, (3) job satisfaction, and (4) demographic characteristics. The results of the study indicated a desire on the part of the majority of hospital pharmacists to organize and bargain collectively, but not at the price of compromising professional principles. It was obvious from the results that the hospital pharmacist had both economic and noneconomic reasons which may account for his positive attitude toward collective bargaining. Items such as salary, fringe benefits, duties performed, promotions, and grievance procedures were obvious sources of discontent. Hospital pharmacists who were males, married, and worked in large hospitals, or who worked in governmental hospitals, were more positive toward collective bargaining than those who were females, unmarried, and worked in small hospitals, or who worked in voluntary hospitals, respectively.

Choich and Hepler (8) undertook a similar study to determine whether hospital pharmacists prefer collective bargaining as a means of influencing the conditions surrounding their practice; both professional and economic issues were examined. Various aspects of job satisfaction and professionalism were studied to determine their relationships to preference for collective bargaining. Data were collected by a questionnaire mailed to a random sample of 2000 active members of the ASHP. The results indicated no strong general preference for collective bargaining among this group of pharmacists, although supervisors and staff pharmacists had a higher relative preference for collective bargaining than did directors and assistant directors of pharmacy; this higher preference was related primarily to economic issues. Dissatisfaction with pay and with the work itself was related most strongly to preference for collective bargaining. Other factors significantly associated with the preference were a lesser belief in professional autonomy, a lesser use of the professional organization as a major work referent, and the type of hospital where employed. Directors and assistant directors indicated a slight preference for collective bargaining with regard to professional activities. Based on their findings, the authors believed that their respondents interpreted the term "collective bargaining" differently from the "collective bargaining" that they presumably voted for in the ASHP referendum. They felt that respondents who use the ASHP as a professional referent tend not to favor collective bargaining but do want to be able to call on the Society for assistance as their bargaining agent if faced with inclusion in a labor union. Additionally, these pharmacists showed a certain naivete about how collective bargaining can be used. They seemed to see collective bargaining primarily in terms of extrinsic issues, e.g., salary, fringe benefits, hours of work. No subsample could be identified in which increased professionalism was associated with increased preference for collective bargaining on professional issues.

REASONS FOR UNION ACTIVITY

The preceding studies are cited as an indication of the attitude of hospital pharmacists toward collective bargaining and unionized activity. But why do some employees join unions?

Bentivegna (9) suggests that the combined pressures of inflation, hospital cost-containment activities, employee concern with job security and professional issues, and publicized contract settlements have all contributed to the creation of a climate favorable to union organizing. In the health care field, union organizing attempts have usually occurred in large hospitals located in major urban areas, particularly on the West Coast, in the industrial northeast, and in the Great Lakes region. Half of all hospitals with collective bargaining agreements are located in six states: New York, California, Michigan, Pennsylvania, Minnesota, and Washington (10). Although union activity seems to be concentrated in a few industrial states, it is beginning to

occur more frequently in small hospitals that are located in cities with few major industries. This activity is increasing, especially in the southwestern, midwestern, and southern states.

Granberg (11), in a presentation to the Iowa Pharmaceutical Association, presented this brief but representative list of reasons:

1. Unfair and harsh treatment by immediate supervisors—the employee acts to "get even."
2. Little, if any, personal recognition—union membership is an employee effort to force recognition.
3. Lack of fair and firm discipline.
4. Fear of job security.
5. Failure to put company personnel policies and employee duties and benefits in writing, e.g., no contract! This represents a lack of trust by the employee in the employer.
6. Lack of recognition for length of service on the job.
7. Failure to sell employees on the advantages and benefits of working for the company.

With these reasons for joining unions in mind, it is possible to list four actions on the part of the employer that may encourage unionization:

1. Downplay employee dissatisfactions.
2. Give employees a minimum of information about the total store management/the goals, sales, profit, etc.
3. Use pressure tactics to manage people—be dogmatic, autocratic, paternalistic.
4. Make all decisions without seeking the advice and opinions of your employees and without letting them know what is going on.

Hacker described some practices that put hospitals in a vulnerable position with regard to unionization (12). These included:

1. Inequitable rotations for weekend, evening, and night-shift workers
2. Irregular and substandard performance appraisal
3. Lack of uniformity among hospital departments in the application of personnel policies
4. Grievance procedures that favor managers and supervisors
5. Lack of opportunities for promotion and transfer within the hospital
6. Lack of leadership for ensuring the rights of employees

According to Rakich (13), factors such as low wages, poor benefits, and job security appear to be among the main reasons for the tendency toward unionization in hospitals. Other factors such as favoritism, lack of communication, and a general deterioration of human relations are not as obvious but are equally important, particularly in the hospital, where there are distinct status differences between occupational groups. When unions have been active in organizing employees of hospitals and other health care facilities, it has been found that issues involving quality of patient care (e.g., the number of doctors in clinics or emergency rooms, improvement of nursing and technician staffs, improvement of X-ray services, availability of physical therapists) are of great concern at all professional levels (14). Salary is the other major issue, although this is far less important at the higher pay levels. Nurses, for example, are much more interested in salary improvement than are the better paid pharmacists, but both groups seek greater impact on institutional decision making.

Robert P. Levoy, Director of Professional Practice Consultants, stated to the ASHP Institute on General Practice of Hospital Pharmacy, "At the outset, it is important to understand what motivates today's employees—the factors that keep workers' morale high and contribute most to job satisfaction." He went on to cite an investigation by the U.S. Chamber of Commerce in which they conducted dual surveys of management and employees' attitudes on the subject of employee priorities in job satisfaction. Ranking by management of the first three of these priorities was (1) good pay, (2) job security, and (3) promotion and growth. The employees' list, however, was quite different. In order of importance, their first three priorities were (1) full appreciation of work performed, (2) feeling "in" on things, and (3) sympathetic help on personal problems. "Job security" was number 4 on their list and "good pay" was number 5 (15).

The fact is that in today's socioeconomic environment money per se and fringe benefits are only a part of the picture. Although the economic features of unionism receive the headlines, the professional elements of the issue are probably the most important in the long run. Historically, before unions can make much progress among professionals, these same professionals must feel that their professional status is threatened by the employment situation.

Should pharmacists become involved in union activities? This is one of the most provocative questions in pharmacy today. Pharmacists should consider all aspects of unionization, because once they join a union it may be difficult to resign. If pharmacists are not satisfied with the specific conditions under the contract negotiated by their union, they may be forced to leave their employment for another position. Unions establish rules for the conduct of their members and these are enforced by monetary fines. Individual prerogatives may be sacrificed for the benefit of the group. The effect of unionization on the profession should be studied closely.

In 1971 a questionnaire was sent to 400 chief pharmacists in hospitals throughout the United States to determine what they think about unions (16). Responses (from 191) indicated that 69% of the chief pharmacists believed unions to be a threat to pharmacy's professional status. Geographically, the chief pharmacists in urban-populated areas were less concerned about the union's threat to pharmacy's professional status than those who were located in the less-populated areas. The survey results indicated that 45% of all respondents felt that pharmacists would participate in strikes if they belonged to unions. Seventy-nine percent felt that belonging to a union in which pharmacy is in the minority will submerge the demands and needs of the pharmacist. Many merge the demands and needs of the pharmacist. Many pharmacists felt that they should not affiliate with unions in which others' interests might be served. The overall survey indicated that 64% of the chief pharmacists felt that unions in pharmacy pose a threat to pharmacy organizations. Since these issues affect the profession of pharmacy, there is still a question as to whether the means employed through unions do justify the end results.

EFFECTS ON THE HOSPITAL

What effect does the union have on the hospital? It would not overstate the case to observe that the relationship of hospitals with their professional personnnel is undergoing profound change and that this change will have tremendous impact on the executive resources and administrative behavior of the hospitals. In 1961, only 4.3% of the nonfederal, nonprofit hospitals had a formal collective bargaining agreement. The total number had increased to 8.1% by 1970 (17). Frenzen's 1978 survey indicates that organizing efforts resulted in collective bargaining agreements with approximately 23% of all hospitals. Approximately one third of the hospital work force is employed in hospitals that have collective bargaining agreements with one or more unions (18).

Since hospitals have been covered under the National Labor Relations Act (NLRA), the National Labor Relations Board (NLRB) has held 423 elections in health care institutions out of 1386 representation petitions filed as of April 30, 1975. Two hundred of these elections were held in hospitals, and unions won 125 (19). Of the ten most active industries with regard to white-collar union organizing in 1980, health services ranked third, with 42 elections. Furthermore, the success rate of 53.6% in white-collar elections was better than the 45% that the unions have been winning in general in recent years (20).

Despite aggressive organizing efforts by labor unions, membership declined slowly from a peak of 25% of the total work force in 1970 to 20% in 1978 (21). The traditional strongholds for unions in the United States are diminishing. The recent recession and foreign competition have affected manufacturing adversely. Deregulation has allowed the entry of nonunion, lower cost competition into the transportation industry. The open-shop movement has decimated organized labor in the construction industry. The service industries, including not-for-profit hospitals, still represent a large, relatively untapped constituency for union organizers who are trying to increase membership.

These figures indicate that at no other time in American history has the hospital administrator more fully felt the impact of the union movement. Faced with increased demand for services, increasing costs, and greater manpower needs, the hospital administrator is affected directly by the trend toward aggressive unionization in the way in which he can cope with these problems. Given the fact that hospitals are labor intensive, and that the level of employment is rising and changing technologies require advanced skills, administrative flexibility in the utilization of personnel is crucial in attempts to minimize hospital costs. Thus, the effect of a union on management's prerogative to control employee activity is of major importance. The disadvantages of the union from the administrator's perspective would center around the effects that unions would have in the hospital organization, particularly in the areas of administrative flexibility, wages, and the possibility of strikes.

UNIONS AND PROFESSIONALISM

Keeping in mind the effects of the union on the profession and the hospital, what is the relationship between professionalization and unions? Haug and Sussman (22) identify professionalization and unionism as two processes by which members of an occupation seek to achieve collective upward mobility. Such combined efforts at job advancement are the analog, on a group scale, of individuals striving for a better job—one with higher pay, better working conditions, more freedom from supervision, and higher community status. Where individual upward mobility is blocked or hindered, occupational incumbents often turn to collective efforts with the same generalized goals of increased earnings, autonomy, and prestige. In short, individuals unlikely to get better work tend to join others similarly situated to make their work better.

Conceptualizing professionalization and unionism as alternative forms of collective upward mobility does not mean there are no differences between the two processes. According to Haug and Sussman, differences can be distinguished in goal priorities and explicit definitions, in strategies of achieving these goals, and in relationships to the public. Workers who choose the union road undertake to gain their ends through a publicized power struggle with specific work systems. Using the mechanisms of collective bargaining with organization pressures, public attitude change through public relations and the press, and occasional strikes, employees may, as a result, receive higher wages, better working conditions, and other benefits. Often, unions are charged with ignoring the public interest in their concern with the interests of their members, and certainly, where public services are involved, as in the hospital, the withdrawal of labor inconveniences the users of these services.

Persons in occupations striving to professionalize are also in a power struggle, but on a societal level. They have, at least in the past, attempted to persuade the public at large, rather than a particular bureaucratic hierarchy, that they are entitled to various benefits. Because of their mysterious specialized knowledge, communal power over members, shared role definitions, and dedication to service, professionals lay claim first and foremost to autonomy and independence on the job, with attendant control over the client, and expect as inevitable secondary benefits both large financial rewards and exalted prestige. Organization takes the form of a professional association rather than a union. Instead of engaging in a power contest between haves and have-nots, the association undertakes to protect and expand the profession's knowledge base, enforce standards of learning, entry, and performance, and engage in similar activities designed to enhance the position of practitioners while simultaneously purporting to protect the welfare of the public in the person of the client. Indeed, professional claims concerning the primacy of the public good over the practitioner's own private benefit might be viewed as a critical difference between the professionalizing and unionizing modes of mobility were it not for considerable evidence that the claims are watered with rhetoric (23).

The roles of the professional association and of the union overlap within the bureaucracy of the hospital. Both groups are moving in the same direction but with different methods and differing philosophies. Differences exist in goal weights as among wages, fringe benefits, and autonomy, the variations in value systems with respect to the public, and the disparity between the pressure tactics used. As professional associations move toward serving as a collective bargaining

agent for their members, these differences create a dilemma for the hospital administrator as he deals with the association on one hand and the union on the other. This issue is particularly relevant to hospital pharmacy, as the following discussion reveals.

ACTIONS OF ASHP

The first recorded actions taken by the ASHP concerning union activities consisted of an Executive Committee vote adopted in January 1961. This Committee reviewed communications from the Colorado Society of Hospital Pharmacists describing efforts by representatives of the Retail Clerks International Association to enroll hospital pharmacists. The Executive Committee then voted to commend the Colorado Society of Hospital Pharmacists for sustaining the professional objectives of pharmacy in adopting a position of opposition to unions for hospital pharmacists in Colorado (24).

In 1964, the ASHP Board of Directors took direct action with regard to unionization of hospital pharmacists when they voted to refer to the Committee on Professional Ethics the request of the Joint Committee with the American Hospital Association that the matter of unionization of hospital pharmacists be studied to determine whether a statement of policy should be issued.

Consideration of this proposal by the ASHP Committee on Professional Ethics resulted in the Society's not taking any action at that time. In 1965, the Secretary of ASHP's Joint Committee with the American Hospital Association reported to that Committee that the only information available at American Pharmaceutical Association headquarters consisted of two reports of the American Pharmaceutical Association Committee on Social and Economic Relations. These reports dealt with union-sponsored pharmacies.

At the 1967 annual meeting, some members of the House of Delegates were interested in formal action by the House with regard to labor relations. After consideration of proposals, it was decided that insufficient information was known, and action adopting a formal position on unions was postponed. In lieu thereof, the House of Delegates adopted the following resolution, which authorized the Society to undertake a national salary survey of hospital pharmacists and to relate the results to the salary of community pharmacists and to other professionals in the hospital: "Resolved that the Society immediately compile statistical factual information regarding present salaries of hospital pharmacists and attempt to relate these to salaries of pharmacists in community and other areas of practice and to other health professionals in the hospital . . ." (25).

The data for this salary survey were gathered by the end of 1968, and the results were compiled and published in the American Journal of Hospital Pharmacy (26).

By late 1968, the union problem in several states, particularly New York, had become acute, and the Board of Directors, at its December 1968 meeting, adopted the following resolutions:

To direct Society staff to study in depth, by engaging in any research that is appropriate, the role the Society should play with regard to the unionization of its members; further,

To present a progress report at the 1969 Montreal Meeting of the Society's House of Delegates if indicated; and,

To direct Society staff to assist the New York State Council of Hospital Pharmacists in whatever manner possible in dealing with matters relating to unions and hospital pharmacists in the State of New York consistent with that which is in the best interests of public welfare, the Society and the Council.

The first resolution was designed to produce an in-depth study of the implications of union activities to the Society. The second resolution was meant to provide assistance to the New York State Council on an interim basis until basic policy could be developed. Pursuant to this second directive, the Society staff has worked closely with the New York State Council. Amendatory language for the Council's constitution was developed to enable it to become active in the labor relations area. The purposes section of the constitution was amended by adding a new section that reads: "To study and promote the economic security of hospital pharmacists in New York State." The Council established, on January 11, 1969, a permanent Committee on Employment Relations to study the union problem and work closely with the Society (27).

The Board of Directors of the ASHP, at its meeting of January 10-11, 1970, voted to engage in collective bargaining by assisting affiliated chapters, on request, in accordance with policies and guidelines as established by the House of Delegates of the ASHP and to adopt the statement, "Economic Status Program of the American Society of Hospital Pharmacists."

This economic status program was placed before the 1970 House of Delegates, but before it was adopted the House wished to obtain a sense of the membership. This vote was taken by mail ballot in the summer of 1970. The membership of ASHP, by a margin of almost 4 to 1, voted to adopt a constitutional change that includes the promotion of the economic welfare of hospital pharmacists as an objective of the ASHP. This objective is in addition to the preexisting professional and scientific objectives of the Society. Along with the constitutional change that was adopted, the members supported, by a vote of 1883 to 603 (over 3 to 1), a policy statement entitled "Economic Status Program of the American Society of Hospital Pharmacists" as proposed by the Board of Directors. On March 29, 1971, this statement was approved by the ASHP House of Delegates by a vote of 101 to 16.

Since the adoption of the ASHP Economic Status Program (ESP), the emphasis has been on assisting affiliated state chapters in developing their own economic status programs that generally incorporate collective bargaining. Annual salary surveys have been conducted.

In his annual report to the ASHP House of Delegates in April 1976, President Eckel stated:

One focal point of ESP activity has been our efforts to obtain exclusive bargaining units for hospital pharmacists under the National Labor Relations Act.

As of August, 1977 three separate bargaining units among professional employees will be considered by the NLRB as appropriate in hospitals: employee physicians, registered nurses, and other professional employees. Employee physicians were included in a ruling on June 29, 1977 (28). Interns and residents were judged

to be students rather than employees and therefore not entitled to protection under federal labor laws (29).

The California Society, with the support of ASHP, is pursuing a test case before the National Relations Board designed to establish this principle. Frankly, we believe the battle will be a long one, but one which we must fight . . . and win. We can no longer safely remain above the battle, nor can we assume that the question is "if" we desire unionization. The question is "whom and when," and if we are to retain control of our economic and professional destiny, we must assure that hospital pharmacists alone determine whether or not they wish to bargain collectively. Remember, we are fighting for the freedom of choice of hospital pharmacists, not for unionism or nonunionism alone. The American Hospital Association has filed a brief requesting the petition from the California hospital pharmacists be dismissed because there are no criteria by which the NLRB can grant pharmacists separate bargaining units without also granting separate units to more than 50 "similarly qualified, equivalently trained health care professional disciplines" (30).

Another significant issue in ESP is the relationship of hospital management to its employees, state chapters, and the Society outside the context of collective bargaining. Lately, many members have voiced to me their concern about potential discontinuation by hospitals of their policy of aid and encouragement of participation in professional organizations. Hospitals, they fear, will be intimidated by the so-called union aspects of the ESP. In a number of professional organizations, there has been a gradual evolution toward programs offering employees the right to deal collectively with their employers. The American Medical Association has recently taken steps to involve itself in traditional employer-employee problems. The American Nurses' Association and other professional organizations have similar programs.

There is recent evidence that the American Hospital Association will adopt a "go slow" policy toward professional associations functioning in the area of economic relations. Eckel has stated:

ASHP is first, last and always a professional organization designed to promote professional goals. Although we have established ESP as one means to promote these goals, our activities in the area of collective bargaining should be viewed as a part of a larger effort to provide improved pharmaceutical services; this is implicit in our wide variety of educational and professional activities. Hospital administrators should and legally can acknowledge this fact in relations with the profession (31).

Robert Greenberg, an attorney for the ASHP, is skeptical about the value of union membership for pharmacists. Mr. Greenberg says that unions seldom acknowledge that paying better wages and benefits to employees should entitle an employer to improved services. It is equally rare, he contends, to find a union that achieves its economic aims and upholds professional standards as well. "A few years ago, many hospital pharmacists were turning to unions," the attorney notes. "But that trend has leveled off and may even show a decline soon. It's because hospital administrators have become more astute in handling personnel. . . . Besides, it's a traumatic step for a pharmacist, who is traditionally a self-employed professional, to start thinking about joining a union" (32).

As Epstein and Stickler suggest, it appears that the hospital administrator may believe he has a dilemma on his hands, involving a choice between unsatisfactory alternatives (33). There have emerged within the modern-day pharmacists' association two separate entities. It is a professional organization engaged with the concerns of health care, including education and training of pharmacists. It is a labor organization with the goals and structure that characterize the traditional representative of employees with respect to hours, wages, and working conditions. Here, the unsatisfactory alternatives would be to treat the pharmacists' association solely under one or the other of its two identities. Nevertheless, as Eckel has stated, the ASHP is not alone in its involvement with the economic status of its members. Actually, among the health professions, nursing has both the most firmly established and most visible collective bargaining program. This tradition dates back to 1934, when the American Nurses' Association developed its Economic Security Program (34). Kralewski states that while nursing has traditionally been the only hospital-based health occupation strongly committed to collective bargaining, pharmacists are strongly oriented to collective bargaining and are rapidly becoming an influential force in the medical care organization. He further stated that it would appear that pharmacy is splitting into two groups—a hospital group and a salaried group involved in traditional drugstore dispensing within large organizational structures.

The evidence indicates that associations will be much more active in the future in collective bargaining agreements, the motivation being not only to serve the needs of their membership, but also to avoid further entrenchment of the union into the profession.

LABOR LAW

Now that we have examined some possible effects of the union on the profession, the hospital, and the professional association, let us review the nation's labor law as it relates to the conduct of the employer-employee relationship.

The NLRA was passed in 1935. Since then it has been amended several times. It is administered by the NLRB, and decisions have been frequently interpreted in the federal courts. Collective bargaining agreements are the basis of the employer-employee relationships, and such agreements delineate the perimeters and substance of the interaction between the union and management. Collective bargaining agreements specify the terms and conditions of employment. Such agreements are enforceable in the courts and usually contain mechanisms such as arbitration for applying provisions to specific circumstances or changed situations (35).

Section 7 of the NLRA guarantees employees the right to engage in self-organization and collective bargaining through representatives of their choice or to refrain from engaging in such activities. Section 8 sets forth broadly worded descriptions of employer and union unfair labor practices. Sections 8(a) and 8(e) state that unfair labor practices for an employer are to:

- Interfere with, restrain, or coerce employees in the exercise of the rights guaranteed in Section 7

- Dominate or interfere with the formation or the administration of any labor organization or contribute financial or other support to it
- Encourage or discourage membership in any labor organization by discrimination with regard to hire or tenure or conditions or employment (A valid "union shop" is an exception.)
- Discharge or otherwise discriminate against an employee because he has filed charges or has given testimony under the act
- Refuse to bargain collectively with representatives designated or selected by the majority of employees in a bargaining unit
- Enter into a "hot-cargo" agreement with a union (The employer promises not to do business with or not to handle or otherwise deal in any of the products of another party.)

Sections 8(b), 8(e), and 8(g) state that unfair labor practices for a labor organization are to:

- Restrain or coerce employees in the exercise of the rights guaranteed in Section 7 or to restrain or coerce an employer in the selection of its representatives for the purposes of collective bargaining or the adjustment of grievances
- Cause or attempt to cause an employer to discriminate against an employee because of his membership or nonmembership in a labor organization (A valid "union shop" is an exception.)
- Refuse to bargain collectively with an employer, provided the union is the designated representative of the majority of the employees
- Engage in certain strikes, secondary boycotts, or other specified types of coercion
- Exact excessive or discriminatory fees or dues under "union shop" agreements
- Cause or attempt to cause an employer to pay for work that is not to be performed ("featherbedding")
- Engage in or threaten recognition or organizational picketing unless certain conditions are met
- Enter into a "hot-cargo" agreement with an employer
- Engage in any strike, picketing, or other concerted refusal to work at any health care institution without giving at least 10 days notice (36)

The Taft-Hartley Act of 1947 (an amendment to the NLRA of 1935) specifically excluded nonprofit hospitals from NLRB coverage. Public Law 93-360, passed in 1974, reversed this position and made nonprofit health care facilities subject to the provisions of the NLRA. Five years after its passage, nearly 4000 hospitals and 1.5 million employees were brought under the jurisdiction of the NLRB (37). Since the labor law is now so expansive and complex, court decisions and NLRB rulings often become the future standards for labor decisions.

Provisions for the use of arbitration to resolve disputes during the life of a contract appear in well over 90% of all collective bargaining agreements (38). Arbitration is a lawful technique making use of an independent third party, the arbiter, for resolving disputes between management and a union in a way that binds both parties to the arbiter's award.

It is frequently accepted as a means of grievance resolution in unionized health care institutions.

Two important points should be stressed relative to arbitration. First, as Kagel suggests (39):

1. The best way to settle a dispute—any dispute—is by negotiation. Most disputes are in fact settled in this way.
2. Arbitration should be the last resort of the parties in the same way the courts should be used as a last resort in a legal controversy.
3. Arbitration should never be used as a substitute for negotiations.

The second major point to stress relative to arbitration revolves around the major service the hospital provides, patient care. Hospital administrators, union representatives, arbiters, and the public probably would agree that hospital employees should be treated fairly. They might also agree that a hospital should be operated with very strict discipline of employees with regard to the care of patients. Conflicts may often arise as to what is the allowable balance between poor employee performance on the one hand and the demands of high-quality patient care on the other. Since these two issues inevitably lead to consideration of the quality of employee training, Krinsky (40) has raised the question, "If the hospital is to be allowed a stricter standard of discipline, is it not imperative, in fairness to the employee and the patient, that the employer be held to a stricter standard in its hiring, training and evaluation procedure?" More concentrated efforts in areas of hiring, training, evaluation, work assignments, and supervision may be required in the future to ensure fair treatment of employees.

To summarize briefly the process of arbitration, if properly designed and implemented and judiciously applied, the procedure can ensure uninterrupted operations where uninterrupted patient care is essential.

UNION TACTICS

How do unions select their organizational targets? What are their strategies of organizing, their tactics for implementation? Metzger and Pointer (41) have outlined the basic approach utilized by union organizers. While unions vary in their strategies of organizing, the common thread throughout all campaigns is the information gathering phase. In most instances, a small committee of employees assists the union in the task. They are usually a group of dissatisfied employees who may well have "invited" the union to come initially. The tactics to be utilized will be largely determined after the facts are assembled. The types of data needed include a complete survey of the physical facilities and employee profile. What is the organizational structure? How many employees are in each department? What is their level of morale? Who are the employees who are sympathetic to the union's cause? From this group of sympathizers, a small committee will develop a theme that will most appeal to the members of the institution. The issue may be wages in one institution; in another it may be unfavorable working conditions.

The first general meeting of employees to be called by the union is a very important one and will be carefully planned in advance. A large turnout of employees is essential as the primary purpose of the initial meeting is to obtain recognition. Preceding the announcement of the meeting, handbills are usually distributed. Concurrent with the distribution of handbills is the effort to sign up employees.

Since the hospital must allow the union reasonable means to communicate with employees, they cannot prohibit distribution of the handbills or solicitation of membership on its premises. These activities may be conducted generally in nonwork areas such as lunchrooms and parking lots during nonwork hours, including lunch hours and rest period.

Unions differ as to the point at which a demand for recognition is made. Thirty percent of the employees must sign authorization cards to obtain a Board-directed election. Many unions wait until their signee list exceeds 50%.

While unions have made decided progress within the health care institution, a hospital administrator can do many things to increase the organization's chances of remaining nonunion. They include intelligent location and acquisition decisions, sensible employer selection and development, sound supervisory training, appropriate no-solicitation rules and other measures to deter a union drive, early detection and response procedures, and an appropriate bargaining-unit strategy. The most important requirement is that the hospital administrator start early (42).

Bice (43) suggests that when confronted with potential union activity, hospital management should carefully collect data on the union and its own labor force. He suggests the data that should be collected be placed into three basic categories: fundamentals, issues, and people.

Generally, the fundamentals cover the tasks being performed, the environment in which employees function, and the policies and programs governing their personal conduct and remuneration for services rendered. The issues relate to those problems and irritants that affect employees while on the job. The sources for those data include both personnel department and department records and personal interviews. Basically, the trick is simply to beat the union at their own game by providing better pay, fringe benefits, and opportunities in advance. Proper information, coupled with competent legal advice, forms the basis of the hospital management's strategy.

Pointer and Metzger (44) indicated one of the major considerations of hospital administrators, legislators, and the consumer-public when addressing the challenge of collective employee activity in a health care facility. This major consideration is the threat of critical service disruption because of the labor-management conflict. Reservations regarding the extension of organizational and collective bargaining rights to hospital employees generally reduce to two connected arguments: (1) the recognition of a union is a direct invitation to strikes and (2) intolerable conditions would be created if critical hospital services were substantially curtailed or eliminated completely because of a strike. Amid all the commotion and concern, they found that work stoppage activity in the hospital industry was relatively slight. Only 2% of the nation's 7172 hospitals experienced work stoppages during 1967. They further found strike activity in hospitals to be relatively concentrated by facility size, geographic location, and control. Generally, facilities that were large, voluntarily or state and locally controlled, and located in the east north central, west north central, and Pacific regions were most likely to experience a work stoppage. Later occurrences of strikes, notably in the Northeast, have indicated the justification of this earlier concern. One recent effort to minimize the detrimental effect of a strike within the institution has been undertaken by the management of Mount Sinai Hospital in New York City (45). They have implemented a computer system to enable the hospital to plan effective staffing rapidly in the event of threatened strikes.

CONCLUSION

The hospital is experiencing a basic change in its traditional employment relations as a result of unionization and collective bargaining. It has not been easy for the administration of the institution to accept these new responsibilities, masking them with its overall commitment to provide high-quality health care service to its patients. Likewise, it has been difficult for the professional employees, including pharmacists, to understand and accept these new aspects of labor relations as they relate to both their professional and personal goals. Adaptation to change will become easier wherever management and labor within the institution realize that they have a mutual relationship; i.e., the origin of quality patient care is to be found in the quality of the employee's work life.

REFERENCES

1. Engle GV, Hall RH: *The Growing Industrialization of the Professions, on the Professions and their Prospects.* Beverly Hills, Sage Publications, 1973, pp 75-88.
2. Bloom BI: Collective action by professionals poses problems for administrators. *Hospitals* 51:168, 1977.
3. U.S. Bureau of Labor Statistics: *Directory of National Unions and Employee Associations, 1973.* Washington, DC, U.S. Government Printing Office, 1974.
4. Unions tighten their grip on pharmacy. *Am Drugg* 173:74, 1976.
5. Unionism in pharmacy. *Am Druggist* 159:15, 1969.
6. Denzin NK, Mettlin CJ: Incomplete professionalization: The case of pharmacy. *Soc Forces* 46:375, 1967-68.
7. Hidde AJ, Covington TR: ASHP members view collective bargaining. *Am J Hosp Pharm* 30:428-435, 1973.
8. Choich R, Hepler CD: Factors related to collective bargaining preferences among hospital pharmacists *Am J Hosp Pharm* 31:456-466, 1974.
9. Bentivegna G: Labor relations: Union activity increases among professionals *Hospitals* 53:132-133, 1979.
10. Frenzen PD: Survey updates unionization activities *Hospitals* 52:93, 1978.
11. Granberg CR: What to do till the union comes. *Iowa Pharm* 28:108, 1970.
12. Hacker RL: Organizational systems for change offer an alternative to unions *Hospitals* 50:45-47, 1976.
13. Rakich JS: Hospital unionization: causes and effects. *Hosp Admin* 18:12-13, 1973.
14. Chamot D: Professional employees turn to unions. *Harv Bus Rev* 54:123, 1976.
15. Levoy RP: How to maintain high staff morale and motivation. *Am J Hosp Pharm* 29:575, 1972.
16. Teplitsky B: What chief hospital Rx men think about unions. *Pharm Times* pp 46-53, 1971.
17. Rakich JS: *op. cit.* p 9.
18. Frenzen PD: *op. cit.* p 93.
19. Sellentin JL: Labor's concerns face management *Hospitals* 50:65, 1976.
20. Kilgour JG: Union organizing activity among white-collar employees *Personnel* 60:21-22, 1983.
21. Berenbeim R: The declining market for unionization. *Conference Board Information Bull* 44:2, 1978.
22. Haug MR, Sussman MB: Professionalization and unionism. *Am Behav Sci* 14:525, 1971.
23. Haug MR, Sussman MB: Professionalization and the public. *Inquiry* 39:57-64, 1969.
24. Anon: Report on unionization of hospital pharmacists and the American Society of Hospital Pharmacists. *Am J Hosp Pharm* 26:506, 1969.
25. *ibid.*
26. Anon: ASHP salary survey, results and evaluation. *Am J Hosp Pharm* 26:253-289, 1969.
27. Anon: Report on unionization of hospital pharmacists and the American Society of Hospital Pharmacists. *op. cit.* p 507.
28. Employee physicians get separate labor bargaining unit certification from NLRB. *Hospitals* 51:17, 1977.
29. State regulation of house staff not preempted, U.S. District Court rules. *Hospitals* 51:22, 1977.
30. AHA urges prompt dismissal of pharmacy petitions for separate bargaining unit representation. *Hospitals* 51:18, 1977.
31. Eckel FM: Toward professional maturity. *Am J Hosp Pharm* 33:675, 1976.
32. Unions, chains vie over loyalty of employee R.Ph.'s. *Am Druggist* 177:18, 1978.
33. Epstein RL, Stickler KB: The nurse as a professional and as a unionist. *Hospitals* 50:45, 1976.
34. Kralewski JE: Collective bargaining among professional employees. *Hosp Admin* 19:35, 1974.
35. Metzger N, Pointer DD: *Labor Relations and Personnel Management in Long-Term Health Care Facilities.* Manual Commissioned by American Health Care Association, 1975, p 40.
36. Miller RL: Anticipate questions, seek answers for adept labor relations efforts. *Hospitals* 50:50, 1976.
37. Dworkin JB, Extejt MM, Demming SR: Unionism in hospitals, or what's happened since 93-360? *Health Care Mgt Rev* 5:80, 1980.
38. Metzger N: The arbitration procedure—part I. *Hospitals* 48:47, 1974.
39. Kagel S: *Anatomy of a Labor Arbitration.* Washington, DC, Bureau of National Affairs, 1961, p IX.
40. Krinsky EB: Problems of discipline and discharge. *Hospitals* 48:49, 1974.
41. Metzger N, Pointer DD: *op. cit.* p 34-38.
42. *ibid.*
43. Bice MO: Building a data base. *Hospitals* 48:77, 1974.
44. Pointer DD, Metzger N: Work stoppages in the hospital industry: a preliminary profile and analysis. *Hosp Admin* 17:9-24, 1972.
45. Ross BT: Computerized system aids staffing in strikes. *Hospitals* 49:50, 1975.

CHAPTER 12

Cost Analysis and Control

DAVID M. ARRINGTON and MARC R. SUMMERFIELD

We have entered a new era in health care reimbursement. Formerly, reimbursement was cost-based. The hospital's main burdens were to provide quality care and to document the costs to the payers. The costs were usually reimbursed.

Insulated from many of the competitive forces that apply to the private sector and fueled by cost-based reimbursement, hospitals had few incentives to contain costs. Meaningful interhospital comparisons of costs and charges were made difficult by variations in mission and patient population. It had become hard to determine how well a hospital was containing costs.

Federal government action initiated the transition from cost-based to prospective reimbursement. The Social Security Act Amendments of 1983 outlined a plan for reimbursing hospitals for the treatment of Medicare recipients. Under the plan, a hospital received a predetermined fee to treat each covered patient. This fee corresponds to the patient's diagnosis. Fees were set for 467 different diagnosis related groups. With few exceptions, the actual cost of care does not modify the amount paid by Medicare. Experts speculate that the other third-party payers will follow with similar plans.

So the challenge is different. A hospital must keep costs at or below the reimbursed amounts. Costs can no longer be *passed through*. Also, if costs are kept below the reimbursed amounts, the hospital may keep part of the difference. The hospitals that provide quality care at the lowest cost will survive. Effective cost control is now a necessity.

TERMS

The terms "cost containment" and "cost control" are used interchangeably, but their meanings differ. Cost containment is the goal of keeping costs at or near their present level—preventing or retarding growth. In contrast, cost control is a process, with a strict set of managerial implications. Both terms can be applied to a program, a department, or a hospital or to the entire health care system.

Managerial *control* is the process that attempts to ensure that actions conform to plans (1). Control in the managerial sense, if used properly, is healthy and necessary. It does not imply power and manipulation as does the lay meaning of the term.

Cost control is the implementation of managerial efforts to achieve cost objectives. It is not arbitrary cost cutting. It is not crisis oriented. Effective cost control is a methodical and continuous process.

The first step in any control process is to establish goals, standards for those goals, and methods for measuring performance. The key word is "plan." The next steps are to measure the performance, to compare the performance with the standards, and to institute corrective action, if necessary (1,2). To summarize—plan, measure, compare, and correct.

Within this framework, there are three types of control methods: *screening controls, steering controls,* and *post-action controls* (1). If approval must be obtained before an activity begins or continues, then a screening control has been implemented. Requiring signatures on expenditures above a certain amount represents a screening control. Screening controls provide an extra margin of safety.

Steering controls monitor ongoing operations to detect deviations and make corrections before an activity is completed. Monthly monitoring of the budget is a steering control. Corrections can be made so as to ensure that yearly expenditures are in line with projections.

Post-action controls measure the results of a completed action. The causes of any deviation from the plan or standard are determined, and the findings are applied to similar future activities. An example of post-action control would be to hasten hospital-wide implementation after a successful demonstration project, e.g., unit dose or IV admixtures.

"Cost reduction" and "cost savings" are two terms related to cost containment and cost control. They are synonymous and imply a real and demonstrated reduction in expenses.

Three related, but often confused, terms are "productivity," "efficiency," and "effectiveness."

Productivity is output per unit input (3). Traditionally, pharmacy output has been defined by the number of "line items," i.e., the number of prescriptions dispensed or requisitions filled. Recently, a more enlightened approach has been proposed that includes two main enhancements, disaggregation of outputs and the concept of weighting (4,5).

Disaggregating outputs involves developing a series of outputs that are more representative of the entire department's activities—distributive and nondistributive, i.e., number of unit doses dispensed, number of IV admixtures filled, number of pharmacokinetic consults, or number of discharge counseling sessions.

Weighting is the method used to equitably recombine the outputs to produce one figure representative of the department's entire output. Commonly, the weighting process involves measuring an average time to perform one unit of each of the outputs. One of the outputs is assigned the value of 1 and others assigned proportionately. The department's total output for a month equals the sum of the products of the number of units performed for each output times the weighting value.

Inputs are usually equated to personnel man-hours. Labor input can also be weighted, by wages, so that the hours put in by pharmacists count more than hours put in by supportive personnel.

Efficiency is commonly defined as the total cost per unit output (3). Productivity improvement is a prime method of improving efficiency and meeting cost objectives, Most discussions of cost control focus on productivity rather than efficiency. Productivity is emphasized because the numerator (output) and the denominator (input) are easily understood, easily measured, and closely aligned with good overall management practices.

Productivity and efficiency usually move in the same direction. If the value of the increased output exceeds the cost of implementing and maintaining the change, an increase in productivity will result in an increase in efficiency (3).

Methods to improve productivity include (1) changing the production process; (2) changing or restructuring entire systems within the organization; (3) changing the quality of mix of labor; (4) changing the quality of the product; and (5) improving employee motivation (1,3,6).

The *effectiveness* of a department is related to how well it achieves its goals. The financial effectiveness of a department is a measure of how well it achieves its financial goals. The cost of operating a unit dose system vs the allowance is a measure of the system's financial effectiveness. The hospital's actual medication error rate, when compared with the desired rate, is a quality assessment and represents a nonfinancial measure of the effectiveness of the unit dose system.

Attempts to reduce or contain costs by improving productivity and efficiency often enter the realm of scientific management—the application of scientific methods to find the best way of doing things. "Best" can be the most productive, most efficient, or most effective. The "things" can be the physical design of the pharmacy, the drug distribution system, the purchasing of pharmaceuticals, or the optimal use of professional and supportive personnel. Methods such as work analysis, work simplification, work sampling, methods improvement, and functional analysis are used (see Chapters 8 and 9).

THE COST CONTROL PROCESS

Step 1: Planning

Planning is the keystone management function. All other functions operate only to carry out the decisions of planning (2). Planning is essential in designing and meeting the financial and nonfinancial objectives of the department. A good plan consists of (1) establishing a goal or set of goals; (2) defining the present situation; (3) identifying the aids and barriers to the goals; and (4) developing a set of actions for reaching the goals (1).

According to Stoner (1), "the fourth step involves developing various alternative courses of action for reaching the desired goal or goals, evaluating these alternatives, and choosing from among them the most suitable alternative for reaching the goal."

Cost-effectiveness analysis measures and compares the cost of implementing and operating alternative approaches to achieving a goal or solving a problem. The purpose is to find the least costly alternative. The drug distribution studies conducted in the 1960s and 1970s were cost-effectiveness studies. Most of the studies showed unit dose to be the most cost-effective system (7).

A companion procedure, cost-benefit analysis, is commonly used to evaluate the value of individual projects. Attempts are made to express all of a program's benefits in monetary terms. The dollar value of the benefits is compared with the cost of implementing and maintaining the program. The program is considered to be "socially valuable" if the ratio is greater than one (8,9). The value of clinical pharmacy services, such as pharmacokinetic monitoring, are conducive to cost-benefit analysis. The reader is referred to Chapter 14 for more on cost-benefit analysis.

Decision making is the selection of a preferred course of action and represents the final stage of planning (10,11).

There are two types of decisions: programmed and nonprogrammed (2,10). Programmed decisions are standing decisions. They guide managers and nonmanagers in repetitive and routine situations and problems. If a particular situation occurs frequently, management should develop an optimal and routine procedure for handling it. A procedure for handling nonformulary requests is an example of a programmed decision. Such procedures can save time and improve productivity, as well as enhance quality and promote uniformity of approach.

Nonprogrammed decisions deal with unusual or unique problems: they are special-purpose decisions dealing with programs, strategies, and budgets. Problems such as how best to use the department's resources require nonprogrammed decisions. Nonprogrammed decisions can be based on analyses such as cost benefit and cost effectiveness or other decision-making tools.

The reader should be aware of the contrast between the traditional and modern approaches to decision making. Whereas traditional approaches rely on habit, judgment, intuition, and creativity, modern approaches rely on mathematical analysis, mathematical models, and computer simulation (1). Quantitative techniques are used to assess the value of each alternative. One example is the use of inventory models such as economic order quantity, designed to balance ordering costs against carrying costs. The aim is to determine optimal order sizes and frequencies for each item (10,12,13).

Modern cost control decisions are often quantitative in nature, but human factors can enter into the decision making. These include the value systems of the decision maker(s), limitations in resources, political implications, and time constraints (10).

The department's budget is a key planning document (see Chapter 15). It is a statement of the financial resources devoted to specific activities over a given period of time. Managers can use budget development as another process to make decisions concerning resource allocation (14).

The budget is also a powerful cost control tool. As the organization engages in its activities, the actual (measured) results are analyzed and compared with the budgeted (planned) results, possibly leading to corrective action. The budget is one of the most powerful cost control tools because of the strong link between the planning and the other control functions.

Step 2: Measurement

The effectiveness of the cost control process depends on the quality and timeliness of the data collected. The data should be concerned with those costs over which the manager has control. They must be presented in a readable, meaningful, and useful form (15).

The monthly data on revenue and expenses forwarded by the hospital's fiscal department to the pharmacy manager can form the base of the department's data collection system. To this data the manager adds workload statistics, drug use and cost data, and hospital indicators. For an in-depth discussion of data-collection systems, the reader is referred to the article by Nold (16).

Data collection is more complex when it involves expenditures for a program or service rather than for a budgeted expense account. Program costs are distributed throughout many expense accounts. The portion of each account—personnel, drugs, and supplies—attributed to the program must be isolated. Work measurement techniques are often used to help identify costs (17).

Step 3: Comparing

After the data are collected, they must be transformed into information. Reports are developed, and the data are analyzed and compared to the standard (18,19).

Financial data can be presented as numbers, graphs, or ratios. Graphs are used to demonstrate trends (19). Both raw data and ratios can be graphed. Nold (19) cites four examples: monthly drug purchases by therapeutic category (Fig. 12.1), monthly drug, personnel, and other expenses vs budget (Fig. 12.2), monthly revenue by charge category (Fig. 12.3), and monthly drug costs per patient day by therapeutic category (Fig. 12.4).

Ratios are used to express two figures from a financial statement as one. The figure can then be compared with a similarly formed ratio from another month, another program, an average, etc (1). Although there are many kinds of ratios commonly used by organizations (e.g., liquidity, debt, coverage, profitability), operating ratios are most common in hospital pharmacy.

Operating ratios measure how well operations are being carried out. One of the common operating ratios in industry is inventory turnover rate (sales/inventory). Ratios commonly used in hospital pharmacy include drug cost per patient day, drug cost per dose, salaries as a percentage of total expenses, and drug costs as a percentage of total expenses. As previously discussed, productivity indicators are ratios that measure the department's output per unit input (20).

Step 4: Correction

If the analysis and the subsequent comparison to the standard indicates that the performance has fallen short, then corrective action is needed. Sometimes the standards will

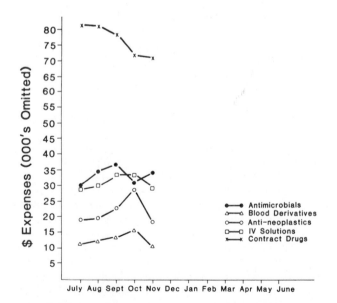

FIGURE 12.1 Monthly drug purchases by therapeutic category. (Reprinted by permission from Nold EG: Financial analysis. *Am J Hosp Pharm* 40:1975-1976, 1983.)

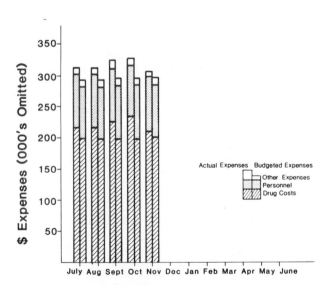

FIGURE 12.2 Monthly drug, personnel, and other expenses vs budget. For each month, the bar on the left represents actual expenses and the bar on the right, budgeted expenses. (Reprinted by permission from Nold EG: Financial analysis. *Am J Hosp Pharm* 40:1975-1976, 1983.)

be adjusted, but more often the activities are modified. Corrective action can involve modifying expenditures, absenteeism, hiring practices, or salary scales. It can also mean adjustments in the use of capital equipment, the use of overtime, or the use of professional and supportive personnel. Some of these approaches will be discussed in the second half of the chapter.

Managers who fail to institute corrective action are merely monitoring performance, rather than exercising control. The emphasis should always be on devising constructive ways to bring performance up to standard, rather than on merely identifying past failures (1).

APPLICATION OF COST CONTROL PROCESS

The earlier part of this chapter concerned itself with the defining of terms and the establishment of baseline knowledge about cost containment and control as well as an introduction to the changing environment of health care. A discussion of the changing health care industry, what opportunities are available/necessitated, and some practical ways to deal with them will be the major focus of this part of the chapter.

For many years, the institutional health care market has been a growth industry; however, public sentiment has recently dictated that the growth phase come to an abrupt halt (21-23). Institutional health care is now considered as a mature industry, with its eroding market share being captured by the home care market (24-33). The reasons for the maturing of the institutional health care market are, on the surface, obscure because technology continues to have major impact in this environment; however, one may speculate that the maturity of this market may have financial roots, i.e., the public is unwilling to devote more of the gross

national product to the financing of health care (34). "Unwilling" seems to be the correct term, since other western countries traditionally devote a higher percentage of their gross national product to health care. The maturing and subsequent shrinking of institutional health care is "the public will."

Each institution has a different "chemistry," and therefore one should establish data bases and approach opportunities that will complement this "chemistry" to optimize success. One assumes that the reader already has an "established system" and that "corrective actions" would be necessary to effect a change.

The "corrective actions" will not be discussed in great detail because, as previously mentioned, they must be tailored to the individual institutions' needs and structure, i.e., "chemistry"; however, there is a listing of suggested readings to complement the treatment of this complex subject.

The overall plan may be defined loosely as increasing cost control within the department of pharmacy services at hospital "X." One needs to do a critical analysis from the outside looking in of how the pharmacy department is viewed in the institution and how the institution is managed. For example, the pharmacy could be viewed as the drug supplier, the supplier of drug-information services, or the controller of the drug-use process in the institution. Each of these establishes the boundaries within which one may render cost control and the opportunity for success; however, if one extends control beyond recognized boundaries, there are "turf issues" that make success difficult and sometimes impossible to achieve. Another example involves hospital organization vs pharmacy organization, i.e., if the hospital has a strong central management focus, then the pharmacy department needs to have the same strong central focus. However, this should not be misinterpreted to mean a one-

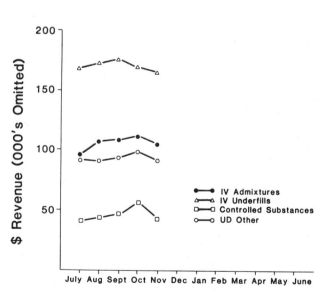

FIGURE 12.3 Monthly revenue by charge category. (Reprinted by permission from Nold EG: Financial analysis. *Am J Hosp Pharm* 40:1975-1976, 1983.)

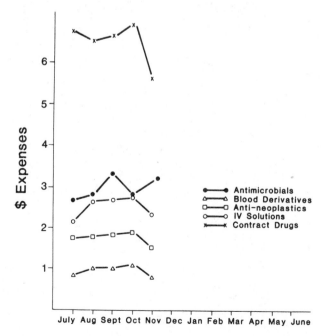

FIGURE 12.4 Monthly drug costs per patient day by therapeutic category. (Reprinted by permission from Nold EG: Financial analysis. *Am J Hosp Pharm* 40:1975-1976, 1983.)

room autocratic department with no satellites and/or little flexibility; it just establishes the overall tone.

A reasonable first step is for the department manager to document the present situation in his/her department using whatever resources are required to make this documentation complete and accurate.

Review this document for aids as well as barriers to success. Make sure that adequate detail is available to assess whether your operation is in compliance with standards linked to accreditation and reimbursement by third parties.

Identify the elements of this document (data base) that present the greatest opportunities for exploitation. This step is a key one because it separates the managers who exercise real control (by taking corrective action) from those who merely monitor performance.

Once the opportunities for exploitation have been identified, set forth a plan for overall direction of the department that is shared at inter- and intradepartmental meetings to gain a firm foundation for action. Staff input into this document is a cornerstone to its long-term success.

In the process of identifying what areas present opportunities for cost reduction, one should give priority to those areas that represent a high percentage of departmental cost. Personnel and drugs/supplies typically represent the two major cost areas, with drugs and supplies typically being 50-70% and personnel/benefits being 20-40% of the budget. Other items generally account for 10-20%. Since drugs/supplies account for a high percentage of pharmacy departmental expenses, consideration must be given to focusing attention in this area.

Drug control must be approached in the correct manner the first time, or else the opportunity for future interventions may be lost. There needs to be a clear definition of what the problem is, with plenty of support data, both financial and clinical; e.g., 80% increase in expense dollars for third-generation cephalosporins, comparing this quarter to prior quarter; no identifiable change in patient mix or physician mix; little apparent wastage; no increase in postsurgical prophylaxis days; no change in hospital's microbiologic flora. Numerous mechanisms (35-43) to handle this and other related problems have been documented in the literature. Some of them include cost improvement (where there is a sharing in the savings achieved with the suggesting party); removal of agent(s) from the formulary so that they are no longer available; requiring third-party approval before therapy is initiated (39); an active education program to promote rational, cost-effective therapy; establishing a listing of drugs that may be chemically different but therapeutically equivalent; reducing the inventory levels of expensive drugs; instituting an active program to reduce wastage; instituting an aggressive drug-purchasing program; increasing security measures to ensure that drug pilferage is at a minimum; ensuring that all vendor discounts are taken; taking advantage of vendor return-goods policies; and reviewing drug handling and storage practices to minimize the incidence of drugs going out of date.

The above-listed mechanisms may be categorized as (1) controlling utilization or (2) controlling procurement or handling practices.

CONTROLLING DRUG UTILIZATION

This area presents the greatest opportunities for savings but also is the most complex. Controlling drug utilization prevents the use of drugs, whereas other techniques involve using them more efficiently. The key elements in this process are the front-line physician, who prescribes drugs for patient use, and the manner in which he/she decides what drugs to prescribe, i.e., drug-ordering habits. Generally recognized factors influencing the physician's drug-ordering habits may include drug company marketing techniques, influential physicians, restrictive drug-ordering policies, or hospital-based counter detailing. The hospital setting is of significant importance in how these factors affect prescribing. In a community hospital, most physicians are in private practice and have already developed many of their drug-ordering habits. By contrast, physicians who have graduated recently from medical school and are participating in advanced training programs, including internships, residencies, and fellowships, are in the process of developing drug-ordering habits that lay the foundation for their career in medicine. Furthermore, if this advanced training site is also a research institution, then new and developing drug technologies will be of significant influence.

Removing drugs from the formulary and not allowing physicians to use them even on a nonformulary basis is the one method that most significantly infringes on the physician's freedom (37). This method should be approached carefully, and significant input from the medical community should occur before final action is taken. The drug(s) to be removed should be reviewed carefully, and their merit or lack of merit in treating the defined patient population should be evaluated thoroughly by physicians who are recognized experts in the field.

Requiring third-party approval before a drug may be used is another mechanism of drug utilization control that is of significant benefit but that also infringes on a physician's normal practice (39). A typical program may require a consultation with a designated "expert" in the field before the drug product may be used. The expert physician would ask the requesting physician questions about the patient and why this particular drug was of greater benefit than similar, noncontrolled drugs. The consultation could include the consultant's examining the patient and reviewing laboratory test results and other pertinent data found in the medical record. The consultant would review his findings with the requesting physician and recommend a course of action. Documentation that the consultation took place would be created, and the drug would be released for physician use.

Education of the medical staff on rational, cost-effective drug therapy has a lot of initial appeal because it is a non-threatening way of changing physician's prescribing habits (39). This type of effort has met with little long-term effect unless there is a constant reminder system used to reinforce the learning objectives. The educational effort can take many forms, including continuing education conferences, newsletters, grand rounds, and journal articles. There is no way to ensure that all medical staff take part in these activities, and therefore, one is usually reaching only a subset of the entire population. A hospital-based, counter-detailing program is used as a reminder system in an educational-based program (37). This counter-detailing team could involve nurses, pharmacists, and physicians. A specific protocol for drug use is formulated, and each member of the team familiarizes him/herself with the details of the protocol and routinely questions physicians who do not follow the protocol. Items covered by the protocol include indications for use of the drug, expected therapeutic outcomes, average duration of therapy, guidelines for dosing and frequency, signs of toxicity or ineffectiveness, and selection of dosage form. The selection of dosage form may have tremendous cost implications. For example, cost differences between the oral and IV route are normally of an exponential magnitude. Certainly, the patient's condition and expected complications of therapy need to play a major role in this type of decision.

Chemically different but therapeutically equivalent drug products have gained interest because of the increased number of similar products, particulary in the antibiotic market. Patented drug items are more costly, justifiably so from the manufacturer's point of view. The manufacturer of a drug product must recover investment cost in order to stay in business; however, a manufacturer may be willing to lengthen the recovery time for investment cost in order to penetrate a market or to increase his share in an existing market. A significant amount of input into decisions of therapeutically equivalent drugs needs to come from the physicians who frequently prescribe drugs. These clinicians often bring up points not previously considered.

A cost-improvement program that provides incentives to people coming up with new and innovative ideas to reduce costs often brings out information that would not have surfaced otherwise. Each of the proposed ideas should be given careful consideration for its merit and practical application. One idea that might have some practical application is using a low-cost drug to alter the elimination of a high-cost drug. By reducing the dose of the expensive drug, you reduce part of the cost and possibly its toxicity. Another example is using two drugs that interact synergistically and thereby reduce the length of therapy and hospitalization. There are also cost-improvement ideas involving controlling the procurement and handling of drugs that will lead to cost savings.

Cost Savings through Controlling Drug Procurement and Handling

Reducing inventory levels may be a reasonable way to reduce drug costs. As an example, if one reduced inventory by $100,000 and invested those dollars in a Treasury bill (assume 10% per year interest), they would earn $10,000 in a year that could be used to offset drug costs. However, this strategy needs to be well thought out to ensure that there are real savings. If, by reducing your inventory, you have to order more frequently, there are a number of hidden costs to consider, including (1) increased number of purchase orders, (2) smaller but more frequent receiving, and associated handling and stocking procedures, and (3) increased number of invoices to be processed. Inventory man-

agement is a science, and the impact of decisions in this area needs to be thought out carefully before implementation. One needs to calculate economic order quantities before arbitrarily reducing inventory levels.

Drug purchasing is an area that offers a high potential for cost savings if handled appropriately (44-52). There are a number of options in this area, including: (1) group purchasing, (2) prime vendor relationship, and (3) direct purchasing from the manufacturer. Each of these options has its merits. A small- to medium-size hospital (<500 beds) may be able to achieve volume discounts not otherwise possible by participating in a buying group. A large hospital may create enough volume to achieve significant savings by buying directly from the manufacturer for a large number of products. However, both the large and small institution may benefit from a ''prime vendor'' concept, in which a wholesaler does significant inventory management and lowers prices for the buyer in order to gain an exclusive contract on the business. The hospital formulary system and the system of purchasing the generic equivalent of brand-name products continue to be major expense-reduction techniques and should be adhered to in an uncompromising manner (53,54). Only with those products for which generic equivalency cannot be demonstrated should the purchase by brand name be considered. Placing the entire drug product line on a bid system, whereby a vendor guarantees supply for a fixed period (usually 1 year) at a fixed price, is an essential element of a purchasing system. The bid system of purchasing guards against frequent price changes. Frequently, companies will bid prices well below published market prices in order to gain the business for a fixed time period. However, if companies bid only their published catalog price but guarantee that price for 1 year, you avoid any price increase that occurs during that time period. The following clause should be included in the contract with the successful bidder (primary vendor): ''If the primary vendor is unable to supply contract items and the purchaser has to obtain supplies from an alternate vendor at a higher cost, the primary vendor must make restitution to the purchaser equal to the net difference.'' This or a similar clause protects the purchaser from unexpected additional expense resulting from a manufacturer's production problems. Other items in purchasing to be carefully considered include (1) vendor discounts and resulting net prices, (2) vendor returned-goods policy and associated credit and service charges, and (3) frequency of deliveries and stock ''outs.''

An active waste-reduction program should be instituted, focusing on areas with a high potential for waste. An IV admixture program is a primary target for waste reduction because of the high dollar cost per unit and the potential for every dose to be customized for the patient. Successful methods of dealing with IV admixture wastage include recycling IV admixtures and standardizing dosages and base solutions. Careful planning of waste-reducing techniques maximizes cost reductions.

Security measures to prevent pilferage must also be actively pursued. Theft of drugs by employees must be considered a reality, and by industry estimates, pilferage represents a major concern. Inventory should be monitored carefully to prevent or minimize pilferage. Theft of drugs by employees must be dealt with in a consistent manner. The usual outcome of theft by employees should be termination and, depending on the extent of involvement, may also include criminal action.

Controlling Personnel Utilization

Personnel costs were identified earlier as being a significant percentage of departmental cost. The two major components of personnel cost are benefits and wages.

Benefits in the hospital industry may normally include the following elements: paid leave, insurance, retirement compensation, FICA tax, educational allowances, savings plans, emergency loans, and hospital discounts. To expedite discussion, benefits will be categorized into those that can be significantly controlled at the departmental level and those that are more centrally controlled. Paid leaves and educational allowances can be controlled significantly at the departmental level and will be discussed further. Paid leave may include holidays, sick time, vacation, funeral leave, military leave, and jury duty. Vacation is the major area in which management can exert significant control because it is handled on a scheduled basis. Managers should minimize the effect that vacation has on productivity by establishing programmed decisions in this area. A well-laid-out procedure on how many people in a specific job category may be on vacation at one time can avoid many problems. Vacation periods involving the summer months and major holiday periods may require special procedures to avoid costly overtime or the required use of temporary employees to cover for employees on vacation. Requesting that employees take a percentage of their allotted vacation in nonpeak periods has many advantages. This non–prime-time vacation policy requires frequent and open communication with employees.

Sick time is another area in which managers can exert significant control. This control should be exercised in a consistent and firm manner. Employees should be fully informed that maintaining constantly good health is the personal responsibility of each employee. When employees become sick, they should seek medical attention and provide the employer with documentation that medical attention was obtained. When employees fail to provide documentation of sickness consistent with hospital personnel practices, they should be counseled and, if appropriate, disciplined. Through the consistent application of procedures regarding employee health, sick time can be minimized.

Educational allowances are usually handled by tuition reimbursement after course work is completed or by paying the expenses of employees attending business-related meetings. A programmed decision should be established to encompass what types of business-related course work will be reimbursed, and boundaries should be set on reimbursed expenses for business-related meetings. In business-related meetings, spending boundaries for items such as transportation, hotel accommodations, meals, and incidentals should be defined carefully.

Wages for employees need to be monitored carefully to ensure equity among employees within the department, the institution, and other institutions doing similar work. Inequity in wage structures discourages employees and can cause a decrease in productivity. Annual salary surveys of your employee recruitment area need to be part of a routine program to ensure wage equity. Of course, if significant shifts in a market occur, a salary survey should be done promptly. Being a market setter in wages offers no advantages and generally decreases the efficiency of the department because the cost per unit of output increases.

Personnel costs and production are closely related and need to be evaluated on the same continuum. Discussion of personnel cost control will focus on three types of changes in production systems and some of the consequential changes in labor mix and employee motivation. The areas to be discussed include computerization (55-58), decentralization, and changing standards. Each of these areas will be reviewed separately for simplicity; however, they may and often do occur simultaneously.

Automating functions, such as a cart replacement unit dose system, necessarily has direct effects on those employees who previously handled tasks on a manual basis. In the planning process for automation, goals need to be defined clearly, and where goals relate to reducing, eliminating, or changing job classifications, up-front and clear communications to the employees involved needs to occur (59). If this communication does not occur on a frequent basis, employees often become demoralized, and productivity drops. Your goal of increasing productivity through automation may be unreachable if this occurs. Clearly define the job skills required of each classification and the number of employees required after automation is implemented in each classification. Then match your current employees and their skills against future requirements and determine the problem areas. Such problems as an excess of low-skill employees usually predominate. Possible alternatives, such as upgrading skills, placing the employees in other positions within the department, or placing them in other, neighboring institutions, need to be considered. Unless one eliminates excesses in the labor force resulting from automation, automation should not be considered an alternative, because it then will add additional cost to the system. The financial decision to automate is not made solely on the ability to eliminate personnel. Other factors should be considered, including the possible benefits of streamlined billing, improved cash flow, decreased errors, increased responsiveness, and decreased length of stay. An integral part of automating involves maximizing efficiency through streamlining production processes. The ability to streamline production processes may come as a direct result of workflow analysis and good planning. "What if" situations need to be analyzed if maximal cost control and reduction are to be realized. An automatic output of the system should be data used to monitor the system (60). Labor standards and standard cost should be employed in the streamlining process to establish a baseline of what the current labor utilization is and what changes have major effect on this utilization pattern (61-67).

Decentralization of pharmacists to the patient care units generally will dictate a higher ratio of pharmacists to supportive personnel. One needs to establish guidelines for cost equivalency between pharmacists and supportive personnel. For example, depending on wage structure, one may hire 1 pharmacist or 1.8 supportive personnel for the same number of dollars. The main issue to consider is the total number of dollars spent for personnel. You may need to adjust the mix of people based on legal or operational requirements. Certain duties can be performed safely or legally only by a pharmacist, while the accomplishment of other responsibilities is more discretionary. For discretionary responsibilities, efficiency should be a primary tool in the decision-making process (68). Decentralizion of pharmacists to the patient care area may result in the increased efficiency of this job classification because of improved employee motivation. You have placed the employee in an environment that enables him/her to use more of his/her education and training by interacting with physicians and nurses. However, decreased productivity may occur if the pharmacist is uncomfortable with the new role. This generally can be avoided through careful communication and planning at the front end. Increased productivity and efficiency are the goals, and changes in the system (decentralization) and personnel mix should be attuned to achieving this result. Decentralization can be—and often is—more costly if it is not planned carefully with measurable goals. Decentralization can be linked closely to a drug utilization effort to achieve maximal cost control/reduction benefit (69).

Changing standards is often a costly process unless the entire system is considered. As mentioned earlier in the chapter, the unit dose distribution system is the most cost-effective system for distributing drugs (7). However, if this system were considered only from the perspective of pharmacy, the result would have been completely different. Each time a change in standard is considered, the total effect on the entire system must be evaluated in order to avoid costly mistakes or to seize cost-reduction opportunities.

Managers must actively seek cost-reducing opportunities, decide which ones to pursue, and determine what to do to make them a reality. Pharmacy departments face a great number of problems and opportunities. Peter Drucker (70) observed that solving a problem merely restores normality, but results "must come from the exploitation of opportunities." This is particularly true in achieving cost objectives. Whether the example is unit dose, drug utilization, formulary management, or decentralization, success depends on assertive management—finding opportunities and concentrating "resources and efforts on them."

REFERENCES

1. Stoner JA: *Management.* Englewood Cliffs, NJ, Prentice-Hall, 1982.
2. Ivancevich JM, Donnelly JH, Gibson JL: *Managing for Performance.* Dallas, Business Publications, 1980.
3. Hepler CD: A primer on productivity. *Top Hosp Pharm Mgt* 1:55-68, May 1981.
4. Levin RH, Letcher KI, de Leon RF, et al: Patient-care unit system for measuring clinical and distributive pharmacy workload. *Am J Hosp Pharm* 37:53-61, 1980.
5. Letcher KI: Performance measurement. In Smith MC, Brown TR (eds): *Handbook of Institutional Pharmacy Practice.* Baltimore, Williams & Wilkins, 1979, pp 88-95.
6. Wolfe AV, Wolfe KJ: Improving department productivity. In Turban E (ed): *Cost Containment in Hospitals.* Germantown, MD, Aspen, 1980, pp 171-176.
7. Summerfield MR: *Unit Dose Primer.* Bethesda, American Society of Hospital Pharmacists, 1983.
8. McGhan WF: Applying cost-benefit/cost-effectiveness analysis to clinical services. In *Symposium Proceedings: Cost Justification of Clinical Pharmacy Services: Strategies for the Eighties.* Sponsored by Pfizer, 1983, pp 8-12.
9. McGhan WF: Cost-benefit and cost-effectiveness: Methodologies for evaluating innovative pharmaceutical services. *Am J Hosp Pharm* 35:133-140, 1978.
10. Robbins SP: *The Administrative Process.* Englewood Cliffs, NJ, Prentice-Hall, 1976.
11. Webber RA: *Management.* Homewood, IL, Richard D Irwin, 1967.
12. VanDerLinde LP: System to maximize inventory performance in a small hospital. *Am J Hosp Pharm* 40:70-73, 1983.
13. Noel MW: Inventory control: A review for hospital pharmacists. *Hosp Pharm* 13:617-631, 1978.
14. William RB: Preparing the operating budget. *Am J Hosp Pharm* 40:2181-2188, 1983.
15. Staley JD: *The Cost-Minded Manager.* New York, American Management Association, 1961.
16. Nold EG: Developing a data-collection system. *Am J Hosp Pharm* 40:1685-1689, 1983.
17. Roberts MJ, Kvalseth TO, Jermstad RL: Work measurement in hospital pharmacy. *Top Hosp Pharm Mgt* 2:1-17, August 1982.
18. Nold EG: Developing reports. *Am J Hosp Pharm* 40:1968-1975, 1983.
19. Nold EG: Financial analysis. *Am J Hosp Pharm* 40:1975-1979, 1983.
20. Strong EP, Smith RD: *Management Control Models.* New York, Holt, Rinehart & Winston, 1968.
21. Egdahl RH: Should we shrink the health care system? *Harv Bus Rev* 62:125-132, January/February, 1984.
22. Reinhardt UE: The health professions' collision course. *Hospitals* 58:96-97, August 1984.
23. Nold EG: Hospital pharmacy financial management: Challenges of the 1980s. *Am J Hosp Pharm* 41:1564-1566, 1984.
24. Curtiss FR: Reimbursement dilemma regarding home health-care products and services. *Am J Hosp Pharm* 41:1548-1557, 1984.
25. Stavro B: Omnicare's aches and pains. *Forbes* 133:74-75, June 1984.
26. O'Donnel KP: Hospital-based home health care: Gaining a competitive advantage where everyone benefits. *Am J Hosp Pharm* 41:147-148, 1984.
27. Swoboda RJ: Home health care: Bane or boon for hospitals? *Am J Hosp Pharm* 41:149-151, 1984.
28. Bishop CT: Home parenteral therapy. *Top Hosp Pharm Mgt* 4:35-42, November 1984.
29. Harris WH Jr: Home parenteral antibiotic therapy. *Top Hosp Pharm Mgt* 4:43-55, November 1984.
30. Pierpaoli PG, McAllister JC III: The evolution of home health care in hospital pharmacy. *Top Hosp Pharm Mgt* 4:1-8, November 1984.
31. Hughes TF: The economics of home health care. *Top Hosp Pharm Mgt* 4:9-15, November 1984.
32. Mackowiak J: Legal issues in hospital-based home health care. *Top Hosp Pharm Mgt* 4:16-25, November 1984.
33. Schneider PJ: Home parenteral nutrition. *Top Hosp Pharm Mgt* 4:26-34, November 1984.
34. Enright SM: Understanding prospective pricing and DRGs. *Am J Hosp Pharm* 40:1493-1494, 1983.
35. Hoffmann RP: A strategy to reduce drug expenditures with a drug utilization review program. *Hosp Pharm* 19:7-11, 1984.
36. Abramowitz PW, Nold EG, Hatfield SM: Use of clinical pharmacists to reduce Cefamandole, Cefoxitin, and Ticardillin costs. *Am J Hosp Pharm* 39:1176-1180, 1982.
37. DeTorres OH, White RE: Effect of aminoglycoside-use restrictions on drug cost. *Am J Hosp Pharm* 41:1137-1139, 1984.
38. Abramowitz PW: Controlling financial variables—changing prescribing patterns. *Am J Hosp Pharm* 41:503-515, 1984.
39. Klapp DL, Ramphal R: Antibiotic restriction in hospitals associated with medical schools. *Am J Hosp Pharm* 40:1957-1960, 1983.
40. Blaufuss JC: Cost containment through active drug-use review. *Top Hosp Pharm Mgt* 1:45-52, November 1981.
41. Leist, ER, Ford DC: Pharmacy strategies for antibiotic review. *Top Hosp Pharm Mgt* 1:53-64, November 1981.
42. Nobel S, Willoughby PW: Drug utilization review for oncology drugs: Background and issues. *Top Hosp Pharm Mgt* 1:65-79, November 1981.

43. Knapp DA, Knapp DA, Michocki RJ, Speedie MK, Jankel CA: Drug prescribing and hospital cost containment. *Top Hosp Pharm Mgt* 2:7-14, November 1982.

44. Pathak DS, Klinger PA: Predictive factors in bid purchasing of antibiotics. *Top Hosp Pharm Mgt* 1:17-28, November 1981.

45. Abramowitz PW: Controlling financial variables—purchasing, inventory control, and waste reduction. *Am J Hosp Pharm* 41:309-317, 1984.

46. McAllister JC: Purchasing and inventory control systems management. *Am J Hosp Pharm* 41:320-322, 1984.

47. Skolaut MW, McAllister, JC: Purchasing and inventory control—past, present, and future. *Am J Hosp Pharm* 41:522-525, 1984.

48. Dedrick, SC, Eckel FM: Assessment of vendors and drug-product selection. *Am J Hosp Pharm* 41:703-708, 1984.

49. McAllister JC: Bid solicitation and contract negotiation. *Am J Hosp Pharm* 41:1164-1172, 1984.

50. Rubin H, Keller DD: Improving a pharmaceutical purchasing and inventory control system. *Am J Hosp Pharm* 40:67-70, 1983.

51. Yost RD, Flowers DM: New roles for wholesalers in hospital drug distribution. *Top Hosp Pharm Mgt* 1:61-67, August 1981.

52. Grimm JE: Practical aspects of selecting a pharmaceutical purchasing group. *Top Hosp Pharm Mgt* 1:49-59, August 1981.

53. Rucker TD: Effective formulary development—which direction? *Top Hosp Pharm Mgt* 1:29-44, November 1981.

54. Daniels CE, Wertheimer AI: Analysis of hospital formulary effects on cost control. *Top Hosp Pharm Mgt* 2:32-47, August 1982.

55. Packer CL: A comparison of hospital data processing costs. *Hospitals* 58:83-86, August 1984.

56. Lockwood WA, Bauman NR: Current and coming technology in hospital pharmacy automation. *Top Hosp Pharm Mgt* 4:1-6, May 1984.

57. Coblio NA: The request for proposal as a tool for computer selection. *Hosp Pharm* 19:79-87, 1984.

58. Gouveia WA: Pharmacy management and the computer. *Top Hosp Pharm Mgt* 1:77-86, May 1981.

59. Kaufman RL: Layoffs, An emerging reality. *Am J Hosp Pharm* 41:296-298, 1984.

60. Adams C, Tuck BA, Hunt ML Jr: Departmental productivity reporting through computerized systems. *Top Hosp Pharm Mgt* 2:47-54, February 1982.

61. Toohey JB, Herrick JD, Trautman RT: Adaptation of a workload measurement system. *Am J Hosp Pharm* 39:999-1004, 1982.

62. Cohen KP: Work simplification: A supervisor's challenge. *Health Care Superv* 2:12-21, October 1983.

63. Covert RP: Management engineering in the hospital environment. *Top Hosp Pharm Mgt* 3:12-19, November 1983.

64. Robertsen JA: Managing for productivity improvement. *Top Hosp Pharm Mgt* 3:17-21, February 1983.

65. Hunt ML Jr, Tuck BA, Adams CT: System to measure the use of pharmacy personnel. *Am J Hosp Pharm* 39:82-85, 1982.

66. Levin RH, Letcher KI, DeLeon RF, McCart GV: Patient-care unit system for measuring clinical and distributive pharmacy workload. *Am J Hosp Pharm* 37:53-61, 1980.

67. Mackewicz DW: Developing a workload measurement system for a decentralized hospital pharmacy service. *Top Hosp Pharm Mgt* 3:22-37, February 1983.

68. Barker KN, Smith MC, Winter ER: The work of the pharmacist and the potential use of auxiliaries. *Am J Hosp Pharm* 29:35-53, 1972.

69. Roberts, AW: Effect on drug costs of implementing decentralized drug distribution. *Am J Hosp Pharm* 40:604-606, 1983.

70. Drucker PF: *Managing for Results*. New York, Harper & Row, 1964.

ADDITIONAL READING

Abramowitz PW, Nold EG: New directions for hospital pharmacy. *Am J Hosp Pharm* 41:724-726, 1984.

Bender FH, DeMatteo CS: Cost containment through P & T committee drug utilization review. *Hosp Formul* 19:699-707, 1984.

Bonney RS: Hospital survival strategies for the 1980s. *Am J Hosp Pharm* 40:1483-1493, 1983.

Bradish RA: Changing an automated drug inventory control system to a data base design. *Am J Hosp Pharm* 39:1502-1505, 1982.

Brakebill JI, Robb RA, Ivey MF, Christensen DB, Young JH, Scribner BH: Pharmacy department costs and patient charges associated with a home parenteral nutrition program. *Am J Hosp Pharm* 40:260-263, 1983.

Caldwell RD, Tuck BA: Justification and operation of a critical-care satellite pharmacy. *Am J Hosp Pharm* 40:2141-2145, 1983.

Check WA: New drugs and drug-delivery systems in the year 2000. *Am J Hosp Pharm* 41:1536-1547, 1984.

Cleverly WO: Strategies for reducing hospital costs. *Drug Ther* 13:68-77, January 1984.

Cohen JE: Reduction in work hours during a period of reduced patient census. *Am J Hosp Pharm* 41:294-296, 1984.

Cowan DZ: Productivity in health care: An overview. *South Hosp* 52:72-78, March/April 1984.

Curtiss FR: Looking beyond DRGs: opportunities for hospital pharmacy. *Am J Hosp Pharm* 41:721-723, 1984.

Curtiss FR: Pharmacy management strategies for responding to hospital reimbursement changes. *Am J Hosp Pharm* 40:1489-1492, 1983.

DiPiro JT, Gousse GC, Kubica AJ: Work sampling to evaluate staff pharmacist productivity. *Am J Hosp Pharm* 36:201-205, 1979.

Editorial: Preparing for prospective pricing. *Am J Hosp Pharm* 40:1479, 1983.

Editorial: Reassessing pharmacy and therapeutics committees. *Am J Hosp Pharm* 41:1527, 1984.

Enright SM: "Procompetition" and the continuing struggle to contain health-care costs. *Am J Hosp Pharm* 40:282-286, 1983.

Enthoven AC: Shattuck lecture—cutting cost without cutting the quality of care. *N Engl J Med* 298:1229-1238, 1978.

Fine DJ, Guild RT, Kleinmann K, Kupersmith J: P & T committee round-table discussion: Eastern region pt. II. *Hosp Formul* 19:561-571, 1984.

Hammel RJ, King CM Jr, Jones TF: Administrative case study: Analysis of a hospital pharmacy's manpower requirements. *Am J Hosp Pharm* 34:969-973, 1977.

Herkimer AC Jr: Strategies for pharmacy management planning and job design. *Top Hosp Pharm Mgt* 3:8-16, August 1983.

Hoffmann RP: Expanding pharmaceutical services through efficient staff scheduling. *Hosp Pharm* 14:192-199, 1979.

Hoffmann RP, Bartt KH, Berlin L, Frank Sr BM: Multidisciplinary quality assessment of a unit dose drug distribution system. *Hosp Pharm* 19:167-174, 1984.

Huber SL, Patry RA, Hudson HD, Godwin HN: Strengthening the formulary system by implementing a drug usage guidelines program. *Hosp Formul* 19:664-668, 1984.

Hunt ML: Use of financial reports in managing pharmacies. *Am J Hosp Pharm* 41:709-715, 1984.

Hyer NL, Wemmerlov U: Group technology and productivity. *Harv Bus Rev* 62:140-148, July/August 1984.

Jones RH: PERT/CPM network analysis: A management tool for hospital pharmacists involved in strategic planning. *Hosp Pharm* 19:89-97, 1984.

Kowalsky SF, Echols RM, Peck F Jr: Preprinted order sheet to enhance antibiotic prescribing and surveillance. *Am J Hosp Pharm* 39:1528-1529, 1982.

Kubica AJ: Cost containment: An overview for hospital pharmacists. *Cur Concepts Hosp Pharm Mgt* 5:4-8, 1979.

Kuntz EF: Hospitals move into home care by striking partnership deals. *Mod Healthcare* 13:116-117, December 1983.

Lee MP: Coping with DRGs: University of California Medical Center, San Diego. *Am J Hosp Pharm* 40:1504-1506, 1983.

Lipman AG: Cost implications of future new drugs. *Hosp Formul* 19:635, 1984.

McAllister JC III, Lindley CM: Strategies for program planning, implementation and control. *Top Hosp Pharm Mgt* 3:72-83, May 1983.

Mehl B: Indicators to control drug costs in hospitals. *Am J Hosp Pharm* 41:667-675, 1984.

Miller DE: Coping with DRGs: Hospital of the University of Pennsylvania, Philadelphia. *Am J Hosp Pharm* 40:1503-1504, 1983.

Nold EG: Financial management of hospital pharmacies. *Am J Hosp Pharm* 40:1339-1341, 1983.

Norvell MJ, McAllister JC, Bailey E: Cost analysis of drug distribution for controlled substances. *Am J Hosp Pharm* 40:801-807, 1983.

Osborne JA: Coping with DRGs: Baptist Medical Center of Oklahoma, Oklahoma City, *Am J Hosp Pharm* 40:1506-1507, 1983.

Phillips DJM, Smith JE: Hospital-based training for pharmaceutical manufacturers' representatives. *Am J Hosp Pharm* 40:1661-1663, 1983.

Quandt WG, Miller DA, Russell KH, Stankiewicz RF: Computerized attendance surveillance to reduce absenteeism. *Am J Hosp Pharm* 41:298-300, 1984.

Roberts RW: Coping with DRGs: Riverside Hospital, Jacksonville, Florida. *Am J Hosp Pharm* 40:1500-1502, 1983.

Scrivens JJ Jr, Magallan P, and Crozler GA: Cost-effective clinical pharmacy services in a veterans administration drop-in clinic. *Am J Hosp Pharm* 40:1952-1953, 1983.

Sebastian G, Thielke TS: Work analysis of an admixture service. *Am J Hosp Pharm* 40:2149-2153, 1983.

Segall LE, Kotzan JA: Comparison of two methods of observing work areas in a hospital pharmacy. *Am J Hosp Pharm* 36:59-63, 1979.

Siegel J, Schneider PJ, Moore TD: Innovative scheduling to maintain clinical pharmacy services despite budget retrenchment. *Am J Hosp Pharm* 41:291-293, 1984.

Smith JE, Phillips DJM, Meyer GE: Diversification strategies for hospital pharmacies. *Am J Hosp Pharm* 41:1788-1791, 1984.

Smith WE: Drug cost containment in the hospital. *Hosp Formul* 13:695-698, September 1978.

Stokes JF: Quality patient care and cost control, too. *Health Care Superv* 21:60-74, July 1983.

Swett TF, Conley DJ: Joint ventures: the theory and practice. *Hospitals* 58:95-100, May 1984.

Templin JL Jr: Productivity and the supervisor. *Health Care Superv* 2:1-11, April 1983.

Thompson JD, Averill RF, Fetter RB: Planning, budgeting, and controlling—one look at the future: Case-mix cost accounting. *Health Serv Res* 14:111-125, 1979.

Trudeau T: A simple work measurement system than can aid in effective production planning. *Hosp Pharm* 15:229-233, 1980.

Upton JH, Crouch JB, Douglas JB: Coping with DRGs: The Moses H. Cone Memorial Hospital, Greensboro, North Carolina. *Am J Hosp Pharm* 40:1496-1499, 1983.

Vaida AJ: Coping with DRGs: Suburban General Hospital, Norristown, Pennsylvania, *Am J Hosp Pharm* 40:1494-1496, 1983.

Wilson CN: Financial tools in evaluating profit and DRG cost determination. *Hosp Pharm* 19:438-439, 1984.

VanDerLinde LP: System to maximize inventory performance in a small hospital. *Am J Hosp Pharm* 40:70-73, 1983.

Wymelenberg S: New accounting system helps control costs. *Hospitals*. 53:68-70, July 1979.

CHAPTER 13

Cost-Benefit Studies

ROBERT A. FREEMAN

Justification of new programs or of any other capital expenditure decision is an important responsibility of a pharmacist-manager. One method that can be used to meet this end is cost-benefit analysis.

Cost-benefit analysis is an analytical decision-making tool that relates the patient care benefits of a health program to the economic costs of producing those benefits. Cost-benefit analysis is, in essence, a method of expressing program benefits and costs in a common denominator, economic value. More specifically, cost-benefit analysis is a way of comparing the economic performance of two or more projects over their expected life cycles.

Individuals who have been involved in the decision-making process of complex organizations will quickly admit that decisions are quite often made on the basis of political pressures. If that be the case, why should anyone bother with cost-benefit analysis? Admittedly, cost-benefit analysis is not the universal antidote for political ills, nor, for that matter, is any other analytical decision-making tool. That admission, however, does not invalidate the technique's applicability.

Cost-benefit analysis can be improved to provide corroborative input into the decision-making process. It should not be, nor was it ever intended to be, the only criterion on which decisions are based. However, if cost-benefit analysis is used as supportive documentation, many of the political objections to a program may be nipped in the bud.

E.J. Mishan, an international authority on cost-benefit analysis, states that the general question cost-benefit analysis answers has two parts (1). First, we want to know whether or not a number of investment projects should be implemented. Additionally, if resources are limited, we need to know which project(s) of a number of otherwise acceptable projects should be implemented.

It is also noted that programs are generally designed to have a more or less permanent effect on a department's service delivery. Hence, one would expect that the benefits of a program are evidenced throughout the life cycle of a project. Similarly, certain aspects of cost are naturally active over this time period.

Since projects have this element of time, it becomes necessary to employ a discount factor to express economic value in the present. Since the value of money is affected by time, it is important to project the expected stream of benefits and cost over the expected life of the project, and subsequently to discount these streams to yield a measure of present economic value.

Empiric determination of a discount rate exceeds the scope of this chapter, and the reader is referred to the works of Klarman (2) and Rice (3) for further insight.

In any event, discounting is a value judgment. One recommendation that might be offered is to employ the interest rate that your institution must pay for acquiring capital funds (4). Using the institution's rate will not cause any unforeseen difficulties unless the rate has been subject to drastic fluctuations.

Moreover, using the institution's rate offers several advantages: (1) the rate is meaningful to your administrator in real dollar terms, (2) the rate is known or easily determinable, and (3) it is convenient.

Calculation of the present value of benefits and costs is somewhat cumbersome, depending on the life of the project. The analysis can be simplified by relying on published interest tables, usually found in finance books, as well as programmable calculators.

COSTS AND BENEFITS

In economic analysis, cost assumes a definition that is somewhat broader in scope than that used in financial statement preparation. In cost-benefit analysis, economic cost is categorized as either direct cost or indirect cost. A direct economic cost is an actual expenditure or outlay attributable to the project. An indirect economic cost is an expense incurred but not actually expended as a result of the project. One example of an indirect cost that does appear on financial statements is depreciation of equipment. In essence, indirect economic costs are important because failure to consider these costs underestimates the true nature of the economic impact of a project.

Direct costs of a project may be further categorized as either investment costs or operating costs (5). Investment costs are those capital expenditures coming about because of the purchase and installation of equipment required by the project. The cost of hiring or training personnel would also be a type of investment cost. These costs are generally borne at the initiation of a project. Operating costs are defined as the stream of expenditures necessary for maintenance of the program. These are generally in the form of personnel costs and equipment service costs.

Although the idea may be somewhat confusing, in certain instances cost may become benefits. Programs dealing with the prevention of a particular illness, for example, have economic costs associated with the treatment of the condition. If a program were not implemented, however, there is an economic cost of doing nothing. In essence, the disease has a cost associated with it, and if the disease were eradicated, society would "benefit" through the reduction in costs attributable to the disease.

Moreover, if resources are utilized improperly or inefficiently, there is an economic cost accruing to society. If a program can be developed that utilizes resources more efficiently or appropriately, society "benefits" through the reduction of costs.

BENEFITS

As indicated, there are instances in which some elements of cost actually appear in the analysis as benefits. Benefits may also come about in the form of revenues received by the institution because of a new program. Benefits may also be in the form of additional output of services measured by their economic value.

The key issue in defining what a benefit is lies in identifying what the objective of the program actually is. Since health programs have the potential of bestowing profuse benefits, it becomes necessary to focus attention on program outcomes and ways of measuring outcomes.

A work of caution should be introduced at this point: cost-benefit analysis does not have a universally accepted protocol established for its application. In fact, it is even difficult to judge whether or not the model has been correctly applied. One criterion that is very important, however, is the element of causality inherently assumed in the model. One assumes in a cost-benefit model that the benefits are "caused" by the project. While this is common sense, its importance cannot be overstated.

APPLICATIONS OF COST-BENEFIT IN HEALTH

A review of the literature reveals that cost-benefit analyses in studying investments in health care have centered along three broad categories of content (6). These content areas are (1) the economic cost of illness, (2) efficiency/effectiveness of service delivery, and (3) return on investment from research and development and education.

Cost of illness studies received considerable emphasis in the 1960s, beginning with works of Klarman (7) and Rice (8). These approaches were directed at establishing the economic value of making public investments to eradicate or prevent certain diseases.

Service delivery has been appraised by cost-benefit analysis to determine the optimal way of providing services given several alternative methods. (In this respect, cost-benefit analysis and cost-effectiveness analysis became quite similar.) A very interesting study is now under way, for example, to determine the optimal way to implement a national strategy for smoking cessation (9). Generally, this

approach rests on basing decisions on the highest benefit-cost ratio.

The third study area has centered on calculating the estimated return on investment of health-related research and development as well as health manpower-training programs (10). For example, the American Enterprise Institute has published a series of books dealing with returns on investment from the pharmaceutical industry (11,12).

THE COST-BENEFIT MODEL

The cost-benefit model may be defined symbolically as follows:

$$NB = \sum_{i=1}^{n} (TB_i - TC_i)$$

where NB = the present value of net benefits; TB = the present value of total benefits over the life of the project; TC = the present value of total project costs over the life of the project; n = the number of years of the project's "life"; and

$$TB_i = \sum_{i=1}^{n} (B_i)(1 + r)^{-t}$$

$$TC_i = \sum_{i=1}^{n} (C_i)(1 + r)^{-t}$$

where B = the total annual benefits of the project; C = the total annual costs of the project; r = the rate of discount; t = the expected life (number of years) of the project.

Hence, the cost-benefit model measures net benefits by subtracting total costs from total benefits. If net benefits are positive, the project is economically viable.

The cost-benefit model requires that we base our decisions on the present value of the streams of benefits and costs discounted by an appropriate interest rate. We have, in essence, standardized our reference point for comparisons by this manipulation. One fact that complicates the analysis is the assumption that costs and benefits occur at continuous rates throughout the life of the project. This, of course, may not be the case and should be accommodated in the analysis.

DECISION-MAKING CRITERIA WITH COST-BENEFIT ANALYSIS

Cost-benefit analysis will provide us estimates of the present value of the net worth of a project. The question now becomes one of how we use this value in decision making.

One application of cost-benefit model is to decide on the desirability of a capital expenditure. We are essentially asking whether the project provides us with any advantage over the status quo. In this type of analysis, the present value of net benefits may be used as a decision criterion. For example, if there appears to be a positive value in implementing the project, we should adopt the project and reach a "go" decision. If the converse be true, our decision would be "no go."

When we are faced with selecting a project from several alternative investments with dissimilar objectives, basing a decision on the present value of net benefits may not be entirely appropriate. We do not always feel comfortable with making decisions on this basis alone.

One basis for consideration rests with the estimation of the benefits-to-cost ratio. With this approach, we would select the project with the highest benefits-to-cost ratio if we are restricted financially to one choice.

The cost-benefit ratio is defined as the present value of economic benefits divided by the present value of economic costs (13). Mathematically, any ratio higher than 1.0 possesses utility to the organization.

Another type of viewpoint that is worthy of mention is marginal cost-benefit analysis. Marginal cost-benefit analysis is concerned with assessing the impact resulting from changing the system. In some instances, marginal cost-benefit analysis provides more important information than does analysis on total costs.

The following example should provide insights into using the benefit-to-cost ratio and marginal analysis. In this hypothetical situation, the chief pharmacist in a 400-bed general hospital is considering a proposal to change the basis for drug charges from the usual method of unit pricing to a per diem method.

Currently, the pharmacy department employs a full-time clerical assistant at the annual expense of $11,000. The chief pharmacist estimates that if he were to adopt the per diem system, the department would only require a half-time assistant for the charging function. In this analysis, he estimates a yearly expense for data processing. His total expense projections for the two systems are as follows:

Cost of Present System*	Year	Cost of Per Diem System*
11,000	01	7500
11,660	02	7950
12,360	03	8427
13,101	04	8933
13,887	05	9469
TC = 62,008		TC = 42,279

*Discounted at a net effective discount rate of 6%.

Benefits from the two systems are the expected patient revenues from the drug products distributed within the pharmacy over the 5-year time period. He obtains these estimates based on simple forecasts of expected revenues from the present system and from the per diem rate. This income stream is discounted at a net effective discount rate of 6%. The estimates of benefits expressed in present value are as follows (revenues were projected with the assumption that bed size remains constant as does average daily census, but average length of stay decreases slightly):

Patient Revenues, Present System	Year	Per Diem Patient Revenues
115,750	01	112,600
114,382	02	111,505
114,382	03	111,505
114,171	04	111,336
113,959	05	111,167
ΣBenefits = 572,644		ΣBenefits = 558,113

The cost-benefit ratios are calculated as follows:

$$(\text{Benefits})/\text{Costs}$$

BC ratio (present system) = 572,644/62,008 = 9.24

BC ratio (per diem) = 558,113/42,279 = 13.20

On this basis, the chief pharmacist would logically elect the per diem system over the present system.

Our chief pharmacist, on further examination, finds that both modifications are similar but will cost an additional $500 for the present system and $450 for the per diem system. Revenues received because of the modification are $28,632 and $27,950, respectively. Using marginal cost analysis to assess this change, he would compute the ratios as follows:

Marginal BC ratio (present system) =
$$28,632/500 = 57.26$$

Marginal BC ratio (per diem) = 27,950/450 = 62.11

Consequently, the decision would not be changed on the basis of marginal cost-benefit analysis. His overall recommendation would be to adopt the modified per diem charging system.

In essence, marginal cost-benefit analysis is employed when we are presented with the need to evaluate potential changes in the project. Marginal cost-benefit analysis provides the decision maker with an evaluation of the incremental costs and incremental benefits.

A third measure for evaluating decisions made through cost-benefit analysis is based on determining the internal rate of return of the project (or, more specifically, the investment). The rate of return on investment allows us to compare competing projects without discounting benefits and costs. It is also a concept that has recognized meaning to persons with financial backgrounds.

As indicated throughout this chapter, we more or less arbitrarily select a discount rate to obtain our measures of present values. In calculating the rate of return, we are actually solving for this rate. The average rate of return on investment is defined as expected average annual net economic benefit divided by average economic investment (14). The average annual net benefit is determined by the total net benefit expected over the life of the project divided by the number of years in the life of the project. Average investment is the expected cost of operating the project at the midpoint in its life cycle.

Using this criterion in our analysis, we would base our decision on the relative rates of return for the potential investments. The project yielding the highest return of investment would be the preferred project, because it utilizes economic resources more efficiently.

We do have to remember, however, that the guiding force of the typical health care institution is not necessarily to maximize the return on the investment. In fact, social desirability may overrule decisions made on this criterion. Therefore, we cannot state definitively that any one of these criteria is preferable. In fact, from the social viewpoint, the net benefit consideration alone is perhaps the most acceptable criterion.

COST-EFFECTIVENESS ANALYSIS

Cost-effectiveness analysis is a technique related to cost-benefit analysis that may prove to be more suitable for the evaluation of alternative programs to accomplish a *single* objective. Cost-effectiveness analysis is also a term subjected to considerable interpretation in the literature. A list of comparable terms might include "life-cycle analysis," "capital budgeting," "investment planning," and "cost-benefit planning."

One distinction between cost-benefit analysis and cost-effectiveness analysis is that cost-benefit analysis examines projects longitudinally, whereas cost-effectiveness analysis is a cross-sectional technique for program review. In cost-effectiveness analysis, we are usually concerned with selecting between or among a series of projects that essentially would accomplish the same objective. In essence we have previously decided that the objective will be attained because it is desirable and are now looking for the best way to accomplish it (15).

It is necessary in cost-effectiveness analysis to be concerned with defining measures of program efficiency or effectiveness. It is essential that we know within reasonable limits how well the objective is accomplished by the number of alternative ways of attaining this objective. Given the levels of success and the costs associated with each alternative, one can then base the decision-making process on efficiency of resource utilization and effectiveness associated with the programs.

For example, if your problem is one of drug distribution, we would examine the various ways that drug products are distributed within the institution and rate each method according to some predetermined criteria (prevalance of medication errors, savings in nursing time, etc). The cost of providing each type of distribution method would then be compared with the level of care associated with each type, and the decision would then follow.

Like cost-benefit analysis, cost-effectiveness analysis requires a certain level of specificity in terms of output specifications and level of performance. Unlike cost-benefit analysis, we are generally dealing with issues of resource utilization at the microeconomic level.

In Chapter 17, one notes that the development of alternative strategies is a major component of the planning process. It would be important to note that cost-effectiveness analysis is an important tool in the planning process and is often evidenced in the evaluative process. Cost-effectiveness analysis is a planning model, as is cost-benefit analysis, but cost-effectiveness analysis has more applicability as an evaluative model.

DECISION-MAKING CRITERIA WITH COST-EFFECTIVENESS ANALYSIS

When using cost-benefit analysis, one is trying to answer questions about the desirability of projects that often have dissimilar objectives. The question that cost-effectiveness analysis attempts to answer is, "Given limited resources, which program, of two or more programs that will otherwise accomplish the same objective, should be implemented?" The issue is now one of effectiveness in objective achievement and efficiency in resource utilization.

There is no one set way to evaluate projects using cost-effectiveness analysis. In any event, the criteria are based on minimization of program cost.

To use cost-effectiveness analysis in program evaluation, one might follow the steps outlined as follows:

1. Identify program costs and outcomes for each program under consideration.

2. Select appropriate measure of program output.
3. Where indicated, project program output and costs.
4. Make recommendation of optimal program on a predetermined criterion (effectiveness-to-cost ratio, rate of return, or efficiency ratio).

Program effectiveness is measured in a number of ways, depending on the objectives of the project. For example, if one of our output measures concerns saving personnel time, the appropriate measure might be "person years" released for other productive activities. Of course, we would assume that the savings in time really do exist, i.e., there are other activities a person could perform, or that the departmental personnel roster can actually be reduced.

For many measures of effectiveness we could express these variables in monetary terms. For example, person years could be expressed in budgetary amounts, or the variable could be left as such. In the latter case, our ratios would take the form of units of time (person years) divided by program costs. This value judgment of appropriate measurement is left to the user's discretion.

SUMMARY AND RECOMMENDATIONS

As a planning tool, cost-benefit analysis has some usefulness to the institutional pharmacist in examing the desirability of investments strategies. There is no universal guide to the applicability, however. Cost-effectiveness analysis has utility in both planning and evaluating ongoing projects. If one were to choose between the two techniques, the more preferable approach would probably be cost-effectiveness analysis, although one must always recognize the errors occurring from improper application of either technique.

With the increasing cost burden of providing institutional services, one should be familiar with the two techniques and decide on the relative appropriateness of each in the planning of the department's growth. It is much easier to justify new approaches in the delivery of pharmaceutical services if the planning effort can be expressed in budgetary figures.

In summary, the techniques of cost-benefit/cost-effectiveness analysis are fairly straightforward. The criteria for evaluation, however, are subject to considerable variation and subjectivity. Cost-benefit analysis will not always provide us with optimal programs. However, one outcome of its application can be the rejection of the worst programs. This, in and of itself, is no minor accomplishment.

REFERENCES

1. Mishan EJ: *Economics for Social Decisions.* New York, Praeger Publications, 1973, p 11.
2. Klarman HE: Applications of cost benefit to health systems technology. In Collen MF (chairman): *Technology and Health Care Systems in the 1980's.* Washington, DC, National Center for Health Services Research and Development, 1973, pp 225-249.
3. Rice DP: *Estimating the Cost of Illness, Health Economics Series.* Washington, DC, U.S. Government Printing Office, No. 6, PHS Publication No. 947-6, 1966, pp 1-107.
4. Wacht, RF: Capital budgeting decision-making for hospitals. *Hosp Admin* 15:14-27, 1970.
5. *ibid.*
6. Dunlop DW: Benefit-cost analysis: A review of its applicability in policy analysis for delivering health services. *Soc Sci Med* 9:133-139, 1975.

7. Klarman HE: Socioeconomic impact of heart disease. *Heart Circ* 2:693, 1964.
8. Rice DP: *op. cit.*
9. Personal communication with author from the American Health Foundation, New York.
10. Hirsh WZ: *Urban Economic Analysis*. New York, McGraw-Hill, 1972, pp 340-346.
11. Schwartzman D: *The Expected Return from Pharmaceutical Research*. Washington, DC, American Enterprise Institute for Policy Research, 1975, pp 23-46.
12. Peltzman S: *Regulation of Pharmaceutical Innovation*. Washington, DC, American Enterprise Institute for Policy Research, 1974, pp 33-500.
13. Smith WF: Cost-effectiveness and cost-benefit analysis for public health problems. In Levey L (ed): *Health Care Administration*. Philadelphia, JB Lippincott, 1973, pp 369-380.
14. Brandt LK: *Business Finance in Management Approach*. Englewood Cliffs, NJ, Prentice-Hall, 1965, pp 379-400.
15. Smith WF: *op. cit.*

CHAPTER 14

Fiscal Planning

JOSEPH A. HARRIS

In 1963 Peter F. Drucker (1) stated, "What is the first duty—and the continuing responsibility—of the business manager? To strive for the best possible economic results from the resources currently employed or available." This statement applies to the health care manager or pharmacy manager as well or better today than in 1963. The acute care hospital is experiencing a maturing and changing market that requires it to be increasingly competitive and efficient in order to maintain its economic viability. With the changing environmental demands being placed on our hospitals, the pharmacy manager will need to develop skills in financial management.

This chapter is structured in a "strategic planning" format. The intent will be to examine format and tools for developing a *fiscal plan* for a hospital pharmacy department. The overall goal will be to ask simple, yet complex questions:

1. Where are we now?
2. Where do we want to go?
3. How do we get there?

These questions will be addressed through external environment analysis, internal environment analysis, formulation of the financial strategy, and monitoring and controlling.

EXTERNAL ENVIRONMENT ANALYSIS

In developing a financial management plan, one of the most important tasks is gaining a thorough understanding of the environment in which the institution and department provide health care services. The environment is considered to be those external factors that have an important influence on performance. An understanding of those factors is essential to making sound financial decisions. This section on external environment is divided into two parts: environment external to the hospital and environment external to the pharmacy department (within the department).

Environment External to the Hospital

Evaluation of the external environment is intended primarily to (1) raise the awareness of the gross health care environment in which the hospital must compete and (2) identify priority issues that a department's financial plan must address or monitor. This section is divided into four areas: (1) trends and issues affecting health care industry, (2) reimbursement systems, (3) pharmacy professional issues, and (4) statistical information.

Each of these areas must be examined from national, regional, state, and local perspectives. The evaluation must be customized to a hospital's needs and wants to meet the institution's size, type, location, etc.

Trends and Issues Affecting the Health Care Industry

Two books, *Megatrends* by John Naisbitt and *In Search of Excellence* by Thomas J. Peters and Robert H. Waterman, Jr., give us insight into the major trends and financial successes that are occurring. Many of these same issues are going to affect financial and personnel management directly or indirectly.

"Societal changes" are influencing the demographics of society. With people relocating more frequently, they are not establishing strong relationships with local health care providers, schools, etc. The population is aging, a factor which will create an increased need for health care services. The public's expectations for good health, more information, increased participation, and more competition has increased with improved education and communication in our society. "Technology" will improve the length and quality of life through the use of computers and microelectronics. These technologies will cause increased awareness of financial issues by both increasing and decreasing health care costs.

How will the health care industry respond to the prevailing trends? Again, the response will be based on local, state, regional, and national factors. Typical responses that will occur in most hospitals will include:

- Programs to contain, avoid, and reduce costs
- Improved financial-monitoring systems
- Creative methods for attracting patients and donations
- Specialization of care
- Corporate formation and restructuring
- Emphasis on ambulatory and preventive programs
- Partnership with the medical staff
- Deregulation initiatives
- Comparative statistics

Programs to Contain, Avoid, and Reduce Costs. The first response in all hospitals will be to contain, avoid, or reduce costs. While the term "cost containment" is not new, hospitals will now pay more than lip service to containment of waste and inefficiencies. Many programs will be eliminated unless the cost-benefit ratio shows a clear advantage for the institution. Programs and products that require ongoing maintenance costs will be curtailed. For example, IV infusion devices requiring special vendor-supplied tubing will be avoided in favor of those that do not require ongoing costs and are not under the complete price control of the device vendor.

Since personnel accounts for 50% of hospital costs, this expense will be more tightly controlled. Programs to measure productivity and quality will be implemented. All personnel will be challenged to improve output, and many positions will be eliminated. Developments or innovations that have increased personnel costs and implemented few automated procedures, as in the move toward primary care nursing, will come under intense scrutiny. The current economy has eliminated the nursing shortage. Now hospital administration, not nursing, will determine the conditions of employment and extent of automation. Social workers, clinical pharmacists, and clinical dietitions will all have to produce cost savings or real revenue in order to gain or retain sufficient staff members.

Improved Financial-Monitoring Systems. Billing and accounts payable are computerized in most hospitals. More financial data will be developed, more financial data-gathering systems will be installed, and more analytical techniques will be employed. Diagnosis related groups (DRGs) alone will require a major change in the classification of data. Financial ratios similar to those used in business will be employed to determine the more profitable diagnoses, physicians, patient types, etc.

Creative Methods for Attracting Patients and Donations. Just as banks and car dealers regularly offer incentives for using their services or products, hospitals will develop methods for attracting and retaining patients. The once cold atmosphere of the patient room will be transformed into a reasonable place to stay while hospitalized. Champagne dinners for new parents, helicopter ambulance services, preferred provider arrangements, and health maintenance organizations will all become more commonplace as hospitals compete for patients with other hospitals and ambulatory patient care centers (APCCs). Hospitals are hiring marketing directors and preparing their administrative teams to respond to change or seek out benefactors for new programs or capital improvements.

Specialization of Care. The entire hospital economy will go through a highly competitive period in which some hospitals will succeed and some will fail. Hospital failures will become a reality in an open, competitive market, just as bank failures now occur. Without state assistance teaching hospitals will be particularly hard pressed to compete while carrying a greater load of medically indigent patients. Hospitals will determine what they do best or where they can make the greatest profit to offset the unprofitable services they are required to retain. Beds will no longer be allocated to physicians on the basis of who can fill them; instead, beds will be filled by physicians who can generate the best return on investment.

Corporate Formation and Restructuring. Hospitals will follow the pattern of major corporations by forming subsidiaries or other business arrangements to maximize profits and minimize liability. The growth rate of these corporations will be matched by other hospital-product vendors now entering the ambulatory care market. Hospitals will follow the same route as drugstores, where we now see a predominance of corporate chains in many areas.

Emphasis on Ambulatory and Preventive Programs. With the decreasing rate of growth and increased competition for inpatient days, hospitals will move strongly toward ambulatory care. The high overhead costs for inpatients, as well as the factors of directives and physician oversupply cited earlier, will eliminate from the market those hospitals without a strong APCC. As Americans grow more "wellness conscious," hospitals will develop prrograms to meet their demands. Sports medicine and athletic conditioning programs are already becoming popular. People will pay a high premium to prevent illness and disease.

Partnership with the Medical Staff. Physicians control most costs within the hospital and determine the types and quantities of patients. Court decisions have ruled that the physician is an employee of the hospital. Hospitals and medical staffs will have no choice but to become partners in providing health care. The "jawboning" of the administrator will be replaced by directives for making patient care profitable instead of charitable. Formularies will experience a great resurgence. Fewer laboratory tests and roentgenograms will be ordered.

Deregulation Initiatives. Health care is one of the most regulated industries. For hospitals to compete effectively and maximize profits, laws will have to be changed. Without the ability to shift costs, hospitals will seek legislative relief from having to treat nonpaying patients or will develop classes of care in which the less financially able patient will receive "equal but separate" care. A special class of care already exists for "VIPs"; this concept will be expanded, and package deals dependent on the level of care and amenities desired (e.g., private room) possibly will develop.

Comparative Statistics. Most comparative hospital statistics now available are inadequate. There are so many internal variables that the statistics really are not comparing common data bases. This will change as standard procedures develop and come into use in all hospitals.

Reimbursement Systems

In developing the pharmacy department's financial plan, administrators must explore the external factors that will directly influence their decisions. They must evaluate the programs, policies and procedures, and individuals that will make financial decisions affecting financial resources.

The DRG system of Medicare and other reimbursement programs that have been instituted or are being proposed will change Medicaid and private insurance reimbursement or already have done so. "All-payer" programs that cover all reimbursement revenue to hospitals have been implemented in New Jersey, Massachusetts, and Maryland. Programs such as preferred provider agreements are being implemented by private industry within state laws, and many other options are being explored.

Professional Issues

This is the most important aspect to explore and understand in terms of your institution. The pharmacy director's prime and exciting responsibility is in the direction of utilization of the hospital and pharmacy's resources to meet the specific *needs and wants* of the institution. The essence of pharmacy management is the analysis of external professional pharmacy issues and presentation of these issues in terms of specific applications to the institution. The pharmacy administration must look for issues in two categories. First among these are issues that will provide improved quality and productivity. Examples might be the improved use of computers in hospital pharmacy practice or direct clinical pharmacist contact with physicians to influence the use of less costly antibiotics.

The second area of evaluation and understanding is *risk* issues. These are the issues that may involve legal risks to an institution and thus have a cost impact. Examples are medication errors and their historical costs in the hospital.

Statistical Information

Most hospital statistics are averaged or aggregate and may or may not fit a given institution or department. Nevertheless, a brief review of some national statistics available for health care and hospital pharmacy practice should be valuable.

The American Hospital Association (AHA) reports health care statistics to institutions primarily through two sources. The AHA Journal *Hospitals* reports *gross* health care statistics, but HAS/Monitrend is a subscriber-based health care statistical information service of AHA that compares the subscriber institution to national, state, and regional hospitals of the same type and size. The services represent 2500 subscribers and are collected and distributed monthly. The sections of the monthly HAS/Monitrend report are:

Executive Summary Section
Nursing Services Section
Ancillary Services Section
Support Services Section
Raw Data Totals
Data Audit Section

An example of the HAS/Monitrend for pharmacy is provided in Figure 14.1. Many state hospital associations report statistical information on a regular basis. Lilly's *Hospital*

Ancillary Services Section
Group Median Data

	Your Prior 3 Month Average	National (A) 915 160 Inst.	State (B) 530 29 Inst.	Regional (C) 1885 24 Inst.	Special (D) 18824 51 Inst.	Variance From Median
1 Pharmacy						
2 Inpt Revenue/Patient Day	49.57	44.19|3	38.46|3	40.76|4	44.81|3	
3 Direct Expense/Patient Day	19.10	17.70|3	18.72|3	17.50|3	17.11|3	
4 Salary Expense/Adj. Patient Day	5.40	5.07|3	5.29|3	7.07|2	5.08|3	
5 Ratio Total Dir. Exp./Revenue	.39	.39|2	.48|2	.43|2	.38|3	
6 Direct Expense Percent	4.65	4.09|3	4.02|4	4.00|H	4.10|3	
7 Outpatient Revenue Percent	5.58	7.08|2	8.84|1	4.69|3	7.24|2	
8 Paid Hours/Adj. Patient Day	.50	.51|2	.53|2	.61|2	.53|2	

Internal Trend Data

	Current Month	Avg. Prior 3 Months Indicator	Avg. Prior 3 Months Raw Data	Same 3 Months Last Year	Percent Change	Average Prior 12 Months
20						
21						
22						
23						
24 Pharmacy						
25 Inpt. Revenue/Patient Day	42.57	49.57	63.948	48.96	1.2	45.50
26 Direct Expense/Adj. Patient Day	26.97	19.10	26.094	18.19	5.0	18.80
27 Salary Expense/Adj. Patient Day	6.14	5.40	7.377	3.21	68.2	4.37
28 Ratio Total Dir. Exp./Revenue	.63	.39		.37	5.4	.41
29 Direct Expense Percent	6.02	4.65	26.094	5.42	−14.2	5.20
30 Outpatient Revenue Percent	8.74	5.58	3.779	3.98	40.2	4.77
31 Paid Hours/Adj. Patient Day	.54	.50	677	.30	66.6	.42

FIGURE 14.1 HAS/MONITREND statistical information service on pharmacy.

Pharmacy Survey (2) is published annually and can be used to compare statistical information to one's institution in a global way.

Another source of statistical comparison is provided by the American Society of Hospital Pharmacists. Michael Stolar, director of Professional and Research Services, is developing an experimental hospital pharmacy management information system, which utilizes its indicators to relate pharmacy product and clinical and administrative services. Preliminary data were published in the *American Journal of Hospital Pharmacy* in November 1983 (3), and it is suggested that hospital pharmacy administrators will find these comparative data of significant value in the future.

Environment External to the Pharmacy Department (Within the Hospital)

The primary intent in evaluating the hospital's internal environment (environment external to the pharmacy department) will be to (1) understand the financial structure and responsibilities within the institution, (2) understand the hospital's financial goals and the policies and procedures for accomplishing them (as the budgeting process), and (3) develop an understanding of the resources available to support our financial planning and the strengths and weaknesses of those resources. This will be accomplished through an analysis of (1) the finance department, (2) the budget, and (3) financial reports.

The Finance Department

The hospital's finance department is the most important source of external information on environmental factors that will influence the pharmacy department's financial activities. The primary function of the finance department and its financial management is to maintain the hospital's viability as the environmental factors change. This function is accomplished through financial and managerial accounting functions. The financial accounting function is the formalized system for reporting the hospital's financial history to the board of directors and government agencies. Managerial accounting is intended to provide financial information that can be used to monitor or make future decisions.

According to Finkler (4), the three broad purposes of an effective accounting system are:

1. Internal reporting to managers, for use in planning and controlling routine operations;
2. Internal reporting to managers, for use in strategic planning, that is, the making of special decisions and the formulating of overall policies and long range plans; and
3. External reporting to the board of directors, government and other outside parties.

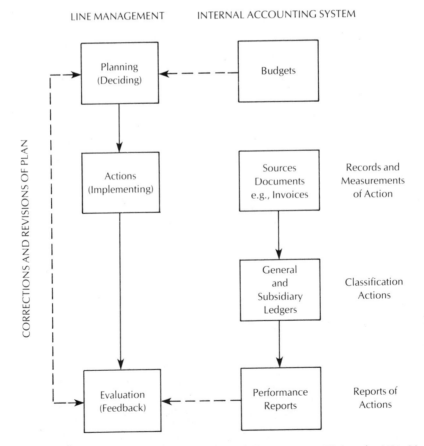

FIGURE 14.2   Management process and accounting. (Reprinted from Horngren CT: *Introduction to Management Accounting*, ed 4. Englewood Cliffs, NJ, Prentice-Hall, 1978, p 5.)

Figure 14.2 shows the nature of the management process and accounting. The primary responsibilities and activities of a hospital finance department are:

1. Planning and maintaining the budget process
2. Keeping proper records to meet external requirements
3. Monitoring and reporting of performance for management purposes
4. Establishing and maintaining relationships with appropriate external organizations, such as governmental agencies and third-party payers
5. Maintaining and advising on policies and procedures and directing financial management to ensure financial performance to meet the hospital's goals and objectives

The primary functions handled within the finance department are:

1. General accounting functions that include accounts payable, cashiering, bookkeeping, financial reporting, and payroll
2. Budgeting for operations, capital, and cash
3. Patient accounting functions that include billing, and collections
4. Reimbursement
5. Other functions, such as cash management and investments, data processing, grants and contracts, internal auditing, management engineering, materials management, medical records, and admitting

The Budget

''A budget is a formal quantitative expression of management plans,'' according to one definition (5). The basic objectives and advantages of a formal budget to any organization, regardless of size or type, are:

1. To formalize in quantitative terms the objectives, policies, and plans for a hospital or any organization
2. To provide a basis for definite expectations and evaluation of financial performance and compel managers to think ahead
3. To provide managers with a tool to control revenue and costs
4. To aid managers in coordinating their efforts by creating a cost awareness that meets the hospital's organizational objectives by harmonizing them with the objectives of the departments

The primary goal of a budget is to meet the financial requirements of an institution, i.e., to meet current operating expenses for operations, education, research, bad debts, charity, etc. The budget's goal is also to meet the hospital's capital needs to maintain current facilities, add new technology, and expand facilities, as well as to maintain both working capital and a reasonable profit.

Budgets may be classified as follows:

1. Master budget
   a. Expense budget
      (1) Personnel budget
      (2) Supply budget
   b. Revenue budget
   c. Financial budget
      (1) Cash budget

(2) Budgeted balance sheet
(3) Budgeted statement of changes in financial position
2. Special budgets
   a. Capital budgets
   b. Performance reports (variance reports)

The expense budget is developed utilizing each hospital's departmental responsibility centers. The revenue budget is developed utilizing revenue- and nonrevenue-generating centers. Hospital management's primary financial objective is to esnure that total revenue is at least equal to total costs.

The expense budget customarily is broken down into personnel and supply costs or labor and nonlabor costs. Development of the personnel budget (salary and wage budget) or the supply of a departmental center is focused on an estimation of the unit's workload and a translation of that workload into personnel requirements to handle that workload efficiently. The supply budget is similarly developed by translating anticipated supply costs to workload projections within a departmental budget center; the revenue budget is generated utilizing data on patient stay and the professional and ancillary services provided. The integration of all these budgets is illustrated in Figure 14.3.

The budget process includes the following steps:

1. Prepare statistical assumptions, including, but not limited to, patient days by service, changes in building gross square feet, introduction of new services and projected dates, number of procedures for the major departments (laboratory, radiology, etc), and number of outpatient visits.

2. Prepare economic forecasts that include salary inflation factors; fringe-benefit inflation factors; inflation factors for supplies and other nonsalary items detailed by major expense item and by department; new developments that may affect the hospital, such as additional physicians leaving the staff, additions to other hospitals in the service area, or major clinics under construction; proposed legislation or government regulations, if they are expected to pass or be

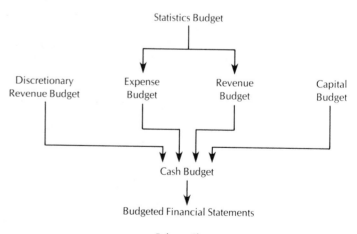

FIGURE 14.3 Integration of budgets. (Reprinted by permission from Rowland HS: *Hospital Administration Handbook.* Rockville, MD, Aspen Systems, p 247.)

implemented; and any other factor that might affect the hospital's income or expenses during the budget period.

3. Distribute budget packages to department heads. These packages will include assumptions, forms, schedules, and historical data for each department. It is best to distribute the packages at a department-head meeting and to have at least 1 hour of formal instruction in budget techniques and accounting constraints.

4. Give technical assistance to department heads as they prepare the first drafts of their budget requests. Prepare budget goals and policies for the period. These will constitute an outline of the financial plan. They may include a targeted net gain or less, a marketing strategy, third-party payer strategy, or any other item that has a bearing on the hospital's finances.

5. Obtain approval of budget assumptions, goals, and policies. Depending on the hospital, this may mean governing board approval, approval by a committee of the governing board, administrative approval, or operating-budget committee approval. Hold departmental budget hearings. Those present should include the controller, the administrator or assistant administrator, and the department head. It is also a good idea to attempt to have a board member present during each budget hearing. This makes the department heads feel that they have been heard, and at the same time provides board members with an excellent opportunity to learn the intricacies of day-to-day hospital operating problems.

6. Prepare typewritten summaries of each budget hearing. These will document promises and statements made between administration and department heads. These summaries will be referred to throughout the year as budget variances are investigated. If the typewritten summaries include personal observations and impressions of the controller, they should be shared only with administration.

7. If these summaries are rather formal and include only factual information, a copy of each summary can be given to the appropriate department head. The format and distribution of budget hearing summaries will depend on the preferences of the controller and the administrator.

8. Summarize the individual department budgets into a first draft of the master budget. After reviewing this for reasonableness, the controller's department summarizes the total budget into a format to be presented to the board or a committee of the board. This presentation will be enhanced by graphs, descriptive narrative, and comparative historical data.

After making revisions mandated by the governing board, the budget is submitted to any relevant outside agency for approval. Many states have a formal rate review process. Others have a required rate and budget review process by a major third-party payer. In addition, Medicare intermediaries require a review of the budget and proposed rates before the start of the fiscal year.

There are several approaches to budgeting, five of which will be discussed: (1) responsibility center budgeting, (2) forcast budgeting, (3) program budgeting, (4) zero-base budgeting, and (5) flexible budgeting.

Responsibility Center Budgeting. Responsibility budgeting recognizes the responsibility centers within an or-

ganization and is generally tailored to the institution's organizational structure. The intent of responsibility budgeting is to provide goal congruence and incentive by tailoring the accounting and budgeting system to make the organizational structure and control system interdependent. Areas of responsibility are broken down into cost centers, profit centers (revenue and expenses), and investment centers (5).

Within the hospital, the responsibility budgeting by the organization structure focuses on control by the department head. The lines of authority and responsibility from the organizational structure plus the chart of accounts for which a responsibility center has control are prerequisites for establishing this type of budgeting system (6).

Responsibility center budgeting and responsibility for those budgets normally are defined by the department head's ability to influence or control costs. Controllability of costs is a matter of degree. Controllable costs are ''defined as any cost that is subject to influence of a given manager of a given responsibility center for a given time span.''(5).

These controllable costs are subject to direct control by the department head. Examples are salary costs and supply costs (drugs, IVs, etc). Noncontrollable costs at the department level are administrative cost allocations, capital depreciation, etc. Responsibility budgeting is one of the primary budgeting methods utilized in most organizations. Expense budgets are developed for each income-generated service. The expense budget is broken down into salary and wage budget and supply budget for each center. The process for developing this type of budget for each responsibility center requires (1) an estimation of the unit's workload, (2) a translation of the workload into resource requirements, and (3) an application of factor prices to estimated resource requirements to derive the expected costs of oerpation.

The revenue budget reflects anticipated income from direct patient care and other operating and nonoperating revenues. Revenues originate from (1) providing stay-specific services, (2) providing ancillary or other professional services to inpatients, and (3) providing ancillary or other professional services to outpatients.

Forecast Budgeting. A critical element in forecast budgeting is the grasp of the upside/downside concept. The upside concept reflects factors that would demonstrate growth or increased demands on services and the cost of providing them. The downside concept would indicate adverse trends or a decline in the demand for services. Forecasting requires a firm grasp of future events, conditions, and the upside/downside impacts in order to determine the measure of budgetary adjustments to be made to previous budgets.

There are basically two types of forecasting methods to consider. These are mechanical and analytical forecasting.

1. Mechanical forecasting, also known as historic forecasting, usually involves a straight percentage increase multiplied across the board. It can be used for yearly projections on demands and services. However, it is best to go back 3 years as the base from which to project.

2. Analytical forecasting employs the upside/downside concept and seeks to project realistic figures based on the impact of demands for services. Critical factors to be considered in forecasting are future events or conditions that will affect situations, people, time, and causative controls.

Program Budgeting. The program budgeting approach focuses on top management's stated (or implied) objectives or program structure (5). The budget and control system is designed to focus resources efficiently to achieve the hospital's goals and objectives. The program structure portrays the hospital's top administration's implementation strategy for these goals and objectives. These programs might include home health care, outpatient surgery, and satellite operations. Once the programs are identified, the budget must be developed to identify activity areas and the evaluation of relative costs and benefits of each. Program budgeting is a strategic technique to achieve an institution's goals by allocating resources for that end.

Program budgeting was an outgrowth of a concept known as planning, programming, and budgeting (PPB), which was experimented with in the 1960s by the federal government and is widely used in state and local government. The steps in the process are as follows:

First, PPB calls for a careful specification and analysis of basic program objectives: What are they really trying to accomplish? The second step is to analyze the output of a given program in terms of the objectives. The third step is to measure the total costs of the program, not just for 1 year, but for at least several years ahead, and not on the basis of the first-year costs alone. The fourth and crucial step is to analyze alternatives. It is competition among alternatives that is crucial. The final step is establishing PPB as an integral part of the budgetary decisions. The programming concept is the crucial link that relates planning to budgeting, converting planning from a paper exercise to an important part of the decision-making process.

Zero-Base Budgeting. Zero-base budgeting arose as a response to the problems of controlling discretionary costs and refers to the practice of having a manager justify his department's activities from the ground up, as though they were being initiated for the first time. Traditionally, proposed budgets have been justified on an incremental basis, i.e., managers have tended to prepare new budgets in terms of changes from last year's budget and results. In contrast, zero-base budgeting gets back to the bedrock questions: Why does this activity or department exist? What are or should be its goals or objectives? Zero-base budgeting complements program budgeting by examining specific expenditure alternatives within a general operational area.

Under the traditional budgeting approach, managers of established activity areas are required to justify any increased funding they seek for the fiscal period. The previous level of funding is accepted as being necessary and represents a portion of the approved expenditure for the budget period. Zero-base budgeting differs from the traditional process in that it requires managers to defend their entire list of budget requests. It mandates that managers develop, evaluate, and ordinally rank alternate approaches to achieving the goals of the unit for which they are responsible. Rather than assessing only the incremental changes in expenditures, zero-base budgeting forces management to evaluate total spending. Once expenditure alternatives are ranked ordinally, management can select those that yield the greatest benefit for the community.

Zero-base budgeting involves two basic steps. The first requires management to identify the objectives of the functional unit, the operational results required to achieve stated goals, alternate approaches to achieving these goals, and the outcomes and resource requirements associated with each. The first phase should be performed by the lowest level of managerial responsibility in the organization. Ideally, the individual who supervises each activity, operation, or task in the functional area should be responsible for developing alternate approaches, outcomes, and resource requirements.

The second step of zero-base budgeting involves an evaluation of the approaches developed earlier. Theoretically, the evaluation is accomplished by developing a rank ordering of the alternatives that is based on cost-benefit or cost-effectiveness analysis. A rank ordering is simply a list of projects arranged so that those with the most favorable cost-benefit or cost-effectiveness ratios appear at the top of the list. Once the ordinal ranking has been constructed, management uses the cost-benefit or cost-effectiveness ratios to develop funding priorities.

The initial ranking of expenditure alternatives should be developed by the managers responsible for specifying the project parameters. Subsequently, managerial personnel at successively higher levels of responsibility consolidate the rankings received from their subordinates and develop their own sets of priorities. Finally, senior management aggregates the subordinates' recommendations into the final ordinal ranking of expenditure alternatives for the institution.

TABLE 14.1 Advantages and Disadvantages of Forecast vs Flexible Budgeting[a]

Forecast (Fixed) Budgeting		*Flexible Budgeting*	
Advantages:	*Disadvantages:*	*Advantages:*	*Disadvantages:*
Traditional approach	Difficult to adjust to actual activity levels	Can be adjusted to reflect actual activity levels	More time consuming
Easily understood	Cannot readily analyze discrepancies caused by changes in volume, price, and activity	Easier to obtain meaningful variance analysis	More costly to implement and monitor
Preparation and reporting time is less than with a flexible budget	Due to inherent limitations, the approach to budget preparation and variance analysis can become haphazard and meaningless	Can serve to more adequately contain costs	Requires additional training
Meaningful only if actual level of activity closely approximates budget		Assists management in identifying the hospital's problems before the fact through the use of budget model applications	Places greater demand on hospital personnel and requires more financial sophistication
		More defensible in rate review, prospective reimbursement, and external price control negotiations	
		More acceptable control tool	

[a]Reprinted by permission from Rowland HS: *Hospital Administration Handbook.* Rockville, MD, Aspen Systems 1984, p 245.

Two specific criticisms of zero-base budgeting are (1) the time and cost involved to do it correctly (this is why many recommend that it be done only every 5 or 6 years) and (2) the fact that budgeting is targeted only at expenses and not revenue.

Flexible Budgeting. Flexible budgeting is a system to tell what it should cost for a specific volume level. This type of budgeting is derived by adjusting the "static" budget to actual work volume achieved. Flexible budgets (also called variable budgets) are prepared for a range of activities and provide a dynamic basis for comparison of changes in work volume. Rowland (6) has provided an excellent review of the process and its advantages and disadvantages, which are summarized in Table 14.1.

BALANCE SHEET DATA AS OF JUNE 30, 1984

ASSETS		LIABILITIES AND FUND BALANCES	
Current Assets	$ 35,479,327	Current Liabilities	$ 16,618,519
Property and Equipment—Net	49,089,431	Long-Term Liabilities	43,788,218
Board Designated Funds	14,295,386	Board Designated Fund Equity	5,289,637
Donor Restricted Funds	6,089,858	Donor Restricted Fund Equity	6,089,858
Other Assets	6,549,549	Operating Fund Equity	39,717,319
Total Assets	$111,503,551	Total Liabilities and Fund Equities	$111,503,551

FIGURE 14.4 Sample balance sheet. (Reprinted by permission from *Annual Report, Finance Department, Sinai Hospital of Detroit, 1985-86*, November 1984.)

To: All Department Heads

SUBJECT: 1985-1986 BUDGET

The 1985-1986 fiscal year is rapidly approaching. The annual budget process associated with the advent of the new year presents us with a unique opportunity to assess both the state of the health care environment and Sinai Hospital's position within it.

We all recognize the significant changes occurring in the health care environment and adjust to the consequences of a fixed price payment system in lieu of the traditional cost reimbursement system. "Competition" and "marketing," concepts long considered the domain of the for-profit sector, are now the focus of intense interest within the not-for-profit health care field. We all strain to learn the newest acronyms of our profession, as PRO's, HMO's, PPA's, PPO's, DRG's and PPS' flood our every conversation. Yet, despite this new environment and its many challenges, we must never lose sight of our commitment to the provisions of high quality health care. Our efforts toward this end can only be met if we maintain a properly paid, productive, efficient work force, and produce an environment in which the patient is viewed as our customer, and these customers are treated with the respect and attention they deserve.

Clearly, there are many areas within our institution which warrant our attention during the forthcoming budget process. First, we must ensure that all employees receive a competitive wage and benefit package, as there is a clear correlation between an employees' wage and their degree of satisfaction with their employment situation. The effort to provide this competitive wage is the key element in our 1985-1986 budget process.

Second, the current reimbursement programs require renewed emphasis upon the provision of services within an ambulatory care setting, thus shifting volume away from the restrictive inpatient reimbursement programs, and into the more efficient outpatient programs, whenever possible.

Third, we must investigate methods to improve the customer relations aspects of our services, so as to complement the clinical expertise afforded all who come to Sinai.

Perhaps not surprisingly, our underlying budgetary strategy concerns the improvement of operational productivity, both within and across departmental lines. Your attention during the preparation of your budget proposals should be focused upon those programs and functions which can lead to an increased efficiency of effort, and a resulting improvement in our ability to provide humane, yet cost-effective, care.

FIGURE 14.5 Directive to department heads relative to budget process. (Figs. 14.5 to 14.13 reprinted by permission from *Budget Packet, Finance Department, Sinai Hospital of Detroit, 1985-86*, November 1984.)

Special Budgets. Capital budgeting concentrates on long-term programs and projects that entail large resource outlays. In health care this historically has been defined as equipment and physical-plant outlays. However, more and more total programs will be evaluated for their long-term cost impact. These and performance report budgets are beyond the scope of this discussion.

Financial Reports

Hospital financial statements, financial indicators, and management reports are routinely generated by the finance department providing management feedback and legal requirements. Statistical reports are also generated for hospitals in general and by individual departments. These sta-

tistical reports are important in day-to-day management.

Financial statements, such as the balance sheet and statement of revenues and expenses, may be produced monthly. The *balance sheet* reports the assets, liabilities, and balances of restricted and unrestricted funds. A sample balance sheet is shown in Figure 14.4. The statement of revenues and expenses (income statement) provides a summation of the hospital's financial operation for a specific period of time.

Financial indicators can be applied to these statements to give a current financial operating status. The most common indicators are liquidity ratios, leverage ratios, and income ratios. Some liquidity ratios follow:

- Current ratio = Current assets/current liabilities: The higher this ratio the better, with common baseline ratio being 2.0.

1985-1986 BUDGET PREPARATION TIMETABLE
Sinai Hospital of Detroit

Friday, Tuesday, Thursday December 7, December 11, and December 13	Presentation of Budget Package to Medical Chairmen, Administrative Staff, and Department Heads.
Thursday January 10, 1985	Deadline for submitting completed budget packages and expense forecasts to the Costs and Budgets Department. Materials not received at this time may not be included in the budget meeting agenda due to timing constraints.
Friday January 18, 1985	Coordinating Council meeting to review calculation of amount available for 1985-1986. Preliminary allocation of amount available to respective Vice Presidents.
Tuesday January 22, 1985	Administrative Staff meeting to review calculation of amount available for 1985-1986.
Wednesday-Friday January 23-25,1985	Meetings to review 1985-1986 capital equipment proposals with Vice Presidents and appropriate administrators and/or Department Heads.
Monday-Friday January 28-February 8, 1985	Meeting between Department Heads and/or Administrators with respective Vice President to review operations budget and allocate amount available.
Week of February 4, 1985	Meeting of Medical Chairman on 1985-1986 capital equipment proposals.
Monday-Wednesay February 11-13, 1985	Time allocated for summarizing capital and operating budget meetings.
Monday February 18, 1985	Meeting of Medical Chairmen to review results of capital and operating budget meetings.
February 19- March 15, 1985	Produce and assemble schedules necessary for the 1985-1986 Budget Presentation Package.
March 18-22, 1985	Review preliminary edition of Budget Presentation Package.
March 25, 1985	Send budget to printer for final production.
April 1985	Capital and operating budget for 1985-1986 to be reviewed and approved by the Finance Committee, Human Resources Committee, and Board of Trustees.
Tuesday April 30, 1985	1985-1986 Board–approved budget submitted to Blue Cross Blue Shield of Michigan and Medicaid.
May 1985	Calendarization of expenses requested from Department Heads.
June 1985	Calendarized expense budgets distributed to all department and administrative staff.

FIGURE 14.6 Example of timetable for budget process.

- Acid test ratio − Cash and marketable securities/current liabilities: The acid test ratio is a tighter measure of liquidity.
- Collection period ratio = Net accounts receivable/average daily operating revenue: This ratio shows the average period of time that accounts receivable are outstanding.

An example of a leverage ratio is:

- Long-term debt to fixed assets = Long-term debt/net fixed assets: This ratio is important in the ability to finance the purchase of new fixed assets—new building, land, etc.

Among income ratios are:

- Markup ratio = Gross patient revenue/operating expense: The markup ratio identifies the number of times the charges are above expenses.
- Deductible ratio = Contractual deductions and provision for uncollectable gross patient revenue: The deductible ratio identifies the revenue that will remain uncollectable.
- Operating margin = Income from operations/total operating revenue: This ratio defines the percentage of collectable revenue after expenses (7).

The accounts receivable report generally represents the largest assets of a hospital. The report is summarized by type of payer into inpatient or outpatient accounts. The following is a list of elements typically included:

1. Billed and unbilled accounts by pay class
2. Accounts receivable by pay class
3. Aging of accounts receivable by pay class
4. Day's revenue in accounts receivable by pay class
5. Accounts receivable by type of patients (inpatients, outpatients, discharged patients)
6. Cash not posted to patient accounts at report date
7. Late charges generated by department and billed by pay class
8. Number of patient accounts receivable aged by pay class
9. Listing of credit balances (or accounts that are due refunds)
10. Collection and delinquent account reports

Cash reports will show the various cash received and disbursements made, generally collected daily and summarized monthly.

INTERNAL ENVIRONMENT ANALYSIS

In this section we will discuss those areas that must be addressed and directly controlled within the hospital pharmacy department. The budget framework and reports, as well as the need for and types of departmental statistics, will be discussed.

The Budget Framework

In this section we will discuss the specific budgeting process for a hospital, policies and procedures, and specific parts that a pharmacy must prepare. We will look specifically

---

To: All Department Heads

SUBJECT: 1985-1986 BUDGET PACKAGE

Accordingly, this budget package introduces "departmental cost per unit of service" which is intended to be a tool in evaluating the departmental operating budget. "Departmental cost per unit of service" was determined by dividing departmental expenses by a measure of department activity such as patient days for a nursing unit. The departmental expenses and activity indicators, as well as the resultant departmenal cost per unit of service for your department for the years 1982-1983 and 1983-1984 and projections for 1984-1985 and 1985-1986 are enclosed. For purposes of the 1985-1986 budget, the yearly expenses, departmental activity level, and departmental cost per unit of service are informational only. But in reviewing the prior year data and the cost projections for 1984-1985 and 1985-1986, you should be prepared to explain any unusual trends and to justify your budget requests in light of this information.

This process is the first step in implementing a flexible budgeting system which allows the departmental budget to adjust with changes in volume and provides more meaningful and timely information to the department manager in terms of their department's cost effectiveness. While full implementation of a flexible budgeting system will take several years, the next step in the process will be to more accurately identify departmental costs which fluctuate with volume, called controllable costs, and those that do not, called fixed costs. Further, it may be necessary to modify the unit of service statistic to one which more accurately reflects departmental volume. It is not considered necessary to fine tune these items at this point as your 1985-1986 departmental budget will not be determined based upon the statistics presented.

This year, it is anticipated that there will be minimal funds available for program enhancements after adjustments for inflationary increases. The development of the 1985-1986 operating expense budget will again be based primarily upon the projected per-case reimbursement level expected under the Medicare DRG payment system but will this year factor in the more restrictive Medicaid per-case reimbursement level anticipated. The overall percentage increase in budgeted expenses is estimated to be 5%. This increase is predicated upon an assumption of 21,500 discharges for 1985-1986 and a slightly declining length of stay. It is to be understood that under a per-case budgeting approach, if either cases decline or length of stay increases, some future adjustment in the budget may be necessary. Therefore, as in last year's package, proposed expense increases must be limited to those of an emergent nature (with explanation) or those that can help reduce expenses in your area.

FIGURE 14.7 Statement of assumptions.

at this budget packet for assumptions, timetable, and forms used for program proposals, personnel budgets, supply budgets, and capital equipment.

The first part of this budget packet is the introduction from top management of the specific issues to be addressed or to be aware of and the strategy for that budget period. An example of such a communication is shown as Figure 14.5. A timetable to be followed by the departments and the hospital as a whole form the next part of the budget packet (Fig. 14.6). It is followed by a statement of assumptions from the finance department (Fig. 14.7).

The kinds of forms used in this process at one hospital are shown in Figures 14.8 to 14.11, with the exception of schedule B, personnel listing and salary.

Capital budget is the last part of the packet to be looked at (Figs. 14.12 and 14.13).

Departmental Statistics and Analysis

The department's statistical reports are broken down from the expense budget into supply (nonlabor) and personnel (labor) costs. The revenue budget is reported at various levels from gross total to decentralized by specific area or unit.

Graphs and statistical analysis may assist in evaluating trends for expenses, revenues, and workload. For example, graphs may be used to show:

1. Drug purchases by therapeutic category
2. Drugs, supplies, personnel, other vs budget or variable budget
3. Revenue by charge category
4. Revenue by DRG category
5. Drug cost per patient day by therapeutic category

1985-1986 BUDGET SCHEDULE A

SINAI HOSPITAL OF DETROIT
DEPARTMENT NAME: PHARMACY
DEPARTMENT NUMBER: 7070

Department 7070 Pharmacy	Class Number	Description	1984-1985 Budget
Salaries and Wages	1	Management—Supervisory	122,444.00
	2	Technicians—Specialists	486,447.00
	7	Residents—Fellows	27,039.00
	8	Non-Phys. Med. Practition.	1,205,171.00
	10	Office Staff	64,724.00
	20	FICA	142,462.00
	21	Overtime	92,026.00
	22	Shift Premium	29,635.00
	26	On-Call Pay	229.00
Total Salaries and Wages			2,170,177.00
Supplies	41	Office & Admin. Supplies	140,000.00
	42	Medical & Surgical Sup.	110,000.00
Supplies	43	Drugs & Pharmaceuticals	4,177,000.00
	44	Intravenous Solutions	1,330,000.00
	54	Dietary—Paper Prods.	1,242.00
	55	Cleaning Prods.	4,000.00
	59	Postage & Frt.	5,118.00
	62	Recruitment	2,949.00
	66	Oth. Minor Equip.	5,163.00
	67	Oth. Supplies & Materials	12,649.00
	94	Repair & Maint. Equip.	2,807.00
	95	Oth. Purch. Services	1,253.00
	101	Licenses & Taxes	125.00
	102	Subscriptions & Books	7,429.00
	104	Travel & Meetings	3,491.00
	106	Rental & Lease Equip.	14,000.00
	112	Ser. To Oth. Organization	−1,695,298.00
Total Supplies			4,121,928.00
			6,292,105.00

FIGURE 14.8 Current budget.

FORMULATION OF THE FINANCIAL STRATEGY

In this section, we will review the questions we asked at the beginning.

1. Where are we now?
2. Where do we want to go?
3. How do we get there?

We will establish our plan and a strategy for accomplishing the plan through a discussion of environmental summary, goals and objectives, alternative analysis and forecasts, and implementation strategies.

Environmental summary

The bulk of this chapter has been targeted at an understanding of the external and internal environmental issues that must be kept in mind for development of a departmental and financial plan. From the analysis, one should know the *needs* and *wants* of those served by the department and those within the department. One should know the financial goals and forecasts of the hospital and the specific objectives that they are addressing. For example, one of the hospital's goals may be to increase outpatient services for the community: a specific objective is set to open two emergency care centers during the next budget year. How will the department address this goal? What financial resources will be needed and what alternative approaches can be taken?

The next important factor to be gleaned from an environmental analysis is the strengths and weaknesses of the hospital and the pharmacy department. These strengths or weaknesses may be the financial position of the hospital or the census and competition within the local area.

Within the pharmacy department, it may be the depth or lack of financial information or the staff's ability to influence the drug use by the medical staff. Also, what are the *opportunities* and *threats* that we must target or avoid in our strategy development? The hospital outpatient goals may allow development of new pharmacy roles in home care or retail services. What is the competition?

Goals and Objectives

This will be the most important and exciting part of plan development. It will form the basis to measure performance next year and next month. The goals and objectives will have to consider as new factors (1) personnel expenses by

---

1985-1986 BUDGET CHANGES—SCHEDULE C
Sinai Hospital of Detroit

DEPARTMENT NAME_____
DEPARTMENT NUMBER_____

This schedule must be completed for all proposed budget reductions/additions. All proposed budget additions must meet one of the following criteria:

(A) Funds requested are of an emergent nature.

(B) Additional funds can be offset by interdepartmental fund transfers.

(C) Sufficient cost savings or additional revenues can be produced by increased efficiencies.

BUDGET CHANGE I

PREPARED BY_____   ADMINISTRATIVE APPROVAL_____   MEDICAL CHAIRMAN APPROVAL_____

FIGURE 14.9 Proposed changes.

1985-1986 BUDGET CHANGES— SCHEDULE D
Sinai Hospital of Detroit

DEPARTMENT NAME_____

DEPARTMENT NUMBER_____

	BUDGET CHANGE I INCREASE (DECREASE)	BUDGET CHANGE II INCREASE (DECREASE)	BUDGET CHANGE III INCREASE (DECREASE)
PERSONNEL COST			
Various Salaries and Wages	_____	_____	_____
020 FICA	_____	_____	_____
021 Overtime	_____	_____	_____
022 Shift Premium	_____	_____	_____
TOTAL PERSONNEL COSTS	_____	_____	_____
SUPPLY AND OTHER COSTS			
041 Office and Admin. Supplies	_____	_____	_____
065 Instrm. & Minor Med. Eqpt.	_____	_____	_____
066 Other Minor Equipment	_____	_____	_____
067 Other Supplies & Material	_____	_____	_____
094 Repairs & Maint.—Eqpt.	_____	_____	_____
095 Other Purchased Services	_____	_____	_____
096 Temporary Personnel	_____	_____	_____
102 Subscriptions and Books	_____	_____	_____
103 Dues and Memberships	_____	_____	_____
104 Travel and Meetings	_____	_____	_____
106 Rental of Lease-Equipment	_____	_____	_____
113 Other Direct Expenses	_____	_____	_____
Other (indicate):	_____	_____	_____
___ _____	_____	_____	_____
___ _____	_____	_____	_____
___ _____	_____	_____	_____
___ _____	_____	_____	_____
___ _____	_____	_____	_____
TOTAL SUPPLY COSTS	_____	_____	_____
GRAND TOTALS	_____	_____	_____

PREPARED
BY_____

ADMINISTRATIVE
APPROVAL_____

MEDICAL CHAIRMAN
APPROVAL_____

FIGURE 14.10   Expense account numbers for proposed changes.

case mix rather than bed size, (2) inventory control and supply costs, (3) shift to outpatient and competitive services, and (4) targeting capital expenses toward the most productive investments.

This is the point at which one must evaluate the hospital and department's mission. Our department's mission statement is: "The provision of pharmaceutical services to assure and advance the safe, effective and appropriate use of medication."

Goals and objectives often are considered to be the same, but goals should be more global and ideal, whereas objectives should be measurable and time defined. An example goal would be to reduce supply costs by 10%; an example objective, to reduce antibiotic use by $10,000 within 6 months.

Once goals are defined, the input of the pharmacy department's staff can greatly influence the definition of objectives. The next step is to define the financial planning and budgeting approach.

Alternative Analysis and Forecasts

For each objective, there are generally many approaches to accomplishing that objective. If not, one probably should examine the objective, since it is specifying the path and not allowing alternatives. (Example: provision of unit dose medication delivery by the most cost-effective method by January 1985. This can be approached centrally or decentrally, by unit pharmacists, floating carts, etc. The answer chosen will depend on the institution.)

1985-1986 BUDGET CHANGES—SCHEDULE E
Sinai Hospital of Detroit

DEPARTMENT NAME_____
DEPARTMENT NUMBER_____

BUDGET CHANGE NUMBER	JOB CLASSIFICATION	FTEs INCREASE (DECREASE)*	BUDGET CHANGE AMOUNT INCREASE (DECREASE)	COMMENTS

*Hours should be indicated in this column if the request relates to overtime, vacation relief, or sick and other relief budgeted amounts.

PREPARED BY_____ ADMINISTRATIVE APPROVAL_____ MEDICAL CHAIRMAN APPROVAL_____

FIGURE 14.11 Personnel detail of proposed changes.

1958-1986 BUDGET INSTRUCTIONS—CAPITAL EQUIPMENT
Sinai Hospital of Detroit

PURPOSE

The Capital Equipment Budget is prepared to enable the hospital to identify situations whereby additions to or replacement of property, plant and equipment are necessary.

DEFINITION OF CAPITAL ITEMS

The Medicare Provider Reimbursement Manual standards for capitalization of purchased items stipulate that it should be capitalized (as opposed to expensed) if:

(A) It has a useful life of two years or more and

(B) The cost of the individual item *exceeds $500*

These guidelines also apply to cost of betterments and improvements that extend the life or increase the productivity of an asset, as opposed to repairs and maintenance that either restore the asset to, or maintain it at its normal or expected service life.

FIVE-YEAR CAPITAL PLAN

For fiscal year 1986-1987 through 1989-1990, separate schedules have been provided for departments requesting capital equipment of individual items having an anticipated cost of *at least $50,000.* Proper preparation of these schedules will assist the Hospital in identifying future capital needs and to appropriately plan with respect to the funds that will be required for such needs.

FIGURE 14.12 Definitions and guidelines.

CAPITAL EXPENDITURE REQUEST   SCHEDULE I
Sinai Hospital of Detroit
Fiscal Year_____

( ) Upgrade—see 8
( ) Replacement—9
( ) Activity increase

1. Description of equipment or improvement requested.   ( ) New program
2. Justification for request.   ( ) Urgent
3. Purchase price $_____ Is lease or rental feasible? (___) Yes (___) No: Annual Rent $_____   ( ) Essential
   Which do you recommend_____ Other minor equipment required?_____ Cost $_____   ( ) Necessary
4. Expected useful live_____years.   Warranty duration_____months.   ( ) Desirable
5. Is a service contract recommended? _____ Annual cost $_____ included in budget?
   _____ Where?_____ Other service arrangements_____ Year needed_____
   Quarter when needed_____
6. Personnel training required?_____ Personnel time savings expected_____ Annual hours_____
7. Additional supplies required?_____ Estimated annual cost $_____
8. What will happen to replaced item? (_____) Sold, estimated price $_____ (_____) Discarded (_____)
   Traded, trade-in allowance $_____ (_____) Remain in area?
9. Age of item replaced (upgraded) _____years: Property tag number_____
10. Expected period of expenditures (_____) July-Sept. (_____) Oct.-Dec. (_____) Jan.-Mar. (_____) April-June

Department number_____   Department head_____   Medical chairman_____

Department name_____   Administrator_____

FIGURE 14.13 Request form.

Implementation Strategies

Various strategies can be taken: (1) diversification, which looks at using strengths and knowledge to move into new areas, or (2) retrenchment, which is to cut back to improve quality and protect what we have and what others can utilize.

To hospital pharmacists, diversification can mean (1) expanding acute care services through management contracts and mergers, (2) developing new services to include long-term care, ambulatory care, occupational health, and preventive and wellness programs, (3) starting other health care businesses, such as consulting and continuing medical education for physicians and nurses, and (4) expanding into non–health care businesses.

MONITORING AND CONTROLLING

Monitoring becomes the last and most important part of the financial planning process. This process show trends and status of the programs and tools in use. It will show the need to change approaches to meet objectives. The following are important rules in collecting data to monitor tools.

Maximize Accuracy. Data should be collected in a manner that minimizes errors. The method for collection should be standardized, and all sources of bias should be eliminated. An external auditor should be able to review the written procedures for data collection and effectively track expenses, revenue, or workload through the system.

Minimize Personnel Time. The data-collection system should be automated wherever possible. When automation is not possible, the personnel time required for collection and processing should be minimized.

Monitor Financial Performance. The financial aspects of each facet of pharmaceutical services should be monitored and analyzed. For example, total departmental revenue should be broken down into discrete components, such as unit dose injections and IV admixtures.

Highlight Trends. The pharmacy director manages on the basis of trends rather than an isolated period of data. The hospital administrator also needs to be aware of trends.

Standard Reporting Periods and Nomenclature. Data should be collected using standards, terminology, and reporting periods that are common to hospitals and pharmacies, with modifications for individual hospitals. The pharmacy should collect, collate, and report data for the same time period as the hospital. While the data collected will be used primarily by the pharmacy for internal management, reports on key factors should be provided to hospital administration on a regular basis. The data will be used for justifying new programs, defending current programs, and analyzing proposed hospital changes. Thus, data need to be collected in a format that is easily understood by both the pharmacy and the administration. Terms unique to pharmacy should be avoided if standard hospital terminology will suffice; data that are understandable only to the pharmacist are of marginal value.

CONCLUSION

There is no single best approach, but a dynamic process of maintaining, defining, and redefining a pharmacy department's goals and objectives for financial management is necessary. Additional assistance can be gained from the references and additional readings suggested at the end of this chapter.

REFERENCES

1. Drucker PF: Managing for business effectiveness. Business classics: fifteen key concepts for managerial success, *Harv Bus Rev* May-June, 1963.
2. *Lilly Hospital Pharmacy Survey, 1984,* Indianapolis, Eli Lilly & Co., 1984.
3. Stolar MH: Description of an experimental hospital pharmacy management information system. *Am J Hosp Pharm* 40:1905-1913, 1983.
4. Finkler SA: *The Complete Guide to Finance & Accounting for Nonfinancial Managers.* Englewood Cliffs, NJ, Prentice-Hall, 1983.
5. Horngren CT: *Introduction to Management Accounting,* ed 4. Englewood Cliffs, NJ, Prentice-Hall, Inc., 1978.
6. Rowland HS: *Hospital Administration Handbook.* Rockville, MD, Aspen Systems, 1984, Chap 16.

ADDITIONAL READING

Christensen CR, Berg NA, Salter MS: *Policy Formulation and Administration,* ed 8. Homewood, IL, Richard D Irwin, 1980.
Nold EB, Williams MS: Financial management. *Am J Hosp Pharm* vols 37-41, 1980-1984.
Stolar MH: National test of an experimental hospital pharmacy management information system. *Am J Hosp Pharm* 40:1914-1919, November 1983.
Trudeau T: *Topics in Hospital Pharmacy Management.* Rockville, MD, Aspen Publications, 1984.

CHAPTER 15

Planning and Forecasting

CHARLES D. HEPLER and ROBERT A. FREEMAN

Planning is that element of a manager's responsibility that is oriented to the future and that is prerequisite to most other managerial functions. Planning is done, poorly or well, by managers at all levels; adequate planning is a fundamental responsibility of all managers. There are many basic orientations to the planning function, for *the future* is a concept that is heavily laden with emotion. Man has attempted to relate the present to the future by a number of emotionally satisfying means, ranging from fatalistic predeterminism to prophecy with intuition, tarot, or tea leaves. This chapter is built on the assumptions that the links between the past, present, and future are discoverable, at least in part, by the application of logic. The methods outlined in this chapter may not provide the emotional satisfaction of other methods, but are recommended to those who are willing to trade emotional satisfaction for the organized uncertainty of science.

PLANNING

The first assumption of this chapter, that the present can influence the future, leads immediately to the concept of planning, which has been defined as (1):

. . . an analysis of relevant information from the present and the past and an assessment of probable future developments so that a course of action may be determined that enables the organization . . . to establish . . . objectives and design means for achieving them.

More briefly, planning is the process of rationally choosing courses of action to maximize the organization's chance of achieving its goals. The three fundamental requirements of planning, therefore, are goals, rationality, and information.

Goal

A goal is a general set of circumstances that is desired for the future, frequently the distant future. Since they are general, goals are frequently difficult to measure precisely. For example, the goals of a hospital might be stated as follows:

. . . to provide a complete range of highest quality health services to its patients in an efficient, personalized, and compassionate manner, and to discharge its public stewardship in advancing medical science and translating it into effective methods of patient care.

Goals are vital to planning because they indicate the purpose and overall direction of organizational effort. Because bureaucracies strive for rationality and logical coherence, the goals of organizational subdivisions should be consistent with the overall goals of the organization. This necessity is sometimes overlooked or misunderstood by a pharmacy director who either is unaware of the hospital's goals or has not promulgated a set of pharmacy departmental goals consistent with the hospital's goals. When such goals are absent, plans produced by the department may be difficult for others in the organization to support for a variety of reasons, e.g., the importance of the plans to the overall goals of the hospital may be unclear, and the plans may, therefore, appear to represent the parochial interests of the pharmacy rather than the broader interests of the hospital.

Goal setting is technically outside the planning process, since planning is directed at goal achievement. Clear goals, nonetheless, are a sine qua non to planning.

The Planning Process and Rationality

Rationality in planning may be advanced by decomposing the planning process into its component steps and then ensuring that each component receives adequate attention. Table 15.1 presents the planning process as consisting of eight essential steps. Planning that omits one or more steps must be incomplete and probably will be ineffective.

The first step in the planning process is the identification and, if necessary, clarification of the goals of the department. This step represents the interface between the ends and means of the department.

The output mix of an institutional pharmacy department consists of multiple kinds of goods and services; therefore, one would naturally expect that the department would have multiple goals. Furthermore, some goals may be more important than others. Since the resources of the department (e.g., manpower, equipment) are usually limited, some form of ranking or goal prioritization must follow.

Goal prioritization is a tentative process of ranking goals in the order of their importance to the department. Numerous criteria can be used to prioritize departmental goals. One

TABLE 15.1 Steps in the Planning Process

1. Goal identification and prioritization
2. Determination of objectives
3. Identification of strategies
4. Selection of optimum strategy
5. Development of functional plan(s)
6. Implementation of functional plan(s)
7. Evaluation of planning effort
8. Revision of planning effort

TABLE 15.2 Objectives and Goals

Characteristics	Goals	Objectives
1. Specificity	General	Very specific
2. Time frame	Long-run	Short-run
3. Scope	Multileveled	Single level
4. Basis	Mission, purpose	Goals
5. Program implications	General	Specific
6. Constraints	Possibility and de- sirability	Available resources

possible criterion is the *centrality* of a departmental goal to the overall goals of the hospital: the departmental goals that are most clearly coincident with institutional goals are given highest priority. Another possible criterion is *immediacy of need* and logical precedence: the department's goals that represent immediate needs and/or are logically prerequisite to other goals are given highest priority. Finally, goal prioritization may consider *resource constraints:* goals that can be achieved with available resources are given higher priority than goals that require substantial budgetary increases. Prioritization may be accomplished democratically within the department, or the director of pharmacy services may make the decisions based on informal input from within the department and from extramural sources such as hospital administration.

Once goals have been identified and prioritized, it becomes necessary to develop objectives. Objectives are similar to goals; both specify a desired state of affairs that should be obtained in a certain period of time. Objectives, however, are more short-term, specific, and measurable than are goals. Objectives are derived from goals and represent definite achievements consistent with those goals.

The differences between goals and objectives are summarized in Table 15.2. It must be noted that setting goals without setting objectives is haphazard; setting objectives without goals is logically contradictory.

Table 15.3 provides the prioritized goal set of a pharmacy department in a mythical, medium-sized general hospital. The subgoals listed were derived from the overall goals of the department that in turn, were derived from the overall goals of Eckes Hospital given earlier in this chapter. These goals do not carry specific time periods or deadlines; in fact they probably would continue as goals even if met. Furthermore, they are rather imprecise. They clearly provide direction, but are less clear about destination. Timetables and specific destinations are provided by objectives. Table 15.4 provides an objective set derived from goal 4. The objectives are arranged in order of logical precedence, include deadlines, and are specific enough to allow a determination of whether or not the objectives were met.

Once an objective set has been developed for each departmental goal, it may be necessary to reexamine the initial priorities that were previously set. We may discover that the amounts of resources required to meet a goal are beyond our capacity. It is always important to remember that goals and objectives are not etched in stone; rather, they can be and should be subjected to constant reappraisal.

A desideratum of goals and objectives is that they must be attainable. Basically, they must be practical and related

TABLE 15.3 Prioritized Goals for Eckes Hospital

Overall goals:	To provide a complete range of highest quality pharmaceutical services to the patients of Eckes Hospital in an efficient, personalized, and compassionate manner and to advance society's knowledge of methods of providing pharmaceutical care.
Goal 1:	To provide pharmaceutical services in an optimally efficient and safe inpatient drug distribution system.
Goal 2:	To establish effective working relationships with other departments of Eckes Hospital.
Goal 3:	To provide opportunities for each pharmacist to develop maximal professional, interpersonal, and administrative competence according to his potential and his interests.
Goal 4:	To provide pharmaceutical products and services at a price that accurately reflects their total cost.
Goal 5:	To encourage applied pharmaceutical research by department members that will improve the quality and efficiency of care at Eckes Hospital and elsewhere.

TABLE 15.4 Objectives Derived from Goal 4

Objective 4.1:	Conduct audit of inpatient drug costs and prices and pharmacy service costs and fees. Target: 12/31/84
Objective 4.2:	Conduct literature search; correspond with other pharmacists regarding methods of changing hospital inpatient for drugs and pharmaceutical services. Target: 2/28/85
Objective 4.3:	Devise and test a pricing method for products and services that accurately reflects total cost. Target: 12/31/85
Objective 4.4:	Propose new pricing method to hospital administration. Target: 3/31/85
Objective 4.5:	Implement experiment with new pricing method. Target: 7/1/85
Objective 4.6:	Monitor performance of new pricing method. Make recommendation to Administration. Target: 12/31/85

to the "real world" of both present and anticipated economic and political constraints.

The objective sets will direct the planning effort toward the identification of strategies or alternative ways to meet the objectives. If there is only one way to accomplish an objective set, the decision-making process becomes quite simple. As the number of alternatives increases, the com-

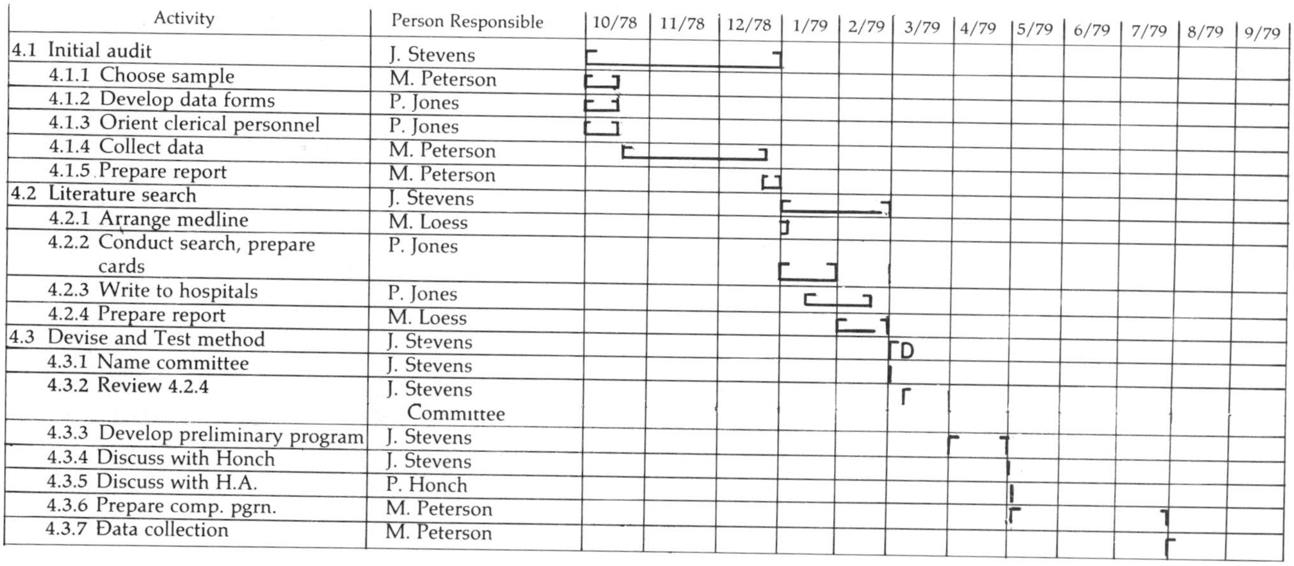

Activity	Person Responsible	10/78	11/78	12/78	1/79	2/79	3/79	4/79	5/79	6/79	7/79	8/79	9/79
4.1 Initial audit	J. Stevens	⌐		¬									
4.1.1 Choose sample	M. Peterson	⌐¬											
4.1.2 Develop data forms	P. Jones	⌐¬											
4.1.3 Orient clerical personnel	P. Jones	⌐¬											
4.1.4 Collect data	M. Peterson		⌐			¬							
4.1.5 Prepare report	M. Peterson				⌐¬								
4.2 Literature search	J. Stevens					⌐		¬					
4.2.1 Arrange medline	M. Loess					⌐¬							
4.2.2 Conduct search, prepare cards	P. Jones						⌐	¬					
4.2.3 Write to hospitals	P. Jones					⌐	¬						
4.2.4 Prepare report	M. Loess					⌐	¬						
4.3 Devise and Test method	J. Stevens						⌐D						
4.3.1 Name committee	J. Stevens												
4.3.2 Review 4.2.4	J. Stevens Committee						⌐						
4.3.3 Develop preliminary program	J. Stevens							⌐	¬				
4.3.4 Discuss with Honch	J. Stevens								⌐				
4.3.5 Discuss with H.A.	P. Honch								⌐				
4.3.6 Prepare comp. pgrn.	M. Peterson								⌐		¬		
4.3.7 Data collection	M. Peterson											⌐	

FIGURE 15.1   Portion of Gantt chart for objective 4.

plexity of decision making also increases. Strategies must be analyzed in light of costs, effectiveness, and goals. This is a difficult, time-consuming process but is also a very important step in the planning process.

After selecting the most practicable strategy, a strategy-specific functional plan, or work program, should be developed. A functional plan is a step-by-step sequential work program that delegates responsibilities and activities to departmental personnel for its conduct. Functional planning involves all of the strategies of "generic" planning with the exception of scope. Planning per se involves or relates to the entire department's activities, while functional planning deals with a discrete activity within the pharmacy's system. Although most planners probably would agree on the necessity for functional plans, there may be less agreement on who should prepare them. Depending on the pharmacy director's managerial philosophy and style, functional plans may be prepared by the director, by the persons responsible for the objectives, or by the persons who will actually carry out the functions. Different individuals may be assigned responsibility for the different objectives in Table 15.4; these individuals, possessing their own special expertise, may be more able to develop functional plans than the individual making the assignments.

Gantt Charts

One very useful technique for functional planning is the Gantt project planning chart (2,3). The Gantt chart is a visual display technique that can be used as a scheduling tool for the entire planning process. The basic chart can be modified to show activities, persons responsible, and the time schedule in graphic form. At any time, anyone in the department can know the progress of the activities simply by looking at the chart.

Figure 15.1 depicts a portion of a Gantt chart for the objectives of Table 15.4. Although it is customary to use separate Gantt charts for objectives and functional plans,

both are included in the figure to exemplify functional plans as well as the Gantt technique itself. Gantt charts must be updated frequently; this can be time consuming unless one of the commercial versions, using pegs, magnets, lights, etc, is employed to monitor a project. Table 15.5 shows the conventional meanings of symbols used in a Gantt chart. Note that activity 4.2.4 (Prepare report on literature search; scheduled for completion by 2/28/85) is behind schedule and that initiation of activity 4.3 will be delayed until 4.2.4 is completed.

Gantt charts alone may be sufficient for scheduling projects such as the one depicted in Table 15.4, where each task has a single immediate predecessor. Many projects, however, involve parallel operations, i.e., two or more tasks stand as immediate predecessors to another task. The development of an IV drug compounding service (IDCS) can serve as an example of such a project. Careful consideration of the abbreviated functional plan (Table 15.5) will elucidate the reason that a target date is given only for the first function, while time requirements in days are given (in parentheses) for the others. It is clear that many functions (e.g., 1.6.2., 1.6.4, 1.6.5) logically can begin any time after 1.6.1 is complete. The target date for the completion of this project need not be 315 days (the sum of the individual function times) after 12/31/84. Furthermore, it is apparent that site renovation (1.6.9) must be completed before major equipment installation (1.6.3) may begin. This project obviously includes parallel operations and would be difficult to schedule with a Gantt chart alone.

TABLE 15.5   Gantt Chart Symbols

Symbol	Meaning
⌐	Scheduled beginning of an activity
¬	Scheduled end of an activity
—	Progress of an activity
V	Current date
D	Activity that may be delayed because earlier activity is delayed

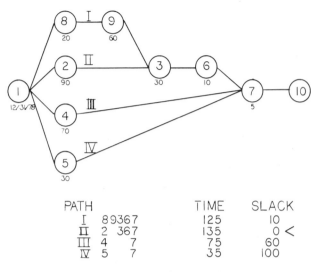

PATH		TIME	SLACK
I	89367	125	10
II	2 367	135	0 <
III	4 7	75	60
IV	5 7	35	100

FIGURE 15.2 Initial network diagram for IDCS plan.

Network Analysis

Network analysis, e.g., the critical path method,* is a technique that is specifically useful for scheduling projects such as the IDCS (4-6). The first step in the critical path method is determining the relationships between all events and depicting them in a network. Figure 15.2 diagrams such a network; it should be carefully compared to Table 15.6. Note that there are four parallel pathways between activities 1 and 10 and that each pathway requires different amounts of time. The pathway that requires the most time for completion (pathway II) is termed the "critical path." The time required for the critical path is the minimal length of time required to complete the project without changing the time estimates; hence, the IDCS project will require a minimum of 135 days after completion of activity 1.

It is possible to prepare a Gantt chart at this point because the necessary scheduling information is now available. The critical path method, however, provides much information in addition to an initial estimate of earliest completion date. The time difference (slack) between any pathway and the critical path is the amount of time that activities along that path can be delayed without delaying the completion of the project. The network in Figure 15.2 includes considerable slack. Note, for example, that activity 5 could be delayed 100 days without delaying the overall project. Observations such as this can be very useful because they suggest the desirability of shortening the time requirements of activities along the critical path and the permissibility of delaying completion of activities that have slack. For example, suppose that it is possible to reassign manpower from activity 4 to activities 2 and 8, to the extent that the time required for activity 4 is lengthened to 100 days, the time required

*One of the earliest network methods, the critical path method, was developed for use in large construction projects at DuPont. The U.S. Navy developed a similar technique, called Program Evaluation and Review Technique, for planning the Polaris Fleet Ballistic Missile Program. The differences between the two techniques fall outside the scope of this discussion. The technique presented here includes elements of both techniques, but will be referred to as the critical path method for simplicity.

TABLE 15.6 Functional Plan for Establishment of IDCS

Objective 1.6 Establish an Intravenous Drug Compounding Service (IDCS)
- 1.6.1 Estimate demand for IDCS in units by area requesting, day, day of week, and season. Target: 12/31/84
- 1.6.2 Determine equipment requirements based on demand (90)
  - 2.1 Types and numbers of devices (15)
  - 2.2 Set specifications for major equipment (15)
  - 2.3 Request bids from potential vendors (30)
  - 2.4 Place orders, receive equipment (30)
- 1.6.3 Install major equipment (30)
- 1.6.4 Determine and provide personnel requirements based on demand (70)
  - 4.1 Determine numbers of personnel needed by type (10)
  - 4.2 Develop employment prerequisites (20)
  - 4.3 Assign existing, and hire new, personnel (30)
  - 4.4 Train new subprofessionals in basic techniques (10)
- 1.6.5 Develop operating procedures for IDCS (30)
- 1.6.6 Develop delivery procedures for IDCS (10)
- 1.6.7 Orient all personnel to IDCS procedures (5)
- 1.6.8 Determine location for IDCS based on demand estimates (20)
- 1.6.9 Renovate IDCS site to conform to environmental control requirements (60)
- 1.6.10 Begin service

for activity 2 is reduced to 70 days, and the time required for activity 8 is reduced to 10 days (Fig. 15.3). The new schedule shows that both paths 1 and 2 are critical and that the time requirement for the project has been reduced by 20 days. Only activities 4 and 5 show any slack now. It may be desirable to reassign additional manpower until no more slack can be eliminated. At this point, an optimal schedule would exist. The schedule could then be displayed on a Gantt chart for project management and control purposes.

Implementation, Evaluation, and Revision

A plan, with all its documents and work programs, is useless unless it is implemented. It is important, therefore, to delegate both authority and responsibility to departmental personnel for the various work programs in the plan. Although planning responsibility may remain with the director of pharmacy services, this person cannot carry out the total process alone.

Evaluation of the plan should properly focus on whether or not the goals and objectives are being met in accordance with the schedule outlined in the plan. There are numerous analytical techniques for program review outlined in this text, and the reader should refer to them. The philosophy of planning evaluation, however, must be based on the first steps of the process: the goals and objectives.

Revision of a planning document is usually mentioned at the end of a list in the planning steps, but this is not its only place in the sequence. In actual practice, revision of goals and objectives and other planning steps can occur at

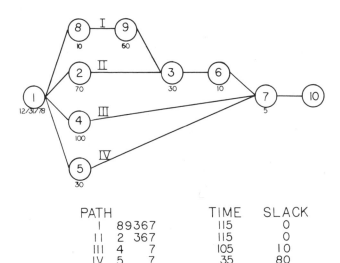

PATH			TIME	SLACK
I	89367		115	0
II	2	367	115	0
III	4	7	105	10
IV	5	7	35	80

FIGURE 15.3 Revised network diagram for IDCS plan.

any phase of the process. Change occurs throughout the conduct of this process, and revisions in priorities should normally be expected.

As indicated previously, planning is continuous. Proper sequencing of activities implies that the process never ends. Hence, planning is a time-consuming, expensive process that requires a commitment not only from departmental personnel but from the hospital administrator as well.

Planning as a formal process has both advantages and disadvantages. The major advantage of planning is that it provides direction and consistency to operations and may help to make daily operation much smoother. Properly developed plans mitigate the uncertainties of the future and reduce the chance that scarce resources may be expended in wasteful or inappropriate directions.

The major disadvantages of planning include the time and expense required for planning itself and for project management. Action-oriented people frequently feel more comfortable "doing" than planning, especially when daily pressures seem to insist that the manager "stop thinking and start acting." The old saw that "it is hard to work on draining the swamp when you're up to your arse in alligators" is an excellent illustration of the interplay of daily pressures to take action and the need to plan for action. The planning process requires a firm commitment of time by all those involved in it. Its success depends greatly on the ability of managers to motivate, coordinate, and control the behavior of others.

Information

The third requirement for planning is information. For convenience in discussion, the information required by planning systems can be divided into two broad classes: control information and demand information.

Control information concerns the operation of the organization itself, e.g., the overall goals and plans of the organization or other departments within the organization. The pharmacy department must consider such information initially when setting its own goals, objectives, and plans and

must remain aware of changes that may require reassessment of its own plans. After a department has developed functional plans, it requires information about the progress of the plans in order to maintain orderly and efficient progress. The Gantt chart shown in Figure 15.1 exemplifies such control information. J. Stevens, the person responsible for activities 4.2 and 4.3, needs to know that a necessary report has been delayed and that prompt corrective action should be considered to prevent the delay of subsequent activities. Stevens also needs information, not on the Gantt chart, about other events in the organization that might necessitate changes in the functional plan or even the objective itself.

Demand information is concerned with matters that are external to the control of the organization, principally the magnitude and nature of the organization's inputs and outputs. In the discussion that follows, demand information will be classified as endogenous, i.e., the inputs and outputs themselves, or exogenous, i.e., social, political, or economic factors that can affect inputs and outputs. Precise distinction between endogenous and exogenous variables depends on frame of reference and is difficult in the abstract. For example, a shift in hospital utilization from inpatient to outpatient service might be endogenous to a hospital-wide analysis but exogenous to a hospital pharmacy analysis, as suggested in the example below. The demand information of primary interest is predicted information about the future. Predictions about the future are, of course, uncertain and hazardous, but nonetheless mandatory for planning.

FORECASTING

One method of managing uncertainty is to use forecasting as a planning tool. Forecasting is defined as the application of quantitative methods to describe the future based on the past. Forecasting rests on the thesis that, although the future is indeterminant, trends that are operative in the present will more or less be operative in the future. If we can identify these relevant trends, we can predict into the future and, hence, reduce uncertainty and its consequences.

The future is likely to be affected by both endogenous and exogenous variables. For most elementary applications, exogenous variables are not mathematically incorporated into the analysis. It is important to remember, however, that omitting these factors may distort projections. Exogenous variables cause problems because they may be responsible for shifts in structure, that is, permanent changes in consumption patterns, attitudes, and the like. This type of shift is likely to be permanent, as opposed to endogenous change, which tends to be temporary and which we can accommodate in analyses.

A reasonable approach is to use formal data analysis to predict the effect of endogenous variables while using another analytical approach, or direct subjective judgment, to account for exogenous variables. Griffith (7) points out that forecasting may be viewed as the interaction of three factors: data, analysis, and judgment, and that the errors of forecasting arise from the same three sources.

Table 15.7 shows selected data from our mythical hospital. These data will be used to demonstrate various forecasting techniques.

TABLE 15.7   Selected Demand Data

Year	Occ	ADC	OPV (1000s)	IPI (1000s)	LVP (1000s)	OPP (1000s)
1970	0.75	225	40.5	262	7.0	10.2
1971	0.79	236	42.9	277	7.2	9.5
1972	0.82	245	46.1	281	6.9	11.9
1973	0.84	251	51.2	286	7.2	12.5
1974	0.84	253	54.5	282	7.1	13.5
1975	0.85	254	57.4	286	7.0	13.3
1976	0.85	254	60.6	284	7.1	14.9

Occ = occupancy rate; ADC = average daily census; OPV = out-patient visits; IPI = inpatient issues; LVP = large-volume parenteral issues; OPP = outpatient prescriptions.

Curve Fitting

Past trends can be used in forecasting by making graphic projections based on simple plot of time series data. Although the practicality of graphic presentation is limited by the ability to physically depict dimensionalities, one can obtain valuable information with this technique.

Suppose, for example, we are interested in forecasting the number of inpatient medication orders received in the pharmacy on an annual basis for the next 2 years. Figure 15.4 shows the plot: inpatient issues rose rapidly in the period 1970-1973, followed by what appears to be a leveling off that is disturbed only by random fluctuations.

As a result, we might speculate that this constancy will continue over the next few years. We would not speculate haphazardly, however. For example, we might observe that average daily census (ADC) has stabilized since 1973, while outpatient visits have increased considerably. We could check to see whether this is relevant by plotting the average daily census against the number of inpatient issues. As Figure 15.5 shows, the points fall fairly close to a straight line that can be drawn through the points by eye, suggesting that ADC is associated with number of inpatient issues. If we believe that ADC will remain stable for the next few years, confidence in our forecast is increased. The *middle dotted line* in Figure 15.4, then, represents the forecast. The two *outside dotted lines* represent high and low estimates, which account for some of the observed random variation. This analysis is a good example of the interplay of endogenous analysis, exogenous analysis, and judgment. In this case, the endogenous variable is inpatient issues (IPI), which we have forecast graphically. Average daily census is, in this situation, exogenous. As outlined above, we have analyzed its relationship with IPI separately and have used judgment in assessing its impact on the forecast. We have also judged the relationship between IPI and another exogenous variable, number of outpatient visits.

Regression

In the real world, it is natural to expect dispersion of data points around whatever smooth line may approximate observed data: curve fitting in such instances will not be perfect. The objective is to find a line that appears to be the best approximation to a data set, for this will increase confidence somewhat when the line is extrapolated into the future to obtain projected values.

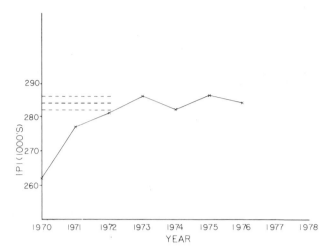

FIGURE 15.4   Time series, inpatient issues (IPI).

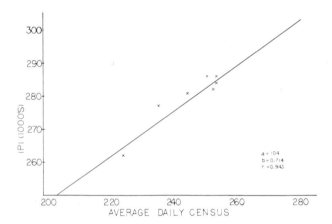

FIGURE 15.5   Regression of number of inpatient issues (IPI) and average daily census.

Regression is a mathematical approach to curve fitting in which the value of some dependent variable (y) is predicted from one or more independent variables ($x_1 \cdots x_n$). Regression models other than two-variable linear models require extensive calculation. In fact, it is seldom efficient to perform multiple regression without using a computer.

The simplest type of regression forecasting uses a straight-line projection of a dependent variable (y) from an independent variable (x), using the bivariate regression equation: y = a + bx.

This model should be familiar from elementary algebra as the equation of a straight line. The values of a and b that provide the best "least-squares" fit of the line to the observed data points may be calculated from the following equation[†]:

$$b = \frac{N\Sigma XY - \Sigma X \Sigma Y}{N\Sigma X^2 - (\Sigma X)^2} \tag{1}$$

$$a = \frac{\Sigma Y}{N} - \frac{b\Sigma X}{N} \tag{2}$$

[†]The notation is an instruction to add, e.g., X = sum of all x values, X^2 = sum of all squared x values.

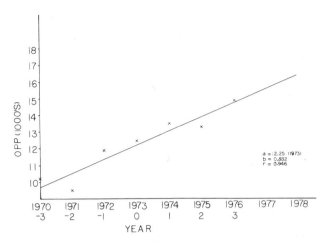

FIGURE 15.6 Time series regression of outpatient prescriptions (OPP).

TABLE 15.8   Rescaling the Time Axis so that $\Sigma X = 0$

Old	1970	1971	1972	1973	1974	1975	1976
New	−3	−2	−1	0	+1	+2	+3

We must recognize that the intercept term, a, refers to 1973, since we rescaled the x axis. The predicted number of outpatient prescriptions in 1978 (5 years beyond 1973) may be readily calculated:

$$\text{OPP (predicted, 1000s)} = 12.25 + (5)(0.832)$$
$$= 16.41$$

Assessing Precision of Estimates

One of the problems with regression equations is that little information is given about the reliability of the model per se. Two statistical values should be calculated for each regression equation and closely examined. The first statistic is the correlation coefficient, which indicates how closely related two variables are by the linear model. The correlation coefficient ranges from −1 to 1; values close to 1 (or −1) indicate a high degree of statistical association. The square of the correlation coefficient, r^2, may be interpreted as the proportion of the total variance in the dependent variable Y which is explained by the functional relationship. One of the objectives of forecasting is to maximize the proportion of explained variance, in order to minimize the errors of prediction. For example, an r^2 value of 0.90 suggests that, unless a shift in exogenous variables should occur, one can predict 90% of future variation by Y by knowing X. The remaining 10% is considered residual, or unexplained, variance.

The correlation coefficient may be calculated with equation 3.

$$r = \frac{N\Sigma(XY) - (\Sigma X)(\Sigma Y)}{\sqrt{[N\Sigma X^2 - (\Sigma X)^2][N\Sigma Y^2 - (\Sigma Y)^2]}} \quad (3)$$

Note that the numerator, and part of the denominator, of equation 3 are the same terms used in the calculation of b in equation 1. If the value of b is already known, it is easier to use

$$r = \frac{bN\Sigma X^2 - (\Sigma X)^2}{\sqrt{N\Sigma Y^2 - (\Sigma Y)^2}} \quad (4)$$

As before, if X has been rescaled so that $\Sigma X = 0$,

$$r = \frac{N\Sigma(XY)}{\sqrt{N\Sigma X^2[N\Sigma Y^2 - (\Sigma Y)^2]}} \quad (3A)$$

or

$$r = \frac{b\sqrt{N\Sigma X^2}}{\sqrt{N\Sigma Y^2 - (\Sigma Y)^2}} \quad (4A)$$

Returning to our effort to relate number of inpatient orders with average daily census (Fig. 15.5), we can use equation 4 to calculate

$$r = \frac{0.714\sqrt{5192}}{\sqrt{7(548106) - (1958)^2}}$$

Freund and Williams (8), in their extensive, nontechnical, discussion of forecasting, recommend a trick that simplifies calculation of the parameters considerably: numbering the years symmetrically around zero. For example, instead of using 1970, 1971, 1972 for x values, we can use −1, 0, +1. This has the advantage that ΣX is zero, so the normal equations simplify to

$$b = \frac{\Sigma XY}{\Sigma X^2} \quad (1A)$$

$$a = \frac{\Sigma Y}{N} = \bar{y} \quad (2A)$$

Regression analysis can improve the precision of the forecasts of inpatient and outpatient pharmacy issues. Calculating the relationship between IPI and ADC with equations 1 and 2 we obtain

$$b = \frac{7(481079) - (1718)(1958)}{7(422388) - (1718)^2}$$
$$= 3709/5192$$
$$= 0.714$$

$$a = \frac{1958 - (0.7144)(1718)}{7}$$
$$= 104$$

Hence, IPI (predicted, in 1000s) $= 104 + 0.714$ ADC. We can use this equation to check the forecast in Figure 15.4. If we expect the ADC to remain stable at about 254 for the forecast period, we can predict that IPI (1000s) $= 104 + 0.714\ (254) = 285$.

Turning to a forecast of outpatient prescriptions (Fig. 15.6), we use equations 1A and 1B. First, we rescale the x axis as shown in Table 15.8. Then we calculate

$$b = \frac{23.3}{28} = 0.832$$

$$a = \frac{85.8}{7} = 12.25$$

$$= \frac{(0.714)(72.056)}{54.57}$$

$$= 0.943$$

$$r^2 = 0.889$$

This is a respectable r^2. It says that about 89% of the variation in inpatient issue volume has been explained by average daily census.

Equation 4A may be used to calculate r for the forecast model of outpatient prescriptions as follows:

$$r = \frac{0.832\sqrt{7(28)}}{\sqrt{[7(1073.3)] - (85.8)^2}}$$

$$= \frac{11.648}{12.307}$$

$$= 0.946$$

$$r = 0.895$$

Again, r^2 suggests that IPP is changing rather consistently with time and that the forecasts are reliable, assuming that no shift in exogenous variables occurs.

Another important statistic in judging the reliability of a forecast is the standard error of estimate. It happens that r can be appreciably influenced by the *ranges* of the variables X and Y. For example, suppose that Y is almost constant over time, so that the calculated value of b is very samll. An example is the large-volume parenteral (LVP) data in Figure 15.7. The extremely small r value (0.069) should not lead to the conclusion that predictions of LVP may be poor. Predictions should be very good: because LVP changes only slightly with time, we can predict future values rather well. The standard error of estimate avoids this difficulty by taking the range of LVP values into account. A convenient computational formula for calculating the standard error of estimate is

$$Sy \cdot x = \sqrt{\frac{\Sigma Y^2 - (a \cdot \Sigma Y) - (b \cdot \Sigma XY)}{N - 2}} \quad (5)$$

Applying equation 5 to our LVP data, we get‡

$$Sy \cdot x = \sqrt{\frac{350.11 - (7.07)(49.5) - (0.00357)(.1)}{5}}$$

$$= 0.123$$

$Sy \cdot x$ may be interpreted as the standard deviation of error around the regression line. The precise use of $Sy \cdot x$ is beyond the scope of this book but may be obtained from most forecasting texts (9). The simplest use is to assess goodness of fit by dividing $Sy \cdot x$ by average Y. For example

$$Y = \frac{49.5}{7}$$

$$= 7.07$$

$$\frac{0.123}{7.07} = 0.017 \ (2\%)$$

---

‡Result is corrected for round-off error.

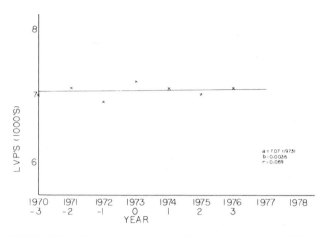

FIGURE 15.7   Time series regression of large-volume parenteral (LVP) issues.

The "error" in the regression line is roughly 2%, certainly evidence of a better fit than was suggested by r = 0.069.

It is important to remember that forecasting is not prophecy and is little more than an educated guess as to what some future will be. More often than not, the forecasts will prove to be more or less inaccurate; yet, absence of forecasting information makes budget preparation and related planning activities more difficult.

Cyclical Change

Once the parameters of a prediction equation are known, it becomes relatively easy to project beyond the data base into the future. As long as cyclical changes do not occur, this type of unadjusted forecasting does not present serious problems. Unfortunately, most time series data such as drug product utilization are subject to seasonal fluctuations. In acute therapy, for example, the utilization of antibiotics, antitussives, and similar drugs may be much higher in the fall and winter quarters than in the spring and summer quarters. When seasonal disturbances are evident, they should be removed before further analysis is performed for the purpose of getting annual estimates. When forecasting within a year, however, seasonal fluctuation must not be ignored or smoothed out. Seasonal disturbances can be reduced or eliminated by using either moving averages or semiaverages (10). These techniques involve separating the data points into groups and then obtaining averages for the groups. A line is then drawn between the average points.

There are other techniques that may be employed to remove seasonal fluctuations. It is important to remember, however, that data manipulations should not be applied indiscriminately.

When data are analyzed on an annual data basis, seasonal fluctuations are usually masked in the aggregate data. When the unit of analysis is monthly or quarterly, cyclical fluctuations are more readily apparent. The key point to watch for in annual data is the problem encountered by shifts in structure from one time period to another. For example, if we were looking at a hospital's inventory level and noted a sudden drop in units stocked, the reason for that drop may be the adoption of a rigid formulary. Hence, the change may be permanent and therefore continue into the future. If an explanation is not apparent, it becomes necessary to look again into the past to obtain a logical explanation.

Most forecasting is on fairly solid ground when projecting into the immediate future. Forecasts for 10-20 years into the future are far less reliable and should be discouraged. Forecasts of this nature can be expected to be subject to shifts in structure because of the effect of exogenous variables.

SUMMARY

Although formal planning and forecasting is an ambiguous, laborious, and sometimes worrisome process, it cannot safely be avoided by a manager. Planning is especially important for managers in hospitals because of governmental mandate and shortages of working capital. The hospital pharmacy manager is faced with the choice either to do his own planning or permit planning to be done for him by higher management. The latter choice may seem a serious abdication of responsibility, especially to younger, better trained hospital administrators. Furthermore, hospital pharmacy planning done by nonpharmacist managers may fail to consider many of pharmacy's newer roles.

Assuming that a hospital pharmacy manager is able and willing to accept responsibility for departmental planning, three final points should be kept in mind. First, hospital management is becoming increasingly complex, and the requisite sophistication of planning grows apace. Second, the hospital pharmacy manager should use the assistance of others in the hospital, e.g., the comptroller's office, in gathering data, and should insist that sufficient data in appropriate formats be routinely collected by the hospital. Finally, the hospital pharmacy manager should ensure that the relationship of his plan to the goals of the hospital is as clear as possible.

REFERENCES

1. Longest BB Jr: *Management Practices for the Health Professional*. Reston, VA, Reston Publishing, 1976, p 60.
2. Buffa ES: *Modern Production Management*. New York, John Wiley & Sons, 1969, p 582.
3. Richards MD, Greenlaw PS: *Management Decisions and Behavior*. Homewood, IL, Richard D Irwin, 1972, p 472.
4. Buffa, *op cit*, chap 8.
5. Griffith JF: *Quantitative Techniques for Hospital Planning and Control*. Lexington, MA, Lexington Books, DC Heath, 1972, chap 8.
6. Bierman H, Bonini CP, Hausman WH: *Quantitative Analysis for Business Decisions*, ed 3. Homewood, IL, Richard D Irwin, 1969, chap 21.
7. Griffith, *op cit*, p 22.
8. Freund JE, Williams FJ: *Modern Business Statistics*. Englewood Cliffs, NJ, Prentice Hall, 1958, chap 18.
9. *ibid*, p 301.
10. *ibid*, p 423.

Management Information Systems

STEPHEN L. PRIEST, JEANNETTE BOUSQUET GOUDREAU,
and JOSEPH M. MORRISSEY

DEFINITION OF INFORMATION RESOURCES

Background

"What's the most useful information resource in your department?" I asked the director of pharmacy. "Well, the patient and drug information system comes to mind first," she responds. "That system provides us with easy retrieval of patient drug distribution history and monitoring information. We use this information resource in dispensing patient medications, utilization review, and in maintaining billing and inventory records."

I direct the same question to the chief admitting officer. "We couldn't live without our registration system," he responds. "It helps us in quick retrieval of a patient's demographic data, including identified congenital diseases, in determining dates of last visits, and in streamlining the registration process to allow patients to enter treatment areas more quickly. It also helps us maintain accurate and timely patient census for usage in such applications as pharmacy, laboratory, and radiology."

The data processing manager answered, "The data base software to monitor and maintain computer usage by application. That, together with the data communications network to each of the hospital's 37 ancillary departments, is probably used more than any other resource we manage."

These responses are typical and highlight several points of view that emerge when trying to define the term "information resources."

First, based on the speciality from which it is approached, the term "information resource" (IR) means different things to different people. Ask every department head in an organization what IRs are and you get as many different answers as there are different department heads.

Although this situation does not help when trying to define terms, still it is a real and quite appropriate situation. Every department has its own objectives. It follows that each department will have its own special needs when using information systems output to meet those objectives. The result is that IR services vary widely across an organization in both form and content.

Another important result is that persons using IRs perceive them primarily as services. IRs are not so much hard-ware and software to the pharmacy as they are services. Without always recognizing the fact, staff are using the output of the IRs that include hardware, software, staff, procedures, and other components.

The pharmacy is most keenly aware of the output provided—the unit dose dispensing schedule, the inventory-on-hand report, the IV preparation list, etc. The "thing" that provides the output, the service, has been called variously the "computer system," the "information system," the "management information system," and the "data processing system." Currently, users perceive that the central computer department is calling this service an "information resource."

Still others relate an IR to a large data base system in which all the hospital's automated data are stored, retrieved, and shared by a multitude of departments.

Finally, to complicate the matter of defining IR further, a new fact of 1980s life must be recognized. While several information systems that exist require IRs provided through centralized computer departments, many information systems can now be entirely selected, installed, and managed by a single department working alone (commonly called "stand-alone" systems). Thus, as various departments identify the need for information systems, the result can be multiple and independent IRs to service those different needs.

What Is an IR?

The pharmacy's perspective is correct. Information systems and information services are the IRs. The computer technician's perspective is also correct. Computer hardware, data bases, and the central IR department itself are the IRs. How can both be correct?

This dilemma is easy to resolve if you consider the point of view of the chief executive officer (CEO). For the CEO, the organizational objectives, not the departmental objectives, are paramount. IRs include all the information services available to the organization to meet its objectives. To the CEO, then, each individual department's information system is an IR, as each had perceived.

But these IR services do not exist in a vacuum. They are made available either through a central IR department, by the pharmacy's own staff, or from a third party outside the organization.

Any internal group that provides IR services should itself be considered an IR. This means that the telecommunications staff and the office automation staff are also IRs.

Further, the most important characteristic linking these various groups is the use of computer technology to provide information services. The tools used—the computers, the telecommunications channels, etc—must also be considered as IRs. Thus, the technician's point of view is also correct.

In summary, these authors consider the term "information resource" to have a twofold meaning. First, IRs include any information service used by the organization. Second, IRs include any internal hardware, software, and staff used to support those information services.

Three interesting facts follow from this definition. First, IRs are a means to an end, tools used to meet organizational objectives. All managers must acknowledge this fact.

Second, our definition includes the traditional information systems, such as pharmacy patient drug dispensing systems. But it is not limited to these; it is open ended. Also included in our definition are the emerging information services such as decision support systems (e.g., financial modeling), office automation (e.g., word processing and spreadsheet), and telecommunications.

Finally, it should be clear that an information system does not necessarily require a computer, although, as a practical matter, the term "information resource" implies the use of the computer.

USERS OF IRs

The User

The terms "end user" and "user" are used interchangeably. These terms imply the ultimate user of the IR service. IR end users are a diverse cross section of an organization: pharmacists, secretaries, technicians, clerks, department heads, senior management, the CEO, etc.

The Used

It is interesting to explore just what it is that end users actually use. The output from the IR is, as you should suspect, information.

We have mentioned the pharmacy's use of information to help answer questions about patient drug utilization or to help make decisions about antibiotic usage. Likewise, the admitting office used the registration system to provide admission schedules and to process patients quickly into the treatment areas. Clearly, what is being used is information, the output from individual management information systems. But there are other kinds of IRs.

Consider the purchasing department that orders supplies by having their microcomputer talk with the IV manufacturer's large-scale computer. In this case, the telecommunications network was being used to exchange information.

While in the first two cases it was the information produced that was ultimately important, in the latter case the resources themselves play the prominent role. Once again, we see that IRs could be thought of as either the service to the user (i.e., the information produced) or the supportive hardware, software, and staff (i.e., telecommunications network).

CONTROL OF PHARMACY IRs

The Past

Economic, technologic, educational, and control constraints once strongly favored centralization of an organization's IRs. This meant that the pharmacy department had little or no control over IRs.

The high cost of computers could not be justified for individual user departments: computers had to be located in one, or very few, physical locations. Computer hardware technology required special environments, such as humidity and temperature control and raised floors, as well as trained and dedicated computer operators. Specialized training in computer programming and systems design was necessary and often was outside the ability of most users; this factor, too, favored centralization of IRs. Managerial control also favored centralization. Organizations wanted to centralize all computer hardware and staff resources in order to maximize usage and productivity of these costly and limited resources.

The Problem

Centralization can sometimes frustrate and isolate pharmacy managers because they thereby are prevented from having first-hand control over management and access to IRs that their department depends on. Centralization can reduce department flexibility and adaptability and may require more money and time to respond to change. Distribution, on the other hand, often increases and expands multidepartment integration requirements. Moreover, few central IR departments can manage effectively and stay current with available software and hardware technology. Yet, many of these newer technologies depend on data bases and other centrally managed technology, such as networking, for their effectiveness.

Alternatives

Today's technology now provides IR and pharmacy management with alternatives to centralization whereby IRs can be distributed and decentralized.

The low cost of micro- and minicomputers and the ease of their operation provides the opportunity for nearly every user to control his/her own IR destiny. Local area networking (electronic linkages that allow multiple and mixed applications to communicate) provide opportunity for both users and central host computers to share the same data bases while offering the managerial independence that both areas desire.

Local area networking allows each application to reside on a separate microcomputer and post and retrieve data from other computers in the network as needed. These new systems will be the key to the pharmacy of the future.

Another distribution alternative is to have remote systems, stand-alone systems. If systems stand alone with no need to interact with other systems and users, then you do not have interface and communication concerns that are present with multiple users. Instead, you have only the operational and resource utilization problems. However, future organizational plans may not favor this alternative for certain applications.

For instance, excessive and costly duplication of data elements in multiple departments using the same data dictionary may favor a central perspective.

Remote clusters may be a feasible distribution alternative. Satellite pharmacies outside the local area of a central inventory may have stand-alone systems for order entry, local inventory, and shipping and receiving while also communicating daily with a host processor for central inventory control, distribution of items from one area to another, and patient billing.

These alternatives are now a consideration because the hardware and system software technology of many new computers require no specially prepared facility or trained operators. User-friendly languages now exist to provide users the opportunity to define, select, and implement many of their own applications and systems.

Definition

Before further discussion on whether IRs should be centralized or distributed, let us first offer another definition to what is meant by ''information resources.'' We will do this by classifying IRs into four categories: (1) management resources; (2) systems analysis and programming resources; (3) computer operations resources; and (4) data base resources. The first category, management resources, pertains to the persons or departments responsible for the planning, policy setting, and prioritizing of applications and even hardware, and their effect on interdepartmental utilization. The second category, systems and programming resources, includes the staff responsible for the definition, design, package selection, programming, and implementation of IR applications. Computer operations resources comprise the third category. This includes the hardware as well as the staff and facilities responsible for the operation of the hardware, including data input, report generation, screen layouts, file and program retention, and file management. The data base resources are the fourth category, which includes the staff responsible for the collection of data and their definition. The manner in which these four resources are allocated and managed throughout an organization determine the extent of centralization/distribution of IRs.

Extreme Centralization

Extreme centralization means that all four resources are controlled by an IR department. This method was preferred in the 1960s and 1970s, when organizations (and their computers) experienced the constraints mentioned above. In this mode, usage and control of IRs are managed through a central IR department and a staff of information specialists. A pharmacy depended on the IR department for accessibility

to the computers, the software, the data bases, and staff resources.

The argument favoring centralization is based on the efficiencies of economics, technology, education, and control that accrue from consolidating computers, facilities, data bases, and IR talent under one central management. Further, centralization can permit unified planning based on organization-wide information needs.

Extreme Distribution

Distributed IRs exist in the extreme sense when the pharmacy department has first-hand and sole control over access to its particular IR need. Today's marketplace makes available turn-key packages that can often be selected and installed with little need for users to have an in-depth understanding of hardware and software concepts. These packages (such as office automation routines) operate on micro- and minicomputers that require minimal operator sophistication. The computer may or may not be physically located and operated in the pharmacy area.

The pharmacy information needs are met through dictionary parameters and data bases that can provide various user-friendly reporting features and optional screens.

Distribution appears to optimize utilization of IRs from the pharmacy perspective.

Solution

Can all the organization's IRs (management, systems/ programming, computer operations, and data bases) be handled solely by the pharmacy—making optimal use of hardware, software, personnel, facility, and data base resources—and still meet the organization's objectives? Should the IRs be centralized under one department and their control and accessibility determined by an IR executive, senior management, or steering committee?

Rather than look at an application in terms of simply IRs, it may be easier to break the resources into four components and to set up criteria and make a decision about each component independent of the other. That is, the pharmacy department, for each application, has the potential to assume responsibility for one, two, three, or all of the four categories of IRs.

The degree of IR responsibility that the pharmacy department can assume, and the decision-making process involved in answering the centralization vs distribution question, is a responsibility that all organizations must recognize and plan for. For a more extensive explanation of the centralization and distribution question, refer to Priest (1).

ROLE OF PHARMACY IN A CENTRAL DATA BASE

It is important for pharmacy departments to put into perspective their role in a hospital-wide patient care system as it relates to IRs. Most organizations are heading toward the concept of a centralized data base, whereby multiple and various departments both utilize and contribute to a centrally located data base. This concept minimizes the incidence of multiple departments collecting and storing individual demographic data (such as a patient's name, age, sex, allergies). It will make identical data available everywhere throughout the organization. Further, data security can be provided through a data base administrator responsible for the integrity and availability of data.

Departments that specialize in maintaining accurate and complete patient data, such as medical records and patient registration, can handle the problems of maintaining accurate census location and demographic data store. This allows other specialized departments, such as pharmacy, to focus on their primary responsibility of providing accurate, timely, and complete drug delivery and information to patients and physicians. No longer does the pharmacy have to maintain separate census and discharge files that are often outdated and incomplete.

A central, or host, data base concept can provide opportunities for the pharmacy that previously were very difficult or impossible to obtain with stand-alone systems. For instance, a central data base that includes laboratory and pharmacy data can provide review of antibiotic usage. When a culture is taken, the prescribed antibiotic can be reviewed to the sensitivity of the organism.

Nursing can order a diagnostic examination that notifies pharmacy of forthcoming drug needs automatically with the examination request. For instance, the ordering of a barium enema may print in pharmacy automatically signaling the need for a bowel prep.

A central data base system can allow the nursing staff to quickly review the patient's medication profile at the nursing station. The potential exists for physicians to prescribe drugs from their offices (given, of course, proper security and identification techniques) and to obtain information regarding adverse reaction potential of a particular drug.

Pharmacy Dependence on Other Departments

As can be seen, the opportunities of a shared central data base are basically endless, and more opportunities are being discovered every day. However, these opportunities also bring a responsibility that was not nearly as recognizable with stand-alone systems. That is, if the admitting office does not maintain an accurate patient census, drugs may be delivered to the wrong areas or not delivered at all. It is of the utmost importance that the pharmacy receive this information in order to dispense medications accurately to the proper nursing units at the correct time. It is also critical to the debit/credit process for patient billing to ensure proper charges for discharged patients.

A central data base system therefore needs full interdepartmental cooperation to ensure that all users of the data base are provided with timely, accurate, and complete patient data. All departments must realize how important it is for each to perform its delicate role.

An example of a central data base system installation that initially caused pharmacy problems was an admitting office discharge procedure that discharged the patient on the central data base prior to the patient's actually leaving the hospital. The pharmacy assumed that the patient was indeed discharged and did not dispense the patient's medication. Because the patient did not actually leave the hospital until early evening and did not receive medication, there was confusion between nursing and pharmacy. Thus, a new discharge procedure was necessary to accommodate the special

needs of the central data base. This one task involved changes in pharmacy, nursing, and admitting procedures to accommodate hospital policy and still use the central data base.

SELECTING THE PHARMACY MANAGEMENT INFORMATION SYSTEM

The Needs List

Prior to beginning the selection process, the pharmacy must assess its department procedures and present distribution system. It is essential that needs and requirements be documented and agreed to by the pharmacy director and other senior pharmacy staff. This process can be preceded by reviewing other hospitals' applications to get a sense of real-world pharmacy software expectations (2). Site visits to these hospitals provide a perspective of opportunities and degree of effort and staff needed for installing systems. The needs list can then be prepared and issued to the in-house IR area or to various software companies for reply (3).

It is important that the needs list not simply duplicate existing manual procedures and reports but indeed satisfy a need by making use of the automated tool. For instance, if the manual system required all physician orders to be delivered directly to pharmacy, the dispensing of the drug, i.e., the need, may now be accomplished by the pharmacist using the computer to enter the drug at the nursing station, thereby decreasing the turnaround time for distribution. Thus, the need is satisfied, and the procedure has taken advantage of the automated system (4).

Evaluation Parameters

The pharmacy needs list can then be compared to what the vendor submits and to what the pharmacy has seen of the vendor's product during the site and vendor demonstration period. Parameters such as costs (software, installation, hardware, training, conversion, and others that should be identified), vendor experience, service record, software adequacy, compatibility with central software and hardware systems, documentation, and training must be listed, and each vendor's product must be compared to the list. This will allow for a more equitable comparison of vendors and product.

The selection of pharmacy IRs is a time-consuming process that should be well planned and include surveys, site visits both to vendors (for demonstrations) and hospitals already using the system, and discussion with present users of the software. A discussion of cost should include total package price, ongoing service contract fees, and fees for additional customization, which most likely will occur once the system is installed. The ongoing service contract must be understood, because many times the customer expects a maintenance contract to include updates, when in fact it is only an "insurance" contract, which says that the vendor will correct program problems, but that almost all updates will incur an additional charge. Additional customization is almost always required for any system and should be included in the budget.

The experience of the vendor, as determined by past installation history, is one crucial parameter used for evaluation. Discussions and visits with hospitals using the vendor will indicate the adequacy of the software, the quality and quantity of service provided, the response time to service, and the effort and staff needed to implement the system.

Site visits to hospitals already using the software can provide invaluable insight into the daily operational concerns for a pharmacy integrated with a host data base system. The experience and opinions of other users allow prospective clients to discuss first-hand the pros and cons of specific features. Several members of the pharmacy staff should take part in the site visit, as well as at least one member of the IR staff. This will allow for a variety of ideas and opinions based on each person's concerns about the system's operation in his/her own area of responsibility.

Even before a final vendor is selected, several implementation concerns should be considered. These include personnel requirements, equipment needs, method of data entry to bring existing files onto the host data base, billing concerns, education and training of the pharmacy staff, and a method of testing the various functions of the software as it compares with the previous or present system. These concerns need to be addressed prior to committing to the software in order for all parties involved within the hospital structure (administration, pharmacy, financial, IR) to realize that the package cost will not be the sole cost of implementing the system. If the cost and time of items such as data entry are not discussed beforehand, then the hospital may not budget for such items as data entry expenses incurred by entering the medication formulary into the host data base. Unplanned costs can delay an installation until additional committee and senior approvals are obtained.

The director of pharmacy should assign at least one person in the department to act as the interdepartment liaison between the IR/vendor and pharmacy staff. This person must have an interest in learning the computer system and a working knowledge of the pharmacy operation. The person must also have training skills and be given some authority to make procedural changes if necessary. Of course, major changes may have to be discussed with senior staff, but the liaison should be able to get senior management support. The person assigned the task of coordinator must "make things happen."

Past computer experience is not absolutely necessary if there is a good working relationship between pharmacy and the IR or vendor staff. This experience will come through getting involved and asking many questions about computer terms, systems analysis, and computer maintenance.

The liaison person should be able to devote the large majority of the work week to the implementation of the computer system for at least a 6-month period in order to meet the plan. A definite timetable must be established at the outset of the implementation to maintain progress and achieve results in the process.

Relating to Both Outside Vendors and/or In-House IR Staff

The aforementioned pharmacy liaison person must be able to establish a viable working relationship with and develop confidence in both in-house IR staff and the vendor staff. Each must feel able to communicate freely and on a regular

basis with reference to any problems that may arise. The vendor staff must rely on this pharmacy coordinator to clearly relay any needs or desires before they can be developed. It is crucial for the in-house IR staff to have a basic working knowledge of the pharmacy software and hardware, or else they will be unable to assist the department effectively in eliminating the occasional "bug" that arrives.

Printers, CRTs, and Form Concerns

A major concern that requires detailed evaluation is the question of how much and what type of hardware equipment will be needed in order for the department to utilize the computer system. The importance of this evaluation cannot be stressed enough by the authors, because a lack of sufficient equipment will serve only to culture frustration in personnel within the department. Parameters such as the daily volume of medication orders, the volume of outpatient prescriptions, routine system maintenance, and the usage requirements for pricing, purchasing, and inventory should be considered carefully when determining the number of terminals (CRTs) required for daily pharmacy operations.

The number and types of printers required can be determined by reviewing the number of lists needed daily as well as the number and types of labels needed and their frequency of usage. For example, separate printers may be necessary for inpatient labels as opposed to total parenteral nutrition (TPN) labels, which are usually larger and used less often than the former. Also, it is necessary to assess the compatibility of printers with the various form types that will be used; this is in reference to weight, thickness, and minimal paper-size requirements of the printer. Each printer has its own features that must be analyzed prior to implementation in order to maximize efficiency and avoid the frustration of using incompatible equipment.

Another major consideration for both printers and CRTs is to standardize as much as possible. Mixing brands or types of equipment makes it difficult for users to change from one to another. Keyboards may be arranged differently on various CRTs, printers may require different ribbons, and form requirements may vary. Using one brand allows for easier replacement with backup hardware and a much simpler training process.

Training Concerns

A well-coordinated training schedule for the department members should be established by the coordinator once he or she is trained by the IR or vendor staff and the testing is complete. Small groups of staff members should be able to review all the system options and experiment with each one that pertains to their daily routine.

Pharmacists more than likely will require a broader scope of training than the technical staff because they will have access to more of the system options (e.g., pharmacists will enter orders in both the IV and unit dose areas and therefore need to have many more functions available to them than the unit dose technicians).

Most important to the overall training process is the emphasis that should be placed on reaching *all* personnel in the department, whether full- or part-time. Failure to do so will result in possible resentment and "fear" of the computer system and its relative mystery. After the system is implemented, a considerable amount of time must be devoted to training new employees as well as to explaining and communicating fully any changes and new features of the system.

An instruction manual composed by the pharmacy coordinator is a necessary tool for all department members, so that they can refer to it when questions arise concerning daily routine. This is also invaluable for reference by new employees in order for them to establish a clear concept of the overall pharmacy operation.

EFFECTIVE STRATEGIES TO INSTALL AND MAINTAIN A PHARMACY IR

Interaction

Not all informations systems have been a success. Many have failed to achieve the advantages that a computerized information system should bring. It has become clear in studying the disappointments and the success stories that the single most critical factor for success is the effective involvement and interaction of the end users and the IR specialists. This is a new world for many users, and it can be a bewildering one because of the complexity and jargon that can often accompany an information system.

The pharmacy staff need to understand the principles of IRs and its own essential role in information system development and use. In the same sense, the central IR department must practice the role of a support department and not dictate the use and restriction of IR systems and services to the users.

Both the pharmacy and IR department staff must understand the roles each plays in the development, use, and evolution of IRs. They must attempt to do this without fear of the jargon that adds to the complexity of information systems. It is critical that all IR users appreciate this basic idea. In order to continuously maintain and use IRs successfully, both the end user and the IR staffs must be held jointly accountable for the information system.

Today, information system opportunities extend beyond the scope of the central IR staff's control. This is cause for both pharmacy and IR staff to examine each other's role and responsibilities in the growth and use of IRs.

No Simple Explanation

There is no simple explanation as how to develop an effective pharmacy system. These authors receive many inquiries from hospitals asking how to design, improve, or implement ways to serve their computer needs. Senior managers and supervisors request that the answers not be in "computerese," but rather in simple language that explains how to plan and maintain an effective computer system.

The only way to develop a successful and usable computer system is for the IR staff to understand more about the pharmacy department than just the required and obvious reports. Likewise, the pharmacy staff must understand more about IRs than simply expecting IR personnel to be experts at mindreading (they are not) who, through a combination of intuition, magic, and mind projection, always know the user's needs with infinite precision (they do not).

Misunderstood Interaction

Many users willingly commit themselves to unstructured, misunderstood, and passive involvement. This means that they understand that they must attend committee meetings and approve numerous memos and reports that define and plan their systems. Further, they believe that the IR department will be responsible for all of the system's planning, training, and implementation, with the user assuming responsibility only for the "acceptance" or "rejection" of the final product. By the same token, to the IR department, programming and system staff involvement often mean working in a rather mechanical manner, literally programming what is requested rather than what is needed or is usable. The IR department does the systems work and pharmacy approves the final product. However, this type of involvement often does not work.

Unstructured Involvement

Unstructured involvement results in IR and vendors spending many hours and dollars on projects that are never utilized. Useless system features result because IR has programmed by the "letter of the law" rather than the "spirit of the law." Projects seemingly can last forever as the pharmacy staff attempts to define and redefine exactly what it wants the system to do, and IR obediently reprograms the additional, forgotten, or misunderstood changes.

Active Interaction

If unstructured and passive involvement does not ensure a successful system, how then do pharmacy and IR personnel arrive at a meaningful, workable system? One method that works, the method which is proposed to both pharmacy and IR, is active interaction.

Interaction can ensure a continual and effective relationship between the IR, vendor and pharmacy department. Interaction means that the user "wears a systems analyst hat" and that IR and vendor communicate in the user's language and ask intelligent questions. It means a complete team approach—the sharing of system analysis responsibility (beginning with project initiation and continuing through implementation), the use of interdepartmental controls, and the sharing of the resulting accolades. Interaction ensures ongoing interdepartmental dialogue.

Interaction means recognizing that automated systems result in changes. Active interaction means that the pharmacy works in harmony with the IR to cause this change to be a planned process, rather than an abrupt interruption.

Initiative

Who takes the initiative in the interaction process? Ideally, interaction occurs when the pharmacy and the IR departments independently assume the responsibility to develop interaction techniques. Both departments have to commit themselves to a successful project regardless of the other's degree of involvement. It is like a successful marriage in which both partners are willing to give more than they receive.

Education

One approach that is valuable as a first step in interaction is education in a formal setting. Pharmacy personnel should be encouraged to attend seminars on the use of computers.

Local colleges and schools offer courses that provide an introduction to data processing (DP) for the user. These courses will introduce the user to the responsibilities involved in using DP services. A formal DP education can remove the mystique of DP and enlighten the user to its potential.

The IR department should also make available formal DP training courses for users within the company. A comprehensive course in introduction to DP will be enlightening to both the user and to IR personnel. The IR instructor will recognize the concerns of the user and can put many fears and misconceptions to rest, and an in-house course will help to promote interdepartmental dialogue.

Viewing the Other's Home

The importance of face-to-face interaction and on-site activities cannot be overemphasized. Many misunderstandings develop when individuals have no idea of the basic elements of a pharmacy's operation. Many organizational procedures are defined by space limitations and equipment needs. Although formal education is the first step in real communication, nothing can substitute for the experience of seeing and touching the real thing. The user might hear the terms "CRT" or "CPU," but these items of hardware become real only when actually viewed and handled. The analyst might hear the terms "unit dose" or "TPN," but these terms of pharmacy become real only when seen through the eyes of the pharmacy user.

Pharmacy staff should ask to visit the IR areas. The IR department can also take the initiative by extending invitations to tour their areas. Often, users "throw the data over the fence" and the reports are "thrown back" with no concept as to what happens regarding program logic, data entry, and computer operations.

A technique that works well is simply to have the pharmacy staff enter data into the computer using their own source documents. A user can become the data entry operator, if only for the moment. The user can see firsthand what happens when source data are illegible or missing: the reasons for control totals become obvious. The tour of the IR area should include a demonstration of the computer's printing actual user reports. This will reveal the time and preparation needed before reports can be delivered. Many people believe that the computer works with the "speed of light" and that 5-page statistical reports for 100 drugs can be printed instantly. An actual demonstration of report preparation brings IR responsibility into focus for the user.

The pharmacy should reciprocate and invite the IR personnel to tour the department to learn why various files are maintained. When viewing the IV preparation area, for instance, IR staff can see the time involved and the knowledge necessary to obtain data prior to terminal input. Discussion with IR of IV preparation and ordering techniques of reports will prove the usefulness of the information. By providing IR with an understanding of the user department, the importance of legible, timely, and accurate reports will become clear.

An expanded version of a pharmacy tour can involve an IR analyst's being assigned temporarily to the department. The analyst can be given responsibility to perform certain tasks; he or she will develop a working dialogue with the user and thus come to understand the pharmacy's work requirements.

Strategy Sessions

It is vital that interaction take place before important committee meetings and planning sessions. When IR staff and user staff get together, they can develop the agenda and discuss the items to be presented. This provides an opportunity to review the appropriate data and reports and the manner in which they are interpreted. Preparation in an informal setting allows for "brainstorming" and an exchange of ideas that might be considered out of place in a full committee setting. Differing points of view and areas of concern of each speciality become apparent and can be accommodated and reconciled to the goals of the group. The end result of these sessions will be formal meetings that run more smoothly and accomplish more objectives. In addition, the parties involved will be more aware of each other's thoughts relative to the optimal operation of the user department.

Attending Pharmacy Staff Meetings

The IR staff can be invited to selected pharmacy staff meetings. If IR understands how systems are to be used, it can assist more effectively in the definition of application features with the ability to "read between the lines" when screens are defined.

Systems Design

Pharmacy should formally document their needs for new or changed system features. Instead of verbally explaining to the IR staff what the feature should be, the feature's format should be put on paper. Discussions aided by a visual document can be understood better by both parties. Some users may even prefer to flow chart the logic that will go into the new or changed feature.

Even small changes in data needs and reports can have major implications for a computerized system. Therefore, it is vital that both users and IR decide whether a change is sufficiently important (i.e., managerially appropriate) to warrant "tinkering" with the system. This aspect of interaction takes into account the amount of work necessary to make the change and will ensure the integrity of the data and reports over time.

System definitions historically were prepared by the IR staff. This resulted in reports looking the way the analyst thought the report should look. Having the pharmacy design screens and reports results in a more usable end product.

There undoubtedly will be changes to the initial designs, and the IR analyst will make suggestions with regard to the logic and reporting formats, but the reports should be what the user feels comfortable with.

Prototypes

Conceptualized system specifications can have their limits. Planning a carefully thought-out system and then trying to maintain its design during actual implementation is difficult, if not impossible, to do in one pass. Many times the pharmacy may not be able to visualize how a system will operate in its final and most effective state. It is the actual "hands-on" experience of manipulating data during entry, retrieval, and reporting that provides both user and IR with convincing understanding of what is really desired and what a system's limitations may be.

Putting up a computer model, whether it be in-house or vendor turn-key software, and allowing the user to "play" with it, can be very effective. Prototype heuristic approaches allow the user to arrive at a workable and understandable system, provide confidence in the system, and speed up the training and implementation process.

Test Data and Calculations

When it is time to approve and accept system program customizations, the pharmacy should be responsible for the final test using their own sample data. In addition, calculations should be tested by the user and compared to manual expectations. For example, when testing the accuracy of a new statistical report, the pharmacy staff can enter a limited number of patients into a test system and then print the test monthly reports to ensure that the system handled the statistics appropriately. If the IR analyst does the final test with his or her own test data, the analyst will check only what appears reasonable from the IR perspective. Most analysts do not have the pharmacy background necessary to be aware of all data input and output possibilities. The pharmacy will be the user of the reports and screens and therefore must confirm the system's accuracy and reasonableness.

Documentation

The pharmacy should prepare all systems manuals and user documents that explain computer systems developed both in-house and from software vendors. The IR analyst can then verify the documentation and reconcile system differences with the pharmacy.

For vendor-provided software, it is the responsibility of the vendor to provide the system documentation. However, it is necessary for users to convert this documentation into procedure manuals for the people working with the system on a day-by-day basis. Vendor-provided manuals are often all encompassing, and most users need only selected instruction for dealing with their unique needs.

Pharmacy-provided documentation, with IR staff review, assures that each department understands the system's functions. Without such an approach, the IR analyst will be the only "expert" on the system. Documentation ensures that the painstaking efforts of all involved will be permanent and will transcend personnel changes in either department.

Parallel Systems

Whenever system changes or "improvements" to existing screens and reports are made, it is important to operate a parallel system for a period of time. This often requires duplicate effort and extensive time demands, but it offers a minimum of risk when going "live" with the new change.

The pharmacy and IR departments must compare the present system with the new system and the cost and risk of ensuring that changes have been made successfully. Often, what appears to be a small system change can have a significant and costly effect on the total system. The uniqueness of many computer programs can lead to unexpected problems if new systems are not verified before implementation.

Some systems do not allow extensive parallels. The response time and complexity of a real-time system may make duplicate input and hardware unreasonable for the user to attempt parallel system comparisons. For this situation, the IR department may develop duplicate sets of application programs, using one set for the live system while the other is for testing programming enhancements. When a change on the test program has been proved acceptable to both the user and IR staff, it can be put into the live system.

For instance, when making a change to a drug order entry system that will require the expiration date to print on a label, the new program change may be tried by the user in a test system to determine whether the change was made properly. Further, the test will also ensure that other features of the system were not affected. Once determined to be acceptable, the new print program can be transferred into the live system.

One method for teaching pharmacy to operate real-time systems is to create test master files for training. For instance, a new pharmacist can learn to enter medication orders by accessing a fictitious patient and then entering drugs as if the patient were active. The system will simulate the actual functions and perform all console lead-throughs without actually updating live files. This method can also be used for ongoing in-house training for new employees.

Written requests commit the department. "Corridor conversations" resulting in immediate IR action often result in IR frustration: the person may simply be asking "can you?" but IR hears it as a "must have" request. Committing a request to writing presents the user with the opportunity to reflect on all of the variables involved.

Troubleshooting

"Troubleshooting" plays an important part in the process of interaction. The IR department must respond quickly and rectify problems that occur in the pharmacy's system, or else pharmacy will seek other alternatives to its problems and lose faith in IRs. Since user staff have been involved in the development of the system from the outset, their knowledge will help focus attention on specific problem areas and save system analyst time. Instead of saying "I don't know what is wrong with this report," an educated user might be able to tell IR, "I think the wrong group of drugs is being extracted."

Work Committee

A successful information system must have continual interaction among the people who will be responsible for using and maintaining it. Establishing work committees that represent the various interests within the hospital promotes user participation and sharing of accountability for the success or failure of the system. A work committee should include staff from the pharmacy, admitting, nursing, medical, and IR department.

Continuing Interaction

The pharmacy department can invite IR personnel to a local, regional, or national allied meeting. Discussions with people from other hospitals will provide IR staff with insight into user needs and concerns. Because of federal and state legislation, many users are now being forced to consider opportunities for computer applications, and all parties can benefit from extended dialogue.

IR and pharmacy departments should participate together in postimplementation cost-benefit studies and continually learn from the experiences gained through the followup studies. These will often reveal benefits not seen in the feasibility study, as well as the absence of benefits that were expected but not realized. Investigation of unrealized benefits may reveal deficiencies in training or implementation methodologies or lack of understanding of the department's operation. Once these deficiencies are recognized, these benefits can be achieved. This knowledge educates the IR and user staffs for future studies and can even generate new feasible studies for additional projects. The bottom line is that, through these studies, the presence of the IRs is justified, the efforts of user staff are justified, and recognition is given to the user and IR departments for a job well done.

Each department can assist the other in gaining understanding of its respective needs by swapping professional literature. An article describing the use of a particular system should be read by personnel from both areas. This review provides ongoing education and possible ideas for additional system features.

Senior Management Interaction

Much has been written about the need for senior management support of users and IR supervisors in the development of computer systems (2,4). Part of this support rests in the realization that some of the already discussed interaction techniques may require extensive time of user supervisors. Senior management may need to authorize temporary user staff or overtime during computer installations. For instance, the installation of a drug inventory function with vendor and item profiles may require that a temporary or independently contracted person be hired for a few months to relieve the supervisor or staff of duties that cannot be handled totally by them during installation.

Evolution of the Information System

There is another phenomenon for pharmacy and IR supervisors to consider in their quest for the "perfect" IR. Individuals involved in a system's development must understand that it is a dynamic and constantly changing process. There is an underlying concept that both user and IR departments must grasp: let it be called the evolution of a conditional IR. The process of implementing an IR is an evolution because this is a stepwise movement toward a goal, a movement in which each step is determined in part by what has preceded it. The term "conditional" is used because an IR can be "perfect" only for a particular point in time and must be capable of change in response to the user's needs and perspective of the system.

A defined IR application is time dependent on a user's current experience, perspective, and position within the organization. At the beginning of a project, IR features are determined by the participant's perspective at that time. With the experience gained and the sophistication developed in using the system, new features become necessary. This cumulative knowledge will, in turn, help both pharmacy and IR staff progress to a point where again more (or less) features are essential. Thus, the system will evolve and change in a pattern that is conditional on the knowledge and perspective of the individuals involved at particular times in the project. The challenge for all participants is to recognize and work within this evolutionary conditional framework.

Changing the Installed Information System

Many of the required procedural changes and uses that accompany a new system require an adjustment period for the user before the full effect of the system can be evaluated. Changes usually require a period of time before the user staff fully integrates the features as their standard operating procedure. During this adjustment time, there may be a minimum of feature changes allowed by IR (except for errors) until the system has been fully installed and used. Once the effect of the system and new procedures is understood, then the user can discuss and request changes through the interaction technique of putting requests in writing.

A realistic compromise concerning immediate system changes can usually be made between the pharmacy and IR. IR can make available a fixed number of systems/programming man-hours for essential system changes within the first month of installation. Thus, the pharmacy will have a set number of IR staff hours available and can determine where these hours should be allocated, and still allow the IR supervisor to remain on schedule with other IR projects. Once the allotted hours are exhausted, the period of adjustment has to be accepted (or else another compromise made with IR). A reasonable adjustment may be 3-6 months.

CONCLUSION

This chapter has attempted to provide the reader with an awareness of how pharmacy relates to the concept of IRs within the hospital organization (5).

The term "information resources" has many definitions as perceived from the area using them. The users of IRs are varied and many.

The question and alternatives associated with controlling the IRs has been discussed. As seen, there is no one "best" solution, and changes in current technology have complicated this decision process even further. An attempt was made to answer this question through defining IR as four areas: management, systems/programming, operations, and data base.

Pharmacy has an essential role in the central data base concept. This chapter demonstrated that there is a vital need for departments to work together and plan (6).

The process of selecting pharmacy IRs can be very complex and requires proper planning and input from central IR management among other departments.

Strategies for an IR installation and its ongoing success were discussed. Allied meetings, systems design, prototypes, work committees, testing, documentation, parallel systems, and troubleshooting problems put into perspective the role of pharmacy and a central IR staff. These strategies are necessary whether one uses an outside vendor or a combination of outside and inside IR staff. People willing to work together are, of course, the essential ingredient for a successful information system (7).

REFERENCES

1. Priest SL: *Managing Hospital Information Information Systems,* Rockville, MD, Aspen Systems, 1982.
2. Swanson DS, Broekemeier RL, Anderson W: Hospital pharmacy computer systems—1982. *Am J Hosp Pharm* 39:2109-2123, 1982.
3. Coblio NA: The request for proposal as a tool for computer selection. *Hosp Pharm* 19:79-87, February 1984.
4. Wareham DV, Johnson SR, Tyrrell TJ: Combination medication cart and computer terminal in decentralization drug distribution. *Am J Hosp Pharm* 40:976-978, 1983.
5. Gouveia WA, Nold E: *Managing Computer Systems: Pharmacy and Other Hospital Departments.* Bethesda, American Society of Hospital Pharmacists, 1983.
6. Martin, J: *An End-User's Guide to Data Base.* Englewood Cliffs, NJ, Prentice-Hall, 1981.
7. Priest, SL, O'Sullivan VJ: The computer is coming, what should I do? *Health Care Superv* 1:75-93, July 1983.

CHAPTER 17

Facility Planning and Design

KENNETH N. BARKER and ROBERT E. PEARSON

This chapter describes the facility planning process, along with the role of the pharmacy (and pharmacist) in this process. The purpose is to prepare the reader for participation in a facilities planning program in a residency or on the job, so that he can then apply this process to the enormous amount of detail involved in a full-scale facility planning project.

This chapter will not offer "standard plans" because of a commitment to the philosophy that such plans do not sufficiently recognize the variation in hospitals and their local needs. The use of "standard plans" also discourages pharmacy planning founded on a thorough in-house study of future needs, functions, and operations that would yield a true picture of the facilities needed.

Topics to be addressed include the factors affecting facility needs, the hospital facility development process, current pharmacy planning, functional programming, the architectural design process, and the process of designing for efficiency and flexibility.

SIGNIFICANCE

Consider this. *If you make a major mistake in planning your pharmacy, you will have to get up and face it, and work in it, every day of your professional life.*

One precept of architecture is that "form follows function." The wisdom of this is seen most clearly in its violation, i.e., when obsolete buildings and fixtures limit the efficiency and effectiveness with which functions can be performed and patients served. The advent of the federal government's prospective pricing program and the encouragement of competition suddenly has placed greater emphasis on the need for efficiency in operations than ever before. Capital investments that offer the prospect of lower operating costs in the short run are in demand and expected to be increasingly so as the rules for government reimbursement of capital costs are clarified. Increased attention to the design of facilities can thus be expected. This will be good news for the pharmacy that is inefficient now and whose administrative pharmacists understand the planning process and can effectively justify what they have and what they need.

FACTORS AFFECTING FACILITY NEEDS

External Factors

The factors affecting the facility needs of an institution are many and varied. Those external to the individual departments include the following. Changes in government or third-party reimbursement systems directly affect planning priorities and resources. The focus on cost containment in hospitals may limit the adoption of new health care technology there, and thus change equipment requirements. Changes in laws, regulation, codes, and standards are important. For example, the number of legend drugs for which the prescription requirements are eliminated ("switched to over the counter") may change drug storage and control procedures. Of great importance will be changes in the hospital's patient mix due to aging and degree of illness. Competition for patients via a demonstrated emphasis on the quality and personalization of care evidenced in layout and design of patient areas is receiving increasing attention. Offering new services demanded by patients must be considered. Bed capacity and projected occupancy are vital to know. Hospital programs and services, e.g., ambulatory and home health care services, may need to be added or expanded. Computerization at the hospital can drastically change the work systems of the individual departments. The demand for better financial management systems, including a focus on cost centers and the creation of "diagnosis related group managers," may change pharmacy accounting procedures and thus the number and nature of the work stations required. Increased hospital attention to productivity measures may result in unfavorable comparisons with comparable pharmacies, prompting changes. Patterns of drug prescription and utilization may result in a decrease in drug prescriptions, thereby decreasing storage needs. Likewise, the rise or decline in alternative therapies may affect drug use, as when drugs replace surgical procedures. The development of new dosage delivery systems, e.g., implanted devices, may create a need for pharmacy space dedicated to the storage of the many new high-tech medical devices involved in drug administration. Trends in other departments, such as the rapid growth and expansion of materials management departments, can have an important effect on many aspects of drug storage and distribution. Any change in hospital mechanical service systems, such as the decision to add a pneumatic tube system, can impact pharmacy greatly. The general trend toward decreased crime may warrant some relaxation of security concerns, thus warranting fewer controls.

Internal Factors

Factors internal to the pharmacy department that influence facilities needs include decisions about the functions to be performed, such as whether a pharmacokinetics laboratory will be added, and the hours of operation. For example, the decision to expand to 24-hour service may necessitate a pharmacy design capable of being operated by a single pharmacist working alone on the night shift, with attendant concerns for the safety of the pharmacist and the security of areas away from view. Changes in work systems, such as the decision to decentralize the distribution process, may result in the need to build satellite pharmacies on the patient care units. Automation, as in the form of computerized accounting, label typing, and automated dispensing machines obviously will have considerable impact in terms of the rearrangement of work flow and consequent changes in facilities. Changes in the utilization of personnel might result in the substitution of auxiliaries for professionals in some cases, necessitating new checking procedures and the need for new "checking stations." Personnel additions obviously must be accommodated in terms of additional work stations, chairs, air-conditioning capacity, etc. Increased emphasis on continuing education and on-the-job training may necessitate special teaching and training areas, which may be shared. A change in hospital policy regarding the investment in inventory to be maintained can drastically change the reserve storage needed. New equipment, such as laminar airflow hoods, will place new demands on utilities and air conditioning.

All of the above demonstrate the great deal of interaction between everything that is happening in the hospital and the facilities in which it happens. All of these factors can have an important influence in determining the design that will be optimal.

Obviously, poorly designed facilities can be a major constraint on the efficiency and effectiveness of pharmacy department operations.

HOSPITAL FACILITY DEVELOPMENT PROCESS

Planning for hospitals is in a period of great turmoil today, mostly because of the federal government's prospective pricing program, which encourages competition. Because hospitals are reimbursed by a flat rate for any given ailment, there is great incentive to redesign inpatient areas for maximal efficiency and for hospitals to specialize in the areas in which they are most efficient, e.g., cardiac care, while dropping other inpatient services entirely. At the same time, the competition for patients has also placed heavy emphasis on making inpatient facilities inviting and attractive to patients. Outpatient (ambulatory) services suddenly became a competitor (rather than a complement) to inpatient services

when the former were excluded from the prospective program. With no lid on outpatient charges and a great financial incentive for minimizing a patient's inpatient stay, great economic pressure is thus exerted on hospitals to substitute outpatient care for inpatient care wherever possible. As a result, the closing of inpatient beds has not been uncommon this last year. The result, at the departmental level, is that many department heads face instructions to cut back on plans (or reduce space) related to inpatient services while developing plans for the expansion of outpatient services (e.g., outpatient dispensing, home health care services).

A separate issue is the availability of capital. How capital expenditures will be reimbursed under prospective pricing systems is not yet resolved, and the process may take several years. Many hospitals are torn between renovating for efficiency and offering the new ambulatory care services needed for survival under prospective pricing, but implement neither because of the problem of raising capital. In summary, it is an extremely difficult time to build or renovate a hospital, and it does seem clear that great changes in hospital construction will occur.

The planning of the pharmacy must proceed as part of the process of designing the rest of the hospital because of the interrelationships described above. All become a part of the hospital's overall facility development process. Each department will be significantly influenced by the needs of the other departments as well as those of the hospital as a whole. It is essential for the chief pharmacist to understand the hospital facility development process if he is to have any influence on it and still be able to perform his duty of seeing that the needs of the pharmacy department are given their proper due, in the proper place, and at the proper time.

The hospital facility development process may be outlined as follows:

1. Marketing plan developed, to identify demand for future services by examining patient mix, services in demand, and income to be generated
2. Competition examined, from both other hospitals and alternative modes of treatment, such as freestanding ambulatory care centers
3. Existing facility resources evaluated, a process which may heavily influence whether to renovate or build anew
4. Financial capability evaluated, focusing primarily on the question of raising capital, a problem made more complex by recent government programs
5. Environmental constraints evaluated, including regulations, legal codes, and local politics
6. "Framework for planning" statement developed, to include hospital mission and role statement, activity projections, priorities, organization plan, schedule, and monitoring and evaluation procedures

All of these concerns are considered as the hospital periodically reformulates its "framework for planning" statement, which is the cornerstone of any specific facility planning project.

The facility planning process, which typically consumes 2-3 years and sometimes longer, includes the stages shown below:

1. *"Framework for planning" statement* developed
2. *Management plan* developed, including examination of the organizational structure of the hospital, review of

individual departments for their capacity to respond to plan changes, and examination of interdepartmental work flows

3. *Analysis of existing facility resources* compiled, including "as-built" plans, space inventory room by room, equipment list showing age and replacement value, site surveys, assessment of structural, mechanical, and electrical systems, code conformity, and traffic patterns

4. *Functional program* compiled, including block diagrams that show department components, flow and traffic relationships, phases in development, new-vs-renovated space, gross cost estimate, and statement of premises and priorities and a series of alternative schematic plans

5. *Architectural schematic plans* drawn, showing layout and design of departments and relationships plus work flow of staff, materials, and patients (includes a brief description of finishes, mechanical and electric systems, and a cost estimate)

6. *Architectural design* developed, adding all other architectural details, including the last review by the users

7. *Construction contract documents* drawn up, including final drawings for regulatory approval and bidding plus the final cost estimate

8. *Construction* begun, including demolition, construction, equipment ordering, and inspection

9. *Occupancy* implemented, including installation of equipment, orientation of staff, moving, evaluation, and follow-up

As the major process described above moves along, it is not difficult to see why a department traditionally thought of as "small" (5% of the typical hospital operating budget) may find that it exerts little control or influence over its own destiny. This need not happen if the pharmacist understands the process and the opportunities it affords him for influence. For example, he can begin by taking every opportunity to assert that, from the facilities planning standpoint, the "pharmacy function" includes drug use control of *all* medications in the hospital and extends far beyond the walls of the pharmacy to include nursing unit design, decisions about hospital communication, transportation, and security systems, etc.

CURRENT PHARMACY PLANNING AND SPACE

Facilities Surveys

In 1982, Stolar (1) conducted a mail survey of a random sample of 931 short-term hospitals employing a pharmacist. The response was 83% (771). He found that a new facility was being planned by almost one-third (30%).

Approximately 49% (49.2%) reported that in the *near* future they would be purchasing major equipment items, particularly computer systems, equipment needed for unit dose, and IV admixture programs.

The 1983 edition of the Lilly Hospital Survey (2), sent to directors of hospital pharmacy and yielding a response rate of about 31% (2169 pharmacists), found that most for-profit and nonprofit hospitals were utilizing slightly larger central pharmacy areas than in the previous year. However, government hospitals with between 100 and 500 beds had somewhat smaller pharmacy quarters when compared to the

TABLE 17.1 Average Central Pharmacy Area[a]

	Average Total Area (sq ft)				
Bed Capacity	Federal	Government	Profit	Private Nonprofit	Average
Under 50	898	286	282	354	363
50-99	1347	607	592	599	611
100-199	2358	1028	745	1149	1099
200-299	2128	1631	1221	1828	1740
300-399	3045	2505	2600	2384	2441
400-499	3981	2070	n/a	2824	2739
Over 499	4469	2736	n/a	4185	3729

[a]Reprinted by permission from Deiner CH (ed): Lilly hospital pharmacy survey, 1983, Indianapolis, Eli Lilly & Company, 1983.

previous year. For-profit hospitals increased the square footage in their central pharmacies by almost 9%.

The space allocated for the average central pharmacy area is shown in Table 17.1. Additional space allocated for ancillary storage of pharmacy-related items occupied 38% of the central pharmacy area in government hospitals, 29% in federal facilities, 20% in for-profit pharmacies, and 23% in not-for-profit pharmacies.

A total of 39.2% (844) of all responding hospitals provided outpatient pharmacy service. Nearly one third of general hospitals and about two thirds of specialized hospitals operated outpatient pharmacies.

Over 90% of federal facilities offered outpatient pharmacy service, and about one third of government and for-profit institutions did so.

Outpatient pharmacies were physically separate from central pharmacy operations in about 26% of those reporting this service. General hospitals and special hospitals differed in this respect, with 17% of general hospitals reporting separate outpatient pharmacy facilities to 43% for specialized institutions.

Satellite pharmacies were reported by 13% (280) of the respondents—6.5% in general hospitals and 37.1% in specialized hospitals. It was not uncommon for the largest specialized institutions to have four or more satellite pharmacies per hospital. General hospitals of similar size had one or two, and, in some instances, three per hospital (2).

A national survey in 1982 by Alexander and Barker (3) based on a stratified random sample with a response rate of 45.6% (844) showed that the pharmacies in the most common types of hospitals (general medical surgical, nonprofit, short-term) occupied about 8 square feet per bed. Pharmacies in government hospitals of all kinds had the most space, while pharmacies in for-profit hospitals had only a little more than half the space of the not-for-profit hospitals. For every hospital type, little correlation between bed size and total pharmacy space was noted. This finding was not as surprising as it may sound, because as hospitals grow in size, new functions are added, while the original functions may not require additional space because of economies of scale (3).

It is impossible to evaluate the *adequacy* of current space allocations in hospital pharmacies without knowing the services they are attempting to provide and the work systems and personnel to be accommodated. For nonprofit hospitals, the space allocations reported are almost exactly the amount of space in the model pharmacy plans for 100-, 300-, and 500-bed hospitals used as illustrations in the 1974 Pharmacy Planning Manual of the Public Health Service. This suggests that these pharmacists could be getting the amount of space they need (although it does not necessarily follow that they are using it well).

The recommended approach to determining pharmacy space needs is the functional planning approach to be described, based on an in-house evaluation of invid-ual hospital needs, rather than relying on comparisons with other pharmacies and other hospitals.

Planning Process

Too often the pharmacist's input in the planning process is minimal. The administrator may call the pharmacist at the last minute to tell him the location and the space that have *already* been determined for the pharmacy. He is then shown a proposed plan, which already has been drawn up by the architect. Another undesirable approach is to contact commercial vendors of pharmacy fixtures and ask them to submit the design for the pharmacy. In recent years, the number of vendors offering hospital pharmacy design services has increased. Such firms can be very helpful *after* needs have been defined, i.e., the functional program has been written. Also, as one would expect, the designs proposed sometimes feature great quantities of the particular line of fixtures the vendor sells.

The planning approach recommended is called *functional planning*. This is an organized and systematic approach based on the architectural principle that states "form must follow function." The implication is that a hospital, along with each department, should be planned from the inside out—with its functional requirements dictating the arrangement, characteristics, and even the appearance of its final structure.

The planning team should include the hospital administrator, the architect, and consultants, plus the department heads. The administrator's role is to define the hospital's goals and to allocate resources. The pharmacist's role is to set forth the objectives and work methods the pharmacy will use in pursuit of the hospital's goals. The architect's role is to translate all of this into architectural plans.

The specific responsibilities of the pharmacist on the planning team are summarized as follows:

1. Set forth the objectives and functions of the pharmacy department
2. Prepare the functional program for the department
3. Serve as the ultimate authority for overseeing compliance with professional and legal standards

When hospital pharmacies are poorly designed, there are usually three reasons:

1. The failure of the administration to involve the pharmacist from the very beginning
2. The failure of the pharmacist to recognize and assume his proper role on the planning team
3. The pharmacist's lack of knowledge about functional planning (particularly functional programming)

The specific steps in planning a pharmacy facility using the functional planning process are shown below. The part of the planning process known as functional programming encompasses steps A through H. Architectural design overlaps functional programming and includes steps G through J.

Steps	*Primary Responsibility of*
A. Identify hospital purpose and goals	Administrator
B. Determine pharmacy goals and objectives	Pharmacist
C. Identify functions	Pharmacist
D. Determine work flow	Pharmacist
E. Identify work areas	Pharmacist
F. Specify requirements for each work area re:	Pharmacist
1. Workload	
2. Equipment and fixtures	
3. Storage	
4. Personnel	
5. Materials handling	
6. Communications	
7. Services	
8. Security	
9. Utilities	
10. Environment	
G. Find optimal arrangement for work areas	Pharmacist/Architect
H. Find optimal locations	Pharmacist/Architect
I. Develop trial schematics (total space calculable here)	Pharmacist/Architect
J. Develop architectureal design	Architect

The functional program will be in the form of a written report, which summarizes the requirements of the pharmacy in quantitative and qualitative terms, i.e., in words and numbers. It does not get into the drawing of plans, which comes after the functional program has been completed.

The purpose of the functional program is to describe individual pharmacy operations and the demands of each on the facility. During the next phase—architectural design—the architect will translate these needs into physical space, equipment, and furnishings. The functional program will show the architect each function the pharmacy intends to perform, i.e., the work flow on a step-by-step basis, so that the needs of each individual worker can be studied. In this way, the performance requirements for each individual work area are communicated to the architect. He should, in turn, consult the pharmacist for proper interpretation of the functional program and ask the pharmacist to react to and evaluate the architect's proposed designs.

FUNCTIONAL PROGRAMMING

The functional program usually begins with a recital of the formal statement of the purpose, goals, and specific objectives of the pharmacy service for the future and then lists the specific functions to be performed. Long-range goals, including those for future growth and expansion plus a timetable for their implementation over the next 5-10 years, should be included. All of the above should already exist in a separate "master plan" document for the department.

Functions

A function is defined as simply "a system of one or more tasks, to serve a stated purpose." A list of typical pharmacy functions is presented below; the terminology used may differ from one pharmacy to another.

1. Reviewing and editing orders
2. Dispensing unit doses to inpatients
3. Extemporaneous sterile compounding (preparation of IV admixtures)
4. Purchasing
5. Storage
6. Administration

The key point is that an effort should be made to identify every specific function to be performed in the new facility, along with the methods and the systems to be used. For example, the type of drug distribution system to be used and whether or not satellites will be built should be known. If such decisions have not been made, then little further progress is possible until they are. Facilities can and should be designed to be flexible (and how to do this is addressed later), but good predictions about future work systems are essential to contain costs.

Questions to Focus Thoughts

Often helpful at this point is a list of questions to stimulate thoughts and force the decisions that must be answered before a physical facility can be designed. Such a list is included in Appendix 17.1. This list may prompt the decision that a *systems analysis* may be needed, for example, which should come *before* the facility design process.

Work Flow Analysis to Identify Work Areas

Work flow analysis is performed to examine what the work flow will be in order to identify all of the tasks along the way. In the new plan, each and every task must have a place where it can be performed, and that place must be properly equipped and have the proper environment. Such places are designated work areas (general and specific). This is a systematic approach to ensure that the plans provide a work area for each and every task.

Work flow analysis for the purpose of facilities design is significantly different from (and less strenuous than) that for systems analysis in that the focus can be limited to only those items having implications for facilities.

The analysis is begun by examining each function to be performed and the work flow involved for each. Work flow can be defined as "the sequence of activities in response to a work order," such as a physician's medication order. The way to begin is to identify each different work order (i.e., anything that causes work to begin), such as a requisition received for filling, or even a "want book" entry indicating that inventory is low and that a purchase order should be initiated.

The way this approach is used to generate a basic list of work areas is illustrated below. In this example, the procedure for the filling of an IV admixture order is listed on the left-hand side. Then, proceeding down the right side, the idea is to stop at each step and try to picture mentally the physical activity that will take place in that step and

then give that mental picture (individual workplace) a generic name, such as "typing station" or "hood." In this way, a list of all the work areas needed is generated.

Task	Work Area
1. Work order received	Pass-through window
2. Label prepared	Typing station
3. Solution, additives, and supplies obtained	Active storage solutions Active storage additives Active storage supplies
4. Assembled/checked in hood	Hood
5. Put in pass-through refrigerator	Refrigerator
6. Waste items discarded	Waste receptable

A work area is defined as "a place where work of a similar nature is performed." A work area may be only a desk, or a counter, or only one section of a long counter, the corner of a room, or the whole room itself. Some work areas typically found in a hospital pharmacy are presented below, where they are organized into general and specific work areas:

A. Dispensing to outpatients
 1. Waiting
 2. Receiving/dispensing
 3. Typing
 4. Medication profile
 5. Filling counter
 6. Communications and references
 7. Weighing
 8. Heating and stirring
 9. Sink
 10. Counseling room
 11. Waste receptacle (see also active storage areas)
B. Order review and editing
 1. Input station
 2. Order review and editing desk
 3. Master file, patient information
 4. Communications and references
 5. Waste receptacle
 6. Active storage, forms

Once all of the work areas needed are identified, you are ready to proceed. The next step calls for the examination of each of these work areas to identify or specify for each the workload, personnel, inventory, and equipment to be accommodated, service and utility needed, etc.

It will be advantageous to first group the work areas to the degree possible. For example, the functional programming specifications for the several specific work areas contained in one small office can usually be combined and considered together under the general work area title for the entire office. This would not be the case in an IV admixture center, for example, where the laminar flow hood would have special utility requirements.

Workload Analysis

The most important determinants of the space requirements of a hospital pharmacy performing a given set of functions are:

1. Workload
2. Equipment and fixtures
3. Storage needs
4. Personnel to be accommodated

It is useful to differentiate between the *extrinsic* workload, which is the external demand on the pharmacy from outside the department, and the *intrinsic* workload, which is that generated from within, as when a drug is prepackaged, creating a need for a label to be typed.

To estimate the workload (whether extrinsic or intrinsic) for any work area, the work units must first be identified. Some typical work units in a hospital pharmacy include the number of physicians' medication orders received for processing, the number of drug information requests, and the number of batches of drugs to be prepackaged. Such workloads may be analyzed and reported in the following ways:

1. The volume per average day
2. The distribution by hour of the day
3. The distribution across a sufficient number of days to include the normal cycles and fluctuations that have implications for facility design

A convenient way to collect workload data is by arranging to have every form time-date stamped as it is processed, for tabulation later. Often such data are already being collected for departmental reports. Otherwise, direct observation may be needed to count and record work units during typical time periods.

When a new facility is planned where none previously existed, the best approach is to examine data from an institution of similar size and with similar programs and services.

Current workload data must be adjusted to reflect changes expected in the future. Formulas for forecasting the extrinsic workload of the pharmacy, based on the past and present number of patient days, for example, are available (4). Adjustments should be made for important trends, asking questions such as these:

1. Does the hospital plan to increase or decrease bed capacity?
2. Will patient mix change?
3. Is the hospital planning to discontinue certain programs, such as obstetrics, or to add others, such as home health care?
4. Will recent medical staff decisions change the number or types of medications ordered in the future?

The study of expected workload will reveal, for example, whether the IV admixture center will require one hood or two and how many typewriters or printers will be needed. Without such information, the final plans might not include a workplace for these extra items of equipment.

Equipment and Fixtures

The cost of equipment may be the single most important cost associated with a new facility. It not only will constitute the greatest portion of the total initial expenditure, but also will be a determining factor in the day-to-day operating expenses of the facility for the long run.

The selection of the equipment for the pharmacy department should be based on an analysis of the work that the equipment is needed to do. Questions relating to *how* the work will be done, e.g., the degree of computerization and automation, must be addressed. If some equipment will be built into purchased fixtures, this also must be known.

The solution is to study the nature of the work at each work area, the volume involved, and the methods to be used. Based on this information, an initial equipment list can be generated. Then, published lists can be consulted for items overlooked (4,5). The purchasing agent will be a source of information about standard items such as office equipment.

A high initial cost should not be a deterrent to the consideration of equipment that has a favorable net effect on operating costs for the long run. A method for determining the most cost-effective alternative is "life cycle costing" (4).

The use of consultants is helpful and justified in the selection of expensive equipment for more complex operations, such as computer applications and unit dose packaging.

The role of the pharmacist is to prepare a proposed equipment list for the pharmacy. Wherever *specialized pharmaceutical* equipment is involved, the pharmacist should, in addition, develop detailed performance standards regarding both the quantity and quality of the output plus the reliability of performance. For example, for a strip-packaging machine, the specifications might include the number of units to be packaged per hour, the minimal acceptable setup and changeover time, and the types of films to be accommodated.

In composing the equipment list, it is important to distinguish between *fixed* and *movable* equipment. Fixed equipment is that which requires installation and becomes attached to the building, such as a fume hood. Movable equipment includes furniture, carts, and typewriters. A separate listing is important, because fixed equipment often is included in the hospital construction contract, whereas movable equipment may be bid on separately.

The physical environment needed to accommodate each piece of equipment must be considered. For example, there must be extra space left around the sides to give access for repairs and maintenance. Some equipment manufacturers will even supply a template to show the access space requirements for each equipment item. Space must be provided for the operator to stand or sit and for the storage of supplies and accessories. Temporary storage space for incoming materials and outgoing products is needed. Trash cans for waste materials sometimes are overlooked.

General characteristics to be sought in all equipment are these: standardization throughout the pharmacy (and hospital); compatibility with existing equipment; modularity; and flexibility. Each of these points will be addressed later.

Remember, every item of equipment ordered is going to have to be put *somewhere*, and the best time to provide a place for it is at the time the facility is being planned.

Storage

Storage fixtures may or may not appear on the final equipment list, as they may be treated as part of construction. However, they should be treated as equipment in the functional program to ensure that they receive proper consideration.

To estimate the type and amount of storage space needed, is it best to actually measure the amount of space currently occupied by all equipment, inventory, supplies, etc. The space now occupied by current stock should be actually measured with a tape measure. This should be done shelf by shelf and drawer by drawer, so that the planner can form a mental picture of the block of space needed to accommodate the contents. Then the average height, width, and depth needed for all of the stock on one shelf, for example, should be estimated. These data then should be broken down by class and summarized three ways: in terms of linear front feet, square feet, and cubic feet. Although such measurements will be approximate, this approach has the important advantage of avoiding the distortion that comes from the common approach of measuring the outside dimensions of existing shelving units, which too often are no longer optimal for the items stored there. When such data are collected by operating personnel, these persons can be instructed to adjust their estimates to reflect the latest developments, including departmental objectives regarding inventory levels.

The results obtained should be presented in the functional program in the form shown in Table 17.2.

Storage requirements may be organized and reported according to the classes of storage as listed below:

A. Frequency of use
1. Most used
2. Lesser used
3. Deep reserve
B. Environmental requirements
1. Air conditioning
2. Refrigeration
3. Freezing
C. Security requirements
1. Controlled drugs (by schedule)
2. Alcoholic beverages
D. Special
1. Disinfectant-proof
2. Autoclave-proof

The reason for this approach is that the compilation of these data in this way makes it possible to enlist the skills of the architects, consultants, fixture vendors, and other outside experts to suggest solutions beyond the storage fixtures traditionally seen in pharmacies. There has been a great need for improvements, and the recent economic pressures to reduce space utilization everywhere have resulted in many new and innovative approaches, all requiring a three-dimensional analysis of space requirements.

The active storage areas of the pharmacy usually include one or more cart-filling stations, arranged in U-shaped alcoves. However, in some centralized operations, carts may also be filled on an assembly-line basis, cafeteria style. Unit dose dispensing systems generally require about 25% more storage space than other systems.

The arrangement of stock should give first priority to placing all of the fast-moving stock together near the front, to minimize pharmacy labor time. Traditionally, most pharmacies have organized their stock by dosage forms, i.e., all oral solids together; all oral liquids, injections, etc. This allows for maximal economy of shelf space, but the value of pharmacy labor wasted is likely to be much greater.

Shelving that is open and adjustable is quite adequate, versatile, and inexpensive. Cabinets and drawers cost considerably more and are generally less efficient to use. Angle-

TABLE 17.2 IV Reserve Storage

Class and Type	Shelf Space Needed for Current Stock Levels		
	Linear ft	Square ft	Cubic ft
IVs and administration sets	198	444	1274
Floor space—pallets	12	42	108
	210	486	1382

adjustable shelving provides gravity feed, thus helping to ensure that drug stocks are replenished from the rear to minimize drug deterioration.

Rotary files for fingertip retrieval of the most used drugs are now used in many pharmacies. However, such rotary files are usually efficient only when no more than two persons are involved in filling prescriptions from the same file. Beyond that point, the one-at-a-time access feature of this type of storage reduces its efficiency.

For bulk storage, rail-mounted storage is recommended for its space-saving feature, i.e., only one aisle space is needed.

Regarding refrigeration, unit dose dispensing systems require a greater amount of refrigerated storage for injectables and liquids. The commercial reach-in type, such as that used in food stores, is preferred by many because it eliminates the labor involved in opening and closing doors.

For reserve and bulk refrigerated storage, the prefabricated cold rooms marketed are in wide use and can be made secure for controlled drugs.

Deep-reserve storage items, such as IV solutions in cartons, often are kept on pallets or on steel shelving in a locked room that may be remote from the pharmacy.

Regarding the storage of controlled drugs, the trend is to emphasize sophisticated electronic alarm systems, rather than sturdier vaults and safes. The regional agent of the Drug Enforcement Administration (DEA) should be contacted for an interpretation of the current regulations and requirements (6).

The problem of storing flammables is familiar to the architect, and he should be the one responsible for complying with all applicable codes and regulations, which vary from state to state. Many hospital pharmacies no longer have their own flammables room. Sealed containers of alcohol eliminate the need in some cases, and in other cases the hospital may provide a flammables room for use by all.

Personnel

The personnel to be accommodated in the pharmacy is another factor of major importance in the design of a new facility.

The architect will need to have documented the number of persons that will be in each area during normal work times as well as peak work periods, so that he can provide adequate working space, the proper number of chairs, the necessary air conditioning capacity, etc. He should be supplied the expected staffing pattern, as well the hours of operation.

Communications

Communication systems needed by the pharmacy should be analyzed, with thought given to not only telephone systems but also telecommunication needs, facsimile reproduction, bulletin boards, and access to all hospital-wide systems.

The pharmacy telephone system should provide separate telephone numbers for business and professional calls, with calls related to patient care answered by a pharmacist directly. Dispensing areas should be designed so that the pharmacist can talk privately on the phone without being overheard. Telecommunication and computer terminals will have special requirements regarding location, space, and utilities that must be checked with the manufacturer.

Materials Handling

The hospital will likely provide a central materials handling system, such as a dumbwaiter or messenger service, for use throughout the hospital for all departments. When planning this system, the architect should be reminded that the pharmacy will be a major user, both for drug products and documents, sending and receiving more units (in unit dose systems) than any other department. Documented for the architect should be the volume of this workload, its distribution by time of day, and size and weight of the largest and smallest units to be transported. He should also be advised that pharmacy has some unique, special requirements such as a rapid response for stat orders and security for controlled drugs during transit.

Before recommending a costly and complicated automated transportation system, the advantages of manual cart delivery and messenger service should not be overlooked. These offer a relatively maintenance-free system, featuring carriers with build-in highly versatile computers (the human brain) for observation, control, recording inventory, feedback, and on-the-spot problem solving. Also, the cost of expanding such systems is minimal.

Care should be taken that all carts will pass through all doors, including elevator doors and passageways, and that they will roll satisfactorily on the type of flooring anticipated.

Services from Other Departments

Services from other departments on which the pharmacy may depend must be identified, so that the architect can locate them as close to the pharmacy as possible. Such services include centralized purchasing, centralized receiving, library, cashier and waiting areas for outpatients, and access to autoclaves.

Security

The hospital pharmacist must deal with security problems at a variety of levels, including the detailed requirements for the various classes for controlled drugs; the regulations for alcohol and alcoholic beverages; regulations regarding prescription legend drugs; and concern for the confidentiality of patient documents—all in addition to the normal security for the protection of the employees and property.

Security considerations may include limiting the number of doors and other means of access to storage areas, the reinforcement of door and wall materials (e.g., requiring that walls be built extended vertically from slab to slab), the quality and types of door locks, electronic controls, and the control of keys (e.g., no master keys).

Visual surveillance of all doors and high-security areas may be needed if the pharmacy is to be manned by one person at night. Automatic door locks, bullet-proof glass, and special alarm systems are being installed in an increasing number of pharmacies.

Now that the general crime level is declining the need for such items may be less. There is concern that such devices too often interfere with the pharmacist-patient interaction, which is important in providing optimal pharmacy service.

Utilities and Environmental Controls

The functional program prepared by the pharmacist should give particular attention to the requirements of the special work areas *unique to pharmacy*. The architect can anticipate the requirements of a normal office, for example, but not for an IV admixture center. He should also be alerted to the need for emergency power for the refrigerators and the security alarm systems.

A data sheet for use in documenting the needs of each work area for utilities as well as other considerations is included in the Appendix 17.2.

Arrangement of Work Areas

Once all work areas are known and the individual requirements of each have been identified, the next step is to analyze and recommend how they should be arranged in relation to each other. Factors to be considered include the flow of products and information, points of input and output, access to fixed or shared equipment (e.g., dumbwaiter), joint use of personnel and equipment, need for visual supervision, and the desire to minimize travel and delay time between work areas.

Those general work areas that probably should *not* be physically separated are order review, distribution, and extemporaneous compounding and packaging. General work areas that may be separated if adequate communications and transportation can be provided are administration, manufacturing and packaging, and bulk storage.

The desired location of the work areas with respect to corridors and elevators should be recorded.

For large, complex facilities there are systematic, quantitative methods for calculating the best arrangement of work areas. Each work area is assigned a number representing the ''degree of closeness'' needed to each of the other work areas (7).

Rendering the Functional Program

The functional program is a written report, composed mostly of tables and diagrams, summarizing the data collected. The architect's first task is to interpret this material and translate it into visual concepts and physical forms. Therefore, every effort to help him through a concise presentation that pinpoints and summarizes the key information will be greatly appreciated.

The table of contents for a typical functional program may include:

1. Purpose of the department
2. Functions
3. Work flow diagrams
4. List of general and specific work areas
5. Workload analysis
6. Furniture and equipment list
7. Storage requirements
8. Other work area requirements
9. Arrangement of work areas

To convey your concepts of area relationships to the architect, include bubble diagrams and sketches.

To begin with it is useful to categorize all pharmacy space into these five major types:

1. Primary activity
2. Support
3. Administrative
4. Educational
5. Research

All space within a hospital may be placed into one of these categories. (NOTE: Some planners include educational and research under administration.)

The recommended approach is to first locate the primary activity spaces, e.g., dispensing, and then locate the appropriate support and administrative spaces. Support space would include all drug storage areas, for example.

The next step may be as simple as drawing the bubble diagram shown in Figure 17.1. A more elaborate approach is to put the name of each general work area on a separate circle cut out of paper and then move these around to find the best arrangement.

Actual sketches may be attempted if the pharmacist is so inclined, although the ideal is to involve the architect at this point and invite *him* to suggest creative solutions to your problems. (The professional architect will appreciate the invitation and the opportunity.)

For sketching, it is particularly valuable to have on hand a schematic drawing showing the area surrounding the probable location of the pharmacy, plus on graph paper to the same scale (e.g., eight to the inch).

ARCHITECTURAL DESIGN PROCESS

Role of the Architect

From the architect's viewpoint, the creative part of a facilities design project represents only about one third of his total effort, but it is "the fun part." This is important to know because it suggest that the best time to capture the architect's personal (and creative) interest in a department is at the very beginning of the design process. If given the opportunity to truly understand the department, he can significantly improve the effectiveness of that department through his designs.

From the architect's viewpoint, the design of any facility involves three major factors: utility, amenity, and expression. Utility simply means it is functional and efficent. A

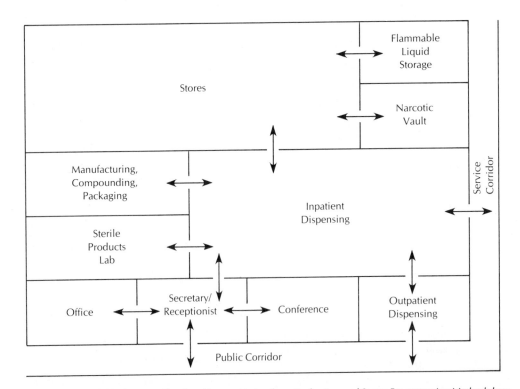

FIGURE 17.1   Bubble diagram. (Reprinted by permission from *Evaluation and Space Programming Methodology Series No. 10: Pharmacy.* Ann Arbor, Chi Systems, Inc, 1979.)

good functional program is the key to helping him address this factor.

The term "amenity" refers to satisfying the human requirements for the people who will work there. Chief concerns are ease of access and movement, personal comfort, and safety and health protection.

The term "expression" means the symbolic aspects or image the facility should project to others when they see it. For example, if the appearance of a dispensing window is to encourage patient counseling, then its design should convey the message that an important pharmacist-patient communication occurs here, the privacy of which must be protected.

A collaborative approach between the architect and the pharmacist can produce designs that encourage the pharmacist to use the best professional practices and that discourages poor practice. For example, to promote personal contact between the pharmacist and patient, the normal working positions of the pharmacist and of the ambulatory patient can be designed to place them face to face in close proximity (without a clerk between them, for example, or a place for a reluctant pharmacist to "hide").

LOCATION AND SPACE

How much total space will the pharmacy need, and where should it be located? These will be among the first questions to which answers will be sought early by the planning team. A good answer requires the comprehensive analysis of pharmacy needs described here, which are then modified and integrated with the needs of other departments by the hospital architect.

To estimate the pharmacy space required, the architect will study the functional program and add space for halls and internal passageways. He will consider the shape and location of available space in the hospital plan. Then, he will develop a set of proposed schematic drawing for all to consider. Once the planning team agrees on one, then pharmacy space needs are determined by measuring the space that plan occupies.

The above description is the best approach and one that unfortunately is not always realized. Too often hospital consultants or architecture firms attempt to use "standard" space allocation formulas without proper attention to the needs of a particular pharmacy function in a particular setting. Hospital pharmacy function and services vary widely, and there have been many important advances in practice; these changes cannot be ignored. Some hospital systems that have gained experience with the design of many hospital pharmacies, all with the same set of predefined functions, have felt they can so standardize departmental space needs that these can be specified in advance of the design of the hospital. Their success if unclear at this time.

The question of the location of the pharmacy should be brought to the attention of the architect and the planning team at the earliest time. This is because it is too common for the pharmacy to be thought of as a department that can be located "almost anywhere" and is therefore given a low priority in the competition for prime locations.

The location of the inpatient pharmacy distribution areas must provide ready and full access to the hospital's materials

handling systems (see previous discussion). When pharmacy satellites are involved, service to those satellites must be adequate and fast. Therefore, it is common to locate the inpatient pharmacy close to the central core of elevators and dumbwaiters, the only exception being if automated horizontal conveyors or automated carts will be used.

If outpatients are to be served, then the outpatient pharmacy dispensing area should be located somewhere along the normal patient traffic flow, perhaps sharing the same waiting room and cashier with the rest of the outpatient clinics. This consideration often necessitates separating the outpatient pharmacy from the inpatient pharmacy, which occurs more frequently as hospital bed size increases.

The location of a drug information center (or any area designed to encourage physician "drop-ins") will need to be located on a route heavily traveled by physicians, such as near the hospital library or a medical staff lounge.

The location of pharmacy satellites varies widely, depending on the specific functions they serve. The ideal location for a general satellite serving a general medical or surgical service is adjacent to or directly opposite the nurse's station (most current satellites are located some distance away only because they were not part of the original plan). All satellites whose function is to dispense drugs in unit dose form to the users should be located to allow face-to-face communications with them, to ensure that the projected benefits of the use of satellites are obtained (see Chapters 32 and 54).

Satellites designed exclusively for clinical pharmacy services should ideally be accessible from both the nurse's station and the physician's work areas.

Satellites designed to serve other pharmacy satellites, such IV admixture production units located in two or three locations throughout a multilevel hospital, should be located to maximize access to the hospital materials handling systems.

Administrative offices may be located separate from the inpatient and outpatient pharmacies. Bulk and reserve inventory can be maintained in remote locations provided the pharmacy controls all access to prescription drug storage areas.

DESIGNING FOR EFFICIENCY

Work Systems

Designing a pharmacy for efficiency includes beginning with an efficient work system that is developed by using a task-oriented approach to design and three-dimensional ("3-D") space planning.

Efficiency is simply the ratio of output (e.g., unit doses dispensed) per resources input (e.g., labor, space). One of the most effective ways to achieve efficiency is to examine work systems at the beginning of the planning process and then design the facility for optimal performance of the new improved systems.

Systems analyses typically begin with flow charting to look for tasks that can be combined, eliminated, or automated [8]. A step beyond this is network analysis (see Chapter 16). Queuing theory and computer simulation models of pharmacy operations can be used to identify mathematically the (theoretically) most efficient operation (9,10), although this can become quite complex.

To illustrate the application of queuing theory, it can be shown that the assembly-line method of dispensing, mostly used by military pharmacies where the task of dispensing is broken down in various elements performed by various personnel in different locations, is efficient only where strict scheduling is possible. The most efficient way to provide service for orders that arrive at random and that require varying periods of time to dispense is to have this done in one place by one person (like McDonalds).

A systems change that can have a great impact on efficiency and on facilities needs is the alteration of the use of personnel, e.g., as when the work of a professional is redesigned and part of it delegated to an auxiliary worker (11,12). For this reason, staffing studies, if planned, should always precede facilities design.

The pharmacist should be aware that it is not unusual for a hospital-wide facility development project to produce the need for changes in pharmacy work systems, which the pharmacist must be wise enough to foresee when planning the pharmacy department. This occurs, for example, when the new hospital design will incorporate the Friesen concept. This is basically a concept for a particular kind of hospital-wide work system. All commodities, including drugs, are required to be delivered on an automatic replenishment basis to the individual patient Nurserver cabinet located outside the patient's room. This relieves the nurse of the necessity of leaving the area and the patient to obtain supplies. The Friesen concept thus would require major changes in the work systems of most pharmacies (13).

The Friesen concept extends beyond the hospital work system to specify that the hospital structure should be specifically designed to facilitate this new work system. This may result in mandatory changes in pharmacy work systems for the efficiency of the hospital as a whole, which the pharmacist must understand and incorporate into his plans for the pharmacy.

Systems changes that have been shown to improve the efficiency of the pharmacy given the proper facility for their performance include prepackaging, standardization of quantities issued, minimization of the variety of inventory items (as possible via a formulary system) mechanization, automation, and improved utilization of personnel.

Task-Oriented Design

In the task-oriented design approach, a facility is viewed as a series of interrelated task centers, and the design of each general work area is based on the specific task to be performed there.

This approach contributes to efficiency through the reduction of travel time, i.e., the number of steps it takes to complete a task. Obviously, if such time can be minimized, the work will be more efficient. Consider the distance traveled in an outpatient pharmacy where the pharmacist must go to the door to receive the prescription, return to get a label typed, put the label on, get an empty container, get the drug, return the stock bottle, and then deliver the prescription to the door.

The travel time involved can be evaluated mathematically by multiplying the number of trips times the distance per trip as shown in Figure 17.2. The total distance traveled per every 100 prescriptions was 2295 feet. To find a better design, one would have to find one that totals less than 2295 feet. (A task-oriented design that reduces the total travel distance to *zero* can be designed by arranging for the pharmacist to do all his work sitting down, with everything within his reach.)

Perhaps the most obvious application of this approach is that already practiced in most pharmacies—the separating of the most used stock from the lesser used stock and the grouping of the former close at hand. The dispensing workplace should be designed to facilitate such a stock arrangement, with first priority placed on this principle instead of grouping drug stock by dosage forms. For convenience in maintaining ampules and syringes on the same shelf as stock bottles, module boxes can be used.

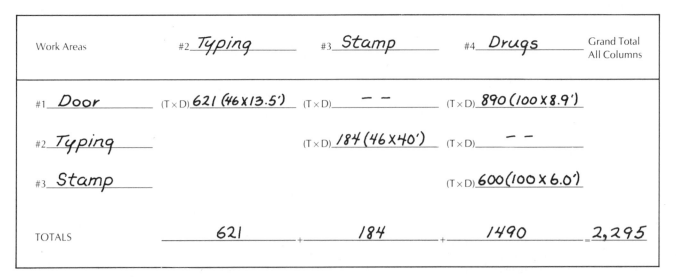

FIGURE 17.2 Efficiency analysis of travel time (travel-trips × distance per 100 work units).

Minimizing motion is another way to improve efficiency through the use of a task-oriented approach. This begins with the recognition of the geometry and mechanics of human movement and proceeds to design the workplace to "fit" the human (see Fig. 8.5). The natural boundaries for human movement are circular, e.g., the hand rotating around a stationary wrist, the forearm rotating around a stationary elbow, and the extended arm and trunk rotating around the waist. Most equipment and building materials are rectangular, but rectangles do not fit the human body very efficiently, since some areas are harder to reach than other areas. The consequences are increased fatigue, lower productivity, and more mistakes. The ideal workplace might theoretically be a three-dimensional circular arrangement. It is not mandatory that equipment be circular in their outside dimensions, but only necessary that the work area itself be so constructed. Such pharmacy fixtures are commercially available (14).

Three-Dimensional Space Planning

The three-dimensional approach to space planning is important for efficiency and space utilization. Every wasted square foot of floor space costs the hospital over $100 to build and many dollars per year to maintain.

Storage needs should be calculated and supplied to the architect and his consultants in terms of three dimensions: linear front feet, square feet, and cubic fee. This will give him the maximal flexibility to explore such space-saving solutions.

An alternative to the use of additional floor space for storage is, for example, vertical space. Considerable attention is being given to exploring such space-saving solutions as storage on suspended balconies, to use the otherwise unusable space near the ceilings in storage rooms.

Rail-mounted shelving is efficient and easy to use. The efficiency comes from the elimination of all aisles between the shelves except one. This aisle can then be "moved" wherever needed by simply pushing apart the two particular shelves, offering access to the item needed.

A third approach, particularly important in the pharmacy where many small items are stocked, is to make maximal use of the space at the back of each shelf and in between shelves. The area for picking of unit doses should be compressed, to minimize travel and motion. To accomplish this, the storage containers for unit dose packages should be designed to take up a minimum of the front-of-the-shelf space; long, thin module boxes are ideal for this. The use of relatively short shelves that are easily adjustable is recommended so that shelves can be placed as close together as possible to further conserve storage space.

DESIGNING FOR FLEXIBILITY

The practice of hospital pharmacy is in a period of great change, with considerable uncertainty about the future. This places a high priority on designing to "build in" flexibility throughout. A recommended approach involves a growth plan, the core concept, and the use of flexible fixtures. Flexible fixtures are those which are modular, interchangeable, movable, and self-contained.

Growth Plan

There should be a growth plan for the pharmacy that provides zones of transition, or space buffers, between the pharmacy and the space external to it. For horizontal expansion, the zone of transition may be an easily movable storage room located in the expansion path. Vertical expansion to another floor is also possible via stairway and elevator, but that is usually more disruptive of work flow and internal control.

Such transition zones should be outlined in the comprehensive master facility plan for the hospital, and it behooves the pharmacist to achieve recognition of his needs in this regard.

The development of the pharmacy growth plan should begin by analyzing future needs at the individual work area level. This is because an increased workload does not affect work areas uniformly. For example, a second typewriter may be needed before a second laminar flow hood, and both before a second refrigerator. The goal is a growth plan that is essentially unidirectional.

Core Concept

The core concept facilitates unidirectional growth by calling for all fixed items to be placed where they will not have to be moved. Examples of such items include plumbing, dumbwaiter, and pneumatic tube stations.

Flexible Fixtures

Truly flexible fixtures will be expandable as the workload increases and adaptable to changes in work methods.

To achieve these goals, all fixtures should modular, to allow additional units to be ordered and inserted as the workload increases. This will make them interchangeable, so that units may be rearranged as work methods change and to allow the substitutions of new upgraded component sections to replace those which have become outmoded or obsolete.

The fixtures should be easily adjustable and not difficult to finish and repair. For example, the storage of drugs in module boxes on adjustable shelves is preferable to casework, cabinets, and drawers. Likewise, prefabricated, expandable cool rooms give greater flexibility than large biologic refrigerators.

Fixtures, including storage shelving, should be movable, although expensive castor and lift systems are not justified for one or two moves a year. Built-in fixtures and custom-built casework should be avoided.

Fixtures should be designed for grouping in *self-contained task centers* for the performance of a particular task in any location to which it may be moved. For example, an ambulatory care pharmacy with two outpatient dispensing task centers should be capable of being separated and each moved to a different outpatient clinic if needed as workload expands.

The use of truly flexible fixtures, as described above, may make it possible for the pharmacy to function using only the quantity of equipment needed for current workloads. (This has advantages for the pharmacist in that the pharmacy can thus minimize its contribution to total costs as a primary cost center). Space for additional equipment can then be "shelled in" for future use. This may be done to accommodate a specific building configuration and/or minimize current capital expenditures while providing for projected workload increases in the future.

IMPLEMENTATION

Preparation

The implementation of the next facilities planning project should begin the day after the facility is occupied. This statement makes the point that facilities planning should be a continuous process. The ideal plan for the facility should be a constantly evolving concept, which is periodically fixed and translated into architectural plans and concrete whenever the opportunity arises. This viewpoint is essential if the pharmacist is to cope effectively with the short deadlines he so often encounters. For example, as noted previously, the first thing asked of the pharmacist will be to recommend the space and location of the new pharmacy, which is not known until the very end of the functional planning process.

Implementation of a facilities design project should begin with reading. Recommended references include the series tentatively entitled *Toward Planning a Better Hospital Pharmacy* to be published in the *American Journal of Hospital Pharmacy;* the out-of-print Department of Health and Human Services publication *Planning for Hospital Pharmacies* still available in many pharmacy school libraries; and the manual *Evaluation and Space Programming Methodology Series Number 10: Pharmacy* published by Chi Systems, Inc. The American Society of Hospital Pharmacists sponsors an Institute on Facilities Planning and Design every 2-3 years. These provide each participant the opportunity to design his own facility under the guidance of the faculty. The current literature of hospital pharmacy should be reviewed for articles such as that by Loeb (15). At least two schools of pharmacy (Auburn and Mississippi) have research programs involving the design of pharmacy facilities.

Visit other hospital pharmacy departments, but be selective. Pick those less than 10 years old or those which have been remodeled recently. In particular, look for those where substantial planning was involved *and* the plan was carried out. Also include bad examples (which will not be difficult to find): researchers have found they often learn more from failures than from "successes."

Politics of Pharmacy Expansion

Once the need for new or modified facilities has become apparent to the pharmacist, he faces the task of convincing those whose support he will need, beginning with the administration. Occasionally this is easy, as when a new facility is being built, but most of the time it is not. Even when it is, it behooves the pharmacist to plan carefully so that he to defend his space later on when cutbacks threaten, as they have since the advent of prospective pricing legislation.

Economics teaches there is no such thing as a "free" lunch, and its corollary is that there is no such thing as "free" space. Space won must then be defended, with the

cost of excess space a negative influence on measures of efficiency and productivity in pharmacy operations.

Space requests that can be cost justified for the pharmacy may nevertheless fail to be competitive with those of other departments. King (16) has recommended the following approaches for competing for space with other departments:

You must evaluate the situation very carefully and ask several questions. Who will ultimately make the space allocation? The administrator? The administrator with the advice and influence of others? If so, who? A committee? If so who is on that committee? How much power or influence does [each member] have over the decision makers? What can yet be done to assure the balance of influence is in your favor? Will the decisions regarding space allocation be made on an objective or a subjective basis? It may be that specific, positive steps will be required to assure your position in the political process, or it may be that your position is already secure once the total situation is analyzed.

In any case, it is important to be assured that your plans for programs and future services have already been discussed and approval has been documented by administration and others involved. You are in a stronger position if the approved plans for these services justify the requirement for additional space rather than developing proposals for services after the space is apparently available.

Having support from various groups from within the hospital such as administration, nursing and medical staff for the projected programs is important, and knowing the space requirement for each specific program is important. In this way if a total space requested is not made available, the projections regarding which programs will have to be cut can be provided before making final space assignments.

Knowing the projected space requirements of the other departments competing for the same area and the known space available will be helpful so as to be aware that cuts will be necessary in the overall program. Knowing whether these decisions will be made on a subjective or objective basis is important to your planning strategy. It may be necessary to incorporate space for Future Achievable Tasks (FAT). If it is apparent that a cut in requested space is necessary, it may take place without a great deal of sacrifice to programs projected for the near future provided the cut can be made from space for future achievable tasks or FAT.

Timetable

Some 2-6 years may elapse between the initial planning and occupancy of your pharmacy. The timing of most of the major deadlines, as the project moves from one stage to the next, will be established by the planning committee: it is essential to know these dates, and to be on the mailing list for updates and changes. There will be many requests to submit lists of equipment to be ordered, the number and type and locations of telephones, and how doors should be keyed and the number of keys needed for each lock, for example. Although such requests may seem trivial, in the aggregate they can be critical to the operation of the pharmacy. It is important to complete such lists by the stated deadlines to allow for the proper review by administrative or technical personnel.

Two tasks that can be begun right away are the securing of "as built" plans and an inventory of current equipment. When remodeling, the new plans must always begin with an assumption regarding the size, shape, and space in the current facility. Too often the "current" plans of the existing facilities are later found to be out of date and inaccurate (e.g., showing walls where none exist or the reverse). A suggested rule is, Remeasure everything; don't assume anything.

An inventory of existing furniture should be conducted to determine which pieces will be replaced vs those to be retained. The list will be used later in the functional planning process described previously. This is the time to reduce the list to only those items that will have a place in the new facility.

The move into the new facility will require a more detailed timetable specific to your department. List everything that will have to be done before, during, and immediately after the move. Organize these items into specific time periods. Loeb used a flip chart method, labeling the sheets with activities that needed to be done each month or week before or after the move. For example, 3 months before the move, verify all telephone orders, complete training session for all employees, and order new medication boxes; have all decentralized substations stocked and setup; and complete all orientation exercises. This exercise will help organize move related functions and place them in a framework of time by which they should be completed. Check the schedule monthly to see that goals are met: if they aren't, reevaluate the schedule (15).

Monitoring Drawing and Construction

Every new drawing of the pharmacy area should be reviewed by the pharmacist line by line for errors. It should not be assumed that because a particular area, e.g., office, has been drawn correctly in the early versions of the plans that this will continue to be the case.

During the time that the interior of the building is being completed, it should be inspected as often as possible. This will allow you to spot possible construction problems which, observed early enough, can be modified without causing extensive and expensive changes or delay. Approximately 3 months before the move, inspect all plumbing, electrical outlets, keys, and locks to make sure they are hooked up and working correctly. Do not forget to look for minor details such as towel dispensers, blackboards, bulletin boards, and coat hooks to make sure they are in place or on order. It is difficult to understate the importance of this.

Personnel Involvement

Whenever a new work area is being designed, the people who will be working in the area should be asked for suggestions and should be allowed to review the final design. They will be able to offer many practical suggestions to help design a more efficient workplace. This also helps to promote a more positive attitude toward the new facility. Employees will be aware of upcoming changes, know why these changes occur, and be willing to accept them better. The larger the share an employee has in the planning and development process, the greater his pride in it. Employees should receive periodic updates as construction progresses and be allowed to tour the construction site.

A program for orientation of employees to the new facility should be undertaken. When major projects are involved, this may include not only printed materials, lectures, and review of the plans, but actual simulation by "walking through" the new work systems planned for the new facility.

It seems to be human nature for personnel to expect new facilities to work perfectly and solve *all* previous problems. They never do, of course, and it is typical for a negative reaction to surface right after the first few days of occupancy. The solution is to first warn employees of this phenomenon in advance to promote more realistic expectations. Then, be sure to provide a mechanism to note and acknowledge problems as they occur and make employees feel confident that these problems are being addressed. A simple device is a log book in which problems can be noted by the employees as they occur each day. At the end of the day, the supervisor should read and initial each entry, to signal to the employee that his problem has been noted. Some problems can be resolved by bringing them back to the group and challenging them to find a way to "make the facility work better under the unexpected circumstances." Given a supportive environment, novel solutions to seemingly insurmountable problems may emerge.

REFERENCES

1. Stolar MN: National survey of hospital pharmaceutical services, 1982. *Am J Hosp Pharm* 40:963-969, 1983.
2. Deiner CH (ed): *Lilly Hospital Pharmacy Survey, 1983.* Indianapolis, Eli Lilly and Company, 1983.
3. Alexander VB, Barker KN: A national survey of pharmacy facilities. Part I: Introduction, space allocation. *Am J Hosp Pharm* (in press).
4. *Evaluation and Space Programming Methodology Series No. 10: Pharmacy.* Ann Arbor, Chi Systems, Inc, 1979.
5. Barker KN: *Planning for Hospital Pharmacies.* HEW Publication No. FRA 74-4003. Rockville, MD, U.S. Department of Health, Education and Welfare, Health Resources Administration, Health Care Facilities Service, 1974.
6. American Society of Hospital Pharmacists: ASHP guidelines for institutional use of controlled substances. *Am J Hosp Pharm* 31:582-588, 1974.
7. Francis RL, White JA: Facility layout and location—an analytical approach, Englewood Cliffs, NJ, Prentice-Hall, 1974.
8. Barker KN, Harris JA, Webster DB, et al: Consultant evaluation of a hospital medication system: Synthesis of the new system. *Am J Hosp Pharm* 41:2016-2021, 1984.
9. Johnson RE, Myers JE, Egan DM: A resource planning model for outpatient pharmacy operations. *Am J Hosp Pharm* 29:411-418, 1972.
10. Myers JE, Hohnson RE, Egan DM: A computer simulation of outpatient pharmacy operations. *Inquiry* 9:40-47, 1972.
11. Barker KN, Smith M, Winters E: A study of the work of the pharmacist and the potential use of auxiliaries. *Am J Hosp Pharm* 29:35-53, 1972.
12. Dostal MM, Daniels CE, Roberts MJ, Giese RM: Pharmacist activities under alternative staffing arrangements. *Am J Hosp Pharm* 39:2098-2101, 1982.
13. Adams RW: Pharmacy services in a 240 bed Gordon Friesen-design hospital. *Hosp Pharm* 14:594, 597-598, 602-603, 606, 1979.
14. Swensson ES: An innovative design in hospital pharmacy facilities. *Am J Hosp Pharm* 28:442-446, 1971.
15. Loeb AJ: Experiences in planning, designing and moving to a new hospital. *Hosp Pharm* 14:441-453, 1979.
16. King CM: Planning facility expansion for pharmacy (letter). *Am J Hosp Pharm.* 39:36-37, 1982.

Appendix 17.1
QUESTIONS TO FOCUS THOUGHTS

A. General

1. Will the inpatient pharmacy activity be operative 24 hours a day? If not, what will be the hours of operation?
2. What provisions will be made for the issue of medications when the pharmacy is closed?
3. How will doctors order medications so that the pharmacy may receive copies of original orders?
   a. Use of NCR or carbon paper
   b. Use of automated devices:
      Direct computer input
      Photocopy
      Telewriter
      Voice recording
      Other
4. How will patient's medication profile (MAR) be maintained in pharmacy and on nursing unit?
   a. Duplicate orders stored together in file
   b. Transcribed onto cards or suitable form
   c. Use of automated devices
5. Will there be a bulk compounding program?
   a. Where and how will the distilled water be obtained?
   b. What type of a sterile area will be required?
   c. What type of a quality control program will be instituted?
6. Will there be a packaging program?
   a. What type of a quality control program will be instituted?
7. What types of pharmacy education programs will be developed?
   a. In-service
   b. Nursing education
   c. Interns
   d. Residents
   e. Technicians
   f. Patients and families
   g. Cooperative clinical pharmacy program with school of pharmacy
8. What type of a pharmacy research program will be developed?
   a. Administrative
   b. Bench type
   c. Clinical
9. Will the pharmacy activity be concerned with radiopharmaceuticals?
   a. Where located?
      Pharmacy
      Radiology
      Other
10. Will there be a drug information center? If so, what will be its:
    a. Function?
       Provision of drug information
          To P&T Committee
          Within pharmacy department
          On patient care areas
          Controlling activities of drug company representatives
          Specific requests (verbal and written)
          Prepared periodical information (bulletins, newsletters, etc)

Poison control
   Respond to calls
   Coordinate poison control with drug information
   Coordinate communications with medical personnel
   Maintain consultant panel
   Coordinate information with treatment center
Investigation drugs
   Literature search
   Review protocols
   Control measures for the hospital
Drug surveillance
   Current and retrospective reviews of all drug practices (drug selection and utilization, adverse actions, drug usage studies)
Education
   Lectures, consultants, surveys, reports, etc
   b. Location?
      Near pharmacy
      Near medical library
      Other
   c. Staff?
      Drug information pharmacists
      Pharmacy residents, interns, students
      Technicians
      Clerks
   d. Hours of operation?
11. What type of a drug distribution system will be employed?
    a. Centralized unit dose
    b. Decentralized unit dose
    c. Combination centralized-decentralized unit dose
    d. Medication administration team
    e. Other
12. If centralized unit dose is employed
    a. How will orders be transmitted to central pharmacy?
       Pharmacy messenger
       Other messenger
       Pneumatic tube
       Drop chute
       Automated device
    b. How will patient medication profiles be maintained?
       Kardex
       Envelope
       Card
       Automated device
    c. How many unit doses are expected to be dispensed per day (assuming that a unit dose may consist of one or more single use packages)?
    d. How are unit doses going to be packaged (procurement of all possible commercially packaged items)?
       Large packaging program
       Small packaging program
       Extemporaneous packaging
    e. How are unit doses going to be dispensed?
       Supervised pickers
       Automated devices

f. How are unit doses going to be prepared for delivery?
Individual patient containers (envelopes, bag, etc)
Individual patient drawers

g. After routine dosage times have been established (e.g., qid, 9,1,5,9; hs, 10 PM), how many dosage intervals are going to be covered by each delivery—or how many deliveries per day will be scheduled?
AM
Noon
Afternoon
Evening

h. What is expected workload of orders to be processed by time of day?
Scheduled
Prn's
IV's
Stat's
Preop's

i. What is expected workload of Rx's or unit doses to be dispensed by time of day?
Scheduled
IV's
Additive
Reconstitution
Compounded

j. How are unit doses going to be delivered?
Pharmacy messenger
Other messenger
Pneumatic tube
Conveyor, dumbwaiter—automatic devices

k. How will unit doses be stored on the nursing units?
Patient drawers in carts
Nurserver
Other location in patient room

l. How will pharmacy be involved with drug administration procedures on nursing units?
Review orders on unit
Review charting
Maintain MAR

m. How will charges be handled?
Nursing unit
Pharmacy

n. How will stat orders be handled?
Sent to pharmacy by automated device (pneumatic tube, conveyor, computer, electrowriter, etc)
Telephone
Picked up by pharmacy messenger
Emergency cart

o. How will narcotics be handled?
Unit dose
Floor stock

p. How will IV additives be handled?
Prepared in advance or on order by pharmacy
Additives sent to nursing unit by pharmacy ready to use
Prepared on nursing unit

13. If decentralized unit dose system is employed:
Satellite pharmacies on nursing units are utilized in this system. Therefore, answer all questions for centralized unit dose system wherever applicable after first answering the following questions:

a. Where will the satellite pharmacies be installed?
b. How many patients will each cover?
c. What will be the operating hours of the satellites?
d. How will the staellites be staffed?
e. What will be the activities of the satellite pharmacist?
Review charts
Consult with physicians on orders
Consult with nurses
Patient interviews
Make rounds with physician
Supervise dispensing and dose preparations on floor

14. If centralized-decentralized unit dose is employed:
After first establishing the extent of use of both systems, answers to the applicable questions for centralized and decentralized unit dose systems should supply all of the information required for establishment of this type of system.

15. If automated dispensing machine systems are employed:
a. What type of an automated dispensing machine system is to be used?
b. How will the automated devices be located?
c. Where will the automated devices be located?
Central pharmacy
Satellite pharmacy
Each nursing unit
Other
d. What type of packages will be used?
e. How will devices be filled?
f. How will automated system be backed up during failures?

16. Will the pharmacy activity include outpatient prescriptions?
a. Who will be entitled to use outpatient services?
Discharged patients only
Anyone
Employees
b. Where will cashier be located?
c. Will there be a separate outpatient pharmacy?
d. Will there be partitioned spaces or offices for pharmacist interviews with outpatients?
e. What procedures will be established for:
Maintenance of outpatient medication profile?
Rx files for outpatients?

B. **Work areas**
1. What are the office requirements?
Chief pharmacist
Assistant chief pharmacist
Other section chiefs
Clerical
Clinical pharmacists (inpatient care areas)
2. Other work spaces required
Inpatient dispensing centralized
Bulk compounding
Packaging
Drug information center
Sterile compounding (including IV additive services)
Editing or order review center
Storage of drugs and supplies (refrigeration, alcohol and other flammable, narcotics and regular active and inactive)
Quality control and research
Education activities
Radiopharmacy
Outpatient dispensing
Cart storage
Staff lockers and lounge area
Waiting areas (inpatient, outpatient, offices)

3. Satellite pharmacy
   Administration
     Office
     Education
     Drug information
   Dispensing
   Compounding
   Editing or order review
   Storage
     Active
     Bulk
     Refrigeration
     Medication cart
     Narcotics

C. Staffing requirements

Decisions arising from considering questions posed in previous sections will bear on factors presented in this section.

1. Based on the drug distribution system chosen, to what extent will nonprofessionals be used?
   a. Label typing
   b. Other clerical duties (filing, record keeping, etc)
   c. Bulk compounding
   d. Packaging
   e. Pickup and delivery
   f. Inventory control
   g. Maintenance of equipment
   h. Housekeeping
   i. Dispensing
   j. Purchasing
2. What supervision will they require?
3. What will be the education and training requirements for nonprofessionals and how will they be trained?
   a. In-house training program
   ɔ. On-the-job training
   c. Formal outside training
4. How will coverage be met during meal hours, days off, vacations, sick leave, etc?
5. With the increasing use of nonprofessionals, what added professional duties will be given to pharmacists?
   a. Patient interviews (admission, discharge)
   b. Maintain patient medication profiles
   c. Edit all medication orders
   d. Discuss drug regimen with physicians
   e. Provide information to interested parties (physicians, nurses, aides)
   f. Supervise medication administration
6. Will there be a clinical pharmacy training program in conjunction with a school of pharmacy; if so, what will be the student/preceptor ratio?
7. If 24-hour service is to be given, how will workload be distributed over the 24-hour period?
8. Will volunteers be used; if so, what chores will they perform? At what hours, on what days?
9. Estimate staffing patterns by class and hours
   a. Full-time pharmacist
   b. Part-time pharmacist
   c. Technician
   d. Clerical
   e. Other

D. Built-in and mechanical equipment requirements

Equipment to be considered herein is limited to that which is build-in or permanently attached to the structure.

1. What mechanical system will be required for carrying supplies and requisition between the inpatient pharmacy and activities?
   a. Pneumatic tube

   b. Dumbwaiter or lift
   c. Elevator
   d. Conveyors
   e. Automatic cart
   f. Other
2. If there is a separate outpatient pharmacy, what will be its needs in regard to the above systems and activities?
3. What will be the preferred pharmacy locations for the desired pneumatic tube and/or conveyor stations?
4. Will the pharmacy activity require gas, vacuum, compressed air and where will the outlets be placed?
5. Where will any special electrical outlets be placed?
6. High-voltage lines?
7. Will there be any special lighting requirements?
8. Will the pharmacy activity require its own still?
9. Will the pharmacy activity require its own autoclave?
10. Where will sinks be required (type and size)?
11. Will any type of special flooring be required? Where?
12. What functional elements and service outlets within the pharmacy activity must be provided with standby power?
13. What special requirements will there be in the sterile area (A/C vents near laminar flow hoods, UV light, etc)?
14. Will any special plumbing fixtures be required? Floor drains?
15. What will be the fixed equipment requirements for each of the following:
    a. Refrigeration
    b. Alcohol
    c. Narcotics and other controlled drugs
    d. Bulk supplies
    e. Active supplies
16. Any special (unusual) cabinet, shelving, and work counter requirements for any areas?
17. Will drinking fountains be required? Where?
18. Bulletin boards? Where? What size?
19. Central vacuum cleaning outlets?
20. Clocks? Where?
21. Signs? Type? Where? Illuminate?
22. Which of the following equipment will be required? Where placed?
    a. Duplicating
    b. Dictating
    c. Transcribing
    d. Labeling
    e. Computer terminals
    f. Calculators
    g. Closed-circuit TV
    h. Files

E. Interrelationships

What will be the interrelationships between the pharmacy activity and the following major activities and groups with respect to the factors listed, as may affect design?

1. Nursing units
2. Administration
3. Medical staff
4. Purchasing
5. Medical surgical supply
6. Business office
7. Personnel
8. Clinical support activities (laboratory, X-ray, surgery, etc)
9. General stores
10. Data management
11. Housekeeping
12. Outpatient activity
    a. Will outpatient pharmacy activity be under separate supervision? (Office area required?)

b. How will outpatient Rx's be filled?

c. Method of payment for outpatient Rx's? (Cashier; in pharmacy?)

d. To what extent will the outpatient department use different stock and therefore require duplicate inventory contract systems, purchasing, charging?

e. Separate waiting areas?

13. Medical records

F. Communications and transport

1. Telephones required? What type? Where placed?

2. Separate intercom system?

3. Tie in to general paging and piped music system?

4. Tie in to emergency alert?

5. What are the bulk materials handling needs of the pharmacy? Vertical? Horizontal? Demand by time of day?

6. What type of transportation system will be used for drug distribution?

   a. Large carts

   b. Patient drawer carts

   c. Automated (automated cart conveyor—pneumatic tube—dumbwaiter)

   d. Other

7. Will there be computer input-output devices in the inpatient and/or outpatient pharmacies, and if so, where located?

G. Location

1. Where should pharmacy activity be located in relation to:

   a. Main entrance and lobby

   b. Outpatient area

   c. Elevators

   d. Information desk

   e. Central stores

   f. Central medical surgical supply

   g. Business office

   h. Physicians' lounge

   i. Loading dock

   j. Other

2. Will there be more than one inpatient pharmacy location (satellites)? Where located?

3. Will there be a separate outpatient pharmacy location? Where located?

4. Will pharmacy be receiving supplies direct from suppliers? Require loading platform, etc?

5. Traffic flow known for all commerce units (people, products, and information units) moving in and out of pharmacy and throughout hospital?

6. When will peak traffic occur relative to above?

H. Environmental requirements

1. Will carpeting be required in any or all areas?

2. Where and to what extent should acoustical treatment be given?

3. What type of temperature and humidity controls will be required?

4. Preferred color scheme by functional areas?

5. Door-keying system and controls?

6. What will be the air filtration requirements?

I. Future requirements

The planning factors most likely to affect future space requirements are listed below. Are higher charges anticipated in any of these during the period for which facility is planned?

1. Number of patients to be served

2. Number of doses administered per inpatient day

3. Whether the operation will remain centralized or decentralized

4. Outpatient services

5. Bulk compounding, non–unit dose packaging and control

6. Storage requirements

7. Number of people working in the area

8. Where IV admixtures are prepared

9. Degree to which medications are provided to nurse in ready-to-administer form

10. The amount of hospital packaging and control required

11. Where drug pricing occurs

12. Size and shape of the unit dose storage containers

13. Extent of automation, use of computers

14. Involvement with drug information

15. Involvement in clinical pharmacy

16. Involvement with education activities

Appendix 17.2 RECORDING OTHER WORK AREA REQUIREMENTS

Data Sheet

SPECIAL WORK AREA REQUIREMENTS

General Work Area No.:_____ Name:_____Date:_____

Special Req. of Specific Work Areas

	No. _____ Name:	No. _____ Name:	No. _____ Name:	No. _____ Name:	No. _____ Name:
Special Requirements					

1. Entrances
   - Needs own entrance, formal
   - Door to outside, utility
   - Near main entrance
   - Near loading dock
   - Other (enter)

2. Personnel to be accommodated
   - Average (circle number seated)
   - Peak (circle number seated)

3. Materials handling system
   - Volume during average period
   - Peak periods
   - Physical dimensions average load
   - Largest load
   - Weight of largest load
   - Minimum transit time, normal orders
   - Emergency orders
   - Service needed:
   - Messenger
   - Pickup area dimensions
   - Cart
   - Parking area needed, space
   - Cart dimensions, LxWxH
   - Signal upon arrival

4. Communications
   - Telephones:
   - Sets, number
   - Type (desk, wall, hands-free)
   - Lines/set
   - Lines
   - Recorders
   - Intercom
   - TV, closed circuit
   - Cathode ray tube display
   - Printout terminal
   - Paging system
   - Security alarm
   - Fire alarm
   - Music
   - Other (enter)

Data Sheet

SPECIAL WORK AREA REQUIREMENTS

General Work Area No.:_____ Name:_____ Date:_____

Special Req. of Specific Work Areas

	No._____ Name:	No._____ Name:	No._____ Name:	No._____ Name:	No._____ Name:
Special Requirements					

5. Special services from other departments
   Data processing
   Duplicating
   Receiving
   General stores
   Inflammables storage
   Materials management
   Sterilization
   Laboratory
   Security
   Other (enter)

6. Security
   Safe, built-in
   Special keys
   Visual surveillance
   Alarm system
   Other (enter)

7. Utilities—electrical
   Outlets, for each give:
       Type
       Voltage
   Control in room
   Explosion proof switches and fixtures
   Emergency power to:
       Refrigerators
       Security alarm systems
   Other (enter)

8. Lighting
   Sunlight excluded
       Controllable
   Tasks at desk level
       Counter level
   Corridor level only
   Special (enter)

Data Sheet

SPECIAL WORK AREA REQUIREMENTS

General Work Area No.:_____ Name:_____ Date:_____

Special Req. of Specific Work Areas

	No. _____	No. _____	No. _____	No. _____	No. _____
	Name:	Name:	Name:	Name:	Name:

Special Requirements

___	___	___	___	___	___
___	___	___	___	___	___
___	___	___	___	___	___
___	___	___	___	___	___

9. Utilities—plumbing
   Water—cold
   Water—hot
   Distilled water
   Special lab drain
   Floor drain
   Other (enter)

10. Plumbing fixtures
    Outlet mounted on sink
    Outlet mounted on wall
    Distilled water outlet
    Gooseneck spout
    Blade handles
    Threaded outlet, with vacuum
       breaker
    Sink
    Lab sink
    Service sink
    Emergency shower
    Other (enter)

11. Mechanical services
    Steam
    Compressed air
    Vacuum
    Gas
    Oxygen
    Other (enter)

12. Environmental requirements
    Air conditioning
    Filtered air, positive pressure
    Temperature (specify range)
    Humidity (specify range)
    Fume removal
    Low noise
    Other (enter)

13. Special comments

CHAPTER 18

Computer Utilization in Institutional Pharmacy Practice

WILLIAM A. GOUVEIA

Computer applications have been developed in each segment of institutional pharmacy practice: drug distribution, management, clinical practice, and ambulatory care. The greatest attention has been given to the management and drug distribution support applications since they have the greatest direct impact on the pharmacy department. Applications to clinical practice have evolved as a component of some drug distribution applications and recently have proliferated on microcomputer systems. Ambulatory applications have been slow to develop since few institutions have outpatient pharmacies; yet some departments have adapted systems designed for community practice to their outpatient pharmacy.

The implementation and use of a computer system in an organization is a continuous process. From the time the use of a computer is considered until the system is implemented, pharmacy personnel at every level in the department must be involved in the process. Implementation of a system changes almost everything the organization does and the way it is done. The system will make changes in the organization, and the organization should constantly make changes in the system. A computer application is seldom completed; maintenance and improvement continue as long as the system is in operation.

THE EVOLUTION OF PHARMACY COMPUTER SYSTEMS

Pharmacy computer systems have evolved since the 1960s when a few experimental projects were developed to determine the potential utility of computers in hospitals and hospital pharmacy (1). In the early 1970s, a few successful applications were developed in specific pharmacy practice areas: outpatient, unit dose, and IV admixture applications (2,3). In the mid- to late 1970s, vendor involvement increased dramatically, both in terms of the number of vendors and in the variety of systems available. In the early 1980s, vendor systems began to receive acceptance in the marketplace, and microcomputers with programs developed by clinical and administrative pharmacists became commonplace in hospital pharmacies. As the 1980s progress, virtually every hospital pharmacy will have at least one system,

whereas many departments will have a number of systems, each designed to meet a specific need.

Mainframe Systems

Large, mainframe computer systems had their origins in the 1960s. These systems have received increased acceptance in the past few years because they provide for an integrated data base whereby all data input by each department is available to other departments. These systems facilitate communication between departments but usually do not provide a great deal of information processing support to individual departments such as pharmacy. A a result, some departments have implemented small dedicated systems to interface with the hospital's mainframe system.

It is likely that such mainframe systems will play a more limited role in the future and may be used primarily for financial functions, whereas a number of smaller departmental systems may be interconnected (networked) to provide the increased functionality provided by the larger systems. This approach allows for each department to select the hardware and software that best meet their needs. Communications networks that allow for the sharing of clinical as well as financial data are becoming commonplace in today's hospitals.

MICROCOMPUTER SYSTEMS

The acceptance of smaller micro- and minicomputer systems has increased as their information processing power and expandability has increased and their cost decreased. User involvement in programming such systems has increased, which often results in a system that more closely meets their expectations.

The development of local area networks (LAN) permits the communication and sharing of data between large and small systems, even those of different manufacturers. This permits the implementation of departmental systems that closely meet a department's operational needs while the need for institutional information communication and integration is met as well.

The key concern of the department manager should be to

assure that each smaller system is well planned in its design and objectives and that it meets a real department need. The same cost-benefit analysis should be done with these systems as has been done with applications on larger systems so that the use of this resource is maximized.

VENDOR SYSTEMS

As vendor systems have increased in variety and in number installed, we can better judge their impact and value in specific institutional settings. Since most of these systems have been designed to meet the needs of a variety of institutions, they may sacrifice utility for flexibility. Many contain features (a wide variety of reports, for example) that are useful in initiating sales interest but are of limited value in the pressures of daily usage in a busy hospital pharmacy.

The claims that have supported the sales of many of these systems, namely, reduced late and lost charges, have decreased the value to institutions under many prospective payment and cost-cap regulations that reduce the benefit of increased revenue generation. Some systems have been designed and programmed before prospective payment regulations were implemented and thus make no provision for the analysis of drug therapy by diagnosis related group (DRG), for example, which is of value to hospitals under prospective pricing methods.

THE PHARMACY INFORMATION MODULE

A model information system for institutional pharmacy is shown in Figure 18.1. This model and its information requirements (Table 18.1) are intended to be as comprehensive as possible. It is likely that such a model need not be implemented in its entirety in a given pharmacy department. Rather, the intention is that the reader select, then establish priorities for, the specific needs of their institution for computer systems.

The boxes in Figure 18.1 signify functions that are performed in hospital pharmacies whether computerized systems exist or not. While most pharmacists could not identify an order entry section of their pharmacy, they probably find that some of the information requirements, i.e., dosage checking, are a routine part of their pharmacy's functions.

Patient information, as shown in Figure 18.1, can come from an automated admission and census system or, in its absence, can be a responsibility of the pharmacy. The formulary file includes the information on drugs stocked by the department, whereas the clinical data base reflects the applications implemented, such as drug interactions screening. Whereas the patient information is not the responsibility of the pharmacy, the formulary and clinical data bases clearly are.

The order entry segment as depicted is the front end of the pharmacy system. Perhaps the most critical part of the system, it determines the nature and accuracy of all other output (4). While order entry implies the capture of complete, legible orders, this segment may also include a considerable amount of quality control. The checking of drug dose, route acceptability, allergy, and drug interactions can be significant aspects of the order entry function. The scheduling and categorization (as new, renewal, or modification of orders) can dictate the nature of other system requirements.

The processing of orders will depend on the needs and priorities of each hospital pharmacy. Orders for IV therapy take longer to process because of their complexity. The computer can contribute to the processing of IV orders by preparing labels and worklists for pharmacy personnel (5). The handling of standard IV drug orders as well as orders for total parenteral nutrition solutions are too complex to be included as part of the unit dose order segment. Therefore, the IV admixture component is usually considered a separate, integrated module within the system.

The unit dose/patient profile applications are the mainstay of hospital pharmacy practice (6). The unit dose system places a significant burden of information handling on pharmacy personnel, as contrasted with the individual prescription system. Patient profile maintenance is time consuming,

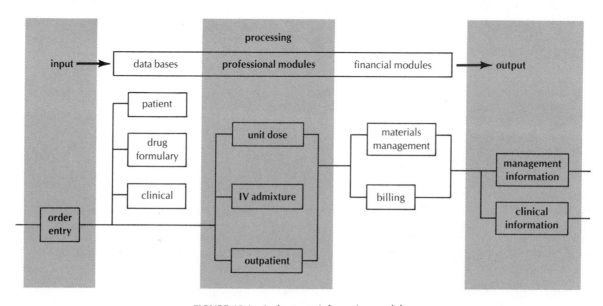

FIGURE 18.1 A pharmacy information module.

and the preparation of unit dose selection lists by a computer can reduce the time as well as the errors associated with unit dose preparation. The preparation of medication profiles can be a major contribution of the system to the medical and nursing staffs since it provides information seldom available in one location in manual systems.

Outpatient pharmacy service is generally limited to larger teaching hospital pharmacies. This situation may change, however, because of the emphasis being given to ambulatory and home care today. Computer applications in the outpatient pharmacy may play a significant role in the determination of drug usage patterns since overprescribing and poor patient compliance may be detected by such systems (7-9).

The financial segment includes the posting of charges, whereas the materials management functions include purchasing and inventory control. A major component of the justification of a system is likely to involve an improvement in the financial picture of the department; thus these modules constitute an important contribution to the system's success.

THE SIZE AND INTEGRATION OF COMPUTER SYSTEMS

Small, dedicated computers are often used to support the pharmacy information module. Functions such as unit dose or IV admixtures have been developed on large as well as small computer systems. Differentiation can be made between the development of a pharmacy module on a large computer and the implementation of hospital information systems (HIS). Most HIS have, as their primary focus, the communication of the medication order from the nursing unit to the pharmacy. Few HIS have provided the in-depth information processing support for the pharmacy as exemplified by the pharmacy module. Thus, some pharmacy departments have purchased a vendor's pharmacy module to handle internal order processing and interfaced the modules with HIS.

The use of small dedicated computers is now state-of-the-art because of their relatively low cost. Greater control by the using department, more reliability and stability of hardware, and independence from a large operating system are among the factors in the success of small systems. In a given hospital, a single large computer system for administrative and accounting applications such as admissions and census, patient billing, and accounts receivable might be connected to a series of computers. A small computer might serve as a communication link to handle data requests from the mainframe and from each dedicated departmental computer. The dedicated departmental computer may or may not be housed within each department but should handle the primary information requirements for that department. Thus, the laboratory computer could request a list of medications for a specific patient from the pharmacy system to determine if a drug may have interfered with a laboratory test. The laboratory computer could also send charges to the mainframe for billing to a specific patient. Institutions

---

TABLE 18.1   Pharmacy Information Module Information Requirements

A. Patient information
  1. Demographic information
  2. Admission discharge and transfer functions
  3. Census listings
  4. Allergy information
B. Formulary data base
  1. Inventory and price data
  2. Drug information
  3. Drug and laboratory interference data
  4. Drug-drug interaction data
C. Order entry
  1. Quality control
    a. Dose check, minimum and maximum
    b. Route acceptability
    c. Drug-drug and drug-lab checking
    d. Drug-specific checks
  2. Order input
    a. Name verification and display
    b. Drug name or code (numeric or mnemonic) entry, generic, trade, or common name
    c. Dose
    d. Route
    e. Frequency
    f. Scheduling, past and future
    g. Duration
    h. Comments
    i. New, renewal, or modification of order
D. IV admixture
  1. Order input (in addition to C2)
    a. Multiple drugs
    b. Total parenteral nutrition solutions
    c. Solution type and volume
    d. Continuous and intermittent

  2. Order review
    a. Solution and drug orders
    b. Current, active orders
    c. Past and current orders
E. Unit dose and patient profile
  1. Order input (in addition to C2)
    a. Regular, prn, and single-dose orders
  2. Order listing
    a. Active order list
    b. All orders list
    c. Medication administration record
    d. Pharmacy fill list
    e. Drug order renewal list
F. Outpatient
  1. Order input (in addition to C2)
    a. Discharge prescriptions
    b. Extended care unit and day hospital prescriptions
    c. Outpatient prescriptions
  2. Order listing
    a. Bottle label
    b. Profile (with or without inpatient medications)
G. Financial/administrative
  1. Inventory listings
    a. Drug status report
    b. Out-of-range report
  2. Controlled substances
    a. Report by drug
    b. Report by patient
    c. Report by nursing station
    d. Inventory, current and biannual

have begun developing networks of computer systems, much like telephone networks, to allow for the sharing of clinical and financial information.

Large computer systems have been the mainstay of hospital financial applications. The success of commercial systems combining financial and clinical systems has been limited. The inherent size and complexity of large systems can limit their reliability and the flexibility of program development. While the integration of information and the development of a common data base can be accomplished with a mainframe computer, this is not always the case. The priority for application development given to individual departments on a mainframe is usually not as high as with dedicated systems. Thus dedicated systems have been developed to meet a need that has not been met with mainframe systems.

To the pharmacist, selection of types or sizes of hardware or of specific programming languages should be less important than the achievement of a functional system for the department. Hardware needs are best determined through careful institutional planning by users and data processing professionals. If an admissions/census system is available on an existing, reliable mainframe computer; if additional terminals and programming time are available; and if the pharmacy obtains a reasonably high priority in systems development, then a mainframe system may be the best route to pursue. A dedicated computer may be feasible if the above is not possible and as long as integration of systems within the hospital is feasible.

OBTAINING A SYSTEM

A pharmacy manager who wishes to obtain a computer system for the department may have to go through a number of steps before the system is available for use in the department. Each manager will have to choose between self-development or selection of a vendor's system. Both routes are presented below. There is some overlap in the development or selection of a system so that the reader might select the components of each that best fits the needs of his hospital.

System Development

The steps involved in the development of a computer system include:

1. Needs assessment
2. Systems analysis
3. Systems design
4. Specification
5. Programming
6. Implementation
7. Maintenance

These steps would be used by a hospital data processing department or computer vendor if a system were to be fully developed. If a system were to be selected from the various vendor offerings available, then needs assessment would be followed by the steps under system selection below and then starting again with implementation and maintenance.

Systems analysis refers to the thorough analysis and documentation of the department's current procedures. This documentation takes the form of numerous flow charts in which activities, personnel involvement, and forms used are indicated. Existing procedures are first documented, and then the new systems are flow charted in a similar manner. During systems design, the systems needed are documented considering the interface between humans and computers, terminals and printers needed, files required, etc. Specification refers to the precise documentation of the format of each display screen, label, report, and form. From this step, the programmer will develop the flow charts of logic and decisions required for the programs. Programming then starts with these detailed charts and the coding (writing of the actual programs), debugging (identifying and then correcting errors in the programs), and documentation of the programs completes the process. The needs assessment, implementation, and maintenance steps are defined below.

The pharmacist's involvement is heavy at the outset of the computer project; is reduced during the specification and programming; and then increases again during the implementation and maintenance steps. The data processing staff should provide the technical direction; the pharmacy staff, professional expertise. Data processing staff involvement will be heavy at first; continue through specification and programming; and then decrease during implementation and maintenance. Clearly, the involvement of both staffs will be required as long as the computer is in operation.

While the pharmacy staff do not have to become computer experts in order to be involved with computer systems, it may be helpful for the data processing or vendor staff to take upon themselves the task of orientation of the pharmacy staff to computer terminology. In turn, the pharmacy staff has the responsibility of preparing the data processing staff to make decisions concerning the pharmacy's system. Thus, orientation in terminology is often necessary—data processing terms for the pharmacy staff and drug terminology for the data processing staff. Common language from the outset will give both staffs a common commitment and understanding. If it is not feasible for the hospital's data processing staff to provide instruction to the pharmacy staff, courses may be taken at a local university.

A pharmacist may feel compelled to learn programming in order to program the system himself. Clearly, it is not necessary for the pharmacist to neglect his pharmacy expertise in favor of data processing knowledge. The time involved is considerable and the effort to become a skilled programmer may not be worth the investment required for a pharmacist. The pharmacist is probably better off relying on the technical expertise of others since the pharmacist has a considerable responsibility for providing professional direction during systems development. It is important to note, however, some pharmacists have successfully programmed, developed, and implemented systems, particularly microcomputer-based systems.

System Selection

The selection of an appropriate system for the pharmacy department is a challenging but rewarding task. The hardware and software packages that vendors offer have a number of variables, each of which can affect the operation of the system. The use of a well-defined and documented procedure for system selection can bring the department's needs in close alignment with the vendor's offering and minimize the risk of implementing a system that will not function to expectation.

The primary steps in the selection of a computer system for the pharmacy include:

1. Needs assessment: During this step a department's systems requirements are determined for functions needed, data storage and retrieval, interfaces with other computer systems, and hardware and terminal devices.

2. Request for proposal (RFP): The RFP is a detailed documentation of the department's requirements to be sent to vendors for their response.

3. Proposal to administration: as a result of the RFP, distribution, and evaluation, a final proposal to hospital administration can be developed in which the cost and benefits of the system selected are documented.

4. Contract development: After a system is selected and the proposal accepted by hospital administration, the final legal contract between hospital and vendor can be developed.

5. Implementation: The department is prepared for implementation, the hardware installed, and software loaded; other departments affected by the system, such as finance and nursing, should be involved in the preparation process as well.

6. Maintenance: The maintenance of the system, both hardware and software, is vital to the smooth functioning of the system over time.

The detailed process for applying the steps above follows.

Needs Assessment

By conducting a comprehensive needs assessment the department manager can (1) know the system functions that should be implemented in their department; (2) be able to determine the vendor's abilities to meet the defined needs of the department; (3) be able to request modification of the vendor system to meet specific needs as required; or (4) be able to change pharmacy procedures to maximize the ability of the system.

The specific components of a needs assessment have been outlined by Nold (10) and include:

1. Hospital and department-specific variables: The number of medication orders, number of beds, number of admissions, transfers and discharges, number and type of personnel involved in each function, and location of each pharmacy dispensing area

2. Personnel: The number and type of personnel and their security levels within the system

3. Data storage: The types of files and the type of data to be stored by the system (e.g., controlled substance requirements)

4. Data retrieval: The type and variety of reports, labels, and lists and which relate to the data stored above should be specified

5. Data transmission: Data transmitted by printed reports, by magnetic tape or disk, or by direct transmission and the need for billing, census, purchasing, and medication order information

6. Hardware: The number and type of terminals and printers consistent with the department's location

Request for Proposal

A RFP is a document developed by the purchaser defining a type of service or product desired. Based upon this document, the potential vendors are requested to provide a written response describing how they propose to deliver the required service and at what price. An RFP is a request for a vendor to present a proposal to provide a product or service (11).

An RFP forms the basis for communication both within the hospital and between the vendor and the hospital. Within the department, the development of the RFP has great value in providing a focus for discussion of how the department's services and procedures can be provided, as well as what the department's priorities are for information services. Within the hospital, the RFP helps the department communicate with administration, finance, medical records, and data processing in terms of what its data processing needs are and how these needs interface with each of the departments. With the vendor, the RFP provides a clear statement of the hospital's requirement so the vendor can assess the capability of their system to meet the hospital needs. Later the RFP can form the basis for the legal contract between the vendor and the hospital.

In the process of development of the RFP, the department's existing manual system should be reviewed and documented. This documentation, which often is in the form of information flow charts, can be compared with the flow charts of the automated system to determine where procedural changes may be required and where functions may be eliminated, thus reducing personnel requirements, for example.

The RFP typically includes the following information: (1) the current data processing system, (2) instructions to the vendor in responding to the RFP, (3) the system specifications, (4) vendor and contractual information requested, and (5) instructions for submitting the final proposal.

Once the RFP is prepared, it should be distributed to qualified vendors (12). Currently, approximately 30 vendors provide pharmacy systems (13). In order to reduce this 30 to a manageable number, a telephone survey might be made to determine which vendors are currently qualified to respond to the hospital's needs. Then the RFP can be distributed, the vendors' responses evaluated, demonstrations of their system solicited, and references reviewed, and sites where the installed system could be planned visited. On the basis of this information, a final list of two or three vendors, in sequence, can be developed (14).

The final RFP should contain a prioritized list of system requirements, with the essential items indicated, and a wish list of items desired but not required included as well.

Vendors should be given 4 to 6 weeks to respond. Their response in writing might be supplemented by a formal presentation at the hospital. If possible, their presentations should be scheduled within a relatively short period of time of one another. A variety of individuals might be included on the evaluation team—from pharmacy, data processing, finance, administration, and possibly nursing. Each vendor should submit a list of client hospitals so that references can be evaluated by telephone initially and by visitation. At each step in the process, it is important to document the vendor evaluations so that the final decision can be made as objectively as possible, particularly since 3 months or more may have passed since the RFP was prepared.

Following vendor selection, a final proposal can be made to hospital administration. This proposal should document the current and proposed systems, a listing of hardware and software required, the results of the vendor selection process, the implementation process, interfaces with other systems and departments, as well as a cost-benefit analysis and a final recommendation to administration (15).

The cost-benefit analysis would take into account the cost reductions in personnel, drugs, and equipment. Depending on the reimbursement to a hospital within a given state, increased revenue obtained from decreased late and lost charges may add to the system's value. Prospective payment systems may alter the need for revenue enhancements, but improved documentation of drugs dispensed may assist in the determination of drug therapy costs. Personnel reductions are a result of a decreased need for label typing, billing, report preparation, keypunching (in the data processing area), manual profile preparation, and/or similar activities.

The costs of a system include:
1. Computer hardware
   a. Purchase/lease
   b. Maintenance
2. Computer terminals
   a. Purchase/lease
3. Computer software
   a. Purchase/lease
   b. Maintenance
4. Site preparation
5. Cable installation

Implementation

Preparation. Preparation is made for both computer equipment and personnel (17). Most small computer systems do not require special site preparation, in particular to control temperature and humidity, as is the case with larger systems. The environment of most pharmacy departments is adequate as long as space is available. For larger systems, space may be sought in the hospital's computer room so the environment is controlled and the computer operations staff is available to operate and maintain the system.

The preparation of personnel requires a great deal of thought and planning. The involvement of virtually all of the pharmacy staff early in the preparation of the RFP, the selection of the vendor, and the proposal to administration will give them a sense of personal commitment to the success of the project.

A variety of policies and procedures may be developed in anticipation of the operation of the system, including daily operations plan, backup, error recovery and documentation, and downtime, scheduled and unscheduled.

Forms must be developed while some existing forms may be modified to accommodate the system. The use of video displays, in place of typewritten forms, is recommended where paper printouts are not necessary.

Many computer installations are guided through the use of the critical path method (CPM) or program evaluation and review technique (PERT) (18) or Gantt charts. These planning methodologies are used to plot each activity re-

quired during the installation process against the time required to complete the task.

Testing System Functions. Systems that are developed for a hospital require extensive testing (19). Vendor-purchased packages that have not been modified require minimal testing. New programs, even those which have been debugged by the programmer, require extensive testing. Testing should be done with real medication orders, at various times during the day, with all the functions available, and at each security level of system user.

Initial testing may be done in the parallel mode, whereby both manual and automated systems are in use. Systems may be placed in operation, following parallel mode, by adding one patient care unit at a time, a pharmacy satellite at a time, or with each new patient admission. The key functions to be tested include:
1. New medication orders
2. Stop orders and order renewals
3. Profile maintenance
4. Dose selection
5. Label and report generation
6. IV orders and labels
7. Backup system
8. Charge function
9. Census

Training. Personnel training might begin while the system is tested in parallel and is required as long as the system is in use in the department. A logical training sequence is preferable, and one or two employees, a pharmacist and a technician, for example, might be assigned this continuing responsibility. Often, some basic information in computer terminology might be provided as well. Training should include orientation to the system in formal, small-group sessions, followed by practical, hands-on training.

The on-line, hands-on training can only be done with a small number of employees who might start with a small number of demonstration patients, then enter simple orders on real patients under careful supervision, and then more complex orders might be entered on a larger number of patients.

The use of training programs, on a personal computer, for example, or the development of a detailed training manual is not recommended, primarily because a great effort is required to maintain such programs or manuals as the primary system changes. Some systems have "help" functions that guide the user as they use the system, in the real programs, through an example of the program functions, by providing immediate access to explanations of program functions.

Maintenance

Systems that are as complex as hospital pharmacy computer systems require a great deal of maintenance of hardware, software, and files (20). Hardware maintenance, including terminals, is usually provided through the hardware vendor by a series of contracts. Contract prices depend on the need for maintenance, 24 hours a day, 7 days a week (the most expensive), to an on-call, labor and parts (the least expensive in the short run), to a variety of options in between.

Software maintenance is required by all systems for as long as they are in use. Extensive or minimal maintenance may be required, depending on the environment in which pharmacy is practiced. Most computer installations will generate a long list of software changes and enhancements requested by the users as they gain experience with the system. These must be prioritized, costed, and approved by departmental, hospital, finance, or data processing management.

File maintenance is vital to pharmacy systems. Some files change infrequently, e.g., physician or pharmacy employee files. Drug interaction files change with some regularity. The primary drug file may change daily or at least weekly to reflect the changes in drug packaging, pricing, formulation, or additions or deletions to the formulary. More than one security level may exist in the pharmacy for file maintenance; however, the number of individuals with authority to modify the files should be severely limited. Other security levels might allow the user to enter orders, others to verify orders, and others to view data only.

THE IMPACT OF A COMPUTER SYSTEM ON PHARMACY PRACTICE

The impact of implementing a pharmacy computer system would be similar to that of any major professional system (e.g., a unit dose drug distribution system). The following factors should be considered:

1. Impact on pharmacy and nursing personnel
2. Impact on departmental finances
3. Impact on material costs such as drug and supplies
4. Impact on quality as measured by medication and dispensing errors
5. The information needs of the pharmacy

There have been few studies of the impact of computers in hospital pharmacy. Nielsen et al (21) found a reduction of about 8 hours per day in the amount of time spent by central admixture personnel in clerical functions. An 11.2% reduction in overall staffing was achieved with that system. In a comparison of a manual traditional system with a computerized unit dose system, Riley et al (22) found a dramatic increase in pharmacy personnel costs ($11,000 for 60 beds for 60 days). Nursing costs were reduced 45%, and the net personnel costs for the two systems showed an increase of $2000 for the unit dose system. This latter study did not measure the impact of the computer system alone since it was implemented at the same time as a unit dose system. Savings in nursing time are seldom realized since nursing payrolls are not usually decreased following the implementation of most pharmacy systems.

The impact of computer systems on personnel time is likely to be centered in three principal areas of pharmacy practice. First, the computer can communicate the order from one location to another. If a hospital does not have logistical support systems (e.g., tube systems), communication of the order using a computer system is not dependent on a messenger.

Second, a system can ensure that the order is complete and legible on input. Whether the order is input by the physician, nurse, or pharmacy personnel, the system can be so structured as to require a complete, legible order. Prob-

lems can be resolved early in the processing of the order, and the physician can often deal with the question at hand before doses of the drug have been administered.

Third, savings can accrue in the area of information processing, particularly in the record keeping associated with profile maintenance. Maintenance of a patient profile—initiation of new orders, discontinuation of orders, and changes in orders—is probably the most labor-intensive task in the pharmacy. Profile maintenance often requires the attention of both pharmacist and technician and is potentially the area of greatest personnel saving in the pharmacy.

The financial impact of a computer system is the basis for the justification of systems in most hospitals. The individual pricing of medications, the posting of charges, and the timeliness of this process can have a major impact on hospital income and cash flow. By using the computer for direct charge input or to generate charges as a by-product of the dispensing process, current prices can be maintained on all drugs as long as the price data in the drug file are current. Charges are not as likely to be lost as they might be in the keypunching process, and on-line systems give some assurance that all information is processed on a current basis. Further, personnel time is saved in keypunching since the pharmacy represents a large volume of individual charges.

The use of the computer for the initial processing of medication orders, the maintenance of profiles, and the subsequent automatic posting of charges to a patient's bill is perhaps optimal. By minimizing the interaction of humans, there can be greater assurance that charges will be posted in an accurate and timely manner. Charges can be a by-product of the dispensing process (where errors are sought out by the pharmacy staff and corrected), which permits the daily posting of charges (if this is institutionally important).

The impact of savings on drug and supply costs may be offset by increased costs for system maintenance. Printed forms may be eliminated and less-expensive data processing paper may be used. Drug cost savings are related to the amount of current inventory and the purchasing data available to the institution before implementation of the system. With the carrying cost of inventory at about 20-25%, a reduction in inventory can be more important today than ever before. If the hospital has satellite pharmacies, the computer may provide current data on the utilization of particular drugs for the patients served by that satellite, for example. The review of drug usage data may permit a more active elimination of drugs from the hospital formulary.

Perhaps the most difficult area to quantify is the value of quality improvements. How much is error rate improvement worth? Do computer systems have an impact on medication errors? What is the value of a legible patient profile? If the hospital has not been able to provide a medication profile to physicians, how much is physician satisfaction worth? These questions are quantifiable only by each individual institution assigning a value to such improvements.

The information needs and what might be termed the "critical information mass" of a pharmacy relates to the size of the hospital, the activity, the census and length of patient stay, the breadth of demand for pharmacy services, and where information bottlenecks occur with the manual system. A long-term psychiatric institution with little patient turnover or medication changes may not be able to justify a computer system for pharmacy. A batch-processing, refill-oriented system might be appropriate for this type of institution.

Larger, acute care institutions with a large house staff, comparatively short length of stay, and high number of medication orders and charges have a high critical information mass and will find that in time they will not be able to provide responsive pharmacy services without computer support. The institutional pharmacist in this case should parallel their justification to that of the comptroller, who would not think of a payroll system without computer support.

Prospective payment methods are still evolving at the state and national level as a new method of hospital reimbursement. While it is too early to know which method, DRG payment per case, for example, will be used on a long-term basis, what is clear is that prospective payment places a much greater demand for more timely and accurate data from clinical and financial departments. The relationship of drug data to each hospital admission will be important to define drug cost as a proportion of hospital cost. Thus, new reimbursement methods place greater demands on department systems, many of which cannot be met easily by manual methods, thus fostering the implementation of computer systems.

A TRANSITIONAL PERIOD

Pharmacy has always been an information-based profession. The amount of information managed by pharmacists increased in the 1960s and 1970s with the advent of the unit dose and IV admixture systems. Clinical pharmacists have concerned themselves with integrating and interpreting medication, laboratory, and diagnostic data. Traditionally, the focus of pharmacy managers has been to justify, select, and implement computer systems (23). Now our concern must shift to the integration of systems and data, and thus we are in a period of transition in terms of information technology—from development and implementation of systems to full utilization of the data collected by them to benefit patients; from acquisition of the system to full benefit of the information processing power that computers can provide; from concern about the details of the hardware and software to the full integration of computer systems into pharmacy practice; and from concern for the features and gimmicks of the software to the implementation of an effective operational system that improves departmental productivity.

Information technology and pharmacy practice are inextricably tied. The investment that pharmacists make in guiding this technology during this period of transition will have significant benefit to our patients, hospitals, and profession.

The author wishes to acknowledge the assistance of Edward L. Decker and Jean M. Mildenberger of the New England Medical Center Pharmacy Department in the preparation of this chapter.

REFERENCES

1. Gouveia WA, Diamantis C, Barnett GO: Computer applications in the hospital medication system. *Am J Hosp Pharm* 26:142, 1969.
2. Knight JR, Conrad WF: Review of computer applications in hospital pharmacy practice. *Am J Hosp Pharm* 32:165-173, 1975.
3. Burleson KW: Review of computer applications in institutional pharmacy—1975-1981. *Am J Hosp Pharm* 39:53-70, 1982.
4. Gouveia WA et al: The pharmacy computer system at the New England Medical Center. *Am J Hosp Pharm* 41:1813-1823, 1984.
5. Lausier M: Computerized hospital information system for an intravenous admixture service. *Am J Hosp Pharm* 34:976-978, 1977.
6. Gousse WL: Computer system for unit dose drug distribution. *Am J Hosp Pharm* 35:711-714, 1978.
7. Madden EE, Vaughan CM, Trahan GJ: Outpatient pharmacy prescription automation. Part two. *Am J Hosp Pharm* 26:151-159, 1969.
8. Weissman AM et al: Computer support of pharmaceutical services for ambulatory patients. *Am J Hosp Pharm* 33:1171-1175, 1976.
9. Wallner JN, Stitt RP: Survey of outpatient pharmaceutical services in university hospitals. *Am J Hosp Pharm* 36:1193-1196, 1979.
10. Nold EG: Computerization needs assessment. *Am J Hosp Pharm* 39:302-306, 1982.
11. Neal T: Developing the request for proposal. *Am J Hosp Pharm* 39:475-480, 1982.
12. Williams FL, Tucker SR: Establishing priorities and distributing the request for proposal. *Am J Hosp Pharm* 39:635-640, 1982.
13. Swanson DS, Brockemeier RL, Anderson MW: Hospital pharmacy computer systems—1982. *Am J Hosp Pharm* 39:2109-2117, 1982.
14. Williams FL, Tucker SR: Evaluating vendor responses. *Am J Hosp Pharm* 39:835-839, 1982.
15. Nold EG: Developing the proposal. *Am J Hosp Pharm* 39:1032-1039, 1982.
16. Entin FJ: Reviewing the contract. *Am J Hosp Pharm* 39:1324-1328, 1982.
17. Thielke TS: Preparing to implement. *Am J Hosp Pharm* 39:1521-1524, 1982.
18. Pathak DS: Appendix: Critical path scheduling and implementation of a computer system in a hospital pharmacy. In Nold E, Gouveia W (eds): *Managing Computer Systems: Pharmacy and Other Hospital Departments.* Bethesda, American Society of Hospital Pharmacists, 1983, pp 309-410.
19. Mildenberger J, Gouveia WA: Managing the implementation of a pharmacy computer system. *Am J Hosp Pharm* 39:1692-1701, 1982.
20. Moore TD, Ruhl NB: System maintenance, problems, and enhancements. *Am J Hosp Pharm* 39:1957-1963, 1982.
21. Nielson CB, Knight JR, Latiolais CJ: Computerized IV admixture services. *Hospitals* 48:113-122, 1974.
22. Riley AN, Derewicz HJ, Lamy PP: Distribution costs of a computer-based unit dose drug distribution system. *Am J Hosp Pharm* 30:213-219, 1973.
23. Gouveia WA, Nold EG: Computer systems planning, development, and impact assessment. *Am J Hosp Pharm* 39:2117-2124, 1982.

CHAPTER 19

Politics and Program Promotion Through Interdepartmental Relations

ROBERT B. WILLIAMS

A few years ago Harry Levinson (1), a well-known consultant in the health care field, said:

It is difficult for people in the medical and allied professions to seek power openly, because they are not supposed to be seeking power if they are dedicated to public service. In a business school, it is all right to say you want to get rich, and be powerful, but if you go to a school of hospital administration, or nursing [or pharmacy], you are supposed to want to serve people. Many people are attracted to these kinds of service roles, because they can deny their less than conscious wish for power, which means that power tends to be exercised in a clandestine fashion. This results in a lot of back-biting, gossip, and other manipulations that are not the best ways for dealing with problems. As people in the hospital learn their professional disciplines, they are placed in managerial positions because of seniority, or because they are the best in a given skill; not because they are the best managers. If it is difficult to manage your own aggressive impulses, then you cannot lead, or manage others very well. You tend to exercise power in subtle subterfuges, which create additional problems.

For some reason, "power" and "politics" are dirty words in hospitals; but power and politics do not come from hospitals—they come from people. Dissect the hospital, cut through the masonry, and what do you find—people. In the context of this chapter, politics is defined as the process by which power and influence are acquired and exercised for the benefit of meeting objectives. Because of our dependence on other people, other departments, and other professionals, pharmacy managers need to be skilled at acquiring and using politics in order to perform their jobs. We are dependent on nurses to communicate with us to ensure timely drug administration, especially with sporadic medication discontinuation, patient transfers, and IV solutions that are ahead or behind schedule. Physicians who do not cooperate in getting discharge prescriptions written on time make the pharmacy look bad when the patient is waiting to go home. The Infection Control Committee needs to lend support to pharmacy's antibiotic drug utilization review program if it is going to be meaningful. And certainly, the hospital administration needs to approve operational and new program budgets if we are going to provide contemporary pharmacy services. And so it goes, dependency on others within the hospital exists to a much greater extent than many of us really realize. Michael Korda (2) said:

You can't learn to acquire power by rules: it has to come from inside; but by following certain rules you can develop an awareness of it. We all have a power potential, but few of us use it, or even know it is there. In more primitive cultures, youths are initiated into the rights of power, sometimes in very complicated ways. The rules are absolute and clear-cut, and must be followed exactly, but they are intended to increase the initiate's awareness of himself—simply carrying out the ritual isn't enough. In certain American Indian tribes, young men bury themselves in pits up to their necks on lowly hills in the desert to learn patience, concentration, and the ability to stay motionless when necessary, however uncomfortable it may be. Survival lies in the ability to control one's body, and one's mind. Our world is not so very different, noisy and complex as it seems, but we are less fortunate than the Indians. We are educated at considerable expense and effort, but no wise teacher prepares us for the world we will face as adults. If we are lucky, we learn how to do a job, but for most people the price of survival is surrender. There is a place for almost everyone in our world, but usually on other people's terms rather than our own. Some of us learn how to succeed, and may even become rich and famous; few learn how to use the world, instead of being used by it.

The purpose of this chapter is to describe how pharmacy managers can use power and politics to their advantage within the hospital, instead of having power and politics use them. Through the understanding of these dynamics, positive interdepartmental relations can be orchestrated in such a way as to help promote pharmacy program development.

SOCIAL PSYCHOLOGY OF HOSPITALS

Hospitals are organizations just like other organizations in the business world. Within the hospital, people behave in ways in which they would not when outside of the hospital setting. They wear uniforms that they would not otherwise wear. They adopt certain styles and formalities in dealing with other people that one does not find elsewhere. Perhaps most important, people's behavior within the hospital shows a selectivity, a restrictiveness, and a persistence that is not otherwise observed in the same people when they are outside the hospital. Since pharmacy managers function within the organizational environment of the hospital, it is important that we understand the social psychology of a hospital. If we view the hospital strictly as a physical system, and do not include the social system, we will always misperceive what is really happening. The hospital organization, then, is truly a social system; one which is contrived by people. As such, hospitals are imperfect systems. They can come apart at the seams overnight, and yet can outlast the very people that created them. The cement that holds our hospitals together is essentially psychologic rather than biologic. Our hospitals are anchored in interpersonal relationships that include the attitudes, perceptions, beliefs, motivations, habits, and expectations of people.

POWER AND INFLUENCE AFFECTS LEADERSHIP

Appointments to positions come from above. Affirmation of positions come from below. In other words, the hospital administrator appoints the pharmacy director, but others within the organization affirm that the person is indeed in a leadership position. Thus, the role of leadership is important to the pharmacy manager in order to benefit from the hospital's political process. The pharmacy manager's leadership ability directly affects the power and influence which that manager will have within the hospital.

Leadership is a process influencing, guiding, and directing the thinking, attitudes, and actions of people aimed at attaining goal-oriented results. In an influential sense, leadership has very little to do with one's position of authority as it relates to the hospital organization chart. A true leader will capitalize on the human resources of the hospital in order to effect change in a positive direction, changes that would otherwise not take place in the absence of the leader.

Power and influence originate from both organizational and nonorganizational sources; from both formal and informal leadership.

PHARMACY MANAGERS NEED POLITICAL SKILLS

We often distrust and question the motives of people in our hospitals who we believe are actively seeking power. This is probably because we have a certain fear of being manipulated by them. Even those who legitimately understand the need for using power and influence are sometimes plagued with guilt feelings because the overall attitude and feeling about power is often negative. Because of this distrust and negative attitude, open discussion and understanding of politics in hospitals never takes place. This misunderstanding is a handicap to pharmacy managers since, in today's complex hospital, the effective performance of most managerial jobs requires one to acquire and be skilled in the use of politics. Understanding the dynamics of politics will significantly increase the performance potential of most managers.

As stated earlier in this chapter, a key distinguishing characteristic of a pharmacy manager is their dependence on a variety of other people in order for them to do their job. This dependence is part of the manager's job because of two organizational facts of life: division of labor and limited resources. Since work within hospitals is divided into specialized areas, we are inherently dependent on division of labor. The limited resources available to these specialized areas further increases our dependency. It follows, then, that to do our job successfully we need to have some control over the people on whom we are dependent. Trying to control others, especially those outside of the pharmacy department, by directing them on the basis of our formal position, simply will not work. It will not work because we are always dependent on some people over whom we have no formal positional authority. For example, many pharmacies are dependent on their purchasing department to get purchase orders out on time and to get pharmaceutical contracts expedited. If this does not happen, there are potential drug outages. When the drugs do get purchased on time and are shipped to the institution, the first place they arrive is on the receiving dock. Should they sit there for an excessive amount of time, the same outage situation could occur. Without the efficient support of a purchasing and receiving department, a basic, but highly dependent position for the pharmacy, the credibility of pharmacy can be significantly weakened.

POWER TYPES

There are four different types of power that can be used to cope with the dependency inherent in our jobs (3). The degree to which the pharmacy manager uses one or all of these power types depends to a large extent on that manager's personal attitudes about power as well as the environment of a given hospital.

The first type of power relates to creating a sense of obligation. Opportunities will be identified for helping others at very little cost to the manager. This help can be as incidental as sending the nursing director a copy of an article you think will help her to solve a current problem she is experiencing. Offering to obtain data for an influential physician conducting an investigational study when the collection of that data will not place additional burden on the pharmacy will likely be viewed by that investigator as a favor he appreciates very much. In turn, it may be a favor that could obligate him to assist you in an important future program.

The second way in which the pharmacy manager can gain power is by building a reputation as an expert. This type of power must be established through visible achievement. This achievement, therefore, must be visible outside of the pharmacy department, and the larger it is, the more visible it will be. Developing programs or procedures that will have an impact on decreased length of stay, improved utilization of laboratory tests, e.g., a pharmacokinetics program, and developing effective bid management procedures for pharmaceuticals to contain costs are examples of visible achievements that will increase the expert reputation of the pharmacy manager in the minds of other influential people throughout the hospital.

The third method of gaining power is to foster personal identification. If people can have a positive identification with the pharmacy manager as a person, a degree of power will be derived from that identification. This requires charisma. This type of power can be used when talking with other influential people about departmental goals, values, and ideals.

The fourth way to attain power is to create a feeling of dependence on other people. Just as the pharmacy manager is dependent on others within the hospital to achieve results, the inverse is true in that the more an individual perceives that they are dependent on the pharmacy, the more they will be inclined to cooperate. There are two methods to create perceived dependence. First, we can identify and acquire the resources that other people require to do their jobs. These resources must not be available to the other people, nor can these resources be available from anyone other than the pharmacy. Examples of this resource could be that of a full-time coordinator for investigational drug services provided by the pharmacy that would greatly assist physicians in acquiring and maintaining high-level investigational studies. Offering a college of pharmacy the resources available through a pharmacy department in order to conduct clerkship education would not only assist the college of pharmacy in meeting its accreditation standards, but could also provide some additional income for the hospital by developing a contract with the college of pharmacy.

A second way to create dependence is by influencing other people's perceptions regarding pharmacy resources. Within the hospital, there are numerous situations in which the pharmacy manager is involved with people who do not continuously interact with the pharmacy, but on whom the pharmacy is still dependent. These people seldom possess hard facts about what the pharmacy's resources really are. Such areas of the hospital that might fall into this category could include voluntary services, laundry, social service, patient transportation, and other departmental services areas having little or no direct involvement with the pharmacy. It might also include individuals within the hospital organization with whom the pharmacy director infrequently interacts, such as the director of laboratory medicine or the chairman of pathology. Under these circumstances, the perception people have regarding the pharmacy manager, or the pharmacy department, may be acquired through tangential or even seemingly insignificant ways. Among these are such issues as dress, manner of speech, arrangement, tidiness and organization of the pharmacy, and the way the pharmacy director's office looks. If the hospital allows departments to print their name on hospital stationery, the department of pharmacy could gain perceived recognition through this simple technique. Numerous other seemingly incidental factors have significant psychologic impact on perceptions.

The successful pharmacy manager will selectively use one or more of these power types to gain a position of power and influence within the hospital. Keen selectivity of these skills is one key to successful interdepartmental relationships.

CHARACTERISTICS OF POWER USERS

There are a number of common characteristics the pharmacy manager must possess in order to be successful in acquiring power and using it to manage the dependence on others (4).

The first characteristic is sensitivity. This sensitivity encompasses the degree to which the manager considers others while he is acquiring and using power. A lack of sensitivity will result in the manager running over people and losing any credibility he may have gained. Using power of any type at the expense of another department will label the pharmacy manager as a user rather than a doer and will destroy his leadership image.

The second characteristic is understanding. The various types of power and methods of influence must be clearly understood before they are used. When and when not to use them will be a skill acquired to be successful.

The development of all the types of power discussed in this chapter is the third characteristic of a successful pharmacy manager. Methods that are more risky than others and that may cause backlash must be avoided in favor of those which are proved and acceptable.

Setting goals and objectives is the fourth characteristic. These will be developed for both the pharmacy department and the pharmacy manager, which will allow both to develop power and influence. Within the hospital, jobs, programs, and developments will be sought after that will use and enhance the political skills of the manager. Depending on the particular hospital setting, this could occur by chairing a cost-containment committee, a quality assurance committee, or other influential bodies. Assuming responsibility for drug administration or IV administration when beneficial to nursing service could broaden the base of power and influence for the pharmacy department.

Power-oriented behavior must be tempered by maturity and self-control. This fifth characteristic is perhaps the most important and can often be overlooked when selfish or single-sighted goals replace those of the department or hospital.

The last characteristic may be the hardest to achieve. Successful pharmacy managers accept the legitimacy of using power to influence people throughout other hospital departments. This legitimacy is acquired because of the positive approach to the political process rather than one of subversion and coercion.

USING POWER TO INFLUENCE DECISIONS AND POLICIES

Using power and influence requires an extensive amount of effort, time, and resources. As such, one is not likely to use power needlessly or wastefully. Furthermore, the potential for success will be enhanced if three conditions exist within the hospital. These conditions are scarcity, criticality, and uncertainty (5).

Scarcity

The power associated with resources has been previously discussed. These resources are usually identified as money, manpower, materials, space, and equipment. In every hospital these resources are unquestionably scarce. With the positive use of power, a pharmacy manager's ability to acquire these resources will be enhanced. Without the use of power, one's ability will be handicapped. Since these resources are scarce in hospitals, the political process flourishes.

Criticality

Drugs are a critical resource. With the increased cost of drugs, they are even becoming a more critical resource. Many pharmacy managers take this fact for granted and do not consciously capitalize on the fact that they already have an inherent power base. By exerting influence on policies and decisions regarding drug control, this influence will be interpreted by others within the hospital as very legitimate. The time and effort exerted to influence policies and decisions regarding a critical resource, in this case drugs, is not only legitimate, but is expected.

Uncertainty

When individuals within the hospital cannot agree about what should be done or how to do a particular task, exercising power and influence will directly affect the decision. The reason for this is quite simple. If there are no clear-cut criteria available to resolve a particular conflict, or problem, then the only way to resolve it comes from the social process, which includes politics. Under conditions of uncertainty, a powerful pharmacy manager can argue his case and usually win it. This is especially true when one is in charge of both scarce and critical resources. By not waiting for someone else to take charge of an uncertain situation, the pharmacy manager has another opportunity to enhance his position within the institution. In the current era of prospective payment systems and their relationships to diagnosis, the faster a pharmacy manager can address the controls necessary to contain or reduce pharmacy-related cost in those diagnosis related groups that lose money for the hospital, the broader will become the base of influence for the pharmacy department.

It is important, therefore, to realize that these three conditions—scarcity, criticality, and uncertainty—exist in every hospital. Because of this fact, the political process comes into play even more so by those individuals and departments who are competing for limited resources.

USING POLITICS FOR PROGRAM PROMOTION

Almost every new program that a pharmacy department wishes to implement will impact to one extent or another on other departments and other people throughout the hospital. The degree to which the pharmacy manager has established his power and influence will greatly affect the outcome of program promotion. The use of the political process within the hospital cannot simply start at the point where a new program is proposed. Rather, it must have been a deliberate and ongoing process, as previously described in this chapter.

Assuming that these political factors have been addressed successfully by the pharmacy manager, there are several points that must be considered to achieve positive program promotion.

Competition

Due to the fact that limited resources exist, and in turn promote the political process, one must establish where the competition is located. If the competition is from a department much larger and more influential than the pharmacy, e.g., the department of medicine or surgery, then the pharmacy will need to critically assess the probability of approval in relation to the political odds possessed by a medical department.

Support

The degree to which a program will be supported is often directly related to the benefits that will be derived by the recipients of the program. If, for example, the pharmacy manager is proposing the addition of an individual to implement an investigational drug services program, the medical staff may view this as significant support for their investigational drug efforts. On the other hand, a director of nursing who feels that drug administration belongs solely within the department of nursing will provide no support to the pharmacy for a drug administration program. Additional areas to review for support are those in which the pharmacy manager has established his power and influence in relation to obligation, expertise, dependence, or personal identification. It is at this juncture that the successful manager will draw on all of the time and effort that has been previously expended in developing a power base. Just as one invests money for future expenditures, so does the pharmacy manager invest time and effort in the political process.

Employee Attitudes

Often the attitude of influential employees within other departments will directly affect the decision makers of that department. For example, if the program being promoted is one that ultimately requires the approval of the chairman of the department of medicine, the previous ''favor'' of assisting an influential physician in his investigational drug studies may have bought a return favor from that physician in helping to convince his chairman that the proposed pharmacy program should receive medical support.

Trade-Offs

Using politics for program promotion may require certain trade-offs. These trade-offs may be seen in terms of time, money, or people. This may mean that the pharmacy manager will have to exercise negotiation skills as well as draw on his political base. For example, showing the director of laboratory medicine that costs for unnecessary laboratory tests can be decreased by supporting the pharmacy's pharmacokinetics program may provide the needed support from laboratory medicine, especially if there are other internal needs that can be met by the cost savings.

The use of politics, then, has no set formula. Rather, the astute pharmacy manager will know which power types to use in relation to the dynamics of his institution and will capitalize on his previous time and effort in developing his base of power and influence.

SUMMARY

Hospital politics is a fact of hospital life. Without it none of us would exist, and hospitals would not exist. Power and politics are not dirty words, but rather are forces to deal with, forces that must be in the managerial armamentarium of the successful pharmacy manager. Politics in this context is the process by which power and influence are acquired and exercised. Whether one has identified politics in the formal way presented in this chapter is secondary to the fact that it must be used within the hospital in order to be successful. By understanding the social psychology of hospitals and how one's leadership within the hospital can affect power and influence, pharmacy managers can acquire the skills necessary to use the political process in program promotion. Without those skills, there is little chance that the political process will be of any value. Equally important are the characteristics that power users possess. By adhering to these characteristics, substantial influence can be exerted on decisions and policies affecting limited resources that are scarce, critical, and uncertain.

To be successful, the pharmacy manager must analyze the hospital, the people in it, their formal and informal positions, and then identify the scarce, critical, and uncertain resources, acquire the power through modes of obligation, expertise, identification, and dependence, and set about legitimizing his authority in the eyes of those around him. By doing so, hospital politics will be one of the pharmacy manager's greatest assets.

REFERENCES

1. American Hospital Association: *Cross-Reference on Human Resources Management.* Chicago, AHA, vol 8, No. 1, 1978.
2. Korda M: *Power! How to Get It, How to Use It.* New York, Random House, 1975.
3. Kotter JP: Power, dependence and effective management. *Harv Bus Rev* 57:129-131, July/August 1977.
4. *ibid.,* pp 135-136.
5. Salancik GR, Pfeffer J: Who gets power and how they hold on to it. *Organ Dynam* 6:13, Winter, 1977.

CHAPTER 20

Professional Staff Management

JAMES C. McALLISTER, LESLIE REUSS MACKOWIAK, and JOHN I. MACKOWIAK

Professional staff management is one of the most complex and challenging responsibilities of today's pharmacist manager. The definition of management, getting work done through others (1), emphasizes that personnel management is the basic means by which organizational objectives are accomplished.

Personnel management is itself challenging, yet the management of professionals is frought with unique complications. Basic requirements for any pharmacy degree and licensure render the professional a well-educated employee who, having met these requirements, may feel that he does not need to be managed. Perhaps these sentiments stem from the very credible focus of the educational system on professional activities and individual performance and accomplishment. Little emphasis is placed on group dynamics to engender teamwork or the achievement of organizational goals.

Professional staff management is made increasingly difficult when one recognizes the influx of ''baby boomers'' into hospital pharmacy practice and examines their nature. This generation has been categorized as being spoiled, requiring constant attention and immediate gratification, and having endless desires for material goods. Indeed, they may sometimes exhibit behavior that reflects an attitude that the institution owes them a job and all the benefits that go with it.

Hepler (2) suggests that behavioral changes have resulted from the professionalization of pharmacy practitioners. They tend to (1) rely on informal and formal collegial associations rather than the management hierarchy for guidance and evaluation; (2) emphasize their ultimate personal responsibility for the service they render; and (3) insist that they be given final authority to choose the exact nature and manner of the services they provide. Managers must consider these assumptions while their management styles and systems are being developed and may need to interact with and through collegial groups as well as individuals. Finally, managers should facilitate professional staff input through participative organizational systems and must ensure that individual and organizational objectives and procedures are well defined and do not conflict.

Professional staff management is likely to become even more difficult in the future. Institutional pharmacy managers will experience pressures to manage more quantitatively as a result of diminishing personnel resources, increased competition among hospitals, decreased utilization of hospital care, and increased availability of computerized management information. The labor-intensity emphasis on technologic advances and productivity enhancements may conflict with a personalized management style, despite the success that has been encountered by managers who have used it. Posey (3) described the potential impact of the influx of baby boomers on hospital pharmacy with respect to the age shift in the practitioner population. These phenomena are likely to compound the obstacles facing the pharmacist manager and warrant continued modification of management styles.

Personnel management is one facet of the *science* of management, a specialty that must be studied and practiced as any other practice specialty. This chapter will provide an overview of management styles, theories, and philosophies and their application to professional staff management. The importance of communication systems for personnel management will be presented. Planning the professional staff management system is presented. A comprehensive departmental plan begins with establishment of job descriptions and assessment of human resource needs. Managing pharmacists begins during the interview and hiring process and is followed by orientation efforts. The professional staff management plan should also facilitate individual staff development, career development and personal growth, and management of stress. Motivation theory and performance appraisal will be discussed and suggestions for enhancing both described. The managers' responsibilities in preparing the professional staff for changes and reconciling intradepartmental conflict are also presented. Management ethics are discussed, including responsibilities the manager has to his staff and commitment to affirmative action and equal opportunity.

MANAGEMENT STYLES

To be effective, a pharmacy manager should use the management planning approach and management style that is the most comfortable and practical (4). Styles are popularly categorized as autocratic or participative and are based on one of several theories—Theory X, Theory Y, or Theory Z.

McGregor's Theory X management assumptions describe employees as being lazy, irresponsible, less than intelligent, resistant to change and requiring close supervision (5). In such an environment, all planning, setting of objectives, and decision making is done alone by the manager. The professional may follow the autocratic manager out of respect for his insight and past successes or as a result of subtle implications of intimidation or fear of retribution. The resultant organization may be characterized by employees who become lazy, lack initiative, and avoid responsibility.

Theory Y managers assume that employees are hardworking, responsible, enjoy their work, work for reasons beyond money, and need only to be supported and encouraged. These managers create opportunities and an environment to encourage peak performance through participative planning and establishment of objectives by all employees. In this environment, managers facilitate self-direction and self-control through an objective-oriented plan resulting in an orgainzation whose employees are relatively satisfied, find their jobs challenging, assume responsibility, and are innovative.

Theory Z organizations are characterized as an extension of a participative management style (6). In such a system, each employee who is affected by a decision is given an opportunity to provide input in the decision-making process.

Several authors have emphasized the importance of the manager's positive or winning attitude as it affects employees and their productivity (7-9). Successful managers are optimistic and enthusiastic, possess a positive self-image, and are self-directed. They are organized, accept responsibility for their action, and are self-disciplined. Finally, today's managers must learn from the past, plan the future, and live in the present, project their best selves, and above all, communicate effectively.

The result of such positive management attitudes was best described by Zellmer (10) as a good place to work—one which crackles with the electricity of enthusiasm and commitment to improving service. Such an environment can be achieved when managers have five basic characteristics—they are open with people, use a team approach to management, give people important work to do, avoid crisis through effective planning, and do not suffer from self-perfectionism.

The nature of professionals, their background, and career goals are probably best served through a participative management scheme. In such an organization, the professional staff manager must exhibit a leadership style compatible with the organization and plan of action. He serves as a role model and sets the tone for achieving departmental goals through the personnel management system. The participative manager must also know his professional staff, their capabilities, and interests—a responsibility that begins during the interview process. To accomplish this, the manager should be approachable, sensitive, and responsive.

The participative professional staff manager must next provide a forum for exchanging information with the pharmacists and develop plans of action with their assistance. Individual tasks or projects are then appropriately delegated to the staff with well-defined limits of freedom and authority. The delegated tasks must be achievable and a date for their completion identified.

The manager should then allow the pharmacist to proceed with the assignment alone, providing general guidance and support on an "as needed" basis. Periodic progress evaluations as well as evaluation of the completed project should be conducted by the manager with the pharmacist. Positive feedback and constructive criticism are the hallmarks for individual professional growth and future motivation.

Perhaps the most difficult behavior for the professional staff manager to exhibit is keeping an open mind and compromising one's biases when evaluating a completed project. As long as the goal has been achieved, he must recognize the accomplishment even though details of the project may not be consistent with the manager's expectations. Essential expectations should have been communicated prior to assumption of the task. Failure to recognize the professional's efforts will likely discourage future participation.

COMMUNICATING WITH PROFESSIONAL STAFF

Communication is the means by which organized activity is unified, enables growth and improvement, and is essential to learning. Since professional staff management involves the achievement of departmental goals through others, communication is the framework on which the personnel management system is built. The pharmacist manager must use written, verbal, and nonverbal forms of communication to effectively manage his professional staff.

Many pharmacists perceive written communication skills as a "gift" which, if absent, cannot be effectively improved. While it may be true that creative writers must have particular aptitudes for their style of writing, the skills involved with utility-based writing used by the pharmacist manager can be acquired (11). Detailed suggestions for improving written communications skills is beyond the scope of this chapter, but the major components of the written communication process are identifying the messages to be conveyed, organizing the thoughts to be presented, converting the thoughts to a written form, and editing the final copy. Once these basic components are understood by the manager, he must become comfortable with a consistent writing style and, most important, he must practice.

Written communications facilitate the presentation of complicated or detailed information and ensure more effective transmission of an accurate message. Written material documents the message for retrospective review and allows careful consideration. The manager must remember, however, that written forms of communication discourage reciprocal communication and limit the amount of information presented.

All of us probably overestimate our verbal and nonverbal communication skills since we inaccurately think of "talking" as communicating. As with written communication skills, the pharmacist manager can significantly improve his skills by studying various techniques set forth by other authors (12,13). Pharmacist managers should also recognize that listening is a critical part of the communication process that is often overlooked, since studies have shown that most people listen at an effective rate of 25%.

Verbal communication enables the transmission of nonverbal messages, since emotional, environmental, and personal factors often modify spoken words. More important, it facilitates reciprocal communication and allows flexibility in the style or content of the material presented, depending on the responses of the listeners. Verbal communications can be intimidating and are also subject to more frequent misunderstandings or misinterpretations. Verbal communication minimizes retrospective consideration of material presented and limits one's ability to communicate detailed data.

The communications system for professional staff management must include methods for both upward and downward communications. Upward communication is the transmission of information from subordinates to managers. The manager must clearly define what he needs to know and establish a means by which the information is communicated. The detail of data transmitted should also be clearly understood by subordinates to prevent unnecessary work and to avoid overwhelming the manager.

Downward communication is the transmission of information from managers to subordinates. The manager should share all information that is essential for the activities of the pharmacist. The amount of data transmitted should give the employee a sense of belonging, provide a means for continuing education, and stimulate more active participation in departmental activities. Sensitive information can be shared, depending on the integrity of the employees, but sometimes must be limited to a "need to know" basis. It is extremely important that the pharmacist manager avoid a situation in which employees find out information from sources outside their peer group—the "we're always the last to know" phenomenon.

The mechanisms by which information is shared by managers and their professional staff vary depending on the size of the staff, their individual responsibilities, their accessibility, and the management style used. Written documents facilitate the transmission of identical information to many people. This may be accommodated by issuing multiple copies of a memorandum or by circulation of a single copy for their review. If the latter method is used, the manager should request readers to initial the circulated copy to verify its review by each individual.

The manager may also request weekly or monthly written reports from their professional staff regarding their activities, suggestions, or observations. These reports should be succinct, highlighting only the basic concepts or comments, and may be a useful adjunct to periodic meetings with the staff. Such a system allows subordinates to systematically pass on useful information and, if mandatory, can be a painless method for teaching pharmacists how to organize their thoughts and improve their writing skills. The pharmacist manager can then request more detailed information on the highest priority items. When this system is used, the manager is obliged to review all the reports, feed back to the employee the most important information, and follow up any unresolved problems.

Periodic staff meetings are an effective way to communicate more information to the professional staff and facilitate clarification of unclear messages. These meetings can be multi-tiered meetings of segregated staffs (e.g., each satellite or major work unit) as well as meetings for the entire staff. Meetings of a subgroup helps engender cohesiveness and sense of purpose within the group and allows them to focus on a unique problem and discuss possible solutions. A meeting of the entire staff allows the transmission of identical data to all and enhances feelings of belonging to the organization. Our experience has shown that a system which employs both types of meetings produces positive results, especially when such meetings are conducted on a regular basis.

The communication system used by the professional staff manager must be consistent with his management style and must meet his own needs as well as those of his staff. It should permit the exchange of necessary information in a timely fashion and should accommodate both upward and downward communication.

HUMAN RESOURCE PLANNING

The most valuable resource in institutional pharmacy is its people, especially its professional staff. Just as in any other facet of pharmacy management, a human resource *plan* is important.

Pharmacists who perform routine distributive functions are generally dissatisfied (13). More diverse roles are emerging for the pharmacist. The workplace is full of change because of limited health care dollars, increasing numbers of graduating pharmacists, and limited upward mobility resulting from large numbers of hospital pharmacy directors and managers under 40 years of age (14). Under these circumstances, strategic planning for human resource management becomes an essential, yet challenging goal for the pharmacy manager.

Human resource development is a relatively new field. One of the best examples of human resource development is in team sports. Everyone is familiar with the football team that strives for a winning program through recruiting, hiring, training, developing, playing, and analyzing its players each year. The coach assesses each player's strengths and weaknesses and assigns that player an appropriate position on the team. Development of the professional staff prepares pharmacists for key positions within the pharmacy. Just as a winning football team needs players with different skills and abilities, pharmacy departments require pharmacists whose skills complement each other to achieve organizational goals.

A human resource plan generally has long-term goals and objectives based on the manager's premises and forecasts. Some literature recommends a 7-year plan as a minimum (15). The internal and external environment of the pharmacy should be reviewed. The human resource plan should facilitate the organization's goals and objectives and coordinate with the overall plan for services. After the scope of services is determined, a compatible organizational structure should be developed based on the preferred management style, spans of control, and centralized vs decentralized decision making. Organizational design studies show that the most successful organizations have a good fit between the organizational structure and the organization's technologies developed to achieve its goals (16). Technologies are the activities, equipment, and knowledge necessary to turn inputs into outputs. Mass production fits well with tall structures. Decentralized pharmacies have a good fit with horizontal structure.

Job Descriptions

A specific job description should be written for each pharmacist role or position. It should list the skills, abilities, and knowledge needed to perform that job adequately. Oral communication skills may be very important for a cardiology clinician who advises physicians on rounds and conducts nursing in-service training. Time management skills and a general knowledge base may be important for a pharmacist in the central distribution area.

Hackman and Oldham (17) identify five characteristics to consider in describing jobs.

1. Skill variety: Degree to which a job requires a variety of activities—also called job breadth
2. Task identity: Job requires completion of whole identifiable pieces of work
3. Task significance: Degree to which the job has a substantial impact on the lives of other people
4. Autonomy: Degree to which job provides freedom, independence, and discretion—also called job depth
5. Job feedback: Degree to which carrying out the work activities required by the job provides individual with direct and clear information about effectiveness of performance.

Increasing the extent to which each characteristic is reflected in the job enhances the level of satisfaction for most pharmacists. It is a challenge for the manager to establish job descriptions with these qualities and still maintain control over services and finances. Massey (18) describes the baby boomers as a "challenger" generation which values experiences, work for self-fulfillment, causes, individualism, and questioning. These correspond to skill variety, task identity, task significance, autonomy, and job feedback. Professionals will demand that their jobs have these characteristics.

Staff Review

The manager must get to know his staff and discover each member's strengths and weaknesses and how they best fit into the organizational design. He should also assist them in developing skills directed toward new roles or improving weaknesses. To increase skill variety and staff flexibility, the manager can rotate pharmacists through different staff positions and work areas.

The manager has the responsibility to ensure that the pharmacist has the skills necessary to meet the responsibility of each position to which he is assigned. Self-analysis and employee tests are available to help the manager assess these skills and abilities. A good job "fit" is important. Job misfit results in unhappy and tense workers (19).

Recruitment, Hiring, and Interviewing

There are many methods by which a manager can recruit a professional staff. These include keeping an applicant file, advertising in newspapers or professional journals, placement services, state pharmacy organizations, American Society of Hospital Pharmacists Midyear placement service, through colleagues, and through schools of pharmacy (20). The method of recruitment used will depend on the level of pharmacist desired, pharmacy budget, and hospital location.

Once the applicants are identified, the interviewing process begins. White (20) lists a traditional strategy that includes four steps in interviewing as (1) putting the applicant at ease, (2) obtaining information from the applicant, (3) giving information about the position, and (4) formally wrapping up the interview. Another interview plan is called targeted selection, or the assessment center method. The basic interview plan has several steps. The interviewing team meets before the interview to decide which assessment dimensions are important for a particular position. Assessment dimensions include leadership, behavioral flexibility, risk-taking, tolerance for stress, and oral communication skills. The interviewing team then formulates questions that will cause the applicant to describe behavior that demonstrates the desired dimensions.

The interview emphasis of this method is on the applicant's past behavior, rather than on their theories, ideas, or reactions to hypothetical situations. Past behavior is the best predictor of future behavior. An example question for a clinical pharmacist where initiative is considered an important dimension might be, "Did you propose any new services in your previous job?" followed by, "Can you give me an example of one?" or "Tell me exactly what you did."

The interviewing team then meets to discuss each applicant's dimensions, validating opinions with examples of the applicant's behavior. This method decreases the potential for halo effects, stereotyping, too rapid decision making, and pressures to fill a position.

Orientation and Training

Once an appropriate applicant is hired, it is important to properly orient the pharmacist to the department since his initial impressions of the organization will become the foundation on which attitudes will evolve. The manager should begin by supplying information on policies, procedures, and philosophies of the pharmacy department and hospital. The manager should then explain the department's goals and objectives, their stage of development, and the departmental expectations of the pharmacist. An organizational chart with names and titles is helpful. Key people need to be identified and available information sources should be described.

The pharmacist comes onto the staff with a professional degree and licensure that identifies that person as a trained professional, because colleges are used as the formal training ground. However, some in-house training may be necessary to introduce the new staff member to the specific services and systems of the institution. While training programs may be expensive, they minimize potential for errors and better prepare the pharmacist to represent the department effectively. A training program improves the potential for the pharmacist to become a successful department member and a valuable resource to the pharmacy.

Development Programs

Professional staff development should be an ongoing part of the strategic plan. The program should be flexible and individualized, since pharmacists may learn at different rates or accomplish behavioral changes more rapidly. The development program can include:

- Personal skills such as communication or creative problem-solving skills
- Interpersonal skills such as team building or issues in pharmacy and technical roles
- Managerial skills such as assessing employee performance or managing conflict
- Clinical skills such as a comprehensive knowledge of cancer chemotherapy or methods for using the Iowa system
- Stress management skills such as training in identifying employee signs of stress

Since most institutional budgets and time are limited for professional staff development programs, the manager must be creative. There are many resources available within most hospitals at no cost, including physician conferences and grand rounds, or programs offered through the institution's personnel department. The personnel department staff should be trained in employee relations and could assist in developing a program for the department. Experienced professional staff can develop programs to teach other staff about their areas of interest, including operations management, clinical skills, or administrative techniques and methods.

Pharmaceutical vendors offer a variety of teaching materials available in the form of films, video cassettes, guest speakers, and programmed learning texts. Public or college libraries may loan out films or materials on management or personal development. National, state, and local pharmaceutical associations as well as schools of pharmacy offer programs and conduct seminars on a wide variety of topics that can assist in professional staff development. Pharmacists should be encouraged to attend these programs when possible.

Freedom from regular duties to attend development programs is difficult, since personnel resources are usually limited. Establishing objectives, direction, and timetables for the development of each employee will help him select the most beneficial programs. Management by objective is a useful management tool to help in accomplishing this.

Career Development

Career development is the responsibility of the individual pharmacist but should be encouraged and supported by the manager. The path-goal theory of leadership states that one of the most important activities of leaders is to clarify the paths to various goals of interest to subordinates. The effective leader forms a connection between subordinate goals and organizational goals. The manager can help bridge this connection through informal counseling and directing or through a more formal career path or ladder.

Schneider and Dzierba (23) discussed a competency-based employee advancement program. Their plan encompasses five pharmacist levels of competency with a point system and specific criteria for advancing from one level to the next. The state of North Carolina pharmacy system has developed a two-track, five-level system for career advancement. They found it important to have separate tracks for clinically oriented and management oriented career development. Each level has a basic skills description (24). Seminars on the "how to's" of career development or skills for

success may also be incorporated in the human resource development programs.

Stress Management

Stress is defined as the nonspecific response of the body to any demand (25). Stress can be classified as positive (eustress) or negative (distress). Some stress can help to motivate an employee. Too much stress can lead to a condition called burnout. Burnout occurs at the end of continuous but distinct stages of maladaptive response to one or more long-term stressors.

People may react to the same stressor (demand) differently and to different degrees. It is ironic that the high achievers who pharmacy managers want to have working for them are the most prone to distress, mainly because of their unrealistic expectations (26).

The main two kinds of stressors are personal stress and stress at work. Sources of stress at work can be intrinsic to the job (time pressures and deadlines). They can also result from the role in the organization (e.g., role conflict), career development (e.g., underpromotion), relationships at work (e.g., threats from below), or organizational structure and climate (e.g., lack of participation) (27). The manager should be aware of these sources of stress and try to minimize these when selecting a management style, creating an organizational structure, writing job descriptions, managing conflict and change, and designing the physical workplace. Stress can also result when professional development is moving too rapidly or too slowly.

The professional staff manager should be sensitive to stress and burnout in himself and the employees and be aware of resources available and measures offered for dealing with them.

In today's competitive health care market, institutional pharmacy managers may look to industry for insight into personnel management. One article (13) summarizes human resource management by stating:

> These increased problems in achieving a "quality level" set of employees have made this HRM strategy, when successfully carried out, a uniquely dynamic competitive weapon. But it is more important than ever to recruit and develop a high-quality group of employees, for companies with a head start are hard to catch. Their good people attract others like them, while conventional organizations have to accept what is left.
>
> Human resource planning can act as a catalyst and an operating mechanism to accelerate the building of an effective work force. Where this is accomplished, people are energized and committed and become the most powerful, fundamental corporate competitive resource of all.

Motivation and Performance

One of the most frequent misconceptions managers have about motivation is that they confuse it with morale. Motivation is the process by which human behavior is activated. It is also concerned with what directs or channels such behavior and how this behavior can be maintained or sustained (28). Morale is a state of mental and emotional well-being that may or may not be related to behavior on the job (29). From research done during the 1950s and 1960s, it became increasingly apparent that workers with high morale were not always productive and high productivity was sometimes found in places with low morale. Thus, the motivation to perform is not synonymous with professional staff morale.

Successful football coaches like the late Vince Lombardi would probably have agreed with this notion. He chose other motivators to increase the productivity of players, and in the end he found that productivity or winning the Super Bowl makes players happy. Achievement often increases morale of employees more than morale increases achievement. Understanding this difference is the first step in increasing productivity. The second step is to understand what motivates or activates professional staff to perform. What drives them to be productive? For a better understanding of this question, it is helpful to turn to the three groups of theories that have been espoused to explain the process: behaviorism, the content theories, and process theories.

Behaviorism simply looks at behavior and its consequences. Everyone who took an introductory psychology course learned about Skinner's operant conditioning (30). A relationship is built between behavior and a positive or negative reinforcement. Omission of the reinforcement or punishment will extinguish a pattern of behavior.

For a number of reasons, the use of positive reinforcers to encourage a behavior and omission of reinforcers to discourage a behavior is preferable to regular use of punishment. Pharmacists punished for being late are more likely to learn not to let the supervisor know they snuck in late rather than to be in on time. They may also become angry or resentful. Punishing the creative but dangerous efforts of an employee may lead to suppressing all creative efforts, even if they are not dangerous.

A number of positive reinforcers have been very effective. In one example using positive reinforcement, when a monthly lottery for a $25 prize was held for all employees with perfect punctual attendance record, sick leave payments were reduced 62% and tardiness and absenteeism reduced 75% (31). To reward good attendance, employees could use their unused sick days to purchase books or attend seminars. Verbal positive reinforcements are also thought to be very effective.

Need theories ask what motivates people. Examples include Maslow's hierarchy of need (32) and Herzberg's two-factor theory (33). The needs include security, love, esteem, personal growth, achievement, responsibility, interesting or challenging work, and autonomy. The important concept in applying the need theories is that each person has a different set of unsatisfied needs that changes over time. As a result, the factors that increase or maintain productivity in one employee may cause a decrease in the motivation of another. It becomes the manager's responsibility to know the professional staff well enough to realize which are motivated or activated by esteem, which by security, or which ones thrive on challenge.

Younger pharmacists may have a very different set of unmet needs than their older counterparts because of their different value structure. Observers feel the baby boomers have a greater need for flexibility, autonomy, and personal growth (34). To satisfy a pharmacist's need for such growth through interesting and challenging work, the manager could rotate staff through different pharmacy areas or provide meaningful additional assignments for employees. Motivation by redesigning a job has been described earlier in this chapter.

Process theories ask how motivation occurs. An example, expectancy theory, may be called a thinking person's theory of motivation. A person's motivation to perform is equal to the employees preference for a set of outcomes (raise, new house, promotion) multiplied by the employee's perception of the chance of the behavior (drug monitoring) being associated with the outcomes, multiplied by the employee's perception of his chance at succeeding at the behavior (affecting drug therapy) (35).

Using expectancy theory to guide a manager's action; communicating the importance of certain behaviors to achieve outcomes; and training, supporting, and encouraging employees to perform the desired behaviors would be expected to increase productivity if the outcomes are desired by the employees.

Regular use of valid performance appraisal instruments assist in communicating the relative importance of behaviors. The instrument should measure the behaviors or outcomes associated with job success. Rarely should instruments measure personality traits of facets that may be related to one's background.

Some form of mutual goal setting, such as management by objectives (MBO), can also be motivating if done properly. To increase productivity, a method of translating the organizations goals into individual goals is necessary. To be effective motivators, the goals should be specific, challenging, and accepted by the staff member. The MBO process should be an ongoing series of meetings between the manager and the pharmacist to monitor his progress, clarify reasons for success or failure, and reestablish of modify goals as necessary (36).

The accuracy of an appraisal should not be taken lightly. The results of the appraisal process may have serious effects on an employee's career, aspirations, and self-esteem. If managers are not confident in their ability to assess an employee's performance of a certain behavior, it would be better not to complete the appraisal than to mislead the employee. If managers use appraisals, it is their responsibility to guarantee their accuracy and provide specific examples to employees when behavior is not what is expected.

Managing Conflict and Change

Sometime managers are called on to resolve conflict between professional staff members. Not only is it difficult to do successfully, but it is often avoided because most managers find it personally stressful. Conflict within an organization should not always be discouraged, since it may reflect an organization in which members are committed to their work. Conflict can create challenges, attention, and may increase effort, whereas lack of conflict may indicate stagnation.

The potential for conflict increases when two people or groups perform similar tasks, have different goals, and must share resources. If pharmacists jointly manage the same technicians, one may want the technician to enter orders into the computer while the other feels he should do work related to inventory control. Since one pharmacist is concerned with short-term patient care goals and the other is more concerned with long-term operations management goals, conflict can be predicted.

In conflict resolution, the manager must always try to get to the source of the conflict and not try for short-term solutions. To do this, the pharmacy manager should not act as a referee and settle the dispute by decree but should facilitate the staff in discussing the problem and identifying a solution. Often this will result in a compromise position and collaboration to resolve the conflict.

Conflict can be functional because it is the predecessor of change. Change enables an organization to adapt to the environment, thereby allowing it to survive. Even though change may be necessary for the organization, resistance from pharmacists often results. Reasons for this include uncertainty of the future, change in familiar comfortable habits, altering interpersonal relationships, or a feeling of powerlessness (37). In handling the change process, most managers rely on one of two methods: communication and education or participation and involvement of employees in the change planning process. Other techniques of change management are support, negotiation, manipulation, or coercion. The last two methods may expedite the change process but may result in future problems with employees. Support is especially useful when staff members have difficulty adjusting to new procedures (38).

Management Ethics

As the health care environment evolves, the hospital pharmacy director is commanding a greater influence within the hospital. Associated with this change is the increasing opportunity to compromise one's managerial ethics. Ethics can be defined as a set of rules and values, often unwritten, which distinguish between right and wrong and describe the moral duty and obligations a pharmacist has to the community.

Management ethics involve decision making and problem solving without compromising professional standards or priorities. During times of emphasis on economies, the professional staff manager must ensure that quality of services is not undermined by excessively reduced resources. For example, a failure to document a verbal order because of time constraints is not an acceptable compromise when staff is limited. Similarly, assumption of professional responsibilities by technicians may not satisfy pharmaceutical service standards. The ethical manager must be realistic in the demands that are placed on their professional staff to achieve organizational goals.

The hiring and promotion of professional staff also must be done ethically. In 1982, 52% of pharmacy students were women (39), whereas the number of female pharmacists increased from 10-25% in the last decade (40). In light of these and other changes, equal opportunity extends beyond the initial hiring process and into opportunity for special training programs and projects, committees, increased responsibilities, and promotions. Managers must ask themselves if they have a true commitment to affirmative action or if they are just following the guidelines and regulations.

Managers are also responsible for complying with the Equal Pay Act of 1963, which requires men and women to be paid equally when they are doing the same job. In the future, managers will also be faced with the issue of comparable worth, which states that an employee's salary should be determined by the complexity of the job, not the demand for the service. Comparable worth is intended to reduce sex discrimination, because jobs predominantly held by women are often paid less than comparable jobs held by men (41). These and other ethical questions will continue to face pharmacy managers as they work to meet society's need for pharmacy services in the future.

CONCLUSION

Professional staff management is a complex responsibility that requires constant awareness, sensitivity, and planning to achieve optimal results. The disparity in size and scope of institutional pharmacy organizations precludes the recommendation of a single management style or system for all situations. Indeed, both autocratic and participative management efforts will be needed on different occasions.

The professional staff manager should recognize that participative management systems are probably the most effective means for managing pharmacists. The ability to actively contribute to the growth or modification of the pharmacy department is frequently motivational and should encourage peak performance. This can only be accomplished through effective communication between the manager and the professional staff. The use of a comprehensive plan for meeting the needs of the organization and its individual members concomitantly is also essential.

The manager of professional staff should realize that failure of an employee to attain individual goals or meet performance standards may reflect the failure of the manager to adequately lead and direct the staff. Optimally, the manager will create a system and an environment in which pharmacists not only have more input in making organizational decisions but also have an incentive to and responsibility for making the system work.

REFERENCES

1. Couch PO: Learning to be a middle manager. *Mgt Dig* 10(2):18-24, 1979.
2. Hepler CD: Professions in modern society: Contract vs. covenant. Pharm Manager 151(3):102-104, 1979.
3. Posey LM: Managing baby-boom pharmacists in the information age. *Am J Hosp Pharm* 41:890, 1984.
4. Herkimer AG: Strategies for pharmacy management planning and job design. *Top Hosp Pharm Mgt* 3(2):8-16, 1983.
5. McGregor D: *The Human Side of Enterprise.* New York, McGraw-Hill, 1961.
6. Ouchie W: *Theory Z: How American Business Can Meet the Japanese Challenge.* Reading, MA, Addison-Wesley, 1981.
7. Waitley DA: *The Psychology of Winning.* Chicago, Nightingale-Conant, 1979.
8. Dubrin AJ: *Winning at Office Politics.* New York, Ballantine, 1978.
9. White SG: Managing the pharmacy manager. *Am J Hosp Pharm* 41:516-521, 1984.
10. Zellmer WA: A good place to work. *Am J Hosp Pharm* 41:889, 1984.
11. Trudeau T: The pharmacy manager as a communicator. Part I: Effective writing. *Top Hosp Pharm Mgt* 2(4):42-55, 1983.
12. Smith TR, Grau M: The pharmacy manager as a communicator. Part

    II: Verbal and nonverbal communications. Top Hosp Pharm Mgt 3(1):50-63, 1983.

13. Stewart JE: Hospital pharmacists' job satisfaction: A review of the data. *Top Hosp Pharm Mgt* 3(1):1-9, 1983.

14. Posey ML: Managing baby-boom pharmacists in the information age. *Am J Hosp Pharm* 41:890, 1984.

15. Skinner W: Big hat, no cattle: Managing human resources. *Harvard Bus Rev* 59:112-116, September/October 1981.

16. Woodward J: *Industrial Organization: Theory and Practice*. London, Oxford University Press, 1965.

17. Hackman JR, Oldham GR: The properties of motivating jobs. In *Work Redesign*. Reading, MA, Addison-Wesley, 1980.

18. Massey M: *The People Puzzle*. Reston, VA, Reston Publishing, 1979.

19. Bartolome F, Evans PA: Must success cost so much? *Harvard Bus Rev* 58:137-148, March/April, 1980.

20. White SJ: Recruiting, interviewing, and hiring pharmacy personnel. *Am J Hosp Pharm* 41:928-934, 1984.

21. *Targeted Selection, A Training Manual*. Pittsburgh, PA, Development Dimensions International.

22. House, RJ, Mitchell TR: Path-goal theory of leadership, *J Contemp Bus* 3:81-97, Autumn 1974.

23. Schneider PJ, Dzierba SH: Competency-based employee advancement. *Top Hosp Pharm Mgt* 3(1):37-49, 1983.

24. *Policy and Procedure Manual*. North Carolina Memorial Hospital, Chapel Hill, NC.

25. Selye H: *Stress in Health and Disease*. Boston, Butterworth Publishers, 1976.

26. Freudenberger HJ: *Burnout: The high cost of achievement*. Garden City, NY, Anchor Press, 1980.

27. Cooper GL, Marshall J: Occupational sources of stress: A review of the literature relating to coronary heart disease and mental health. *Occup Psychol* 50:49, 1976.

28. Steers RM, Porter LW: *Motivation and Work Behavior*. New York, McGraw-Hill, 1979, p 6.

29. Gray JL: *Supervision*. Boston, Kent Publishing, 1984, p 142.

30. Skinner BF: *About Behaviorism*. New York, Vintage, 1976.

31. Hampton DR, Summer CE, Webber RA: *Organizational Behavior and the Practice of Management*. Glenview IL, Scott, Foresman, 1982.

32. Maslow AH: A theory of human motivation. *Psychol Rev* 50(4):29-47, 1943.

33. Herzberg F, Mausner B, Syndermon B: *The Motivation to Work*, New York, John Wiley & Sons, 1959.

34. Anon: Baby boomers push for power. *Bus Week* 2:52-62, July 1984.

35. Vroom VH: *Work and Motivation*. New York, John Wiley & Sons, 1964.

36. Locke EA, Shaw KN, Soari LM, Latham GP: Goal setting and task performance. *Psychol Bull* 90:125-152, 1981.

37. Byron RL: Resistance to change. *Curr Concepts Hosp Pharm Mgt* 2:6-8, 1980.

38. Kotter JP, Schlesinger LA: Choosing strategies for change. *Harvard Bus Rev* 57:106-114, 1979.

39. Chasin SH: Enrollment report on professional degree programs in pharmacy, fall 1982. *Am J Pharm Educ* 47:275-288, 1983.

40. Nice FJ, Schondelmeyer SW, Bootman JL: Women in pharmacy management—why not? *Am Pharm* NS24:214-219, 1984.

41. Seligman D: Pay equity is a bad idea. *Fortune* 110(9):133-140, 1984.

ADDITIONAL READING

Drucker PF: *Management: Tasks, Responsibilities, Practices*. New York, Harper & Row, 1974, p 111.

Harold K, O'Donnel C: *Essentials of Management*. New York, McGraw-Hill, 1974, p 1.

Knapp ML: *Nonverbal Communication in Human Interaction*. New York, Holt, Rinehart & Winston, 1972.

Noel MW, Bootman JL: *Hospital Pharmacy Human Resources Management*. Bethesda, Aspen Systems, 1985.

Personnel management series. *Am J Hosp Pharm* 41:318-319, 516-521, 928-934, 1173-1177, 1361-1366, 1567-1573, 1824-1828, February-September, 1984.

Russell C et al: *Interpersonal Communication in Pharmacy*. New York, Appleton-Century-Crofts, 1982.

CHAPTER 21

Financial Fundamentals

HAROLD M. SILVERMAN

Hospital pharmacy managers must have an appreciation of the basics of finance in order to be effective as planners and administrators in today's increasingly complex institutional environment. Certainly, we are faced with decisions related to finance and/or accounting on a daily basis.

Understanding these principles and knowing how to use them to our benefit will strengthen our overall management skill and increase our effectiveness, especially when dealing with administrative staff members. The purpose of this chapter will be to review and introduce some fundamental concepts of finance and accounting and to illustrate their application to institutional pharmacy.

FUNCTION OF ACCOUNTING

When asked the function of their accounting departments, many institutional pharmacy managers will simply reply, "harassment." Despite this seemingly practical point of view, the basic function served by accounting is to provide information about monetary matters. Three of the basic ways in which we use the principles of accounting will be reviewed.

Accountability

Accounting is most commonly used by management to ensure that organizational monies are disbursed appropriately and efficiently. Accounting provides a mechanism for allowing institutional management to monitor how monies are allocated and spent. Have we responsibly allocated our budgets? Have we remained within the allowed expenditure allocations for drugs, other supplies, personnel, books and journals? Accounting systems allow us to see that money is used in a manner that is both proper and efficient.

Outside Information

Accounting systems provide information about the overall health of the organization to employees, creditors, stockholders, and others outside the institution. This information takes the form of an annual report or statement that serves as a means to communicate the financial health of an institution to interested parties. Who might be interested in this kind of information? The answer to that question depends on the corporate organization of your hospital. As recipients of public monies, all institutions must provide information on their financial status to regulatory agencies and third-party payors. A for-profit institution must supply this information to current and potential investors; voluntary nonprofit institutions must provide financial information to benefactors, public agencies, and others who are potential supporters of the institution. Public or tax-supported institutions, such as county or state hospitals, must provide this information to financial underwriters and others seeking to support the activities of the institution through the purchase of long-term debt notes or bonds. States, municipalities, and other governmental jurisdictions that run hospitals or medical centers often seek to obtain capital financing through the issuance of bonds. The ratings of these bonds, which serve as a mechanism for establishing their value, will be affected by the status of the institution, as reflected by financial information.

Program Analyses

Accounting furnishes the raw data for program analysis. The bases for determining the potential value of a new program and evaluating the viability of an existing program can usually be found in one kind of financial information or another.

In the hospital, a host of opportunities exist for analyzing, evaluating, and implementing both new and old services can be derived from financial information. Fortunately, pharmacy managers have not been faced with performing such analyses on a continuous basis, but the need to do so arises often enough that an understanding of the fundamentals of accounting is helpful in carrying out this responsibility. However, the recent change from a retrospective to prospective reimbursement method implemented by the Medicare system heralds a major change in all reimbursement methods because of the likelihood that other payors will implement similar systems or adopt similar standards. The changes in reimbursement have forced hospital pharmacy managers to reevaluate many existing programs and forced a harder look at new proposals. Since the implementation of the Social Security Act Amendments of 1983 (PL 98-21), many studies have appeared in the pharmacy literature that document effective approaches to cost justification and/or analysis of services.

Naturally, financial information is not the only tool used

in program analysis, but financial analysis plays a major role in the process, which will be reviewed in the section ''Cost Analysis'' later in this chapter.

ORGANIZING ACCOUNTING DATA

Financial information can be arranged by any of four major systems. Each has a different application, but, as a hospital pharmacy manager, you will be exposed to all of them. These parameters are not specific and many organizations employ a mixture of all four categories.

The most widely used method is tracking financial information by *account*. In this system, all monies spent for a common purpose are grouped into a single account, and all those authorized to allocate funds for that purpose draw their monies from the account.

Another approach is to allocate funds by *program*. Program allocations could be made to an entire pharmacy department, or they could be made to individual segments of a pharmacy department, depending on management's approach. The advantage of program allocation is that it makes tracking the efficiency of a program (in financial terms) relatively easy.

Financial information can also be organized by *source of funding*. This approach uses grants or other funding sources as the basis for their organization. This approach is most useful where grants or other third-party funding sources are the prime source of revenue.

The fourth approach to organizing financial information is to use the *responsibility center*. Simply stated, the responsibility center approach tracks its money by monitoring the people responsible for spending it.

The vast majority of institutions utilize a combination of these systems. Thus, a pharmacy department may be considered a responsibility center, but the accounts used to organize financial information about the pharmacy are common to all departments that have the ability to spend money. Also, special grants or other restricted funds are maintained in separate accounts, but the allocation of these funds usually conforms to the same standards that are used to allocate other, unrestricted funds of the institution.

ACCOUNTING ASSUMPTIONS

When dealing with accounting information, several basic assumptions are made. It is important that all accounting information conform to these assumptions because, as such, they provide a basis for the confidence we place in accountants and the profession of accountancy.

1. The information provided deals only with monetary facts.

2. The data provided applies to a specific period of time, usually no more than a single year at a time. Summary reports may, of course, cover a longer period of time.

3. For purposes of accounting, the organization and those who run it are separate entities. Only the organization is the focus of the accounting statement, although the picture presented by the financial report people will reflect directly on those who run it.

4. We assume that the organization is a going concern. It is fiscally viable and will be in existence next year.

5. Item costs are shown at actual, not current, value. Item costs may be defined as the cost of each item of the organization's property.

DEFINITIONS

Like pharmacy, the profession of accounting has its own language. It is important to understand some of the more commonly used terms because they appear in the accounting literature and documents so frequently. Some of the basic definitions to learn are:

revenue   Money earned by an organization for services rendered.

expenses   Money used to acquire resources or provide services for the organization.

cash equivalents   Items owned by the organization that are to be converted into cash in the near future. Some examples are accounts receivable as items of revenue and accounts payable as items of expense.

assets   Resources owned by an organization.

liabilities   Resources owed by an organization.

equities   Organizational interest remaining after liabilities (monies owed) have been subtracted from assets. In nonprofit organizations, this is called the ''fund balance.'' In the for-profit organization, it is called ''profit.''

ACCOUNTING STATEMENTS

In any organization, there are four basic kinds of financial statements that might be rendered, revenues and expenses, balance sheet, fund balances, and changes in financial position.

The statement of revenues and expenses is a periodic summary of the money earned (revenue) and spent (expense) by the organization based on the organization's total resources, not just its cash flow. This is an operating report. That is, it reflects the operations of the organization for the period in question, usually 1 month. The statement of revenues and expenses is also summarized at the end of 3 months (a quarterly report), at the end of the 6-month period (a semiannual report), and at the end of the year (the annual report). This is the most common financial statement with which a department manager will work because it is an operating report.

The balance sheet, also known as a statement of financial position, reflects the total financial condition of an organization by including all assets and liabilities. The difference between assets and liabilities is known as the fund balance, or profit.

The statement of fund balances is a brief annual summary of what factors have contributed to a change in the fund balance from one year to the next. For example, the fund balance may have increased because of increased revenues, decreased expenses, or transfers between funds that are not reflected in the operations statement, or statement of revenues and expenditures.

The statement of changes in financial position is rendered together with the statement of fund balances and is intended to explain to shareholders or other interested parties all changes in the balance sheet, other than those in the fund balance.

When a statement is prepared, certain basic rules are followed. Accounting rules are based on the concept that assets always must equal liabilities; if the equation does not balance, something is wrong. Every transaction must have a debit (assets or expenditures increase, liability or fund balance, or revenue increase). When analyzing an accounting transaction, follow these steps:

1. Identify the accounts involved. There may be more than two!
2. Determine which accounts are to be debited and which are to be credited.
3. Ascertain the amounts involved in the transaction.

To illustrate the analysis of a transaction, let us look at what is involved when a hospital buys and then pays for medication it has purchased:

1. Hospital buys medication:
   a. Debit the account called "supplies expense"
   b. Credit "accounts payable"
2. When bill is paid 3 weeks later:
   a. Debit "accounts payable"
   b. Credit "cash"

ACCRUAL ACCOUNTING

What is the accrual concept? Accrual methods are used by organizations that must recover the costs of operation from their users, as do hospitals in providing patient care services. It is important for institutional pharmacy managers to understand the accrual concept simply because most hospitals use it. In fact, most organizations, regardless of the service or business they are in, use accrual accounting in the purchasing of supplies. The basic differences between accrual and cash accounting lie in how they recognize an expense. The accrual concept recognizes an expense as a worker performs a service and looks at economic performance. Contrast this approach with cash-basis accounting, which only recognizes an expense when the bill is paid and looks at payment.

For example, if you order $10,000 worth of serum albumin and only $5000 is paid in the current period (usually 1 month), the remaining $5000 is recognized as an accrued expense because the hospital already has the full use of the whole $10,000 worth of supplies. Nonprofit organizations use the accrual system, rather than the cash-basis system, because it presents a complete record of all transactions within a given time period. All supplies ordered are recorded as an accrued expense when the goods are received and a liability for payment exists.

If your hospital operates on a cash basis, it would not recognize the full $10,000 worth of serum albumin during the first month. It would only recognize $5000 because that was all it had paid for.

Actually, accounting departments in most institutions keep both cash-basis and accrued books. This is done because the information provided by both approaches is valuable to different people served by the accounting department. Insiders are more interested in a cash-basis accounting analysis because it tells you about *cash flow*, or the actual balance of what came in vs what was spent. People outside the organization are more interested in an accrued statement because it takes all resources into account, both those realized and expected.

Purchase orders for goods or services not yet received should not be taken as an accrued expense because the organization has not yet gained use of the supplies or services they represent.

ANALYZING A FINANCIAL STATEMENT

The ability to understand, interpret, and project the financial condition of an organization depends on your ability to analyze its financial statement. While financial statement analysis is a well-developed art for business and the for-profit sector, it is less well defined for the nonprofit and service sector. In analyzing a financial statement, some of the questions you should ask are: Is the organization financially solvent over the short term (this year and next)? How financially solvent is the organization over the long term (beyond next year)? How stable is the organization's revenue base? How fast are organizational expenses increasing and which ones are rising at the fastest rate?

One conducts a financial analysis by comparing current figures with those of the previous year or by comparing the figures presented by two organizations within the same industry. Both methods of analysis require consistency of accounting practices between the periods and/or organizations being compared. If accounting methods are inconsistent or major changes in the organization take place, you cannot draw a valid conclusion as to its overall financial condition.

The following are basic steps in analyzing a financial statement.

Look at Revenue

When does the organization recognize revenue? This is not as critical an issue for nonprofit corporations as it is in the for-profit sector. The nonprofit sector does not tie revenue as closely to expenses as a for-profit organization, which insists that revenue be the leading factor, with costs tying themselves into the revenue. In a nonprofit organization, costs are often the leading factor and revenues tie themselves into known costs. Three criteria by which you may determine when the organization recognizes revenue are:

1. The objectivity of the revenue source. In other words, is the source of revenue a realistic one in terms of the industry and the customers normally dealt with by the institution.
2. Performance of a critical action by the organization that indicates a service has been rendered. In the case of a hospital, the critical event is the rendering of care, administration of medication, taking an X-ray, doing a blood test, etc.
3. The collectibility of the revenue. Is the patient covered by insurance or is he self-paying? If he is covered by insurance, has the patient's policy been verified as valid for the current condition and is this an insurer that normally does business with the hospital? If he is a self-pay patient, what steps have been taken to assure collectibility of the revenue? This is a key issue for many hospitals, particularly those serving an inner city population. Several institutions

have had to seek special support from local government to continue operations when the percentage of uncollectible revenue became overwhelming. A few have even been forced to close or reorganize under the bankruptcy laws.

Look at Expenses

When does the organization recognize an expense? Expenses should be matched with revenues. An incurred cost should not be recognized as an expense if its associated revenue has not been recognized.

On the other hand, if an obligation, such as vacation accruals (time earned but not used) or interest expense (owed but not yet paid), has been incurred by an organization, the associated expense should be recognized and not deferred to a later period.

Determine Common Size Ratios

Common size ratios are merely expressions of the amount of money in each account presented as a percentage of the whole. The addition of common size ratio data to a financial statement makes it easier to spot trends or major differences in financial data from one period to the next.

Examine Sources of Revenue and Expense

Examining the sources of organizational revenues is an important part of any financial statement analysis. Both the sources of revenue and types of organizational expense should be relatively stable from one period to the next. Stability of revenue and expense sources can be taken as a general indication of organizational stability. Trends or sudden changes in either revenue or expense should be identified and explained.

Perform Ratio Analyses

A variety of ratios are useful in financial statement analysis.

Liquidity or Solvency Ratios

These provide a measure of an organization's ability to meet its short-term obligations. There are three kinds of liquidity ratios, the current ratio, which measures current assets vs current liabilities; the quick ratio, which compared quick assets, those that are readily convertible to cash, against liabilities; and the total ratio, which compares total assets against total liabilities. Each of these ratios can indicate that the organization is solvent or the final value is greater than 1. Liquidity ratios are a useful way of getting an overall picture of an organization and denote a trend, especially when comparing financial data between two different periods.

Structure Ratios

Structure ratios are the most significant because they measure the various sources of revenue and expense and can be

developed quickly form statements providing common size data. The specific ratios to be used depend on the specifics of the organization being analyzed. For example, ratios can be developed to measure each of the various revenue sources against the total organizational revenue. In the hospital, structure ratios might be developed for each of the various third-party providers, private contributions, corporate contributions, government grants, private grants, and private pay patients.

You can also develop structure ratios for individual items of expense, comparing each item against the total expense. Or you might compare one type of expense against the total of that type of expense, e.g., you might want to compare pharmacist salaries against total salaries. The value of structure ratios lies in watching for changes or trends from one period to the next.

Performance Ratio

The performance ratio indicates the cost of each unit of service provided and how much revenue is supplied by each dollar of assets needed to maintain the organization in a functional state. It is calculated by dividing total units of service (patient days, prescriptions filled, etc.) by assets necessary to provide those services. The performance ratio is valuable because it tells you, in gross terms, the value of organizational assets needed to provide each unit of service. If tracked from one period to the next, it can supply valuable information on changes and trends in productivity, where increased productivity is defined as reducing the amount of assets needed to provide a unit of service.

Fund Sources and Uses Ratios

These ratios measure the sources and uses of an organization's accumulated funds against total revenue or assets. One interesting ratio divides organizational liabilities by total assets, as an indicator of the amount of other people's money being used by the organization. Another divides total long-term debt by the net amount invested in plant and equipment, as an indicator of how long-term debt is being used by an organization. A high ratio (approaching 1) indicates that long-term debt is being used for building or fixed assets. A low ratio indicates that long-term debt is being used for other purposes.

Surplus Ratios

Surplus ratios indicate profits (or increases in the fund balance) on 1-year and cumulative bases. These ratios compare the total surplus, or deficit, with total assets; the total accumulated surplus, or deficit, with total assets; and the total accumulated surplus, or deficit, with total liabilities.

These ratios are intended to look at the cumulative surplus or deficit of an organization and are often taken as an overall indication of the financial health of an organization.

Use Statement of Changes in Financial Position

This statement is provided to inform you of major changes in the sources or uses of organizational funds. Net changes in working capital (current assets less current liabilities) or cash available to the organization are important indicators of an organization's liquidity.

This statement answers two very important questions: Where does the organization get its money and what does it do with it? As such, it provides you with a good indication of the current direction of the organization and how it has changed over the past year.

THE AUDITOR

Auditing is the process of comparing what actually happened with what should have happened. It assesses compliance with accounting standards, legal requirements, and performance (i.e., operational efficiency or program effectiveness). Most institutions employ auditors who, acting as independent agents, perform internal audits of any of the various departments or sections of the hospital. The internal auditor should provide an impartial evaluation of operational efficiency, effectiveness, and conformance to organizational standards and should be particularly helpful to line managers within the organization in helping them reach their goals.

External audits are performed by outside organizations to provide assurance to interested third parties that everything is going well. External audits are useful because they can be used to attest to the organization's efficiency to outside agencies and potential grantors and to improve organization public relations.

One of the more common audit procedures experienced by pharmacy managers is the *performance audit*. The performance audit measures compliance with organizational goals and fiscal efficiency. The auditor attempts to assess the quality of services provided while balancing this against the cost of providing such services. Performance audits can be expected to:

- Focus on organizational goals
- Settle intraorganizational disputes
- Set nonfinancial goals
- Put pressure on operating managers
- Emphasize cost efficiency and cost-cutting programs

COST ANALYSIS

Cost analysis is used to answer three basic questions. How well am I doing? What problems need my attention? How can I best accomplish the job at hand?

Hospitals are labor-intensive organizations providing service activities; therefore, the major inputs to and outputs of programs cannot always be inventories accurately. How much is patient care worth? What is the value of relieving a patient's pain or avoiding a drug side effect? How should the total of all manpower be allocated to each program or service carried out by a pharmacy service?

Just as output is difficult to measure, the establishment of operational goals is equally difficult. Performance, too, is often hard to measure in the absence of a profit-and-loss situation. Because program participants often have multiple objectives they want to achieve, detached and objective analysis becomes a complex matter.

Hospitals are highly political organizations. The influences of sociopolitical forces also makes the assignment of

costs or the determination of relative priorities less straightforward than in the noninstitutional or for-profit segment.

Finally, hospital accountants are trained in traditional fiduciary accounting, a fact that often hinders their acceptance or understanding of much of what goes on in the institutional environment. Like most other things in the hospital, this too is changing, but at a slow pace.

All of these problems are faced by hospital pharmacists seeking to justify new services or retain existing ones on a cost-effectiveness basis. The justification of such services as unit dose distribution and IV admixtures have already been accomplished and much background material on these appear in the literature. However, cost analysis has not yet been adequately studied by pharmacists seeking to justify new clinical service programs or to retain existing programs. This issue is made more complex by the imposition of prospective reimbursement on American hospitals.

Cost analysis techniques are used every day by hospital pharmacy managers and can be applied in three different ways.

Routine Operations

The first application of cost analysis is in planning and controlling routine operations. Cost analysis can help determine your operational goals, decide when they are to be accomplished, and designate the resources, programs, and services to be used in achieving them. Furthermore, cost analysis is helpful in evaluating the efficiency of current services and programs and the efficiency and effectiveness of various sections within an organization. For example, cost analysis can be used as a tool to assess such activities as drug distribution, satellite pharmacies, clinical service programs, packaging operations, and IV admixture systems.

Long-Range Planning

The second major application of cost analysis is in long-range planning and policy determination. This should be of definite interest to the institutional pharmacy manager because of its usefulness as an aid in selecting strategic goals, formulating overall policy direction, and setting guidelines that control the acquisition, disposition, and use of major resources. Moreover, cost analysis is of definite benefit in developing both new services and the research and development strategies needed to implement them. Where would we be today without the cost analyses of unit dose and other contemporary services. Some have utilized this tool to evaluate clinical services and other innovative practice programs, but more work must be done in this before they, too, may be widely accepted and implemented.

Determining Cost and Price of Department Services

Cost analysis is useful in such day-to-day activities of the institutional pharmacist as inventory valuation, reimbursement and pricing, and determining service costs for control purposes. Several characteristics of the modern institutional environment make cost analysis somewhat complicated.

Defining Terms

Before we go any further, it will be useful to define some basic terms that are used in the cost analysis and cost measurement.

Cost. A cost is defined as any resource foregone to achieve a goal. The concept of cost is most easily understood when we use money to buy something, although it is impossible to be consistent in our definitions of cost for every situation. The money we spend is our foregone resource, and the goods or services purchased is the goal to be achieved. We can broaden this concept a bit further by thinking of other resources that might be foregone to achieve a goal. For instance, in allocating our time each day, we are "spending" a valuable and irretrievable resource. Hopefully, the time spent at work and at play is allocated appropriately to allow us to achieve preset goals.

Cost can also be measured as a lost opportunity. What else could you have done with the resources at hand because of a previous decision to allocate costs in a certain way?

Cost Objective. A cost objective is any activity for which separate cost measurement is desired. These can, and usually are, set at almost every level of the organization and certainly influence the way resources are allocated. Cost objectives might reflect an overall institutional philosophy, the goal of a particular member of the administrative staff, a departmental goal, or a personal goal. Cost objectives might be reflective of different medications, medication groups (antibiotics, antineoplastics, etc.), or diagnostic groups for which cost information is compiled.

Cost Accumulation. Cost accumulation is the establishment of an organized and systematic system for the collection of cost data. Costs can be accumulated in any of a number of ways. Traditionally, they are collected within institutional accounting systems and by department managers and others.

Cost Allocation. Cost allocation is the process during which specific accumulated costs are identified and assigned to specific cost objects. For example, the cost of operating departments, such as engineering or housekeeping, that serve an entire institution but have no way of billing a patient for their services are routinely allocated among other hospital departments that utilize their services via a formula devised to equitably allocate costs. In the case of engineering, it might be according to work performed, and in the case of housekeeping, it might be according to the number of square feet of floor space occupied. Other departments might use different measures, such as the number of employees or total hours of operation each month.

Variable Costs. Variable costs are those that vary according to a level of activity or volume of work. In the case of a department of pharmacy, some variable costs are the cost of drugs, cost of packaging supplies, some labor costs (overtime, premium time, etc), and the cost of those services directly related to carrying on pharmacy operations.

Fixed Costs. A fixed cost is one that remains relatively unchanged during a given time period, despite wide variations in activity. Some costs that might be considered fixed are postage and other costs of operating a departmental office, departmental research and education, building depreciation, utilities, the cost of a departmental library, and travel and educational expenses.

Committed Costs. These are fixed costs incurred by the institution regardless of the level of activity to be carried out. Some costs that might fall into this category are building depreciation, rent, insurance, and salaries of some key personnel. A fixed cost becomes a committed cost when it is absolutely essential to the institution's existence. Noncommitted fixed costs are considered *discretionary fixed costs* and are usually among the first to be cut in a cost-containment program.

Mixed Costs. In real life, the cost of most items is mixed. That is, one component of the cost behaves as a fixed cost and another behaves as a variable cost. For example, the cost of pharmacy personnel is variable because the need for staff fluctuates directly with the volume of work to be done. On the other hand, it is fixed for a given time period because staff are permanent employees of the institution and are not usually employed with the understanding that they can be paid on an "as needed" basis. The cost of basic pharmacy staff is fixed, unless permanent alterations are made.

HOW ARE COSTS MEASURED?

Costs can be measured in several different ways. The most widely used approach, known as the *industrial engineering method,* concentrates on finding the most efficient means and resource combination to achieve a specific level of input and output. It can be used if there is a definite relationship between input and output and all activities can be outlined in detail.

The kinds of activities best suited to the industrial engineering method are work measurement, time and motion studies, systems flow charting and engineering, and detailed activity analysis. It cannot be readily applied if the output from an activity is difficult to describe in physical terms, if relationships are impractical to observe or define, or if activities cannot be identified in terms of a particular input as leading to given levels of output. The industrial engineering method can be used to measure such activities as the number of requisitions filled by a technician, the number if medication cassettes or doses filled per unit time, and the number of seconds it takes to enter a medication order into a computer system.

Another approach to cost measurement is the statistical method. This technique involves the application of statistical methodology (regression analysis) to current figures to project what the future holds or what would have held under unchanging circumstances. The wide availability of microcomputer technology and "what if" spreadsheet programs such as Visicalc, Supercalc, and others to any institutional manager have brought statistical analysis within the reach of all.

Break-even Analysis

Once costs have been measured, the data are often used for operational planning via break-even analysis. "Break even" is the point at which your net income is zero, where income equals expenses. For this type of analysis, it is essential to know both fixed and variable costs associated with a given activity. Costs are then projected against revenue to determine the break-even point.

Another way of calculating the break-even point is by dividing fixed costs by the total contribution margin per unit. The total contribution margin is the difference between total revenue and total variable costs. The total contribution margin per unit is calculated by dividing the total contribution margin by the activity level.

$$\text{Total contribution margin} =$$
$$\text{Total revenue} - \text{Total variable costs}$$

$$\text{Contribution margin per unit} = \frac{\text{Total contribution margin}}{\text{Activity level}}$$

$$\text{Break even point} = \frac{\text{Fixed costs}}{\text{Contribution margin per unit}}$$

In a hospital, where revenue is often fixed and predefined, we can project the level of service to be provided for dollars allocated. It is possible to use break-even analysis for a new program or service. If the method of contribution margin is used to calculate your break-even point, you must know all fixed and variable costs and apply them accordingly. The unit of service must be defined before you can complete the calculation. It can be number of patient days, prescriptions filled, consultations provided, patients seen, or any other measure you wish to provide, as long as it can be directly related to the program at hand.

Also, break-even analysis can be used in the situation where a certain prescribed level of service must be provided by the pharmacy. By working backward, you can project fixed and variable costs necessary to provide the prescribed services and determine the revenue necessary to break even. Your break-even point can change with patient mix, reimbursement type, and under the latest prospective reimbursement regulations, diagnosis mix because of differences in fixed and variable costs as well as differences in the level of reimbursement for each patient.

COST ACCOUNTING

Cost accounting systems trace object costs by accumulating departmental costs and applying them to units of work, or output. This system, also called *cost application* or *cost absorption,* is useful for determining the cost of a product or service and maintaining responsibility and control. Some of the terms used in cost accounting are as follows:

direct materials   Raw materials that become an integral part of the final product and can be conveniently assigned to specific physical units. Usually, this cost is variable, depending only on the cost of materials.
direct labor   All labor that is an integral part of the production and can be assigned specifically and conveniently to a given unit of output. This is also a variable cost, depending on the value and amount of labor applied to production.
overhead   All other costs that can be assigned to a specific unit of work and are neither direct material or direct labor. The overhead may include costs that are fixed (do not change), variable, or mixed.

In service-oriented organizations, such as the institutional pharmacy, cost accounting systems have certain character-

istics. First, in such functions as clinical or distributive services, the output is typically something that cannot be physically inventoried. Other functions such as packaging, some aspects of IV admixture programs, and some aspects of drug distribution systems deal with an output that is physical in nature and can be readily inventoried.

Second, the service output is multidimensional and cannot be measured in a single quantitative unit. The process leading to the provision of the service is labor intensive, and direct materials play a lesser role in production. The application of inputs directly to service output is difficult, since production formulas measuring such relationships do not exist.

Finally, many costs cannot be controlled because they are either fixed costs that are committed or are mixed and do not vary directly with output or production.

Differences in service or product costing methods center largely around how the input costs are assigned to the various outputs. Product costing, such as packaging, production, bulk compounding, and cost per dose of distribution, is largely an averaging process because it is neither practical nor possible to trace each cost to a specific unit of output or job. It can be argued that many management control functions do not require detailed tracing of costs. The two following examples will serve to illustrate the different types of costing methods available.

Job Order Costing

Job order costing is used when the product is identifiable by unique batches, jobs, or projects. Costs are assigned to functions or programs listed in detail. Direct materials and direct labor costs are traced by means of source documents such as requisitions, work orders, and time records. Overhead is assigned by measuring the area (square feet) of floor space used by each program or by determining the cost of fringe benefits assignable to each person involved.

In the institutional pharmacy, job order costing can be applied to the routine "production" functions common to all pharmacies. Some of these are purchasing and inventory control, manufacturing and/or packaging, and routine unit dose or traditional drug distribution programs where records are maintained by patient or by the amount of time spent by personnel on each activity. If such records are not kept, job order costing is impossible because you will be missing a major cost component from the analysis.

Process Costing

Process costing, generally used when there is a continuous and uniform mass production of "like units" assigns costs based on a broad averaging method. Total departmental costs are accumulated for a given period in relation to the total number of units processed. The total cost is then divided by the number of units to obtain a broad-based average unit cost.

Process costing may be used where the rate at which units of service are provided is too high to allow staff to stop and record their time, such as in an assembly line type of operation. The cost information obtained from this kind of analysis is really just a broad average of all costs applied to the major "product" of the department. In the case of the department of pharmacy, this might be applied to obtaining an overall cost per prescription filled. Process costing can be extremely misleading because it ignores the appropriate allocation of costs between different kinds of services provided by a department.

Normal Costing and Standard Costing

Cost accounting systems can be further defined by product costing valuation principles. In *actual cost systems,* the costs actually incurred are assigned directly to services or products.

In *normal cost systems,* actual direct materials and labor costs are assigned to products or services, but actual overhead costs are not. Instead, a predetermined overhead rate is used.

In *standard cost systems,* the cost of a given product or service is based on predetermined standard usages and rates. Such systems are also useful not only for service costing, but also for management control purposes. Three types of standard costs are:

1. Basic standards. These long-term, generally unchanging averages provide a base for comparison of actual costs over the years with the same standard. Changes in technology and other circumstances often make these standards less useful in the nonprofit environment.

2. Ideal or optimal standards. Based on the level of efficiency that could be achieved under ideal circumstances, these standards are useful only when they can provide a psychologic incentive for achieving increases in productivity. If the standards are unattainable, they can turn out to be a negative influence on the work force.

3. Currently attainable standards. Reflecting management's estimates of what cost levels are achievable under an efficient set of operating conditions, currently attainable standards should be used when standard cost systems are applied. These standards allow for lost time, production breakdowns, product spoilage or loss, or other unusual problem situations.

In many systems, costs are allocated among departments, sections, or segments of the organization. This is done to predict the economic impact of specific planning and control decisions; stimulate managers to make more efficient use of resources and promote a higher level of understanding of and commitment to organizational goals by department heads; compute income costs and profit contributions made by various segments of the organization; and to compute rates for governmental and other third-party payors.

Step-Down Costing

One of the most frequently used methods of cost allocation is the step-down method, in which costs allocated with nondirect patient service areas, such as cafeteria and plant maintenance, are allocated to direct patient service areas such as pharmacy and laboratory. Costs are assigned by the relative rate at which direct service areas make use of nondirect areas. Since the services of nondirect areas are used by employees of direct areas in the course of doing their jobs, allocation is often made on a per employee basis,

assuming that all employees utilize nondirect service areas equally. The highest cost nondirect service centers are allocated first.

In another version of the step-down method, the operating costs of nondirect service areas are spread equally over all direct service areas, regardless of the number of employees.

BUDGETING

Budgeting, an activity carried out by virtually all pharmacy managers, can serve several different purposes. Technically, a budget is a formal quantitative expression of the plans and/or intentions of management. A budget may be expressed in terms of dollars and cents, but it also can be expressed in terms of units of work to be performed, productivity, etc.

Purposes of a Budget

Why should we bother to prepare a budget? There are three very good reasons for having a budget:

- The process of preparing the budget provides a forecast or plan of what can be expected in the upcoming operating period.
- It serves as a communication device between all levels of the organization.
- Managers at all levels are forced to think ahead and make operating choices.

These three important purposes of the budget are of almost daily concern to institutional pharmacy managers. No one who has ever been involved in budget deliberations and planning can deny that the entire tone of an organization is affected by *plans or forecasts of future activity*. Staff personnel are quick to pick up the sense of management's attitudes about their and the organization's future. Positive attitudes will be sensed and adopted as staff looks forward to new systems, projects, and maybe even personnel. On the other hand, a negative attitude or plan on the part of top management for a particular department or section will be immediately translated into forecasts fo doom and gloom for the future of everyone concerned. The final decision to implement or deny a new service or the plans of a particular operating department can either be incredibly uplifting or devastating to the personnel involved, whose entire world may be altered as a result of the decision.

The budget is certainly a *stimulus to communications* between all levels of the organization because of its impact on everything done by the organization. Another aspect of the importance of the budget as a tool for communications is the role of the budget as a coordinating tool. It provides top management with a concise, although admittedly narrow, evaluation of a manager's performance in terms that are readily understandable: has he or she stayed within or exceeded the allotted budget? Naturally, there should be more to the evaluation of a manager's performance than mere budget adherence, but the manager who remains within budgeted guidelines or who can readily account for any differences in operational terms is always respected and may be given the benefit of the doubt in other discussions.

The mere presence of an approved organizational budget *forces managers to think ahead, plan and make choices to facilitate the accomplishment of departmental and organizational goals while remaining within budgetary guidelines.* One illustration of how management is forced to plan ahead by budgetary limitations is the formulary process and drug product selection. One of the major purposes of the formulary and drug product selection is to provide the most appropriate and current drug therapy while conserving institutional dollars. To some, these goals may seem at odds, but the decisions to be made by members of the Pharmacy and Therapeutics Committees and pharmacy management must address the questions of whether newly proposed drugs offer a significant therapeutic advantage or will be frivolous additions.

Using a Budget

How can we *use* a budget? It is important to differentiate the reasons for having a budget (above) from the ways to use the budget, because we, as managers, may have no choice as to why the budget process is implemented. But learning how we can use the budget may enable us to significantly improve our status within the organization.

Budgets can be used to anticipate future needs and events, an especially important activity in day-to-day management of the institutional pharmacy. One of the most important things to be considered when preparing a new budget is what new therapies, treatment programs, or service programs are to be implemented by the institution in the upcoming period and how will these affect our department. For example, if your ambulatory service center is to undergo a remodeling, will pharmacy be affected? If so, will we have to add dollars to specific areas of our budget to allow for this remodeling? If pharmacy is not directly affected, will the remodeling affect our patient load. If it is to be temporarily reduced during the remodeling period, pharmacy will be indirectly affected because of a reduced demand for services. This may translate into lower drug costs, reduced revenue, and a reduction in the need for personnel to staff the facility during the remodeling period.

Another type of projection that should be considered for budget planning is to attempt to assess the impact of drugs you expect to be released during the upcoming period and the possible impact of those drugs on your budget. Will they be added to the formulary. If so, will they replace a current medication or be added without corresponding deletions? Will they affect hospital stay, potentially reducing overall revenue?

Budgets are used to set departmental goals and objectives that are both achievable and in line with those of the institution. This is an important consideration when proposing new or future budget allocation. It would be senseless to establish goals for the department of pharmacy that are not achievable in the current or future operating environment or to establish a goal that was not consistent with the stated goals of the institution.

For instance, while it is always desirable for a department of pharmacy to conduct ongoing research, the funding of such a program might not be feasible either because of the conditions under which the institution is forced to operate or because such a program is inconsistent with the established goals of the hospital. On the other hand, it may be possible to establish a trimmed down research program or a program limited to the investigation of a specific area of practice. Another way to approach the establishment of a departmental research program is to begin with a project funded by an outside source.

Another institutional pharmacy program that may be difficult to establish in some institutions because of operating conditions or institutional goals is a pharmacy internship or residency. If the institution does not include education as one of its major goals, it may be difficult to convince hospital administration to fund such a program. If, however, you can demonstrate that the addition of a pharmacy intern or resident to your staff will provide significant benefit to the institution through improved planning, operating efficiencies, or special services to be provided, you may be able to justify such a position and still be within the established framework of operating efficiency and institutional goals.

Budgets can be used as *tools for selecting programs to help achieve goals efficiently and to choose resource combinations that help achieve operational efficiency.* In this context, efficiency can be defined as the achievement of maximal output per dollar of cost or, conversely, minimizing the input necessary to achieve maximal output. If budgetary guidelines are used to help select programs and choose the combinations of institutional resources necessary to achieve the maximal output for minimal levels of input, you will be more likely to achieve your goals and remain consistent with those of the institution.

Budgets help conduct *ongoing performance evaluation* of a department, section, or individual worker. This is one of the most widely used applications of the budget. Virtually every manager from the chief executive officer down to line supervisors is judged by his or her adherence to established budgetary criteria. Naturally, there are other criteria on which management and supervisory personnel are evaluated, but adherence to budgetary guidelines is important, especially if the manager being evaluated gave significant input into or was responsible for establishing the budget in the first place. More information on the use of budgets as evaluation tools can be found in the section on ''Performance Management'' below.

Finally, budgets are *helpful in calculating prices to be charged for services and setting reimbursement rates.* This is a function not usually dealt with by pharmacy managers. However, the changing reimbursement environment may force this issue to be one of greater interest and involvement among institutional pharmacists. Most institutions employ a reimbursement specialist to calculate the process to be charged and negotiate reimbursement rates.

Budget Types

There are several types of budget. The most often used is the so-called *master budget,* which usually represents the total operating budget for an institution's activities over the period of one fiscal year.

Operating master budgets include estimates of revenue, production or service units, and an administrative budget. The budget for production or service units (prescriptions filled, orders processed, consultations completed, drug information questions) can be further subdivided into materials (drugs, packaging materials, supplies, forms, etc), direct labor, and indirect overhead costs.

Another type of master budget is the *financial budget*. The financial budget consists of cash budgets needed to plan for cash flow and financial statement budgets, in which individual programs or departments are budgeted to keep track of their revenue and expenses.

Special-purpose budgets also deserve a mention here. Some examples of special-purpose budgets are capital expenditure budgets and multi-year budget projections. Each has a specific application and is utilized only in limited situations. For example, the capital equipment budget usually represents the organization's future plan for purchases of capital equipment, often defined as equipment with an expected life of at least 5 years and costs more than a minimal amount, usually $250. Capital equipment budgets allow large dollar expenditures to be planned for future years and provides both administrators and reimbursement agencies with the knowledge needed to program these expenditures over a period of several years.

How Budgets Are Structured

Budgets may be structured in a variety of ways, but the most common approach is to characterize an item of expenditure according to whom the payment is actually made. Major budget areas within an institutional pharmacy, therefore, might include such items as salaries, drugs (often broken down to different categories or types), other supplies, equipment, books and journals, travel and other educational expenses, and contract services.

Other possible budget structures might include function, program, or organizational subunit. Functional budgets might allocate expenses to registered pharmacists, supportive personnel, inpatient supplies, ambulatory care supplies, and administrative expenses. Program budgets might allocate expenses to such categories as unit dose distribution, IV admixture services, clinical practice, and ambulatory care. Budgets written by organizational subunit might allocate expenses to individual satellite pharmacies, the drug information center, pharmacokinetics laboratory, and departmental administration. As you can see, the possibility of considerable overlap exists between the various approaches. However, the most important factor in selecting a budget method and following through with that method is a clear definition of each category and the expenses to be included in those categories.

Budget Preparation

In most organizations, budgeting is carried out in a prescribed manner according to standardized procedures. Each department and/or functional area is provided with a specific set of guidelines on the standard method of budget preparation used within the institution. The traditional approach for budgets structured by either expense item or organizational unit is to simply apply an incremental increase or decrease to each line item in the budget.

In the *incremental approach* to budget preparation, the first step is to extrapolate next year's level of spending from last year's and to vary the result by comparing the level of activity given in the old budget with that anticipated for the new year. The second step is to adjust line items for inflation, new contract settlements, or other new circumstances projected to affect existing activities. The third step is to apply the necessary increments to individual line items for new projects or programs.

After preliminary budget figures are prepared, a *sensitivity analysis* should be performed by changing some parameters and determining the potential impact of those changes on the budget. What would we like to change about current operations and how will this affect our budget? Computerized spreadsheet programs such as Visicalc, Calcstar, and others are particularly useful here, since they can automatically calculate the budget impact and save many hours of arduous calculation.

Especially important here is the concept of "budgetary slack." Slack is represented by items within a budget that do not have a direct relationship to operations but provide some of the motivations found in the for-profit sector, such as educational expenses, travel, secretaries, office space, and equipment. Budgetary slack is important to maintain because losing it can lead to losing employees who have lost the benefits to which they have become accustomed.

Most budgets fall short in forecasting the public's demand for services and assessing the impact of inflation, factors that are essentially impossible to predict. Thus, it becomes impossible to accurately budget for supplies that are directly affected by demand or inflation. All you can do is make your best guess and hope that it is close.

Other Budgeting Approaches

Since the vast majority of institutional pharmacy managers are involved in traditional budgeting systems, minimal consideration will be given to other systems and philosophies. However, they should be given theoretical consideration since an understanding of the philosophy behind these methods can help to fully appreciate the approach being used in your own institution. Also, it may be possible to integrate one of these philosophies into the traditional approach.

Evaluative Budgeting. Cost-benefit benefit analyses are used extensively for new or comprehensive programs. This philosophy is employed in traditional systems when attempting to justify a program. The evaluative approach can be applied to a budget structured by function, in which case it is known as *performance budgeting*. When evaluative budgeting is applied to budgets structured by organizational unit, the process is known as *responsibility center budgeting*. When applied to budgets structured by program, the result is *zero-based budgeting* (ZBB) or *program, planned budget systems (PPBS)*. While ZBB rejustifies all budget expenses each year and makes no predetermined judgments of need, services, or expense, *PPBS* makes an explicit attempt to define organizational goals and objectives (programs) and to fund them individually.

Negotiative Budgeting. When the negotiative approach is applied to budgets structured by organizational unit, the result is management by objective (MBO). In this approach, both the operational and fiscal objectives of each organizational unit are renegotiated for each budget period and mutually agreed on by both department manager and administrator. If MBO is applied within a department, the objectives must be agreed upon by the department head and individual section managers or supervisors.

Negotiative budgeting requires a complete alteration of management style, since the major emphasis in this system is placed on the role of negotiation and bargaining, as opposed to evaluation. If the department head is a more skilled negotiator, he or she will always achieve their goals under this system, because the final negotiated conditions will always be within reach. If, on the other hand, the administrator is the more skillful negotiator, more may be achieved within a given department.

Uncontrolled MBO systems will lead to behavioral alterations aimed at achieving goals or getting around agreed on objectives. The key to this system is to be certain that the evaluation and negotiation process is fair and complete. The standards agreed on should be midway between the desires of administrator and department head.

CAPITAL BUDGETING

The purpose of capital budgeting is to plan and control programs and projects athat have an impact on costs and revenue in more than a single year's operations, in terms of either costs or benefits. Therefore, capital budget preparation is intimately linked to long-range planning programs.

In hospitals, capital budgets are useful for several purposes that are not of major interest to most pharmacy managers, such as calculating the annual cost impact of the department of buildings and grounds. However, capital budgets can be of use to institutional pharmacy managers in evaluating the overall effectiveness of programs, calculating investment in or the cost of research or training programs, evaluating the use of new equipment or facilities, and performing cost-benefit analyses of programs or departmental activities.

Capital expenditures can be evaluated by using one of three possible models: payback, the net present value, or the internal rate of return.

The *payback model* is the simplest to use, simply dividing the total cost by the annual cash savings generated by the equipment, assuming that some savings are apparent. The project that "earns" back its cost in the shortest time is the most desirable because it offers the least risk. The drawback of this approach is that it does not weigh the value of dollars from one year to the next.

In the *net present value method* of evaluation, calculate the difference between the aggregate discounted benefits minus aggregate discounted costs, using the discount rate at a minimum acceptable rate. Then, select the project yielding the best net present value. If a piece of equipment costs $50,000 and has a useful life of 5 years, the net present value would be calculated as shown in Table 21.1, assuming a discount rate of 10% each year.

When using the *internal rate of return method*, calculate the discount rate that makes the aggregate discounted benefits equal to the aggregate discounted costs. If the calculated value exceeds the minimum acceptable rate, the project should be accepted. The internal rate of return method does not take the useful life of the equipment into account; thus,

TABLE 21.1 Calculating Net Present Value

Year	Amount of Investment	Weighted Value (10% Discount)
0	(50,000)	−50,000
1	10,000	10,000 × 0.9 = 9,000
2	10,000	10,000 × 0.81 = 8,100
3	10,000	10,000 × 0.72 = 7,200
4	10,000	10,000 × 0.65 = 6,500
5	10,000	10,000 × 0.58 = 5,800

Total benefit = 36,600
Net present value after 5 years = −13,400

it is not as useful as the other approaches to evaluating a piece of capital equipment.

$$\text{Internal rate of return (\%)} = \frac{\text{Average yearly benefit}}{\frac{1}{2} \text{ total investment}}$$

PERFORMANCE MEASUREMENT

A prime objective of many financial system is to build in tools for measuring managerial performance according to the degree of adherence to a budgetary plan; achievement of stated goals with regard to units of work, expense, or revenue (as in MBO) or other performance criteria. In many cases, nonadherence or nonachievement of goals is outside of the manager's control. For example, an institutional pharmacy manager may be faced with an unpredicted change in direct costs of medication and supplies, an unforeseen need for additional personnel because of increased demand for services, increased use of high-cost medications because of the introduction of a new drug that replaces an older, less expensive one, and a change in the hospital's patient mix or the introduction of new procedures, both of which can directly affect pharmacy costs.

One must also be aware of changing practice standards. Existing performance criteria may become outdated and no longer reflect day-to-day pharmacy practice. The alert institutional manager is familiar with these changes in practice standards and is able to account for them and their effects on performance criteria.

Management control may be defined as the process used by managers to ensure that resources are obtained and effectively used in the accomplishment of an organization's goals. Effectiveness relates to your ability to produce the expected results, efficiency in achieving effectiveness with minimal input, or it can also refer to the greatest output per unit of input. Both concepts are extremely difficult to measure but are essential to management control.

The basic management control systems found in any organization are personnel and payroll, financial reporting systems, physical assets control, establishing and achieving program objectives, and ensuring compliance with all applicable legal and regulatory requirements. These systems should ascertain that the results intended are achieved on schedule and efficiently. This requires a statement of goals (or plans) and subsequent evaluation of how these goals are to be reached. Planning takes place at three levels in any organization:

1. Strategic planning to determine the overall direction of the entire organization
2. Management planning to achieve program goals that are generally related to the overall strategic plan
3. Operational planning to see that departments or other operational areas perform their functions in a manner that is consistent with the rest of the organization.

Management control requires measurement and feedback, so that problems requiring a solution can be identified and acted on. Measurement systems are established and operated mainly by accounting staff members, who should see that they are fair to all groups within the organization and that all areas have goals that are congruent with those of the overall organization.

CONCLUSION

The move toward a national prospective payment program by the Social Security Ammendments of 1983 has established a precedent from which there will be no turning back. Hospital reimbursement for Medicare services have been altered in virtually every state of the union and other insurance providers are trying to install systems that incorporate many of the same cost-reducing mechanisms as are incorporated into the new Medicare regulations, hoping to reduce their own payments per admission.

The initial year of prospective payment has been one of uncertainty for many and marked by a plethora of articles in the literature documenting the competitive environment that now exists in American hospitals. With resource limitation, many departments are competing for limited funds. The successful pharmacy manager will be the one who is able to employ sophisticated financial techniques and prove his or her need for a portion of those limited resources. It is hoped that the material presented in this chapter will help to provide a basis from which the student can begin learning those techniques.

ADDITIONAL READING

Abramowitz PW: Controlling financial variables-changing prescribing patterns. *Am J Hosp Pharm* 41:503-515, 1984.

Abramowitz PW: Controlling financial variables-purchasing, inventory control, and waste reduction. *Am J Hosp Pharm* 41:309-317, 1984.

Bergen SS, Roth AC: Prospective payment and the university hospital. *N Engl J Med* 310:316-318, 1984.

Bonney RS: Hospital survival strategies for the 1980s. *Am J Hosp Pharm* 40:1483-1488, 1983.

Curtiss FR: Pharmacy management strategies for responding to hospital reimbursement changes. *Am J Hosp Pharm* 40:1489-1492, 1983.

Enright SM: Understanding prospective pricing and DRGs. *Am J Hosp Pharm* 40:1493-1494, 1983.

Ginzburg PB, Sloan F: Hospital cost shifting. *N Engl J Med* 310:893-898, 1983.

Grauer DW: Improving a hospital pharmacy department's profitability. *Am J Hosp Pharm* 40:1183-1187, 1983.

Hunt ML: Use of financial reports in managing pharmacies. *Am J Hosp Pharm* 41:709-715, 1984.

Leaf A: The doctor's dilemma—and society's too. *N Engl J Med* 310:718-720, 1984.

Lee HE: Coping with DRGs: Evanston Hospital, Evanston, Illinois. *Am J Hosp Pharm* 40:1508-1509, 1983.

Lee MP: Coping with DRGs: University of California Medical Center, San Diego. *Am J Hosp Pharm* 40:1504-1506, 1983.

Mcphee SJ, Myers LP, et al: Cost containment confronts physicians. *Ann Intern Med* 100:604-605, 1984.

Mehl B: Reimbursement mechanisms for hospital services. Part 1. *US Pharm* 11:H1, 1983.

Mehl B: Reimbursement mechanisms for hospital services, Part 2. *US Pharm* 12:H1, 1983.

Mehl B; Reimbursement mechanisms for hospital services, Part 3. *US Pharm* 1:H1, 1984.

Miller DE: Coping with DRGs: Hospital of the University of Pennsylvania, Philadelphia. *Am J Hosp Pharm* 40:1503-1504, 1983.

Osborne JA: Coping with DRGs: Baptist Medical Center of Oklahoma, Oklahoma City. *Am J Hosp Pharm* 40:1506-1507, 1983.

Roberts RW: Coping with DRGs: Riverside Hospital, Jacksonville, Florida. *Am J Hosp Pharm* 40:1500-1502, 1983.

Speranzo AJ: Financial management of hospitals. *Am J Hosp Pharm* 41:935-941, 1984.

Stolar MH: Description of an experimental hospital pharmacy management information system. *Am J Hosp Pharm* 40:1905-1913, 1983.

Stolar MH: National test of an experimental hospital pharmacy management information system. *Am J Hosp Pharm* 40:1914-1919, 1983.

Suzuki NT, Pelham LD: Cost benefit of pharmacist concurrent monitoring of cefazolin prescribing. *Am J Hosp Pharm* 40:1187-1191, 1983.

Turnbull RH, Ashby DM: Coping with DRGs: Harper-Grace Hospitals, Detroit, Michigan. *Am J Hosp Pharm* 40:1499-1500, 1983.

Upton JH, Crouch JB, Douglas JB: Coping with DRGs: The Moses Cone Memorial Hospital, Greensboro, North Carolina. *Am J Hosp Pharm* 40:1496-1499, 1983.

Vaida AJ: Coping with DRGs: Suburban general hospital, Norristown, Pa. *Am J Hosp Pharm* 40:1494-1496, 1983.

Vladek BC: Medicare hospital payment by diagnosis related groups. *Ann Intern Med* 100:576-591, 1984.

Williams RB: Preparing the operating budget. *Am J Hosp Pharm* 40:2181-2188, 1983.

Zilz DA, Nold EG: Health care trends influencing financial management of hospital pharmacies. *Am J Hosp Pharm* 40:1532-1536, 1983.

CHAPTER 22

Management Aspects of Prospective Payment

JAMES M. HETHCOX

Enactment of the Social Security Act Amendments of 1983 effected the movement of Medicare inpatient reimbursement from a cost-based, retrospective system to a fixed, diagnosis-specific, prospective payment system. This change, described as dramatic, revolutionary, catastrophic, transposed the financial incentives that molded hospital decision making for two decades.

We have come through a time when . . . the development of the acute, general hospital was the end-all of the system, when more manpower of all kinds . . . more new drugs, more new equipment, with ''more'' being the key phrase, were seen as necessary (1).

With health care consumers (business, government, third-party payers, etc) becoming more prudent purchasers, future reimbursement plans—regardless of form—may be expected to embody financial stimuli for all providers to limit the consumption of health care services. ''Today, business and government are saying 'too much!''' ''The price is too high!'' ''We may not need all this!'' (1)

Successful institutional pharmacy management demands an understanding of the current environment, especially the financial incentives and their role in hospital decision making.

THE HOSPITAL ENVIRONMENT

Today's hospital milieu is complex and dynamic, with numerous external forces impacting the hospital—governmental regulation, competition, consumer demands, and reimbursement (Table 22.1). For our purposes, attention will be focused on reimbursement, or more specifically, on prospective payment.

A shift in society's health care priorities, from access to and quality of care to cost of care, has recently been witnessed. Formerly, the provider (e.g., the hospital) unilaterally determined the quality of care; however, a payer has been quoted as saying, ''Quality is what I say it is and to me if a hospital is licensed and accredited, it provides quality care'' (2). Clearly, providers making decisions regarding quality also must now consider the cost.

The Tax Equity and Fiscal Responsibility Act (TEFRA), diagnosis related groups (DRGs), and other prospective pay-

ment systems reflect a continued progression toward the long-term goal of reducing health care costs. For a score of years, hospitals were financially rewarded for providing and spending more. Today, incentives encourage the judicious expenditure of limited resources. Financial risks have been shifted from payer to provider, and hospitals will now be rewarded for reducing costs.

This reversal of incentives affects both hospital decision making and professional behavior. The primary element in hospital decision making is no longer revenue maximization; it now is minimization of expenses. For example, expensive inpatient services will, where possible, be replaced by less costly ambulatory services (e.g., outpatient and home care), and services will be provided at a competitive, acceptable level (the necessary will be distinguished from the superfluous). Stress will be inevitable as these cost-control decisions conflict with our professional perceptions relative to access to and quality of care.

TABLE 22.1 External Forces Impacting the Hospital

- Government regulation
- Accreditation and licensure requirements
- Reimbursement and cost constraints
- Capital formation
- Competition
  —Physicians
  —Alternative providers
  —Multihospital systems
  —''Consumers'' (e.g., coalitions)
- Physician surplus
  —Migration of physicians to rural areas with modification of established referral patterns
  —Entry of physicians into financially attractive endeavors for delivery of care external to the hospital (e.g., freestanding ambulatory surgical and minor emergency facilities)
  —Entry of physicians and hospitals into joint ventures
- Demographic changes
  —Aging population
  —Mobile population (e.g., urban to rural; region to region)
- Consumer demands
  —Technology
  —Ambulatory versus inpatient services
  —Lower costs
- Liability risk

The hospital's response to reimbursement changes will depend on the hospital's financial situation, structure, and general environment. Initial concentration on the reduction and containment of expenses (when staffing may be reduced, benefit programs may be modified, and programs having an unfavorable benefit to cost ratio may be eliminated) will be supplanted by the more complex, long-term response of strategic planning. Results of the latter may include diversification, restructuring, marketing, control of technology, joint ventures, etc (3,4).

For success in today's environment, hospitals must effectively manage overall operating costs while producing additional income. Prerequisites will include leadership, innovation, creativity, risk-taking, and application of sound management principles (3). Hospitals must analyze the present, project the future, and respond in a timely, creative manner (4). Some will be winners; others will be losers.

THE HOSPITAL PHARMACY ENVIRONMENT

The 1960s and 1970s were evolutionary for institutional pharmacy practice. The development and implementation of more comprehensive, progressive pharmacy services were reflected in the fiscal growth of the pharmacy department. Several factors that contributed to this growth are readily identifiable (5,6):

- Emphasis on improved quality of care and on efficiency in overall hospital operations
- Reimbursement incentives
- Introduction of more effective, more expensive pharmaceuticals
- Advances in pharmacy education
- Labor substitution with pharmacy staff to offset shortages of other staff (e.g., nurses)

Programs having potential to either enhance the quality of care or generate additional revenue could be justified with very little consideration of costs since the expense could be passed to the payer. Today, however, with the hospital's financial incentives reversed, the pharmacy must justify existing programs as well as new programs in economic terms—not just in terms of quality.

No longer can we simply show that our pharmacy services increase the level of patient care or reduce medication errors. No longer can we simply save nursing time or show how pharmacists can take drug histories better than physicians (7).

Investment of hospital resources must now be justified by the satisfaction of an institutional need or by a favorable ratio of benefits to costs. Although proven performance and credibility relative to a manager's stewardship may continue to influence the allocation of resources, the pharmacy manager's proposals and justifications must be "better conceived, written, and documented" than those of other managers if the pharmacy department is to compete effectively for the institution's stinted funds (1). The program development process in Table 22.2 may be helpful in developing and presenting winning proposals and justifications.

If regressive actions (e.g., personnel reductions and curtailment or elimination of services) are to be avoided when reductions in operating costs are mandated, pharmacy management must otherwise have a favorable impact on the

TABLE 22.2 Program Development

- Identify the concept.
- Develop (1) the philosophy and goals and (2) objectives (1-year and 5-year, if practical); correlate these to the institution's goals, objectives, and strategic plans (the program should satisfy an institutional need).
- Define (1) the program components and (2) the operating responsibilities (overall as well as for each component).
- Develop an implementation plan, including a timetable.
- Prepare budgets: (1) revenue (develop a charge schedule and forecast volumes), (2) expense (consider personnel, minor equipment, supplies, operating overhead, etc), and (3) capital (consider major equipment, construction or modification of facilities, etc); if possible, identify sources of capital funding.
- Identify the benefits and other impacts—positive and negative—of the program (be willing to take losses and make sacrifices to maximize overall profitability).
- Provide additional justification (e.g., results of a literature search and experiences of others).
- Develop a marketing plan.
- Develop an evaluation methodology for assessing the success or failure of the program.
- Formally submit a proposal—well written and documented—to the institution's decision makers/resource allocators when the program is compatible with the institution's needs and capabilities.

TABLE 22.3 Strategic Planning

- Define your present position (e.g., current mission, goals, objectives).
- Analyze the external and internal environmental trends and projections for factors affecting the organization's mission and/or success.
- Assess the barriers (threats) and opportunities, the organizational strengths and weaknesses, and the ability to manage change.
- Identify strategic alternatives and select strategies.
- Market (gain acceptance of) strategies.
- Develop tactics to carry out strategies.
- Implement strategies and tactics.
- Monitor, measure, and evaluate impact of strategies.

institution's system of drug-use control.* Strategic planning may be useful in such situations as well as in the identification and implementation of new, financially advantageous endeavors (e.g., an outpatient pharmacy). This planning process is outlined in Table 22.3.

PROSPECTIVE PAYMENT AND THE PHARMACY MANAGER

Prospective payment has challenged all hospital managers to enhance the profitability of the institution. Simply, for the pharmacy manager, this challenge calls for more effective management of costs and production of nontraditional revenues. Today's successful pharmacy manager must practice sound fiscal management and demonstrate both a business and a professional acumen in decision making.

Budgeting

Sound fiscal management implies the routine analysis of revenues and expenses, including comparisons to the bud-

---

*The sum total of knowledge, understanding, judgments, procedures, skills, controls, and ethics that assures optimal safety in the distribution and use of medication (8).

get. Because pharmacy revenues and expenses generally correlate to institutional volumes (e.g., patient days or discharges), it is essential for the pharmacy manager to develop and utilize a flexible budget in our fluid environment. With access to more sophisticated hospital information systems, these budget correlations should also reflect consideration of the institution's case mix (e.g., by major diagnostic categories [MDCs] or DRGs).

As attention is now focused on the reduction and/or control of costs and as pharmacy charges have historically been set for budgetary considerations unrelated to the actual cost of providing the product or service, it is imperative that the pharmacy manager undertake a determination of the true costs of departmental products and services. The cost of a product, for example, should include the cost of the product itself, the personnel expense required to produce an average unit of the product, supply and material costs, and other overhead allocations.

Staffing

The days of expanding hospital pharmacy manpower have passed, at least for the near future. Services imposing significant personnel demands (e.g., unit dose distribution, IV admixture services, decentralization) will be closely reexamined. The pharmacy manager must be prepared to not only justify these services but also to accept staffing reductions during periods of declining institutional volumes.

In view both of the above and the current emphasis on efficiency and increased productivity, it is incumbent on the pharmacy manager to develop systems for ongoing, concurrent monitoring of workload and productivity. Standards (e.g., patient care units or relative-value units per manhour) and staffing guides (e.g., as utilized by nursing in various patient care workload schemes) should be established. Staffing should then be matched to the workload (part-time staff might provide needed scheduling flexibility). Also, comparisons between current and past performances and between similar departmental sections should be routinely analyzed for unfavorable variances.

The pharmacy manager should also evaluate the ratio of supportive staff to professional staff and, in so doing, the assignment of departmental tasks. For obvious financial reasons, increased utilization of supportive personnel should be explored; however, compliance with legal, licensure, and accreditation requirements must not be compromised. Similarly, computerization and other automation should be considered where cost effective.

Recent studies have shown that "workers at all levels who continually face new jobs will be more vital, more productive, and more satisfied with their work . . . even though the changes in job . . . are entirely lateral" (9). Thus, cross-training of employees might provide the pharmacy manager with greater versatility within the department while also deterring job-related burnout. The cost of providing such additional training must, however, be recognized.

The pharmacy manager should also consider implementation of a merit-based performance appraisal system and establishment of employee quality circles. Both have po-

tential to stimulate greater efficiency in departmental operations.

Purchasing

Drug costs recently have represented approximately 5% of the hospital's total expenses (5) and roughly two thirds of the direct expenses of the pharmacy department. Regrettably as Zilz and Nold (5) state, "most pharmacists still do not have an appreciation for the financial impact of inventory carrying costs, addition of new items to the formulary, [and]change in turnover rates. . . ."

Clearly, a major objective of the pharmacy manager should be to minimize the department's cost of goods sold (i.e., to minimize the cost per unit purchased) while assuring the quality of the pharmaceuticals purchased. This can be accomplished, in part, through utilization of a drug buyer, contract pricing, participation in group purchasing and prime vendor programs, and application of other successful principles of the materials manager.

Drug Buyer. For improved efficiency, the pharmacy manager should delegate to one individual responsibility for daily purchasing tasks. It is recommended that this buyer, for salary considerations, not be a pharmacist; further, the buyer might be assigned to the purchasing department rather than to the pharmacy department. However, ultimate responsibility for drug procurement (e.g., vendor selection) should rest with the pharmacist.

Contract Pricing. The pharmacy manager must take measures (e.g., use of a drug buyer) to ensure utilization of available contracts if the full benefit of contract pricing is to be enjoyed. If unused, contract prices represent only an unrealized potential for savings (10).

Group Purchasing. Participation in group purchasing—especially through a large, committed-volume group—should result in more attractive contract pricing and should be investigated by the pharmacy manager. Additionally, through the economies of scale realized in group purchasing, each participant's administrative costs (e.g., costs of requesting, analyzing, and awarding bids) should be reduced.

Prime Vendor. Utilization of a progressive pharmaceutical wholesaler as a drug-depoting, prime vendor offers the pharmacy manager a proven approach to improved inventory management. Such a program should result in reduced inventory (both in physical volume and dollar value), reduced carrying costs, increased inventory turnover, and reduced administrative costs (e.g., processing of fewer purchase orders and payment of fewer vendor accounts).

Other Principles of Materials Management. The pharmacy manager should consider additional principles of the materials manager to reduce the cost of goods sold. These might include:

- Product standardization (e.g., IV administration equipment)
- Stock exchange systems for extradepartmental inventory areas (e.g., anesthesia, emergency department, surgery)
- Computerization (e.g., utilization of a fully automated inventory management system or utilization of computer-generated activity or velocity reports from a departmental system or a prime vendor's system)

- Prompt processing of vendors' returns
- Prompt payment and taking of vendors' cash discounts

Formulary Management

Although not addressed in the previous discussion, formulary management affords the pharmacy manager one of the most effective approaches to controlling the department's cost of goods sold. However, unlike the purchasing activities reviewed above, formulary management requires a strongly cooperative effort (typically via the Pharmacy and Therapeutics Committee) of the medical staff, the hospital administration, and pharmacy management and staff in balancing therapeutic and financial concerns.

A progressive approach to formulary management is recommended. For example, emphasis might initially be focused on seldomly prescribed or duplicate products and then be shifted to a more critical evaluation of therapeutic classes or categories. An alternative approach, one perhaps capable of initially producing greater financial benefits, would be to target those major drug categories experiencing a proliferation of products; attention would be concentrated on the cost effectiveness of older products, recognizing, however, that acquisition cost alone does not reflect a drug's cost effectiveness nor lack thereof.

Components of formulary management are illustrated by:
- Generic and therapeutic substitution
- Automatic stop orders (e.g., for antibiotics prescribed for surgical prophylaxis)
- Prescribing restrictions (e.g., written requests for nonformulary items and countersigning for restricted drugs)
- Drug protocols (e.g., a protocol for use of hetastarch vs albumin in cardiopulmonary bypass procedures)

Drug Utilization Review

Consumption of pharmacy resources, more specifically drugs, has primarily been determined by the physician's prescribing pattern. Drug utilization review (DUR) therefore provides the pharmacy manager another useful tool with which to favorably impact costs. Like formulary management, DUR requires the active participation of a supportive medical staff and may also be the responsibility of the Pharmacy and Therapeutics Committee.

Among the elements considered in DUR are the necessity, the appropriateness (e.g., dosage and route of administration), and the cost effectiveness of the therapy. For maximal benefit, DUR must correlate clinical and financial data (e.g., clinical outcome and total cost of therapy, not just drug costs); as hospital information systems become more sophisticated, as well as more prevalent, this task will become less formidable.

Retrospective DUR is primarily useful for the identification of areas warranting scrutiny. Initially, review might be concentrated on the more expensive drugs and/or those diagnoses having high drug costs. Drug usage should be monitored and prescribing patterns reported (e.g., by diagnosis and/or by physician and ultimately by diagnosis by physician).

Possible indicators to be monitored retrospectively include (10):

- Average length of stay
- Number of drugs/patient
- Number of doses/patient
- Number of therapeutic classes/patient
- Drug cost/patient

Variances among members of the medical staff and/or a medical staff department should be closely analyzed. Additionally, comparisons to regional and/or national data should be incorporated into the review as such data become available.

Concurrent review permits prompt intervention and problem resolution (e.g., timely conversion from parenteral to oral therapy). An effective approach to concurrent review might involve concentration on a specific diagnosis or drug; all orders for such would be reviewed daily with appropriate recommendations made to the prescriber.

Protocol development reflects a prospective DUR activity. In this activity, for example, a treatment algorithm might be designed to achieve overall cost effectiveness in therapy.

Medical Staff Education

If efforts to control drug costs are to be successful, the medical staff must be kept informed. Formulary decisions, results of DUR, etc should be regularly communicated to the physicians, including house staff; examples of vehicles for such communication include newsletters, group presentations, and consultations by pharmacists. Additionally, where possible, cost information (e.g., comparisons of alternative therapies) should be accessible to physicians via computer.

Systems Assessment

The pharmacy manager should continuously scrutinize departmental operations for cost effectiveness. This scrutiny should reflect a "back to basics" approach in which all functions, including the routine, are carefully examined (11). Whenever costs are considered to be excessive, all components (i.e., personnel, equipment, supplies, overhead) should be assessed and one or more manipulated (e.g., functions automated or waste reduced) to produce the desired improvement. When issues are interdepartmental in scope (e.g., standardization of IV concentrations or wastage of IV admixtures), joint committees (e.g., a pharmacy-nursing committee) should be considered.

Drug administration should be included in the functions examined. The following generalizations illustrate this point:

- Nonscheduled drugs have lower associated costs (i.e., purchasing, storage, distribution, administration costs) than do controlled substances.
- Drugs requiring fewer doses (via the same route) result in lower administration costs; oral products result in lower administration costs than do parenteral products.
- Secondary IV vehicles vary considerably in cost (e.g., mini-bags greater than mini-bottles greater than manufacturers' "piggybacks").
- The operating cost of an electronic IV delivery device that requires a captive administration set is greater than that of one that does not require a special set.

Also, the pharmacy manager should not overlook the importance of minimizing lost charges. As long as some payers pay charges, lost charges have obvious revenue implications; furthermore, the need to know what resources have been consumed exists regardless of payer status.

Computerization

The previous discussion relative to systems assessment would be incomplete without acknowledgment of the potential for the computer to enhance the efficiency of many departmental operations. Additionally, computerization is needed for the collection and processing of data required for effective departmental management in today's environment. Although a review of computer applications in hospital pharmacy practice is beyond our scope, a tabulation of some of the more common applications is presented for illustration:

- Distribution applications (e.g., order entry, profile maintenance, printing of lists and labels)
- Billing and expense reporting
- Purchasing and inventory management
- Controlled drug record keeping
- Clinical applications (e.g., drug interactions screening, pharmacokinetics)
- Drug utilization review
- Drug information
- Management applications (e.g., workload, productivity, staffing determinations)

Clinical Services

Clinical pharmacy services that encourage more cost-effective therapy are clearly compatible with the financial incentives of prospective payment. Such services should, in fact, serve as an interface between the administrator's concern for cost and the physician's concern for quality.

It has been suggested that the clinical pharmacist's contributions might have even greater financial than clinical impact (5). However, the pharmacist must assume an aggressive, participative role at the point of prescribing. This process is facilitated by decentralization since the pharmacist is more readily available for consultation.

Examples of clinical services worthy of the pharmacy manager's consideration are:

- Physician consultations (e.g., relative to cost effectiveness of alternative therapies and other prescribing considerations)
- Patient teaching (e.g., discharge consultations and training for home therapy, such as home parenteral nutrition)
- Drug information services
- Pharmacokinetic services
- Patient monitoring (e.g., pharmacist-conducted patient follow-up per an established treatment protocol, as in an anticoagulant clinic)
- "Postadmission" surveillance of new formulary additions

Those activities (e.g., patient teaching) which have the potential to reduce hospital admissions will be even more important under a capitation form of prospective payment.

TABLE 22.4   Managing Under Prospective Payment

- Develop an appreciation of the hospital's external environment.
- Develop a basic comprehension of the reimbursement system, but don't overly concentrate on details. Reimbursement is dynamic; however, future reimbursement systems will address a common goal—a reduction in health care costs.
- Develop an understanding of the hospital's internal environment:
  —Identify institutional strategies, and anticipate actions.
  —Analyze the environment continuously due to its fluidity.
  —Participate in aggressive, two-way information exchange.
- Support the institution:
  —Assess the departmental philosophy for institutional compatibility.
  —Develop a complementary departmental mission.
  —Identify departmental implications of institutional strategies, and develop complementary strategies and tactics.
- Strive for ongoing improvement in resource management, taking a panoramic perspective to drug-use control.
- Avoid crisis management; don't take action solely for action's sake.
- Be an innovative leader who takes controlled risks.

Diversification

As stated previously, the pharmacy manager has been challenged not only to more effectively manage costs but also to produce nontraditional revenues for the institution. One approach to the latter is diversification, as illustrated by:

- Ambulatory care services
- Outpatient pharmacy services (e.g., a retail pharmacy)
- Home care programs (e.g., enteral and parenteral nutrition, antibiotic therapy, chemotherapy)
- Surgical supply sales
- Durable medical equipment (rent, lease, sale)
- Manufacturing (e.g., for other hospitals and pharmacies)†
- Drug assay services
- Patient teaching programs (e.g., for diabetics)
- Consultation services (e.g., DUR and departmental management)
- Drug information services
- Clinical research

The requirements for start-up and operating capital are significant for several of the above programs and services. Therefore, the pharmacy manager might wish to explore joint ventures (e.g., with a pharmaceutical vendor).

CONCLUSION

Changes in the hospital environment—especially those reimbursement changes that reversed the hospital's financial incentives—have dramatically altered hospital decision making. A dual challenge to more effectively manage costs and to produce nontraditional revenues has been presented to the pharmacy manager of today. The successful manager, in responding to this challenge, must practice "opportunity management"—creating opportunities and strengths from the problems and weaknesses of the present (12). Table 22.4 summarizes an approach for such success.

Some habits, customs, and sacred cows may have to be

---

†This activity has clear implications relative to the Food and Drug Administration and Good Manufacturing Practices.

sacrificed or compromised, but such is inevitable on the road to progress. Creativity, ingenuity, and sound fiscal management will be the successful bywords (13).

REFERENCES

1. Lachner BJ: Cost justification from the administrator's viewpoint. In *Proceedings of the Symposium on Cost Justification of Clinical Pharmacy Services: Strategy for the Eighties.* New Canaan, CT, Mark Powley Associates, 1983, pp 2-7.
2. Bonney RS: Hospital survial strategies for the 1980s. *Am J Hosp Pharm* 40:1483-1488, 1983.
3. Enright SM: Understanding prospective pricing and DRGs. *Am J Hosp Pharm* 40:1493-1494, 1983.
4. Anon: DRGs: Positive view is vital to coping. *Hosp Pharm News* 2:1, 3, February 1984.
5. Zilz DA, Nold EG: Health-care trends influencing the financial management of hospital pharmacies. *Am J Hosp Pharm* 40:1532-1536, 1983.
6. Abramowitz PW, Nold EG: New directions for hospital pharmacy. *Am J Hosp Pharm* 41:724-726, 1984.
7. Williams RB. Introduction. In *Proceedings of the Symposium on Cost Justification of Clinical Pharmacy Services: Strategy for the Eighties.* New Canaan, CT, Mark Powley Associates, 1983, p 1.
8. Brodie DC: Need for a theoretical base for pharmacy practice. *Am J Hosp Pharm* 38:49-54, 1981.
9. Ouchi WG: *Theory Z.* New York, Avon Books, 1981, p 28 (paperback edition).
10. Curtiss FR: Pharmacy management strategies for responding to hospital reimbursement changes. *Am J Hosp Pharm* 40:1489-1492, 1983.
11. Upton JH, Crouch JB, Douglas JB: Coping with DRGs: The Moses H. Cone Memorial Hospital, Greensboro, North Carolina. *Am J Hosp Pharm* 40:1496-1499, 1983.
12. Williams RB: Introduction. In *Proceedings of the Symposium on Hospital Pharmacy Management in the '80s: Planning, Managing and Marketing with Limited Resources.* New York, Pfipharmecs Division of Pfizer Inc, 1984, p 3.
13. Lee HE: Coping with DRGs: Evanston Hospital, Evanston, Illinois, *Am J Hosp Pharm* 40:1508-1509, 1983.

CHAPTER 23

Contract Pharmacy Services

FREDERIC R. CURTISS

Hospital officers are turning increasingly to outside contractors to manage certain hospital departments. Food service is more likely to be contracted than any other hospital department, followed closely by housekeeping (1). Approximately one in five hospitals in the United States have contracts for one or both of these two services. The number of hospital clients using pharmacy management companies in 1982 was 363, up more than 25% from 1981, and following a gain of 16% in 1981 over 1980 (2). At a total number of 363 contracts nationwide, pharmacy departments in hospitals are as likely to be managed by an outside contractor as the emergency room, laundry, plant operations/maintenance, cardiopulmonary diagnostics, and respiratory therapy departments.

Pharmacy management companies are relatively limited in number, with a total of only 13 companies in 1982. Three companies dominate the market, possessing 78% of the pharmacy contracts. The largest pharmacy management company, HPI Health Care Services, Inc.,* held 37% of all pharmacy contracts in 1982.

BACKGROUND

Hospital pharmacy practice has evolved rapidly in the last three or four decades. Prior to the discovery of antibiotics and other major therapeutic advances in the 1930s and 1940s, the role of drug therapy in hospital care was relatively unimportant. As drug therapy became a more significant part of patient care, the role of the hospital pharmacist also became more important. Correspondingly, by the 1950s, pharmacy departments became more common in hospitals; 59% of hospitals maintained a pharmacy department in 1956 (3). By 1975, two thirds of U.S. hospitals maintained a pharmacy department with a (full-time) registered pharmacist (4). The evolution of the hospital pharmacist's role was summarized by the study Commission on Pharmacy in 1975: pharmacy practice had evolved into a "knowledge system"; many of the drug compounding and preparation functions had been assumed by the pharmaceutical industry, and the pharmacists were increasingly involved in direct patient care, including communication of drug information and education of physicians (5). Pharmacists became more responsible for the oversight and performance of the entire

*Formerly HPI Hospital Pharmacies.

drug use process: (1) identifying the patient's problem, (2) determining the patient's history of drug use, (3) prescribing, (4) selection of drug product, (5) drug dispensing, (6) education and counseling of the patient, (7) drug administration, (8) drug therapy monitoring, (9) drug use review, and (10) drug education of health professionals (6).

By the late 1970s, *comprehensive hospital pharmacy services* had come to mean pharmacist involvement in the entire drug use process and implementation of specific systems and services (7):
1. Unit dose drug distribution systems
2. Centralized IV admixture programs
3. Clinical pharmacy services

With the use of more potent drugs through the 1950s and greater use of the IV route of drug administration in the 1960s and 1970s, it became increasingly apparent that comprehensive pharmacy services were not a luxury in hospitals but a necessary part of patient care. Published reports of medication errors began appearing in the 1950s (8-10). Later research studies showed that even patients in university teaching hospitals were not protected from medication errors and that one in every six doses was administered in error (11,12). Another study reported a medication error rate of 18%, which reached 31% when wrong time of administration was counted as an error (13). Subsequent studies confirmed the high incidence of medication errors in hospitalized patients (14-17).

In addition to the medication error rates that established the need for greater control of drug distribution systems by pharmacists, the need for comprehensive pharmacy services was further evidenced in studies examining adverse drug reactions. Adverse drug reactions are defined as the unintended and undesirable, noxious effects of drugs used for diagnostic, prophylactic, or therapeutic purposes. A summary report of nine studies conducted over a 15-year period show that up to 7% of all hospital admissions are due to adverse reactions; and as many as one in five patients experience an adverse drug reaction while hospitalized (18). More recently, adverse drug reactions have been found to be the most common type of iatrogenic illness in hospitalized patients (19).

The need for comprehensive pharmacy services, including more active pharmacist involvement in drug prescribing, has been underscored by several studies that found less than optimal prescribing decisions to be common: widespread use of largely ineffective drugs (20), irrational dosage amounts or combination therapy (21-23), and a preference for newer agents of greater expense and sometimes higher toxicity but not necessarily higher efficacy (24). Unnecessary, costly, and dangerous prophylactic antibiotic use in hospitalized patients has been documented, with only 10% of patients receiving appropriate prophylactic antibiotic therapy (25). Further evidence of misprescribing was found in a study of 10,700 prescriptions, which revealed 1130 errors and a physician noncompliance prescribing rate of 14.38% (26).

Therefore, several factors conspired to highlight the need for and functioning of the pharmacist as the watchdog of drug prescribing. Accordingly, pharmacist responsibility expanded beyond drug distribution to direct patient care services now described as "clinical pharmacy." *Comprehensive* hospital *pharmacy services* now denote (1) a complete unit dose drug distribution system, (2) a pharmacy-based IV admixture program, (3) pharmacy quality assurance program, (4) clinical pharmacy services, and (5) full-time pharmacist and pharmacy management.

WHY CONTRACT PHARMACY SERVICES?

Personal familiarity with more than 300 hospital pharmacy contracts and a review of the literature show that hospitals contract with pharmacy management companies for many reasons besides achieving implementation of comprehensive pharmacy services in a timely and efficient manner. Pharmacy department management services and contracts have grown for the following reasons:

1. Shortage of hospital pharmacists, particularly in remote geographic areas
2. Difficulty in retaining competent pharmacy personnel and achieving continuity in pharmacy department services
3. Insufficient hospital pharmacy knowledge and experience among available pharmacy personnel
4. Inadequate management training among available hospital pharmacists
5. Unsatisfactory performance of in-house staff in achieving pharmacy department objectives
6. Accreditation, certification, and other regulatory pressures
7. Need for greater drug use control to contain drug diversion or reduce medication dispensing and administration errors
8. Physician demands for certain clinical pharmacy services such as pharmacokinetic dosing, patient education, and drug information services
9. Hospital administration demands for drug formulary development
10. Unavailability of sufficient nursing staff
11. Respond to nursing staff demands relating to a need for greater confidence in the pharmacy department and drug distribution responsibilities
12. Improved financial performance of the pharmacy department, including reduction in lost charges and greater control of acquisition costs
13. Insufficient capital to refixturize, purchase new equipment, or otherwise modernize the pharmacy department
14. Specific hospital personnel management objectives such as evaluation of staff performance or termination of certain personnel
15. Need to control uncertainty in the organization relative to its environment
16. Personality conflicts and other organizational politics
17. Need for reallocation of available in-house management resources to other responsibilities and problem areas in the hospital
18. Purchase of certain specialized technical and professional services unavailable elsewhere

Trained and experienced hospital pharmacists are in short supply, and many hospitals located in remote geographic areas have no access to hospital pharmacists at all. Disregarding aspects of education, training, and experience of pharmacist manpower, the Department of Health and Human Services (DHHS) reports that approximately 3000 counties in the United States have less than the number of pharmacists required to serve the population (27). On a regional basis, the Northeast has the fewest pharmacists per person, 60.8 pharmacists per 1000 population, while the North-Central United States has an average of 67.7 pharmacists per 1000 population.

Hospitals in many remote areas have experienced difficulty in recruiting and retaining competent hospital pharmacists. Often, small hospitals have had to turn to local community pharmacists to perform drug purchasing, inventory control, and oversee the drug distribution process on a part-time basis. Generally these community pharmacists lack sufficient hospital pharmacy knowledge and experience. Even if otherwise competent in pharmacy and clinical practice, comprehensive pharmacy systems and services require the participation and oversight of full-time pharmacist, properly trained in hospital pharmacy practice.

Whether full- or part-time, the pharmacy staff in a given hospital may exhibit unsatisfactory performance in achieving certain pharmacy department objectives, be they financial, drug use control, clinical, or other. Certainly, the implementation of comprehensive pharmacy services in hospitals is still incomplete, with many hospitals not reaching this professional practice standard. As late as 1978, only 24.3% of all hospitals had both unit dose drug distribution systems and pharmacy-based IV admixture programs (28). By 1982, only 7.4% of all U.S. short-term hospitals had implemented full-scope, comprehensive pharmacy services, including at least three clinical pharmacy programs (29). Inadequate training of pharmacists in hospital practice and a lack of management expertise appeared to be the most important obstacles to the implementation of comprehensive pharmacy services in U.S. hospitals (30). The problem of insufficient management training among hospital pharmacists is also reflected in the results of a survey of over 400 hospital administrators in 1978, which noted inadequate communication of the benefits of the unit dose drug distribution system to hospital administrators by pharmacists (31).

Small hospitals are particularly prone to incomplete implementation of necessary pharmacy services. The Council on Professional Affairs of the American Society of Hospital

Pharmacists recently addressed the poor quality in scope of pharmacy services in many small hospitals and concluded, "A primary cause of this problem was the inadequate understanding of hospital pharmacy practice by administrators and pharmacists in these facilities" (32).

Drug use control is the fundamental responsibility of any hospital pharmacy. The need for better drug use control has increased with the advent of more potent drugs and with recognition of the variance in patient response to certain agents, particularly those drugs which exhibit pharmacokinetic differences among patients. Effective drug use control begins with getting the right drug to the right patient in the right dose and in the right form of administration at the right time. In other words, drug use control begins with an effective and responsive drug distribution system. Failure of hospital drug distribution systems to protect patients continues to surface, and as recently as 1982, a call for widespread adoption of unit dose drug distribution systems in hospitals was dramatized at a coroner's inquest into a death in a Toronto hospital (33). The jury found that the death was due to a drug administration error, which could have been prevented had a unit dose system been operational in the hospital. The jury went on to recommend that the government help finance implementation in hospitals without unit dose systems.

The need for greater control of the entire drug use process and the adoption of broader standards and practice recommendations for hospital pharmacy has put further strain on the already short supply of trained hospital pharmacists. Practice standards now require the pharmacy to evaluate the appropriateness of prescribed drug therapy, including analysis of the effectiveness of drug therapy and general drug utilization review (DUR), as well as consultation with physicians, nurses, and other health practitioners (34). Other minimum standards require maintenance of a medication profile for each patient, review of the appropriateness of all physician medication orders by a pharmacist prior to dispensing, preparation of all sterile products (including IV admixtures, piggybacks, and irrigating solutions) by pharmacy personnel, provision of drug information to patients as well as staff, preparation of an operations manual governing all pharmacy functions, development and maintenance of a drug formulary for the hospital, etc. Moreover, the same pharmacy standards apply to all hospitals, regardless of size. Accreditation, certification, and other regulatory demands relating to these practice standards have in many cases precipitated hospital contracts with pharmacy management companies in order to correct deficiencies quickly and efficiently.

Pharmacy management companies have developed particular proficiency in implementing complete unit dose and IV admixture systems in hospitals. The large pharmacy management companies operate "implementation teams," which have the necessary experience and capability to implement these complete drug distribution systems within 4-6 weeks of the start of the contract. These implementation teams are not as encumbered by personality conflicts and other barriers as in-house pharmacy staff when implementing changes in drug and IV distribution systems and in the pharmacy department. Implementation teams can achieve in a matter of days what may take years to accomplish by in-house staff pharmacists. As late as mid-1982 experts were still citing examples of in-house pharmacists needing up to 2 years to merely obtain approval from hospital administrators to *begin* implementation of a unit dose system or a pharmacy-based IV admixture program (35).

Once these complete drug and IV distribution systems are operational and other management controls are in place, the pharmacy department operations are typically turned over to a director of pharmaceutical services employed by the management company to operate the pharmacy under the terms of the contract. Since the drug and IV distribution systems are operated under specific policies and procedures and according to performance standards, dramatic changes can occur in the correction of former problems having to do with drug diversion, medication administration errors, etc. Pharmacist reconciliation of the drug dispensing record with the medication administration record (MAR) helps detect, correct, and often prevent medication administration errors and requires accountability for all drug doses leaving the pharmacy. Drug diversion through pilferage is also made more difficult. Pharmacist reconciliation of the dispensing record and MAR to the patient billing document helps to further control drug loss due to wastage, as well as virtually eliminate lost charges and thereby improve the financial performance of the pharmacy.

Aside from the need for hospitals to implement comprehensive pharmacy services, sometimes made more acute as a result of deficiencies indentified by regulatory agencies, hospitals may turn to pharmacy management companies to satisfy physician or nursing staff demands. Nurses may demand greater confidence in the pharmacy department in its performance of drug distribution tasks. Physicians may demand clinical pharmacy skills in pharmacokinetic dosing, patient education, or drug information. Also, pharmacy contracts may be consummated as a result of a shortage of nursing staff. A complete unit dose system and centralized IV admixture program can save as much as 14-17 minutes or more of nursing time per patient day (0.23-0.28 nursing hours per patient) compared to traditional drug distribution and IV admixtures prepared by nurses (36). Clearly, comprehensive pharmacy services substitute pharmacy labor for nursing staff shortages.

Nursing payroll is typically the largest single line item expense in hospitals. Increasing nursing productivity and managing this expense item are of obvious importance to hospital officers. Nursing-management negotiations regarding labor issues may include demands having to do with working conditions and responsibility associated with drug distribution. In some cases, hospital contracts with pharmacy management companies may come about to meet certain nursing staff demands such as a more reliable and responsive drug distribution system and greater confidence in the pharmacy department. Rapid correction of deficiencies by a pharmacy management company may help avoid a strike or unionization of nurses.

The financial performance of the pharmacy department is a major factor in many hospital pharmacy contracts. Often, the profitability of the pharmacy department (i.e., excess revenue over department expense) can be improved dramatically by a pharmacy management company, simply through a reduction in lost patient charges. Reconciliation of the pharmacy dispensing record with the nursing MAR and the patient billing document on a regular and timely basis ensures that all doses are accounted for and charged properly and that each patient is charged only for those doses actually administered. Greater pharmacy department productivity, reduction in drug costs associated with drug diversion due to pilferage, and reduced drug acquisition costs can further improve the financial performance of the pharmacy department under a management contract. Finally, the large pharmacy management companies have considerable experience in the development of drug formularies, which have financial implications for hospitals as well as a salutary effect on patient care through more appropriate drug prescribing.

The large pharmacy management companies are proprietary organizations with greater access to capital than most community, nonprofit hospitals. New hospitals and hospitals short of cash or otherwise experiencing difficulty in obtaining affordable debt financing can still refixturize and update the pharmacy department via a management contract. Capital costs incurred by the contractor in purchasing equipment, replacing fixtures, and modernizing the pharmacy department are amortized over the term of the contract and financed via pharmacy revenues. Also, when the management contract includes complete control of the hospital's drug inventory, the hospital can benefit from an immediate cash infusion on valuation of the drug inventory and its purchase by the contractor.

Pharmacy management companies are attractive to some hospitals seeking to meet certain personnel management objectives such as performance evaluation of pharmacy personnel. The large management companies have the necessary resources to evaluate staff performance and productivity and can make specific recommendations to hospital officers. These studies can be used to make informed personnel changes and to justify these changes. Less often, a hospital may enter a pharmacy contract in part to terminate certain personnel or otherwise carry out difficult personnel management decisions that it might not otherwise achieve.

Resolving personality conflicts and dealing with organizational politics are an important part of the successful management of any organization. Hospital care is not immune from personal ego needs, personality conflicts, and other problems of an emotional as opposed to rational nature. While we might all hope that patient care needs and the desire to deliver effective medical services in an efficient manner would transcend such emotional factors, this is not always the case. Indeed, territorial battles are almost guaranteed in an industry where functional areas are protected by licensure and other certification mechanisms, down to specific and discrete patient care tasks. Territorial conflicts and other emotional factors can so embroil pharmacists that they become incapable of achieving objectives such as implementing a complete unit dose drug distribution system and other comprehensive pharmacy services. Pharmacy management companies have a distinct advantage in overcoming these obstacles via a broad knowledge and experience base in personnel management and the ability to tap an extensive personnel resource pool. For example, if a personality conflict surfaces between the director of pharmacy services or any other pharmacy staff person and the director of nursing or other influential hospital personnel, the pharmacy contractor can reassign pharmacy staff among hospitals, virtually overnight if necessary. Conflict situa-

tions can be analyzed and personalities assessed to best match pharmacy personnel with the needs in any given hospital. Perhaps a pharmacist or support person of a different age, sex, ethnicity, training and experience, personality type, communication skills, or other factor may be able to mesh better with nonpharmacy personnel in the hospital to resolve the conflict and to achieve objectives in a timely manner.

Indeed, this ability to transfer pharmacy personnel among hospitals is an important factor in the ability of large pharmacy management companies to attract and retain the best hospital pharmacists, even in remote hospitals. That is, many pharmacists, particularly young practitioners, are attracted to pharmacy management companies to achieve a level of geographic and professional mobility while enjoying the stability of remaining with a single organization.

From a more philosophical perspective, organizations are usually not capable of generating all of the resources and functions necessary to maintain themselves over time (37). Access to trained personnel and continuity of management contribute to organizational stability. This access to resources increases predictability for the organization and reduces environmental uncertainty (38). Management contracts and other interorganizational relationships can be viewed as a strategy to reduce uncertainty and dependence, in order to manage a changing environment and to achieve organizational stability (39).

A myriad of other human resource factors may contribute to a decision to contract with a pharmacy management company. For example, perhaps a relatively acute need arises within a given hospital to focus existing in-house management resources. A pharmacy management contract removes responsibility for day-to-day management from hospital officers and thereby permits concentration of available in-house management resources to other responsibilities and problem areas. Also, some small hospitals may be simply unable to attract sufficient management talent to oversee all hospital operations. A contract with a large pharmacy management company carrying a reputation for success can ameliorate a management shortage at levels above the pharmacy department.

Finally, large and small hospitals alike may at times experience the need for certain specialized technical or professional services that may not be available elsewhere except through a large management company. By virtue of shared resources and economies of scale, a large management company can attract leaders in various fields and those individuals with the greatest expertise. These individuals may be involved in the development and provision of the most progressive services such as comprehensive quality assurance programs (40) and clinical pharmacy certification programs (41). This level of expertise would simply be unavailable to most hospitals except through such a management contract with a large company.

CONTRACT TERMS AND SCOPE OF SERVICE

Large pharmacy management companies have the capability to implement comprehensive and progressive pharmacy services in a rapid but orderly and nondisruptive manner. Indeed, most hospital pharmacy contracts specify the time frame for implementation of specific services, usually no more than 60 days from initiation of the contract. Contractors may even guarantee certain performance standards for various systems and services in the terms of the contract.

Not all pharmacy contracts involve "full-scope" comprehensive services, however. Sometimes hospitals will purchase discrete, limited services, and the contract terms will of course vary accordingly. For example, a hospital may contract with a management company only to perform an analysis and evaluation of the hospital's current drug delivery system and pharmacy operations. The contractor may be responsible only for identifying deficiencies and making specific recommendations for correction of the deficiencies. The service would probably be performed within a specified time frame for a fixed fee amount, like any other consultant management service. The fee would generally be paid to the contractor in one lump sum on completion of the study and submission of a written report. Alternately, portions of the fee may be paid at various stages of the study or in part of periodic reevaluation points such every 6-12 months.

Limited-scope contracts may involve the purchase of one or more specific services, such as:

1. Personnel search and successful placement of the director of pharmacy services, other staff pharmacists, or support personnel
2. Backup support services to assure continuity of service, particularly in small hospitals in remote areas, during times of illness or unexpected leaves of absence of existing pharmacy personnel, or to protect against other threats to continuity of pharmacy service
3. Productivity and efficiency studies and evaluations
4. Drug formulary development
5. Development of policy and procedures manuals for pharmacy operations
6. Drug purchasing
7. Inventory control
8. Drug information and/or staff (and "in-service") education
9. Pharmacy quality assurance programs, including periodic assessment and evaluation
10. Retrospective DUR studies
11. Analysis of lost pharmacy charges or other financial performance of the pharmacy department
12. Analysis of drug diversion within the hospital

Generally the term "limited-scope" pharmacy contracts is not used to refer to relationships between hospitals and community pharmacists in which the community pharmacist is employed by the hospital for a few hours each week to do such things as check inventory, purchase and stock drugs, and otherwise meet minimum accreditation standards. In some small hospitals, community pharmacies may be involved in certain drug distribution responsibilities, including, in some cases, actually dispensing medications to hospital patients from the community pharmacy. These arrangements may not involve formal contracts and are more commonly referred to as "consultant pharmacist services."

Limited-scope pharmacy contracts are held by both large and small companies. Most full-scope pharmacy contracts are held by the large pharmacy management companies, but small companies may also provide full-scope pharmacy services, and in a few instances a hospital will contract with a second hospital for limited- or full-scope pharmacy services.

Comprehensive pharmacy systems and services require the participation and oversight of a full-time pharmacist, properly trained in hospital pharmacy practice. Full-scope pharmacy contract services would include most or all of the following: (1) complete unit dose drug distribution system, (2) complete pharmacy-based IV admixture program, (3) comprehensive quality assurance program, (4) daily reconciliation of patient charges with the pharmacy drug dispensing profile and the nurses' MAR, (5) in-service education of nurses, physicians, and other health professionals, (6) concurrent monitoring of patient drug profiles to check for drug interactions, adverse drug reactions, and inappropriate drug prescribing, (7) complete pharmacy staffing, including personnel recruitment, selection, education, training, and fringe benefit expenses, (8) professional and technical support, including backup pharmacists and technicians to ensure continuity of services, (9) management and supervisory support services provided by regional and home office personnel, (10) research and development, including innovations in drug delivery, electronic data processing, and clinical pharmacy services such as pharmacokinetic analyses and drug dosing, (11) purchase of entire pharmacy department inventory and remodeling and refixturization to permit implementation of unit dose and IV admixture programs, (12) management training and education programs for staff pharmacists and support personnel, (13) drug information services, including periodic newsletters, (14) full-time pharmacist service, including 24-hour on-call coverage, (15) periodic management reports to hospital administration, (16) development of hospital-specific pharmacy policies and procedures manuals, (17) pharmacist participation in hospital committees such as the Pharmacy and Therapeutics (P&T) Committee and Utilization and Review Committee, (18) retrospective DURs, and (19) drug therapy consultations with nurses and physicians.

Each of the services identified above may be specified to varying degrees in the contract. Alternately, each service is explained in greater detail in the "proposal for services." This document is generally prepared following an on-site analysis and evaluation of the hospital's present drug distribution system and pharmacy operations. Following the on-site visit, often referred to as a "feasibility study," the proposal is prepared, including an explanation of the deficiencies detected and the proposed systems and services to correct the deficiencies. A contract may be negotiated between the management company and the hospital subsequent to presentation of the results of the on-site study and analysis of the proposal for services. Elsewhere, Fink (42) has described some of the liability and other legal issues associated with hospital pharmacy contracts. Under the terms of the full-scope pharmacy contracts, the management company assumes responsibility for essentially all pharmacy services and department operations. However, the hospital cannot of course abrogate ultimate responsibility for the quality of care rendered to patients in the hospital and, by necessity, must provide certain services and facilities necessary for complete pharmaceutical services. As with the responsibilities of the pharmacy contractor, the responsibilities of the hospital should also be specified in the contract and may include the following:

1. Nursing staff responsibilities, including the actual administration of drug to patients, updating patient MARs, and cooperation with the pharmacy department in reconciling the dispensing record to the MAR

2. Allocation of physical space for the pharmacy department, unit dose cabinets, and exchange carts in the nursing units and other parts of the hospital and space requirements for the night drug storage locker

3. Billing and collecting pharmacy charges and deductions from revenue associated with contractual allowances to third-party payers and bad debts

4. Preparation of appropriate claim forms, cost reports, and other documents for third-party payers and any other necessary interactions with these parties

5. Day-to-day housekeeping and other maintenance services of the pharmacy department and related space operated by the contractor in the hospital

6. Local telephone, power, and other utility services

7. Receiving and storage space and perhaps some limited services associated with these functions of the contractor in managing pharmacy inventories

Pharmacy management companies are paid for their services in several ways, ranging from fixed annual management fees, generally paid in monthly amounts, to revenue-sharing arrangements in which the contractor and the hospital share in the pharmacy department revenue in a specified proportion, e.g., 50% of the pharmacy department revenue to each. While most hospital-pharmacy management company financial arrangements will involve one of the following methods, some contracts may incorporate two or more of these methods:

1. Annual management fee, including all drug costs, salary, and other operating expenses.

2. Management fee with a pass through of drug costs to the hospital. The cost pass through may be calculated from the management company's actual acquisition costs (AAC), average wholesale price (AWP), discounted AWPs such as estimated acquisition costs (EAC), or via some other price schedule.

3. Management fee tied to hospital census or volume of activity, e.g., management fee per patient day, per patient case, per diagnosis related group (DRG).

4. Unit service charge (SC) in which the hospital is charged for each unit dose dispensed by the pharmacy to patients or to the nursing unit. The SC amount is usually calculated from some multiple factor times the cost of the medication, e.g., $1.2 \times$ AWP.

5. Revenue-sharing agreements in which the hospital and the management company share, in specific portion, the patient charge for the medication dispensed. For example, a particular unit dose of medication may have an AWP cost of $0.90 and the hospital employs a patient charge schedule of three times AWP, yielding a patient charge of $2.70. If the revenue-sharing arrangement specifies the portion as hospital, 60%, and pharmacy contract, 40%, the pharmacy contractor is paid $1.08 for dispensing this unit dose of medication ($0.40 \times$ $2.70).

Except for the revenue-sharing type of arrangement, a hospital's pharmacy price schedule is essentially independent of the financial arrangement with the pharmacy contractor. Most hospitals finance pharmacy services through a markup on the cost of medication actually dispensed to the patient, using the AAC, AWP, EAC, or some similar basis. Customary markup multipliers range from 2.5-4.0 times the drug cost. These drug cost "multiples" are generally supplemented by minimum patient charges such as $0.75 for an oral solid unit dose, $1.00 for a oral solid controlled substance, and $3.00 for an injectable medication. The minimum amount is charged to the patient when the cost of the medication times the multiplier is less than the minimum amount. "Minimum" patient charges are conceptually sound, and thereby ethical, since this method recognizes that there is a service cost associated with dispensing a unit dose of medication that is relatively fixed and independent of the actual product cost of the medication.

Regardless of the type of financial arrangement between the pharmacy management company and the hospital, the patient price schedule should be determined by the hospital without any element of control by the contractor. However, the pharmacy management company will generally have responsibility for maintaining the patient price schedule and for updating the schedule periodically.

The precise terms of a contract will be unique to a given hospital–management company arrangement. The financial arrangement and scope of services of the contract will result from negotiations between the management company and the hospital. Depending on the unique circumstances in a given hospital, the pharmacy management company may assume certain financial risks in providing pharmacy services to the patients and staff of the hospital. For example, in the financial arrangement specified in No. 1 above, a pharmacy management company would assume a considerable degree of risk having to do with drug utilization, including the use of expensive medications. In this arrangement, the pharmacy management company may limit its risk through certain conditions, specified in the contract, such as adjustment for fluctuating patient case mix (or severity of illness) or a maximum aggregate *drug cost* as a percent of the total fee paid by the hospital to the contractor, e.g., 50% of the management fee.

Conversely, the hospital would assume a considerable degree of risk associated with the total cost of the pharmacy contract in the service charge (SC) arrangement (No. 4 above). In this case, the total amount paid to the pharmacy management company would depend on drug utilization, determined of course by drug prescribing, and the possible use of expensive medication. A hospital may try to limit this element of financial risk by specifying certain conditions in a contract such as a maximum amount to be paid to the contractor, determined on a per patient day or per patient case basis; e.g., up to but not more than $40 per patient day.

Other terms of the financial arrangements between hospitals and pharmacy management companies may include provisions such as a cash discount for prompt payment by the hospital to the contractor, an adjustment factor for third-party contractual allowances to the hospital, or other deductions from revenue such as bad debts, as well as a myriad of other factors. The management company may also specify a minimum profit amount to the hospital such as $10 per patient day or $75 per patient case. This amount would be calculated from the average amount of pharmacy revenue per patient day less the average amount paid to the management company per patient day, perhaps less the amounts having to do with deductions from revenue. For example, a pharmacy contract guarantees a minimum pharmacy department gross margin of $40 per patient day for the hospital. Actual total pharmacy revenue from patient charges for a given fiscal period equals $1 million divided by 12,500 total patient days, yields $80 per patient day. Pharmacy (SC) charges for the same fiscal period totaled $600,000, or $48 per patient day. In this example the pharmacy management company would be obligated to return $100,000 to the hospital ($8 per patient day times 12,500 patient days) under this financial guarantee.

Often a pharmacy management company can implement full-scope pharmacy services in a hospital and finance these services without raising patient prices, solely through gaining control of lost pharmacy charges (43). Inadequate record keeping and insufficient reconciliation result in lost patient charges of as high as 30%. Alternately, patient revenue may be enhanced without increasing patient prices through (1) updating drug costs in a more timely manner, (2) greater consistency in patient pricing, or (3) reducing interdepartmental transfers of medications, i.e., drugs charged to nursing units rather than individual patients.

GOVERNMENT REGULATIONS AFFECTING PHARMACY MANAGEMENT CONTRACTS

All Medicare and Medicaid regulations that affect hospital operations and the provision of patient care may of course affect directly or indirectly the management of the pharmacy department by a contractor. Also, state and federal regulations regarding drug distribution and controlled substances are generally recognized as the responsibility of the pharmacy management company. However, the following five regulations are of particular note and will be discussed here:
1. Medicare conditions of participation
2. Maximum allowable cost (MAC) limits
3. Prudent buyer concept
4. Prohibition against revenue-sharing arrangements
5. Access to books and records of subcontractors

The Medicare Conditions of Participation affect pharmacy contractors and in-house pharmacy services alike. The conditions are those requirements that hospitals must meet in order to participate in the Medicare and Medicaid Program (Titles XVIII and XIV of the Social Security Act). These conditions were first published in 1966, and on June 20, 1980, HCFA published a notice of proposed changes in Subsection 485.25 of Subpart C of the standards pertaining to pharmaceutical services.

The Conditions of Participation are used by Medicare intermediaries to accredit approximately 1500 of the 6700 short-term hospitals in the United States. Most of these are small, rural hospitals. The rest of the 6700 hospitals are accredited by the Joint Commission on Accreditation of Hospitals (JCAH), and JCAH standards supersede the Medicare Conditions of Participation for accreditation purposes. In early 1983, HCFA published proposed rules, which if finalized will grant hospitals much greater flexibility in meeting the Medicare standards for accreditation (44). The proposed changes included relaxation of standards for pharmaceutical services.

Part 19 of the Code of Federal Regulations specifies that the cost of drugs and related medical supplies furnished by providers to Medicare beneficiaries "shall not exceed the amount a prudent and cost-conscious buyer would pay for the same item" (45). This reasonable cost limitation is generally referred to as "the prudent buyer concept." Part of the prudent buyer regulation states that for purchases made on or after the effective date of the final MAC determinations, the allowable cost for any multiple-source drug for which a MAC has been established may not exceed the lowest of: (1) the actual cost, (2) the amount that would be paid by a prudent and cost-conscious buyer for the drug if obtained from the lowest priced source that is widely and consistently available within a provider's service area, whether sold by generic or brand name, or (3) the MAC. The only exception to the MAC limitation occurs when a physician certifies that in his medical judgment a specific brand name drug is medically necessary for a particular patient. The individual patient's name and the particular drug prescribed must be clearly identified and the certification made in the physician's own handwriting. There is also one *exemption* to the MAC regulations for unit dose drug distribution systems, including pharmacy-based medication dispensing records and profile monitoring, when operated by a pharmacy management company (46). Hospital drug distribution systems overseen and otherwise managed by community pharmacies are not included in this exemption.

The government appears intent on continuing the MAC program for drugs dispensed by community pharmacies to Medicaid recipients. However, the MAC program as applied to hospital services has been superseded by the Medicare Prospective Payment System (PPS), which reimburses hospitals at a prospective fixed price per DRG (per Medicare discharge). Medicare PPS is effective for Medicare payment of hospital services commencing with each hospital's new cost-reporting period beginning on or after October 1, 1983. The Medicare DRG prices are paid by HCFA without regard to actual costs of the provider institution or actual patient charges. Hence, determination of "reasonable costs" by Medicare intermediaries is no longer necessary since hospitals now have a strong financial incentive to be "prudent" in purchasing products and services, including drugs and medical supplies, in order to control their costs at a level less than or equal to the DRG prices (47).

Two additional federal regulations have particular relevance to hospital pharmacy departments operated by management companies. Section 109 of the Tax Equity and Fiscal Responsibility Act (TEFRA) passed by Congress in 1982 prohibited payment for services provided to hospitals (or hospital patients) by contractors and paid by hospitals on the basis of "a percentage (or other proportion) of the provider's charges, revenues, or claim for reimbursement" (48). This provision of TEFRA would seem to exclude percentage contracts and revenue-sharing arrangements between hospitals and contractors, including pharmacy management companies. However, due to language in the statute having to do with exceptions to this prohibition, HCFA encountered difficulty in writing regulations to implement this section of TEFRA. Also, new financial incentives inherent in Medicare PPS supersede the perceived need for HCFA to police the cost-control behavior of hospitals. Consequently, regulations to implement the prohibition of revenue-sharing arrangements have not been written by HCFA, and hence the prohibition is unenforceable.

Section 952 of P.L. 96-499, The Omnibus Reconciliation Act of 1980, required HCFA to write regulations prohibiting reimbursement for the cost of services provided to hospitals by subcontractors unless the contract included a clause allowing the secretary of Health and Human Services and the comptroller general ". . . access to the contract and to the subcontractor's books, documents, and records necessary to verify the costs of the contract" (49). Final regulations published on December 30, 1982, made this requirement retroactive to all contracts entered into or renewed after December 5, 1980. The access clause requirement pertains to all contracted services, including legal services, management and consultant services, etc, wherein the annual cost of the contract in $10,000 or more. The $10,000 threshold amount may be increased to $50,000 (50).

As with other HCFA regulations pertaining to most "reasonable cost" determinations by Medicare intermediaries, the perceived need for monitoring and enforcement of the access to subcontractors' records was transcended by the Medicare prospective payment system.

REFERENCES

1. Johnson DEL: Contract management shared services survey. *Mod Healthcare* 13(8):89-95, 1983.
2. Johnson DEL, Punch L: Contract management and shared services. *Mod Healthcare* 12(7):103-112, 1982.
3. *Hospitals* (Guide Issue) 31:Part 2, Table 16, p 399, Table 23, p 412, August 1957.
4. Stolar MH: National survey of selected hospital pharmacy practices. *Am J Hosp Pharm* 33:225-230, 1976.
5. American Association of Colleges of Pharmacy: *Pharmacists for the Future*. Ann Arbor, Health Administration Press, 1975, pp 49-59.
6. McCleod DC: The drug use process. In McCleod DC, Miller A (eds): *The Practice of Pharmacy*, Cincinnati, Harvey Whitney Books, 1981, pp 11-15.
7. Tanner DJ: Comprehensive pharmaceutical services in an 85-bed hospital: A one-year evaluation. *Am J Hosp Pharm* 34:486-490, 1977.
8. Byrne AK: Errors in giving medications. *Am J Nurs* 53:829-831, 1975.
9. Schlosberg E: Sixteen safeguards against medication errors. *Hospitals* 32:62, 1958.
10. Safren MS, Chapanis A: A critical incident study of hospital medication errors. *Hospitals* 34:32-34, 1960.
11. Barker KN, McConnell WE: The problems of detecting medication errors in hospitals. *Am J Hosp Pharm* 19:360, 1962.
12. Barker KN, Heller WM: The development of a centralized unit dose dispensing system for UAMC. Part VI: The pilot study—medication errors and drug losses. *Am J Hosp Pharm* 21:609, 1964.
13. Barker KN: The effects of an experimental medication system on medication errors and costs. *Am J Hosp Pharm* 26:388-397, 1969.
14. Parker PF: Unit dose systems reduce error, increase efficiency. *Hospitals* 42:65, 1968.
15. Owyang E, Miller RA, Brodie DC: The pharmacist's new role in institutional patient care. *Am J Hosp Pharm* 25:316, 1969.
16. Best DF, Jr: An integrated pharmacist-nurse approach to the unit dose concept. *Am J Hosp Pharm* 25:397-407, 1968.
17. Smith WE, Mackewicz DW: An economic analysis of the PACE pharmacy service. *Am J Hosp Pharm* 27:123-126, 1979.
18. Stewart RB: Adverse drug reactions in hospitalized patients. *Pharm Intern* 1:77-79, April 1980.
19. Steel K, Gertman PM, Crescenvi C, et al: Iatrogenic illness on a general medical service at a university hospital. *N Engl J Med* 304:638-642, 1981.
20. Temin P: *Taking Your Medicine: Drug Regulation in the United States*. Cambridge, MA, Harvard University Press, 1980.
21. Castle M, Wilfert CM, Cate TR, et al: Antibiotic use at Duke University Medical Center. *JAMA* 237:2819-2822, 1977.
22. Scheckler WE, Bennett JV: Antibiotic usage in seven community hospitals. *JAMA* 213:264-267, 1970.
23. Stewart RB, Cluff LE, Philip JR (eds): *Drug Monitoring: A Requirement for Drug Use*. Baltimore, Williams & Wilkins, 1977.
24. Maugh TH II: A new wave of antibiotics builds. *Science* 214:1225-1228, 1981.
25. Fry DE, Harbrecht PJ, Polk HC: Systemic prophylactic antibiotics. *Arch Surg* 116:466-469, 1981.
26. Ingrim NB, Hokanson JA, Guernsey BG, et al: Physician noncompliance with prescription writing requirements. *Am J Hosp Pharm* 40:414-417, 1983.
27. Anon: *Supply and Characteristics of Selected Health Personnel*. DHHS Publication No. (HRA) 81-20. Health Resources Administration, Division of Health Professions Analysis, Bureau of Health Professions, Hyattsville, MD, June 1981.
28. Stolar MH: National survey of hospital pharmaceutical services—1978. *Am J Hosp Pharm* 36:316-325, 1979.
29. Stolar MH: National survey of hospital pharmaceutical services—1982. *Am J Hosp Pharm* 40:963-969, 1983.
30. Haas M: Comprehensive pharmacy services in the small hospital. In McCleod DC, Miller WA (eds): *The Practice of Pharmacy*, Cincinnati, Harvey Whitney Books, 1981, pp 440-457.
31. Dorman MR, Brown TR, Smith MC, et al: Do administrators' views show why hospitals do or don't use unit dose? *Hospitals* 52:107-109, 1978.
32. Anon: Report of the Council on Pharmaceutical Affairs of the American Society of Hospital Pharmacists. *Am J Hosp Pharm* 38:1207, 1981.
33. Anon: Coroner's jury advocates unit dose. *ASHP Newsletter* 15(12):3, 1982.
34. Anon: Minimum standards for pharmacies in institutions. *Am J Hosp Pharm* 34:1356-1358, 1977.
35. Chase P: Assessment of pharmaceutical services in the small hospital. *Am J Hosp Pharm* 39:864-865, 1982.
36. Marshall G: Clinical program may effect savings. *Hospitals* 48:79, 80, 102, December 1974.
37. Aldrich HE, Pfeffer J: Environments of organizations. In Inkeles A (ed): *Annual Review of Sociology*, vol 2. Palo Alto, CA, Annual Review, 1976.
38. Zuckerman HS, Wheeler JRC: Management contracts: Strategy for organizational stability. *Health Care Mgt Rev* 7(4):45-51, 1982.
39. Longest BB, Jr: An external dependence perspective of organizational strategy and structure: The community hospital case. *Hosp Health Serv Admin* 26(2):50-69, 1981.
40. Horowitz KN, Lamnin L: Design and implementation of a quality assurance program for pharmaceutical services. *Am J Hosp Pharm* 37:82-84, 1980.
41. Talley CR: Certification program for clinical services developed by HPI Hospital Pharmacies. *Am J Hosp Pharm* 38:1418-1420, 1981.
42. Fink JL: Liability issues relating to contract pharmaceutical services. *Am J Hosp Pharm* 40:2188-2190, 1983.
43. Anon: Why some hospitals are turning to contract pharmacies. *Am Druggist* 175(2):21-25, 1977.
44. Medicare and Medicaid Programs. Conditions of participation for Hospitals. 42 CFR Parts 405, 480, 482, 483, 484, 485, 487, 488. Proposed Rule. *Fed Reg* 48(2):299-315, 1983.
45. Cost of Drugs and related medical supplies. Prov. Reimb Manual, Part I, Section 2119, as reported in Para. 5923 of the *Comm Clearing House Medicare and Medicaid Guide*, vol 1, pp 1951.6-52.
46. Methodology for comparing prices: Unit dose. Prov. Reimb. Manual, Part I, Section 2119, as reported in Para. 5923.61 of the *Comm Clearing House Medicare and Medicaid Guide*, vol 1, pp 1951, 14, 1951.15.
47. Medicare Program; Prospective payment for Medicare inpatient hospital services; Final rule. *Fed Reg* 49(1):233-339, 1984.
48. H.R. 4961, Tax Equity and Fiscal Responsibility Act of 1982, Medicare and Medicaid Spending Reductions, as passed by Congress on August 19, 1982. *Medicare and Medicaid Guide*, extra edition No. 361, August 24, 1982, Chicago, Commerce Clearing House.
49. Medicare Program: Access to books, documents, and records of subcontractors. Final rule. *Fed Reg* 47(251):58260-58270, 1982.
50. Reg. Sec. 420.300-304, Subpart D, Access to books and records of subcontractors. *Medicare and Medicaid Guide*, Para. 20,906G, pp 8361.14-8363, Chicago, Commerce Clearing House.

Drug Information and Drug Actions

ASSIMILATION AND PROVISION OF COMPREHENSIVE INFORMATION ON DRUGS AND THEIR ACTIONS

Fundamental to the pharmacist's contribution to health care is his knowledge of drugs and their actions. The pharmacy department is the primary source of information concerning drugs. The pharmacy must maintain the appropriate information sources and develop mechanisms for evaluating information and transmitting it to the institution's professional staff and to the patient.

The pharmacist must have the ability to use his basic science knowledge and his knowledge of the effects of drugs on biologic systems in assessing such determinants of drug action as absorption, distribution, metabolism, and excretion of a drug; drug interactions with other drugs, foods, or diagnostic agents; effects of a disease state on the drug's action; and miscellaneous patient and drug variables. Thus, the pharmacist practicing in an institution must be knowledgeable in chemistry, pharmacology, toxicology, pathophysiology, pharmaceutics, therapeutics, and patient care techniques, and he should have some background in the social sciences.

CHAPTER 24

Searching and Organizing the Professional Literature

G. EDWARD COLLINS

The hospital pharmacist is presented with many challenges in today's practice. One of the most exciting is the increasing responsibility for assuring the intelligent and safe use of drugs. In order to assist the physician in bringing new advances in medical care to patients, continued education and an approach to therapy that is flexible enough for the utilization of new techniques and drugs are required. At the same time, one must be cognizant of the rapidly rising cost of health care and take this fact into consideration when developing safe and effective therapeutic alternatives. The pharmaceutical scientist and the clinical pharmacologist cannot determine the place for medical advances in actual patient care; this responsibility remains with the practitioners who care for patients on a day-to-day basis. Walton (1) states that there are two prerequisites for performing this responsibility:

1. Reliable evaluation of the potential therapeutic and toxic effects of these drugs must be achieved through competent clinical investigation.
2. The results of such clinical studies must be rapidly, completely, and accurately communicated to the practitioner who uses the information.

As one of the users of this information, the hospital pharmacist is presented with a significant challenge. In 1984, the Excerpta Medica data base added 65,000 new articles concerning drugs. In total, 400,000 articles are cited in this data base, which contains significant information relevant to health care, medicine, and related sciences. Additional citations can be found in other data bases. Relevant literature is published in more than 3500 biomedical journals worldwide.

In addition to size, another problem faces the practitioner who keeps abreast of changes in this vast field. The quality of the professional literature continues to be suspect. Several authors in the late 1950s and 1960s drew attention to the varying quality of scientific literature (2,3). More recently, Fletcher and Fletcher (4) evaluated clinical research reported in general medical journals. They found that over a 30-year (1946-1976) period the frequency of studies with weak research designs had increased. DerSimonian et al (5) also evaluated the quality of reports appearing in major medical journals. These authors determined the frequency of reports

concerning what they considered important aspects of design and analysis in clinical trials reported in the *New England Journal of Medicine, Lancet, British Medical Journal,* and *Journal of the American Medical Association* during 1979 and 1980. Of 11 items that the authors believed were critical to the evaluation of the aspects of design and analysis, they found that clinical trials reported in *New England Journal of Medicine* reported 71% of those items; *Journal of the American Medical Association,* 63%; *British Medical Journal,* 52%; and *Lancet,* 46%. The authors believed that these were major deficiencies. Evaluation of the scientific literature is addressed in Chapter 25.

The staggering size and varying quality of the professional literature require that the hospital pharmacist develop a greater sophistication in his understanding of the organization of this literature and in his ability to critically evaluate the data presented.

ORGANIZATION OF THE LITERATURE

In order to effectively use the professional literature, one must first understand how it is organized. Professional literature is best thought of as a pyramid that is divided into three sections (Fig. 24.1).

The base of the pyramid represents the primary literature. Primary literature provides the broad base for development of the rest of the professional literature. Primary literature contains original reports of scientific studies on which the knowledge of drugs and therapeutics is built. By nature, it is the largest and most current of the information sources, and periodical journals are its most common format. Use of the primary literature has the advantages of providing access to the original data from a study as well as having the most current information. The greatest disadvantages are the size and varying quality of the literature.

Indexing and abstracting services make up the secondary sources. These publications provide the user with concise tools for gaining access to the primary literature. There are several secondary sources useful for providing access to the primary literature; no single service is all inclusive. The subjects covered and the completeness of indexing are reflected in the type and number of primary sources that are

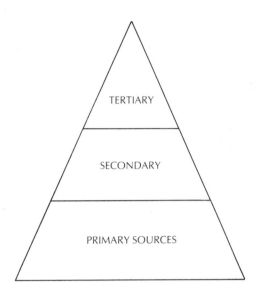

FIGURE 24.1 Pyramidal structure of the professional literature.

covered. Not all material from a publication may be selected for indexing. Secondary sources also differ in several respects. These sources all provide some type of indexing of the primary literature; however, not all of them provide abstracts of the cited material. Abstracts are useful in selecting articles that need to be more closely examined. Secondary sources also differ in the time between appearance of a document in the primary literature and its inclusion in the secondary source. This is referred to as "lag time." For some services, the "lag time" may be as short as several weeks, and in others, it may be as long as several months. Effective use of a secondary source requires that one be familiar with all of these differences.

The top of the pyramid depicts the tertiary sources. These include textbooks, monographs, compendia, handbooks, and published symposia. They represent the condensation of basic facts originally published in the primary literature. Because tertiary sources make up the smallest section of the scientific literature, they offer the advantage of being the easiest to use. Their size, however, presents two significant limitations. To prepare these sources, basic data have been evaluated, interpreted, and reduced to a manageable form. In doing so, the author may have lost some of the original meaning of the data. Tertiary sources also suffer from "lag time." Several years may pass before some facts make their way into the tertiary literature. In the meantime, new information may be discovered, rendering the source out of date almost at the time of publication. To compensate for this deficiency, the user must have some familiarity with primary literature in the field.

SEARCHING THE LITERATURE

Before beginning a search of the literature, it is essential to thoroughly define the question to be answered. This is done by classifying the question according to one of several classification schemes. Classification of the question by type (stability, pharmocology, drug interaction, indication, etc) and expertise of the requester (physician, pharmacist, etc)

aids in the interpretation of the request and stimulates the necessary questions useful for obtaining appropriate background information. In addition, it is often useful to discuss the question with the individual who has posed it. Therefore, the question can be refined, and the individual searching the literature has a complete understanding of the question. A complete analysis of the question to be answered allows one to narrow the scope of the search to save time; classification of the question allows the search to be directed to those sources most likely to contain the sought-after information; and a well-defined question allows the responder to tailor the reply to meet the specific needs of the requester.

The search should be approached in a systematic manner and is usually initiated through the use of tertiary literature. Tertiary sources are usually the most readily available and the easiest to use. They are also the sources with which most individuals are familiar. Every hospital pharmacy should have a core selection of major textbooks (Table 24.1). Additional resources should be selected based on the type and scope of services offered, as well as available financial resources. Selection of tertiary sources also depends on the proximity of larger health science libraries. One must also be prepared to purchase new editions when published; however, before purchasing any textbook, if at all possible, it should be completely evaluated to ensure that it will meet anticipated needs. If the question has been well defined, it may be possible to direct the search to specific sources. The following publications have been classified according to the type of information they are most likely to contain.

No single tertiary source will have all the necessary information. Some texts are useful for locating more than one type of information. To facilitate the search, each pharmacist should be thoroughly familiar with the type of information contained in each reference.

Tertiary Resources

Identifications/Availability

American Drug Index: Billups NF, Billups SM (eds), JB Lippincott Co (annual). Alphabetical listing of drugs by trade, generic, and chemical name. The trade name entry includes manufacturer, chemical or generic name, package size, dosage form, strengths,

TABLE 24.1 Recommended Hospital Pharmacy Library: Core Collection

1. *The Pharmacological Basis of Therapeutics*
2. *American Hospital Formulary Service Drug Information*
3. *Facts and Comparisons*
4. *Drug Interactions*
5. *Handbook of Nonprescription Drugs*
6. *Handbook of Clinical Drug Data*
7. *AMA Drug Evaluations*
8. *Manual of Medical Therapeutics*
9. *Harrison's Principles of Internal Medicine*
10. *Dorland's Illustrated Medical Dictionary*
11. *Clinical Laboratory Medicine*
12. *Handbook of Injectable Drugs*
13. *Guide to Parenteral Admixtures*
14. *Approved Prescription Drug Products with Therapeutic Equivalence Evaluations*

and uses. Generic and trade names are cross-indexed. Includes directory of manufacturers.

Facts and Comparisons: Kastrup EK (ed), Facts and Comparisons Division, JB Lippincott Co (monthly supplements). Comparative product information for drugs with same indications, including relative cost and availability. Also includes brief discussion of pharmacology, uses, and cautions.

American Druggist Blue Book: Lee FH (ed), Hearst Corp (annual). Provides information by trade name, giving manufacturer, package size, dosage form, and cost. Extensive list of manufacturers and telephone numbers.

Drug Topics Red Book: Knipping WJ (ed), Medical Economics Books (annual).

Physicians's Desk Reference: Medical Economics Books (annual). A collection of drug package inserts. Also includes list of manufacturers and telephone numbers. Provides approximately 1000 pictures of different drugs.

Pharm Index: Skyline Publishers, Inc (monthly supplements). Indexed by trade names, generic names, manufacturer, and therapeutic use. Each update includes monographs of new chemicals, new dosage forms, new indications, discontinued items, products which are to be marketed in the future, and product cost. Also includes review articles on drug classes.

United States Adopted Names (USAN) and USP Directory of Drug Names: Griffiths MC (ed), United States Pharmacopeial Convention, Inc (annual). Alphabetical listing of USAN cross-referenced to trade names and synonyms. Provides pronunciation, formula, chemical names, CAS registry number, and therapeutic category.

Martindale, The Extra Pharmacopoeia: Wade A (ed), The Pharmaceutical Press (5 years). Extensive list of international products with monographs. Referenced. Now available full-text on-line computer.

Merck Index, An Encyclopedia of Chemicals and Drugs: Windholz M (ed): Merck and Co, Inc (8 years). Description of the physical and chemical properties of approximately 10,000 substances. An entry includes alternative name, trade name, formula, toxicity, therapeutic category, and references.

Index Nominum: Laboratory of the Swiss Pharmaceutical Society of Zurich (annual). Alphabetical listing of generic and trade names of internationally available drug products.

Handbook of Nonprescription Drugs: Griffenhagen GB (ed), American Pharmaceutical Association (2-4 years). The best single guide to nonprescription drugs. Extensive tables and monographs detailing the scientific data on over-the-counter products.

Drug Compatibility and Drug-Drug Interactions and Drug–Laboratory Test Interactions

Handbook on Injectable Drugs: Trissel LA, American Society of Hospital Pharmacists (2-4 years). Provides extensive information on the physical and chemical characteristics as well as the compatibility of individual drugs.

Guide to Parenteral Admixtures: King JC, Cutter Laboratories, Inc (supplements). Alphabetical listing of drugs and their compatibility with other drugs and fluids.

Drug Interactions: Hansten PD, Lea and Febiger (2-3 years). Descriptions of drug-drug interactions including the interaction, mechanism, clinical significance, management, and references. Also presents interactions of drugs and laboratory tests, clinical significance, and references.

Adverse Effects/Toxicity

Meyler's Side Effects of Drugs: Dukes MNG (ed), Excerpta Medica distributed by Elsevier Science Publishing Co, Inc (an-

nual). Extensive listing of drugs by therapeutic class and reported side effects. Well referenced.

Drug-Induced Ocular Side Effects and Drug Interactions: Fraunfelder FT, Lea and Febiger. The first text devoted to this subject. Well referenced.

Drugs, Chemicals and Blood Dyscrasias: Swanson M, Cook R, Drug Intelligence Publications. Thorough review of the adverse hematologic effects of drugs and chemicals. Referenced.

Hepatotoxicity: The Adverse Effects of Drugs and Other Chemicals on the Liver, Zimmerman HJ, Appleton-Century-Crofts. Extensive review of the published data on drug-induced hepatoxicity. Well referenced.

Clinical Toxicology of Commercial Products, Gosselin RE et al., Williams and Wilkins Co (6-7 years). Excellent source. describes the manifestations and treatment of acute poisonings. Comprehensive listing of ingredients of commercially available products. Well referenced.

Handbook of Poisoning: Prevention, Diagnosis, and Treatment: Driesbach RH, Lange Medical Publications (2-3 years). Concise reference on the subject. Both short- and long-term toxicities are presented. The brevity of the text may require supplementation with other references.

Pharmacology and Disease Treatment

There are many reference texts which could be selected for this section. Those most commonly available and those with the greatest potential value have been selected. Other specialty references may be useful for some practice environments.

The Pharmacological Basis of Therapeutics: Goodman LS, Gilman A (eds), Macmillan Publishing Co (5 years).

Clinical Pharmacology: Basic Principles in Therapeutics: Melman KL, Morrelli HF, Macmillan Publishing Co.

Harrison's Principles of Internal Medicine: Thorn GW, et al, McGraw-Hill Book Co (4 years).

Current Therapy: Conn HF (ed), WB Saunders Co (2 years).

Current Medical Diagnosis and Treatment: Krupp MA, Chatton MS (eds), Lange Medical Publications (annual).

Manual of Medical Therapeutics: Campbell JW, Frisse M (eds), Little, Brown & Co.

Handbook of Nonprescription Drugs: Griffenhagen GB (ed), American Pharmaceutical Association.

Principles and Practice of Infectious Diseases: Mandell GL, et al, John Wiley & Sons, Inc.

Clinical Disorders of Fluid and Electrolyte Metabolism: Maxwell MH, Kleeman CR, McGraw-Hill Book Co.

Heart Disease, A Textbook of Cardiovascular Medicine: Braunwald E, WB Saunders Co.

Pediatric Therapy: Shirkey HC, CV Mosby Co (2-4 years).

American Hospital Formulary Services Drug Information: American Society of Hospital Pharmacists (annual with supplements). Provides comprehensive, reliable data about drugs in monograph format. Allows for quick comparison of drugs with similar therapeutic use. Recently redesigned for easier use. Now available in full text on-line computer.

AMA Drug Evaluations: American Medical Association, Department of Drugs, John Wiley and Sons, Inc (3 years). Authoritative text reviewing therapeutic categories of drugs. Critical in nature and referenced.

Diagnostic Laboratory Tests

Clinical Laboratory Medicine: Ravel R, Year Book Medical Publishers, Inc (4 years).

Todd-Sanford-Davidsohn, Clinical Diagnosis and Management by Laboratory Methods: Henry JB, WB Saunders Co.

Miscellaneous

Handbook of Clinical Drug Data: Knoben JF, et al, Drug Intelligence Publications.

USP DI, Volume I, Drug Information for the Health Care Provider: Volume II, Advice for the Patient: United States Pharmacopeial Convention, Inc (annual).

Approved Prescription Drug Products with Therapeutic Equivalence Evaluations: Food and Drug Administration (annual with supplements). A must for pharmacists and others who are responsible for drug product selection.

Applied Therapeutics: The Clinical Use of Drugs: Katcher S, Young LY, Applied Therapeutics. A unique format of questions and answers organized in chapters on a broad range of therapeutics. Well referenced and indexed.

If the desired information is not found in the tertiary literature, the secondary literature must be employed to locate relevant articles in the primary literature. Abstracting/indexing services should not be used as a final source of information. Although tempting, abstracts should not be relied on as an accurate assessment of the results of clinical studies or other research published in the primary literature. These services are only tools to assist in locating the necessary primary literature.

There are many secondary sources. As with tertiary sources, there is no single most appropriate indexing/abstracting service. To effectively use them, one must be familiar with the characteristics of each service (Table 24.2). In addition, each service has developed its own specialized vocabulary to assist with indexing and retrieval. The assistance of a qualified librarian is invaluable when conducting extensive searches of the professional literature.

Secondary Resources

Adverse Reaction Titles: Excerpta Medica (monthly). Citations, approximately 4000/year, including original papers, preliminary communications, reviews, editorials, letters to the editor, and abstracts of papers presented at congresses are included if they contain significant information on (1) the complications, side effects, and undesirable reactions produced by drugs or other biologically active substances in man or experimental animals, (2) experimental toxicology and teratology to the extent that clinically used drugs are investigated, and (3) suicide, attempted suicide, drug abuse, and accidental overdose.

TABLE 24.2 Abstracting Indexing/Services for the Professional Literature

	Publication Cycle	Approximate No. of Journals Reviewed	Lag Time	Frequency of Index	Citations Per Year	Available on Microfiche	Available On-Line Computer
Clin-Alert	Semimonthly	800 +	1-2 mo	Quarterly, cumulative, year-to-date	300	No	No
Current Contents Clinical Practice	Weekly	790 +	2-6 wk—varies with title	Weekly, triannual, cumulative	129,400 journal and book articles	No	Yes (SCISEARCH-SCI on-line)
de Haen, Adverse Drug Reactions and Interactions System	Quarterly	1,250	1-4 mo	Quarterly, cumulative, year-to-date	3,000	Yes	No
de Haen, Drugs in Research	Bimonthly	1,250	1-2 mo	Bimonthly, cumulative, year-to-date	10,000	Yes	No
de Haen, Drugs in Use	Quarterly	1,250	1-4 mo	Quarterly, cumulative, year-to-date	8,000	Yes	No
Excerpta Medica, Adverse Reaction Titles	Monthly	3,500	2-4 mo	Monthly	4,000	No	Yes
Excerpta Medica, Drug Literature Index	Semimonthly	3,500	2-4 mo	Monthly	62,000	No	Yes
Index Medicus	Monthly	(Approx) 2,700	2-4 mo (1-3 mo on-line)	Monthly, annual, cumulative	250,000	No	Yes
Inpharma	Weekly	1,500	3 wk–2 mo	Monthly, semiannual, annual cumulative	2,300	No	No
International Pharmaceutical Abstracts	Semimonthly	600	2-5 mo	Monthly, semiannual, annual cumulative	7,000	Yes	Yes
Iowa Drug Information Service	Monthly	155	1-4 mo	Monthly, cumulative annual cumulative	14,000	Yes	Yes (special searches)
Reactions	Bimonthly	1,500	1-2 mo	Quarterly, annual cumulative	1,000	No	No
Science Citation Indexes	Bimonthly	3,320	2-6 wk—varies with title	Bimonthly, annual cumulation	565,000 journal and book articles	No	Yes
Unlisted Drugs	Monthly	700-800		Semiannual, annual cumulative, biannual cumulative	2,500	No	No

Drug Literature Index: Excerpta Medica (twice monthly). Citations, approximately 62,000/year, are indexed if they contain significant information on (1) the effects of drugs, related compounds, and naturally occurring substances on biologic substances, (2) clinical studies on drug action, (3) pharmacokinetic studies, (4) structural analysis, synthesis, and determination methods of drugs, hormones, and other substances known to have an effect on a biologic substrate, and (5) substances, the chemical structural formulae of which indicate they may have an influence on a biologic substrate, even though the paper does not report any study of this influence.

INPHARMA: ADIS Press International Inc (weekly). A comprehensive indexing/abstracting service designed to provide a rapid current awareness and alerting service to major reports on drugs and therapeutics. Content includes coverage of important research and development drugs, summaries of major drug trials, selected papers on clinical pharmacology, summaries of major literature reviews, and comprehensive bibliographies of newly marketed drugs.

Reactions: ADIS Press International Inc (approximately every 2 weeks). A significant indexing/abstracting service providing a rapid alerting service to important case reports and incidence studies. Content also includes coverage of abuse and dependence studies with therapeutic drugs, reports of the effects and treatment of poisonings, and summaries of major literature reviews on clinical drug toxicity.

Clin-Alert: Science Editors, Inc (semimonthly). An abstracting service intended to acquaint the health professional with abstracts of reports concerning exceptional situations encountered with the use of modern therapeutic agents and procedures. Included are reports of adverse drug reactions, drug interactions, and related therapeutic hazards.

de Haen, Drugs in Research: Paul de Haen International, Inc (bimonthly). Provides, on microfiche, standardized, structured reports of investigational drugs involved in preclinical studies as well as those involved in clinical studies. Contains approximately 10,000 reports/year.

de Haen, Drugs in Use: Paul de Haen International, Inc (quarterly). Provides, on microfiche, standardized, structured reports of drugs involved in clinical studies, regardless of the world marketing status of the drugs. Contains over 8000 reports/year.

de Haen, Adverse Drug Reaction and Interaction System (ADRIS): Paul de Haen International, Inc (quarterly). Provides, on microfiche, standardized, structured reports of adverse drug reactions and drug interactions excerpted from clinical studies of both investigational and approved drugs. Contains approximately 3000 reports/year.

International Pharmaceutical Abstracts (IPA): American Society of Hospital Pharmacists (twice monthly). A comprehensive abstracting service to the world's pharmaceutical and medical literature. Abstracts are divided into 25 sections that cover subjects from clinical, practical, and theoretical literature as well as economic topics. Approximately 7000 records/year. Available in print and through international on-line computer systems. Data base covers more than 600 worldwide publications.

Iowa Drug Information Service: Iowa Drug Information Service (monthly). A unique information storage and retrieval service that provides not only the index, but the complete microfiche of the article from 155 medical and pharmaceutical journals. Articles relevant to drug therapy are indexed and microfilmed monthly, giving the subscriber systemized access to the article through generic drug name index or disease classification index. The complete service, which began in 1966, contains over 190,000 microfilmed articles.

Index Medicus: National Library of Medicine (monthly). One of the most comprehensive indexing services in the world. Published monthly as a bibliographic listing of references to current articles from approximately 2600 of the world's biomedical journals. Included are subject and author sections and a separate bibliography of medical reviews. Approximately 250,000 citations annually.

Science Citation Index (SCI): Institute for Scientific Information, Inc (bimonthly). Citations, approximately 505,000 journal and back articles annually. It is comprised of three related portions: the Source Index, the Permuterm Subject Index, and the Citation Index. Each one indexes items from all issues of the SCI source journals. Journals from all disciplines are represented. Citations may be accessed by name of author, organization or geographic location, subject knowledge, or a particular reference (citations).

Unlisted Drugs: Unlisted Drugs (monthly). Identifies and describes all newly reported compounds and products that are not listed by name, manufacturer, and composition in the latest editions of common drug reference compendia. Each month, approximately 200 new drugs are described. Each entry includes name, composition, manufacturer, activity, reference, structure, dosage, and synonyms.

Current Contents, Clinical Practice: Institute for Scientific Information (weekly). Provides access to the tables of contents of the latest journal issues from over 790 of the world's journals. Complete bibliographic information is provided for ordering reprints. Also included is an index to all significant words from every title.

Recently many of the secondary literature services have made their data bases available for on-line searching by computer (Table 24.3). This new technology has enhanced the ability to rapidly and accurately search these data bases. As with manual searches, the assistance of a medical librarian is helpful when attempting complicated, intricate

TABLE 24.3 On-Line Data Bases of the Pharmaceutical and Medical Literature

1. International Pharmaceutical Abstracts: Produced by the American Society of Hospital Pharmacists; searching through Dialog, BRS, NLM (TOXLINE). Data base covers more than 600 worldwide publications from 1970 to present.
2. RngDoc. Produced by Derwent Publications Ltd; searching through SDCIS. Data base offers detailed abstracts of journal articles on drugs. Approximately 1000 abstracts are published per week.
3. Medline. Produced by the National Library of Medicine (NLM); searching through Dialog, BRS, NLM. Approximately 3000 biomedical journals are covered with retrieval back to 1966 on-line. Medline is the on-line version of Index Medicus. NLM also produces other data bases including TOXLINE, Registry of Toxic Effects of Chemical Substances (RTECS), Toxicology Data Bank (TDB), CANCERLIT, CANCERPROS, CLINPROT, and POPLINE.
4. Excerpta Medica. Produced by Excerpta Medica; searching through BRS and Dialog. Data base includes citations and abstracts to the contents of 3500 journal titles from 1975 to present. Comprehensive coverage of pharmaceuticals and foreign medical literature. The data base is used to provide 43 printed abstracting journals and two bibliographies: *Drug Literature Index* and *Adverse Reactions Titles.*
5. BIOSIS Previews. Produced by BioScience Information Service; searching through BRS, Dialog, and SDCIS. The on-line data base of Biological Abstracts and Biological Abstracts/PRM. Monitors publications in the life science, including journals, books, government reports, and meeting proceedings.
6. Pharmaceutical News Index (PNI). Produced by Data Courier, Inc.; searching through Dialog. Data base includes FDC Reports. References cover personnel, finances, management decisions, new product development, government regulatory activities, and health legislation.

TABLE 24.4 Major On-line Vendors of Literature-Retrieval Systems

1. Bibliographic Retrieval Services (BRS)
   BRS Customer Service
   1200 Route 7
   Latham, NY 12110
   (800)833-4707
   (518)783-1161 (New York)
2. Dialog Information Services, Inc.
   Marketing Department
   3460 Hillview Ave.
   Palo Alto, CA 94304
   (800)227-1927
   (800)982-5838 (CA)
3. Medlars Management System
   National Library of Medicine
   8600 Rockville Pike
   Bethesda, MD 20209
4. SDC Information Service (SDCIS)
   System Development Corporation
   2500 Colorado Ave.
   Santa Monica, CA 90406
   (800)421-7229
   (800)352-6689 (CA)

searches. Four major vendors currently provide methods for searching the major data bases relevant to the practice of pharmacy (Table 24.4). Several authors have provided a complete review of this topic (6-9).

Many hospital pharmacies, particularly those with drug information services, have acquired the necessary hardware and software to conduct searches. Certainly the cost of hardware and the time necessary for searching must be carefully evaluated, but the advantages that can be gained with on-line literature searching are many. In-depth searches of several data bases can be accomplished in the same time that only a limited search can be performed manually. On-line searching efficiency can be improved by attendance at courses offered by several of the vendors of these services. Of the vendors offering on-line services, Dialog provides access to the largest number of data bases and is easiest for the novice to use. In addition to time savings, on-line searching improves the completeness of the literature used to formulate a response.

On-line computer capabilities offer other advantages as well. Specially designed current awareness searches are available through several data base publishers. For those with specialty practices, this offers an excellent way to stay abreast of publications in a particular field. Complete texts of journals and several tertiary sources are now available for on-line searching and review. Currently the number available are limited, but the concept of ''paperless library'' is not far from reality.

REFERENCES

1. Walton CA: The problem of communicating clinical drug information. *Am J Hosp Pharm* 22:458-463, 1965.
2. Schor S, Karten I: Statistical evaluation of medical journal manuscripts. *JAMA* 195:13, 1966.
3. Laties VG, Weiss B: A critical review of the efficacy of meprobamate in the treatment of anxiety. *J Chronic Dis* 7:6, 1958.
4. Fletcher RH, Fletcher SW: Clinical research in general medical journals. A 30-year perspective. *N Engl J Med* 301:180-183, 1979.
5. DerSimonian R. et al: Reporting on methods in clinical trials. *N Engl J Med* 306:1332-1337, 1982.
6. Tousignaut DR: Online literature retrieval systems: How to get started. *Am J Hosp Pharm* 40:230-239, 1983.
7. Kruse KW: On-line searching of the pharmaceutical literature. *Am J Hosp Pharm* 40:240-253, 1983.
8. Knodel LC, Bierschenk NF: Selective use of online literature searching by a drug information service. *Am J Hosp Pharm* 40:257-259, 1983.
9. Schneiweiss F: Use and cost analysis of online literature searching in a university-based drug information center. *Am J Hosp Pharm* 40:254-256, 1983.

ADDITIONAL READING

Beatty WK: Searching the literature and computerized services in medicine. Guides and methods for the clinician. *Ann Intern Med* 91:326-332, 1979.
Davis NM: Drug information requests—the top of the iceberg. *Hosp Pharm* 5:4, 1970.
Walton CA, et al: Drug literature utilization: Selection, evaluation, and communication. In Blissitt CW, et al (eds): *Clinical Pharmacy Practice*. Philadelphia, Lea & Febiger, 1972, pp 374-406.
Watanabe AS et al: A systematic approach to drug information requests. *Am J Hosp Pharm* 32:1282-1285, 1975.

Publishers

ADIS Press International, Inc., 401 South State St., Newtown, PA, 18940.
American Pharmaceutical Association, 2215 Constitution Ave., NW, Washington, DC 20037.
American Society of Hospital Pharmacists, 4630 Montgomery Ave., Washington, DC 20014.
Appleton-Century-Crofts, 25 Van Zant St., East Norwalk, CT 06855.
Applied Therapeutics, Inc., PO Box 1903, Spokane, WA 99210.
BioScience Information Service, 2100 Arch St., Philadelphia, PA 19103.
Cutter Laboratories, Inc., 3900 Manchester Rd, St. Louis, MO 63144.
The C. V. Mosby Co., 11830 Westline Industrial Dr., St. Louis, MO 63141.
Data Courier, Inc., 5161 River Road, Bethesda, MD 20816.
Derwent Publications Ltd., Rochdale House, 128 Theobalds Rd., London WC1X 8RP, England.
Drug Intelligence Publications, 1241 Broadway, Hamilton, IL 62341.
Elsevier Science Publishing Co., Inc., Division of Biomedical Division, 52 Vanderbilt Ave., New York, NY 10017.
Excerpta-Medica, Inc., PO Box 3085, Princeton, NJ 08540.
Facts and Comparison Division, JB Lippincott Co., 111 W Port Plaza, Suite 423, St. Louis, MO 63146.
Food and Drug Administration, 5600 Fishers Lane, Rockville, MD 20857.
Hearst Corporation, 224 W 57th St., Room 307, New York, NY 10019.
Institute for Scientific Information, Inc., 3501 Market St., Philadelphia, PA 19104.
Iowa Drug Information Service, The University of Iowa, Westlawn, Box 330, IA 52242.
JB Lippincott Co., East Washington Square, Philadelphia, PA 19105.
John Wiley & Sons, Inc., 605 Third Ave., New York, NY 10158.
Lange Medical Publications, Drawer L, Los Altos, CA 94022.
Lea & Febiger, 600 S Washington Square, Philadelphia, PA 19106.
Little, Brown & Co., 34 Beacon St., Boston, MA 02106.
Macmillan Publishing Co., Inc., 866 Third Ave., New York, NY 10022.
Medical Economics Books, 680 Kinderkamack Rd., Oradell, NJ 07649.
Merck & Co., Inc., PO Box 2000, Rahway, NJ 07065.
McGraw-Hill Book Co., 1221 Avenue of the Americas, New York, NY 10020.
National Library of Medicine, 8600 Rockville Pike, Bethesda, MD 20209.
Paul de Haen International, Inc., 2750 S Shoshone St., Englewood, CO 80110.
Raven Press, 1140 Avenue of the Americas, New York, NY 10036.
Science Editors, Inc., 149 Thierman Lane, Louisville, KY 40207.
Skyline Publishers, Inc., PO Box 1029, Portland, OR 97207.
The Pharmaceutical Press, 1 Lambeth High St., London SE1 7JN, England.
Unlisted Drugs, Box 401, Chatham, NJ 07928.
US Pharmacopeial Convention, Inc., USP Publication Services Department, 12601 Twinbrook Pkwy., Rockville, MD 20852.
WB Saunders Co., W Washington Square, Philadelphia, PA 19105.
Williams & Wilkins Co., 428 E Preston St, Baltimore, MD 21202.
Year Book Medical Publications, Inc., 35 E Wacker Dr., Chicago, IL 60601.

CHAPTER 25

Literature Evaluation

HAZEL H. SEABA

Practicing pharmacists are probably most concerned with evaluation of clinical studies and clinical surveys of a drug's pharmacology or some aspect of the drug's use in therapeutics. Clinical studies and surveys are the primary resource used by pharmacists to gather information for rational drug prescribing and effective drug use. Once the primary literature for any topic is identified and retrieved, the next step, evaluation, is often approached with hesitancy. Whatever the source of this hesitancy and whatever the strengths of one's educational background, evaluation can be accomplished with skill by all pharmacists. Literature evaluation is approaching published studies and surveys with the goal of understanding what the research accomplished and concluding how this knowledge relates to current therapeutics.

A published study should bring the reader logically through the rationale for the study, the protocol (plan) under which the research was executed, the results of the study, and the significance of those results. The reader must give attention to each part of the study, and final assessment is based on his or her judgment of the reasonableness of each part of the research.

BASIC ELEMENTS OF CLINICAL STUDIES

Objective and Purpose

Investigators begin research with an objective to be achieved or a question to be answered. The research objective may involve describing a situation of interest, e.g., describing the clinical course of a disease process or characterizing the attitude of a group of individuals. Alternatively, the investigator's purpose may concern analytical research. Analytical research investigates cause-effect relationships (1). Regardless of the purpose of the research, however, the investigator's objective needs to be clearly stated. If a research report does not state the objective in the introduction or purpose section, the reader may find it in the summary or conclusion.

If a cause-effect relationship is to be investigated, the researcher should clearly state the problem to be addressed in the investigation. Following statement of the problem, the specific question or questions to be answered are identified. Clearly stating the question is an important step that sets the clinical stage for decisive answers (2). The reader's overall responsibility in literature evaluation is to determine how well the author realized the objective or answered the question.

The diagnostic and prognostic parameters of the population to whom the research is targeted are specified in the objective; thus, the reader is provided with a statement of who is represented in the study. The objective for analytical research further describes the treatment, therapy, or procedure to be applied to that part of the population participating in the research. The indicators that the investigator uses to observe and measure the treatment outcome are identified and correlated with the population's original characteristics. Last, the outcome that the investigator hopes to achieve is stated.

In the objective, the investigator hypothesizes the relationship between the treatment and the outcome. He or she then tests the relationship and hopefully discovers the true influence of the treatment (cause) on the subjects' outcome (effect). To quantitate the relationship and provide a means for analyzing the outcome, a statistical hypothesis is used. Clinical investigators frequently express the statistical hypothesis in the form of a null hypothesis. The null hypothesis states that there is no value, worth, or difference between the tested situations. The investigator, through experimental and mathematical methods, generates data that will allow the investigator to either concede or reject the null hypothesis.

Population and Sample

Simply stated, the population is a group of patients or items to which the investigator wishes to apply the research results. The entire population can rarely, if ever, be studied. Thus, the investigator has to choose a limited number of individuals from the entire population to study, i.e., a sample. If the research results are to be applied to the population, the sample must be a reliable substitute for the larger population. Investigators, then, are confronted with some risk of making a sampling error, which is the difference between how the entire population responds and how the sample responds. The population must be clearly defined, and the sample must adequately represent the entire population. The reader thereby knows the targeted population by the characteristics that describe the sample.

With the targeted population in mind, the sample is selected; however, not all selection factors are completely under the investigator's control. In clinical research, selection control can be particularly difficult to achieve. Individuals have diverse reasons for seeking medical care, choosing a specific doctor or hospital, and consenting to participate in a research study. If the investigation depends on referrals from other doctors or hospitals, many factors determine who is referred. Surveys may depend on medical records for their population sample. Retrieval factors, such as completeness of the medical record data base, access to the data base, and completeness of the information in the record determine the representation of a medical record sample. These subject selection factors are potential sources of selection bias.

To control bias (prejudice that causes the sample to be different from the defined population) the sample must be selected by diagnostic inclusion criteria that are appropriate for the condition or disease. When the study involves prevention or prophylaxis, each member of the sample must be susceptible to and exposed to whatever situation the researcher wanted to prevent. Subject characteristics such as sex, age, weight, economic and geographic status, coexisting diseases, use of other treatments or drugs, and the severity, extent, and duration of the disease may influence the patient's response to the investigative treatment. As potential prognostics, these characteristics must be considered at the time the target population is identified and the sample eligibility established. The sample is most likely to truly represent the population if it is randomly chosen, i.e., all members or items of the population have some chance of being chosen.

The investigator may not have access to the entire population and, therefore, cannot choose a random sample. If the investigator does not choose a probability (nonzero chance of being selected) sample, bias may enter the study. A "chunk" sample describes a nonrandom sample convenient for the investigator's research. The "chunk" sample individuals are members of the population who are available for research, but may not represent the population. A "volunteer" sample (self-selecting) is also a convenient group to study but may not indicate how the "nonselecting" group would respond to the same investigation. The reader, through pharmaceutical and medical judgment, must determine how closely the sample will predict the response of the targeted population.

The number of individuals or items selected for the sample is determined by several factors, including the amount of risk the investigator is willing to take that whatever is measured could occur by chance; the magnitude of the difference between treatments or situations to be measured (the smaller the difference, the larger the sample size must be); and the amount of assurance the investigator wants that the research will show valid, statistically significant results. The appropriate sample size can be fixed at the start of the study or can be determined at some point during the research when the investigator has enough data to reach a reasonable conclusion (sequential design).

Design, Sample Allocation, and Control

Clinical studies may be described as being prospective (start and look forward) or retrospective (start and look backward). These adjectives apply to two separate aspects of clinical investigation. First, the manner in which the subject data are collected may be prospective or retrospective. If the investigator designs the procedure by which the data are recorded and controls its collection, the study data are prospective. If the investigator collects the data from records that were compiled independently prior to the study, the study data collection is retrospective. Second, the group to be studied may be observed either prospectively or retrospectively in time. In a prospective study the subjects are chosen, the treatment is applied, and the observable events are then followed, such as cure or incidence of side effects. In a retrospective design, the subjects exhibiting the effect, cure, or side effect are chosen, and the investigator then determines which subjects had the disease or used the treatment. The first observes cause-to-effect and the last observes effect-to-cause. Patients who are followed prospectively have been called cohorts and those who are followed retrospectively have been called cases or trohocs.

The retrospective trohoc study design, case control study, is more vulnerable to reliability and validity threats than prospective cause-to-effect studies. The reader's judgment of the retrospective case control study should be based on the study's ability to convincingly show whether or not the cause (disease, drug, etc) has been used by the subjects and whether or not the subjects are a representative sample of the total population. The control group (discussed below) should be selected with specified inclusion criteria (3,4).

The concept of control is basic to scientific research, and several different concepts of control have been developed. Feinstein (5) has outlined three: the idea of regulation, the control period, and the idea of comparison. The concept of regulation control distinguishes a clinical trial or experiment from a survey, cohort study, and case control study. In a survey or cohort study, the investigator does not decide what treatment the subjects will undergo, whereas in an experiment, the investigator does decide. Thus, in the clinical trial the investigator controls allocation of the sample members to the study treatments. In the survey or cohort study and the case control study, sample members have either been allocated to the treatment groups before the study begins or they are allocated to the treatment groups by someone other than the investigator. Quality control, as applied to the production of pharmaceuticals, is a regulatory control. Controlling the environment of the research study is also a regulatory control; not losing patients for follow-up and maintaining patient compliance are environmental controls. Second, the control period describes the qualification period during which subjects are tested or interviewed for their ability to meet the criteria of the study. The stabilization period, which may be used to record baseline test values, is a control period. A washout control period occurs between treatment periods in a crossover design study. The investigator should explain to the reader the length of the treatment period and the choice of whether or not to use a placebo during the washout. The third concept, control as a comparison, is necessary for the investigator to conclude that the treatment, prophylaxis, or procedure was responsible for the observed effect. Comparison controls available to the researcher are:

1. No treatment. The treated group is compared to a

group that is the same in every respect except it receives no treatment. This study design demands that there be no measurable placebo effect associated with the treatment.

2. Patient-his-own-control. Patients serve as their own controls when they are observed for a period of time and then the experimental treatment or procedure is applied. The pretreatment state is then compared to the treated state of the patient. Unless the treated or posttreated state is a high-order pharmaceutical or medical "breakthrough," the study results are suspect. Subjects used as their own controls cannot substitute for a true control.

3. Intrasubject control. In some clinical studies, it is possible to compare treatments or compare treatment to placebo in the same patient. Comparing different treatments in corresponding areas of the body (finger joints, eyes, ears, etc) may be possible if the areas are equally diseased and the treatment only affects the local area.

4. Placebo. The comparison group receives a "treatment" identical in all respects to the real treatment except it is inactive. A "treatment" placebo must resemble the active dosage form in all characteristics that the subject can discern, such as taste, color, odor, and appearance. The placebo, inactive pharmacologically, elicits psychologic and physiologic responses.

5. Active treatment. Active treatment controls are used when it is impossible or unethical not to treat a group of subjects. Comparative efficacy information for a new drug is obtained by using an older standard drug as an active control.

6. Case control or matched control. In retrospective studies, in which patients who already exhibit some effect are followed in search of a cause, the subjects are matched with a control who does not exhibit the effect. The investigator seeks a control for each subject who is comparable both demographically and clinically. The goal is to establish comparable susceptibility to the effect in the subjects and controls. The controls are often chosen to match such subject demographic variables such as age, sex, socioeconomic class, and race. Clinical variables, such as family history, medication history, health status, hospitalization, or ambulatory status, should be considered for matching (6).

Matching may also be used to select controls for surveys or cohort studies. To improve the comparability between the study's treatment groups, the investigator may seek a matched control for each member of the intervention group. Again, both demographic and clinical characteristics are considered for matching. Generally, less than four variables are matched.

7. Historical control. The historical control is data generated at a previous time. Historical controls have been employed in studies of diseases or conditions that are predictable in their natural history, signs, symptoms, and mortality rate. The ability of the historical control to describe the current group in all respects except treatment is often open to doubt. The major concerns are changes wrought by time and the reliability of the original recorded data. Time influences the population susceptible to and exposed to diseases and the diagnostic and health care available. Medical records suffer changes in disease classification schemes and completeness of patient prognostic data. Despite the problems inherent with the historical control, under circum-

stances where the disease condition is rare or there is pressure to quickly obtain comparative efficacy information for a promising new treatment, it may be used (7,8). When compared with the results of randomized controlled clinical trials, the historical control trial appears to have some bias in the direction favoring the experimental treatment over the control treatment (9,10).

8. Crossover design control. Crossover exists when one group of subjects receives sequential treatments and another group receives the same treatments in the opposite order. All subjects receive both the experimental treatment and the control treatment in sequence. If there is not an adequate washout period between the treatments, the patients will not return to baseline status, and bias may influence the study's outcome due to carryover effects. The period of time between treatments has to be short enough not to allow a change to occur in the natural course of the disease or subject parameter being measured but long enough to allow the pharmacologic, physiologic, and psychologic effects of each treatment to disappear.

As crossover designs compare the outcome of each treatment on each subject, the precision of the outcome measurements is greater than that obtained from a parallel group study. This crossover design feature is particularly advantageous for comparative bioavailability studies of healthy subjects. Use of the crossover design to assess drug efficacy in diseased subjects, however, requires justification. This is done by showing that the subjects return to baseline status prior to each treatment period and that there was no carryover effect from one treatment period to the next (11).

9. Strata control. Qualitative comparability of the study groups may be improved with strata control. Before the subjects are assigned to groups they are stratified for subject variables that are capable of influencing the results of the investigation. The individuals in each strata are assigned to the treatment groups. Each treatment group is thus assured of an adequate representation from each strata. Age, sex, weight, and severity of disease may be stratified when they are known to affect the outcome of a disease process (prognostic stratification).

The reader may indeed wonder how to judge the appropriateness of the investigator's choice of a control. The logic employed to determine which control is appropriate is based, according to Feinstein (12), on four factors: potency, relativity, multiplicity, and concurrency of the treatment and control. Potency of the treatment or procedure is the first factor. For drug studies the choice of the drug's dosage and administration rate is a potency decision. The dosage regimen should be reasonable to test the relationships stated in the study's objective. If the investigation involves a comparison, the three other factors are also of concern. The second factor, relativity of the investigation, considers to what control the treatment should be compared. An efficacy study requires a placebo or no-treatment control, whereas an efficiency study requires that the treatment be compared to an established or standard treatment. Constituents, those ingredients which are administered with the active treatment, are also of concern in a comparison study. For pharmaceuticals the constituents are the "inactive" ingredients that are present in the dosage form. For drug comparisons the constituents should be the same for each treatment group.

The environment in which the treatments or procedures are delivered should be the same for all groups. Environment describes the care and attention the groups receive from the investigators. Multiplicity, the third factor, considers the number of treatments to be compared and also influences the choice of a control. For example, a study comparing an oral drug preparation to an intramuscular drug preparation may require a control (placebo) for both the oral and the intramuscular preparation. A combination investigational treatment consisting of two active drugs may require an active control for each drug. The last factor, concurrency, or whether or not the study subjects received their individual treatments at the same time, affects the comparability of the treatment groups. Crossover studies, studies in which treatments are employed in stages, and studies in which treatments are separated by long periods of time may not be able to assure treatment group comparability. These studies require justification that one treatment does not affect the success of the next and that the disease state of the subjects has not changed with time.

After choice of control, the next concern is the method by which treatments or procedures are assigned to members of the study sample. In patient-his-own-control studies, case control studies, cohort or survey studies, and historical control studies, the assignment has been made by someone other than the investigator. Other study designs provide the investigator with more opportunities for assuring the comparability of the treatment groups and thus improving the study's validity. Randomized allocation to the treatment and control groups provides the investigator with several advantages (13). Randomized allocation means that each subject in the study has a nonzero and independent chance of receiving the study treatments. Randomized assignment of sample subjects to various treatment groups provides the best assurance that no treatment group is biased with subjects having particular characteristics. The treatment groups also tend to be balanced for subjects with various prognoses. Some of the prognostic indicators may be known and some may not. Last, randomization of subjects to the groups assures the validity of employing statistically significant tests to compare the treatment outcomes. The randomized clinical study is useful to determine the efficacy of a treatment or the relative efficiency of more than one therapeutic treatment. However, some therapeutic questions cannot use this powerful design. Studies concerning the treatment of rare disease states do not lend themselves to randomization as there are too few individuals available for research. Also, ethical considerations preclude randomized clinical trials to determine adverse events such as teratogenicity or carcinogenicity.

Adaptive allocation methods may also be used to determine which treatment a subject receives (14,15). In contrast to fixed randomized allocation, adaptive allocation procedures change the subject's probability of being assigned to the treatment groups as the study progresses. In an adaptive design study, the treatment that a newly recruited subject receives is dependent on the subjects already in the study. Assignment of the subject's treatment is determined either by the balance of subjects already in treatment groups (baseline adaptive allocation) or by the response of individuals who entered the study first (response adaptive allocation).

The response adaptive allocation design assumes that subjects who enter the study have the same characteristic responses to the treatments. This design hopes to give the largest number of subjects the best treatment. Since the responses of previous subjects must be known before the next subject can be allocated, the design suffers when the subjects' responses do not occur in a short period of time. Also, the design demands that only one response be measured to determine how successful the treatments are before admitting the next subject.

The investigator has to be concerned not only with the initial comparability of the treatment groups but also with the comparability of the treatment groups throughout the study. To this end the investigator has to ensure that all the participants will remain available for observation or examination at the times specified in the protocol and for the necessary duration of time. Subjects in the comparative groups should be examined or observed with equal regularity and duration so that all events have the same opportunity for detection. Both the sample subjects and the investigator or observer should adhere to the study regimen of treatment, observation, examination, and data collection. The reader may wish to expand his or her understanding of research design. Chapter 40 provides further material, including a discussion of the criteria used to assess a causal relationship and the ability of research designs to establish and maintain reliable and valid measurements and procedures.

Data Collection

Before collecting any data the investigator must clearly define what is to be measured or observed. These definitions are necessary so that problems associated with choosing, observing, and classifying the study events are controlled (16). This control allows the study data to be assessed and validated and the results reproduced.

The quantity that is actually measured or observed is called a variable. As its name implies, the value of a variable can vary. There are several different scales available to assign measurement values to a variable. Metric variables are ranks with equal intervals between the ranks, e.g., 1, 2, 3. Ordinal variables are graded ranks with an unequal interval between the ranks, e.g., mild, moderate, severe. Nominal variables are not graded or ranked, e.g., eye color, hair color. Existential variables describe the presence or absence of an item or are expressed as yes or no.

The evidence or data collected may be termed "hard" or "soft." "Hard" data describe measurements or observations that can be made with little subjective judgment. "Soft" data require subjective judgment and interpretation. Because of its objectivity, it is easier to establish the reliability of "hard" data. Whereas the "hard" data measurements may be preferred because they can be evaluated with greater confidence, the importance of "soft" data measurements such as pain relief or quality of life is not diminished.

The most important evidence or data collected by the investigator is an index to the research and is called the index variable(s). Index variables may be used to determine sample eligibility. The study's results are an analysis of the index variables. An index variable may be expressed numerically (metric) or further categorized to an expression with clinical meaning, e.g., ordinal variables such as abnormally high, normal, or too low. The investigator should inform the reader if a measurement reflects a single observation or if multiple observations were averaged or summed. The conclusion of the study may be based on the outcome of a single index variable, or index variables may be combined to express a more complex total situation. The combination of index variables may consider each variable equal and combine the variables with Boolean logic (and, or, not). Alternately, the variables may be weighted and the combination index is a sum of individual weighted variables.

Combining variables requires sound clinical judgment and logic. The reader has to determine the physiologic and clinical relevance of the variables. Since "hard" data are more easily defended and considered more reliable, the investigator may choose index variables which, although reliable, may not directly reflect the objective of the study. The index variables should be suitable for the objectives of the study and measure what the investigator wanted to measure.

The manner in which data are collected also influences the reliability of the results. The investigator is obligated to show that the methods of observation or measurement are standard throughout the study and are reproducible. Bias can be generated by both the individual responsible for measurement and by study subjects. The best attempts to be objective can become unknowingly biased if either the subject or observer knows which treatment the subject is receiving. A double-blind study, in which both the subject and the observer do not know which treatment the subject is receiving, eliminates this bias. If possible, separate individuals should administer the treatments and execute the measurements or observations. If only the subject is blinded, the study is single-blind.

After the study is underway and data are being collected, events do not always happen as planned. If the subject has to administer a treatment or make an observation, the possibility of noncompliance exists. Whether or not missed doses and lost observations are included in the raw data is a matter requiring the investigator's judgment. The treatment or procedure may cause unexpected adverse effects in individual subjects. Subjects with disease conditions may experience serious decline in their health. In these two instances, ethical considerations preclude further participation, and the subjects may be withdrawn from the study. Particularly in studies of long duration, subjects may drop out on their own accord and be "lost to follow-up." Prophylaxis is the best management of this data loss, and efforts should be taken to find these individuals. Although the investigator cannot protect the protocol from all interruptions or collect perfect data, the interruptions and imperfect data should be pointed out to the reader and the manner in which these factors are handled in the analysis explained.

Data Analysis

The objective of research is to observe and measure changes or differences that occur in the index variables because of the treatment under study. Measurement of change over time requires pretreatment data collection. Data collected during and after the treatment or procedure can be contrasted to pretreatment data and the change expressed in several ways. Change expressed as trend is plotting the data measurements and fitting a line or curve to the data points. Variables with graded ranks (ordinals) may be used to compare the pre- and posttreatment results in clinically relevant terms, such as better, worse, or the same. In comparison studies, the change measured in the treatment group is compared to the change occurring in the control group. If the investigator is interested only in the difference between the index variable outcome of the treatment group and the control group, then pretreatment measurements are not needed.

The analysis of the results of a clinical study generally consists of a descriptive statistical analysis and an inferential statistical analysis. First, the data are summarized by descriptive statistics. Descriptive statistical analysis presents the central tendency of the data (mode, median, mean) and the dispersion of the data (range, percentile, standard deviation). The measurement scale of the variables (metric, ordinal, nominal, existential) dictates which measure of central tendency or dispersion is appropriate. Descriptive statistical analysis characterizes either the difference between the change in the treatment group and the control group or the difference between the outcome variable of the treatment group and the control group. Descriptive statistical analysis is an evaluation of the data for the study groups only.

The second step, inferential statistical analysis, is an extrapolation of the study results to the larger target population. Inferential statistical analysis allows the reader to evaluate the generalizability of the research results. So far, the analysis of clinical studies and surveys has not required a knowledge of statistics. Statistical manipulation cannot rectify errors made in the design and execution of the research. Thus, clinical knowledge, logic, and judgment applied to evaluation of research are extremely valuable. The knowledge required to determine the most appropriate statistical test to apply to the data is beyond the scope of this chapter. However, knowledge of basic terms and definitions can provide insight to these mathematical manipulations.

Many inferential statistical tests are based on the criteria that the sample is a random sample of the population. If the sample was not or could not be chosen randomly, statistical tests requiring random samples cannot be utilized for analysis. Another assumption common to many statistical tests is normal (Gaussian) distribution of the data. As normal distribution may not occur in patient-related data, the investigator may attempt to normalize the data via a mathematical transformation or use another method of analysis that does not require the assumption of normality (nonparametric).

Earlier, the null hypothesis was presented as a tool for testing the hypothesis of a study. The null hypothesis states that the treatment is of no value or that there is no difference between treatments (17,18). The null hypothesis may be either true or false and the investigator, after the analysis of the data, will either concede or reject the hypothesis (Table 25.1).

The opportunity exists for making two different errors: type I or type II. The probability for making a type I error is called alpha (α) and the probability for making a type II error is called beta (β). If a type I error is made, the null

TABLE 25.1   Null Hypothesis Decision Table

Investigator's Decision	Null Hypothesis	
	True	*False*
Concede	No error	Type II error or β
Reject	Type I error or α	No error

hypothesis is rejected when indeed it was true. This means a worthless treatment has been declared useful. A type II error means a treatment that is truly useful has been declared worthless. Type I errors are most detrimental to ethical professional practice; however, they cannot be completely eliminated, as the null hypothesis would have to be conceded each time to have zero type I errors. The probability (*P* value) of making a type I error is calculated, and the decision to concede or reject the null hypothesis is based on the magnitude of this probability. Thus, the less the α value (*P* value), the lower the probability of making a type I error. Frequently, α values of *P* less than or equal to 0.01 or 0.05 are used to declare the results of the study statistically significant. Mainland (19) suggests a working definition of significance of "probably indicating something that would rarely occur as the result of chance alone." Thus, if the difference between the treatment group outcome and the control group outcome is statistically significant, the null hypothesis is rejected and it is concluded that the difference is probably real and would rarely occur as a result of chance alone.

When the null hypothesis cannot be rejected, i.e., the calculated *P* value is greater than the established α, the reader needs to evaluate β (20,21). Conceding the null hypothesis does not mean that the comparison treatments are equivalent. It only means that this particular research study failed to find a difference between the treatments. Whereas "negative" trials (*P* value >0.05) can mean that there is very little difference between the treatments tested in the trial, it can also mean that a type II error has occurred. There are several factors that contribute to the probability of making a type II error. The ability of a clinical trial to find delta (Δ), a difference between treatments of a given size, is partially dependent on the size of the trial sample. Thus, "negative" trial results may be caused by an inadequate sample size.

Establishing and recruiting an adequate sample size is an important step for investigators. Before beginning a trial, the investigators choose α and β levels and establish Δ, the smallest clinically important difference between treatments that they want to detect. With these values, the appropriate sample size is calculated. If the calculated sample size is not achievable, then a greater risk of making a type II error may be accepted and/or a larger Δ adopted.

As with all methods of analysis, the null hypothesis is not without problems and criticisms (17,18). It can be used to determine the significance of only one objective, be it an objective based on a single variable or several variables. To achieve the single index for analysis, the combination of variables may sometimes seem contrived from the viewpoint of clinical judgment. By its definition the null hypothesis shows only differences in treatments or procedures, not

similarities. Establishing the significant *P* value as 0.05 or less is common but still an arbitrary cutoff point. We might consider whether or not results with *P* values greater than 0.05 are clinically useful.

Pharmacists whose curriculum did not include basic statistics and who wish to evaluate further the statistical analyses utilized in clinical research may be guided by surveys describing the relative frequency of use of statistical tests in pharmacy and medical journals (22-25). The results of these surveys suggest that the descriptive statistical procedures of mode, median, mean, and range, percentage, standard deviation, and inferential statistical procedures of *t*-test, and chi square account for approximately 75% of the statistical analyses found in pharmacy and medical journals. An understanding of these procedures would provide a reasonable background for evaluation of statistical analyses by pharmacists. Chapter 42 discusses many of the important concepts necessary to evaluate statistical analyses.

Conclusion

The final obligation of the investigator is to draw a conclusion from the research that allows the research to make a contribution to pharmaceutical and medical practice. The reader's responsibility is to evaluate the conclusion with respect to the entire study.

The concepts of clinical and statistical significance deserve careful consideration by both investigators and readers. Anello (26), in his discussion of this topic, said, "Statistical significance tells nothing about the quality of planning or execution of an experiment, nothing about the biological or clinical meaning of difference in numbers, and nothing about whatever was alleged to cause the difference." Statistical significance is not a direct measure of clinical significance. The application of research results to practical, therapeutic situations should be made with this distinction in mind.

Federal drug legislation requires that drug therapies be proved safe and efficacious prior to marketing. Pharmacists' literature evaluation is frequently concerned with safety and efficacy. Although the Food and Drug Administration (27) has defined their interpretation of "adequate and well-controlled clinical investigations," we do not have a definition of what constitutes safety and efficacy. As pointed out by Feinstein (28), our problems with these two concepts are multiple and not easily solved. The possibility of statistically significant results not being clinically significant has already been mentioned. Delta, the clinically significant difference between treatments in comparative studies, is determined by judgment. To obtain an overall picture of efficacy, it may be important to consider the effect of drug therapy on several signs and/or symptoms of a disease process. However, statistical tests can only assess the response of one variable or index. If multiple variables are combined to generate a single index variable, the combination must withstand close clinical scrutiny. With pharmaceutical agents we need to consider not only pharmacologic efficacy but also the therapeutic efficacy. Demonstration of pharmacologic efficacy by itself does not allow for the deduction of therapeutic efficacy. Also, the interaction of a patient with health care professionals is complex and cannot or may not be

TABLE 25.2   Results of Therapeutic Literature Evaluation Studies

Study	Result
1951 Ross (29)	63% of 100 articles had no or inadequate control
1961 Badgley (30)	41.5% of 103 articles had a problem(s) with derivation of conclusion
1964 Mahon, Daniel (31)	94.6% of 203 articles did not meet all four validity criteria
1966 Schor, Karten (32)	47.5% of 295 articles were judged not acceptable
1968 Reiffenstein et al (33)	83.1% of 367 articles did not meet all four validity criteria
1970 Lionel, Herxheimer (34)	32.6% of 141 articles were judged not acceptable
1978 Ambroz et al (36)	66% of 172 randomized controlled trials were judged less than well executed
1979 Horwitz, Feinstein (4)	46% of 85 case controlled studies were not adequately compliant with 12 methodologic criteria
1980 Mosteller et al (40)	76% of 132 randomized controlled trials did not adequately report on five important pieces of information
1982 Der Simonian et al (42)	44% of 67 comparative trials did not adequately report on 11 criteria
1982 Venulet et al (43)	39% of 5737 adverse drug reaction articles did not provide information to calculate incidence of adverse reactions
1983 Tyson et al (44)	90% of 86 studies did not fulfill criteria to justify their treatment/management conclusions
1984 Evans, Pollock (45)	80% of 45 articles were judged to have doubtful clinical significance

clearly distinguished from the patient's interaction with drug therapy. The common expression of safety, "do the benefits outweigh the risks?" does not provide firm direction for literature evaluation.

QUALITY OF PUBLISHED THERAPEUTIC RESEARCH

It is of course impossible to achieve perfect design, data, analysis, and conclusions in the real world of pharmacy and medicine. The goal is evaluation of research with guidance from sound clinical judgment and common sense. The responsibility of the reader to judge the reliability and validity of clinical research reports and to evaluate the generalizability of research results cannot be abrogated to journal editors or referees. There has been substantial evidence, beginning in 1951 and continuing into the present, that research reports with incomplete documentation, poor design, questionable data collection methods, inappropriate statistical analyses, or indefensible conclusions are published (4,21,29-45). There have been at least 19 separate evaluations of segments of the medical and pharmacy literature. Whereas earlier evaluation studies tended to consider any therapeutic study or report that appeared in selected journal issues, several recent studies have concentrated on a specific topic in therapeutics, e.g., cancer therapy (40), adverse drug reactions (43), therapy for pregnant women and newborn infants (44), and antibiotic prophylaxis for surgical abdominal wound infections (45). Sources of the articles evaluated were primarily U.S., Canadian, or British journals. The majority of the evaluation studies used a checklist of important design and/or analysis criteria to judge the acceptability of the reports and studies. Methods used in these various evaluation studies are different, and the operational definitions of an acceptable or valid clinical study are also different. Despite these limitations, the outcomes from 13 studies are presented in Table 25.2.

Several authors limited their assessment to the statistical analyses performed in the evaluated articles. Gore et al (35), White (37), and Glantz (38) specifically evaluated the inferential statistical analyses in the journal issues they reviewed. These authors found that 44-61% of journal articles that used inferential statistical analyses had at least one error of commission or omission in the statistical analysis. Studies with "negative" (not statistically significant) outcomes have also been evaluated for the appropriateness of the conclusions. Freidman et al (21) and Reed and Slaichert (41) evaluated the ability or power of negative-outcome clinical trials to support the negative outcome. Freidman et al (21) found that about 69% of the 71 randomized controlled trials evaluated had a greater than 20% risk of missing a true 50% therapeutic improvement. Reed and Slaichert (41) found that 60-84% of the 2619 tests in 355 articles from six journals had a greater than 20% risk in missing a relatively large treatment difference. The possibility that a clinical trial with negative results had a sample size inadequate to detect even a relatively large difference between treatments should always be considered.

Overall, criteria used to judge clinical studies may have become more stringent over the years; however, the results of these evaluations are still disheartening. Clinical study results are the foundation of therapeutic decisions. The shortcomings of clinical research identified by these studies should alert health professionals to the care required in all literature evaluation activities.

REFERENCES

1. Feinstein AP: Clinical biostatistics, XLIV. A survey of the research architecture used for publications in general medical journals. *Clin Pharmacol Ther* 24:117-125, 1978.
2. Fredrickson DS: The field trial: Some thoughts on the indispensable ordeal. *Bull NY Acad Med* 44:985-993, 1968.
3. Feinstein AR: Clinical biostatistics, XX. The epidemiologic trohoc, the ablative risk ratio, and 'retrospective' research. *Clin Pharmacol Ther* 14:291-307, 1973.
4. Horwitz RI, Feinstein AR: Methodologic standards and contradictory results in case-control research. *Am J Med* 66:556-564, 1979.
5. Feinstein AR: Clinical biostatistics, XIX. Ambiguity and abuse in the twelve different concepts of 'control.' *Clin Pharmacol Ther* 14:112-122, 1973.
6. Hayden GF, Kramer MS, Horwitz RI: The case-control study, a practical review for the clinician. *JAMA* 247:326-331, 1982.
7. Gehan EA: Comparative clinical trials with historical controls: A statistician's view. *Biomedicine* (Special Issue) 28:13-19, 1978.
8. Cranberg L: Do retrospective controls make clinical trials "inherently fallacious?" *Br Med J* 2:1265-1266, 1979.

9. Sacks H, Chalmers TC, Smith H: Randomized versus historical controls for clinical trials. *Am J Med* 72:233-240, 1982.

10. Sacks HS, Chalmers TC, Smith H: Sensitivity and specificity of clinical trials, randomized *v* historical controls. *Arch Intern Med* 143:753-755, 1983.

11. Hills M, Armitage P: The two-period cross-over clinical trial. *Br J Clin Pharmacol* 8:7-20, 1979.

12. Feinstein AR: Clinical biostatistics, III. The architecture of clinical research. *Clin Pharmacol Ther* 11:432-441, 1970.

13. Byar DP, Simon RM, Friedewald WT, et al: Randomized clinical trials, perspectives on some recent ideas. *N Engl J Med* 295:74-80, 1976.

14. Simon R: Adaptive treatment assignment methods and clinical trials. *Biometrics* 33:743-749, 1977.

15. Hill C, Sancho-Garnier H: The two-armed-bandit problem: A decision theory approach to clinical trials. *Biomedicine* (Special Issue) 28:42-43, 1978.

16. Feinstein AR: Clinical biostatistics, IV. The architecture of clinical research (cont.). *Clin Pharmacol Ther* 11:595-610, 1970.

17. Feinstein AR: Clinical biostatistics, V. The architecture of clinical research (concl.). *Clin Pharmacol Ther* 11:755-771, 1970.

18. Mainland D: Statistical ward rounds—17. *Clin Pharmacol Ther* 10:714-736, 1969.

19. Mainland D: Statistical ward rounds—18. *Clin Pharmacol Ther* 10:867-900, 1969.

20. Feinstein AR: Clinical biostatistics, XXXIV. The other side of 'statistical significance': alpha, beta, delta, and the calculation of sample size. *Clin Pharmacol Ther* 18:491-505, 1975.

21. Freiman JA, Chalmers TC, Smith H, et al: The importance of beta, the Type II error and sample size in the design and interpretation of the randomized control trial, survey of 71 "negative" trials. *N Engl J Med* 299:690-694, 1978.

22. Feinstein AR: Clinical biostatistics, XXV. A survey of the statistical procedures in general medical journals. *Clin Pharmacol Ther* 15:97-107, 1974.

23. Moore R, Smith MC, Liao W, et al: Statistical background needed to read professional pharmacy journals. *Am J Pharm Educ* 42:251-254, 1978.

24. Hayden GF: Biostatistical trends in *Pediatrics:* Implications for the future. *Pediatrics* 72:84-87, 1983.

25. Emerson JD, Colditz GA: Use of statistical analysis in *The New England Journal of Medicine. N Engl J Med* 309:709-713, 1983.

25. Anello C: Considerations of significance—clinical and statistical. In McMahon FG (ed): *Importance of Experimental Design and Biostatistics.* Mount Kisco, NY, Futura, 1974, p 5-14.

27. U.S. Food and Drug Administration. Hearing regulations and regulations describing scientific content of adequate and well-controlled clinical investigations. *Fed Reg* 35:7250-7253, 1970.

28. Feinstein AR: Clinical biostatistics, IX. How do we measure "safety and efficacy?" *Clin Pharmacol Ther* 12:544-558, 1971.

29. Ross OB: Use of controls in medical research. *JAMA* 145:72-75, 1951.

30. Badgley RF: An assessment of research methods reported in 103 scientific articles from two Canadian medical journals. *Can Med Assoc J* 85:246-250, 1961.

31. Mahon WA, Daniel EE: A method for the assessment of reports of drug trials. *Can Med Assoc J* 90:565-569, 1964.

32. Schor S, Karten I: Statistical evaluation of medical journal manuscripts. *JAMA* 195:1123-1128, 1966.

33. Reiffenstein RJ, Schiltroth AJ, Todd DM: Current standards in reported drug trials. *Can Med Assoc J* 99:1134-1135, 1968.

34. Lionel NDW, Herxheimer A: Assessing reports of therapeutic trials. *Br Med J* 3:637-640, 1970.

35. Gore SM, Jones IG, Rytter EC: Misuse of statistical methods: Critical assessment of articles in *British Medical Journal* from January to March 1976. *Br Med J* 1:85-87, 1977.

36. Ambroz A, Chalmers TC, Smith H, et al: Deficiencies of randomized control trials (abstract). *Clin Res* 26:280A, 1978.

37. White SJ: Statistical errors in papers in the *British Journal of Psychiatry. Br J Psychiatry* 135:336-342, 1979.

38. Glantz SA: Biostatistics: How to detect, correct and prevent errors in the medical literature. *Circulation* 61:1-7, 1980.

39. Hibberd PL, Meadows AJ: Information contained in clinical trial reports. *J Inform Sci* 2:165-168, 1980.

40. Mosteller F, Gilbert JP, McPeek B: Reporting standards and research strategies for controlled trials, agenda for the editor. *Controlled Clin Trials* 1:37-58, 1980.

41. Reed JF, Slaichert W: Statistical proof in inconclusive 'negative' trials. *Arch Intern Med* 141:1307-1310, 1981.

42. DerSimonian R, Charette LJ, McPeek B, et al: Reporting on methods in clinical trials. *N Engl J Med* 306:1332-1337, 1982.

43. Venulet J, Blattner R, von Bulow J, et al: How good are articles on adverse drug reactions? *Br Med J* 284:252-254, 1982.

44. Tyson JE, Furzan JA, Reisch JS, et al: An evaluation of the quality of therapeutic studies in perinatal medicine. *Obstet Gynecol* 62:99-102, 1983.

45. Evans M, Pollock AV: Trials on trial, a review of trials of antibiotic prophylaxis. *Arch Surg* 119:109-113, 1984.

ADDITIONAL READING

Bulpitt CJ: *Randomised Controlled Clinical Trials.* The Hague, Martinus Nijhoff, 1983.

Byar DP, Simon RM, Friedewald WT, et al: Randomized clinical trials, perspectives on some recent ideas. *N Engl J Med* 295:74-80, 1976.

DerSimonian R, Charette LJ, McPeek B, et al: Reporting on methods in clinical trials. *N Engl J Med* 306:1332-1337, 1982.

Fletcher RH, Fletcher SW: Clinical research in general medical journals, a 30-year perspective. *N Engl J Med* 301:180-183, 1979.

Freiman JA, Chalmers TC, Smith H, et al: The importance of beta, the Type II error and sample size in the design and interpretation of the randomized control trial, survey of 71 "negative" trials. *N Engl J Med* 299:690-694, 1978.

Friedman LM, Furberg CD, DeMets DL: *Fundamentals of Clinical Trials.* Boston, John Wright, 1982.

Horwitz RI, Feinstein AR: Methodologic standards and contradictory results in case-control research. *Am J Med* 66:556-564, 1979.

Ingelfinger JA, Mosteller F, Thibodeau LA, et al: *Biostatistics in Clinical Medicine.* New York, Macmillan, 1983.

Larsen RJ: *Statistics for the Health Sciences.* Columbus, Ohio, Charles E Merrill, 1975.

Riegelman RK: *Studying a Study and Testing a Test, How to Read the Medical Literature.* Boston, Little, Brown, 1981.

CHAPTER 26

Development and Implementation of Drug Information Services

ANN B. AMERSON

The minimum standards for pharmacies in institutions, developed by the American Society of Hospital Pharmacists (ASHP), identify the evaluation and dissemination of comprehensive information about drugs and their usefulness to the institution's staff and patients as a prominent component of pharmaceutical services. Standard IV (Drug Information) and Standard V (Assuring Rational Drug Therapy) both address philosophies and functions that encompass drug information services. With this responsibility recognized, it then becomes a matter of the degree to which the services can be formalized and justified within the pharmacy department.

The mechanism used by some institutions is establishment of a formal drug information service or center. This concept was first developed in 1962 and over 20 years later still remains a viable, useful approach to accomplishing this responsibility. The origin, growth, and development of drug information centers have been reviewed (1). This chapter focuses on considerations in development of drug information services.

DEFINING DRUG INFORMATION SERVICES

Examining the current practice is one way to define drug information services. Drug information centers provide a number of different services that are now established (Table 26.1). Brief comments about each of these services are in order.

Answering Questions. Provision of drug information on demand is one of the first services usually considered. This type of service allows the inquirer to have specific information needs met in a timely fashion. Information resources can be concentrated in a central, accessible location with personnel available for answering questions. Although some investment is necessary to establish this service, centralizing resources avoids unnecessary duplication. The expertise of individuals may be more fully developed and efficiently utilized when the individuals are routinely involved in providing the service. The number and types of questions and callers are often used to measure success and requires appropriate documentation.

Pharmacy and Therapeutics Committee Activities. The Pharmacy and Therapeutics (P&T) Committee is a committee of the medical staff with the director of pharmacy (or his designee) usually serving as secretary. Pharmacy participation on this committee can involve preparing agendas and/or minutes, providing drug evaluations, and influencing institutional drug use policies. Involvement in these activities is increasingly important with the implementation of payment by diagnosis related groups (DRGs) (2-4). Institutions with a relative lack of formulary control have recognized the necessity of greater selectivity and are moving to develop or improve formularies. The opportunity exists for leadership from pharmacy with the avenue for developing these activities already established. The cost savings that can result underscore the importance and need for these activities.

Once a formulary is developed, maintenance is required. Formulary maintenance includes revision, printing, and distribution. Since these functions are closely tied to P&T Committee activities, they represent a logical and necessary component of communicating committee actions to the medical staff. Availability of a current formulary should facilitate appropriate utilization of drugs within the institution.

Publications. Efforts to communicate information on drug use policies and current developments that influence drug selection are an important component of drug information services. Most often newsletters are published to accomplish this, but other techniques have been utilized to convey certain kinds of information. For example, pocket-sized cards

TABLE 26.1 Drug Information Services

1. Answering questions
2. P&T Committee activity
   a. Drug evaluations and drug use policies
   b. Formulary development and maintenance
3. Publications—newsletters, bulletins, journal columns
4. Education—in-service programs, students
5. Drug use review
6. Investigational drug activity
7. Coordination of reporting programs
8. Poison information

can be developed that focus on a class or group of agents that provide information to aid in appropriate selection. Publications within an institution are used to complete a cycle of discussion, decision, communication, and implementation. Factors to consider in developing a newsletter are discussed in Chapter 31.

Dissemination of information outside the institution is important. Exchange of newsletters facilitates communication of differing approaches to the same problems and promotes information sharing. Publishing columns in state and national pharmaceutical journals is another means of sharing information.

Education. Involvement in this activity varies considerably depending on the resources within the institution and whether or not the institution is a teaching facility. Since the minimum standards for institutional pharmacies identify a responsibility to both health professionals and patients regarding drug information, needs and resources for both groups should be evaluated and prioritized. A program for development and dissemination of information for discharge counseling is an example of a drug information service for patients. In-service programs for various groups can be coordinated as a drug information service and involve a continuing commitment. A primary reason for development of a formal center is for teaching pharmacy students and training residents. Teaching other health professional students is another possibility.

Drug Use Review. Increasingly important, drug use review may be tied to P&T Committee activities or may be involved with other medical staff committes such as infection control. A successful program requires planning, coordination, and interaction with the medical staff. Drug information service involvement can include the literature support for development of criteria and participation in data gathering and analysis.

Investigational Drugs. In a facility where investigational drugs are regularly used, appropriate emphasis must be given to having the proper information available to all health professionals involved with their use. Various approaches to provide this service depend on the resources of the institution. The drug information service can provide the necessary liaison between the Institutional Review Board, the P&T Committee, and the pharmacy. The responsibility of coordinating the acquisition, development, and dissemination of appropriate information for investigational drugs is a drug information service. Regardless of how often investigational drugs are used, a procedure should exist to ensure information is available.

Coordination of Reporting Programs. National programs such as the Food Drug Administration Adverse Drug Reaction Reporting Program (ADRRP) and the Drug Product Problem Reporting Program (DPPRP) depend primarily on the initiation of reports by individuals. Coordination of this process in an institution from a central place facilitates consistency and completeness in reporting. Since both of the programs involve drugs, this function can be included as a drug information service.

Poison Information. This area may be viewed as a specialized component of drug information that has some different requirements. A decision to provide this service requires a substantial commitment of resources, personnel,

and time for an effective program. This service is discussed in more detail later.

Drug information services are defined primarily from a functional viewpoint. Inclusion of all or most of these functions should result in a total program as provided by a drug information center. However, certain drug information functions can be identified, developed, and implemented as part of a pharmacy service without a formally established drug information center.

In the environment where a formal drug information center or service exists, these functions or activites should be melded together into a program with goals and a philosophy. In the event the resources cannot be committed to a total program, certain functions may be identified and incorporated as part of the pharmacy service. Although the next section will discuss developing drug information services from a program standpoint, the same principles generally apply to selection of a specific function for initiation.

DEVELOPMENT

Establishing Goals. When developing drug information services, needs should be identified and prioritized. The target audience(s) should be recognized and the geographic intent identified. Will services be limited to the institution, or will they encompass an area outside the institution? What are the specific needs of the target audience? Will drug information services be part of a comprehensive clinical services program, or will they be the primary source of clinical activity? The determination of these factors assists in establishing short- and long-term goals and objectives in the areas of service, education, and research. A good service program in drug information can be freestanding or an essential support program for clinical services. A good service program is necessary for an effective teaching program. The role in research activities can be variable, from assisting in development of protocols to design and initiation of significant funded research. The primary needs identified will also establish the relative emphasis given to each of the three areas.

Justification. With increasingly tight resources in health care, justification of new services as well as established services is essential. Some priorities of the drug information specialist, the pharmacy director, and the hospital administrator may differ and each party should recognize this. For example, the drug information director may feel that day-to-day information requests should be top priority. For the pharmacy director and hospital administrator, however, information provided to the P&T Committee for developing a formulary or a drug use review program may have a higher priority. Recognizing that compromise may be necessary, the drug information specialists and pharmacy directors should work together to develop appropriate priorities and schedules for implementation. Certainly, the pharmacy director will have to be in full support of the proposed services when presenting the request to hospital administration.

When preparing justification, the needs of the target audience and the services to meet these needs should be identified. In this process, support from potential users of the service should be generated to confirm the needs. Medical staff and/or nursing support would be crucial for services initiated within an institution and should be sought in written form.

Another source of justification may be formal statements or guidelines adopted by such groups as the ASHP. Currently, statements exist on the Hospital Pharmacist and Drug Information Services, The Formulary System, The P&T Committee, and Guidelines for Formularies. Recognition of services by national organizations can be used as an additional source of justification. Requirements imposed by the Joint Commission on Accreditation of Hospitals may provide another avenue of justification. These might include activities such as a drug use review.

In the justification process, cost factors must also be addressed. In general, most aspects of drug information services are viewed as incurred costs to the department. The acquisition and maintenance of the resources require a continuing budgetary commitment in addition to personnel expenses. Opportunities for the service to generate revenue should be assessed. These could result in the form of a charge for questions, investigational drug services, outside consulting, or subscription services to other institutions (1). In general, these charges do not generate enough revenue to support the total cost of the service (5).

Another way to approach the cost justification issue is examination of potential dollar savings resulting from the activities of the service. These are most likely to be formulary activities such as reducing the number of products and the selection of therapeutic equivalents. These savings, however, can be significant (6).

DETERMINATION OF NEEDED RESOURCES

Developing a budget proposal requires assessment of needs for space, personnel, equipment, and information sources. In an existing facility, requirements for space should be estimated even though space for operation may be identified only after the program is approved. Any anticipated renovation costs should be included in the budget. For a new facility, such cost is unnecessary, but space requirements should still be identified.

Some considerations in the identification of space include the work environment, accessibility to a medical library, and teaching programs. Space that is located out of the mainstream of pharmacy operations and is conducive for information retrieval and evaluation without significant noise distractions is desirable. Accessibility to medical library services may be an important consideration where choice of space is available. A medical library also may provide a source of space, since several drug information centers are located within medical library facilities. If the teaching of pharmacy students is a major component, the space requirement increases. Tatro (7) has recommended some guidelines that consider the number of people staffing the center and space requirements for information storage and retrieval. A drug information center staffed by one full-time equivalent pharmacist and secretary should contain a minimum of 840 square feet.

Factors to consider in estimating personnel requirements include the scope of services expected. If several functions are initiated and, particularly, if a significant educational component is involved, commitment of at least one individual's time is necessary. For the function of answering questions, it is important to have someone available to respond to calls during the hours of operation. Unless combined with a poison center, most centers operate on a standard daytime schedule with coverage provided after hours through a 24-hour pharmacy service or on-call personnel. Arrangements for additional coverage may include utilization of staff pharmacists, residents, and/or students. These individuals require appropriate training and orientation. Adequate secretarial services should be available, the need being determined by the scope of services proposed.

Equipment needs include office furniture (desks, files, shelving), typewriter or word processor, microfiche reader/printer, and telephones. Computer systems for on-line literature retrieval should be evaluated and can be used cost effectively (18). As more data bases (e.g., Drugdex, American Hospital Formulary Service) are offered on-line, the utility of a personal computer should be evaluated.

Factors important in selecting information sources include the scope of references needed, availability of existing resources, and financial investment required. Information resources can be divided into references, journals, and secondary literature sources. Each component must be evaluated against existing resources as well as identifying opportunities to acquire certain resources on a no-charge basis. For example, a number of publishers provide complimentary copies of certain journals to the drug information service and/or the pharmacy director. In evaluating the existing institutional library services, the opportunity for cooperation in resource acquisition can be explored as well as the kinds of library services available (e.g., reprints, current awareness program, computer retrieval services). If a medical library is readily available (within walking distance), this can reduce the need for certain types of resources such as journals and secondary literature sources. Some references may also be acquired by the library that will not need duplication in the drug information center (e.g., references dealing with foreign products). Computer retrieval services are generally available through medical libraries, and the need for this resource should be evaluated. Development of a close working relationship with library personnel will provide mutual benefits for both parties.

The financial requirements for information resources involve both the initial investment and maintenance costs. The initial investment is incurred in acquiring adequate resources. After the first year, costs will continue for maintenance and updating reference resources. The investment and maintenance requirements for journals and secondary literature sources are similar in that they are annually recurring costs. For reference sources, the initial investment usually exceeds the maintenance costs.

PLANNING FOR IMPLEMENTATION

Once approval is obtained and an implementation date is set, policies and procedures for operation should be developed. These include a statement of the service's general philosophy and identification of the specific role in various activities within the department. Procedures for handling phone calls should be developed along with forms for documentation, particularly if several people will be involved in providing this service. Since a number of people may be involved in provision of on-line service, a training program, encompassing both competency in utilization of resources and procedural matters, would help ensure consistency. Notifying the target audience about implementation of the service, particularly the function of answering questions, is a key element. Methods that might be used to announce the new service would be use of a newsletter (if already established); a separate announcement that is distributed, posted, and/or mailed; letters to key individuals; and in-service training for various groups of the target audience.

If the decision is made to implement a large-scale service with a variety of activities, priorities concerning the order of implementation are also needed. Assessment of the most pressing needs may indicate that the formulary and P&T Committee aspect requires immediate priority with a newsletter to physicians to communicate the on-going activities in this area. Implementation of on-line services may have to wait until these other activities are established.

DOCUMENTATION AND EVALUATION

In the present environment of cost containment, documentation and evaluation of the service's activity, quality, and cost benefit are essential. This applies to new services being instituted as well as to established services. Increasingly, reevaluation of established programs will be undertaken, with cuts likely for activities that are not well documented.

For services provided, documentation of the activities is the easier process addressed. Useful documentation includes the number and kinds of callers, types of questions, copies of newsletters and publications, and copies of the formulary and P&T Committee information. The number of calls provides an indication of growth (in a new service) or stability (in an established service) but does not measure total productivity (1,7). Other statistics such as the number of monographs prepared for the P&T Committee help reflect a broader scope of activity. More than likely, demonstration of impact and effectiveness will also be necessary.

Measuring user satisfaction through questionnaires or follow-up calls is one means of documenting services and their value. If payment is made for services and use remains stable or grows, this would be an indication of the service's value. Most important would be demonstration of benefits vs cost. One example where this concept can be applied would be cost savings from formulary input and direction. Another would be the effectiveness of drug information service efforts to educate physicians about drug costs. Assessment of use before and after such efforts may indicate cost savings as well as the effectiveness of the particular tool (newsletter, cost card, etc).

Finally, attention should also focus on the quality of services, developing some mechanism to periodically review the accuracy and timeliness of information provided, and whether or not it has an impact on patient care. Various methods have been used to assess these aspects (1).

POISON CONTROL SERVICES

Poison control centers were developed before drug information centers, with the first center established in 1953

(9). Such centers proliferated rapidly, with more than 600 centers identified during the 1960s. However, resources were not distributed or utilized with any consistency, as coordination and direction were lacking (10). Development of regional centers, with the first in 1971, has led to a decline in the total number of centers. In 1983, 385 centers or services were listed. In 1978, the American Association of Poison Control Centers (AAPCC) published criteria for regional poison control centers that served as further impetus to their development (11). At the end of 1982, there were 26 centers designated as meeting AAPCC criteria (9). A recent evaluation comparing information provided by regional and nonregional centers found that regional centers provided better and more consistent information (12).

Interestingly, poison control services have been mandated in some states by statutes (9). Although this happened very early in their history (1957 in Connecticut), this trend is more recent, with state statutes becoming more comprehensive in their requirements. The AAPCC criteria seem to have influenced the degree of comprehensiveness. Specific poison control statutes exist in 13 states with a joint drug information center mandated in five (9).

Some of the most important requirements identified for a regional poison control center include a 24-hour service, a toll-free telephone number, community education activities, and a case-reporting system (9). Veltri (10) has described in some detail the necessary considerations for staffing, space, information resources, and funding in a regional poison control center. Readers are referred to this article for specific details.

The combination of drug and poison information functions into one center deserves comment. As previously indicated, this has been mandated by statute in a few states. In the last survey of drug information centers, the number affiliated with a poison control operation had increased to 36 (37.5%) of the 96 centers reporting (1). The combination of two such services has some advantages and disadvantages. The obvious advantages for both programs include reduced costs and space requirements. As discussed by Troutman and Wanke (13), in the combined situation, the drug information service will usually benefit from the communication and data-management equipment as well as the increased staffing of the poison control center. The poison control center operation benefits from the literature search and evaluation skills of the drug information specialist.

Potential disadvantages in combining services include lack of development of maximal skills of staff members in either discipline and possible disputes over areas of responsibility. Since poison information calls usually require more immediate response, drug information inquiries may be unduly neglected unless appropriate priorities are identified. Poison information providers, particularly nonpharmacists, may feel added pressure in having to respond to drug information inquiries. Potential disadvantages to both services, however, could be avoided with appropriate recognition and action.

FUTURE DRUG INFORMATION PRACTICE

Drug information centers will continue to evolve and mature much like poison control centers. Regionalization of services provided by drug information centers needs evaluation and, if feasible, criteria should be established for regional centers. Specific drug information functions such as P&T Committee support are important in the institutional setting, and pharmacists, in general, should improve their ability to function in this area.

The Special Interest Group (SIG) on Drug and Poison Information of the ASHP has provided an opportunity for interaction of practitioners in these areas. Many SIG activities have focused on drug information practice. The development of criteria for a specialty residency in drug information by the SIG, which was approved by the ASHP Board of Directors, is a positive indicator for the future (14). This training program will supply a core of individuals with specialized training in the area, a source of personnel that has been lacking (15). A recent survey indicated 12 drug information training programs with 10 of these seeking accreditation under the specialty standard (16). The SIG activities have addressed other areas such as minimum standards and quality assurance. Minimum standards for personnel, physical facilities, organization, resources, and services were discussed by the SIG and have been incorporated as the basis for qualification of the site for residency training. Quality assurance guidelines (not an official ASHP guideline) were developed by the SIG in 1980 to offer technical assistance to ASHP members. Continued activities of this nature will provide needed leadership for a maturing drug information practice.

In the future, the number of drug information centers may increase but not as rapidly as in the past 10 years. The opportunity and/or demand for some drug information services will be increased. This allows the individual pharmacist a more active role in determining drug use policy and an opportunity to fulfill some of the responsibilities identified in the minimum standards. Services provided by centers will undergo some reevaluation and possible reorganization to better meet the changing needs, but drug information services will remain an important component of pharmacy practice.

REFERENCES

1. Amerson AB, Wallingford DM: Twenty years' experience with drug information centers. *Am J Hosp Pharm* 40:1172-1178, 1983.
2. Vaida AJ: Coping with DRGs: Suburban General Hospital, Norristown, Pennsylvania. *Am J Hosp Pharm* 40:1494-1496, 1983.
3. Upton JH, Crouch JB, Douglas JB: Coping with DRGs: The Moses H. Cone Memorial Hospital, Greensboro, North Carolina. *Am J Hosp Pharm* 40:1496-1499, 1983.
4. Lipman AG: TEFRA and the P&T Committee (editorial). *Hosp Formulary* 18:365, 1983.
5. Rosenberg JM: Drug information centers: Future trends. *Am J Hosp Pharm* 40:1213-1215, 1983.
6. Shielding drug information centers from budget cuts. *ASHP SIGNAL* 7:36, 1983.
7. Tatro DS: Establishing a drug information service. *Top Hosp Pharm Mgt* 2(1):74-86, 1982.
8. Schneiweiss F: Use and cost analysis of online literature teaching in a university-based drug information center. *Am J Hosp Pharm* 40:254-256, 1983.
9. Russell SL, Czajka PA: Comparison of poison control statutes in the United States. *Am J Hosp Pharm* 41:481-484, 1984.
10. Veltri JC: Regional poison control services. *Hosp Formulary* 17:1469-1486, 1982.
11. The American Association of Poison Control Centers: Regionalization criteria. *Vet Hum Toxicol* 20:117-118, 1978.
12. Thompson DF, Trammel HL, Robertson NJ, et al: Evaluation of regional and nonregional poison centers. *New Engl J Med* 308:191-194, 1983.
13. Troutman WG, Wanke LA: Advantages and disadvantages of combining poison control and drug information centers. *Am J Hosp Pharm* 40:1219-1222, 1983.
14. ASHP supplemental standard and learning objectives for residency training in drug information practice. *Am J Hosp Pharm* 39:1970-1972, 1982.
15. Pearson RE: Drug information specialists—an endangered species? (letter)? *Am J Hosp Pharm* 32:783, 1975.
16. Kirkwood CF: Residency programs in drug information. *Am J Hosp Pharm* 41:145-146, 1984.

CHAPTER 27

Adverse Drug Reactions

RONALD B. STEWART

Adverse drug reactions (ADRs) have been defined by the World Health Organization as "any response to a drug which is noxious and unintended, and which occurs at doses used in man for prophylaxis, diagnosis, or therapy" (1). Estimates hold that about one million patients are hospitalized, and as many as 140,000 deaths occur in the United States every year as a direct result of medications prescribed by physicians or those purchased over the counter (2).

Many patients also experience ADRs during hospitalization. Careful monitoring of drug therapy by pharmacists can result in detection of drug-induced disease, and often these drug-induced diseases can be prevented. Pharmacists also have an important responsibility to report ADRs to the Food and Drug Administration (FDA).

NATURE AND SCOPE OF DRUG-INDUCED DISEASE

The percentage of patients who experience an adverse reaction to drugs in the hospital, with few exceptions, has ranged between 10% and 20% (Table 27.1) (3-12). Differences between these observed prevalences apparently reflect differences in populations studied, criteria for evaluating ADRs, and surveillance techniques. Most ADRs that occur in the hospital are minor. Sixty to seventy percent of reported ADRs include minor gastrointestinal disturbances, rash, itching, drowsiness, insomnia, weakness, headache, tremulousness, muscle twitching, and fever. In all intensive

prospective studies, the majority of ADRs resulted from the pharmacologic effects of drugs and have usually been well-known toxic effects or side effects. Therefore, it has been suggested that by more careful prescribing, dosage regimen selection, and drug monitoring many reactions experienced by patients could be prevented.

The incidence of patients admitted to hospitals has been the subject of several large prospective studies. Caranasos et al (5) monitored 6063 admissions to a medical service during a 3-year period and observed that 2.9% of admissions resulted from drug-induced illness. Miller (6), in a similar study of 7017 medical patients, found 3.7% of admissions were either caused by or strongly influenced by an ADR. In both of these studies, the drugs found to lead to hospitalization were similar (Table 27.2). More recently, ADRs leading to hospitalization in elderly patients have been studied. Williamson and Chopin (13) monitored 1998 consecutive admissions to 42 geriatric medicine departments in England, Wales, and Scotland and found ADRs present at the time of hospitalization in 15.3% of elderly patients taking prescribed medications. In 209 (10.5%) of these patients, it was thought that an ADR contributed to the need for admission, and in 55 patients (2.8%), the drug was the sole cause. These studies have been concerned only with drug-induced illness and have not included admissions resulting from inappropriate drug therapy prescribed by physicians or from noncompliance with prescribed therapeutic regimens.

TABLE 27.1 Incidence of Adverse Drug Reactions (ADRs)

Author	No. of Patients Studied	Patients Experiencing ADRs in Hospital		Patients Admitted with ADRs	
		No.	%	No.	%
Gardner and Watson (3)	939	99	10.5	48	5.1
Bergman et al (4)	229	49	21.4	—	—
Caranasos et al (5)	6063	—	—	177	2.9
Miller (6)	7017	—	—	260	3.7
Smith (7)	900	97	10.8	35	3.9
Hurwitz, Wade (8,9)	1160	118	10.2	58	5.0
Ogilvie, Ruedy (10)	731	132	18.0	48	6.6
Levy et al (12)	2499	—	—	103	4.1
Levy et al (12)	2399	—	—	167	5.7

McKenney and Harrison (14) studied 216 patients admitted to a 100-bed general medical ward of a large teaching hospital to document all drug-related hospital admissions. They found that 59 (27.3%) patients were admitted with a drug-related problem, and the most common cause was ADRs (11.1%). Noncompliance, inadequate drug therapy, drug misuse, and drug overdose accounted for 16.2% of the admissions. Stewart et al (15) used a similar methodology to investigate drug-related admissions to an inpatient psychiatric unit and found 41.7% of all admissions were related to drug problems. Over half (52%) of these drug-related admissions resulted from drug abuse, whereas drug overdose, side effects, and noncompliance accounted for 16%, 12%, and 20% of admissions, respectively. This work suggests that when all drug-related problems are considered, they represent a major public health problem.

Estimates of morbidity, mortality, and cost of drug-induced illness to patients in this country abound in the medical literature (1,16-19). Direct costs of ADRs include the cost of hospitalization and treatment. A factor that has largely been ignored in calculating costs of ADRs is the indirect cost sustained by the community as a consequence of lost contributions by the individual to the gross national product as a result of temporary or permanent disability. Mach and Venulet (20) found that in many instances the indirect cost may exceed the direct cost by tenfold.

Smith and Visconti (21) estimated the cost of ADRs during a three-month study of drug-induced disease on a medical service of a major teaching hospital. The population studied comprised 685 patients and, of these, 149 acquired at least one ADR during hospitalization; 86 of these patients had some type of ADR present on admission. Economic data gathered with relationship to ADRs were direct costs, including costs of detection, of avoiding ADRs, and of the treatment associated with the reaction. Indirect costs included premature death, loss of work associated with the reaction, permanent disability, and/or increased susceptibility to other drug-induced and natural conditions. Direct and indirect costs to these patients resulting from drug-induced disease was estimated to be $160,156.

Since most studies have been conducted on adult medical wards in university hospital settings, it is impossible to project the precise impact of drug-induced illness on morbidity and cost. However, the available evidence would suggest the problem represents a major public health hazard.

ROLE OF THE PHARMACIST IN ADVERSE DRUG REACTION MONITORING

In recent years, hospital pharmacists have developed new roles in the clinical environment. These new roles include acquiring drug histories on newly admitted patients, discharge counseling and patient education, nutritional support services, pharmacokinetic dosing services, and drug monitoring. These new activities, coupled with the traditional function of control and distribution of medications from a central location, make pharmacists ideally suited to monitor and report ADRs occurring in health care institutions.

Over the last decade pharmacists have taken a leadership role in designing and implementing systems to monitor and report ADRs. Pharmacists have assumed this role both in the United States and in many other countries (22-25).

Pharmacists are required by the Joint Commission on Accreditation of Hospitals (JCAH) to develop written policies and procedures governing the safe administration of drugs (26). The JCAH states that "medication errors and drug reactions shall be reported with written procedures. This requirement shall include notification of the practitioner who ordered the drug. An entry of the medication administered and/or the drug reaction shall be properly recorded in the patient's medical record. Hospitals are encouraged to report any unexpected or significant adverse drug reactions to the Hospital Reporting Program of the Federal Food and Drug Administration and to the manufacturer" (26).

The American Society of Hospital Pharmacists (ASHP) included ADRs in its "Statement of Hospital Drug Control Systems" (27). The JCAH and the ASHP provide the following standards relating to ADRs:

1. A written procedure for recording and reporting ADRs should be developed.
2. ADRs should be reported immediately to the practitioner who ordered the drug.
3. Records of the episode should become part of the patient's chart and of the pharmacy's records.
4. ADR data collected from the institution should be reviewed and evaluated.
5. The Pharmacy and Therapeutics Committee (P&T Committee) should review reported ADRs.
6. ADRs should be reported to the FDA and the drug manufacturer.
7. Published reports of ADRs should be distributed to the medical and nursing staffs.

TABLE 27.2   Common Drugs Causing Hospitalization of Medical Patients

Caranasos et al (5)[a]		Miller (6)[b]		Levy et al (12)			
				Jerusalem		Berlin	
Drug	No. of Times Cited	Drug	No. of Times Cited	Drug	% of All Reactions	Drug	% of All Reactions
Aspirin	25	Digoxin	41	Ampicillin	7.7	Digoxin	27.5
Digoxin	24	Aspirin	24	Digoxin	6.8	Analgesic compound	12.0
Warfarin	12	Prednisone	15	Furosemide	4.9	Warfarin	6.6
Hydrochlorothiazide	11	Warfarin	9	Quinidine	4.9	Insulin	6.6
Prednisone	8	Guanethidine	5	Aspirin	4.9	Oral hypoglycemics	4.2

[a]6063 patients.
[b]7017 patients.

8. Proper steps should be taken to reduce the incidence of ADRs within the institution.

Many uses have been identified for the information gained by hospital ADR reporting programs. The information can (1) provide a measure of the quality of care, (2) protect against liability, (3) measure potentially correctable drug-related problems, (4) measure clinical nurses' and physicians' observations of ADRs, (5) identify new, unusual, or serious ADRs to the FDA, and (6) serve as an educational tool to increase awareness of drug effects (28).

MONITORING DRUG THERAPY FOR ADVERSE DRUG REACTIONS

Pharmacists may participate in monitoring activities on an individual patient basis or by monitoring large patient populations. Several publications are available to assist pharmacists in techniques of individual patient monitoring (29,30). Methods to increase detection, evaluation, and reporting of ADRs in hospitals have also been described in the literature.

Detection and evaluation of ADRs have often been criticized because identification of these problems lacks adequate definition and operational criteria. Several guides or algorithms have been published to assist pharmacists and physicians in determining the likelihood of the occurrence of ADRs (31,32).

Methods to monitor for ADRs have been classified as retrospective and prospective surveillance.

Retrospective Surveillance Methods

These systems usually employ some method of reviewing the patient's medical record either at the time of or after discharge from the hospital.

Patient Chart Check-Off

This system requires each physician, when completing a chart, to fill out an ADR notification sheet. A sheet is completed for every patient discharged, and the medical record is not considered complete by the medical records department until the ADR sheet is completed. If the patient has experienced an ADR while under the care of a physician, it is noted on an alerting form, which is forwarded to the individual responsible for reporting the ADR. The patient's record is then reviewed to obtain complete information concerning the circumstances of the reaction. Although this system has been shown to increase reporting, it is not as effective as prospective surveillance (33,34). A variation of the notification card system is placement of a short form on each medication cart. The form is used to document both ADRs and medication errors. In this system, the nurse has primary responsibility for detection, and the pharmacist is responsible for compiling and reporting these drug-related problems. These problems are presented monthly to the P&T Committee, which is responsible for identifying trends and finding solutions to the problems (35).

Chart Screening

This method involves retrospective scanning of patients' charts and is supplemented from progress notes and phy-

sicians' orders. This system provides much more information than voluntary reporting and can be accomplished by supportive personnel. It was demonstrated in one study that one technician with minimal training can scan charts of all patients discharged from a 700-bed hospital (36).

Retrospective reporting systems have several disadvantages. It is often difficult to be sure of all circumstances surrounding an ADR after a patient has been discharged. The patient is not available for questioning or examination, and the physician has responsibilities to other patients. In these reporting systems, it is likely that the majority of ADRs experienced by patients will not be reported by health professionals.

Prospective Surveillance Methods

A more satisfactory method of documenting ADRs is through a prospective surveillance system that monitors patients and reports ADRs while the patient is hospitalized. There are several advantages to this. Circumstances surrounding a suspected ADR can be thoroughly investigated. Physicians, other health professionals, and even the patient can be interviewed to determine whether or not the observed sign or symptom is likely to have resulted from a medication. If necessary, a challenge dose of the medication may be administered or additional laboratory studies can be ordered to confirm a reaction. In prospective studies, steps can be taken to ensure that ADRs experienced by patients are recorded and reported by health professionals. These programs can also be designed to provide active feedback of information that can be used by the hospital staff to prevent the occurrence of drug-induced disease.

Voluntary Reporting by Physicians

This method is based on the voluntary cooperation by physicians (and other members of health professions) working in institutions to complete an ADR form after noting a reaction. Observations on ADRs are forwarded to a collecting center (FDA) where reports are analyzed.

Voluntary reporting systems provide surveillance of wide geographic areas and large numbers of patients at risk. In this country, for instance, there are 200,000 potential physician observers monitoring over 200 million patients. Advantages of the voluntary system are that it is relatively easy to manage, its operating costs are small, and it covers a broad range of drugs and all types of pathologic and therapeutic environments. Voluntary reporting may be erratic, incomplete, and of questionable reliability; however, patterns of drug-induced disease may be recognized when several reports of a new ADR are submitted by more than one physician to a national center.

The importance of voluntary reporting of ADRs was underscored by Rossi et al (37). They observed that none of the phase IV studies designed for three drugs (cimetidine, cyclobenzaprine, prazosin) detected any new ADRs. Nearly all new ADRs induced by these drugs resulted from information submitted by physicians through voluntary reporting (37).

In 1982, the General Accounting Office described what it thought was one of the best hospital ADR reporting programs (38). The pharmacy is the central collection point for

ADR forms in this hospital. Forms completed by any health professional detecting an ADR, are sent to the pharmacy. The forms, containing the patient's social security number, date, and type of reaction, are followed-up by a physician identified as an ADR monitor. A hospital ADR committee, composed of at least four physicians, the pharmacy director, and nursing and administration representatives, meets monthly to review reports. This committee forwards selected reports to the FDA and publishes selected reports in a hospital newsletter or pharmacy journal (39).

Intensive or Comprehensive Drug Monitoring

Undesirable effects of drugs have often been recognized only after long clinical experience. For example, it took nearly 80 years to identify aspirin as a frequent cause of gastric hemorrhages (40). Several studies have employed an epidemiologic approach to the study of ADRs with the purpose of providing more rapid identification of drug-induced disease. Two of these studies, the Boston Collaborative Drug Surveillance Program and the Gainesville Drug Study Program, have been operational for nearly 10 years and have collected information on a combined total of more than 50,000 patients (22,23).

Intensive drug monitoring programs provide standardized types of information for all patients. Information is collected on a large population of patients exposed to medications and includes the dose and duration of exposure. In these systems, both numerator (patients reacting) and denominator (patients exposed) are known, and therefore, rates of reactions can be calculated. This information is usually correlated with demographic data (age, sex, race) and other pertinent information such as laboratory test values, height, weight, and associated disease states.

Records from these systems are more complete, and follow-up is facilitated. Within these programs prospective studies of specific medications or clinical events can be undertaken. These programs provide the potential to conduct in-depth studies of ADRs previously identified by less sophisticated systems of voluntary reporting.

Intensive drug monitoring systems are expensive, requiring the time of personnel who acquire and process data, computer technology, and an identifiable population at risk. These programs are usually limited to university teaching hospitals where the variety of medications used has been restricted through a hospital formulary, and disease states may not be representative of those seen in community hospitals. Methods employed have been described in several texts (22,41).

Several references are available to the pharmacist for aid in monitoring patients for ADRs. These are listed below with a brief description of their contents.

1. *American Hospital Formulary Service* (42). The new hard-bound version of this text was first published in 1984. It contains a comprehensive listing of drugs, including dosage forms, indications, and ADRs. An extensive listing of ADRs of individual drugs is also provided.

2. *Monitoring for Drug Safety* (41). This book provides a worldwide overview of postmarketing surveillance in general patient populations, specialized monitoring programs (i.e., hospitals, national registries, poison information), and techniques and principles of epidemiology. The importance of the media, patients, doctor, industry, and government in drug monitoring is the topic of other chapters.

3. *Drug Effects in Hospitalized Patients* (23). This book is divided into two parts. Part I contains four introductory chapters discussing methods of studying drugs, interpretation of surveillance data, and methodology of the Boston Collaborative Drug Surveillance Program. Part II presents efficacy and toxicity data collected by the Boston study on 22 drug categories.

4. *Drug-Induced Blood Disorders* (43). This comprehensive text deals with various aspects of ADRs relating to hematology, including mechanisms, diagnosis, reporting, and prevention of these effects. The remainder of the text discusses major drug-induced blood disorders, including aplastic anemia, agranulocytosis, and thrombocytopenia.

5. *Drug Monitoring: A Requirement for Responsible Drug Use* (22). The first eight chapters discuss responsibilities of the public, the professions, and the pharmaceutical industry for drug monitoring. Chapters 9 through 16 discuss methods currently utilized in the United States and abroad to monitor ADRs. Chapters 17 through 24 describe results from the University of Florida drug monitoring program.

6. *Meyler's Side Effects of Drugs* (44). This text contains a comprehensive discussion of ADRs presented by drug category. It is well referenced and documented and is probably the most comprehensive reference text available on the subject of drug-induced disease. Since 1977, *Side Effects of Drugs Annual* has been published to provide a critical and up-to-date review of new information relating to ADRs and drug interactions (45). The annual can be used independently or as a supplement to *Meyler's Side Effects of Drugs*.

7. *Textbook of Adverse Drug Reactions* (45). The first four chapters deal with history, pathogenesis, assessment, and detection of ADRs. The remaining 25 chapters focus primarily on an organ system approach in reviewing ADRs. The last chapter discusses medicolegal aspects and implications of ADRs.

8. *Iatrogenic Disease* (47). This text provides an organ system approach in reviewing diseases induced by drugs (skin disease, blood dyscrasias). Its purpose is to summarize available knowledge on drugs that induce specific disease states. Specific chapters are devoted to monitoring concepts, epidemiology, and drugs in breast milk. A companion text, *Iatrogenic Diseases Update 1981,* has been published to update the original text (48).

9. *Adverse Effects of Antiepileptic Drugs* (49). This text presents a comprehensive review of anticonvulsant drug-induced disease and specific side effects of the individual antiepileptic drugs. It lists sources of clinical information on adverse effects of these drugs, identifies areas in need of further investigation, and suggests guidelines to minimize side effects of drug therapy with anticonvulsants. Fifteen chapters discuss diseases induced by antiepileptic drugs (organ system approach) and 12 chapters are devoted to specific antiepileptic drugs and their side effects.

RECENT DEVELOPMENTS AFFECTING ADR MONITORING

Impacts of diagnosis related groups (DRGs) on the problem of ADRs at this time are unclear (49). Over the years much information on short-term ADRs has been obtained by monitoring hospitalized patients. In the 1970's, the average hospital stay on the inpatient medical wards was about 8 days, thus providing an adequate time period to monitor patients for short-term ADRs. DRGs are expected to greatly reduce hospital stays and, therefore, there will be less opportunity to observe patients for ADRs. Better systems of monitoring for ADRs after hospitalization will be needed.

Availability of microcomputers will enable many hospital pharmacists to begin their own drug monitoring programs. With the use of microcomputers, essential clinical data, and drug use information, ADRs can now be easily obtained and stored at the ward level. Trend analysis on drug use and ADRs is now within easy reach of the practicing pharmacist as a result of computers.

PREVENTION AND CONTROL OF DRUG-INDUCED DISEASE

When treating patients with medication, the goal is to employ the most effective agent to treat a condition while minimizing hazards of therapy. Several principles should be followed to prevent drug-induced illness. First, one should be knowledgeable about the patient's medications. Second, when another medication is prescribed, it is important to have a thorough understanding of its pharmacology. Third, one should be knowledgeable concerning characteristics of the patient himself. Finally, the patient should be given as few medications as possible. Each of these principles will be considered briefly to illustrate how they contribute to the prevention of drug-induced disease.

Before a new drug is prescribed for a patient, it is important to identify medications previously prescribed for that patient. This usually requires a careful medication history or availability of a patient medication profile to identify the use of both prescribed medications as well as over-the-counter preparations. The history should also include any allergies to medication. Knowledge about the patient's medications should prevent duplication of agents with similar pharmacologic activity or administration of medications to patients who may be unable to tolerate the drug. In addition, the history may be used to identify clinical manifestation attributable to medications.

A thorough knowledge of a drug's pharmacology, including its mechanism of action, metabolism, excretion, and dose, is essential. Few medications have narrow ranges of action. For example, chlorpromazine has been shown to have sedative, antipsychotic, α-adrenergic blocking, and anticholinergic effects as well as other properties. Such knowledge is helpful in preventing various drug interactions.

One must also have a knowledge of the patient characteristics that may influence his or her response to medication. These include age, history of previous drug intolerance, status of renal and liver function, and concomitant diseases. It is also important to determine how the patients perceive their illness, how much they know about their medication, and their ability to comply with prescribed therapy.

One of the more important principles in prevention of drug-induced illness is the use of only those medications that are absolutely essential. Studies have shown that as the number of medications administered to a patient increases, the number of ADRs increases at a disproportionately higher rate.

Pharmacists can make significant contributions to the goal of improving the efficacy of drug therapy and decreasing its risks. A constant awareness of the hazards of drug therapy and careful consideration of risk to benefit ratio when using medications are essential.

REFERENCES

1. International drug monitoring. The role of the hospital—a WHO report. *Drug Intell Clin Pharm* 4:101-110, 1970.
2. Talley RB, Laventurier MF: Letter *JAMA* 229:1043, 1974.
3. Gardner P, Watson J: Adverse drug reactions: A pharmacist-based monitoring system. *Clin Pharmacol Ther* 11:802-807, 1970.
4. Bergman HD, Aoki VS, Black HJ, et al: Advantage of a unit dose drug distribution system in surveillance of adverse drug reactions. *Clin Toxicol* 5:404-411, 1972.
5. Caranasos G, Stewart RB, Cluff LE: Drug induced illness leading to hospitalization. *JAMA* 228:713-717, 1974.
6. Miller RR: Hospital admission due to adverse drug reactions. *Arch Intern Med* 134:219-223, 1974.
7. Smith JW, Seidl LG, Cluff LE: Studies on the epidemiology of adverse drug reactions. V. Clinical factors influencing susceptibility. *Ann Intern Med* 65:629-640, 1966.
8. Hurwitz N: Predisposing factors in adverse reactions to drugs. *Br Med J* 1:536-539, 1969.
9. Hurwitz N: Admissions to hospital due to drugs. *Br Med J* 1:531-536, 1969.
10. Ogilvie RI, Ruedy J: Adverse drug reactions during hospitalization. *Can Med Assoc* 97:1450-1457, 1967.
11. Steel K, Gertman PM, Crescenzi C, et al: Iatrogenic illness on a general medical service at a university hospital. *N Engl J Med* 304:638-642, 1981.
12. Levy M, Kewitz H, Altwein W, Hildebrand J, et al: Hospital admissions due to adverse drug reactions: A comparative study from Jerusalem and Berlin. *Eur J Clin Pharmacol* 17:25-31, 1980.
13. Williamson J, Chopin JM: Adverse reactions to prescribed drugs in the elderly: A multicare investigation. *Age Ageing* 9:73-80, 1980.
14. McKenney JM, Harrison WL: Drug-related hospital admissions. *Am J Hosp Pharm* 33:792-795, 1976.
15. Stewart RB, Springer PK, Adams JE: Drug related admissions to an inpatient psychiatric unit. *Am J Psychiatry* 137:1093-1095, 1980.
16. Melmon KL: Preventable drug reactions—causes and cures. *N Engl J Med* 284:1361-1368, 1971.
17. Medical News. *JAMA* 220:1287-1288, 1972.
18. Stetler CJ: Letter. *JAMA* 229:1043-1044, 1974.
19. Karch F, Lasagna L: Adverse drug reactions: A critical review. *JAMA* 234:1236-1241, 1975.
20. Mach EP, Venulet J: The economics of adverse drug reactions. *WHO Chron* 29:79-84, 1975.
21. Smith MC, Visconti JA: Research Report on the "cost" of the 1962 drug amendments. *Inquiry* XI:61-64, 1975.
22. Stewart RB, Cluff LE, Philp J: *Drug Monitoring: A Requirement for Responsible Drug Use.* Baltimore, Williams & Wilkins, 1977.
23. Miller RR, Greenblatt DJ: Drug Effects in Hospitalized Patients. New York, John Wiley & Sons, 1976, p 346.
24. Berbatis CG, Eckert GM: Positive aspects of monitoring of drug therapy. *Aust J Hosp Pharm* 6:153-155, 1976.
25. Busto U, Naranjo CA, Ruiz I, et al: Drug monitoring: The University of Chile clinical hospital experience. *Am J Hosp Pharm* 36:596, 1979.
26. Joint Commission on Accreditation of Hospitals. *Accreditation Manual for Hospitals.* Chicago, JCAH, 1983.
27. American Society of Hospital Pharmacists statement on hospital drug control systems. *Am J Hosp Pharm* 31:1198-1207, 1974.
28. Jones JK: Assessment of adverse drug reactions in the hospital setting: considerations. *Hosp Formulary* 14:769-775, 1979.
29. McKenzie MW, Pevonka MP, et al: The pharmacists' involvement in the long term care facility. *J Am Pharm Assoc* 15:18-20, 1975.
30. Pulliam CC: Therapeutic judgment. *Am J Hosp Pharm* 31:385-387, 1974.
31. Kramer MS, Leventhal JM, Hutchinson TA, et al: An algorithm for

the operational assessment of adverse drug reactions. I. *JAMA* 242:623-632, 1979.

32. Hutchinson TA, Leventhal JM, Kramer MS, et al: An algorithm for the operational assessment of adverse drug reactions. II. *JAMA* 242:633-638, 1979.

33. Cluff LE, Thornton GF, Seidl LG: Studies on the epidemiology of adverse drug reactions. 1. Methods of surveillance. *JAMA* 188:976-983, 1964.

34. Nelson RW, Shane R: Developing an adverse drug reaction reporting program. *Am J Hosp Pharm* 40:445-456, 1983.

35. Trudeau T: Pharmacy questions and answers. *Hosp Top* 58:42-47, 1980.

36. Canada AT: Adverse drug reaction reporting: A practical program. *Am J Hosp Pharm* 26:18-20, 1969.

37. Rossi AC, Knapp DE, Anello C, et al: Discovery of adverse drug reactions. *JAMA* 249:2226-2228, 1979.

38. Report to the Secretary of Health and Human Services: *FDA Can Further Improve Its Adverse Drug Reaction Reporting System.* U.S. General Accounting Office, Gaithersburg, Md, 1982.

39. Jacinto MS, Kleinman K: Hospital pharmacy program for reporting adverse drug reactions. *Am J Hosp Pharm* 40:444-445, 1983.

40. Meyler L, Peck HM: *Drug Induced Disease,* vol 3. Amsterdam, Excerpta Medica, 1968, p 1.

41. Inman WHW: *Monitoring for Drug Safety.* Philadelphia, JB Lippincott, 1980.

42. *American Hospital Formulary Service.* Bethesda, Md, American Society Hospital Pharmacists, 1984.

43. Grunchy de CC: *Drug-induced Blood Disorders.* Oxford, Blackwell Scientific Publications, 1975, p 204.

44. Dukes MNG: *Meyler's Side Effects of Drugs,* vol 9. Amsterdam, Excerpta Medica, 1980.

45. Dukes MNG: *Side Effects of Drugs Annual 8.* Amsterdam, Excerpta Medica, 1984.

46. Davies DM: *Textbook of Adverse Drug Reactions.* London, Oxford University Press, 1977.

47. D'Arcy PF, Griffin JP: *Iatrogenic Diseases,* ed 2. London, Oxford University Press, 1979.

48. D'Arcy PF, Griffin JP: *Iatrogenic Diseases.* London, Oxford University Press, 1981.

49. Schmidt D: *Adverse Effects of Antiepileptic Drugs.* New York, Raven Press, 1982.

50. Bonney RS: Hospital survival strategies for the 1980's. *Am J Hosp Pharm* 40:1483-1488, 1983.

CHAPTER 28

Drug Interactions

PHILIP D. HANSTEN

Intense interest in the topic of drug-drug interactions began in the mid-1960s following the publication of a symposium in the Proceedings of the Royal Society of Medicine (1). In the late 1960s and early 1970s, pharmacists enthusiastically embraced this "new" field of study but with varying results. It soon became obvious that many patients receiving interacting drug combinations did not manifest the expected adverse response. This resulted in some pharmacists and physicians reaching the premature conclusion that, in general, drug interactions were clinically unimportant. We now know that drug-drug interactions can indeed cause significant untoward consequences but that many interactions do so only in the presence of certain predisposing factors. As in many other areas of human endeavor, oversimplification of the problem resulted in an easy but inappropriate answer. The current challenge facing pharmacists and physicians is to identify patients who are actually at risk of developing adverse drug interactions and to take actions that will minimize the likelihood of such adverse events. This is not an easy task, but pharmacists in institutional practice are in an excellent position to address this problem.

MISCONCEPTIONS ABOUT DRUG INTERACTIONS

In addition to erroneous conclusions regarding the general clinical importance of drug interactions, a number of specific misconceptions have arisen. These misconceptions may result in inappropriate action or inaction on the part of health professionals. An understanding of these principles is important in developing institutional pharmacy systems designed to address the drug interaction problem.

1. Misconception: "Due to high awareness of drug interactions by health professionals, we are close to the irreducible minimum for adverse effects from drug interactions." This may be true for a handful of well-known drug interactions but is certainly not the case for drug interactions in general. The average level of sophistication of health professionals regarding drug interactions is simply not sufficient to allow this conclusion. Available evidence from epidemiologic studies and the experience of drug interaction exerts indicate that the majority of adverse drug interactions that occur in patients are not even diagnosed as such, let alone prevented.

2. Misconception: "Only 20 or 30 drug interactions are of clinical importance, so one can learn those and forget the rest." There are several flaws in this statement. First, clinical evidence clearly indicates that at least 150 drug interactions have caused adverse effects in some patients. Thus, the task is not so much selecting the *interactions* which are potentially clinically important, but rather the *patients* who are predisposed to developing adverse drug interaction effects. Second, even if there were only 20-30 important drug interactions, available data are insufficient to determine which interactions should be placed in this category. Moreover, the "top 30" could vary considerably, depending on the type of patients and many other factors.

3. Misconception: "The large number of clinical studies on certain drug interactions have allowed us to predict the likely magnitude of the interaction response in specific patients." Unfortunately, this is not yet possible. If a study of 20 patients shows that drug A produces a mean increase of 50% in serum levels of drug B, this does *not* mean that the patient receiving these two drugs is likely to have about a 50% increase in drug B serum levels. The outcome of drug interactions is highly variable from patient to patient. Thus, mean values from the literature can usually be used only as rough guides to estimate the magnitude of the interaction in a specific patient.

4. Misconception: "When one realizes that a patient is receiving an interacting drug combination, it is usually necessary to substitute a noninteracting drug for one of the drugs to avoid adverse effects." One may *choose* to substitute a noninteracting drug as the most appropriate course of action, but it is seldom *necessary*. The adverse effects of interacting drugs can usually be prevented by adjusting the doses of one or both drugs, adjusting dosing times, or simply monitoring the patient more closely.

5. Misconception: "Drug interaction mechanisms are largely of academic interest with little bearing on the resolution of drug interaction problems in specific patients." Knowledge of the mechanisms by which a given drug interaction occurs may be quite useful in determining the likely time course of the interaction. We know, for example, that it may take 10 days to 2 weeks for maximal enzyme induction to occur, whereas maximal enzyme inhibition may occur in a matter of hours. Furthermore, displacement of one drug from plasma protein binding by another drug tends to produce only a temporary increase in the pharmacologic

response of the displaced drug. Knowledge of drug interaction mechanisms can also enable rational selection of methods to avoid the interaction. An obvious example would be separation of administration times of two drugs when the drug interaction mechanism is inhibition of gastrointestinal absorption of one drug by the other.

6. Misconception: "When a patient is stabilized on a given drug and a drug is added which increases or decreases the effect of the stabilized drug, it is usually necessary to prophylactically adjust the dose of the stabilized drug." This may be necessary under certain circumstances such as interactions involving drugs with a narrow therapeutic index. However, in many cases it is possible to simply add the interacting drug and monitor for the need to adjust dosage. When doses are adjusted at the same time that the interacting drug is started, one introduces two perturbations to the system simultaneously. This may result in delays in determining whether the interaction occurred in the patient and may also delay selection of the new adjusted steady-state dose of the drug affected by the interaction. This is especially true if one does not completely understand the time course of the interaction in question.

7. Misconception: "The adverse effects of drug interactions generally occur rapidly." There are a few drug interactions that produce adverse effects within minutes or hours, especially if the mechanism is pharmacodynamic addition or antagonism. However, the vast majority of adverse results from drug interactions occur only after several days or more. This fact should be considered when designing methods of notifying prescribers of potential interactions in their patients. In most cases, a written notification within a day or two would be sufficient.

PITFALLS IN EVALUATION OF DRUG INTERACTION LITERATURE

Evaluation of the original literature on drug interactions can result in erroneous conclusions unless one is careful to avoid certain pitfalls. Examples of these pitfalls and suggestions for avoiding them are described below.

1. Failure to allow sufficient time for the interaction to develop. This error has caused considerable confusion regarding several interactions. For example, the ability of tricyclic antidepressants to inhibit the antihypertensive response to guanethidine takes place over several days. Thus, early short-term studies failed to detect the interaction, and it was several years before the true nature of the interaction was elucidated.

2. Inappropriate extrapolation of interactions from one member of a drug class to all members of that class. Although some drug classes probably interact in a fairly homogeneous way (e.g., thiazide diuretics), for many other drug classes the individual agents may interact differently because of differences in elimination pathways or other factors.

3. Inappropriate evaluation of the significance of case histories. This pitfall can take at least two forms. First, one or two cases of a possible interaction can be interpreted as proof that an interaction exists. Conversely, *failure* to find evidence of an interaction in a few patients receiving a given combination is sometimes interpreted as proof that an in-

teraction does *not* exist. Both of these conclusions may be premature.

4. Extrapolation from short-term studies to conditions of multiple dosing. Again, both false positive and false negative results may occur. In some cases single-dose studies indicate that an interaction occurs, but the interaction is not seen with long-term use of the drugs. Conversely, single-dose studies may fail to reveal an interaction that takes several days or more to develop.

5. Failure to realize that more than one mechanism may be involved. Many interactions take place as a result of two or more mechanisms. Failure to realize this can result in inappropriate assessment of the likely time course of the interaction and selection of inappropriate methods to circumvent the interaction.

6. Failure to consider the effects of dose. Most drug interactions are dose related, with the magnitude of effect being greater at larger doses of one or both drugs. Accordingly, there is usually a threshold dose, below which no interaction occurs. For example, quinidine doses of below 400-500 mg/day have minimal effects on serum digoxin concentrations. Thus, one should carefully consider the effects of the dose when evaluating drug interaction information.

7. Inappropriate extrapolation of data from healthy subjects to the patient population. Studies in healthy subjects are invaluable in the investigation of drug interactions. However, diseases may predispose patients to, or protect patients from, the adverse effects of given drug interactions. Thus, studies in healthy subjects, in the absence of accompanying data from patients, may result in false negative or false positive results.

MONITORING FOR DRUG INTERACTIONS IN THE INSTITUTIONAL PHARMACY SETTING

The goals of drug interaction monitoring are threefold: first, one needs to identify the patients who are receiving drug combinations that can potentially interact; second, one needs to determine which of the patients receiving interacting drugs are likely to be at risk of developing adverse consequences from the interaction; and third, one needs to take action that will minimize the likelihood of adverse consequences.

Computers are absolutely essential to efficient monitoring of drug interactions in the institutional pharmacy setting. Computers, however, can handle only the first of the three goals of drug interaction monitoring, i.e., the identification of those patients receiving potentially interacting combinations. Computers contribute relatively little to the vital tasks of assessing the risk of adverse events in patients receiving interacting drugs and determining a course of action that will minimize the risk.

A number of design features should be considered when one is preparing or purchasing computerized drug interaction systems. For example, it is important to account for the fact that drug groups or classes may not interact in a homogeneous manner. The gastrointestinal absorption of both tetracycline and doxycycline is reduced by iron preparations. However, the metabolism of tetracycline is not affected by concurrent administration of enzyme inducers as is doxycycline. Thus, the computer program should not consider all tetracyclines as one homogenous interacting drug class. Also, combination products should be entered into the system so that each interacting component of the product can be considered. Furthermore, provisions should be made to avoid excessive duplicate interaction alerts for a given patient when a drug is reordered or when doses are changed. It is also necessary to program the system to account for route-dependent drug interactions such as those for which only the oral form of a drug interacts.

An important decision regarding the drug interaction data base concerns the number of interactions to be included. As mentioned previously, one cannot select 20 or 30 "important" drug interactions and expect to detect most of the clinically significant problems. Conversely, inclusion of over 200 drug interactions generally results in so many interaction alerts that they are soon ignored. The optimal number of interactions to be included will vary depending on the goals of the systems. However, in most cases, 100-150 interactions have proved to afford a reasonably complete system without an excessive number of interaction alerts. Choosing the specific interactions to be included is another difficult task and requires consideration of factors such as the severity, immediacy, and predictability of the interaction as well as local drug-use patterns. Furthermore, some interacting drug combinations occur so frequently that including them in the data base may result in an excessive number of alerts. In such cases, alternative methods of addressing the problem may be indicated, such as education of prescribers through newsletters or conferences.

Institutionalized patients may be at greater or lesser risk of the adverse effects of interactions than other patients, depending on the situation. Factors increasing the risk of adverse interactions in institutionalized patients include the generally increased number and severity of diseases and the correspondingly increased number and toxicity of medications to treat those diseases. On the other hand, some interactions such as those involving oral anticoagulants may be less likely to produce adverse effects in a hospitalized patient in whom the anticoagulant response is carefully monitored than in an outpatient who is not monitored as closely. As another example, enzyme inducers such as barbiturates appear less likely to interfere with the therapeutic effect of high-dose, short-term corticosteroids in a hospitalized patient than the carefully titrated long-term use of corticosteroids in an outpatient with a chronic disease such as rheumatoid arthritis, asthma, or systemic lupus erythematosus.

Because of the large volume of new information published on drug interactions, the data base should be updated at least twice each year. This would allow timely incorporation of new interactions as well as modification of interactions already present in the data base. Some computerized drug-interaction systems have been marketed with inadequate mechanisms for updating the data base; thus, one should ask specific questions regarding how often will the data be updated. One should also determine who will make the updates and whether they are qualified to do so. Finally, one should ask for the criteria that are used to select new interactions for inclusion in the system. This is an important consideration, because the uncritical addition of drug in-

teractions can transform a workable system into a monster that issues interaction alerts at the slightest provocation.

Another design decision for a drug interaction data base concerns whether or not to divide the interactions into categories or classes of importance. There are both advantages and disadvantages that attend such categorization of drug interactions. On the negative side it has been argued that placing interactions into categories of importance is somewhat arbitrary since the available information on most interactions is incomplete. Moreover, it is clear that a given interaction may cause a serious adverse effect in one patient with certain predisposing factors and have no effect in another patient who is not so predisposed. Thus, the use of categories inevitably results in some overestimation and underestimation of the clinical importance of interactions in specific patients. On the positive side, placing interactions into categories gives the user a rough initial estimate of the potential severity of the adverse effect. Furthermore, the disadvantages of using categories stated above can be largely overcome if the user is aware of these limitations and understands the importance of evaluating each case individually. It is the author's opinion that for a computer system, two categories are sufficient. One category should include interactions that are truly of major importance based on their severity, immediacy, and predictability. The other category can include all other interactions considered important enough to warrant inclusion in the system.

ASSESSING THE CLINICAL IMPORTANCE OF DRUG INTERACTIONS IN SPECIFIC PATIENTS

Once the pharmacist has been alerted to the fact that a patient is (or soon will be) receiving an interacting drug combination, two difficult questions remain: Is this patient at significant risk of developing adverse effects from the interactions? If yes, what can be done to minimize the risk? Experience has shown that most pharmacists and physicians cannot efficiently answer these questions with currently available tools. It is virtually impossible for health professionals to remember all of the conditions that may affect the risk or management of every drug interaction of potential clinical importance. Thus, we are experimenting with methods that may help pharmacists to rapidly assess the likelihood that an interaction will occur, and determine ways that the adverse effects of that interaction may be circumvented. One of the most promising devices is the decision table (2,3). The decision table is similar to a flow chart or algorithm but is more compact and allows one to see more clearly the relationship between various conditions and possible actions. Decision tables also eliminate the repetition of action recommendations, which are frequently necessary with the standard algorithm format.

Table 28.1 represents an example of a decision table for the interaction of β-adrenergic–blocking agents and epinephrine.

TABLE 28.1   Decision Table for β-Adrenergic Blockers and Epinephrine[a]

Once it has been determined that a patient is (or may soon be) receiving an interacting drug combination, two important questions need to be addressed. Is this patient potentially at risk of developing the adverse consequences of the interaction, and if so, what can be done to minimize the likelihood that these adverse effects will occur? For most interactions, many variables need to be addressed in order to answer these questions, a time-consuming process. In order to facilitate this decision making process, we have begun to use decision tables. The decision table is similar to an algorithm or flow chart, but is more compact and depicts more clearly the relationship between the various conditions and the possible actions. Further, decision tables eliminate the repetition of action recommendations which is often necessary with the standard algorithm format. To use the following decision table, begin with the "Conditions" portion of the table in the upper left-hand corner. The first condition is "Method of Epinephrine Administration." Read from left to right to locate the method of epinephrine administration (i.e. locally, inhalation, injection). If the epinephrine is to be administered "locally," read down to below the heavy horizontal line to the section entitled "Clinical Consequences or Action Required." In the box where an "X" appears, read back across to the far left-hand column (in this case, "A clinically important interaction is unlikely"). If the method of epinephrine administration is by "inhalation," return to the second Conditions box in the far left-hand column entitled "Type of beta blocker," then read to the right and choose the appropriate column, "non-selective" or "cardioselective." If the beta-blocker under consideration is "non-selective," two "Xs" appear in this column in the "Clinical Consequences or Action Required" section, both of which are applicable. Thus, by isolating the conditions which pertain to the specific patient situation, one is guided to the appropriate column with "Xs" to indicate which Clinical Consequence or Action Required statements apply. The footnotes allow explanation and additional information without excessively cluttering the decision table itself. It should be noted that drug interaction decision tables such as this are an aid to clinical judgement, not a substitute for it. Thus, they should be used only by those who can evaluate the applicability of the Clinical Consequences or Action Required statements to the specific patient in question.

BETA-ADRENERGIC BLOCKERS AND EPINEPHRINE

Non-selective beta-blockers inhibit the beta-stimulatory effect of epinephrine, leaving unopposed alpha stimulation which may result in hypertension. The bronchodilation produced by epinephrine may be inhibited by non-selective beta-blockers, and possibly also by large doses of cardioselective beta-blockers.

Conditions	Method of epinephrine administration	Locally	Inhalation		Injection (For systemic effects)		
	Type of beta-blocker (See footnote 2)		Non-selective	Cardio-selective	Non-selective		Cardioselective
	Indication for epinephrine use.				Anaphylaxis	Other	
Clinical Consequences or Action Required	A clinically important interaction is unlikely.	X_1					
	Epinephrine-induced bronchodilation may be inhibited. Consider changing to a cardioselective beta-blocker. (See footnote 2)		X_3				
	The patient's blood pressure may increase, especially if epinephrine doses are repeated. You should now monitor the patient's blood pressure.		X				
	Epinephrine-induced bronchodilation may be inhibited somewhat with large doses of the beta-blocker.			X			X
	The patient is likely to be resistant to favorable effects of epinephrine.				X_4		
	An acute hypertensive reaction may occur. Use conservative doses of epinephrine and monitor blood pressure carefully.					X	
	Hypertensive reactions to epinephrine do **not** appear likely with cardioselective beta-blockers.		X_5				X_5

1. Significant interaction is unlikely when epinephrine is being used for only local effect.

2. Cardioselective beta-blockers include atenolol (Tenormin), metoprolol (Lopressor), and acebutolol. Non-selective beta-blockers include alprenolol, nadolol (Corgard), oxprenolol, pindolol (Visken), propranolol (Inderal), sotalol, and timolol (Blocadren).

3. The bronchodilation of other beta-agonist sypathomimetics may also be inhibited.

4. In patients with anaphylaxis, who are receiving non-specific beta-blockers, the hypotension and bronchoconstriction may not respond adequately to epinephrine injections. Such patients may require vigorous supportive care, including careful attention to volume replacement.

5. Metoprolol (even when used in doses of 200-300 mg/day) appears to have minimal effect on the pressor response to epinephrine. It seems likely that other cardioselective beta-blockers would behave similarly, but little clinical information is available.

[a]Reprinted by permission from Hansten PD: Beta-adrenergic blockers and epinephrine. *Drug Interactions Newsletter* 3:41-44, 1983.

REFERENCES

1. Symposium Number 7: Clinical effects of interaction between drugs. *Proc R Soc Med* 58:943-998, 1965.
2. Holland RR: Decision tables: Their use of the presentation of clinical algorithms. *JAMA* 233:455-457, 1975.
3. Hansten PD: Utilization of drug information in pharmacy systems. In Fokkens O et al (eds): *Medinfo-83 Seminars*. Amsterdam, North Holland, 1983, pp 123-125.

ADDITIONAL READING

Hansten PD: *Drug Interactions,* ed 5. Philadelphia, Lea & Febiger, 1985.

Hansten PD (ed): *Drug Interactions Newsletter*. Spokane, Applied Therapeutics (monthly).

Hartshorn EA: *Drug Interactions Update*. Bethesda, Md, American Society of Hospital Pharmacists, 1983.

Mangini RJ (ed): *Drug Interaction Facts*. St Louis, Facts and Comparisons Inc. (Quarterly).

Rizack MA: *Medical Letter Handbook of Drug Interactions,* 1983. New Rochelle, NY, Medical Letter, 1983.

Stockley E: *Drug Interactions*. Oxford, Blackwell Scientific Publications, 1981.

CHAPTER 29

Utilization of Clinical Laboratory Data*

JACK M. ROSENBERG and INGO S. KAMPA

Laboratory tests are biochemical, chemical, or physical methods of measuring biologic or physiologic functions of the body. They are an important part of health care and have become indispensable for routine screening and the diagnosis of disease. Added to these roles is their value in managing patients. They are used routinely to assess compliance, monitor both the efficacy of prescribed treatment and the advent of adverse or toxic reactions, and, at times, to help determine the drug of choice.

Moreover, recent innovations confirm that the importance of laboratory procedures in health care is still growing. In diabetology, for example, patients may now monitor blood glucose levels at home and immediately contact the physician if therapeutic adjustments are necessary. Day-to-day glucose control is thus improved. In the laboratory, periodic assessment of a diabetic's glycosylated hemoglobin values—hemoglobin molecules to which glucose binds—reflects the patient's glucose status for the preceding few months and thus the quality of disease control.

As the same time, the proliferating numbers of tests and corresponding increases in costs mandate a conservative approach. Tests must be ordered appropriately and performed and interpreted correctly. Results of initial screening or diagnostic tests usually suggest the specific follow-up tests necessary for a definitive diagnosis.

THE PHARMACIST'S ROLE

All pharmacists, at least to a certain extent, are involved in monitoring patient care, and a growing number now have input into the management of patient therapy. Thus, all pharmacists should have an appreciation of why laboratory tests are used and of the information to be gained from them. Moreover, drugs may influence the results of laboratory tests in a variety of ways. Considering that the area of the pharmacist's unique expertise is drugs, some knowledge of their impact on testing results is a natural extension of the pharmacist's knowledge base.

By virtue of their pharmacologic and toxicologic properties, many drugs can alter body functions, which will be reflected on laboratory tests. When drugs are known to cause such effects, patients receiving any of these agents on a long-term basis must be monitored periodically to detect any altered functions.

For example, the mechanism of action of thiazide diuretics causes potassium to be excreted from the body. If exogenous supplementation is overlooked or inadequate in patients with normal renal function, symptoms of deficiency may appear. Monitoring potassium concentrations should therefore be routine whenever these agents are administered. The aminoglycosides provide an example of toxicologic effects; they are known to cause nephrotoxicity in some patients. Although a variety of factors have been suggested as influencing the appearance of this toxicity (e.g., age, gender, duration of therapy, dosage administered), none has been proved conclusively. Thus, predicting which patients are at greatest risk is not always possible. Patients receiving aminoglycosides therefore require periodic renal function studies to detect any diminished function. Similarly, the antiepileptic carbamazepine may depress bone marrow function in some patients; periodic blood counts are used to detect any significant decrease in blood cells and thus the need for alternate therapy. (Unfortunately, the advent of some serious drug effects cannot be predicted by monitoring; e.g., aplastic anemia that sometimes occurs in patients receiving chloramphenicol is not preceded by identifiable blood changes.)

Drugs and their metabolies may also interfere with some testing methods in vitro. One such example would be a drug that interferes with a reagent used in a particular test. The risk here is that therapy might be adjusted based on an incorrect result. The effect of penicillin, cephalosporins, tetracyclines, vitamin C, and other drugs on the copper reduction test for urinary glucose is a well-known example, as is the potential of phenothiazines to cause either false positive or false negative immunologic urine pregnancy test results.

Because pharmacists have a fuller appreciation of the actions of medications, they are in a good position to anticipate and advise on such interactions. The number of drugs potentially capable of affecting laboratory tests both in vivo and in vitro is too enormous to list in this chapter. Both the package insert and a competent reference source

---

*Portions of this chapter are adapted from Rosenberg JM, Kampa IS: Common laboratory data, Part I. *Wellcome Trends in Hospital Pharmacy*, vol 5, No. 9 (July), 1983; and Kampa IS, Rosenberg JM: Common laboratory data, Part II. *Wellcome Trends in Hospital Pharmacy*, vol 5, No. 10 (August), 1983. By permission of Park Row Publishers, New York, and Burroughs Wellcome Co., Research Triangle Park, NC.

(such as Hansten's *Drug Interactions* or the United States Pharmacopeia's *Drug Information for the Health-Care Provider*) will be of use in identifying a particular drug's effect on laboratory test results.

In selected settings, pharmacists may be asked to suggest therapeutic alternatives if the results of laboratory assays indicate some impairment of the functional capacity of the organs of elimination and metabolism. For instance, a physician may wish to avoid a drug that is excreted largely unchanged or as an active metabolite by the kidneys in a patient with compromised renal function and may ask the pharmacist's help in selecting a therapeutic equivalent that is metabolized in the liver. If no such alternative exists, the appropriate dosage reduction or dosing-interval extension, or both, of the renally excreted drug may be mathematically determined.

A knowledge of laboratory data is important for another reason: laboratory testing has become so much a part of the fabric of health care that a basic understanding of it has become essential for comprehending and evaluating the literature and prescribing information. Added to these clinical considerations is a practical one: any pharmacist who lacks such an appreciation will be at a disadvantage in discussions with other health care professionals and unable to maintain a coequal relationship.

GENERAL PRINCIPLES

Laboratory evaluations are employed for a variety of reasons. Screening tests are done routinely when patients are admitted to the hospital or during a yearly physical examination to detect any problems that may not be clinically apparent or to confirm a suspicion of underlying disease. Additionally, tests may be used in screening large numbers of people for a particular disease, for instance, the use of urine glucose testing during a mass program to detect diabetes. (Any patients with positive urinalysis test results would then undergo a 2-hour postprandial glucose assay or a glucose tolerance test, or both, to confirm the presence of diabetes.) A physician who suspects renal dysfunction could confirm its presence from the results of the BUN and serum creatinine levels or by determining the creatinine clearance.

Aside from their screening or diagnostic role, laboratory evaluations are frequently used in managing or monitoring the course of an illness or treatment of a particular disease. The daily use of urine glucose testing by insulin-dependent diabetics and the periodic monitoring of blood glucose by the physician are well-known examples. Similarly, patients receiving oral anticoagulants require routine determinations of prothrombin time. As has been shown, the onset of a variety of toxic and adverse reactions can be determined by laboratory testing.

Therapeutic drug monitoring, the measurement of drug concentrations in the serum or plasma, is now used routinely to individualize the dosage of certain agents. Many drugs that can cause serious or even life-threatening side effects are now known to exhibit relatively narrow therapeutic ranges. That is, serum levels maintained within a fairly narrow range (that varies from drug to drug) will produce optimal therapeutic drug benefits with little risk of toxicity. Levels below this range will not provide optimal disease control, whereas levels above the therapeutic range heighten the risk of toxic side effects. Further complicating therapy with these drugs is the fact that the serum concentration that results from a dose cannot be predicted accurately. Measuring steady-state concentrations of the drug thus helps establish the optimal dose for a particular patient and allows the clinician to maintain each patient's serum concentrations within an efficacious range. Moreover, toxic reactions with some of these agents (e.g., phenytoin and digoxin) may mimic a recurrence of the underlying disease; in these cases, differentiating the cause of symptoms can be difficult. Here, assaying the serum drug concentrations will provide the clinician with objective data on which to base therapeutic decisions.

LABORATORY PROCEDURES

Laboratory tests are generally conducted on biologic fluids—usually serum, plasma, whole blood, and urine. Other fluids such as cerebrospinal fluid and synovial fluid may also be used in today's clinical laboratory. Procedures for the nearly 800 tests in use in the clinical laboratory include enzymatic assays, colorimetric procedures, flame emission and absorption techniques, specific ion electrodes, radioimmunoassays, radioassays, enzyme immunoassays, fluorescent immunoassays, nephelometric determinations, high-pressure liquid chromatography, and electrophoretic techniques. The variety of techniques and the vast number of analytes assayed results in a variety of ways to express data. It is therefore important to examine both the numerical answers and the units in which the results are expressed when laboratory data are analyzed and compared. The pharmacist should become familiar with the normal values and how they relate to the results of an individual's laboratory test. The normal ranges supplied by the laboratory are specific for the methods used and the analytical units in which they are expressed.

Laboratory tests can be performed individually or in groups. Test groups usually refer to a battery of tests for a specific organ or disease evaluation. For example, a thyroid test group usually includes a tetraiiodothyronine (T_4), thyroid-stimulating hormone (TSH), and a triiodothyronine uptake (T_3U) essay. All three test procedures are related, and this relationship determines the thyroid status of the patient. There are also large screening procedures or profiles that are routinely performed on patients or are part of annual physical checkups. These screening procedures have often adopted the name of the instrument by which they are performed. Thus, a SMAC profile is a set of up to 40 different tests performed on a sequential multi-analysis computerized (SMAC) instrument. Others are the SMA-12, SMA-6, and SMA-18 profiles performed on a Technicon sequential multi-channel analyzer (SMA). However, in recent years, there has been a move away from the multi-test profiles in favor of the more specific organ-related or disease-related profiles. The use of laboratory computers now makes it possible to assemble tests from many instruments for grouping into many varieties of specific profiles.

INTERPRETING RESULTS

Results of biochemical profiling must be placed in clinical perspective. Normal ranges are usually based on the statistical concept of random or normal distribution. The mean value of the analyte $\pm$ 2SD is considered the normal range and includes 95% of a population. Since, by design, 5% of a clinical laboratory's results will fall outside the normal range, abnormal findings may be artifactual. Further testing is therefore necessary to confirm or exclude underlying disease when results are abnormal. In this respect, it should be remembered that underlying organ-system disease is often reflected by a pattern of abnormal tests. For example, when renal impairment exists, the BUN and creatinine levels should both be elevated. The elevation of a single value in such cases is suspicious. Such results must be verified by repeat or confirmatory testing or, in some cases, by the patient's history.

A variety of factors, including gender, age, time since last meal, specific foods ingested, timing of the sample, and even some diagnostic and therapeutic procedures, may also affect test results. Concentrations of substances in the body are dynamic, and significant diurnal variations are often the case. (Overnight fasting with blood drawn early in the morning attempts to normalize these variations.) For example, if a person undergoing a triglyceride determination has fasted only 6 hours instead of the recommended 10-12 hours, the results are likely to be affected. Certain parameters are more responsive to diurnal variation and food intake than others. Creatinine levels seldom vary no matter when the sample is drawn, whereas a random glucose concentration may vary considerably depending on the subject's diet, amount of exercise, and even the degree of stress.

Individual differences among patients (e.g., age, gender, race, diet) may also affect the interpretation of test results. The so-called normal ranges for analytes are often determined from specimens obtained from young, healthy individuals. When, for example, test data from elderly patients—who have altered metabolic and excretory functions—are compared to normal ranges, differences can be observed that are not related to the presence of disease. Often the normal ranges of analytes in children also vary substantially from those of adults for many components.

The patient's diet can affect many values. Eating a high-protein diet elevates BUN and uric acid levels, for instance; laboratories that serve affluent communities may adapt to this variance by altering the upper limit of normal on the BUN and uric acid determinations. As with drugs, some foods may interfere directly with laboratory tests. For example, foods containing high amounts of serotonin can elevate 5-hydroxyindolacetic acid.

Diagnostic and therapeutic procedures sometimes alter concentrations of a substance—a digital prostate examination, for instance, may raise serum acid phosphatase levels; intramuscular injections may damage cells, causing potassium, lactic dehydrogenase (LDH), creatinine phosphokinase (CK), and glutamic oxaloacetic transaminase (SGOT) to be released into the bloodstream. Just as abnormal results may be erroneous, normal results must occasionally be viewed with suspicion. A "normal" serum calcium value in a patient with documented hypoalbuminemia should be a matter of concern, for example, because calcium binds primarily to albumin. The "normal" value in this case actually suggests excessive levels of ionized calcium.

Improper storage or transport of samples may also yield spurious results. For example, the hemolysis of a whole blood sample that has been allowed to stand renders the sample useless for assaying glucose and LDH, among other analytes. Improper collection of the specimen may also negate the results. This is usually seen in a 24 hr urine specimen, where not all samples have been saved. Technical errors by laboratory personnel, especially in transcribing results, are a frequent source of erroneous findings. Even the assay itself may be at fault occasionally, usually because reagents are outdated or have been stored or prepared improperly. In this respect, it is prudent to note that laboratory results are only as good as the laboratory that furnishes them. Occasional errors are always possible of course, but it should be remembered that the competence of clinical laboratories can vary greatly. Then, too, some tests such as hormonal assays may be difficult to perform even with high-skilled personnel.

CLINICAL RELEVANCE

The clinical value of a test is related to its specificity and sensitivity. The degree of a test's sensitivity is assessed by the percentage of positive results it yields in patients who have a specific disorder. For example, assays for phenylketonuria are highly sensitive; virtually all patients with this genetic metabolic error yield positive results. Unfortunately, the sensitivity of some assays improves only as the underlying disease progresses: early in the disease process the physiologic aberrations are apparently not pronounced enough to measure. For example, about 72% of patients with advanced colon cancer will have a positive result on the carcinoembryonic antigen (CEA) test versus only about 20% of those who are in the early stages of the disease.

As assay's specificity is determined by the percentage of negative results normal patients achieve. Assays for phenylketonuria are highly specific as well as sensitive, since over 99% of normal individuals will yield a negative result. The CEA assay is variably specific; about 3% of nonsmoking individuals will have a false positive result, whereas 20% of normal smokers will have a false positive finding. As a general rule, routine evaluations are extremely sensitive but relatively nonspecific. That is, they readily demonstrate altered concentrations of a particular substance or substances, thus suggesting some impairment, but they do not identify the specific disorder. The concepts of sensitivity and specificity are sometimes combined and expressed as the efficiency ratio of a particular test. For example, LDH is elevated in hepatic dysfunction and after a myocardial infarction. Although LDH assays are 100% sensitive, their efficiency actually falls in the lower 70% range because they do not distinguish the underlying cause of the elevation. (Indeed, even when liver disease is strongly suspected, the specific hepatic dysfunction remains to be determined.) LDH isoenzymes are used to establish the underlying disorder.

BIOCHEMICAL PROFILING

A discussion of the hundreds of laboratory tests now performed is beyond the scope of this chapter. We will concentrate on those evaluations that are routinely performed on blood and urine. The analyte is given followed by its normal range and the common method of determination.

Glucose (70-100 mg/dl—Hexokinase)

Glucose is an important energy source for all tissue cells. Some tissues, such as the brain and spinal cord, depend entirely on glucose as their source of energy. Blood glucose is a continuous variable. It is elevated following the ingestion of carbohydrates. This elevation is reduced to a normal level by the removal of glucose from the blood by various tissues (e.g., hepatic, adipose, muscle) for both immediate energy use and storage. When the blood glucose level falls between meals, it is supplemented by the release of glucose stored in tissue (hepatic glycogen). Additionally, glucose is produced in tissues such as the liver by a process called gluconeogenesis. All of these processes are controlled by a variety of hormones, the principal ones being insulin and glucagon. Malfunctions of these hormone systems result in an abnormal increase or decrease of blood glucose.

Hyperglycemia. Diabetes mellitus is the most common cause of hyperglycemia. It results from either a decrease in the insulin that is available or a reduction of insulin's ability to function properly in the removal of glucose from the blood. Besides an elevated blood glucose, its common biochemical abnormalities are an increased 2-hour postprandial glucose concentration and an abnormal diabetic glucose tolerance curve. (In the glucose tolerance test, glucose is administered, usually orally, and blood glucose levels, obtained over a period of 3-5 hours, determine the curve.) Other, less frequent causes of hyperglycemia are Cushing's syndrome (hyperplasia of the adrenal cortex, which results in large increases in glucocorticoid release caused by hypersensitivity to carbohydrates or amino acids such as leucine. It may also result from insulinoma (islet cell adenoma of the pancreas). Diabetics may be at risk for hypoglycemia, usually because exogenous administration of the hormone is excessive, because they have missed a meal (thus reducing carbohydrate intake), or because their insulin requirements have changed.

Blood Urea Nitrogen (7-22 mg/dl—Enzymatic)

BUN, although a misnomer, is taken to mean serum urea. Urea is produced by the liver from ammonia that is derived from the deamination of amino acids. Because urea is reabsorbed and then excreted by the kidneys, BUN concentrations are indicative of renal function; elevated BUN levels are seen in many types of kidney disease. The BUN concentration may be toxic, a condition called uremia.

Elevated BUN concentrations may also be seen in such conditions as congestive heart failure, where reductions in the circulating blood volume cause decreased renal perfusion. High-protein diets and disease-related destruction of cellular proteins will also increase BUN levels.

Low BUN levels are normally seen in individuals who have a negative nitrogen balance, i.e., during periods of growth, pregnancy, and starvation.

Creatinine (0.8-1.3 mg/dl in Males; 0.6-1.0 mg/dl in Females—Jaffé)

Intramuscular creatine phosphate is a high-energy compound stored in skeletal muscles and other tissues. It is converted to its catabolic end product, creatinine, in the muscles. Creatinine is then released into the bloodstream and excreted by the kidneys, primarily through glomerular filtration. The amount of creatinine produced during a 24-hour period is stable and does not depend on protein or water intake or urine production, all factors that can modify other renal function tests. Increased blood creatinine levels thus indicate impaired renal function. Low creatinine levels have no clinical significance.

The creatinine clearence (125 ml/min in males; 110 ml/min in females) is often obtained to determine the glomerular fitration rate and thus the degree of kidney dysfunction. It is calculated by comparing the serum creatinine concentrations obtained over a given time with the amount of creatinine excreted in the urine during that period.

Uric Acid (3.0-7.1 mg/dl in Males; 2.6-5.6 mg/dl in Females—Uricase)

Nucleic acid catabolism results in the breakdown of purine to uric acid, which is excreted by the kidneys. Uric acid is usually assayed to confirm a diagnosis of gout, an inherited disorder characterized by high serum uric acid concentrations and the deposition of urate crystals around the joints. Elevated uric acid levels also occur in kidney disease because of the impaired excretion. Despite this, uric acid concentrations do not provide an accurate index of kidney function.

Acidotic metabolic states promote reabsorption of uric acid by the kidneys, thus increasing serum concentrations. Additionally, diseases characterized by marked cellular destruction—certain types of cancer, pneumonia, and the toxemias of pregnancy—also increase uric acid levels.

Low uric acid levels are not indicative of disease. They may result from a benign genetic disorder, xanthine oxidase deficiency, in which uric acid synthesis is impaired. Aggressive treatment for gout may also decrease uric acid concentrations.

Bilirubin (1.5 mg/dl Total, 0.4 mg/dl Direct—PNB)

Bilirubin is a waste product produced from the breakdown of hemoglobin. This occurs primarily in the spleen where red cells are destroyed. Unconjugated bilirubin is then transported via the bloodstream to the liver, where it is conjugated with glucuronic acid and excreted in the bile. The conjugated bilirubin is known as direct bilirubin, whereas total bilirubin refers to the sum of the unconjugated and conjugated forms.

Either accelerated destruction of red cells or decreased excretion of bilirubin via the bile, or both, can result in increased total bilirubin concentrations. Obstruction at any point in the bile duct may cause reabsorption of conjugated bilirubin into the bloodstream, increased direct and total bilirubin levels, and jaundice. The inflammatory response that accompanies such diseases as acute viral hepatitis may contribute to the obstruction of bile canals, thus also increasing concentrations of direct and total bilirubin.

Jaundice may also result from disease-induced destruction of hepatic cells; the hepatocellular destruction reduces the liver's capacity to convert unconjugated to conjugated bilirubin, thus imparing excretion and increasing total bilirubin concentrations. Similarly, the cellular necrosis and scarring that accompany cirrhosis of the liver reduce the number of functioning hepatic cells, which impedes conjugation and increases total bilirubin levels.

Cholesterol (120-130 mg/dl, 0-19 Years; 120-240 mg/dl, 20-29 Years; 140-270 mg/dl, 30-39 Years; 150-310 mg/dl, 40-49 Years; 160-330 mg/dl, 50-59 Years—Enzymatic)

Although blood cholesterol concentrations may be altered in a variety of disease states, the major reason for assaying this lipid lies in its presumed relationship to atherosclerosis. High cholesterol levels correlate positively with coronary heart disease. In addition to total cholesterol, high-density lipoprotein cholesterol (HDA-cholesterol) and low-density lipoprotein cholesterol (LDL-cholesterol) are also measured. High levels of HDL-cholesterol are thought to be beneficial, whereas high levels of LDL-cholesterol are thought to increase the risk of atherosclerosis.

High serum cholesterol concentrations may also be seen in chronic liver disease, kidney disease, diabetes mellitus, and hypothyroidism. Low levels of the lipid are observed during starvation and hyperthyroidism.

Electrolytes

Depending on their migration in an electrical field, electrolytes are classified as either anions or cations. Proper electrolyte balance is critical for sustaining life, since this balance affects nearly all metabolic processes. Electrolytes maintain osmotic pressure and proper pH, participate in enzyme reactions, and regulate the proper functions of heart and skeletal muscle.

Sodium (135-145 mmol/L, Ion-Specific Electrode)

Sodium, the most plentiful electrolyte, is maintained in high concentrations in the extracellular fluid and in low concentrations intracellularly. (Potassium concentrations are a mirror image—high intracellular and low extracellular concentrations.) The cell membrane contributes to maintaining this homeostasis by preventing the exchange of sodium and potassium. In normal individuals, the kidney maintains the correct sodium concentration by excreting excessive amounts consumed. In the unlikely event of insufficient exogenous sodium, the kidney conserves body sodium by reducing the amount excreted.

Hypernatremia. Excessive sodium concentrations may result if the body's water stores are depleted, since the kidney's ability to concentrate urine in the presence of depleted water stores is limited. Insensible water losses through the

lungs, skin, and stool aggravate the condition. Should water starvation continue, the kidneys' compensatory ability to increase sodium excretion proportionately may be overwhelmed, resulting in hypernatremia. Mineralocorticoids may increase serum sodium concentrations by promoting sodium retention by the kidney. In certain diseases of the adrenal gland, most commonly adrenal tumors, excessive mineralocorticoid production occurs and serum sodium increases.

Characterized by low or absent levels of antidiuretic hormone (ADH), diabetes insipidus causes large water losses, resulting in hypernatremia.

Hyponatremia. Decreased serum sodium levels do not always reflect body stores of the cation. In dilutional hyponatremia, the extracellular fluid has expanded with no concomitant increase in sodium; thus, patients are edematous. Dilutional hyponatremia is seen in cirrhosis, congestive heart failure, and nephrosis and may also be caused by aggressive administration of osmotically active solutes (e.g., albumin).

Hyponatremia that reflects a concomitant decrease in body stores can result from aggressive diuresis, sweating that is followed by replacement of water but not salt, and gastrointestinal losses. Diabetic ketoacidosis, for instance, causes hyponatremia secondary to nausea and vomiting. Other causes are sodium-wasting renal disease and Addison's disease (in which the loss of adrenal hormones, including aldosterone, causes large losses of urinary sodium) and inappropriate secretion of ADH (in which the physiologic stimuli to cease ADH production go awry).

Potassium (3.5-4.5 mmol/L—Ion-Specific Electrode)

The most abundant of the intracellular cations, potassium is contained primarily within muscle tissue. Because potassium is measured in the extracellular fluid, its values are only a small fraction of the sodium values. These concentrations are critical, however, because potassium controls the excitability of nerve and muscle fibers, including those of the heart.

Hyperkalemia. Excessive potassium blood levels can reduce the excitability of nerve and muscle fibers. Concentrations in the serum may become elevated in the later stages of renal disease and may result in complete renal shutdown. Any trauma that causes cellular damage also elevates serum potassium levels, as the damaged cells spill potassium into the extracellular fluid; hemolytic anemia causes hyperkalemia in this fashion, as do burns and crush injuries. Overuse of potassium supplements may also increase serum levels.

By causing sodium depletion, Addison's disease correspondingly increases blood levels of potassium, despite the fact that large amounts are being excreted renally. (Insulin treatment reverses this action, but potassium replacement is necessary.)

Hypokalemia. Blood concentrations of potassium that are below the optimal range tend to increase the excitability of nerve and muscle fibers. Dietary potassium deficiency is infrequent. Prolonged gastrointestinal losses through vomiting and diarrhea are a common cause of hypokalemia, as is long-term self-medication with laxatives. Diuretic therapy may also promote hypokalemia, and periodic monitoring of potassium levels should be performed. Less frequent causes of reduced serum potassium include Cushing's syndrome, in which excessive adrenal hormones are produced, and tumor of the adrenal gland (Conn's tumor).

Carbon Dioxide (22-32 mmol/L—CO₂ Electrode)

Sometimes called bicarbonate, CO_2 is the body's primary mechanism for eliminating acid, vast quantities of which are generated during energy production. Thus, CO_2 contributes to maintaining pH within normal limits. Although the CO_2 concentration in the blood may be the first clinical suggestion of a dysfunction in the acid-base balance, full appreciation of the acid-base status of an individual requires other information—plasma pH, buffering capacity, hemoglobin concentrations, P_{O_2}, and P_{CO_2}. Moreover, because acid-base balance must remain within a fairly narrow range to sustain life, the body maintains this balance at all costs. Thus, an abnormal CO_2, even as the first diagnostic clue, suggests a long-standing defect, and serious damage may have already occurred.

Decreased CO₂. During hyperventilation, increased amounts of CO_2 are lost, resulting in decreased blood levels and increased pH. The underlying etiology is overstimulation of the part of the brain that controls breathing; anxiety and toxic substances can provoke hyperventilation. In the metabolic acidosis of diabetic coma, both CO_2 and pH are decreased. The rapid metabolism of fatty acids overwhelms the body's ability to excrete them by normal mechanisms, resulting in concentrations of acid in the plasma. In shock, another form of metabolic acidosis, glucose is not completely metabolized because of the oxygen deficit; this results in excessive lactic acid levels.

Increased CO₂. Respiratory acidosis, which is accompanied by decreased pH values, results from lung diseases that impair CO_2 excretion. In metabolic alkalosis, which can result from loss of the stomach's acid contents, both pH and CO_2 are elevated. Such loss can occur through prolonged vomiting, excessive self-medication with sodium bicarbonate, overzealous gastric suction, or vigorous diuretic use (when potassium and chloride are not adequately replaced).

Chloride (97-108 mmol/L—Coulometric)

Like sodium, chloride is maintained predominantly within the extracellular fluid, and it is thought to maintain the electrical neutrality of the blood.

Hyperchloremia. Excessive elevations of chloride can be seen in metabolic acidosis, kidney dysfunction, Cushing's disease, and hyperventilation.

Hypochloremia. Diabetic ketoacidosis, massive diuresis, and excessive gastrointestinal losses through prolonged vomiting or diarrhea deplete blood stores of chloride. Hypoventilation, heat exhaustion, and Addison's disease also promote excessive chloride excretion.

Blood Proteins

Total proteins can be divided into albumin and globulin fractions. These can be further divided into many fractions by electrophoresis. The specific proteins in the various fractions can be identified and quantitated by various chemical and immunochemical means.

Albumin (3.8-4.8 gm/dl—BCG)

The most plentiful blood protein, albumin comprises from 52-68% of total protein. It contributes nearly 80% of the serum colloid osmotic pressure. Severe deficiencies decrease osmotic pressure and may cause edema and transudation. Decreased levels may result from chronic liver or kidney disease. Malnutrition and malabsorption may also reduce albumin concentrations. (Many substances, including some drugs, are carried in the bloodstream bound primarily to albumin. Since the unbound portion of a drug is responsible for its pharmacologic activity, fewer binding sites in the bloodstream could result in excessive free levels.) Increased albumin levels, which are seen in dehydration and hemoconcentration, are not clinically significant.

Globulins (1.5-3.8 gm/dl—Electrophoresis)

Globulins consist of α_1, α_2, β, and γ fractions. Decreases in globulin concentrations occur through the same mechanisms that cause albumin deficits. Chronic infection or rheumatoid arthritis raises immunoglobulin levels. Discrete patterns that identify the underlying etiology can be discerned by electrophoresis. Spiking of one or several of the immunoglobulins in the γ group suggests a diagnosis of multiple myeloma, a fatal malignancy. Any abnormalities of the γ-globulin fraction require further laboratory studies, such as the quantitation of the immunoglobulins (IgA, IgM, IgG) as well as other specific proteins. Decreased globulin concentrations can result from tumor of the thymus, impaired hepatic production, or genetic defects.

Calcium (8.7-10.2 mg/dl—o-Cresolphthalein Complex)

Only about 1% of total body calcium circulates in the bloodstream; the balance is contained in the bones and teeth. Of this 1%, the unbound portion, or ionized calcium, is thought to be more important physiologically. It is usually not measured directly, but estimations are made based on the amount present in the serum and from the pH of the blood. Calcium is important in transmission of nerve impulses, in maintaining normal contractility of muscles, as a cofactor in certain enzyme reactions, and in coagulation of the blood.

Hypercalcemia. To maintain calcium homeostasis in the bloodstream, parathyroid hormone regulates release and uptake of calcium by bone. Thus, uncontrolled, exaggerated release of parathyroid hormone—seen in tumors of the parathyroid gland—causes excessive bone losses of calcium and corresponding elevations in the serum levels. Hypercalcemia also occurs in Paget's disease, in various cancers that have metastasized to bone, and in multiple myeloma. Elevated serum calcium levels may arise secondary to the use of thiazide diuretics and also accompany some respiratory diseases because of altered CO_2 tension concentrations.

Hypocalcemia. Vitamin D deficiency is probably the most common cause of hypocalcemia, but it also occurs in malabsorptive states, kidney disease, with overuse of over-the-counter aluminum antacids, and in hypoparathyroidism.

Phosphorus (2.5-4.9 mg/dl—PMAPS)

Normally, serum phosphorus concentrations are inversely related to the calcium levels. Because of this relationship, phosphorus is usually elevated in those diseases that cause hypocalcemia and decreased in those conditions that cause hypercalcemia.

Hyperphosphatemia. Commonly seen in renal insufficiency, hyperphosphatemia also accompanies hypervitaminosis D and hypoparathyroidism. Serum phosphorus elevations are also seen occasionally in hyperthyroidism. Blood concentrations of phosphorus are higher during periods of growth; thus, children normally have higher levels than adults.

Hypophosphatemia. In certain malabsorptive syndromes, the intestine is unable to absorb either calcium or phosphorus, with the result that serum concentrations of both are lowered.

Enzymes

The amounts of enzymes present in the blood depends on a variety of factors, such as the rate of enzyme secretion, catabolism, altered enzyme synthesis, and tissue injury. When the latter occurs, enzymes found in the tissue cells are released, and large increases are seen in the bloodstream. Since cells contain more than one enzyme, certain patterns of enzyme elevation are seen in tissue injuries.

Alkaline Phosphatase (50-136 IU/L—p-NPP)

Alkaline phosphatase, which catalyzes the hydrolysis of organic phosphate monoesters, is present in osteoblasts, liver, kidney, intestinal lining, and placenta. Increased levels are clinically significant and may be seen in bone fractures and such bone diseases as hyperparathyroidism, osteomalacia, primary and secondary bone tumors, and Paget's disease. Any space-occupying hepatic lesion will elevate alkaline phosphatase levels; elevated concentrations may also be an early sign of bile-duct obstruction. Obstructive jaundice also elevates serum levels of the enzyme. Alkaline phosphatase is normally elevated during periods of growth and pregnancy. The actual source of an elevated alkaline phosphatase concentration can be identified by alkaline phosphatase isoenzyme determinations.

Lactic Dehydrogenase (100-190 IU/L—UV 340 nm)

LDH, which catalyzes lactic and pyruvic acids, is present in most body tissues. Increased blood concentrations of LDH are seen following myocardial infarction, all types of liver disease, skeletal muscle disease, and hemolytic anemia. Screening tests for LDH are sensitive but not specific; differing patterns of its five isoenzyme fractions allow identification of the physiologic source. For example, LDH isoenzyme 1 is increased following myocardial infarction,

whereas LDH isoenzyme 5 is increased in hepatic disease. Some caution must be exercised in evaluating increased LDH isoenzyme 1, however, since any condition that causes red cell destruction, including hemolytic anemia and accidental hemolysis, will also elevate the isoenzyme.

Glutamic Oxaloacetic Transaminase (25-41 IU/L— UV 340 nm)

Although a determination of serum glutamic oxaloacetic transaminase (SGOT) is ordered commonly, the correct name of this enzyme is aspartate aminotransferase (AST). It catalyzes the formation of glutamic acid and is found in the liver, heart, kidney, pancreas, and skeletal muscle. Determinations of AST are commonly used to monitor patients exposed to potentially hepatotoxic drugs. AST is elevated in infectious hepatitis, toxic hepatitis, infectious mononucleosis, cirrhosis of the liver, hepatic cancer, after myocardial infarction, in skeletal diseases, and in kidney diseases. Isoenzyme determinations are not yet clinically practical.

Glutamic Pyruvic Transaminase (3-36 IU/L—UV 340 nm)

Again, a determination of serum glutamic pyruvic transaminase (SGPT) is often ordered, but the enzyme's correct name is alanine aminotransferase (ALT). It is found in high concentrations in the liver, and thus, elevations are useful for diagnosing hepatic disorders. Excessive levels are seen in infectious hepatitis, obstructive jaundice, and cirrhosis. ALT may also be elevated in myocardial infarction, although it is seldom used diagnostically for this purpose. It can also be used to monitor patients who have been exposed to potentially hepatotoxic drugs.

Gamma Glutamyl Transferase (5-55 IU/L in Females; 15-85 IU/L in Males—γ-GPNA-HCl)

Assays of this enzyme, which is believed to assist amino acid transport through the cell, have largely replaced SGPT determinations. γ-Glutamyl transferase (GGT) is found in large amounts in the liver; it is a very sensitive indicator of obstructive liver disease and is sometimes used in screening programs for cirrhosis. Pancreatic disease occasionally causes serum GGT levels to rise.

Creatinine Phosphokinase (21-215 IU/L in Females; 35-232 IU/L in Males—UV 340 nm)

A catalyst in energy production, CK is distributed in muscle tissue throughout the body. Thus, elevations are seen in any muscle disease—myocardial infarction, muscular dystrophy, etc. Traumatic muscle damage—including intramuscular injections of such irritating drugs as chlorpromazine, digoxin, and the cephalosporins—also increases blood CK concentrations. There are three isoenzymes of CK, designated MM, MB, and BB. The normally occurring isoenzyme is MM. When cardiac damage occurs, CK-MB is released into the bloodstream. This isoenzyme is specific for cardiac muscle; hence, its presence confirms myocardial infarction.

HEMATOLOGY

The most common hematologic laboratory procedure is the complete blood count (CBC). The cellular components of blood consist of red blood cells (RBCs), white blood cells (WBCs), and platelets. Hemoglobin (the substance that carries oxygen) is contained within the red cells.

Red Blood Cells (4,000,000-5,400,000/mm³ in Females; 4,400,000-6,300,000/mm³ in Males)

The number of RBCs indicates the hemoglobin and thus the oxygen-carrying capacity of the blood. Anemia can be caused by a reduction in the number of red cells, reduced size of the red cells, or a reduction in the amount of hemoglobin contained within the red cells. A reduced number of red cells indicates anemia and/or loss of blood due to bleeding.

Increased numbers of red cells indicate that the patient may be suffering from polycythemia vera.

Hemoglobin (12-16 gm/dl in Females; 14-18 gm/dl in Males)

Hemoglobin (Hgb) is a heme-protein contained within the red cell, the main function of which is the transport of molecular oxygen to tissue cells. Reduced quantities of hemoglobin indicate anemia. Hgb can be reduced because of a decreased quantity in the red cells, often caused by iron deficiency or other factors that interfere with its synthesis or because of a decreased number of actual red cells.

Hematocrit (35-40% in Females; 42-52% in Males)

The hematocrit (HCT) is the actual volume of the red cells in a unit volume expressed as the percent. If a column of 10 cm of blood is centrifuged, the liquid portion of the blood (the plasma) is separated from the cells. If the red cells occupy 5-cm of the 10-cm tube, the hematocrit is 50%. A low HCT indicates either a reduced number or size of red cells or increased plasma volume. Anemia caused by a reduction in the number of RBCs or periods of bleeding results in decreased hematocrit.

Red Blood Cell Indices

The blood indices are the mathematical calculations derived from the RBC, hemoglobin, and hematocrit results.

Mean Corpuscular Volume (80-99 μ³)

The mean corpuscular volume (MCV) indicates the average size of the red cell. Some forms of anemia are distinguished based upon the size (volume) of red cells. Anemias caused by chronic blood loss are usually normocytic, whereas iron-deficiency anemia is microcytic and pernicious. (Anemias that do not affect red cell volume also exist, e.g., decreased hemoglobin.)

Mean Corpuscular Hemoglobin (27-34 pg)

Mean corpuscular hemoglobin (MCH) indicates the mean amount of hemoglobin contained within a red cell. Various anemias are associated with a reduction in hemoglobin (hypochromic) in the red cell. Increased hemoglobin in red cells (hyperchromic) is also encountered. Both are detected by the MCH.

Mean Corpuscular Hemoglobin Concentration (29-34%)

The mean corpuscular hemoglobin concentration (MCHC) is similar to MCH, except that it expresses the hemoglobin content of the red cell as a percentage of the overall red cell volume.

Platelets (150,000-400,000/mm³)

The amount of platelets indicates the ability of the blood to clot. Reduced amounts (150,000/mm³) increase the danger of internal bleeding or inhibit the activity of blood to clot following a traumatic injury. Increased amounts (often >1,000,000/mm³) are seen following splenectomy.

Erythrocyte Sedimentation Rate (10-20 mm/hr)

The erythrocyte sedimentation rate (ESR) is a measure of the separation of cells from the plasma over a 1-hour period. It is a nonspecific indicator of most inflammatory processes.

White Blood Cells (5,000-10,000/mm³)

WBCs consist of many varieties of cells that are identified by the differential count. Increased WBCs are usually an indicator of infection. The specific type of WBC that is increased can identify the class of pathogen (bacterial versus viral) or indicate other, usually serious, diseases (e.g., leukemia).

A reduced number of white cells indicates an individuals' impaired immunologic response to infection or other diseases. This is often seen following radiation therapy or chemotherapeutic cancer treatments and in transplant patients receiving immunosuppressive drugs.

Differential Count

The differential count demonstrates the percentages of the various white cells on a blood smear. Usually 100-200 cells are counted.

Neutrophils (60-70%). An increase in these cells is usually seen in response to bacterial infection. There are a variety of neutrophils; one can see a gradation of young, unsegmented (band) cells to older, highly segmented neutrophils. During the initial early stages of infections, the number of unsegmented neutrophils increases. This is known as a shift to the left, whereas the presence of highly segmented neutrophils is known as a shift to the right. The latter condition is rarely seen.

Lymphocytes (20-30%). Increased numbers of lymphocytes are usually seen during viral disorders. In various lymphocytic leukemias, very early lymphocytes (lymphoblasts) are seen, and the overall percentage of lymphocytes in these patients can rise above 90%.

Eosinophils (0-7%). This type of neutrophil contains red-staining granules. Eosinophils are usually elevated in allergies and skin irritations as well as in parasitic disorders. Eosinophilia can also result from drug-hypersensitivity reactions and malignancies, including Hodgkin's disease.

Basophils (0-1%). These neutrophils contain granules that stain a very dark blue. Basophils are usually elevated as a result of heavy-metal poisoning, chronic myeloid leukemia, myelofibrosis, and polycythemia vera. Decreased numbers of basophils are difficult to detect because of the minute quantities present.

Monocytes (0-6%). Monocytes are elevated during recovery from acute infections and agranulocytosis. They are also elevated during mycotic, rickettsial, protozoal, and viral infections and during subacute bacterial endocarditis.

URINALYSIS

Although a variety of biochemical tests may be performed on urine, the initial screen consists of an examination of its appearance. Tests for abnormal components include protein, glucose, blood, ketones, and bile pigments. Grossly, urine is examined for color, concentration, and pH. Colors ranging from pale yellow to deep gold are normal, with the shade depending on the concentration of solutes. Blood, hemoglobin, degradation products, and bilirubin and its metabolites may all cause color distortions. Abnormal color is not an absolute indicator of pathology, however. A variety of exogenous substances—including foods, drugs, and vitamins, may discolor urine.

The specific gravity of the urine suggests the kidney's concentrating ability. Normally, specific gravity ranges from 1.002 to 1.025, with the latter value reflecting maximal concentrating ability. Fresh urine samples from normal individuals are acidic. Although alkaline urine may indicate a disease process (e.g., urinary tract infection or systemic alkalosis), it may also result from assaying an aged specimen.

It should be remembered that assays of urinary values of substances may not be as precise as serum determinations. For example, it is documented that many diabetics have renal glucose thresholds significantly higher than nondiabetics.

A microscopic examination of the urine is also conducted. From 10-55 ml of urine are centrifuged, and the sediment—either stained or unstained, or both—is examined microscopically for the presence of a variety of structures. We will discuss only the most important of these.

White Blood Cells

The presence of 0-2 WBCs/high-power field is normal. Increased quantities indicate the presence of an infection.

Red Blood Cells

A small amount (0-2 RBCs/high-power field) is also normal. Increased numbers indicate hematuria.

Casts

The presence of casts in the urine generally suggests various types of kidney disease. Often, kidney disease or its severity may be discerned by the type of cast present (hyaline casts, watery casts, etc.). However, the presence of casts per se is not necessarily indicative of renal disease; their clinical significance must be interpreted in light of other information.

Bacteria

The presence of a large number of bacteria in a fresh, uncontaminated sample is diagnostic of urinary tract infection.

Crystals

A large variety of crystals can also be seen in the urine specimen. They may impart a cloudy appearance to a fresh-voided specimen. As with casts, their presence alone does not necessarily suggest disease. Some crystals are natural and benign.

SUMMARY

This chapter serves as a brief guide to the appropriate use of many laboratory assays now available. The clinical value of the tests in routine screening, diagnosis, and management is explained, with emphasis on the pharmacist's role. Correct interpretation of the tests is also discussed. Biochemical profiling of such analytes as glucose, BUN, creatinine, uric acid, bilirubin, and cholesterol is explained, and the clinical significance of alterations of these analytes in the bloodstream is discussed. Additionally, biochemical profiles of the electrolytes, blood proteins, calcium, phosphorus, and enzymes are described, as are normal values and clinical significance of alterations of these substances in the bloodstream. The hematology section examines the value of RBCs, hemoglobin, and hematocrit, blood indices, platelets, WBCs, and the differential count as barometers of a patient's status. The section on urinalysis describes the clinical significance of the gross appearance of the urine, as well as its microscopic examination.

ADDITIONAL READING

Bondy PK, Rosenberg, LE: *Metabolic Control and Disease*. Philadelphia, WB Saunders, 1980.

Henry B: *Clinical Diagnosis and Management by Laboratory Methods*. Philadelphia, WB Saunders Co, 1978.

Maxwell MH, Kleeman CR: *Clinical Disorders of Fluid and Electrolyte Metabolism*. New York, McGraw-Hill, 1979.

Meites S: *Pediatric Clinical Chemistry*. Washington, DC, American Association for Clinical Chemistry, 1977.

Tietz NW: *Clinical Guide to Laboratory Tests*. Philadelphia, WB Saunders, 1983.

Tietz NW: *Fundamentals of Clinical Chemistry*. Philadelphia, WB Saunders, 1976.

CHAPTER 30

Pharmacotherapeutic Considerations During Nutrition Support

PAUL W. NIEMIEC, Jr., and TIMOTHY W. VANDERVEEN

The practice of nutrition support has rapidly evolved into a multidisciplinary effort in order to provide a rational, cost-effective, and sophisticated approach to nutrition by relying on the distinctive professional expertise of each discipline. The pharmacist has assumed an important developmental role in clinical nutrition, contributing pioneering efforts in the areas of:

1. Parenteral and enteral nutrition formula compounding and distribution, including aspects of stability, compatibility, sterility, formula design, storage, and quality control
2. Cost-effective product utilization and selection
3. Technologic development of nutritional products and delivery systems
4. Administrative planning
5. Provision and coordination of ambulatory nutrition support services
6. In-service education
7. Metabolic monitoring of nutritional response
8. Pharmacotherapeutic/pharmacokinetic considerations during nutrition support

A careful review of medication therapy should be an integral part of patient monitoring during nutrition support and an important responsibility of the pharmacist involved in a multidisciplinary team effort. Intensive monitoring of drug therapy in nutritionally supported patients has revealed conflicts that were previously unrecognized or given only superficial attention by nutrition support services and other services involved with patient care. "Nutrition tunnel vision" has at times led us to reach inappropriate conclusions and make changes in nutritional therapy without full realization of the contribution of concurrent drug therapy. For instance, enteral nutrition is frequently discontinued because of suspected formula intolerance. However, careful evaluation of the circumstances surrounding the gastrointestinal (GI) disturbance may incriminate one or more medications as etiologic factors (1).

A review of classic drug-nutrient interactions, including drug-induced nutritional deficiencies and appetite suppression, has been published by Roe (2). Drug therapy may induce specific nutrient deficiencies or cause appetite suppression, altered taste perception, and impaired nutrient absorption, metabolism, and excretion. Medication-induced nutritional deficiencies may develop slowly without overt clinical symptoms, and diagnosis may require sophisticated laboratory analysis or radiologic examination. Consequently, although many possible deficiencies have been described (2), the actual incidence and clinical significance of many of these remain unclear.

Limited attention has been given to practical considerations in drug-nutrition interrelationships despite the frequency of medication therapy in hospitalized patients. It is the intent of this chapter to focus on practical drug-nutrient conflicts that are believed to be clinically important and have been observed to reoccur during monitoring of nutrition support therapy. In many cases, conflicts involve well-known pharmacologic effects of drugs that simply require reinterpretation to the patient who is also receiving nutritional support. Frequently, these conflicts have resulted in avoidable complications, inappropriate therapeutic maneuvers, or discontinuation of nutrition support.

Medications may have a significant impact on interpretation of the response to nutrition support by altering nutrient substrate utilization or laboratory indices, as well as necessitating therapeutic maneuvers to avoid conflicts. Therapeutic maneuvers to anticipate include electrolyte supplementation in excess of anabolic requirements, aggressive monitoring of serum and urine electrolytes, and modification of nutritional formula design and rate of administration.

Since pharmacologic and nutrition support are often administered simultaneously, it is essential to provide each modality in a safe, compatible, and efficacious manner. Recognition and anticipation of potential drug-nutrition support conflicts and therapeutic maneuvers by performing a medication history and daily medication profile review are important components of nutritional assessment and metabolic monitoring.

The remainder of this chapter will address practical pharmacotherapeutic and pharmacokinetic considerations during nutrition support.

DRUG ADMINISTRATION VIA ENTERAL NUTRITION DELIVERY SYSTEMS

Enteral feeding tubes represent convenient avenues for medication administration. Consequently, enteral feeding systems are frequently utilized simultaneously for nutrition support as well as drug delivery.

Medication administration by the enteral route may induce formula intolerance and/or result in less than optimal drug absorption. The compatibility and stability of numerous medications after mixture with enteral formulas are relatively unknown and require investigation. Cutie et al (3) evaluated the physical compatibility of three enteral formulations with 52 commonly used medications. The authors evaluated the mixtures immediately after mixing for viscosity and pH changes or separation and found many pharmaceutical preparations other than acidic syrups to be reasonably compatible. They emphasized the fact that their study did not determine chemical stability. Little is known concerning medication availability from enteral feeding systems and drug absorption during continuous nutrient infusion or during the luminally malnourished state.

Reports have suggested an apparent interference of oral phenytoin absorption by continuous enteral feedings (4,5). Varying influences of divalent ions and nutrient substrates on phenytoin absorption have been noted (6-9). Studies demonstrating food alteration of drug absorption have generally been performed in healthy subjects receiving regularly scheduled meals. Extrapolation of the results of these studies to patients receiving continuous enteral nutrient infusions requires a gigantic leap of faith. These and other practical administration problems necessitate an in-depth evaluation of drug administration practices in hospitalized patients receiving enteral nutrition support.

Destruction of sustained-release oral dosage forms by crushing to facilitate their administration via enteral feeding tubes is therapeutically inappropriate. Although this may appear to be common sense, attempts are made to crush and administer Theo-Dur and Procan SR tablets through feeding tubes. Administration of these dosage forms in this manner may result in higher than expected peak serum concentrations and subtherapeutic concentrations later in the dosing interval. Table 30.1 lists selected products that have been formulated for sustained release. Substitution of a liquid form or non–sustained-release product is necessary in this

TABLE 30.1   Selected Sustained-Release or Delayed-Release Drug Products

Dimetapp Extentabs
Donnatal Extentabs
E.E.S.
E-Mycin
Feosol Spansules
Fero-Gradumet Filmtabs
Klotrix
Procan SR
Quinaglute Dura-Tabs
Quinidex Extentabs
Sinubid
Slow-K
Theo-Dur

situation and may require more frequent dosing. Transition from parenteral to enteral nutrition therapy will frequently necessitate reassessment of the most optimal means of administering drug therapy.

The administration of crushed tablets or capsule contents via large-bore nasogastric tubes may cause no problems, but small-bore feeding tubes are more prone to occlusion. Particles may adhere to the inside of these tubes and aggregate or react with the enteral formula causing occlusion. If occlusion occurs, nutrition support will be interrupted until patency is restored or a new feeding tube is passed. Feeding tube occlusion may result in aberrant serum glucose control during insulin therapy or in a delay in reestablishing nutritional support, especially in patients in whom difficulty has been experienced with feeding tube placement or transpyloric migration. Although manipulation of the feeding tube may restore patency, occluded tubes must generally be removed and replaced. The incidence of feeding tube occlusion due to medication administration can be minimized by thoroughly pulverizing the solid dosage form, preparing a medication slurry, and flushing the tubes with warm water or saline solution before and after medication administration. Substitution of a liquid dosage form or avoidance of drug administration by this route will minimize feeding tube occlusion.

The increasingly popular use of enteral tube feedings (10) and development of sophisticated packaging and distribution systems (11-13) should be accompanied by due regard for the risks of bacterial contamination of enteral formulas or equipment by feeding system manipulation (14-20). Contamination of formulas with *Enterobacter cloacae, Pseudomonas aeruginosa, Escherichia coli*, and *Klebsiella* species has been demonstrated, with logarithmic growth occuring at room temperature but not under refrigeration or freezing (14). The consequences of formula contamination may be amplified during transpyloric feeding or H_2-receptor antagonist therapy, since the normal antibacterial defense mechanism of gastric acid is either bypassed or suppressed (21). Uniform standards for storage and handling of enteral products do not currently exist (14). Consequently, use of an enteral feeding system for medication delivery must be conducted with due regard for this contamination potential.

Patients requiring insulin therapy during enteral nutrition require careful monitoring of insulin administration and enteral formula infusion. Failure to adjust insulin administration according to changes in the feeding regimen caused by formula intolerance or feeding tube occlusion will result in undesirable serum glucose fluctuations. Administration of insulin on a regularly scheduled basis or the use of long-acting insulins during enteral nutrition predisposes the patient to hypoglycemia if the feeding is interrupted.

DRUG ADMINISTRATION VIA PARENTERAL NUTRITION DELIVERY SYSTEMS

Parenteral nutrition solutions have generally not been used as ''drug-delivery vehicles'' because of limited compatibility information, caution concerning drug mixture with proteinaceous substances, and concern for bacterial contamination associated with additional mixtures. Drug mixture with parenteral nutrition solutions may facilitate management of patients with severe fluid restriction, limited peripheral venous access sites, and those receiving home nutrition support (22). Correlation of drug dosage and nutrient requirements with solution infusion rate necessitates a cautious and responsible approach. Further research in this area should document chemical stability and pharmacologic effectiveness after admixture. Distinction should be made pertaining to medication admixture as a large-volume parenteral solution or during administration by coinfusion or auxiliary medication infusion unit. Medications documented to be chemically stable in model parenteral nutrition formulas include cimetidine (23), aminophylline (22), and metoclopramide (24). For more specific information, the reader is referred to a recent review of compatibility information pertaining to nutrient and drug mixture with parenteral nutrition solutions (24). Cyclic administration of parenteral nutrition solutions has been employed to provide a 6-hour ''window'' for central vein infusion of incompatible medications such as amphotericin B (25).

MEDICATION-INDUCED CHANGES DURING NUTRITION SUPPORT

Major classes of medications that interact with nutrition support include (1) antibiotics, (2) diuretics, (3) corticosteroids, (4) antacids, (5) oral electrolyte solutions, and (6) chemotherapeutic agents. Medication-induced changes observed during nutrition support include (1) GI disturbances, (2) electrolyte imbalances, (3) fluid disturbances, (4) alteration of glucose metabolism, (5) alteration of protein metabolism, and (6) acid-base disturbances. Table 30.2 presents a compilation of the most common medication-induced changes observed during nutrition support.

Gastrointestinal Disorders

Nausea, vomiting, and diarrhea are criteria used to evaluate tolerance to enteral nutrition. Although these symptoms often indicate intolerance to feeding formulas, they are common side effects of medication therapy. Many clinicians have the preconception that enteral feedings are poorly tolerated, and the onset of signs or symptoms of intolerance often results in discontinuation of the feedings rather than consideration of other possible causes.

Medications may cause various GI disorders, including nausea and vomiting, altered bowel motility, obstruction, ulceration, bleeding, and malabsorption syndromes. Epidemiologic surveys have suggested that 20-40% of all adverse drug reactions involve the GI tract (26). The package insert of many drugs includes various GI disturbances as possible side effects of therapy. Although numerous drugs have been implicated in the cause of GI disturbances, those most frequently associated with GI abnormalities include antibiotics, oral electrolyte solutions, analgesics, antacids, stool softeners, and iron salts (26). Adverse GI reactions may be caused by a drug's mechanism of action (guanethidine), drug toxicity (digoxin), or a direct irritant effect (iron salts) on the gastric or small bowel mucosa (26). In some cases, side effects may be independent of dosage or may resolve with continued therapy.

TABLE 30.2   Medication-Induced Changes During Nutrition Support

Medication-Induced Change	*Clinical Observation*
Electrolyte imbalances	Altered renal/GI excretion; inherent drug content
Antibiotics	
Ampicillin, carbenicillin, ticarcillin	↓ Serum K
Amphotericin B	↓ Serum K, Mg
Diuretics	
Furosemide, ethacrynic acid	↓ Serum Na, K, Mg, Ca, Zn, Cl
Thiazides	↓ Serum K, Mg, Zn; ↑ serum Ca
Spironolactone	↑ Serum K
Corticosteroids	↓ Serum K, Ca, PO_4; ↑ serum Na
Antacids	
Mg-containing	↑ Serum Mg (severe renal failure)
Al-containing	↓ Serum PO_4
Cisplatin	↓ Serum Mg, other electrolytes
Glucose/insulin	↓ Serum K, Mg, PO_4 (anabolism)
Alteration of glucose metabolism	Altered cellular uptake and insulin effectiveness
Corticosteroids	Hyperglycemia, glucosuria
Diuretics	Hyperglycemia
Alteration of protein metabolism	Antianabolic effects
Corticosteroids	↑ BUN, ↑ UUN; negative nitrogen balance
Diuretics	Factitious ↑ BUN with hypovolemia
Tetracycline	
Alteration of acid-base balance	Function of electrolytes and acid lost in daily fluid losses
Corticosteroids	Metabolic alkalosis
Diuretics (furosemide, ethacrynic acid)	Metabolic alkalosis
Cimetidine, ranitidine	Inhibitory effect on gastric acid secretion decreases volume and acid loss secondary to nasogastric suction, blunting tendency to metabolic alkalosis

BUN, UUN = blood and urinary urea nitrogen, respectively.

Nausea and Vomiting

Drug-induced nausea and vomiting may result from a direct GI irritant effect and stimulation of the vomiting center (potassium chloride, iron salts), stimulation of the medullary chemoreceptor trigger zone (morphine), or drug toxicity (digoxin) (27). This nonspecific symptom may also be associated with disorders such as pancreatitis or ileus. Additionally, psychologic duress related to hospitalization, the act of medication ingestion, or excessive rates of enteral feeding administration may result in nausea and vomiting. In an attempt to identify the cause of these symptoms, the patient's drug therapy, clinical status, and nutrition support must be reviewed.

Enteral tube feedings are frequently blamed for nausea, vomiting, and cramping. New-onset nausea or vomiting following previously successful continuous feeding is not infrequently found to be coincidental with bolus medication administration (potassium supplements, analgesic elixirs) via the nasogastric tube. Recognition and reevaluation of the method of drug administration may permit successful reinstitution of tube feeding while minimizing the risk for aspiration. Likewise, a thorough medication history and

TABLE 30.3 Drugs Frequently Associated with Nausea and Vomiting (29,30)

L-Asparaginase	Erythromycin	Nitrogen mustards
Caffeine	Ibuprofen, related compounds	Penicillamine
Carmustine	Imidazole carboxamide	Phenylbutazone
Cephalexin	Indomethacin	Potassium chloride
Cholestyramine	Iron salts	Quinidine
Cisplatin	Isoxsuprine	Reserpine
Clofibrate	Levodopa	Salicylates
Colchicine	Lithium	Sulfonamides
Cyclophosphamide	Lomustine	Sulfonylureas
Daunomycin	Mefenamic acid	Tetracycline
Digitalis compounds	Mitomycin C	Theophylline
Diethylstilbestrol	Narcotic analgesics	Trimethoprim-sulfamethoxazole
Doxorubicin	Nitrofurantoin	

profile review may provide reasonable suspicion of drug toxicity based on pharmacokinetic assessment or drug-drug interaction. For example, since phenytoin is characterized by a narrow therapeutic range and nonlinear pharmacokinetics, a prior dosage increase or change in bioavailability may result in phenytoin toxicity (28). Medications frequently associated with nausea and vomiting are listed in Table 30.3.

Diarrhea

Diarrhea may be characterized by an increase in stool frequency, volume, or water content. Diarrhea is a common finding in hospitalized patients, especially in those with significant malnutrition. Diarrhea associated with enteral nutrition therapy may be multifactorial in nature and difficult to assess. Administration of a concentrated feeding formula at an excessive rate early in the therapy of a nutritionally depleted patient may result in diarrheal stools. Diarrhea may also be caused by abnormal intestinal water and electrolyte transport, altered GI motility, nutrient or bile acid malabsorption, increased osmotic solute loads, enteral formula contamination, and viral gastroenteritis. Pathologic processes such as diabetes mellitus, hyperthyroidism, and short bowel and blind-loop syndromes may also be associated with diarrhea. A secretory diarrhea of fluid and electrolytes may result from altered mucosal permeability associated with inflammatory bowel disease, bacterial overgrowth, laxatives, radiation enteritis, and bile acids (31,32).

A commonly reported complication of drug therapy is diarrhea. Drug-induced diarrhea may be caused by a medication's chemical irritant effect, alteration of bowel flora, overdosage, or hypertonicity. The incidence and severity of diarrhea may be influenced by medication dosage and method of administration, disease state, and nutritional status. Medications frequently cited as having the potential to induce diarrhea are listed in Table 30.4. Those most commonly associated with diarrhea include magnesium hydroxide-containing antacids, laxatives, broad spectrum antibiotics, quinidine, guanethidine, alkylating agents, colchicine, lactulose, and sorbitol (26,30,33). Selected descriptions of drug-induced diarrhea follow.

Oral Electrolyte Solutions. Enterally administered potassium and magnesium salts can induce diarrhea on the basis of medication hypertonicity. Evidence also suggests that saline laxatives may stimulate release of the hormone cholecystokinin-pancreozymin, which increases the secretory activity of the GI tract (34). Diarrhea associated with potassium chloride elixir is generally caused by the method of administration (see under "Osmolality of Medications").

Magnesium salts have multiple uses as cathartics, antacids, and electrolyte replacements. Since they serve many roles, their use as antacids lulls one into overlooking their inherent cathartic properties. Malnourished patients appear to be particularly sensitive to magnesium catharsis. Magnesium salts are poorly absorbed from the small intestine; consequently, an osmotic diarrhea can result as a function of magnesium dosage. Magnesium hydroxide (Milk of Magnesia) is frequently employed as the "house laxative"; yet numerous antacid products also contain considerable amounts of magnesium in combination with aluminum hydroxide. The effect of antacids on GI motility is dependent on magnesium and aluminum content and antacid dosage. High-dose antacid therapy can present significant amounts of magnesium ion to the intestinal tract. Alternating magnesium- and aluminum-containing antacids on an every-other-dose basis often reduces the tendency toward diarrhea. Because of poor magnesium bioavailability, 30-40 mEq/day of magnesium sulfate would have to be administered enterally as an electrolyte supplement to provide 5-12 mEq of magnesium ion systemically. Since the usual cathartic dosage of magnesium sulfate is approximately 125 mEq, a fine line exists between effective supplementation and effective

TABLE 30.4 Medications Frequently Associated with Diarrhea (26,30,33)

Alkylating agents	Erythromycin	Methyldopa
Ampicillin	5-Fluorouracil	Neomycin
Antacids	Guanethidine	Penicillamine
Antimetabolites	Iron salts	Phenylbutazone
Cephalexin	Isoxsuprine	Phosphate salts
Clindamycin	Lactulose	Potassium salts
Clofibrate	Laxatives	Propranolol
Colchicine	Lincomycin	Quinidine
Corticosteroids	Magnesium salts	Reserpine
Digitalis compounds	Mefenamic acid	Sorbitol
Dioctyl sodium sulfosuc-	Methotrexate	Tetracycline
cinate		

catharsis. Because of the above considerations and the fact that diarrhea begets further hypomagnesemia, it may be more feasible to supplement a severely hypomagnesemic patient with parenteral (IM, IV) magnesium sulfate.

Antibiotics. Antibiotics have traditionally been associated with diarrhea on the basis of altering bowel flora and causing local GI irritation. Some authors have suggested that administration of Lactinex granules via the feeding tube may help restore balance to the intestinal flora (35). Depending on the antibiotic used, dosage, and report cited, the incidence of antibiotic-induced diarrhea may vary from 1-30%. Diarrhea secondary to antibiotics (ampicillin, clindamycin) may also be independent of dose or route of administration. Antibiotics associated with severe diarrhea and/or pseudomembranous colitis include ampicillin, cephalexin, chloramphenicol, clindamycin, lincomycin, penicillin G, and trimethoprim-sulfamethoxazole (30,36). Antibiotic-induced colitis is generally accompanied by a profuse, watery diarrhea (with or without blood) that occurs during drug therapy, but onset of diarrhea may, in some cases, be delayed for several weeks after drug discontinuation.

Other Medications Causing Diarrhea. Lactulose is a nondigestible disaccharide that produces an intentional and sometimes severe, watery diarrhea when given in pharmacologic dosages. Fermentation of unabsorbed sugar by intestinal bacteria results in lactic acid production, GI irritation, and diarrhea. Lactulose therapy often interferes with attempts at successful enteral feeding. Likewise, the use of sorbitol as a vehicle for Kayexalate administration serves as a laxative.

Colchicine is a known inhibitor of intestinal epithelial cell mitosis and disaccharidase activity. Colchicine therapy may result in nausea and vomiting, nutrient malabsorption, diarrhea, and intolerance of milk and refined sugar products (32). Because of biliary recycling of the parent compound, adverse GI effects may be seen following oral or parenteral administration. Avoidance of milk, refined sugar in the form of fruit juices, etc and enteral formulas containing lactose or sucrose may allow for a successful enteral approach to the patient receiving colchicine.

A GI intolerance to quinidine usually occurs during initiation of therapy independent of serum concentration and may be transient in nature with continued therapy. The sympatholytic action of guanethidine results in a comparative excess of parasympathetic innervation of the GI tract resulting in increased GI motility and diarrhea in some patients. Severe diarrhea from guanethidine may require symptomatic treatment and medication discontinuation. Nausea, vomiting, and less commonly, diarrhea following oral or parenteral administration of digoxin is usually associated with overdosage and may be reflective of toxicity.

Other drugs rarely reported as causing diarrhea, but observed to be associated with onset of diarrhea in selected cases, include spironolactone, cimetidine, and furosemide. Diarrhea resulting from cimetidine administration is generally reported as mild and transient, but recent reports have cited a seemingly associated, persistent diarrhea occurring after 7-10 days of oral cimetidine therapy (37-39). Furosemide may decrease water and electrolyte absorption in the small intestine, accounting for diarrhea observed in patients receiving high dosages (40). In addition, the sucrose content

of various medications may be participatory in an osmotic diarrhea in some infants and patients with bowel resections (see ''Sucrose Content of Medications''). Since the cause of diarrhea is often difficult to identify, a special effort should be made to temporally associate medication administration and enteral nutrition with observed changes in bowel motility.

Osmolality of Medications

The osmolality of enteral formulas varies and is a function of nutrient sources and concentration (41). Formula osmolality must be considered in relation to GI tolerance during enteral nutrition, with tolerance also dependent on the rate and method of formula administration, feeding tube location, and individual patient differences. In general, formulas exceeding 500-600 mOsm/kg must initially be diluted to avoid inducing an osmotic diarrhea secondary to a hypertonic load.

Feeding tubes represent convenient avenues for medication administration and electrolyte replacement. Significant GI intolerance in the form of nausea, vomiting, and diarrhea is associated with the administration of undiluted, hypertonic oral electrolyte solutions and medications via feeding tubes (1). Although hypertonic electrolyte replacement solutions are generally well diluted prior to oral or parenteral administration to avoid toxicity (42,43), this is not always practiced with potassium administration by feeding tubes. Dilution of a dosage of 10% potassium chloride (KCl) elixir (3000 mOsm/kg [1], Table 30.5) in 8 ounces of water or juice for administration through the feeding tube is seldom viewed as practical at the time of administration, especially since this may represent the fluid equivalent of several hours of continuous tube feeding. Flushing a dosage of KCl elixir with 10-20 ml of fluid through the feeding tube would still present the GI tract with a hypertonic bolus. The small intestine is especially sensitive to hypertonic medications and osmolar loads, and administration of undiluted KCl elixir via the feeding tube directly into the duodenum or jejunum can be expected to potentiate significant drug-induced intolerance. A GI irritation with subsequent diarrhea may further contribute to stripping of the intestinal mucosa and perpetuate a malabsorption cycle.

Electrolyte supplementation by parenteral means or by appropriate dilution and mixture with the enteral formula is preferable to bolus administration of undiluted solutions via the feeding tube (1). Table 30.6 presents derived linear regression equations that predict formula osmolality after

TABLE 30.5　Selected Osmolalities of Electrolyte Solutions (1)

Electrolyte Solution	mOsm/kg
KC1 elixir, 10% (sugar free)	3000
KC1 injection (2 mEq/ml)	3600
K phosphate injection (3 mmol P/ml)	5450
Na acetate injection (2 mEq/ml)	3980
NaCl injection (4 mEq/ml)	7090
Na phosphate injection (3 mmol P/ml)	4650
NaHCO$_3$ injection (1 mEq/ml)	1730

the addition of typical electrolytes found physically compatible for 24 hours in full-strength Isocal. Additions of varying amounts of 10% KCl elixir to Isocal, Ensure, and Sustacal generated the following linear regression equation for predictions of formula osmolality following KCl admixture (1):

Final osmolality (mOsm/kg) =
2.0 (mEq KCl elixir 10%/liter formula) +
Original formula osmolality

In addition, the high osmolality of antibiotic suspensions and numerous oral medications (1,44,45) administered repeatedly in bolus dosages via feeding tubes may have an impact on apparent GI intolerance and drug absorption, especially in infants and severely malnourished patients. Table 30.7 presents determined osmolalities of selected antibiotic suspensions and oral liquids (1). Many oral medications have osmolalities in excess of 2000 mOsm/kg, with contributing factors to hypertonicity including pharmaceutical vehicles and additives such as sucrose, sorbitol, ethanol, and propylene glycol. In contrast, the osmolality of many injectable medications is significantly less (44,45), and this has prompted suggestions to administer medications parenterally if possible or consider the use of selected injectable forms for enteral administration (44,45). Serious concern and speculation has been raised about a suspected correlation between necrotizing enterocolitis and GI illness with the administration of hyperosmolar feedings (>400 mOsm/kg) and hypertonic medications in premature infants (45-47). Although conflicting data exist, animal studies suggest that infusion of hypertonic glucose, sodium bicarbonate, and high concentrations of ampicillin into the mesenteric artery can result in intestinal necrosis (48). The seriousness of this matter warrants extensive attention and investigation. Until more information is available, however, it would seem prudent to limit the administration of oral medications in hypertonic form to infants as much as possible. Alternative administration suggestions include (1) dilution of oral medications prior to administration, (2) use of the IV route when feasible, and (3) administration of

selected injectable products enterally (45). Routine admixture of medications to enteral formulas to neutralize medication hypertonicity cannot be recommended at this time, pending specific study of drug stability and availability from enteral tube feeding systems.

Sucrose Content of Medications

Atrophy of intestinal microvilli and deficits in brush border disaccharidase activity may accompany protein calorie malnutrition (32,49-55). Carbohydrate intolerance secondary to lactase, sucrase, or maltase deficiency is frequently associated with GI disorders such as celiac sprue, tropical and nontropical sprue, gastroenteritis, postgastrectomy, and irritable colon syndromes (56). Diarrhea and environmental insults in the form of intestinal infection, surgery, or drug therapy may cause structural and functional damage to the mucosal surface with temporary deficits in digestive enzyme activity (52).

Because of potential disaccharide-induced formula intolerance, both pediatric and adult enteral formulas are available without sucrose and lactose. However, many oral drug suspensions, solutions, and elixirs contain sucrose as a flavoring agent. Polypharmacy can result in the administration of high sucrose loads, and medicinal sucrose may in some cases represent 20-40% of an infant's daily carbohydrate intake.

It has been our observation that medications containing sucrose may affect apparent tolerance of enteral formulas in patients with suspected sucrase deficiency or deficits in intestinal absorption of glucose. Certain patients may al-

TABLE 30.6 Osmolality of Full-Strength Isocal after Electrolyte Addition (1) (Per Liter Formula)

Additive	Regression Equation
K acetate injection (KAc)	y = 2.1 (mEq KAc/liter) + b[a] (r = 0.99)
KCl elixir (sugar free)	y = 2.0 (mEq KCl/liter) + b[a] (r = 0.99)
K phosphate injection (KP)	y = 1.0 (mEq KP[b]/liter) + b[a] (r = 0.99)
Na acetate injection (NaAc)	y = 2.1 (mEq NaAc/liter + b[a] (r = 0.99)
NaCl injection	y = 1.9 (mEq NaCl/liter) + b[a] (r = 0.99)
Na phosphate injection (NaP)	y = 1.6 (mEq NaP[b]/liter) + b[a] (r = 0.99)
NaHCO₃ injection	y = 1.0 (mEq NaHCO₃/liter) + b[a] (r = 0.99)

[a]Original Isocal osmolality determined to be 281 mOsm/kg.
[b]K phosphate and Na phosphate addition expressed in terms of mEq K and Na content.

TABLE 30.7 Osmolalities of Selected Antibiotic Suspensions and Oral Liquids (1)

Antibiotic Suspension or Oral Liquid	Concentration	mOsm/kg
Aldactone suspension[a] (Searle, Chicago)	25 mg/5 ml	2245
Bactrim suspension (Roche, Nutley, N.J.)		4560
Ceclor suspension (Eli Lilly, Indianapolis)	250 mg/5 ml	2430
V-Cillin K suspension (Eli Lilly, Indianapolis)	250 mg/5 ml	2995
E.E.S. suspension (Abbott, North Chicago)	200 mg/5 ml	4475
Keflex suspension (Dista, Indianapolis)	250 mg/5 ml	2445
Lasix oral solution (Hoechst-Roussel, Somerville, N.J.)	10 mg/5 ml	3938
Pathocil suspension (Wyeth, Philadelphia)	62.5 mg/5 ml	2980
Principen suspension (Squibb, Princeton)	250 mg/5 ml	3070
Prostaphlin oral solution (Bristol, Syracuse)	250 mg/5 ml	2420
Tagamet liquid (Smith Kline & French, Philadelphia)	300 mg/5 ml	4035
Utimox suspension (Parke-Davis, Morris Plains, NJ)	250 mg/5 ml	1775
Neutra-Phos oral solution (Willen Drug, Baltimore)	16.7 mgP/5 ml	250

[a]Prepared extemporaneously with methylcellulose as a suspending agent.

ready be maximally absorbing a given amount of glucose in their diet prior to the introduction of a sugar-containing medication. Sensitivity to sucrose appears to occur more frequently during initiation of enteral feeding in severely malnourished patients, infants, or patients with resected bowels.

Brush border enzymes such as sucrase have an extremely short half-life in terms of hours (57), with intestinal sucrase activity being diet-responsive and declining significantly within 2-5 days of ingestion of a low carbohydrate diet (53,58). This time response corresponds to the estimated time for intestinal epithelial cell turnover in the small in-testine (58). A dose-dependent, inverse relationship between unabsorbed sugar and intestinal transit time has been demonstrated in malnourished infants, with improvement of glucose, sucrose, and lactose absorption after 2 months of high-protein feeding (55). Prior to restoration of functional enzyme activity, which is promoted by luminal nutrition (32,54,55), disaccharide malabsorption can result in an osmotic and fermentative diarrhea, with severity being a function of carbohydrate dosage and degree of sugar digestion (52).

Table 30.8 provides a list of the sucrose content of various medications. Attention to temporal relationships among GI symptoms, feeding and concurrent medication administration, and an awareness of a medication's sucrose content and inherent capability to induce diarrhea may help to clarify the cause of a recent change in bowel motility.

Chemotherapy-Induced Gastrointestinal Toxicity

Cancer chemotherapeutic agents cause significant GI toxicity due to the rapid turnover time of intestinal cells. Anorexia, nausea, vomiting, and mucosal ulceration may be dose-limiting to chemotherapy and impair adequate nutritional intake (59,60). Virtually all antineoplastics are capable of causing nausea, vomiting, and diarrhea, with GI toxicity usually abating a few days after completion of a course of therapy. Doxorubicin-cyclophosphamide combinations, cisplatin, vinblastine, and bleomycin are notorious for causing severe GI toxicity.

Table 30.9, adapted from Donaldson and Lenon (59), lists various chemotherapeutic agents known for causing GI toxicity. In addition, chronic radiation therapy may adversely affect nutritional status, depending on the cumulative dosage received and specific organs irradiated. Radiation tolerance doses generally range from 3000-6000 rads, depending on the organ involved (59). Radiotherapy may cause dysphagia, nausea, and vomiting, esophagitis, taste alterations, ulceration, enteritis, colitis, obstruction, diarrhea, nutrient malabsorption (abdominal irradiation), and decreased intestinal disaccharidase activity. Symptoms may

TABLE 30.8 Sucrose Content of Various Medications

Product Name	Form	Sucrose Content (g/5 ml)
Aquasol A	Drops	0
Aquasol E	Drops	0
Bactrim	Suspension	2.5
Benadryl	Elixir	1.5
Betapen-VK	Suspension	2.8
Ce-Vi-Sol	Drops	0
Cefaclor	Suspension	3.0
Chloromycetin	Suspension	1.5
Cleocin	Suspension	1.5
Compazine	Syrup	3.5
Dilantin	Suspension (30 and 125 mg/5ml)	1.0
Dynapen	Suspension	2.3
Elixophyllin	Elixir	0
E.E.S.	Drops, solution	1.5
Fer-In-Sol	Drops	2.0
Feosol	Elixir	0.8
Gantrisin	Suspension	3.5
Ilosone	Suspension	1.6
Ilosone	Liquid	2.0
Ilosone	Drops	0.3
Keflex	Suspension	3.0
Lanoxin	Elixir	2.2
Larotid	Suspension	2.2
Lasix	Oral solution	0
Mycostatin	Suspension	2.5
Phenobarbital	Elixir (Lilly, Phillips-Roxane)	0.6
Poly-Vi-Sol	Drops	0
Polycillin	Suspension	1.9
Polymox	Suspension	2.5
Potassium Chloride	10% oral solution (Phillips-Roxane)	0
Principen	Suspension	3.2
Prostaphlin	Oral solution	2.3
Septra	Suspension	3.7
Slophyllin-80	Syrup	0
Tagamet	Suspension	2.0
Tegopen	Suspension	2.4
Tempra	Syrup	3.0
Tempra	Drops	1.2
Theolair	Elixir	2.5
Theragran	Liquid	0
Tri-Vi-Sol	Drops	0
Tylenol	Elixir (120 mg/5ml)	3.0
Tylenol	Elixir (160 mg/5ml)	1.5
Tylenol	Drops	0
Unipen	Oral solution	2.5
Utimox	Suspension	1.7
Veetids	Suspension	2.8
V-Cillin K	Suspension	3.0

TABLE 30.9 Gastrointestinal Toxicity of Antineoplastic Agents (59)

Anorexia, nausea, vomiting	Carmustine
	Cisplatin
	Cyclophosphamide
	Daunomycin
	Doxorubicin
	Hexamethylmelamine
	Imidazole carboxamide
	Lomustine
	Mitomycin C
	Nitrogen mustards
	Streptozotocin
Ileus	Vinca alkaloids
Stomatitis	Bleomycin
	Dactinomycin
	Doxorubicin
	5-Fluorouracil
	Methotrexate
	Vinblastine
Pancreatitis	L-Asparaginase

persist for several weeks following completion of radiotherapy. The subsequent administration of actinomycin D or doxorubicin has been reported to reactivate latent radiation effects (59). Aggressive cancer therapy with combinations of antineoplastics or in combination with radiation can be expected to potentiate GI toxicity and complicate an enteral approach to nutrition. Specific antidiarrheal therapy and continuous rather than bolus enteral feeding may assist in improving tolerance.

Constipation

Constipation should be assessed in relation to a patient's usual bowel habits. During enteral nutrition, constipation must be differentiated from a pathologic obstruction that may preclude the safe use of the GI tract until the obstruction is resolved. Constipation may result from drug therapy, mechanical obstruction of the GI tract, colon spasms, prolonged bed rest, or numerous pathologic conditions including severe infections, cerebrovascular accident, and colon cancer. Any agent or pathologic process that decreases intestinal motility or alters innervation of the intestinal musculature has the potential to induce constipation. Ileus may result from intestinal muscle paralysis (adynamic), contraction (dynamic), or mechanical obstruction and is generally associated with abdominal pain, distention, and persistent fecal vomiting in addition to constipation. Ileus may be secondary to drug therapy (e.g., tricyclic antidepressants, anticholinergics, antipsychotics), recent surgery or anesthesia, severe infection, diabetes, spinal cord injuries, tetanus, hypomagnesemia, or cystic fibrosis. Enteral formula administration in the presence of ileus increases gastric fluid residual volumes and the risk of regurgitation and aspiration.

Drug-induced changes in intestinal motility may be caused by varying mechanisms. Constipation is frequently associated with use of narcotic analgesics as a result of the following mechanisms: increased gastric, small intestinal, and colonic tone; increased ileocecal valve and anal sphincter tone; decreased gastric, pancreatic, and biliary secretions; decreased peristaltic contractions and sensory reflex for defecation; delayed gastric emptying; and increased reabsorption of intestinal water. Despite some development of tolerance to these effects, chronic narcotic use is usually accompanied by constipation. Narcotic-induced constipation may be relieved by the use of bulk-forming laxatives (e.g., Metamucil). Tricyclic antidepressants, phenothiazines, antihistamines, and anticholinergics reduce peristalsis because of their anticholinergic properties. Aluminum hydroxide-containing antacids (e.g., Amphojel, ALternaGEL)

cause constipation because of their aluminum content, and this may be alleviated by alternating or substituting their administration with magnesium-containing antacids (e.g., Maalox). Medications commonly associated with constipation are shown in Table 30.10.

Metoclopramide reportedly facilitates an increase in gastric emptying and pyloric sphincter relaxation (61-63) and may be helpful in gastroparesis associated with tumor burden, diabetes, and postoperative gastric atony (64-69). Controlled observations are needed to establish the drug's efficacy in facilitating enteral feeding tube placement and enteral nutrition in association with parenteral nutrition or postoperative ileus (61,70).

In addition, obstruction of the GI tract by medication mass (bezoar) has been attributed to hydroscopic bulk laxatives, cholestyramine, nonreabsorbable aluminum-containing antacids, ascorbic acid tablets, and Isocal feedings (71-78). Although rare, this complication may be associated with intestinal perforation and peritonitis and has necessitated exploratory laparotomy and bowel resection. Case reports concerning medication bezoars usually show predisposing factors to exist that may influence the risk for intestinal obstruction. Pathologic factors include intestinal malrotation or displacment, vagotomy, and poor hydration. Concurrent anticholinergic or narcotic therapy may have been participative by decreasing intestinal secretions and motility. Insufficient fluid administration with bulk laxatives may predispose to GI obstruction. Aluminum hydroxide-induced obstruction has been reported in renal failure patients receiving repeated, high antacid dosages for control of hyperphosphatemia (76). Despite the rarity of medication bezoars, the implications are sufficiently serious to warrant consideration in the predisposed patient.

The patient receiving enteral nutrition should have bowel frequency monitored regularly. Medications predisposing a patient to constipation should be noted, especially in chronically bedridden patients. The use of appropriate laxatives on a short-term basis may be required in chronically inactive patients if there is no evidence of functional obstruction or intestinal pathology.

Electrolyte Imbalances

Medications may alter a patient's electrolyte status through their inherent electrolyte content or their effects on electrolyte absorption or excretion. Recognition and identification of drug-induced changes in electrolyte balance will facilitate appropriate interpretation of patient response to nutritional support. Consideration of this subject is critical, since morbidity and mortality have been directly attributed to drug-induced electrolyte imbalances (79).

Electrolyte imbalances are primarily caused by diuretics, antibiotics, corticosteroids, and antineoplastics, but chronic use of laxatives and antacids have also been associated with electrolyte aberrations (79,80). Tables 30.11 to 30.16 summarize various reported electrolyte imbalances associated with drug therapy. Where possible, a proposed mechanism is cited and referenced, although such mechanisms may be controversial or multifactorial in nature. Selected examples follow, illustrating common examples of drug-induced electrolyte imbalances observed during nutrition support.

TABLE 30.10 Drugs Commonly Associated with Constipation

Al-containing antacids	Ganglionic blockers
Anticholinergics	Iron salts
Antihistamines	Kayexalate resin
Antipsychotics	Narcotic analgesics
Calcium salts	Tricyclic antidepressants
Cholestyramine resin	Vinca alkaloids
Clonidine	

TABLE 30.11 Selected Drugs Reported to Affect Sodium (Na) Balance

Drug	Proposed Mechanism
Hypernatremia	
Amphotericin B	↑ Renal water loss
Cholestyramine	Na content; osmotic diuresis (79)
Corticosteroids	Aldosterone-like Na retention (81)
Demeclochlortetracycline	↑ Renal water loss; suppression ADH action (79)
Lactulose	↑ Fecal water loss (79,82)
Laxatives	Dehydration
Lithium	↑ Renal water loss; suppression ADH action (79)
Mannitol	Renal water loss greater than natriuresis, accompanied by ↓ water intake (79)
Penicillin G sodium	Na content with impaired renal function (79)
Saline infusions	Na content (79)
Sodium bicarbonate	Na content (79)
Hyponatremia	
Captopril	
Cisplatin	Renal tubular defect (83)
Diuretics	↓ Renal tubular Na reabsorption; volume depletion-ADH release (84,85)
Intravenous fat	Pseudohyponatremia-lipemic serum sample
Lithium	↑ Natriuresis
Mannitol	Osmotic extracellular water shift
Carbamazepine	
Chlorpropamide	
Chlorthalidone	
Clonidine	
Cyclophosphamide	
Ibuprofen	Inappropriate ADH secretion-like syndrome; potentiation of ADH (79,80)
Morphine	
Thioridazine	
Tolbutamide	
Vincristine	

ADH = Antidiuretic hormone.

TABLE 30.12 Selected Drugs Reported to Induce Hyperkalemia

Drug	Proposed Mechanism
Antineoplastics	Lysis of tumor cells (86,87)
Arginine HCl	Intracellular K displacement by arginine (79)
Captopril	↓ Urinary excretion
Indomethacin	↓ Urinary excretion, secondary hypoaldosteronism (79)
K penicillin G	K content and rapid IV administration; high doses during renal failure (43)
Mannitol	Cellular K leak (88)
Oral K supplements	Concurrent renal impairment and/or spironolactone (79,80)
Salt substitutes	Inherent K content (79)
Spironolactone	Antagonism of aldosterone; ↓ distal renal tubule K secretion, concurrent renal impairment and/or K supplementation, catabolism, hemolysis, or diabetes (79,84,85,89)
Succinylcholine	Cellular K leak (79)
Triamterene	↓ Distal renal tubule K secretion (84,85,90)

Hyponatremia in Association with Hypoalbuminemia and Malnutrition

Sodium balance is subject to numerous variables including organ function, degree of hydration, total daily sodium intake (diet, IV fluids, and medications), as well as daily excretory losses. Hyponatremia and edema are frequently associated with hypoalbuminemia. Severe malnutrition is often characterized by a relative total body sodium excess, high intracellular sodium concentrations, and lower than "normal" extracellular fluid sodium concentrations. Serum sodium concentrations ranging from 128-134 mEq/liter are frequently observed in severe malnutrition and may be physiologic in that setting. Attempts to correct serum levels to the "normal" range by salt administration in the hypoalbuminemic patient may increase serum hydrostatic pressure and result in "third-spacing" of fluids and edema formation.

Determination of total daily sodium intake, including that from medications and IV solutions (Tables 30.17 to 30.18), may reveal an excessive sodium load being presented to the protein-malnourished, edematous patient. An example of such a calculation is illustrated in Table 30.19. Total daily sodium intake amounted to 423 mEq or 9.7 g (equivalent

TABLE 30.13   Selected Drugs Reported to Induce Hypokalemia

Drug	Proposed Mechanism
Aminophylline	↑ Distal renal tubule K secretion (79)
Acetazolamide	↑ Distal renal tubule K secretion
Amphotericin B	Renal tubular defect, K wasting; distal renal tubular acidosis (91,92)
Ampicillin (high dose)	Nonreabsorbable anion theory; ↑ distal renal tubule K secretion (93)
Carbenicillin	Nonreabsorbable anion theory; ↑ distal renal tubule K secretion (94-98)
Chlorthalidone	↑ Distal renal tubule K secretion (84,85)
Cisplatin	Renal tubular defect; hypomagnesemia (83,99)
Corticosteroids	↑ K mobilization from tissues and K renal excretion (81,100)
Epinephrine	Intracellular K shift
Ethacrynic acid	↑ Distal renal tubule K secretion (84,85)
Furosemide	↑ Distal renal tubule K secretion (84,85)
Glucose	Anabolic shift of K intracellularly
Gentamicin (multiple course)	Renal tubular defect, K wasting, hypomagnesemia (101,102)
Insulin	Anabolic shift of K intracellularly
Kayexalate resin	Cation exchange with ↑ fecal K elimination
Laxatives	Diarrheal losses and secondary hyperaldosteronism
Licorice	Mineralocorticoid activity of glycyrrhizic acid resulting in ↑ K renal excretion
Lithium	Distal renal tubular acidosis (79)
Levodopa	↑ Renal excretion (79)
Mannitol	↑ Distal renal tubule K secretion (79)
Metolazone	↑ Distal renal tubule K secretion
Nafcillin	Reported dose-related ↑ urinary K excretion (103)
Penicillin G sodium (high dose)	Nonreabsorbable anion theory; ↑ distal renal tubule K secretion (104)
Salicylates (chronic, high dose)	↑ K renal excretion
Sodium bicarbonate, bicarbonate precursors (citrate, acetate, lactate)	Intracellular K redistribution with metabolic or respiratory alkalosis (79)
Thiazide diuretics	↑ Distal renal tubular K secretion (84,85)
Ticarcillin	Nonreabsorbable anion theory; ↑ distal renal tubule K secretion (94-98)

TABLE 30.14   Selected Drugs Reported to Alter Phosphate (PO_4) Balance

Drug	Proposed Mechanism
Hyperphosphatemia	
PO_4-containing laxatives	Chronic ingestion (with renal compromise)
Intravenous PO_4 salts	Overcorrection of hypophosphatemia (with renal compromise)
Hypophosphatemia	
Acetazolamide	↑ Renal excretion (79)
Al-containing antacids	↑ Binding of PO_4 (dietary and GI secretions) within GI tract; ↑ fecal PO_4 elimination (usually in setting of low PO_4 intake or chronic diarrheal losses) (105,106)
Calcitonin	↑ Renal excretion; ↑ skeletal uptake (107)
Corticosteroids	(108)
Epinephrine	↑ Cellular uptake (107,108)
Ethacrynic acid	↑ Renal excretion (107)
Furosemide	↑ Renal excretion (107)
Glucagon	↑ Renal excretion (79)
Glucose	↑ Insulin secretion with anabolic, intracellular PO_4 shift; oxidative phosphorylation of glucose; phosphaturia accompanying glucosuria (107-110)
Insulin	Anabolic, intracellular PO_4 shift
Saline infusions	↑ Renal excretion (107)
Sodium bicarbonate	↑ Renal excretion; ↑ cellular uptake and glycolysis (79,107)
Thiazide diuretics	↑ Renal excretion (107)
Vitamin D excess	↑ Intestinal Ca absorption

to 24 g sodium chloride), of which a large portion was coming from ticarcillin. The authors have observed severely hypoalbuminemic patients who were receiving as much as 23 g of sodium per day and were in frank anasarca.

Clinically important quantities of sodium may be delivered in a combined fashion to the patient with compromised renal, cardiovascular, hepatic, or nutritional status. Monitoring sodium balance by accurately accounting for total daily intake, physical assessment of the patient, observation of body weight changes, and assessment of 24-hour or spot urinary electrolytes will facilitate rational electrolyte modifications of enteral and parenteral formulas. High-dose synthetic penicillins, corticosteroids, and hypotensives can have a major impact on patient fluid and sodium balance as a result of inherent electrolyte content (antibiotics) or increases in renal tubular sodium and fluid retention (corticosteroids, hypotensives). On the other hand, overly aggressive therapy of edematous patients with potent natriuretic diuretics (>1 kg weight loss/day) such as furosemide may result in severe hyponatremia and seizures. Hyponatremia due to diuretic therapy is generally considered rare unless accompanied by severe dietary restrictions of sodium. Thiazide-induced natriuresis is generally self-limited with continued therapy because of proximal renal tubule readjustment to maintain sodium balance (84,85).

Alterations of Potassium Balance

Potassium balance can be influenced by numerous physiologic events, nutritional support, and drug therapy. Hypokalemia may represent depletion of body potassium

TABLE 30.15 Selected Drugs Reported to Alter Magnesium (Mg) Balance

Drug	Proposed Mechanism
Hypermagnesemia	
Mg-containing antacids	GI absorption of Mg (bioavailability = 15-30%) with concomitant renal impairment
Mg-containing salts	
Spironolactone	↓ Renal excretion, concurrent renal impairment
Hypomagnesemia	
Amphotericin B	Renal tubular defect (91,92)
Cisplatin	Renal tubular defect; persistent renal Mg leak (83,99,111-113)
Digoxin	↑ Renal excretion, Mg wasting (107,114)
Ethacrynic Acid	↑ Renal excretion, Mg wasting (84,85,114)
Furosemide	↑ Renal excretion, Mg wasting (84,85,114)
Gentamicin, tobramycin (multiple course)	Renal tubular defect, Mg wasting (115-118)
Insulin	Anabolic intracellular shift (107)
Laxatives	↑ GI losses (119)
Mannitol	↑ Renal excretion (79,114)
Saline infusion	↑ Renal excretion (107)
Thiazide diuretics	↑ Renal excretion (may need other predisposing factors) (84,85,114)

TABLE 30.16 Selected Drugs Reported to Alter Calcium Balance

Drug	Proposed Mechanism
Hypercalcemia	
Androgens	Associated with cancer activation (107)
Ca salts, antacids	Excessive intake
Chlorthalidone	
IV fat	Pseudohypercalcemia (120)
Lithium	↓ Urinary Ca excretion (79)
Tamoxifen	
Thiazide diuretics	↓ Urinary Ca excretion (84,85)
Vitamin D analogues	↑ Intestinal calcium absorption, ↑ bone resorption (79)
Vitamin A	Chronic ingestion of ≥50,000 units/day (79)
Hypocalcemia	
β-Adrenergic blockers	↓ Parathyroid hormone action (79,107)
Blood transfusions	Transient Ca complexation with citrated blood (79)
Calcitonin	↓ Bone absorption (107)
Cimetidine	Impaired parathyroid function (79,107)
Cisplatin	Renal tubular defect, hypomagnesemia (79,83,99)
Colchicine	↓ Parathyroid hormone secretion, action (107)
Corticosteroids	↓ Intestinal absorption, ↑ urinary excretion, ↓ bone absorption (81,107,121)
Ethacrynic acid	↑ Renal excretion
Furosemide	↑ Renal excretion, ↓ parathyroid hormone secretion, action (84,85)
Gentamicin (multiple course)	Renal tubule defect resulting in magnesuria, possible secondary hypocalcemia (115,117)
Glucagon	(107)
Heparin	Pseudohypocalcemia (122)
Mithramycin	↓ Bone resorption (79,107)
PO$_4$-containing laxatives	Chronic ingestion of large doses (79,107)
PO$_4$ supplementation	Overly aggressive IV supplementation, Ca complexation (79,107,123)
Phenobarbital	Altered vitamin D metabolism (79,107)
Phenytoin (chronic use)	Altered vitamin D metabolism (79,107)
Theophylline	(107)
Sodium nitroprusside	(107)

stores, anabolism, and increased GI losses as a consequence of diarrhea, vomiting, nasogastric suction, fistulas or drainage, renal tubular losses as a consequence of altered tubular transport (renal tubular acidosis), diuretic therapy, and high-dose penicillin therapy. Hyperkalemia may be related to compromised renal function, catabolic trauma, metabolic acidosis, multiple blood transfusions, and reabsorption of GI blood. The total available potassium load from whole blood transfusions varies as a function of storage time, with

TABLE 30.17   Sodium Content of Various IV Solutions

IV Solution	Na/liter (mEq)	Na/liter (g)
Sodium chloride, 0.2%	34	0.8
Sodium chloride, 0.45%	77	1.8
Sodium chloride, 0.9%	154	3.5
Lactated Ringer's solution	124-137	2.8-3.2
Normal serum albumin, 5%	32	0.7
Normal serum albumin, 25%	130-160	3.0-3.7
Plasma protein fraction	130-160	3.0-3.7

TABLE 30.18   Inherent Electrolyte Content of Antibiotics

Antibiotic	Sodium Content (mEq/g)		Potassium Content
Ampicillin	2.9		
Azlocillin	2.2		
Carbenicillin	4.7		
Cefamandole	3.3		
Cefazolin	2.1		
Cefotaxime	2.2		
Cefoxitin	2.3		
Ceftizoxime	2.6		
Cephalothin	2.8		
Cephapirin	2.4		
Cephradine	6.0	(with sodium carbonate)	
	0	(sodium free)	
Chloramphenicol	2.2		
Methicillin	2.9		
Metronidazole	28.0		
Mezlocillin	1.85		
Moxalactam	3.8		
Nafcillin	2.9		
Oxacillin	2.8		
Penicillin G sodium	10.0	mEq/5 mil. units	
Piperacillin	1.85		
Ticarcillin	5.2-6.5		
Penicillin G potassium			8.5 mEq/5 mil. units

TABLE 30.19   Calculation of Daily Sodium (Na) Intake in Hospitalized Patients

Source	Amount/24 hr	Na Content	mEq Na/24 hr
NaCl, 0.9%	1.2 liters	154 mEq/liter	185
Sustacal	2.4 liters	39 mEq/liter	94
Ticarcillin	24 g	6 mEq/g	144
			423

approximately 10 mEq/liter and 20 mEq/liter available after 10 and 21 days, respectively (124). In addition, hyperkalemia may be an artifact of red blood cell or platelet hemolysis associated with blood sampling methodology. Drug-induced hyperkalemia may result from the use of potassium-sparing diuretics, potassium supplements, salt substitute overuse, inherent drug-potassium content, or chemotherapeutic lysis of tumor cells.

Hypokalemia. Drug-induced intracellular potassium shifts (e.g., insulin) and increased renal potassium losses (e.g., diuretics, corticosteroids, high-dose penicillins) in association with anabolic nutrition support and/or GI potassium losses may precipitate a rapid and severe hypokalemia requiring aggressive intervention. Anticipation of these events, especially in the malnourished patient, is complemented by careful monitoring of serum and urinary electrolytes.

The administration of high-dose penicillin therapy may result in significant urinary wasting of potassium, necessitating aggressive potassium supplementation ($\geq$ 60-100 mEq KCl/day) to combat hypokalemia (93-98). Carbenicillin and ticarcillin have been reported to act as nonreabsorbable anions in the distal renal tubule, promoting a dose-dependent urinary potassium excretion and hypokalemia (94). This may be accompanied by a secondary metabolic alkalosis aggravated by urinary acid losses. Other penicillins (e.g., ampicillin, penicillin G sodium) may act in a similar manner when given in high dosages (93,103,104). Although nafcillin has an extrarenal pathway of excretion, an apparent association between nafcillin administration and urinary potassium wasting consistent with one published report has been noted on occasion (103). It has been theorized that redistribution of body potassium stores may also be contributing to the development of penicillin-induced hypokalemia (96). Whatever the specific mechanism(s) of action, the following seem to be consistent observations concerning the effects of high-dose ($\geq$ 20 g/day) ticarcillin or carbenicillin therapy on potassium balance in adults:

1. Urinary potassium excretion and predisposition to hypokalemia increase markedly within the first 24-72 hours of therapy.
2. Urinary potassium losses may vary from 50-250$^+$ mEq/day.
3. Serum potassium concentrations decline more rapidly in patients with low potassium baselines (<3.5 mEq/liter), often declining below 3 mEq/liter without aggressive supplementation.
4. Despite hypokalemia, marked urinary potassium excretion persists throughout penicillin therapy, requiring continued supplementation.
5. Resolution of potassium wasting usually occurs within 48 hours of antibiotic discontinuation.
6. The induced hypokalemia seems somewhat nonresponsive to spironolactone therapy.
7. Concurrent corticosteroid therapy increases observed potassium wasting.

Serum potassium decreases of 10-30%/day may be observed in conjunction with carbenicillin dosages of 400-500 mg/kg/day. Use of therapeutically equivalent but comparatively lower molar dosages of ticarcillin may modify the degree of renal potassium wasting observed.

Clinicians must anticipate the need for additional potassium supplementation in excess of anabolic requirements and plan the route of administration when a patient is to start receiving carbenicillin or ticarcillin therapy. Some clinicians institute potassium supplementation at the outset of carbenicillin/ticarcillin therapy after assessing renal function. Depending on the daily dosage of potassium chloride required to maintain adequate serum levels, supplementation may be provided intravenously or by dilution in the feeding formula. During enteral nutrition therapy, large daily requirements for potassium may necessitate parenteral replacement rather than formula supplementation to ensure continued tube feeding tolerance. Avoidance of using parenteral nutrition solutions to provide all potassium requirements until potassium balance is stabilized will help to prevent costly wasting of nutrition formulations. (The same is applicable to insulin admixture.)

With the exception of the potassium-sparing diuretics (e.g., spironolactone, triamterene), diuretics have the infamous distinction of causing hypokalemia. The extent of diuretic-induced potassium loss varies with diuretic potency and clinical status of the patient. Hypertensive patients chronically treated with thiazide diuretics seldom have a total body potassium deficit exceeding 200 mEq (5% body stores). Although isolated patients receiving thiazides may experience an extensive kaliuresis associated with dietary sodium restriction, dietary sources of potassium will usually be sufficient to avoid significant hypokalemia. Patients treated with potent diuretics such as furosemide and ethacrynic acid may have a more extensive kaliuresis and be more predisposed to the development of hypokalemia (84,85). Patients with malnutrition, congestive heart failure, cirrhosis, and ascites who are treated with potent diuretics are particularly prone to severe hypokalemia. This patient population may already have severe total body potassium deficits prior to a diuretic insult on potassium balance.

Hyperkalemia. Hyperkalemia is a potentially serious complication of therapy with potassium-sparing diuretics such as spironolactone, and it may occur when spironolactone is used alone or in combination with thiazide diuretics (85,89). Hyperkalemia is usually associated with the presence of other predisposing factors such as coadministration of potassium supplements, salt substitutes, high endogenous potassium loads due to tissue catabolism or hemolysis, diabetes, or compromised renal function (i.e., creatinine clearance < 50 ml/min). Spironolactone is contraindicated in severe renal failure because of its inhibitory effects on renal tubular potassium secretion and sodium-potassium exchange. Because of the half-life of spironolactone's active metabolites, maximal therapeutic effects of the drug are not seen for 2-3 days with continued dosing. Onset of hyperkalemia may be insidious, and potassium levels should be monitored closely when initiating therapy or during a change in clinical status. In the absence of predisposing factors, however, problems are not usually observed with spironolactone-induced hyperkalemia.

Alterations of Calcium and Magnesium Balance

Diuretic therapy may alter calcium and magnesium balance. Thiazide diuretics reportedly decrease urinary calcium excretion up to 40% from baseline, and elevated serum calcium levels may be observed after a week of therapy (84,85). These effects may be transient and are generally not clinically significant unless there is preexisting hypercalcemia (e.g., neoplasm, hyperparathyroidism). On the other hand, diuretics such as furosemide and ethacrynic acid increase urinary calcium excretion and may lower serum levels.

Severe hypomagnesemia is characterized by both decreased serum and urinary magnesium concentrations (125,126). Predisposing factors include magnesium-deficient nutrition support, malabsorption, chronic alcoholism, pancreatitis, and chronic or excessive GI fluid losses from vomiting, diarrhea, nasogastric suctioning, and lower bowel or biliary fistulas (107,119,125). Medications associated with clinically significant hypomagnesemia are listed in Table 30.15 and include diuretics (84,85,114), aminoglycosides (115-118), amphotericin B (91,92), and cisplatin (83,99,111-113).

Significant magnesium depletion may be observed in patients treated chronically with thiazide diuretics, furosemide, and ethacrynic acid (30,128). The fact that significant magnesium depletion may occur with these diuretics has largely been ignored by clinicians and should be reemphasized. Recent reports have demonstrated the essentiality of magnesium in the restoration of intracellular potassium concentrations by potassium supplementation (127,128) and cited the association of kaliuresis and phosphaturia with magnesium deficiency. Coexisting deficits of magnesium and potassium are frequently observed in chronic alcoholism, malnutrition, hyperaldosterone states, and patients with GI losses (107,119).

Cisplatin-Induced Electrolyte Imbalances

Cisplatin nephrotoxicity may be characterized by acute tubular necrosis (ATN) or more subtle effects on renal tubular function. Cisplatin-induced ATN may result in elevations of serum urea nitrogen, creatinine, potassium, and phosphate (113). Nephrotoxicity may also be characterized by persistent renal magnesium wasting and hypomagnesemia with accompanying hypokalemia and hypocalcemia (83,111,112). A renal tubular defect allowing for a selective magnesium "leak" is hypothesized, with preliminary evidence indicating that magnesium loss is unrelated to changes in glomerular filtration rate or cisplatin dosage. Diuretics, saline diuresis, and aminoglycosides may further enhance renal magnesium losses. Hypokalemia and hypocalcemia have been attributed to a deficiency of magnesium by various mechanisms, and replacement of all three ions may be needed chronically to restore body stores, normalize serum levels, and facilitate glucose utilization.

Amphotericin B–Induced Electrolyte Imbalances

Amphotericin B disrupts normal cation exchange in the distal renal tubules resulting in renal tubular acidosis and urinary potassium wasting. Hypokalemia commonly occurs in association with renal tubular acidosis but may be evident within the first 2 weeks of therapy independent of renal tubular acidosis. Urinalysis may reveal an alkaline urine pH and the equivalent of 100-200 mEq of potassium lost per day. In addition, serum magnesium levels are frequently observed to decrease with amphotericin B therapy and must be closely monitored (91,92).

Antacid-Induced Electrolyte Imbalances

Antacids may be associated with clinically significant alterations in phosphate and magnesium balance due to their specific cation content. Profound and serious hypophosphatemia may occur within 24-48 hours of initiating nutrition support with inadequate phosphate supplementation (107-110,129). With normal renal function, adult patients generally require $7-10^+$ mmol of phosphate per 1000 nonprotein kcal (107,129). Predisposing factors to severe hypophosphatemia (serum concentration < 1 mg%) include severe protein-calorie malnutrition, diabetes mellitus, chronic alcoholism, pancreatitis, sepsis, respiratory alkalosis, and therapy with aluminum-containing antacids (105-108). Aluminum-containing antacids bind both dietary and intestinally-secreted phosphate (107), with phosphate-binding capacity being a function of aluminum content. When comparing similar antacid volumes, the phosphate-binding capacity for various antacid products is quantitatively related as follows: ALternaGEL, Basaljel, Gelusil-II, Maalox TC, Mylanta-II > Gelusil, Gelusil M, Maalox, Maalox Plus, > Amphojel, Mylanta, > Riopan, and Riopan Plus (130).

The GI absorption of magnesium during chronic therapy with magnesium-containing antacids (150-300 ml/day) in patients with significant renal compromise (creatinine clearance ≤ 20 ml/min) may result in hypermagnesemia and magnesium intoxication (126).

Glucose Intolerance and Insulin Usage

Numerous factors may alter glucose tolerance during nutrition support, including diabetic predisposition, disease process, hormonal state, potassium and phosphate status, glucose infusion rate change, cellular glucose oxidation rate, and medications. Glucose intolerance is frequently observed in association with sepsis-stress-steroids or uremia and may serve as an early warning of sepsis prior to observed elevations in white blood cell count or body temperature. The pancreatitic patient may have a highly unpredictable response to a glucose load, depending on extent of organ compromise.

Maximal cellular glucose utilization rates of 7 mg/kg/min have been reported in surgical patients receiving parenteral nutrition (131). Glucose infusion rates in excess of 6-7 mg/kg/min may contribute to an increased incidence of hyperglycemia, fatty liver infiltration, and excessive carbon dioxide production without benefiting further energy production (131). Highly stressed or septic patients may not tolerate glucose infusion rates in excess of 4-5 mg/kg/min (132). Exogenous insulin administration in these patients may normalize serum glucose without improving cellular glucose oxidation (132).

Selected medications that may alter glucose metabolism by inhibiting peripheral glucose utilization or pancreatic insulin secretion are listed in Table 30.20. Corticosteroid-induced glucose intolerance is discussed further under "Cor-

TABLE 30.20 Medications Potentially Affecting Glucose Metabolism (133,134,137-140)

Clinical Observation	
Hyperglycemia	*Hypoglycemia*
Bumetanide[a]	Anabolic steroids
Chlorpromazine[a]	Clofibrate
Chlorthalidone	Disopyramide[a]
Clonidine[a]	Fenfluramine
Colchicine[a]	Guanethidine[a]
Corticosteroids	Haloperidol[a]
Dextran-40,75[c]	Insulin
Diazoxide	Pentamidine
Dopamine	Propranolol, β-blocker class (highly
Epinephrine	variable effects)
Ethacrynic acid (highly variable effects)	Sulfonylureas
Furosemide	
Isoproterenol	
Lithium carbonate	
Metolazone	
Nifedipine[a,b]	
Phenytoin[a,b]	
Prazosin[a]	
Probenecid	
Propranolol (highly variable effects)	
Theophylline	
Thiazide diuretics	
Triamterene	
Verapamil[a,b]	

[a]Limited or conflicting reports, further substantiation needed.
[b]May apply only to noninsulin-dependent diabetics.
[c]False increase by o-toluidine methods.

ticosteroid-Induced Changes." Temporal association of medication administration with a change in glucose status may necessitate a reevaluation of intracellular electrolyte status, insulin dosage requirements, and glucose infusion rate. Possible medication interference with interpretation of urine glucose concentrations must also be considered (133,134).

Regular insulin may be administered by admixture in parenteral nutrition solutions, via subcutaneous or IV sliding-scale coverage, or by a separate, continuous low-dose insulin infusion. Short-acting, regular insulin is preferred during continuous nutrition support because longer acting insulins may predispose the patient to hypoglycemia if alimentation is unexpectedly interrupted. Intravenous administration of insulin is the preferred route in critically ill patients since subcutaneous injections may be poorly or erratically absorbed. Numerous variables affect the pharmacokinetics of insulin adsorption to glass and plastic surfaces of parenteral nutrition delivery systems (24), but up to 50% adsorptive loss may occur (135). Albumin addition is not recommended for the purpose of decreasing insulin adsorption to these delivery systems, since overall adsorption may only be decreased marginally and patients can be successfully titrated to clinical response without the costly use of albumin (24). A reasonable approach in titrating adult insulin requirements during parenteral nutrition includes (1) judicious addition of 50% of the previous day's sliding-scale insulin requirements to the next day's parenteral nutrition solutions (avoiding hypoglycemia) and (2) addition of in-

TABLE 30.21 Medication-Induced Acid-Base Disorders (79,141,143)

Drug	Proposed Mechanism
Metabolic alkalosis	
Ampicillin	↑ Renal hydrogen secretion (93)
Blood, packed RBC	Metabolism of citrate anticoagulant to bicarbonate (citrate mEq/unit = 17 blood, 5 packed RBC) (79,141)
Carbenicillin	↑ Renal hydrogen secretion (79,94,97,141)
Corticosteroids	↑ Renal hydrogen secretion, ↑ renal bicarbonate reabsorption, hypokalemia (79,81)
Ethacrynic acid	↑ Renal hydrogen secretion, ↑ renal bicarbonate reabsorption, hypokalemia, hypovolemia, hypochloremia (79,141,143)
Furosemide	Same as ethacrynic acid
Ringer's lactate solution	Large volumes—bicarbonate precursor
Sodium bicarbonate, acetate, citrate, lactate	Source of alkali, bicarbonate precursors
Thiazide diuretics	↑ Renal hydrogen secretion, ↑ renal bicarbonate reabsorption (79)
Ticarcillin	↑ Renal hydrogen secretion (79)
Metabolic acidosis	
Acetazolamide	↓ Renal acid secretion (transient), ↑ renal bicarbonate excretion (79,148-150)
Amiloride	↓ Renal hydrogen secretion (151)
Ampicillin	Diarrheal bicarbonate losses (79)
Amphotericin B	Distal renal tubular acidosis (rare systemic acidosis) (91,143)
Cholestyramine resin	↑ Intestinal bicarbonate loss via chloride-bicarbonate exchange (79)
Clindamycin	Diarrheal bicarbonate losses (79)
Colchicine	Diarrheal bicarbonate losses (79)
Laxatives	↑ Intestinal bicarbonate loss (79)
Sodium nitroprusside	Lactic acidosis secondary to cyanide toxicity (79)
Spironolactone	↓ Renal hydrogen secretion (152)
Sulfamylon	Carbonic anhydrase inhibitor (79,141)
Tetracycline	Antianabolic ↑ uremia in renal compromise (79)
Toxins (methanol, ethylene glycol, salicylates, paraldehyde)	Accumulation of organic/inorganic acids (79,141)
Cimetidine, ranitidine	Inhibitory effect on gastric acid secretion decreases volume and acid loss secondary to nasogastric suction, blunting tendency to metabolic alkalosis (144-147)

sulin to parenteral nutrition formulas in increments no smaller than 5 units (24). Insulin requirements frequently decrease with resolution of infection, improvement of uremia, and during continued hemodialysis. Renal insulin metabolism and excretion is diminished during renal failure (136); thus, a prolonged insulin half-life necessitates a cautious use of lower insulin dosages. Appreciation of these dynamic variables will help to avoid costly wasting of formulas due to excessive insulin addition.

Acid-Base Imbalances

Many primary and compensatory pathophysiologic factors affect acid-base status during nutrition support (141). In addition, excretion of an acid load may be compromised in the protein-malnourished patient secondary to speculated deficits in renal ammoniagenesis (142). Table 30.21 lists selected drug-induced acid-base disturbances. Patients receiving cimetidine or ranitidine during nutrition support may be less susceptible to metabolic alkalosis induced by nasogastric suctioning, since the volume of gastric acid loss is decreased with these agents (144-147).

Medication Fluid Volumes

Polypharmacy and colloid-crystalloid administration frequently limits the fluid volume that can be allocated for nutrition support in the critically ill, fluid-restricted patient. Totaling daily fluid input including medication volumes and daily sodium intake from all sources (IV fluids, nutrition support, medications) will frequently reveal a shocking discovery in the edematous patient. In an attempt to limit fluid intake, it is desirable to optimize medication fluid volumes

as much as possible. There is a general lack of information concerning medication administration by central vein (153) as well as maximal medication concentrations that may be given by this route without inducing toxicity. In general, Food and Drug Administration approval for antibiotics and other injectables involves drug concentrations that are intended for peripheral vein administration, thus conforming to administration methods used in clinical trials.

Until more information becomes available, the clinician can attempt to reasonably limit medication fluid volumes by identifying maximal drug concentrations that ensure solubility and are approved for administration. Selected medication fluid volumes, adapted from Rapp et al (154) and Trissel (155) are presented in Table 30.22. Efforts to modify medication volumes must be coordinated with the pharmacy admixture service.

Corticosteroid-Induced Changes

Corticosteroids have a marked impact on nutritional status, assessment, and therapy because they influence carbohydrate, protein, and fat metabolism as well as fluid and electrolyte balance (81,121,156). It is important to anticipate the toxic effects of acute therapy and recognize the metabolic changes induced by chronic therapy. The biologic spectrum of effects is dependent on glucocorticoid and mineralocorticoid potencies, dosages used, duration of therapy, and preexisting patient status.

Glucocorticoids stimulate gluconeogenic enzymes and promote hepatic gluconeogenesis from circulating amino acids. They produce a state of "insulin resistance" by inhibiting insulin binding to peripheral receptor sites, thus decreasing glucose utilization by interfering with cellular

TABLE 30.22   Selected Medication Fluid Volumes (154,155)

Medication	Maximal Concentration/Rate Recommended for Peripheral Line Injection	Comment
Acetazolamide	500 mg/5 ml, over 1-2 min	
Acyclovir	7 mg/ml, over 60 min	
Amikacin	Dose/100 ml, over 30-60 min	Smaller, nonapproved volumes have been used, i.e., dose/15 ml over 30 min
Aminophylline	No dilution required, maximal rate 25 mg/min	Available 25 mg/ml
Amphotericin B	0.1 mg/ml, over 4-6 hr	Nonapproved concentrations up to 0.3 mg/ml have been administered by central vein; documentation needed
Ampicillin	1 g/10 ml, over 10-15 min	
Azlocillin	1 g/10 ml, over 5-30 min	
Bumetanide	Dose over 1-2 min	Available 0.25 mg/ml
Carbenicillin	1 g/5 ml, over 2-15 min	
Cefamandole	1 g/10 ml, over 3-30 min	
Cefazolin	1 g/10 ml, over 3-30 min	
Cefotaxime	1 g/5 ml, over 3-30 min	
Cefoxitin	1 g/5 ml, over 3-30 min	
Ceftizoxime	1 g/10 ml, over 3-30 min	
Cephalothin	1 g/10 ml, over 3-30 min	
Cephapirin	1 g/10 ml, over 3-30 min	
Cephradine	1 g/10 ml, over 3-30 min	
Chloramphenicol	1 g/10 ml, over 1-30 min	
Cimetidine	300 mg/20 ml, over 1-20 min	
Clindamycin	300 mg/50 ml, over 10 min	Must be diluted prior to infusion
Dexamethasone Na phosphate	Dose over several minutes	Direct IV administration; available 4 mg/ml
Diazepam	No dilution required, maximal rate 2 mg/min	Available 5 mg/ml
Digoxin	Dose over 1-5 min	Direct IV administration; available 0.1 and 0.25 mg/ml
Erythromycin gluceptate	500 mg/100 ml, over 20-60 min	
Erythromycin lactobionate	500 mg/100 ml, over 20-60 min	
Ethacrynic acid	50 mg/50 ml, over several minutes	
Furosemide	No dilution required	Available 10 mg/ml
Gentamicin	Dose/50 ml, over 30-120 min	Smaller, nonapproved volumes have been used, i.e., dose/15 ml over 30 min
Hydralazine	No dilution required	20 mg/ml
Hydrocortisone Na succinate	No dilution required, 100 mg/2 ml, over 1 min; ≥500 mg over 10 min	
Meperidine	10 mg/ml, infuse very slowly	Available 25-100 mg/ml
Methyldopa	100 mg/10 ml, over 30-60 min	
Methylprednisolone Na succinate	No dilution required, maximal rate 50 mg/min (high-dose therapy over 10-20 min)	
Metoclopramide	10 mg/2 ml, over 1-2 min	
Metronidazole	500 mg/100 ml ready to use, over 60 min; 500 mg/62.5 ml IV, over 60 min	IV form requires pH neutralization
Mezlocillin	1 g/10 ml, over 3-30 min	
Miconazole	Dose/200 ml, over 30-60 min	Dose + 50 ml, over 60 min by central vein with fluid restriction (manufacturer)
Morphine	Dose slowly	Direct IV administration; available 8, 10, and 15 mg/ml
Moxalactam	1 g/10 ml, over 3-30 min	
Nafcillin	1 g/15 ml, over 5-60 min	
Netilmicin	Dose/50 ml, over 30-120 min	
Oxacillin	1 g/20 ml, over 10-30 min	
Penicillin G, potassium	¼ daily dose/unstated volume, over 60-120 min	Administration rate dependent on K content
Phenytoin	No dilution required, maximal rate 50 mg/min	Available 50 mg/ml
Piperacillin	1 g/5 ml, over 3-30 min	
Procainamide	Dose at maximal rate 50 mg/min	Available 100 mg/ml and 500 mg/ml (*must be diluted*)
Quinidine gluconate	16 mg/ml at 1 ml/min	Available 80 mg/ml
Tetracycline	500 mg/100 ml, infuse slowly	
Ticarcillin	1 g/4 ml, infuse slowly	
Tobramycin	Dose/50 ml, over 20-60 min	Smaller, nonapproved volumes have been used, i.e., dose/15 ml over 30 min
Trimethoprim/sulfamethoxazole	5 ml/75 ml, over 60-90 min	Fluid restriction 5 ml/50 ml, 2-hr expiration (manufacturer)
Vancomycin	500 mg/100 ml, over 20-30 min	Some recommend 60 min infusion time vs histamine-like reaction
Verapamil	No dilution required, maximal rate 5 mg/min	Available 2.5 mg/ml; administer dosage over minimum 3 min in elderly
Vidarabine	450 mg/1000 ml, over 12-24 hr	Do not refrigerate, prewarming may facilitate dissolution; in-line filter recommended

glucose uptake despite augmented serum insulin concentrations. Corticosteroid-induced amino acid mobilization from muscle and liver provides a ready substrate for hepatic glycogen formation and deposition (156). Acute corticosteroid therapy induces hyperglycemia in nondiabetic patients, and diabetic patients frequently need upward titration of insulin requirements. With chronic therapy some degree of adaptation usually occurs in both diabetic and nondiabetic patients, and serum glucose concentrations return toward pretreatment values (157-159). The duration of corticosteroid-induced hyperglycemia appears to be dose related, with peak serum glucose concentrations occurring approximately 8 hours after drug administration (160).

Corticosteroids other than dexamethasone possess varying degrees of mineralocorticoid activity and act on the distal renal tubules to enhance sodium reabsorption and increase potassium and hydrogen excretion (156,161). Excess mineralocorticoid administration clinically presents as mild hypernatremia, increased extracellular fluid volume with edema, hypokalemia, and metabolic alkalosis (81,121,156,161). In addition, urinary calcium, phosphate, and zinc excretion may be increased (162). The intensity of the pharmacologic effects may be enhanced by hypoalbuminemia (161) and other medications. Larger doses of hydrocortisone may increase renal sodium reabsorption only transiently despite continued therapy, but smaller dosages have been associated with persistent sodium retention and kaliuresis (160).

The catabolic and antianabolic effects of chronic corticosteroid therapy can result in severe muscle wasting, atrophy of lymphatic tissues, osteoporosis from loss of bone protein matrix, thinning of the skin, decubitus formation, and negative nitrogen balance (121,163-165). These agents may also interfere with wound healing, suppress growth, and induce muscle weakness and myopathy (81,121). Interestingly, with routine vitamin status screening, the authors have observed a 50% incidence of severely depressed serum retinol concentrations in patients chronically treated with steroids.

Corticosteroids promote a redistribution of fat from peripheral to central sites and an increase in total body fat content, as characterized by the classic cushingoid manifestations of moon facies, pendulous abdomen, and buffalo hump. They have also been associated with fatty liver infiltration, hyperlipidemia, increased serum cholesterol levels, and marked hypertriglyceridemia, with the lipid profile resembling that of a poorly controlled diabetic (121,166,167). Corticosteroids may facilitate the lipolytic effects of epinephrine and norepinephrine on adipose tissue (156).

Anthropometric standards have not been established for steroid-treated patients. Baseline anthropometric measurements and laboratory tests are important so that the patient may serve as his/her own control for future evaluation of nutritional status. Beware the "moon face" that may "mask" the malnourished individual lying under the bedsheets. In addition, corticosteroids possess dose-related, reversible immunologic depressant effects on thymus-derived T lymphocytes (involved in cell-mediated immunity) and bone marrow–derived B lymphocytes (involved in antibody production) (81,121,165). Consequently, these drugs interfere with delayed hypersensitivity skin testing and may produce false negative results. Corticosteroids acutely enhance

TABLE 30.23   Nutritional Assessment Findings in Patients Receiving Chronic Glucocorticoid Therapy

Serum electrolytes	Micronutrient status
↑ Sodium	↓ Serum/RBC zinc
↓ Potassium, phosphate, calcium	↓ Serum vitamin A
Glucose metabolism	Anthropometric/physical findings
↑ Serum/urine glucose	Edema
Protein metabolism	↑ Body fat
↑ BUN, UUN	Moon facies
Negative nitrogen balance	Impaired wound healing
Fat metabolism	↓ Arm muscle circumference
↑ Serum cholesterol	Negative skin tests
↑ Serum triglycerides	Osteomalacia

intravascular to extravascular redistribution of lymphocytes, resulting in lymphocytopenia that is independent of nutritional status (161). In addition, corticosteroid-induced leukocytosis may be differentiated from the leukemoid reaction of infection, since the latter is accompanied by an increase in immature band forms and toxic granulation (168).

Clinical patient findings during corticosteroid therapy are summarized in Table 30.23. These frequently include (1) elevated fasting serum glucose concentrations, (2) elevated BUN and BUN:serum creatinine ratios proportional to the degree of catabolism and renal compromise, (3) altered electrolyte and trace mineral status, (4) persistent negative nitrogen balance (4-6 g/day), and (5) decreases in serum and urinary creatinine paralleling muscle wasting and decreased creatinine production. Acute steroid therapy in seriously ill and injured patients has been shown to increase urinary urea nitrogen and creatinine excretion (169). In practice, a cautious approach to initiating nutrition support and achieving estimated caloric requirements in the steroid-treated patient should include the following:

1. Judicious use of insulin and potassium supplementation to facilitate glucose utilization and potassium homeostasis
2. Use of low-sodium feedings
3. Use of optimal protein-calorie percentage formulas to improve nitrogen balance without causing excessive ureagenesis (170,171)
4. Close daily monitoring to include weight change, intake and output, and serum and urine electrolytes

The clinician must anticipate the relative glucocorticoid and mineralocorticoid properties of the various corticosteroids and plan therapeutic maneuvers during nutrition support to avoid serious metabolic aberrations. For instance, the use of a potent mineralocorticoid can be expected to increase the risk for a hypokalemic metabolic alkalosis, which may further impair the respiratory status of a patient during nutrition support. Substitution of an equivalent dosage of a less potent mineralocorticoid may facilitate the use of more standard electrolyte additives to a parenteral nutrition formula.

Nephrotoxicity

Recognition of potentially nephrotoxic medications taken prior to admission and during hospitalization in conjunction with prospective monitoring of renal function facilitates modification of nutrition formula design to prevent excessive ureagenesis. Selected medications associated with acute or chronic nephrotoxicity include aminoglycosides, amphotericin B, cisplatin, pentamidine, radiographic contrast media, lithium, and certain analgesics (172). Additive nephrotoxic effects may result from combined use of antibiotics such as aminoglycosides, vancomycin, and amphotericin B. Dynamic changes in the creatinine and urea clearance rates in critically ill patients necessitate nutritional formula design manipulation of caloric density, protein-calorie percentage (171), or energy-nitrogen ratio (173), to maintain BUN concentrations < 100 mg% or BUN:serum creatinine ratios < 20:1 + 10.

Hypoprothrombinemia

It has been theorized that broad-spectrum antibiotic therapy, especially with agents that undergo extensive biliary secretion, causes hypoprothrombinemia by inhibition of vitamin K-producing intestinal bacteria (174,175). Not all antibiotics that achieve high biliary concentrations have been associated with an increased incidence of hypoprothrombinemia. Furthermore, there is no evidence in humans that the bacterial forms of vitamin K (menaquinones) are related to prothrombin synthesis or are absorbed from the GI tract (176,177).

Hypoprothrombinemia and bleeding disorders have been reported in patients receiving the cephalosporin antibiotics cefamandole (175,178,179), moxalactam (180,181), and ceftriaxone (182). Although the mechanism for the hypoprothrombinemia is in dispute (175,176,183-185), these cephalosporins and cefoperazone share a common 1-methyl-5-thiotetrazole side chain that has resulted in a dose-dependent inhibition of hepatic prothrombin synthesis in an animal model (176,184,185). Moxalactam may also impair platelet function (186) in addition to possessing hypoprothrombinemic properties. Other antibiotics associated with a dose-dependent impairment of platelet aggregation and prolonged bleeding times include penicillin G, ticarcillin, and carbenicillin (174,187-189).

The onset of cephalosporin-induced hypoprothrombinemia usually occurs within 4-6 days and is responsive to administration of fresh frozen plasma. Although it has been reported that the hypoprothrombinemia is responsive to vitamin K administration (179,190), the delayed recovery (within ≥ 24 hours) is atypical of a true vitamin K deficiency (185). Patients with a history of poor dietary intake should be closely monitored for cephalosporin-induced hypoprothrombinemia. Clinical correlates associated with greater risk for bleeding include malnutrition, renal failure, and surgical trauma (190).

PHARMACOKINETIC ALTERATIONS DURING MALNUTRITION AND REPLETION

The diverse pathophysiologic changes that can occur during protein-calorie malnutrition support the contention that drug response and disposition may be altered during malnutrition (191-193). Numerous alterations in GI physiology collectively favor a potential decrease in rate and extent of oral drug absorption (191). Deficits in lean body mass and changes in the extracellular fluid and fat compartments and the circulating protein pool may modify a drug's volume of distribution or alter the intensity of pharmacologic response (191,192). Consequently, interpretation of therapeutic serum drug concentrations (e.g., phenytoin) may differ in the malnourished state. Although alterations of metabolic enzyme systems and hepatic drug clearance are anticipated, the overall effect of malnutrition on liver function and drug clearance is complex and difficult to quantitate. The net pharmacologic effect may reflect additive or opposing contributions of altered enzyme activity, hepatic blood flow, and protein binding. In addition, manipulation of dietary components may induce or alter hepatic enzyme activity (194-198). Nonuniform changes in renal function have been observed during malnutrition (191,199-201), and interpretation of estimated creatinine clearance by currently available predictive formulas may have to be qualified in cachectic patients.

Despite evidence suggesting altered pharmacokinetics in malnutrition, there is a distinct lack of systematic, well-controlled studies relating to drug disposition and response in malnourished humans. Study design limitations have included use of small sample sizes and single-dose studies, lack of control groups or replicate assays, failure to address statistical significance, and dependency on animal models or pediatric kwashiorkor patient models. Before-and-after nutritional rehabilitation studies of drug disposition generally fail to define criteria for "nutritional recovery." In addition, there is little reason to assume that pharmacokinetic alterations will be similar in kwashiorkor and marasmus, thus definitive, descriptive criteria for the type and severity of malnutrition must be included in the study design. Further confounding matters is the likelihood that malnutrition can seldom be isolated as the sole pathology affecting drug response, since coexisting factors include primary organ compromise, body-mediated stress responses, and drug-drug interactions. Subclinical malnutrition may present the researcher with a spectrum of subtle and sequential changes affecting pharmacologic response. It is likely that varying degrees of malnutrition have already been included as a covariable in many existing pharmacokinetic studies in chronically ill patients. Although there is a lack of practical knowledge and application in this area (191), an accumulating body of pharmacokinetic data in animal and human studies is raising provocative questions.

Body Composition and Organ Function Changes During Malnutrition and Repletion

Efforts are under way to understand the effects of short-term and chronic malnutrition on organ mass and function. It is apparent that protein-calorie malnutrition may cause major losses of structural and functional organ protein that may alter the efficiency of drug handling. Chronic starvation in humans results in decreases in kidney, liver, and cardiac size and protein content paralleling body weight loss (202). Studies in animal and human starvation demonstrate swelling and atrophy of hepatocytes, decreased microsomal protein, enzyme and phospholipid content, and 25-40% losses of liver protein mass (202). Starvation-induced losses of cardiac protein mass and muscle fiber diameter in dogs has resulted in deficits in myocardial function that respond slowly to refeeding (202). Disruption of the functional integrity of the GI tract during luminal malnutrition results in malabsorption and diarrhea that may perpetuate a vicious cycle of gut mucosal stripping, continued malabsorption, and negative nitrogen balance. Studies in pediatric protein-malnourished patients suggest functional deficits in renal function that are responsive to refeeding (200), whereas limited study in malnourished adults provides conflicting information (191,199,201).

Drug absorption during malnutrition has received minimal attention. In practice, absorption is frequently assumed, but variable absorption is suspected because of increases in GI motility or altered bioavailability. There is an almost absolute lack of information pertaining to drug absorption during continuous enteral feeding (4,5), which may pose different bioavailability conditions than those in absorption studies conducted in healthy volunteers eating regularly spaced meals. In addition, the clinician may be lulled into a false sense of security in assuming adequate drug absorption during nasogastric suctioning. Enteral provision of nutrients results in villous regeneration and increases in mucosal absorptive surface. The impact of mucosal regeneration on drug absorption is largely unexplored.

Nutritional repletion is associated with resolution of edema, increases in serum proteins and active body cell mass, and redistribution of extracellular fluid to the intracellular compartment, all of which may influence drug volume of distribution. Elwyn et al (203) used radioisotopes to compare body water changes in critically ill postoperative patients and patients with chronic wasting disease vs controls. They found significant distortions of extracellular (ECW) and intracellular (ICW) water in both patient groups, with ECW increases of 4 and 5 liters in postoperative and marasmic patients, respectively. Response to parenteral nutrition for 18 ± 10 days in nine patients resulted in a mean ECW decrease of 2 liters with redistribution to the intracellular compartment. Consequently, patients with protein or protein-calorie malnutrition may have a larger than normal volume of distribution per body weight for drugs that distribute primarily to extracellular fluids (e.g., aminoglycosides), and volume of distribution may subsequently change upon refeeding. In the authors' experience, aminoglycoside volume of distributions often vary from 0.3-0.4 liter/kg in malnourished adult patients, with lower than expected peak serum aminoglycoside concentrations achieved after standard dosing per body weight.

Multiple animal and human studies evaluating liver function in starvation reveal a marked and rapid decrease in hepatic microsomal enzyme content and activity consistent with the morphologic changes observed in the starved liver (198,202,204-207). Refeeding has promoted increases in liver microsomal protein, enzyme, and lipid content in animal studies (192,198,206-208). Starvation in animal models has resulted in a decreased rate of metabolism for barbiturates, morphine, and chlorpromazine with resultant increases in sleep time (192,204,209). Interestingly, a high-carbohydrate diet has been reported to transiently "stun" the mixed-function oxidase system in animal models and decrease barbiturate metabolism (209,210). Both oxidative and conjugative pathways of drug metabolism may be compromised in malnutrition and responsive to refeeding, as determined in human studies by decreases in antipyrine (211-216) and propranolol (213) hydroxylation and chlor-

amphenicol (216-218) glucuronidation. Potential impairment of these metabolic pathways during malnutrition supports a cautious approach with respect to drug dosing intervals used for theophylline, phenytoin, diazepam, morphine, barbiturates, propranolol, quinidine, and chloramphenicol. A reported decrease in indocyanine green body clearance in protein-depleted patients (202,219,220) is suggestive of decreased hepatic blood flow and possible impaired clearance of flow-dependent drugs such as morphine, lidocaine, propranolol, theophylline, and verapamil. Increased bromsulphalein retention during malnutrition (221) suggests possible modification of the efficiency of biliary drug excretion, with the effects of parenteral nutrition-associated cholestasis on enterohepatic drug recycling unknown.

The influence of dietary manipulations of carbohydrate, protein, and fat on theophylline and antipyrine kinetics has provided some intriguing information (194-196) and raised important questions concerning the impact of nutrition support and nutrition formula design on theophylline therapy. These dietary crossover studies demonstrated a statistically significant decrease in theophylline half-life during high-protein feedings, suggesting a possible protein-inductive effect on the cytochrome P-450 system. Conversely, a high-carbohydrate/low-protein diet was observed to increase theophylline half-life threefold vs the high-protein diet (196). A high-fat diet was not observed to alter theophylline or antipyrine body clearance (195).

Reports of parenteral nutrition-associated nephromegaly (222) and protein-induced renal tubular hypertrophy (223) raise provocative questions concerning drug renal clearance during nutritional repletion. Additionally, serum creatinine may be inappropriately low and represent a poor index of renal function in patients with severe deficits in lean body mass. Regression equations used to conveniently estimate creatinine clearance on the basis of serum creatinine (224-226) have not been derived in malnourished subjects who frequently excrete less than 10-15 mg/kg/day of urinary creatinine (Cr_u). Comparison of measured vs estimated creatinine clearance in 78 patients excreting $\leq$ 14 mg/kg/day Cr_u revealed a statistically significant overprediction of creatinine clearance by 7-14 ml/min dependent on regression formula used (unpublished observations of the authors).

Buchanan et al (227) used pooled kwashiorkor serum to determine that drug protein binding was not as deranged as might be anticipated. However, it may still be prudent to observe severely hypoalbuminemic patients for a more intense initial pharmacologic response to highly protein-bound drugs that possess low hepatic extraction ratios (e.g., phenytoin, warfarin).

Numerous potential pharmacokinetic alterations are suspected during malnutrition, but overall drug handling is complex and dependent upon the interactive influences of the drug's chemical properties, the type and severity of malnutrition, and the impact of malnutrition on intrinsic hepatic drug clearance, cardiac output and liver blood flow, glomerular filtration rate, and protein binding. Nutritional repletion may facilitate gradual improvement or alteration of the pharmacokinetic processes of absorption, distribution, metabolism, and excretion. Pharmacokinetic description represents an invaluable tool for the future study of dynamic

TABLE 30.24   Pharmacokinetic Studies in Malnutrition and Feeding

Drug	Dosage Form	Population	Alteration
Absorption			
Cefoxitin	IM	Pediatric PM	Unaltered (228)
Chloramphenicol	Oral suspension	Pediatric PCM	Delayed but increased (216-218)
Penicillin G	IM	Pediatric PM	Unaltered (229)
Phenytoin	Oral suspension	Neurosurgical patients	Decreased during continuous enteral feeding (4)
Phenytoin	Capsules	Obstetric patients	Decreased during continuous enteral feeding (5)
Sulfadiazine	Tablets	Pediatric PCM	Delayed (216)
Tetracycline	Capsules	Adult PCM	Unaltered (230)
Tetracycline	Capsules, oral solution	Adult PCM	Decreased (231)
Tobramycin	IM	Pediatric PM	Unaltered (232)
Distribution			
Gentamicin	IV	Pediatric PM	Increased Vd with refeeding (233)
Gentamicin	IV	Pediatric PCM	Increased Vd/weight vs controls (234)
Phenylbutazone	Oral powder	Adult PCM	Increased Vd/weight, decreased protein binding (238)
Theophylline	IV	Pediatric PM, PCM	Increased Vd vs controls (235)
Metabolism			
Antipyrine	IV, oral solution, capsules	Adult, pediatric PCM	Decreased hydroxylation (211-213, 216)
Antipyrine	Oral solution	Pediatric PM	Decreased hydroxylation (214,215)
Antipyrine	Oral solution	Healthy adult subjects	Increased metabolism by high-protein diet (195)
Chloramphenicol	Oral suspension	Pediatric PCM	Decreased glucuronidation (216-218)
Phenylbutazone	Oral powder	Adult PCM	Increased Vd/weight, decreased protein binding (238)
Propranolol	Oral tablet	Adult PCM	Decreased hydroxylation (213)
Sulfadiazine	Tablets, IV	Adult PCM	Increased acetylation (237)
Sulfadiazine	Tablets	Pediatric PCM	Decreased acetylation (216)
Theophylline	Elixir	Healthy adult subjects	Increased metabolism by high-protein diet (195)
Theophylline	Tablet, suspension	Pediatric asthmatics	Increased metabolism by high-protein diet, decreased by high-carbohydrate diet (196)
Theophylline	IV	Pediatric PM, PCM	Nonsignificant decreased clearance vs controls (235)
Excretion			
Gentamicin	IV	Pediatric PM	Increased with nutritional repletion (233)
Gentamicin	IV	Pediatric PCM	Unaltered vs controls (234)
Penicillin G	IV	Pediatric PM	Increased with nutritional repletion (236)

PM = protein malnutrition; PCM = protein-calorie malnutrition; Vd = volume of distribution.

organ function changes occuring during malnutrition and repletion.

The results of selected pharmacokinetic studies in humans during malnutrition or refeeding are summarized in Table 30.24.

REFERENCES

1. Niemiec PW, Vanderveen TW, Morrison JI, et al: Gastrointestinal disorders caused by medication and electrolyte solution osmolality during enteral nutrition. *J Parenter Enter Nutr* 7:387-389, 1983.
2. Roe DA: Interactions between drugs and nutrients. *Med Clin North Am* 63:985-1007, 1979.
3. Cutie AJ, Altman E, Lenkel L: Compatibility of enteral products with commonly employed drug additives. *J Parenter Enter Nutr* 7:186-191, 1983.
4. Bauer LA: Interference of oral phenytoin absorption by continuous nasogastric feedings. *Neurology* 32:570-572, 1982.
5. Hatton RC: Dietary interaction with phenytoin. *Clin Pharm* 3:110-111, 1984.
6. Chapron DJ, Kramer PA, Mariano SL, et al: Effect of calcium and antacids on phenytoin bioavailability. *Arch Neurol* 36:436-438, 1979.
7. Garnett WR, Carter BL, Pellock JM: Effect of calcium and antacids on phenytoin bioavailability (letter). *Arch Neurol* 37:467, 1980.
8. Melander A, Brante G, Johansson O, et al: Influence of food on the absorption of phenytoin in man. *Eur J Clin Pharmacol* 15:269-274, 1979.
9. Johansson O, Wahlin-Boll E, Lindberg T, et al: Opposite effects of carbohydrate and protein on phenytoin absorption in man. *Drug-Nutr Interact* 2:139-144, 1983.
10. Vanderveen TW: Pharmacy involvement in enteral nutrition. *Am J Hosp Pharm* 40:857-859, 1983.
11. Giudici RA, Prendergast BD: A centralized pharmacy enteral tube feeding packaging and distribution system. *Nutr Support Serv* 2:41-49, 1982.
12. Fagerman KE, Flaska L, McCamish MA, et al: Mechanized bulk production of enteral diet: a comparison with manual methods of preparation. *Hosp Pharm* 17:374-379, 1982.
13. Fagerman KE, Dean RE: Bulk production and freezing of elemental enteral feedings. *Nutr Support Serv* 3:8-11, 1983.
14. Fagerman KE, Paauw JD, McCamish MA, et al: Effects of time, temperature, and preservative on bacterial growth in enteral nutrient solutions. *Am J Hosp Pharm* 41:1126-1136, 1984.
15. Furtado D, Parrish A, Beyer P: Enteral nutrient solutions (ENS): in vitro growth supporting properties of ENS for bacteria. *J Parenter Enter Nutr* 4:594, 1980.
16. Allwood MC: Microbial contamination of parenteral and enteral nutrition solutions. *Acta Chir Scand* [Suppl] 507:383-387, 1981.
17. Casewell MW, Cooper JE, Webster M: Enteral feeds contaminated with *Enterobacter cloacae* as a cause of septicemia. *Br Med J* 282:973, 1981.
18. Gill KJ, Gill P: Contaminated enteral feeds. *Br Med J* 282:1971, 1981.
19. Hostetler C, Lipman T, Geraghty M: Bacterial safety of reconstituted continuous drip tube feeding. *J Parenter Enter Nutr* 6:232-235, 1982.
20. Baldwin BA, Zagoren AJ, Rose N: Bacterial contamination of continuously infused enteral alimentation with needle catheter jejunostomy—clinical implications. *J Parenter Enter Nutr* 8:30-33, 1984.
21. Giannella RA, Selwyn BA, Zamcheck N: Influence of gastric acidity on bacterial and parasitic enteric infections. *Ann Intern Med* 78:271-276, 1973.
22. Niemiec PW, Vanderveen TW, Hohenwarter MW, et al: Stability of aminophylline injection in three parenteral nutrient solutions. *Am J Hosp Pharm* 40:428-432, 1983.
23. Tsallas G, Allen LC: Stability of cimetidine hydrochloride in parenteral nutrition solutions. *Am J Hosp Pharm* 39:484-485, 1982.

24. Niemiec PW, Vanderveen TW: Compatibility considerations in parenteral nutrient solutions. *Am J Hosp Pharm* 41:893-911, 1984.

25. Reed MD, Lazarus HM, Herzig RH, et al: Cyclic parenteral nutrition during bone marrow transplantation in children. *Cancer* 51:1563-1570, 1983.

26. Stewart RB, Cluff LE: Gastrointestinal manifestations of adverse drug reactions. *Am J Dig Dis* 19:1-7, 1974.

27. Guyton AC (ed): *Textbook of Medical Physiology,* ed 5. Philadelphia, WB Saunders, 1976, pp 899-900.

28. Tozer TN, Winter ME: Phenytoin. In Evans WE, Schentag JJ, Jusko WJ (eds): *Applied Pharmacokinetics. Principles of Therapeutic Drug Monitoring.* San Francisco, Applied Therapeutics, 275-314, 1980.

29. Bramble MG, Record CO: Drug-induced gastrointestinal disease. *Drugs* 15:451-463, 1978.

30. Dukes MN (ed): *Meyler's Side Effects of Drugs,* ed 9. Amsterdam, Excerpta Medica, 1980.

31. Pietrusko RG: Drug therapy reviews. Pharmacotherapy of diarrhea. *Am J Hosp Pharm* 36:757-767, 1979.

32. Gray GM: Drugs, nutrtion, and carbohydrate absorption. *Am J Clin Nutr* 26:121-124, 1973.

33. Cluff LE, Caranasos GJ, Stewart RB: *Clinical Problems with Drugs.* Philadelphia, WB Saunders Co, 1975.

34. Harvey RJ: Saline purgatives act by releasing cholecystokinin. *Lancet* 2:185, 1973.

35. Kaminski MV, Freed BA: Enteral hyperalimentation: Prevention and treatment of complications. *Nutr Support Serv* 1:29-40, 1981.

36. George WL, Sutter VL, Finegold SM: Antimicrobial agent-induced diarrhea—a bacterial disease. *J Infect Dis* 136:822-828, 1977.

37. Field R, Meyer GW: Diarrhea from cimetidine. *N Engl J Med* 299:262, 1978.

38. Ruddell WS, Losowsky MS: Severe diarrhoea due to small intestinal colonisation during cimetidine treatment. *Br Med J* 280:273, 1980.

39. Triger DR, Slater DN, Goepel JR, et al: Systemic candidiasis complicating acute hepatic failure in patients treated with cimetidine. *Lancet* 2:837-838, 1981.

40. MacKenzie JF, Cochran KM, Russell RI: The effect of frusemide on small intestinal absorption of water and electrolytes. *Gut* 15:831, 1974.

41. Chernoff R: Enteral feedings. *Am J Hosp Pharm* 37:65-74, 1980.

42. Hultgren HN, Swenson R, Wettach G: Cardiac arrest due to oral potassium administration. *Am J Med* 58:139-142, 1975.

43. Mercer CW, Logic JR: Cardiac arrest due to hyperkalemia following intravenous penicillin administration. *Chest* 64:358-359, 1973.

44. Ernst JA, Williams JM, Glick MR, et al: Osmolality of substances used in the intensive care nursery. *Pediatrics* 72:347-352, 1983.

45. White KC, Harkavy KL: Hypertonic formula resulting from added oral medications. *Am J Dis Child* 136:931-933, 1982.

46. Book LS, Herbst JJ, Atherton ST, et al: Necrotizing enterocolitis in low birth weight infants fed an elemental formula. *J Pediatr* 87:602-605, 1975.

47. Willis DM, Chabot J, Radde IC, et al: Unsuspected hyperosmolality of oral solutions contributing to necrotizing enterocolitis in very-low-birth-weight infants. *Pediatrics* 60:535-538, 1977.

48. Book LS, Herbst JJ: Intra-arterial infusions and intestinal necrosis in the rabbit: Potential hazards of umbilical artery injections of ampicillin, glucose, and sodium bicarbonate. *Pediatrics* 65:1145-1149, 1980.

49. Leleiko NS, Murray C, Munro HN: Enteral support of the hospitalized child. In Suskind RM (ed): *Textbook of Pediatric Nutrition.* New York, Raven Press, 1981, pp 357-374.

50. Campos JM, Neto UF, Patricio F, et al: Jejunal mucosa in marasmic children. Clinical, pathological and fine structural evaluation of the effect of protein-energy malnutrition and environmental contamination. *Am J Clin Nutr* 32:1575-1591, 1979.

51. Brunser O, Castillo C, Araya M: Fine structure of the small intestinal mucosa in infantile marasmic malnutrition. *Gastroenterology* 70:495-507, 1976.

52. Kretchmer N: Biology of carbohydrate intolerance in children. In Suskind RM (ed): *Textbook of Pediatric Nutrition.* New York, Raven Press, 1981, pp 475-482.

53. Rosensweig NS, Herman RH: Control of jejunal sucrase and maltase activity by dietary sucrose or fructose in man. *J Clin Invest* 47:2253-2262, 1968.

54. Greene HL, McCabe DR, Merenstein GB: Protracted diarrhea and malnutrition in infancy: Changes in intestinal morphology and disaccharidase activities during treatment with total intravenous nutrition or oral elemental diets. *J Pediatr* 87:695-704, 1975.

55. James W: Intestinal absorption in protein-calorie malnutrition. *Lancet* 1:333-335, 1968.

56. Gray GM, Fogel MR: Nutritional aspects of dietary carbohydrates. In Goodhart RS, Shils ME (eds): *Modern Nutrition in Health and Disease,* ed 6. Philadelphia, Lea & Febiger, 1980, pp 99-112.

57. Olsen WA, Korsmo H: The intestinal brush border membrane in diabetes. *J Clin Invest* 60:181-188, 1977.

58. Rosensweig NS, Herman RH: Time response of jejunal sucrase and maltase activity to a high sucrose diet in normal man. *Gastroenterology* 56:500-505, 1969.

59. Donaldson SS, Lenon RA: Alterations of nutritional status. Impact of chemotherapy and radiation therapy. *Cancer* 43:2036-2052, 1979.

60. Shils ME: Nutritional problems induced by cancer. *Med Clin North Am* 63:1009-1025, 1979.

61. Albibi R, McCallum R: Metoclopramide: Pharmacology and clinical application. *Ann Intern Med* 98:86-95, 1983.

62. Pinder R, Brogden R, Sawyer P, et al: Metoclopramide: A review of its pharmacological properties and clinical use. *Drugs* 12:81-131, 1976.

63. Ponte C, Nappi J: Review of a new gastrointestinal drug: Metoclopramide. *Am J Hosp Pharm* 38:829-833, 1981.

64. Snape WJ, Battle WM, Schwartz SS, et al: Metoclopramide to treat gastroparesis due to diabetes mellitus. *Ann Intern Med* 96:444-446, 1982.

65. Shivshanker K, Bennett R, Haynie T: Tumor-associated gastroparesis: Correction with metoclopramide. *Am J Surg* 145:221-225, 1983.

66. McClelland R, Horton J: Relief of acute, persistent postvagotomy atony by metoclopramide. *Ann Surg* 188:439-447, 1978.

67. James W, Hume R: Action of metoclopramide on gastric emptying and small bowel transit time. *Gut* 9:203-205, 1968.

68. Arvanitakis C, Gonzalez G, Rhodes J: The role of metoclopramide in peroral jejunal biopsy. *Dig Dis Sci* 21:880, 1976.

69. Christie D, Ament M: A double-blind crossover study of metoclopramide versus placebo for facilitating passage of multipurpose biopsy tube. *Gastroenterology* 71:726-728, 1976.

70. Davidson E, Hersh T, Brunner R, et al: The effects of metoclopramide on postoperative ileus. *Ann Surg* 190:27-30, 1979.

71. O'Malley JM, Ferrucci JT, Goodgame JT: Medication bezoar: Intestinal obstruction by an Isocal bezoar, *Gastrointest Radiol* 6:141-143, 1981.

72. Lloyd-Still JD: Cholestyramine therapy and intestinal obstruction in infants. *Pediatrics* 59:626-627, 1977.

73. Poley JR: Cholestyramine and intestinal obstruction. *Pediatrics* 61:332, 1978.

74. Cohen MI, Winslow PR, Boley SJ: Intestinal obstruction associated with cholestyramine therapy. *N Engl J Med* 280:1285-1286, 1969.

75. Potyk D: Intestinal obstruction from impacted antacid tablets. *N Engl J Med* 283:134-135, 1970.

76. Townsend CM, Remmers AR, Searles HE, et al: Intestinal obstruction from medication bezoars in patients with renal failure. *N Engl J Med* 288:1058-1059, 1973.

77. Hurley JK: Bowel obstruction occuring in a child during treatment with aluminum hydroxide gel. *J Pediatr* 92:592-593, 1978.

78. Vickery RE: Unusual complications of excessive ingestion of vitamin C tablets. *Int Surg* 58:422-423, 1973.

79. Cadnapaphornchai P, Taher S: Drug-induced fluid and electrolyte disorders. In Anderson RJ, Schrier RW, (eds): *Clinical Use of Drugs in Patients With Kidney and Liver Disease.* Philadelphia, WB Saunders, 118-135, 1981.

80. Nanji AA: Drug-induced electrolyte disorders. *Drug Intell Clin Pharm* 17:175-185, 1983.

81. Bond WS: Toxic reactions and side effects of glucocorticoids in man. *Am J Hosp Pharm* 34:479-485, 1977.

82. Nelson DC, McGrew WR, Hoyumpa AM: Hypernatremia and lactulose therapy. *JAMA* 249:1295-1298, 1983.

83. Bjornson DC, Stephenson SR: Cisplatin-induced massive renal tubular failure with wastage of serum electrolytes. *Clin Pharm* 2:80-83, 1983.

84. Beck LH: Edema states and the use of diuretics. *Med Clin North Am* 65:291-301, 1981.

85. Davies DL, Wilson GM: Diuretics: Mechanism of action and clinical application. *Drugs* 9:178-226, 1975.

86. Fennelly JJ, Smyth H, Muldowney FP: Extreme hyperkalemia due to rapid lysis of leukaemic cells. *Lancet* 1:27, 1974.

87. Muggia FM: Hyperkalaemia and chemotherapy. *Lancet* 1:602-603, 1973.

88. Makoff DL, DaSilva JA, Rosenbaum BJ: On the mechanism of hyperkalemia due to hyperosmotic expansion with saline or mannitol. *Clin Sci* 41:383-393, 1971.

89. Greenblatt DJ, Koch-Weser J: Adverse reactions to spironolactone. A report from the Boston Collaborative Drug Surveillance Program. *JAMA* 225:40-43, 1973.

90. Walker BR, Capuzzi DM, Alexander F: Hyperkalemia after triamterene in diabetic patients. *Clin Pharmacol Ther* 13:643-651, 1972.

91. Maddux MS, Barriere SL: A review of complications of amphotericin-B therapy: Recommendations for prevention and management. *Drug Intell Clin Pharm* 14:177-181, 1980.

92. Medoff G, Kobayashi GS: Strategies in the treatment of systemic fungal infections. *N Engl J Med* 302:145-155, 1980.

93. Gill MA, DuBe JE, Young W: Hypokalemic, metabolic alkalosis induced by high-dose ampicillin sodium. *Am J Hosp Pharm* 34:528-531, 1977.

94. Lipner HI, Ruzany F, Dasgupta M, et al: The behavior of carbenicillin as a nonreabsorbable anion. *J Lab Clin Med* 86:183-194, 1975.

95. Klastersky J, Vanderkelen B, Daneau D, et al: Carbenicillin and hypokalemia. *Ann Intern Med* 78:774-775, 1973.

96. Tattersall M, Battersby G, Spiers A: Antibiotics and hypokalemia. *Lancet* 1:630-631, 1972.

97. Cabizuca SV, Desser KB: Carbenicillin-associated hypokalemic alkalosis. *JAMA* 236:956-957, 1976.

98. Stapleton FB, Nelson B, Vats TS, et al: Hypokalemia associated with antibiotic treatment. *Am J Dis Child* 130:1104-1108, 1976.

99. Lyman NW, Hemalatha C, Viscuso RL, et al: Cisplatin-induced hypocalcemia and hypomagnesemia,. *Arch Intern Med* 140:1513-1514, 1980.

100. Shenfield GM, Knowles GK, Thomas N, et al: Potassium supplement in patients treated with corticosteroids. *Br J Dis Chest* 69:171-176, 1975.

101. Holmes AM, Hesling CM, Wilson TM. Drug-induced secondary hyperaldosteronism in patients with pulmonary tuberculosis. *Q J Med* 39:299-314, 1970.

102. Cronin RE, Bulger RE, Southern P, et al: Natural history of aminoglycoside nephrotoxicity in the dog. *J Lab Clin Med* 95:463-474, 1980.

103. Mohr JA, Clark RM, Waack TC, et al: Nafcillin-associated hypokalemia. *JAMA* 242:544, 1979.

104. Brunner FP, Frick PG: Hypokalemia, metabolic alkalosis and hypernatraemia due to "massive" sodium penicillin therapy. *Br Med J* 4:550-552, 1968.

105. Shields HM: Rapid fall of serum phosphorus secondary to antacid therapy. *Gastroenterology* 75:1137-1141, 1978.

106. Lotz M, Zisman E, Barter FC: Evidence for a phosphorus depletion syndrome in man. *N Engl J Med* 278:409-415, 1968.

107. Zaloga GP, Chernow B: Calcium, magnesium and other minerals. In Chernow B, Lake CR (eds): *The Pharmacologic Approach to the Critically Ill Patient.* Baltimore, Williams & Wilkins, 1983, pp 530-561.

108. Knochel JP: The pathophysiology and clinical characteristics of severe hypophosphatemia. *Arch Intern Med* 137:203-220, 1977.

109. Weinsier RL, Krumdieck CL: Death resulting from overzealous total parenteral nutrition: The refeeding syndrome revisited. *Am J Clin Nutr* 34:393-399, 1980.

110. Craddock PR, Yawata Y, Van Santen L, et al: Acquired phagocyte dysfunction: A complication of the hypophosphatemia of parenteral hyperalimentation. *N Engl J Med* 290:1403-1407, 1974.

111. Blachley JD, Hill JB: Renal and electrolyte disturbances associated with cisplatin. *Ann Intern Med* 95:628-632, 1981.

112. Schilsky RL, Anderson T: Hypomagnesemia and renal magnesium wasting in patients receiving cisplatin. *Ann Intern Med* 90:929-931, 1979.

113. Gonzalez-Vitale JC, Hayes DM, Cvitkovic E, et al: The renal pathology in clinical trials of cis-platinum (II) diamminedichloride. *Cancer* 39:1362-1371, 1977.

114. Rude RK, Singer FR: Magnesium deficiency and excess. *Ann Rev Med* 32:245-249, 1981.

115. Bar RS, Wilson HE, Mazzaferri EL: Hypomagnesemic hypocalcemia secondary to renal magnesium wasting. A possible consequence of high-dose gentamicin therapy. *Ann Intern Med* 82:646-649, 1975.

116. Chernow B, Zaloga GP, Pock A, et al: Aminoglycoside-induced hypomagnesemia: A prospective study. *Clin Res* 30:863A, 1982.

117. Finton CK, Chernow B, Bjorkland S, et al: Gentamicin-induced hypomagnesemia. *Crit Care Med* 10:220, 1982.

118. Patel R, Savage A: Symptomatic hypomagnesemia associated with gentamicin therapy. *Nephron* 23:50-52, 1979.

119. Main AN, Morgan RJ, Russell RI, et al: Magnesium deficiency in chronic inflammatory bowel disease and requirements during intravenous nutrition. *J Parenter Enter Nutr* 5:15-19, 1981.

120. Giacoia GP, Krasner J: Interference of intravenous lipid emulsion with the determination of calcium in serum. *Am J Med Tech* 45:767, 1975.

121. Dujovne CA, Azarnoff DL: Clinical complications of corticosteroid therapy. *Med Clin North Am* 57:1331-1342, 1973.

122. Godolphin W, Cameron EC, Frohlich J, et al: Spurious hypocalcemia in hemodialysis patients after heparinization. *Am J Clin Pathol* 71:215-218, 1979.

123. Winter RJ, Harris CJ, Phillips LS, et al: Diabetic ketoacidosis. Induction of hypocalcemia and hypomagnesemia by phosphate therapy. *Am J Med* 67:897-900, 1979.

124. Simon GE, Bove JR: The potassium load from blood transfusion. *Postgrad Med* 49:61-64, 1971.

125. Juan D: Clinical review: The clinical importance of hypomagnesemia. *Surgery* 91:510-517, 1982.

126. Massry SG, Seelig MS: Hypomagnesemia and hypermagnesemia. *Clin Neph* 7:147-153, 1977.

127. Dyckner T, Wester PO: Ventricular extrasystoles and intracellular electrolytes before and after potassium and magnesium infusions in patients on diuretic treatment. *Am Heart J* 97:12-18, 1979.

128. Whang R, Aikawa JK: Magnesium deficiency and refractoriness to potassium repletion. *J Chronic Dis* 30:65-68, 1977.

129. Thompson JS, Hodges RE: Preventing hypophosphatemia during total parenteral nutrition. *J Parenter Enter Nutr* 8:137-139, 1984.

130. Gambertoglio JG, Mangini RJ, Robinson DC: Kidney diseases. In Katcher BS, Young LY, Koda-Kimble MA (eds): *Applied Therapeutics. The Clinical Use of Drugs.* San Francisco, Applied Therapeutics, 1983, pp 551.

131. Wolfe RR, O'Donnell TF, Stone MD, et al: Investigation of factors determining the optimal glucose infusion rate in total parenteral nutrition. *Metabolism* 29:892-900, 1980.

132. Burke JF, Wolfe RR, Mullany CJ, et al: Glucose requirements following burn injury. Parameters of optimal glucose infusion and possible hepatic and respiratory abnormalities following excessive glucose intake. *Ann Surg* 190:274-285, 1979.

133. Koda-Kimble MA, Rotblatt MD: Diabetes mellitus. In Katcher BS, Young LY, Koda-Kimble MA (eds): *Applied Therapeutics. The Clinical Use of Drugs.* San Francisco, Applied Therapeutics, 1335-1414, 1983.

134. Hansten PD: *Drug Interactions.* Philadelphia, Lea & Febiger, 1979, pp 349-365, p 449-455.

135. Weber SS, Wood WA, Jackson EA: Availability of insulin from parenteral nutrient solutions. *Am J Hosp Pharm* 34:353-357, 1977.

136. Rabkin R: Effect of renal disease on renal uptake and excretion of insulin in man. *N Engl J Med* 282:182-186, 1970.

137. Furman BL: Impairment of glucose tolerance produced by diuretics and other drugs. *Pharmacol Ther* 12:613-649, 1981.

138. Carter BL, Small RE, Mandel MD, et al: Phenytoin-induced hyperglycemia. *Am J Hosp Pharm* 38:1508-1512, 1981.

139. Strathman I, Schubert EN, Cohen A, et al: Hypoglycemia in patients receiving disopyramide phosphate. *Drug Intell Clin Pharm* 17:635-638, 1983.

140. Raia JJ, Patton LR, Klein RA, et al: Prolonged hypoglycemia during pentamidine therapy. *Clin Pharm* 2:505-506, 1983 (letter).

141. Narins RG, Emmett M: Simple and mixed acid-base disorders: A practical approach. *Medicine* 59:161-187, 1980.

142. Klahr S, Tripathy K, Lotero H: Renal regulation of acid-base balance in malnourished man. *Am J Med* 48:325-331, 1970.

143. Kaehny WD: Pathogenesis and management of metabolic acidosis and alkalosis, In Schrier RW (ed): *Renal and Electrolyte Disorders.* Boston, Little, Brown, 79-120, 1976.

144. Barton CH, Vaziri ND, Ness RL, et al: Cimetidine in the management of metabolic alkalosis induced by nasogastric drainage. *Arch Surg* 114:70-74, 1979.

145. Rowlands BJ, Tindall SF, Elliott DJ: The use of dilute hydrochloric acid and cimetidine to reverse severe metabolic alkalosis. *Postgrad Med J* 54:118-123, 1978.

146. Doherty NJ, Sufian S, Pavlides CA, et al: Cimetidine in the treatment of severe metabolic alkalosis secondary to short bowel syndrome. *Int Surg* 63:140-142, 1978.

147. Finkelstein W, Isselbacher KJ: Cimetidine. *N Engl J Med* 299:992-996, 1978.

148. Dickinson GE, Myers ML, Goldbach M, et al: Acetazolamide in the treatment of ventilatory failure complicating acute metabolic alkalosis. *Anesth Analg* 60:608-610, 1981.

149. Miller PD, Berns AS: Acute metabolic alkalosis perpetuating hypercarbia. *JAMA* 238:2400-2401, 1977.

150. Bear R, Goldstein M, Phillipson E, et al: Effect of metabolic alkalosis on respiratory function in patients with chronic obstructive lung disease. *Can Med Assoc J* 117:900-903, 1977.

151. Wan HH, Lye MD: Moduretic-induced metabolic acidosis and hyperkalemia. *Postgrad Med J* 56:348-350, 1980.

152. Gabow PA, Moore S, Schrier RW: Spironolactone-induced hyperchloremic acidosis in cirrhosis. *Ann Intern Med* 90:338-340, 1979.

153. Ivey MF, Adam SM, Hickman RO, et al: Right atrial indwelling catheter for patients requiring long-term intravenous therapy. *Am J Hosp Pharm* 35:1525-1527, 1978.

154. Rapp RP, Wermeling DP, Piecoro JJ: Guidelines for the administration of commonly used intravenous drugs—1984 update. *Drug Intell Clin Pharm* 18:218-232, 1984.

155. Trissel L (ed): *Handbook on Injectable Drugs.* Washington, American Society of Hospital Pharmacists, 1983.

156. Haynes RC, Murad F: Adrenocorticotropic hormone; adrenocortical steroids and their synthetic analog; inhibitors of adrenocortical steroid biosynthesis. In Gilman AG, Goodman LS, Gilman A (eds): *The Pharmacologic Basis of Therapeutics.* New York, Macmillan, 1980, pp 1466-1496.

157. Perley M, Kipnis DM: Effect of glucocorticoids on plasma insulin. *N Engl J Med* 274:1237-1241, 1966.

158. Woods JE, Zincke H, Palumbo PJ, et al: Hyperosmolar nonketotic syndrome and steroid diabetes. *JAMA* 231:1261-1263, 1975.

159. Miller SE, Neilson JM: Clinical features of the diabetic syndrome appearing after steroid therapy. *Postgrad Med J* 40:660-669, 1964.

160. Kishi DT: Disorders of the adrenals. In Katcher BS, Young LY, Koda-Kimble MA (eds): *Applied Therapeutics: The Clinical Use of Drugs.* San Francisco, Applied Therapeutics, 1983, pp 1275-1295.

161. Chin R, Chernow B: Corticosteroids. In Chernow B, Lake CR (eds): *The Pharmacologic Approach to the Critically Ill Patient.* Baltimore, Williams & Wilkins, 1983, pp 510-529.

162. Flynn A, Strain WH, Pories WJ, et al: Rapid serum zinc depletion associated with corticosteroid therapy. *Lancet* 2:1169-1171, 1971.

163. Harman JB: Muscular wasting and corticosteroid therapy. *Lancet* 1:887, 1959.

164. Rasmussen H, Bordier P, Kurokawa K, et al: Hormonal control of skeletal and mineral homeostasis. *Am J Med* 56:751-753, 1974.

165. Claman HN: Corticosteroids and lymphoid cells. *N Engl J Med* 287:388-395, 1972.

166. Plotz CM, Knowlton AI, Regan C: The natural history of Cushing's syndrome. *Am J Med* 13:597-614, 1952.

167. Soffer LJ, Iannaccone AL, Gabrilove JC: Cushing's syndrome: A study of 50 patients. *Am J Med* 30:129-146, 1961.

168. Shoenfeld Y, Gurewich Y, Gallant LA, et al: Prednisone-induced leukocytosis: Influence of dosage, method and duration of administration on the degree of leukocytosis. *Am J Med* 71:773-778, 1981.

169. Schiller WR, Long CL, Blakemore WS: Creatinine and nitrogen excretion in seriously ill and injured patients. *Surg Gynecol Obstet* 149:561-566, 1979.

170. Cogan MG, Sargent JA, Yarbrough SG, et al: Prevention of prednisone-induced negative nitrogen balance. Effect of dietary modification on urea generation rate in patients on hemodialysis receiving high-dose glucocorticoids. *Ann Intern Med* 95:158-161, 1981.

171. Vanderveen TW, Niemiec PW: Parenteral nutrition. In Herfindal E (ed): *Clinical Pharmacy and Therapeutics,* ed 3. Baltimore, Williams & Wilkins, 1984, pp 25-42.

172. Cronin RE: Antimicrobial agent nephrotoxicity. In Anderson RJ, Schrier RW (eds): *Clinical Use of Drugs in Patients With Kidney and Liver Disease.* Philadelphia, WB Saunders, 1981, pp 54-65.

173. Mirtallo JM, Kudsk KA, Ebbert ML: Nutritional support of patients with renal disease. *Clin Pharm* 3:253-263, 1984.

174. Hochman R, Clark J, Rolla A, et al: Bleeding in patients with infections. *Arch Intern Med* 142:1440-1442, 1982.

175. Fainstein V, Bodey GP, McCredie KB, et al: Coagulation abnormalities induced by beta-lactam antibiotics in cancer patients. *J Infect Dis* 148:745-750, 1983.

176. Lipsky JJ: N-Methyl-thio-tetrazole inhibition of the gamma carboxylation of glutamic acid: possible mechanism for antibiotic-associated hypoprothrombinaemia. *Lancet* 2:192-193, 1983.

177. Shearer MJ, McBurney A, Barkhan P: Studies on the absorption and metabolism of phylloquinone (vitamine K₁) in man. *Vitam Horm* 32:513-542, 1974.

178. Hooper CA, Haney BB, Stone HH: Gastrointestinal bleeding due to vitamin K deficiency in patients on parenteral cefamandole. *Lancet* 1:39-40, 1980.

179. Rymer W, Greenlaw CW: Hypoprothrombinemia associated with cefamandole. *Drug Intell Clin Pharm* 14:780-783, 1980.

180. Holt RJ, Gorrochategui M, Perez C: Hypoprothrombinemia associated with moxalactam treatment of a septic sternoclavicular arthritis due to citrobacter diversus. *Drug Intell Clin Pharm* 15:288, 1981.

181. Weitekamp MR, Aber R: Prolonged bleeding times and bleeding diathesis associated with moxalactam administration. *JAMA* 249:69-71, 1983.

182. Haubenstock A, Schmidt P, Zazgornik J, et al: Hypoprothrombinaemic bleeding associated with ceftriaxone. *Lancet* 1:1215-1216, 1983.

183. Bruch K: Hypoprothrombinemia and cephalosporins. *Lancet* 1:535-536, 1983.

184. Lipsky JJ, Lewis JC, Novick WJ: Production of hypoprothrombinemia by moxalactam and l-methyl-5-thiotetrazole in rats. *Antimicrob Agents Chemother* 25:380-381, 1984.

185. Lipsky JJ: Mechanism of the inhibition of the gamma-carboxylation of glutamic acid by N-methylthiotetrazole-containing antibiotics. *Proc Natl Acad Sci USA* 81:2893-2897, 1984.

186. Au JP, Geiger GS: Thrombocytopenia associated with moxalactam administration. *Drug Intell Clin Pharm* 18:140-142, 1984.

187. Brown CH, Natelson EA, Bradshaw W, et al: The hemostatic defect produced by carbenicillin. *N Engl J Med* 291:265-270, 1974.

188. Shattil S, Sanford J, Bennett JS, et al: Carbenicillin and penicillin G inhibit platelet function in vitro by impairing the interaction of agonists with the platelet surface. *J Clin Invest* 65:329-337, 1980.

189. Bang NU, Kammer RB: Hematologic complications associated with beta-lactam antibiotics. *Rev Inf Dis* 5:380-393, (suppl), 1983.

190. Ansell JE, Kumar R, Deykin D: The spectrum of vitamin K deficiency. *JAMA* 238:40-42, 1977.

191. Krishnaswamy K: Drug metabolism and pharmacokinetics in malnutrition. *Clin Pharmacokinet* 3:216-240, 1978.

192. Buchanan N: Drug kinetics in protein energy malnutrition. *S Afr Med J* 53:327-330, 1978.

193. Brock JF: Dietary protein deficiency: It's influence on body structure and function. *Ann Intern Med* 65:877-897, 1966.

194. Kappas A, Anderson KE, Conney AH, et al: Influence of dietary protein and carbohydrate on antipyrine and theophylline metabolism in man. *Clin Pharmacol Ther* 20:643-653, 1976.

195. Anderson KE, Conney AH, Kappas A: Nutrition and oxidative drug metabolism in man: Relative influence of dietary lipids, carbohydrate, and protein. *Clin Pharmacol Ther* 26:493-501, 1979.

196. Feldman CH, Hutchinson VE, Pippenger CE, et al: Effect of dietary protein and carbohydrate on theophylline metabolism in children. *Pediatrics* 66:956-962, 1980.

197. Campbell TC: Nutrition and drug-metabolizing enzymes. *Clin Pharmacol Ther* 22:699-706, 1977.

198. Campbell TC, Hayes JR: Role of nutrition in the drug-metabolizing enzyme system. *Pharmacol Rev* 26:171-197, 1974.

199. Klahr S, Alleyne GA: Effects of chronic protein-calorie malnutrition on the kidney. *Kidney Int* 3:129-141, 1973.

200. Alleyne GA: The effect of severe protein calorie malnutrition on the renal function of Jamaican children. *Pediatrics* 39:400-411, 1967.

201. Srikantia SG, Gopalan C: Renal function in nutritional edema. *Ind J Med Res* 47:467-470, 1959.

202. Grant JP: Clinical impact of protein malnutrition on organ mass and function. In Blackburn GL, Grant JP, Young VR (eds): *Amino Acid Metabolism and Medical Applications.* Boston, John Wright, 1983, pp 347-358.

203. Elwyn DH, Bryan-Brown CW, Shoemaker WC: Nutritional aspects of body water dislocations in postoperative and depleted patients. *Ann Surg* 182:76-85, 1975.

204. Dixon RL, Shultice RW, Fouts JR: Factors affecting drug metabolism by liver microsomes. IV. Starvation. *Proc Soc Exp Biol Med* 103:333-335, 1960.

205. Kato R: Effects of starvation and refeeding on the oxidation of drugs by liver microsomes. *Biochem Pharmacol* 16:871-881, 1967.

206. Norred WP, Wade AE: Dietary fatty acid induced alterations of hepatic microsomal drug metabolism. *Biochem Pharmacol* 21:2887-2897, 1972.

207. Wade AE, Norred WP: Effect of dietary lipid on drug-metabolizing enzymes. *Fed Proc* 35:2475-2479, 1976.

208. Campbell TC, Hayes JR: The effect of quantity and quality of dietary protein on drug metabolism. *Fed Proc* 35:2470-2474, 1976.

209. Strother A, Throckmorton JK, Herzer C: The influence of high sugar consumption by mice on the duration of action of barbiturates and in vitro metabolism of barbiturates, aniline and *p*-nitroanisole. *J Pharmacol Exp Ther* 179:490-498, 1971.

210. Jansson I, Schenkman JB: Studies on three microsomal electron transfer enzyme systems. Effects of alteration of component enzyme levels in vivo and in vitro. *Mol Pharmacol* 11:450-461, 1975.

211. Homeida M, Karrar ZA, Roberts JC: Drug metabolism in malnourished children: A study with antipyrine. *Arch Dis Child* 54:299-302, 1979.

212. Narang RK, Mehta S, Mathur VS: Pharmacokinetic study of antipyrine in malnourished children. *Am J Clin Nutr* 30:1979-1982, 1977.

213. Obel AO, Vere DW: Antipyrine and propranolol disposition in malnutrition. *East Afr Med J* 55:20-24, 1978.

214. Buchanan N, Davis M, Danhof M, et al: Antipyrine metabolite formation in children in the acute phase of malnutrition and after recovery. *Br J Clin Pharmacol* 10:363-368, 1980.

215. Buchanan N, Eyberg C, Davis MD: Antipyrine pharmacokinetics and D-glucaric excretion in kwashiorkor. *Am J Clin Nutr* 32:2439-2442, 1979.

216. Mehta S, Chander KN, Sharma B, et al: Disposition of four drugs in malnourished children. *Drug Nutr Inter* 1:205-211, 1982.

217. Mehta S, Kalsi HK, Jayaraman S, et al: Chloramphenicol metabolism in children with protein-calorie malnutrition. *Am J Clin Nutr* 28:977-981, 1975.

218. Mehta S, Nain CK, Sharma B, et al: Steady state of chloramphenicol in malnourished children. *Ind J Med Res* 73:538-542, 1981.

219. Paumgartner G, Probst P, Kraines R, et al: Kinetics of indocyanine green removal from the blood. *Ann NY Acad Sci* 170:134-147, 1970.

220. Pollack DS, Sufian S, Matsumoto T: Indocyanine green clearance in critically ill patients. *Surg Gynecol Obstet* 149:852-854, 1979.

221. Kinnear AA, Pretorius PJ: Liver function in fatal kwashiorkor. *S Afr Med J* 31:174-175, 1957.

222. Cochran ST, Pagani JJ, Barbaric ZL: Nephromegaly in hyperalimentation. *Diagn Radiol* 130:603-606, 1979.

223. Brenner BM, Meyer TW, Hostetter TH: Dietary protein intake and the progressive nature of kidney disease: The role of hemodynamically mediated glomerular injury in the pathogenesis of progressive glomerular sclerosis in aging, renal ablation, and intrinsic renal disease. *N Engl J Med* 307:652-659, 1982.

224. Cockroft DW, Gault MH: Prediction of creatinine clearance from serum creatinine. *Nephron* 16:31-41, 1976.

225. Jelliffe RW: Creatinine clearance: Bedside estimate. *Ann Intern Med* 79:604-605, 1973.

226. Mawer GE, Knowles BR, Lucas SB, et al: Computer-assisted prescribing of kanamycin for patients with renal insufficiency. *Lancet* 1:12-15, 1972.

227. Buchanan N: Drug-protein binding and protein energy malnutrition. *S Afr Med J* 52:733-737, 1977.

228. Buchanan N, Mithal Y, Witcomb M. Cefoxitin: Intravenous pharmacokinetics and intramuscular bioavailability in kwashiorkor. *Br J Clin Pharmacol* 9:623-627, 1980.

229. Buchanan N, Hansen JD, VanderWalt LA, et al: Chloramphenicol metabolism in children with PCM. *Am J Clin Nutr* 29:327-328, (letter), 1976.

230. Raghuram TC, Krishnaswamy K: Influence of nutritional status on plasma levels and relative bioavailability of tetracycline. *Eur J Clin Pharmacol* 12:281-284, 1977.

231. Raghuram TC, Krishnaswamy K: Tetracycline absorption in malnutrition. *Drug-Nutr Inter* 1:23-29, 1981.

232. Buchanan N, Eyberg C: Intramuscular tobramycin administration in kwashiorkor. *S Afr Med J* 53:273-274, 1978.

233. Buchanan N, Davis MD, Eyberg C: Gentamicin pharmacokinetics in kwashiorkor. *Br J Clin Pharmacol* 8:451-453, 1979.

234. Bravo ME, Arancibia A, Jarpa S, et al: Pharmacokinetics of gentamicin in malnourished infants. *Eur J Clin Pharmacol* 21:499-504, 1982.

235. Eriksson M, Paalzow L, Bolme B, et al: Pharmacokinetics of theophylline in Ethiopian children of differing nutritional status. *Eur J Clin Pharmacol* 24:89-92, 1983.

236. Buchanan N, Robinson R, Koornhof HJ, et al: Penicillin pharmacokinetics in kwashiorkor. *Am J Clin Nutr* 32:2233-2236, 1979.

237. Shastri RA, Krishnaswamy K: Metabolism of sulphadiazine in malnutrition. *Br J Clin Pharmacol* 7:69-73, 1979.

238. Krishnaswamy K, Ushasri V, Naidu AN: The effect of malnutrition on the pharmacokinetics of phenylbutazone. *Clin Pharmacokinet* 6:152-159, 1981.

CHAPTER 31

Communicating Drug Information

RONALD P. EVENS

The hospital pharmacist shares with those who create, investigate, market, prescribe, administer, and regulate the use of therapeutic agents an irreducible obligation to introduce into patient care the maximum extent of the scientifically proved knowledge of drug capabilities and limitations.

The pharmacist's role in drug information communication was recognized and promulgated by the American Society of Hospital Pharmacists (ASHP) in 1968 (1). This position paper further outlines the performance criteria of the drug information specialist, for which the pertinent aspects concerning communication follow (2):

. . . 3. He possesses verbal and written communications skills, which enable him to contribute effectively to intra- and inter-institutional dialogue relative to pharmacotherapeutic information. 4. He has the capacity for substantial contributions to the continuing education of all health professionals. 5. He is involved directly or indirectly in patient care with drugs as a contributor to its continuing quality. In addition, the knowledge and skills prerequisite to drug information practice are delineated further in detail in the society's guidelines for the specialized residency in drug information.

In order to fulfill these responsibilities of service and continuing education, the gap has to be bridged between the drug literature, which is already vast in volume and continually spiraling, and the persons in need of information, i.e., practitioners such physicians, nurses, dentists, other pharmacists, and the patient. Burkholder (3) stated that "drug information as a product has no usefulness until it is communicated to those who have need for it. . . ." The solution to this communication problem is the retrieval, formulation, and dissemination of accurate, reliable, objective, and applicable drug knowledge in the appropriate clinical context, to the correct location, for the right practitioner, and within a reasonable time frame.

The development of "drug information communications and services" has been muddled by uncertainty and wide variation in their descriptions, but definitions of each component term can provide insight into their actual requirements for pharmacy practice. Information can be defined as knowledge, news, advice, and instruction. Communication involves dissemination, report, message, transference, and enlightenment. Service is aid, promotion, support, and backup. Therefore, a composite of the above definitions for these three terms more completely delineates their appli-

cations in pharmacy practice, e.g., the support of other clinicians through dissemination of drug knowledge and advice describes a drug information communication.

This chapter's content is based on four aspects: (1) the aforementioned responsibilities identified by the ASHP, (2) the above-noted professional challenge to deliver drug information, (3) the previously stated description of communication requirements, and (4) the lack of and need for specific delineation of drug information communications in the pharmacy literature. The first discussion of communication principles and techniques provides guidelines and suggestions for improving professional dialogue. Then, the following types of communication are presented: drug information inquiry-responses (I/R), Pharmacy and Therapeutics (P&T) Committee monographs, pharmacy bulletins and newsletters, and direct patient interactions. For each of these, prototypes are discussed, their content is examined, and the approach in their preparation and dissemination is delineated.

COMMUNICATION PRINCIPLES

The pharmacist's first step in communicating drug information requires professional self-assessment and program planning. The purchase of resources and an announcement of service availability constitute an inadequate scheme to initiate such communications, since such an ill-devised simplistic plan leads to a lack of acceptance or even resistance, underutilization, or possibly failure. Therefore, the subsequently outlined preparations serve to facilitate the hospital pharmacist's communication of drug information by creating a practical stepwise method of implementation adaptable to most institutions:

1. Determine institutional information needs based upon hospital size, "in-house" medical-surgical services (e.g., trauma, obstetrics, chronic care, etc), pharmacy service sophistication (e.g., unit dose, IV additives, pharmacokinetics), nursing staff, and the type of medical practitioners (e.g., house staff, private physician, practitioner-educators, specialists).

2. Evaluate existing literature and reference resources available in the pharmacy and hospital libraries.

3. Assess the pharmacy personnel's education, training, and experience.

4. Obtain support documents of national professional standards, e.g., American Hospital Association Standards for Accreditation of Hospitals (4), the position paper on "The Hospital Pharmacist and Drug Information Service's" (1), and The Report of The Study Commission on Pharmacy, "Pharmacists for the Future" (5).

5. Procure precedents of similar institutions' programs in drug information communication (6-8).

6. Outline direct or indirect benefits to the patients and especially drug utilization review process. This latter clinical service has achieved high priority for hospital pharmacies to foster cost-effective drug prescribing under austere new federally mandated funding schemes for health care.

7. Establish program objectives tailored to a hospital's services, patient population, and information needs.

8. Prepare a budget for resources, supplies, and personnel.

9. Solicit medical and nursing practitioner support from individuals in concurrence with new pharmacy functions.

10. Acquire hospital administrative approval.

11. Conduct a pilot program for a specific physician group or nursing unit, documenting questions provided and user (practitioner) evaluation.

12. Institute the complete drug information communication program with prior announcement to the target population, indicating purpose, content, and benefits with sample questions, bulletins, or monographs.

A properly conceived, effective system of information dissemination is dependent on skills employed in communications. Effective drug information communication is based not only on unique existing or retrievable knowledge, but also on one's ability to disseminate that knowledge (format, content, technique). The subsequent six points elucidate general characteristics that are prerequisites for all types of pharmacy communications: first, credibility and patient safety are dependent upon the accuracy of the information. "Communication is more serious here than in any other area, since human health and life are involved. . ." (9). Therefore, the most current and correct clinical information is required that directly applies to the specific problem. Second, objectivity in literature review and analysis ensures that responses will present the facts and appropriate conclusions, including all sides of a controversy. The facts in context will often speak for themselves. The pharmacist's opinion and assessment are additional commentary. Third, the reliability of communications is established by repeated provision of useful drug information to practitioners. The inquirer should expect a similar level of sophistication for each question posed. It is important to promote a scope and level of service that can continually be provided on a daily basis. Fourth, efficiency in communications necessitates a rapid response time frame adapted to the emergence of the situation. Check with the inquirer concerning the response time needs if it is not readily apparent, and then establish priorities for question or monograph processing. If a delay is inevitable, progress with the question should be communicated to the inquirer with the expected time of completion. Fifth, awareness and comprehension of patient care needs, the activities and routine problems of a nursing unit, and the practitioners' busy schedule in the institution create an appropriate sensitivity

to adapt interprofessional communications to the patient care setting. Sixth, professionalism and courtesy in all communications obviously enhance their acceptance by practitioners.

A verbal or written communication should be a carefully organized discussion of applicable statements, i.e., complete in considering all salient clinical aspects but concise by eliminating extraneous, tangential, or excessive phraseology or data. The ideal communication should possess the following characteristics: (1) objective summaries of the drug literature; (2) condensation of literature from multiple resources without repetitive statements from each; (3) drug literature evaluation comments outlining the major attributes or deficiencies in the literature content or methods of reporting; (4) sufficient documentation providing the actual evidence to support any general statements; and (5) conclusions of the pharmacist, based on the literature data, its evaluation, and personal experiences. In general, this content should be adapted to the institution's needs (e.g., private vs teaching hospital, general care vs specialty hospital such as cancer chemotherapy, acute vs chronic care) and the inquirer's needs (physician-student, intern, resident, attending, private, or specialized nurse, pharmacist, respiratory therapist, etc).

DRUG INFORMATION INQUIRY—RESPONSE COMMUNICATION

For the communication of drug information to a practitioner in reply to specific questions, there are three types of pharmacy providers: the retriever, the informant, or the consultant. They constitute three levels of service within a spectrum of professional skills, expertise, and sophistication of service. The misconceptions concerning these different levels of activity were aptly described by Walton (10) as follows:

We are confronted immediately with the necessity of determining exactly what one means when he suggests that the pharmacist be a "consultant." In most cases, a careful analysis of the proposals oftentimes reveals nothing more than the notion that all practicing pharmacists should equip themselves with voluminous files of catalogs and product information cards so they may serve as encyclopedic reservoirs of facts, which might otherwise be provided by an intelligent receptionist prossessing the same stockpile.

The retriever recovers or procures information from previously catalogued literature, library journals, drug company data, or textbooks. This information is usually transmitted verbatim, and/or bibliographies or photocopies are supplied upon request. The professional expertise is limited to selective retrieval of appropriate literature data for a clinical problem. This level of drug information function suffices for initial pharmacy involvement in communications but is equivalent to the medical reference librarian's function to provide bibliographies or references. This retrieval of knowledge and data should be the base from which the informant and consultant pharmacist functions are developed. At the next level, the informant selectively retrieves the drug information, evaluates and interprets the literature, and provides an answer to a question. Then, as well as performing the informant functions, the consultant confers with the inquirer to solicit a complete patient data baseline, discusses the problem, deliberates over the alternative solutions, and provides conclusions, advice, and/or recommendations (a consult).

A drug information communication starts with proper assessment of the problem to ascertain the clinical context of the situation, i.e., obtain a brief disease history and drug history, as well as to clarify the question. When this is efficiently and accurately solicited, which is usually not volunteered, the pharmacist can prepare a drug information response that will be stylized to the therapeutic situation. For example, to a "what is the dose of amikacin" question, an apparently correct response of "7.5 mg/kg every 12 hours" could be completely wrong if the patient has renal failure.

Communications in response to specific questions include verbal exchanges and written reports. All questions should be communicated verbally in direct telephone or face-to-face dialogue as soon as possible. If an intermediary professional is used to disseminate a verbal response, the pharmacist should exercise care to ensure an understanding of the posed question and complete comprehension of the reply by the intermediary so that accurate transmission of the information is ensued without significant reinterpretation. By tactfully asking the intermediary to state his or her comprehension of the response, the pharmacist can ascertain the accuracy of information transmitted by this courier.

When the pharmacy resources and expertise exist, written reports should follow up the verbal reply to document the communication for the user and provide a more complete, sophisticated consultation service. In addition, these reports can potentially generate patient charges for this new pharmacy service. The two primary types of written responses are interprofessional memoranda and patient chart notes, which may be pharmacy notes on pharmacy records attached to a chart, direct chart entries in the patient's progress notes, or official consultation records. A pharmacy program of notation and consultation is described by Bell et al (11). The appropriate format of communication is dependent on the institution's medical record policies (American Hospital Association Standards for Accreditation of Hospitals—Medical Records [12]), the type of information requested, and the receptivity of the medical practitioners for paramedical personnel involvement in drug therapy. A discussion of the pros and cons of solicited and unsolicited pharmacist entries in patient charts is described by Davis (13).

The content of a drug information communication in response to specific inquiries is described in the subsequent idealized outline. A pharmacist's individual reply should adapt as much as possible to this content within the limitations of his drug information service objectives, professional skills and experience, and information needs. Specific adaptations of responses will be described following this outline:

1. Question summary: The original question is repeated to establish the problem under consideration.

2. Data baseline: The information solicited from the inquirer is delineated, i.e., the clinical context of the response including pertinent patient identification (e.g., weight, age, sex), drug data (e.g., dosage regime, prior therapy, concomitant therapy), and disease data (e.g., severity, duration, pattern and presentation of primary problem, complications, concomitant diseases, organ function).

3. Information summary: The literature is abstracted, compiled, interpreted, condensed, and correlated accurately, completely, and concisely, with specific summary comments.

4. Documentation: Sufficient specific data are provided to support the above statements, since this is the evidence to substantiate summary points and later conclusions. Also, this enhances the credibility and validity of the response, since the correspondent will seldom retrieve and read the documents summarized. This evidence would encompass incidence or response rates, exemplary case reports, numbers of patients involved, and dosage regimes.

5. Evaluation: In order to establish the validity of the clinical information, the pharmacist critiques the literature, identifying significant major attributes or deficiencies in patient selection, design of dosage regimes, control of bias (e.g., blinding, placebo, randomization, crossover techniques), significance of results, appropriateness of monitoring parameters, or relevance and accuracy of conclusions.

6. Conclusions: The author's judgments from the clinical trials are noted with reasonable qualifying remarks based on the drug literature evaluation. The pharmacist's opinions and conclusions should also be enclosed, which may differ due to variable clinical data from multiple resources and the evaluation.

7. Recommendations: Extrapolation of the literature data to the clinical problem under review absolutely necessitates collection of a complete patient data base. This prevents a right answer to a question from becoming inaccurate when it is out of context.

8. Information sources: The references should be listed with appropriate differentiation into text, journals, company, or testimonial types. This affords further credibility, documentation of accuracy, and future retrieval when required.

9. Background discussion: Descriptions of disease states or pharmacology are included only when they are necessary to substantiate drug indications or actions, or when the pharmacist perceives a lack of user knowledge in these areas. Care is necessary to avoid indirect insults to the intelligence of a practitioner requesting information. See Appendix 31.1 for sample questions.

In an early dissertation by Kelsey (14), lack of adaptation of information was described as a primary problem associated with the dissemination and utilization of drug information. Therefore, the previously cited content of a drug information communication and its length should be tailored to the specific situation. Seven additional guidelines are provided for the preparation of a written drug consult in response to drug information questions.

First, in differentiating verbal and written activities, a verbal communication is a synopsis of the information summary, documentation, evaluation, conclusions and/or recommendations, and a citation of the references. In a written report, the question summary and initial data baseline are additionally necessary, since they establish the context of the response in the absence of a verbal dialogue between practitioners.

Second, the scope of the question affects the type and volume of the information summary, documentation, and conclusions for communications. Requests for specific data, e.g., absorption or side effects, narrow the discussion to fewer principles necessitating a brief report, but a general information question, e.g., drug descriptions or therapeutic alternatives, broadens the points of consideration and length of a reply.

Third, the type of question adjusts the content of a drug information response. The subsequent question categories are listed with specific considerations that require assessment during the initial processing of a drug problem and may become inclusions in a response:

1. Identification or availability: Foreign or USA product? Country of origin? Substitute desired? Old or new drug? Investigational? Indication? Other names? Label or bottle available?

2. Pharmaceutical preparations: Ingredients? Admixture technique? Stability (vehicle, temperature, pH, duration, concentration)? Solubility? Preservatives?

3. Drug interactions: Physical or therapeutic? Other drugs? Mechanism? Incidence? Patient reactions? Management? Sequence of administration? Dose relationship?

4. Adverse effects: Side effect—idiosyncrasy or allergy? Incidence? Severity? Progression? Duration? Amount of drug exposure (dose, duration, prior exposure)? Temporal sequence? Drug or disease interference? Presentation? Management? Dose-response?

5. Poisoning or overdose: Age? Patient size? Patient presentation? Route or site of exposure? Quantity of toxin? Duration of exposure? Time lag up to call for help? Prior drug therapy? Lavage and/or emesis? Antidote? Management? Location?

6. Dosage: Loading, induction, or maintenance? Dose, frequency, or duration? Equivalent drug? Dose-response? Diet?

7. Administration: Route? Rate? Volume? Concentration? Special equipment? Precautions?

8. Biopharmaceutics: Absorption, distribution, metabolism, or excretion? Bioavailability, disintegration, or dissolution? Drug blood levels? Drug tissue levels? Half-life? Protein binding? Dose-pharmacokinetic change? Diet? Age? Vascular blood flow?

9. Indications: Goals of treatment—Acute or chronic? Prophylaxis, cure, or palliation? Contraindications?

10. Efficacy: Time of response (onset, duration)? Percentage of responders? Degree of response? Tolerance? Number of patients (case reports or common use)? Specific type of patients? Monitoring parameters?

11. Pharmacology: Mechanism of action? Animal vs human data? Structure-activity relationships?

Fourth, the intended application of the information alters the orientation of the content. For example, an academic or personal inquiry by a practitioner is intended for general background knowledge with future applications. In contrast, a patient management problem requires correlation of specific clinical data to a specific clinical problem.

Fifth, the availability of information determines the length and content. When there is a dearth of literature, the few case reports and/or clinical trials are completely described, and limited conclusions are drawn with qualifications for the paucity of data. When a wealth of data exists, all of the clinical trials cannot be reviewed and abstracted because of practical restraints of time for work and space for response. Therefore, my personal "2-4-6 literature rule" is recommended for drug information responses; i.e., when supporting a singlepoint that is consistently reiterated in the lierature with little disagreement, two references are good and minimal, fur are excellent and maximum, but six are excessive.

Sixth, the degree of controversy expands the discussion in direct proportion to the number of opposing opinions introduced. Clinical data are presented for each claim, and the conclusions must assess each argument and judge the consensus of the evidence.

Seventh, adaptation of resources can be helpful by utilizing references with which the practitioner is most familiar, e.g., pediatricians—*Pediatric Therapy, Manual of Pediatric Therapy, Pediatric Clinics North America*. Last, the response time frame to a question is tailored to the situation; an emergency vs clinic patient in waiting room or at home, vs inpatient management, vs academic questions. If it is not readily apparent, the pharmacist should query the requester in order to establish time frame priorities for responses. See Appendix 31.1 for four sample questions that address drug administration, side effects, identification, and efficacy.

PHARMACY AND THERAPEUTICS COMMITTEE MONOGRAPHS

The P&T Committee must examine the merits and limitations of new drugs in contrast to existing formulary agents, so that optimal patient care with drugs will be provided at the lowest possible cost. The deliberations should be based on objective, factual information, i.e., controlled clinical trials, and the proved consensus of worldwide clinicians. The pharmacist should not take an adversarial role by preparing a document to refute the claims of a physician requesting the drug. Confrontation breeds conflict and contempt and raises issues of objectivity. In addition, there may be other attributes of the new drug not elucidated by the requesting physician. Therefore, the pharmacy should communicate a monograph that compiles and analyzes the world's literature, fully characterizing this new drug's advantages and disadvantages. Drug information communication directed to the P&T Committee include both the written document to be described in the subsequent material and a verbal presentation. During P&T Committee meeting, a verbal synopsis of the monograph would highlight the significant differences, pro and con, between this new agent and the institution's present medications. In addition, the pharmacist should be prepared to respond to members' questions concerning the literature's and monograph's description of the drugs.

In the preparation of a monograph, the pharmacist usually is providing the full and key information on which the committee physicians, who are unfamiliar with this new drug, will formulate a decision for optimal patient care. The package insert is not an objective review and is frequently incomplete in characterizing the degree of efficacy or incidence of side effects. The only other information available to the P&T Committee is the initial brief request for the drug by one physician, and perhaps, individual members may have read a clinical study about the drug. Therefore, a monograph encompasses salient pharmacologic, therapeutic, toxicologic, and economic aspects of the drugs' utilization in medical practice, in accordance with the following outline:

1. Background information (optional): A very brief description of the manifestations of the disease process that are amenable to treatment establishes the context in which the drugs will be contrasted and/or an analysis of the monitoring parameters of the drugs' actions may explain difficulties or limitations in comparing published clinical investigations.

2. Identification: The two drugs' pharmacologic and/or chemical categories or ingredients are established as well as dosage forms and manufacturer.

3. Mechanisms of desired drug actions—new mechanisms are identified to justify a possibly unique role of a new drug.

4. Indications and contraindictions (Food and Drug Administration approved and otherwise, because drugs placed openly on formularies will be used for any potential use).

5. Efficacy: The percentage and degree of patient response to therapy for each indication.

6. Biopharmaceutical parameters: Absorption, distribution, metabolism, excretion, blood levels, and tissue levels (if applicable).

7. Dosage and administration: Averages and ranges up to maximum effective doses.

8. Side effects and toxicity.

9. Cost: Economic impact is expressed fully by last year's expenditure for the number of doses dispensed of the replaced drug vs projected cost of the new drug for the same number of doses and anticipated expenditures for the new drug, which may experience greater utilization due to improved safety and efficacy.

10. Conclusions: Summarization of advantages and disadvantages.

11. Recommendation: When the evidence is overwhelmingly one-sided in favor of drug addition or rejection, a recommendation is superfluous. In situations where variable positive and negative information is elucidated for the new drug, the pharmacist forwards his professional opinion or judgment based on the literature's content and its evaluation. This can be accomplished in written adjunctive recommendations or in a verbal presentation at the P&T Committee meeting.

In the preparation of a monograph (see Appendix 31.1), several techniques and helpful hints are presented in the following discussion and in Snyder's article discussing concise communications (15). First, the monograph is a comparison of the properties of new drugs against present formulary drugs for the purpose of choosing between them and not just a review article. When a new drug is a unique entity, i.e., the sole treatment for a health problem, a review discussion is sufficient. Second, two approaches for the organization of information provide equally appropriate methods to contrast the two drugs: (1) the above categories of information constitute the outline and main sections of the monograph, and then, the drugs are contrasted under each with follow-up comparative conclusions; or (2) each drug is separately examined considering each category, and the comparative conclusions follow these two discussions.

Third, the information within each category of the monograph should incorporate the following three aspects of content: (1) abstracts of the clinical trials compiling, correlating, and condensing this literature into summary statements; (2) documentation of such generalizations with representative examples of clinical trials or case reports from any clinical trials that are used for monographs (data include doses, numbers of patients, response or incidence rates); and (3) evaluation of the clinical data's strengths and weaknesses, providing an assessment of its validity (editorial comments about the poor study design in clinical trials will appropriately alter the impact of that data).

Fourth, the concentration of discussion in a monograph will depend on the major points of differentiation between the new and possibly replaced drugs. If the only distinctions involve biopharmaceutical parameters, the other information categories are briefly reviewed, but half of the document may discuss these most important differing considerations. If there is disagreement concerning the drugs' efficacy, greater concentration of discussion is required to completely elaborate these differences but not at the sacrifice of inadequately delineating other sections. If there are contrasting advantages or disadvantages between the two drugs in almost every category, a balanced discussion is prepared.

Fifth, the length of a P&T Committee monograph should be practically limited to two to three single-spaced or four double-spaced typed pages, which affords a maximum quantity of information in the smallest amount of space. It is difficult to condense the literature to this small quantity, but such conciseness without sacrificing completeness is favored by P&T Committee members in their considerations of drug admission to a formulary. Lengthy documents require more time to read and digest and create the possibility of never being read in the first place.

Sixth, the references for a monograph should be the primary literature, journals and periodicals, so that a worldwide consensus of clinicians and researchers can be assessed and provided through their drug investigations. It must be the most current literature available, representing the most efficacious and safest therapeutic measures. The volume of literature condensed in a monograph varies with the availability and complexity of information, but 15-50 literature citations is a reasonable guideline, since that amounts to approximately two to five journal articles per category noted in the monograph outline. As cited in the previous discussion of inquiry responses, the degree of controversy similarly will alter the volume of commentary.

The last point of discussion for a P&T Committee monograph is the appropriate timing for dissemination of the communication. The members should receive the monograph about 5-7 days prior to the meeting, so that it will be recently read by the members in their preparations for the meeting.

PHARMACY BULLETINS AND NEWSLETTERS

These communications serve two primary purposes: (1) continuing education (CE) through information dissemination and (2) official notice of new pharmacy policy, programs, procedures, or drug utilization. The types of communications vary with the target population from a general topic, generic communication for institution-wide distribution, to specialized newsletters for phamacists (intradepartmental), nurses, or physicians with adaptation of the content to their information needs.

The subsequent list of items generally constitutes the standard content of bulletins:

1. Drug reviews: Complete reviews of medical/pharmaceutical literature for new formulary drugs; brief reports of drug ingredients, e.g., Shohl's solution; newly marketed drugs from package insert or text information; discussions of drug groups, e.g., salt substitutes, insulins; and biopharmaceutical reviews, e.g., food and drug absorption or drug metabolism

2. Abstracts: Summaries of significant journal articles in an abstract that describes the purpose of the trial, patient population, drug regimes, results, and author's conclusions with or without a subsequent reviewer's critique

3. Announcements: Drug distribution and procedures or innovations, new pharmacy laws, P&T Committee decisions concerning policy and new drug admissions, presentation of CE films provided by pharmaceutical companies, and drug shortages

4. Drug use problem as noted in the literature: Drug administration, e.g., IM phenytoin, IV iron-dextran; new side effects, e.g., nonsteroidal anti-inflammatory drugs and renal failure; bioavailability, e.g., variable digoxin tablet absorption

5. Sample drug information inquiries previously answered

6. Bibliographies of current review articles

A review of 50 pharmacy newsletters indicates that 60-70% contained P&T Committee actions, therapeutic uses of drugs, abstracts of literature articles, new drug reviews, and reviews of therapeutic groups. Also, 40-50% of these newsletters contained drug abuse data, adverse reactions or interactions, and legislative information (16).

The initiation of newsletters as pharmacy communications requires these administrative steps: (1) hospital administrator's approval of the new service and/or educational programs; (2) medical director concurrence when provided for and directed to medical practitioners; (3) nursing director agreement for pharmacy-nursing bulletins. The prior consent and support of administrators with a joint announcement of the program affords a better acceptance of the newsletters by the information user. Five practical points concerning the content and preparation can maximize the effectiveness and utilization of the newsletters: (1) a well-organized content, (2) concise and direct statements, (3) complete information (who, what, when, where, why, how), (4) avoidance of demands, complaints, or reprimands that alienate practitioners, and (5) pertinent topics to the practice of the target population (15-17). A precaution against plagiarism is also warranted. If a document is reproduced verbatim, permission must be obtained from the author and/or publisher holding the copyright. In addition, an interprofessional document has no room for comical content that detracts from its drug information intent.

PATIENT-PHARMACIST DRUG INFORMATION COMMUNICATIONS

The consumer of drugs, i.e., the patient, should be the recipient of drug information to ensure proper drug administration and comprehension of a drug's desired benefits and untoward effects. The pharmacist is a provider of this information through verbal counseling and written information inserts with drug dispensing.

The content of these communications depends upon the patient's information needs as follows:

1. Self-administration encompasses reinforcement of directions for use, adjunctive procedures in administration of a drug, and maximum dosage guidelines, e.g., the importance of continual administration of antibiotics during asymptomatic periods to ensure a cure or antihypertensives to maintain blood pressure control and improved absorption through adjunctive measures, e.g., concomitant food abstinence with penicillins or water consumption with sulfas.

2. Precautions should forewarn patients of potential side effects without scaring them in order to avoid noncompliance because of bothersome unexpected symptoms. Also, potential common drug interactions should be noted to preclude toxicity or lack of efficacy, e.g., warfarin and aspirin. Limitations on physical activities require notation with any sedative, vision-impairing agent, or motor-suppressing drug.

3. Drug knowledge provided to patients creates an informed, more compliant patient through comprehension of a drug's action and rationale. The areas of consideration are simplified mechanisms of drug action, indications for the drug's use, time frame of drug activity correlated to the drug regimen and patient response, and storage requirements to optimize drug shelf-life (e.g., refrigeration). An exemplary resource to provide this patient counseling information is the card file system. Further assistance can be obtained from the *Drug Consultation Guide* (18).

A complete description of patient interviewing techniques and recording forms, e.g., discharge summary and medication history, are available elsewhere (19-21). The subsequent list summarizes the significant considerations and relationships in pharmacist-patient communications:

1. The pharmacist should identify himself and briefly indicate his purpose.

2. The patient should be put at ease, since he may be anxiety prone in his ill state.

3. The patient's situation as a sick person who possibly fears his disease and/or treatment and its effect on his societal roles and responsibilities should be understood.

4. The pharmacist should possess empathy or concern for the patient's well-being, without sympathy, which is negative and demeaning.

5. A professional attitude and demeanor should be presented to enhance the patient's perception of the pharmacist's contribution to drug therapy.

6. A patient, good listener is required to better understand the patient's concerns and questions.

7. The pharmacist should control the interview to maximize time devoted to each patient and minimize excessive or peripheral patient responses.

8. Questions should be phrased in an open-ended format to prevent yes or no answers, which fail to elucidate the incidence of severity of problems or degree of comprehension of comments.

9. Phrases that connote a negative, demeaning, or sympathetic attitude, which ''turn off'' the patient to counseling should be avoided.

10. Only positive and minimal nonverbal communication through gestures or facial expressions should be provided.

11. Privacy of dialogue and counsel without interruption should be answered.

12. The pharmacist should be prepared for spontaneous, unanticipated patient reactions, e.g., aggression, silence, or crying.

One form of written communication from a pharmacist to a patient is the patient package insert, which is intended to educate the patient to improve compliance (22). Its content includes the generic and trade names of the drug, a general description of its purpose, instructions for self-medications, precautions for drug-drug, or drug-food interactions, side effect precautions with their tolerance and management, storage requirements, refill instructions, and overdosage warnings with its treatment. The style and format should stimulate and facilitate the patient's reading and comprehension. Legibility requires bold print and symbols to subdivide content and attract attention. Readability requires beief, concise, specific topical sentences with key words in layman's terms at the patient's educational level but without overly simplistic or childish phraseology. An example of such inserts is found in a loose-leaf text publication by Griffith (22).

SUMMARY

The communication of drug information is a cornerstone of professional interaction in pharmacy as the technical dispensing functions are assimilated by ancillary personnel. This chapter is devoted to describing the types of communication presently transmitted by pharmacists. It elaborates upon the problems in their provision and provides suggestions to improve their content, validity, credibility, and acceptance.

REFERENCES

1. American Society of Hospital Pharmacists: The hospital pharmacist and drug information services. *Am J Hosp Pharm* 25:318-382, 1968.
2. American Society of Hospital Pharmacists: ASHP supplemental standard and learning objectives for residency training in drug information practice. *Am J Hosp Pharm* 39:1970-1972, 1982.
3. Burkholder DF: The future of the hospital pharmacist in drug information services. *Am J Hosp Pharm* 24:216-219, 1967.
4. Joint Commission on Accreditation of Hospitals: *Pharmaceutical Services, Standards for Accreditation of Hospitals*. Chicago, American Hospital Association, 1976, pp 143-184.
5. American Association of College of Pharmacy: *Pharmacists for the Future, the Report of the Study Commission on Pharmacy*. Ann Arbor, Health Administration Press, 1975.
6. Collins GE, Lazarus HL: *The Drug Information Services Handbook*. Acton, MA, Publishing Sciences Group, 1975.
7. Burkholder D: Operation of the drug information services at the University of Kentucky Medical Center. *Am J Hosp Pharm* 22:48-51, 1965.
8. Rosenberg JM: The drug information center at Mercy Hospital Rockville Center. *NY Hosp Pharm* 3:5-7, 1968.
9. Pearson E, Salter FJ, James C, et al: Michigan regional drug information network, part one: Concept. *Am J Hosp Pharm* 27:912, 1970.
10. Walton CA: The problem of communicating clinical drug information. *Am J Hosp Pharm* 22:459-463, 1965.
11. Bell JE, Grimes BJ, et al: A new approach to delivering drug information to the physician through a pharmacy consultation program. *Am J Hosp Pharm* 27:29-37, 1970.
12. Joint Commission on Accreditation of Hospitals: Purposes of the Patient Medical Records, Standards for Accreditation of Hospitals. Chicago, JCAH, 1976, p 93.
13. Davis NM: A question: Should pharmacists make permanent entries on patients' charts? *Hosp Pharm* 11:336-350, 1976.
14. Kelsey FE: The problems associated with the dissemination and effective utilization of drug information. *Am J Hosp Pharm* 22:30-31, 1965.
15. Snyder JD: Ten commandments for concise communications. *Hosp Form Mgt* 4:16-18, 1969.
16. Teplitsky B: What particular subjects are discussed in pharmacy newsletters? *Pharm Times* 40:36-37, 1974.
17. Schultz WL, Dendick ST: Pharmacy newsletters: A needed service. *Hosp Pharm* 10:146-147, 1976.
18. Maudlin R, Young L: *Drug Consultation Guide*, ed 3. Drug Intelligence Publications, Hamilton, IL, 1976.
19. Froelich RE: Understanding the patient: Preliminaries to the interview. In Blissit CW, Webb OL, Stanaczek WF (eds): *Clinical Pharmacy Practice*, Philadelphia, Lea & Febiger, 1972, p 89-96.
20. Covington TR: Interviewing and advising the patient. In Francke DE, Whitney HAK Jr (eds): *Perspectives in Clinical Pharmacy*, ed. 1. Hamilton, IL, Drug Intelligence Publications, 1972, pp 212-228.
21. Stanaczek WF, Carlin HS: Patient dismissal. In Blisset CW, Webb OL, Stanaczek WF (eds): *Clinical Pharmacy Practice*, Philadelphia, Lea & Febiger, 1972, pp 299-319.
22. Griffith HW: *Drug Information for Patients*. Philadelphia, WB Saunders, 1978.

Appendix 31.1
SAMPLE DRUG INFORMATION INQUIRIES: WRITTEN RESPONSES

1. Re: Iron-Dextran IV Administration

INQUIRY: Can iron-dextran be given by means of an infusion?

Although the company package literature (1) describes only a slow IV push of 1 ml or less per minute or IM scheme of administration with undiluted drug, the preferred technique is dilution in several hundred milliliters (e.g., 200-300 ml) of normal saline (NS) solution and infusion over 30-60 minutes, as noted by the *Manual of Medical Therapeutics (2)*. An initial test dose (0.25 ml) is necessary to detect potential allergic anaphylactic reactions. Since most untoward reactions occur within the first few minutes of infusion, Newcombe (3) administered iron-dextran at an initial rate of 10 drops/min for 20 minutes followed by 45 drops until the solution was completely administered. The maximum strength of iron-dextran in NS solution is 5%. This administration method is supported by Hanson and Hendeles (4) in their review of IV iron-dextran therapy.

REFERENCES

1. *Physicians' Desk Reference*, ed 38. Oradell, NJ, Medical Economics, 1984, p 1336.
2. Boedeker EC, Dauger JH (eds): *Manual of Medical Therapeutics*, ed 23. Boston, Little, Brown, 1980, p 283.
3. Newcombe R: *J Ther* 1:20, 1966 (per Martindale: *The Extra Pharmacopoeia Abstract*).
4. Hanson DB, Hendeles L: *Am J Hosp Pharm* 31:592, 1974.

2. Re: Tetracylines—Fetus

INQUIRY: What is the time frame for fetal dental toxicity of tetracycline in a pregnant woman (3 months) who has gonorrhea?

REPLY: The chelation of tetracycline with calcium and the mineralization of deciduous teeth, in utero, from about the fourteenth week of gestation create the potential for teeth discoloration prior to eruption (1). Thirteen case reports of yellow or yellow-brown discoloration and fluorescence of childrens' teeth followed maternal consumption of tetracycline during gestation (2-7). The daily dosage varied from 0.5 to 1 g, and total ingestion ranged from as little as 3 to 21 g. In a recent clinical trial, doxycycline was given to 43 women during early pregnancy. At 1 year of age, all the children were reported to be normal (8). A retrospective review of the dentitions of 94 children whose mothers, took tetracycline during pregnancy (average of 1 g/day × 15 days) noted only 13 of 94 cases of discoloration (9). The incidence was associated with time of gestation, i.e., 1-14 weeks' exposure, 0 of 7; 15-24 weeks, 0 of 47; 25-28 weeks, 1 of 15; and 29-40 weeks, 12 of 25. Definitive association of tetracycline to abnormal dentition was established by Genot et al (10) in a double-blind, matched-pair, placebo-controlled trial. In 41 pairs of pregnant women receiving 14-22 g of tetracycline or placebo, their 1- and 2-year-old offspring had 63% vs 7% stained teeth, respectively, and 73% vs 54% fluorescence. In 48 vs 61 children, 3-5 years old, dental staining was 72% vs 0%, respectively (10). Again, there was an association with time of administration during pregnancy and duration of administration as follows:

Trimester	Weeks Drug Taken	+ 1-2 yr	+ 4-5 yr
1	6	0/2	0/2
2	2	0/2	1/4
3	6	21/23	25/33
3	2	3/3	8/9
3	6	6/7	14/16

Therefore, in this case of a pregnant woman at 3 months of gestation, tetracycline could be used for a 2-week course of treatment or less without tetracycline deposition in fetal dental tissues. If therapy is required for over 2 weeks during the second trimester or for any length of time in the third trimester, fetal tooth discoloration is very likely. In the context of this case, the Centers for Disease Control recommends erythromycin, 1.5 g po for the first dose and then 0.5 g qid × 4 days, as the oral substitute for penicillin-allergic patients in the treatment of gonorrhea (11).

REFFERENCES

1. Anon: *Lancet* 1:917, 1966.
2. Harcourt JK, Johnson NW, Storey E: *J Oral Biol* 7:431, 1962.
3. Rendle-Short JJ: *Lancet* 1:1188, 1962.
4. Kutsher AH, Zegarelli EV, et al: *JAMA* 184:586, 1963.
5. Swallow JN: *Lancet* 2:611, 1974.
6. Kline AH, Blattner RJ, Lunin M: *JAMA* 1844:178, 1964.
7. Anthony JR: *Postgrad Med* 48:165, 1970.
8. Horne Jr HW, Kundsin RB: *Int J Fertil* 25:315-317, 1980.
9. Toaff R, Ravid R: *Lancet* 2:281, 1966.
10. Genot MT, Goaln HP, et al: *J Oral Med* 25:75, 1970.
11. *Morbid Mortal Wkly Rep* 23:341, 1974.

3. Re: Identification of Wood Rose Seeds

INQUIRY: What are the psychoactive components of Wood Rose seeds that are being used as agents of abuse?

The Wood Rose plant is a member of the genus *Ipomoea* (G. Sullivan, personal communication, 1978). Several species within this genus contain hallucinogenic alkaloids. The total content of these alkaloids is approximately 0.05%, with D-isolysergic acid amide being the principal psychoactive compound. Also, D-isolysergic acid and D-lysergic acid methylcarbinolamide are present but in lesser quantities (1).

REFERENCE

1. Claus EP, Tyler VE, Brady CR: *Pharmacognosy*. Philadelphia, Lea & Febiger, 1979, p 280.

4. Re: Bleomycin—Warts

INQUIRY: Can bleomycin be used to treat cutaneous warts refractory to conventional therapy?

REPLY: Bleomycin sulfate (Blenoxane, Bristol Laboratories) is an injectable antineoplastic agent that shows efficacy in the treatment of warts, although it is not an approved indication by the FDA. This drug activity relates to its initial Japanese use for cutaneous neoplasms (1). Bleomycin is a water-soluble glycopeptide mixture derived from *Streptomyces verticullus* (2). An enzyme metabolizes and deactivates bleomycin through hydrolysis of an ammonia group in all body tissues except the lung and skin (2). Since metabolism is very slow in the skin, the drug can accumulate in the skin to cytotoxic levels that can potentially cause beneficial suppression of abnormal growths or cutaneous reactions. Lesions do not occur after oral use until the total dose exceeds 100 mg. In wart therapy, a total dose of 1-2 mg is employed by local injections directly into the cutaneous wart to avoid skin reactions (3-8).

Seven studies have been conducted with 1200 patients (over 1600 warts) receiving direct bleomycin injections into the skin and show a cure rate of 49-100% (3-9). Warts at all body sites respond well, although plantar and mosaic warts do not respond as well, perhaps because of their size and greater resistance. Bremer (3) and Koenig and Horwitz (10) stated that the best response occurred in warts refractory to prior therapy, which was supported by Cordero et al (5) and Shumer and O'Keefe (8). Two controlled trials comparing bleomycin to a placebo control solution show 0% cure rates (95 warts) (7,8) for placebo vs 81% cures (151 warts) (8) and a 99.7% (1052 warts) response rate (7). However, one Danish trial with 108 warts produced the opposite results with placebo in saline solution or oil superior to or the same as bleomycin in placebo or oil (23% and 44% vs 13% vs 42%, respectively) (9). The variation in responses from 50-100% could be attributed to different injection techniques, doses in volume or number, and types of warts. The negative results of the Danish study in contrast to all the other consistent positive results has no apparent explanation.

The administration of bleomycin for warts employs direct injection of small doses, about 0.1-0.3 mg, into the wart, usually at the base. The number of injections depends on the size of the wart. Usually, only one or two treatments are necessary for a cure, given at a biweekly or monthly interval. The maximum total doses are 1-2 mg. The bleomycin solution is diluted to 15 mg in 15 ml (0.1%) and cooled to near freezing.

Side effects are minimal with the local direct injections of bleomycin into warts. No scarring occurred (3-9). Slight burning or mild pain often occurred on injection (3,5,8,9). Hyperpigmentation occurred in two trials (4,7) and not at all in five others. It was mild, around the warts, infrequent, and reversible. No systemic reactions were noted in three studies.

CONCLUSION: Intralesional injection of bleomycin can successfully cure warts in most cases with only one to two treatments given 2 to 4 weeks apart. Warts recalcitrant to conventional therapy also respond well. The one negative study creates the need for additional placebo comparative studies to confirm the earlier two comparative and four open trials. Toxicity has been minimal in frequency and mild in severity with slight pain or burning the only significant reaction.

REFERENCES

1. Mishima Y, Matunaka M: *Acta Derm Venereol* 52:211, 1972.
2. Goodman L, Gilman A, et al: *The Pharmacological Basis of Therapeutics,* ed 6. New York, Macmillan, 1980, p 1993-1995.
3. Bremer RM: *Cutis* 18:284, 1976.
4. Abbott LG: *Aust J Derm* 19:69, 1978.
5. Cordero AA, Guglielmi HA, Woscoff A: *Cutis* 26:319, 1980.
6. Hudson AL: *Arch Derm* 112:1179, 1976.
7. Shumach PH, Haddock MJ: *Aust J Dermatol* 20:41, 1979.
8. Shumer SM, O'Keefe EJ: *J Am Acad Dermatol* 9:91, 1983.
9. Munkvad M, et al: *Dermatologica* 167:86, 1983.
10. Koenig RD, Horwitz LR: *J Foot Surg* 21:108, 1982.

Appendix 31.2
SAMPLE PHARMACY AND THERAPEUTICS COMMITTEE MONOGRAPH

PHARMACY AND THERAPEUTICS COMMITTEE MONOGRAPH (LEVODOPA AND CARBIDOPA)

Background

The pathophysiology of parkinsonism is related to disturbed neurotransmission in the CNS (1-4). Neuronal nerve endings, which originate in the substantia nigra and terminate in the corpus striatum, contain high concentrations of dopamine. Under normal conditions, dopamine is an inhibitory cerebral catecholamine in this nigrostriatal pathway that exerts control over muscular activity and coordination. Acetylcholine is the neurotransmitter in the basal ganglia responsible for excitatory activity opposing dopamine's action. In parkinsonism, the balance between these neuronal messengers is disrupted by depletion of cerebral dopamine levels (as little as 10% of normal) (4), especially in the striatum, which results in excitatory cholinergic CNS override. The subsequent clinical sequelae involve abnormal skeletal muscle activities, e.g., the frequently observed triad of bradykinesia, rigidity, and tremor. Also, normal functional capability is frequently impaired, with an inability to perform the daily activities such as eating, dressing, walking, and washing.

Levodopa

Usage. Levodopa is the cornerstone of parkinsonism therapy to provide the catecholamine precursor and replace the depleted stores of dopamine. Levodopa readily traverses the blood-brain barrier, whereas it is relatively impervious to dopamine. Treatment necessitates a prolonged induction phase with gradual dosage increments over 1-2 months. This permits tachyphylaxis to develop gradually to the untoward reactions, especially gastrointestinal, which limit the rate at which optimal dosage is attained. The therapeutic end point is the individualized balance between optimal response as evidenced by control of rigidity, bradykinesia, and tremor vs excess toxicity. The patient response is usually observed by the following sequence of alterations: improved well-being and vigor, alertness and freer movements, loss of rigidity, gradually lessened tremor, and dyskinesia (2).

Biopharmaceuticals. Upon oral administration, levodopa is metabolized primarily in the periphery to dopamine (about 95%) by the enzyme aromatic L-amino acid decarboxylase, which is located in the liver, gastrointestinal tract, heart, lung, and kidney (1-5). A peak level of 0.5 to 2.5 μg/ml is achieved in 1-2 hours with a half-life of about 45 minutes (6). Elimination of dopamine is a metabolic process to phenolic acids and homovanillic acid (60%), amines, and amino acids. The maintenance dosage requirements average about 5-6 g/day (range 3-8 g) in four to eight divided doses (1-3).

Side Effects. These toxic signs include gastrointestinal changes (nausea, vomiting, anorexia), psychiatric changes (agitation, insomnia, confusion, nightmares), infrequent hypotension, and the most important dose-limiting reactions, dyskinesias, (grimacing, finger flexion, extension, and involuntary movements of hands, feet or head) (1-4).

Summary. From these data, the limitations of levodopa therapy become evident as follows:
1. Large oral doses
2. Dose-limiting gastrointestinal toxicity
3. Delayed, slow-onset of action
4. Side effects on multiple organ systems, especially CNS

Carbidopa-Levodopa

Mechanism. An approach to minimize these limitations involves the combination of an enzyme-blocking drug, e.g., MK485 (19) and RO4-4602 (20), to prevent peripheral metabolism and levodopa, which is exemplified by Sinemet, which contains carbidopa (MK-486, L-alpha methyldopa-hydrazine) and levodopa. Because of carbidopa's structural similarity to dopa and its inability to pass the blood-drain barrier, the peripheral decarboxylation of levodopa is solely inhibited, enhancing levodopa's cerebral penetration and concentration and lowering the systemic toxicities secondary to peripheral dopamine (7-10). The levodopa plasma levels are elevated 5- to 10-fold and the biologic half-life is prolonged, which permits dosage reduction of levodopa to about 20% of its original quantity (7-10,13).

Efficacy. The clinical literature is replete with documentation of the administration and indications for this combination therapy (11-18), but these results must be weighed against the common, unavoidable limitations created by utilization of subjective criteria to evaluate drug-induced responses. For example, the patient's symptomatic manifestations and observer's assessments are formulated into rating scales of patient disabilities, e.g., total disability (Northwestern University Disability Scale), functional disability, physical examination for the cardinal triad of signs, and aggregate of motor functions. Under these circumstances, levodopa was compared to the carbidopa-levodopa combination in double-blind, placebo-controlled trials by Fermaglich et al (11) (10 patients), Marsden et al (12) (40 patients), Mars (13) (25 patients), Mones (14) (37 patients), Fermaglich (15) (40 patients), Markham et al (16) (20 patients), Holden et al (17) (10 patients), and Glasgow et al (18) (23 patients). Their results indicate equivalent or slightly greater control of parkinsonian signs. Also, the onset of action was enhanced, frequently within 1-2 weeks for the combination drug. Last, since pyridoxine is a cofactor in the metabolism of levodopa, concomitant pyridoxine (e.g., multiple vitamins) will increase its destruction and complicate therapy. Carbidopa circumvents this problem by blocking the peripheral metabolism of concomitant levodopa (21,22).

Side Effects. Significant amelioration of the nausea and vomiting complications was observed (11-18). This action is based upon a reduction of peripheral dopamine reaching the vomiting centers and, consequently, yields attainment of therapeutic levodopa levels in a greater proportion of the patient population. The CNS side effects, primarily dyskinesia, were not reduced and possibly were earlier in onset and of greater intensity. In addition, there is a suggestion of an accelerated onset of the ''on-off'' phenomenon which is an unpredictable abrupt cessation and later return of levodopa response that may persist for hours or days.

Conclusion

The subsequent conclusions have been forwarded in these clinical reports for the combination in comparison to levodopa:

1. The intolerable nausea, vomiting, and anorectic complications are minimized.

2. The dosage of levodopa is reduced up to 80%.
3. Onset is more rapid, i.e., 1-2 weeks vs 1-2 months.
4. Psychiatric CNS side effects are not altered.
5. Dosage-limiting dyskinesias are at least equivalent or greater with the combination.
6. Response to levodopa therapy is not significantly altered with the combination.
7. The late complication of the ''on-off'' reaction is potentially enhanced (more data are required).
8. The combination product avoids the levodopa-pyridoxine drug interaction.

REFERENCES

1. Brogden RN, Speight TM, Avery GS: *Drugs* 2:262, 1971.
2. Yahr MD, Duvoisin RC: *N Engl J Med* 297:20, 1972.
22. Fahn S: *Neurology* 24:431, 1974.
23. *Drug Topics Red Book,* Oradell, NJ, Medical Economics, 1983.

COMMENT: The above monograph properly presents summary commentary and evaluation, but clinical data from representative trials are lacking, e.g., degree of responses and incidences of side effects, with both drugs.

Product Formulation, Packaging, and Distribution

DEVELOPMENT AND CONDUCT OF A PRODUCT FORMULATION AND PACKAGING PROGRAM

Frequently, the institutional pharmacist must respond to the need for special dosage forms and formulations not available commercially. Not infrequently, this also involves a knowledge of appropriate packaging. An adequate understanding of the principles involved in the formulation and preparation of pharmaceutical dosage forms is needed. This involves the concepts of biopharmaceutics, bioavailability, pharmacokinetics, pharmaceutics, stability, physiochemistry, kinetics, microbiology, quality assurance, and techniques of medication administration. In some instances, as in the case of intravenous admixtures and total parenteral nutrition, the pharmacist must also be familiar with patient variables such as electrolyte and fluid balance, and such factors as personal hygiene, environmental control, and equipment performance. Similar concepts hold true in radiopharmacy. Furthermore, the pharmacist must be able to evaluate the economic factors involved including the cost of labor, raw materials, space, equipment depreciation, and other items of fixed overhead.

CHAPTER 32

Medication Distribution Systems

KENNETH N. BARKER and ROBERT E. PEARSON

One of the primary responsibilities of the institutional pharmacy practitioner is drug distribution. Currently the major portion of a pharmacist's (and pharmacy technician's) time is spent in drug distribution, including IV admixture preparation. In hospitals with over 200 beds, this occupies 71-74% of their time, compared to 16% spent in management tasks and 10-13% in clinical practice (1). Many administrators as well as other professionals view drug distribution as the primary reason for a pharmacist's existence, and poor performance in this area can undermine support for all other pharmacy programs.

To ensure that patients receive the correct drugs at the proper time, the pharmacist must be responsible for the distribution and control of all drugs used within the institution, including controlled substances (e.g., narcotics), investigational drugs, and those brought in by patients. This responsibility includes procurement and maintenance of adequate supplies throughout the hospital; review of the prescriber's original order prior to dispensing; routine review of patient medication profiles; establishment of procedures and controls to ensure the dispensing of all drugs in unit dose (ready for administration) form; their distribution to the patient's bedside along with the appropriate drug use information; and all compounding, manufacturing, packaging, and labeling of drugs. The pharmacist must also prepare drug formulations needed but not commercially available when feasible (2). The extension of the pharmacist's responsibility for control of drug distribution and use throughout the hospital (i.e., to produce and maintain all medication order information routinely used by the physician and nurse) is growing in importance as increasing computerization makes this feasible.

DEFINITIONS

The following definitions differ in some cases from those used by others but are believed to be the most useful for presenting this material in a logical fashion.

unit dose   A physical quantity of a drug product ordered by a prescriber to be administered to a specified patient at one time, in ready-to-administer form with no further physical or chemical alterations required.
NOTE: By definition, essentially every dose in every institution is in dose form at the time it is administered.

unit dose package   A package containing one unit dose, labeled to identify the contents and including all distribution control information such as patient name, and location and date and time that the medication is due. Drug use information may or may not be included.

single unit package   A package that contains one discrete pharmaceutical dosage form (e.g., one tablet, one 5 ml volume of liquid). A single unit package may be a unit dose package if it happens to contain the particular dose of drug ordered for one patient and is properly labeled (see definition of unit dose package).

drug distribution system   A system that has as its purpose the selection, acquisition (from the manufacturer), control, storage, dispensing, delivery, preparation, and administration of drug products in health care institutions in response to the order of an authorized prescriber. Synonyms: Medication distribution system, drug management system, drug delivery system.
NOTE: A unit dose drug distribution system is one in which all drug products are in unit dose form. The step in the system (e.g., dispensing) at which they are put in this form is not specified.

unit dose dispensing system (type of distribution)   A drug distribution system in which all doses are in unit dose form at the time they are dispensed.

dispensing   The act of a pharmacist in supplying one or more drug products to (or for) a patient, usually in response to an order from an authorized prescriber, utilizing his professional knowledge, judgment, and skills to assess the patient and the drug and then plan, develop, control, and monitor the maintenance and delivery of the drug along with the information needed for its proper storage and administration (3).
NOTE: By definition, in a unit dose dispensing system all doses are put in unit dose form by a pharmacist. Thus, every patient is assured that every unit dose he or she receives has been prepared for administration under the supervision of a pharmacist.

drug distribution control (DISCON) information   Information necessary to control the distribution of a unit dose package so that it is delivered as ordered to the right patient, at the right date, and the right time.
1. An order validated by a pharmacist
2. A description of the unit dose ordered
3. The time and date that the unit dose is due to be administered
4. The identification and location of the patient
5. The transportation instructions
6. The drug use (e.g., administration) instructions

7. Labeling, both in route and in temporary storage locations
8. Feedback signaling deviations from the performance standards for the above.

drug use information   Information needed to administer the dose and assess the response. (DISCON information is excluded.)

a system   An aggregate of two or more physical components and a set of disciplines or procedures by means of which they function together for a stated purpose.

STEPS IN DRUG DISTRIBUTION

The drug distribution system in the broadest sense can be summarized as a chain of 12 steps, beginning at the drug manufacturer and ending at the patient's bedside, as shown below.

At the manufacturer:
1. Order processing
2. Production and filling
3. Shipping

At the pharmacy:
4. Ordering/receiving
5. Storing
6. Preparation for dispensing (includes compounding, measuring, packaging, labeling)
7. Dispensing
8. Transportation to nursing unit

On the nursing unit:
9. Ordering/receiving
10. Storing
11. Preparation for administration (includes compounding, measuring, packaging, labeling)
12. Administration to patient

Within the hospital, steps 4-12 constitute the hospital drug distribution system.

RELATIONSHIP TO CLINICAL FUNCTION

Although the subject of clinical functions and activities has been dealt with in another chapter, their articulation with the drug distribution functions and activities is so close, and the literature on the relationship between the two has been so confusing, that the following is offered for clarification.

Figure 32.1 illustrates the distribution function as distinguished from the clinical function(s). Those clinical activities that relate to the formulation of the prescriber's orders to initiate drug therapy include history taking, participation in physicians' rounds, consulting, and prescribing on protocol. Those clinical activities that relate to the use of the drug after it arrives in unit dose form include chart monitoring, pharmacokinetic monitoring, and patient counseling. Those activities in between, which are directed toward supplying (1) the ordered unit dose, (2) the control (DISCON) information needed to ensure that it arrives as intended, and (3) the drug use information needed by the user, all constitute activities of the distribution function.

Figure 32.1 also graphically illustrates the way in which pharmacists have literally expanded their role (in both directions) in drug therapy beyond the distribution function that used to be their sole concern (4).

The relationship between the distribution and clinical functions may be summarized most simply by stating that the pharmacist's role in drug therapy lies in drug distribution and use, and that the clinical function related to the "use" part but includes the selection of the drug to be distributed and used.

DEMAND

Drug distribution systems exist because there is a demand for individual doses accompanied by administration information to be delivered at specific times, in specific forms, and to specific patients. It is the pharmacist's responsibility to meet that demand, and to do so he must study and understand it.

By Time of Day

The demand for doses to be given originates at the tip of the physician's pen (or light pen) when he writes an order in the patient's chart. The frequency distribution of the demand thus created is illustrated as follows: an order calling for doses "tid" written at 9:32 AM would (appear to) call for the first dose to be given immediately and the subsequent two doses to be administered at equal intervals (e.g., 5:32 PM and 1:32 AM) over the next 24-hour period. This might be ideal from the standpoint of the patient's therapy, but if all orders were handled this way, the nurse could not group them for better efficiency and control. As a practical matter, the nurse is typically subject to so many interruptions, she would seldom be free to administer each dose at the exact time called for by the order.

The first of many compromises between the regimen actually ordered and that actually delivered occurs here. With-

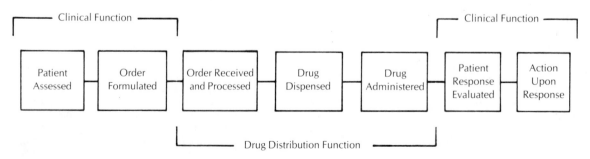

FIGURE 32.1   Drug distribution function vs clinical function.

in each hospital there exists a standard dosing schedule (whether formally recognized or not) that dictates for a given patient care unit the hours at which doses based on orders for specified regimens will be given. For example:

tid   9 AM–1 PM–5 PM

bid   10 AM–10 PM

q6h 9 AM–3 PM-9 PM–3 AM

It is assumed that the physician is aware of this schedule when he writes the order (not always true), and that he accepts the fact that the first dose will be given at the next regularly scheduled time for that regimen. If the physician wants the patient to receive the first dose immediately, he must typically write *"now,"* in which case the second dose will be given at the next regularly scheduled time.

Until such time as individualized automated bedside dispensing systems (or self-care systems) become widespread, it seems likely that the use of such standardized dose schedules will remain. Their importance to the pharmacist is that *they alter and essentially define the distribution curve of the demand for doses by time of day,* and thereby the workload of the nurse and pharmacist who must respond.

The derived demand for regularly scheduled doses in a 300-bed reference hospital (data from which will be used throughout this section for purposes of illustration) is shown in Figure 32.2 for the medical, surgical, and pediatric units, respectively. Note that this demand is characterized by tremendous peaks at 4-hour intervals (necessitating the use of a semilog scale in this chart) plus several lesser peaks at other times. Some manipulation of the shape of this demand can be accomplished by adjusting the standard dosing sched-

ule, and some hsopitals have tried using different schedules on different floors. However, the latter increases confusion among nurses transferring between floors and thus increases the risk of error (5).

The demand for nonregularly scheduled (nonroutine) doses is quite different and is illustrated for the reference hospital in Figures 32.3 and 32.4. Such orders include "stat" (immediately), "prn" (as needed by the patient), and "preop" (just prior to surgery) as shown. Perhaps the most striking characteristic of the demand for nonroutine doses is its relative smoothness (in the aggregate), with the exception of the prn doses ordered "hs" (hour of sleep).

By Dosage Form

Since all doses are ultimately destined for direct administration to the patient, they must either be in ready-to-administer form or only require modifications that lie within the skills and abilities of the personnel who will be responsible for administering them. Examples of the tasks required, for example, include measuring (withdrawing) the proper volume of drug from an ampule; deciding that two tablets of a drug as it comes from the manufacturer are required to constitute one unit dose; dissolving powder for injection in a suitable solvent; adding two or more drugs to an IV admixture; maintaining the sterility of injectables; protecting drug stability from attack by light or room temperatures; interaction of the dose with the temporary container or syringe; and the inspection of the drug and injection device for signs of defects.

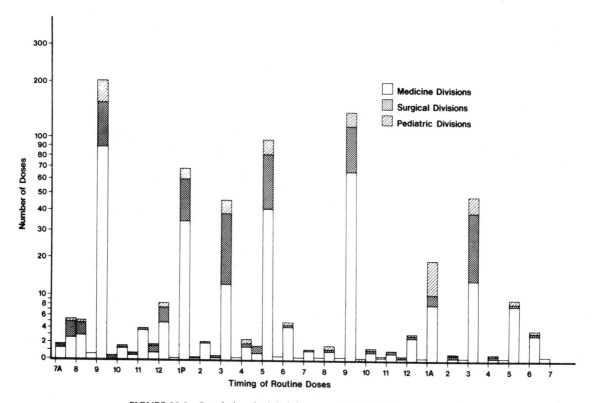

FIGURE 32.2 Regularly scheduled doses in a 300-bed reference hospital.

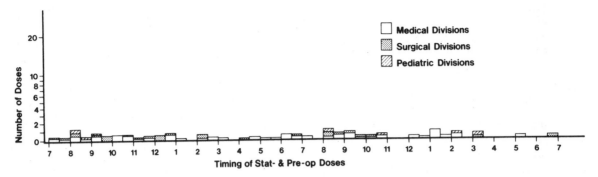

FIGURE 32.3   Nonregularly scheduled stat and preop doses in a 300-bed reference hospital.

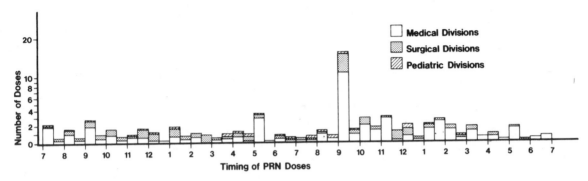

FIGURE 32.4   Nonregularly scheduled prn doses in a 300-bed reference hospital.

By Delivery Requirements

To deliver doses to specific patients requires knowledge of the location of all patients in the hospital and a method of positively identifying each patient whenever a dose is due. This in turn creates a demand for labeling, not only for the drug but also in order to identify the patient and his or her location.

HISTORICAL RESPONSE

The ways in which hospitals have attempted to respond and meet the demand for the distributon of unit doses may be analyzed and summarized in terms of the way they have provided for each of three fundamental elements: (1) the production of the unit doses, (2) the mechanism for their storage and delivery, and (3) the communications involved in controlling the drug distribution process.

Production of Unit Dose

The "production" (or preparation for administration) of the unit dose from the bulk drug product might, in theory, occur anywhere along the chain of steps beginning with the pharmaceutical manufacturer and ending with the nurse who administers the unit dose. Historically, the trend has been to move backward down the chain. Originally, each unit dose was prepared on an individual basis at or near the patient's bedside by the administering nurse 1-2 hours prior to need. Then, as evidence accumulated that the results were inadequate, the response was to move this production pro-

cess back down the steps in the distribution system—first from the individual nurse to the nurses' station, then to a central nursing area, to the pharmacy, and finally to the manufacturer (e.g., Tubex). The strategy in every case was to concentrate the workload in one location and thereby achieve the economies of scale that make improved controls economically feasible.

In practice, the nurses first turned the production of the unit doses over to a "medication nurse" who specialized in this task and then, later, to a centralized nursing medication team (some specializing in IV therapy alone). Next, some such teams arranged to prepare their unit doses near the pharmacy where they could be checked by a pharmacist before release. With the advent of unit dose systems, unit dose production was moved further back down the chain into the pharmacy. Now the number of drug products that can be purchased prepackaged in single unit (if not unit dose) form from the pharmaceutical manufacturers is increasing steadily (6), and most pharmacies report that they seek to buy all drugs prepackaged in this way (1).

Storage and Delivery

The mechanisms for the storage and delivery of unit doses (including their precursors) have evolved in a similar way. Once, drugs were all stored in hospital "drug rooms," accessible to all nurses and with minimal controls. In response to demonstrated problems (e.g., inventory losses, faulty charges) drug stocks were increasingly centralized to improve control—moving them first from an open drug room to individual medication rooms on each nursing unit, with the main stock kept in the pharmacy, and finally to unit dose systems where all stock is retained in the pharmacy (or at a pharmacy substation or cart) until just prior to use.

When most drugs were maintained in bulk quantities (floor stock) on the nursing units, the individual nurse was the mechanism for storage and delivery, totally and solely responsible for meeting the unit dose demand by getting the raw ingredients from her floor stock of drugs and producing the unit dose at the time of need. Thus, the nurse was the individual on the "front line," confronting the unit dose demand. The rest of the storage and delivery mechanism was relatively simple; the pharmacy functioned essentially as a drug wholesaler, and its main function was to respond to the nurse's order for restocking, which occurred only 2-3 times a week.

From the viewpoint of the pharmacy, the workload under this system (which still exists in some hospitals) was comfortable if unchallenging. With a comprehensive floor stock and total responsibility for unit dose production, the nurse faced the unit dose demand essentially alone, buffering the demand on the pharmacy to a point that the pharmacist seldom encountered an order that demanded immediate attention or that could not be temporarily delayed for batching or other convenience.

Later, to improve control, certain drugs were selected to be dispensed in multiple-dose form on an "individual prescription basis." This helped the nurse by labeling a specific container as containing the particular drug product to use in producing unit doses for a specific patient. At the same time, however, it transferred some of the work "back down the chain" to increase the pharmacy workload.

Finally, as it became clear that existing mechanisms for storage and delivery were placing demands on nurses they were unable to meet, the response was to lighten the burden by again transferring more tasks further down the chain to the pharmacy. The unit dose concept, emerging in 1961 (7-12), held the pharmacy responsible for the storage of all drugs. For example, before the reference hospital implemented a unit dose dispensing system, the percent of the total dollar value of all drug inventory in the hospital that was stored on the nursing units was about 50%; afterward, this dropped to less than 5%. The unit dose concept also held the pharmacy responsible for the delivery of all unit doses at the time of need. Thus, the pharmacy was finally brought in contact with and exposed to the "full force" of the true unit dose demand, facing, for example, a need to prepare and then deliver all drugs in unit dose form 1-2 hours prior to need. As many as 14 deliveries a day to most nursing units seemed indicated (Figs. 32.2 to 32.4). In centralized systems, the great increase in the frequency of deliveries necessitated the consideration of elaborate courier and automated delivery systems. In decentralized systems, elaborate satellites (subpharmacies) were built on each nursing unit to reduce delivery times.

Communications for Controlling Distribution

As the responsibility for more and more aspects of the production, storage, and distribution of unit doses has become increasingly centralized further down the chain of steps constituting the drug distribution system, there has been a predictable increase in the need for improvement in the communications for controlling unit dose delivery. When nurses were responsible for almost all of the storage, production, and delivery (not to mention administration), they generally relied upon a system of handwritten nursing medication records (e.g., Kardex), temporary "traveling" labels (medicine cards), and memory. The disclosure of the inadequacies of such methods focused increased attention on the need for improved control communications. Today, the communication methods that control unit dose delivery are increasingly being provided via computers and automation and feature the increased involvement of the pharmacist.

Inadequacies of Traditional Systems

The drug distribution systems of today have evolved largely in response to the inadequacies of the systems of the past as they were revealed over the years. Criteria by which they were measured and found wanting included (1) quality, (2) efficiency, (3) control of inventory, (4) utilization of personnel, (5) lost inventory, and (6) lost charges.

Quality

The generally recognized measure of the quality of a hospital medications system is the medication error rate—defined in general as the percent of stated administered doses that deviate from the physician's orders, as measured by the observation method developed by Barker (13) and McConnell and Juran and Dingham (14). Errors are viewed as outcome measures of the drug distribution system, and each error is viewed as an incident of system failure. In 1961, the initial use of this method, in which a pharmacist/observer accompanies the nurse and witnesses the administration of each dose, led to the disclosure that errors were occurring at a rate 1422 times the number being reported voluntarily on incident reports, or roughly one error per patient per day excluding wrong time errors. Similar findings were subsequently obtained in hospital studies of various types and sizes in the United States (5,15-20), the United Kingdom (21), and Canada (22,23). The most recent studies have continued to produce generally comparable results, demonstrating that the problem of medication errors has not yet been solved in many hospitals (24-27).

A current list of the factors that have been shown to be associated with high medication error rates is presented in Table 32.1. One factor for which a relationship with errors has been repeatedly sought without success is the pharmacologic category of the drug.

At an early time, it was concluded that the following problems lay at the root of the inadequacies of the then-current systems:

1. The utilization of systems (e.g., floor stock, patient prescription) inadequate for coping with the increasing complexity of unit dose distribution

2. The utilization of personnel (e.g., nurses) inadequately trained for the preparation of doses for administration

Recognized as contributing to the complexity of drug distribution and resulting in errors were (1) the use of con-

TABLE 32.1 Factors Statistically Associated with Error Rates

1. Work shift (e.g., day shift)
2. Medical service (e.g,, pediatric dosage errors)
3. Order type (e.g., dosage error involving doses ordered stat)
4. Dosage form (e.g., oral liquids, injections)
5. Nurse's medication workload (e.g., higher workloads)
6. Selected psychologic characteristics of the nurse (e.g., nurses prone to specific error types, visual impairment)
7. The extent of measurements and calculations required (a direct relationship)
8. Confusing drug nomenclature (e.g., Diamox and Dymelor)
9. Automatic stop orders (e.g., initiated unknown to prescriber)
10. Controls system on dated items
11. Proper temperature in refrigerators
12. Review of patient charts
13. Separation of internal and external liquids
14. Number of different doses patient was receiving (a direct relationship)
15. Presence of outdated or deteriorated medications
16. Adequacy of the supply of emergency drugs
17. Posting of conversion charts (for converting from metric to apothecary and vice versa)
18. Recording of adverse drug reactions
19. An active pharmacy and therapeutics committee
20. Type of distribution system (e.g., unit dose vs others)

fusing and misleading drug nomenclature by pharmaceutical manufacturers; (2) the use of abbreviations too abbreviated to discriminate or too parochial to communicate to all; (3) the use of two measurement systems—metric and apothecary; (4) the use of handwritten (and thus sometimes illegible) communications; (5) the lack of discipline over the order entry task to ensure that all orders received are clear, complete, and not contradictory to other orders; (6) the necessity for multiple handwritten transcriptions of orders; and (7) the use of verbal orders (5,11).

Efficiency

Efficiency is defined here as the ratio of input to output, with input measured as dollars invested in labor and inventory and the output measured in terms of doses delivered correctly. Problems with quality that may be expected to have an impact on efficiency (by reducing the denominator) have been mentioned earlier.

The nursing shortage (recurring periodically) first prompted the examination of whether or not the distribution and administration of medications consumed nursing time that might otherwise be saved, transferred to another level of employee, or computerized (28,29). The discovery that nurses' medication-related activities consumed approximately 45% of their time (30) and that 16% of this time was spent on paperwork alone (31) fueled the conclusion that more efficient systems could be devised.

Utilization of Personnel

The system demanded of the nurse a better educational background than the typical nurse of the time (e.g., diploma program RN) possessed and failed to utilize the only worker present with the needed expertise, i.e., the pharmacist, for the preparation of doses for administration (10). The typical pharmacists in smaller hospitals (200 beds or less) of one state were found to spend only 5.5-17.3% of their time on tasks truly requiring the expertise of a pharmacist (32).

Inventory Losses

Existing distribution systems were found to be subject to inventory losses due to pilferage and wastage of drugs from the large store of drugs kept on nursing stations as "floor stock." One early study found that drug losses from nursing unit stocks represented 34% of the total dollar value of drugs (at acquisition cost) administered that year (33). A study in 20 hospitals reported an estimated loss of $77.63 per bed annually in 1961 dollars (34).

Lost Charges

At the root of the inadequacies of systems regarding the capturing of charges was the fact that systems tended to rely on nursing personnel to protect the hospital's drug inventory and collect the charges. This was done despite the recognition that nurses did not view this as one of their primary functions. They received no formal training in financial matters and hospital accounting systems were unable to audit their performance, the reason being the peculiar difficulties of identifying the specific units of drug inventory after the drug products entered the process of conversion into unit doses.

Model for a New System

The recognition that existing systems of drug distribution were fundamentally inadequate and becoming more so as the prescribing of drugs for hospitalized patients steadily increased coincided with hospital pharmacists' search for new roles in the early 1960s. In the early 1960s, interdisciplinary research teams were organized and supported by large federal grants (e.g., over a million dollars to the University of Arkansas Medical Center) to develop alternative systems (33,35). These concentrated efforts resulted in the design of model or ideal systems, which in turn served as patterns for the development of systems that were as advanced as they were practical (i.e., from the standpoint of technology, economics, hospital politics) for their time (19,33,35).

The model developed, installed, and evaluated at the University of Arkansas Medical Center was unique in demonstrating and evaluating in a single, unified system: (1) the unit dose dispensing concept in its purest form, apart from clinical activities, (2) the editing center concept, and (3) the use of automated data processing equipment.

Theory

The approach in the development of this model was to study the inadequacies of existing systems and then synthesize a new, improved system based on the theoretical principles summarized below:

1. *The law of requisite variety.* This law of cybernetics states that a system will tend to go out of control on every attribute not subject to control and on every subsequent attribute downstream. This suggests that the approach to an

error-free system is the painstaking consideration of the control of each and every step. (Some controls may cost more than the effect they produce is worth—a value judgment of the type that ultimately leads to the question: What is it worth to achieve zero errors?)

2. *Simplification*. The most efficient and reliable system is generally the one with the fewest links, all other things being equal.

3. *Standardization*. This is usually the first recommended step to improve data integrity in the face of a system containing a great variety of attributes. To standardize is to simplify per se.

4. *Mechanization and automation*. Machines can do certain kinds of tasks more accurately (e.g., print, transcribe) and efficiently (e.g., calculate, measure doses in large quantities) than people can.

5. *Specialization*. Generally, the worker who specializes in specific tasks will become more expert and more efficient in those tasks, and the economies of scale make it possible to provide specialized workplace, equipment, and controls that in turn will contribute to his or her productivity and effectiveness.

6. *Improved utilization*. In particular, the education and training required by each job must not exceed that of the worker assigned to do it.

7. *Centralization*. Concentrating all like work in one place offers the economies of scale and increased controls that become achievable through the application of machines, specialization, the improved utilization of key personnel, the standardization of procedures, and a specially designed work environment.

Application

From the general principles stated above, the following principles specific to drug distribution systems were derived:

1. All drugs should be dispensed in unit dose packages (see under "Definitions").

2. All unit doses (packages) should be retained in the pharmacy and delivered to the patient's bedside only at the time they are due.

3. All medication orders should be edited in the pharmacy before going into effect, and all DISCON information should come from this (one) source.

In the model system, all drugs were dispensed in unit dose package form, including narcotics, IV additives, ointments, and ophthalmics, excluding only the emergency box items, mouthwash, and disinfectants. This simplified nurses' involvement in drug distribution by relieving them entirely of the step of preparing unit doses for administration. That task was transferred and centralized in the pharmacy. There, all doses were prepared and labeled by standardized and mechanized procedures in specially designed areas under the supervision of a pharmacist and were subject to controls fully as rigorous as those at a pharmaceutical manufacturer. Single unit packages purchased from the manufacturer were used whenever possible, but these were always adjusted and relabeled as necessary to put them in unit dose package form before dispensing.

The net result was that the nurse found every dose delivered ready for administration at that moment.

All drugs were retained in the pharmacy, open and staffed around the clock until 2 hours before doses were due. Automated data processing equipment sorted all orders 14 times/24-hour day to identify those with regularly scheduled doses due, according to a standardized dosing schedule. This made it possible to dispense no more than one unit dose of a particular drug to a specific patient at one time. This greatly simplified the nurse's responsibility for the timing of doses, and in the case of those nonregularly scheduled doses, where the timing requires a nursing judgment (e.g., prn, preop, and stat orders), the work in obtaining the dose was limited to picking up a special phone and asking the pharmacist to send it.

All unit dose packages were dispatched by automatic dumbwaiter/conveyor, courier, and/or pneumatic tube.

All medication orders were transmitted to the pharmacy via copy through the pneumatic tube. There they were edited before being activated. In the editing process, all drug nomenclature, abbreviations, terminology, dosage measurement systems, and administration instructions were standardized; all incomplete orders were completed; any conflicts with existing orders were resolved; and it was confirmed that the unit dose called for was in inventory and could be dispensed. For further simplification, the description of the unit dose prescribed was rewritten to match the standardized labeling on the unit dose to be dispensed.

The centralization of the editing function permitted the use of automated data processing equipment, standardized procedures, and improved utilization of personnel by assigning this work to a pharmacist with education training and experience better suited to this task than the nurse.

Every transcription of the order required for use by anyone in the hospital was then produced automatically from one source only via a printer at that location. This included a drug summary form sent to the nursing unit and updated as needed, which replaced the nurses Kardex and medicine cards; the medication administration record in the patient's chart; the patient's medication profile in the pharmacy; and the labeling on the envelope in which each unit dose was dispensed. The latter was used by the picker in filling the order and by the pharmacist (and later the nurse) in checking the fill.

Every unit dose was dispensed in its own individual envelope. These were generated at each filling time by the automated data processing equipment and contained the complete edited order on the front, including the patient's name, identification number, and date and time that the dose was due. Their use eliminated the need for carts and cassettes, which must travel twice the distance (i.e., must be returned for filling), require the extra step of cleaning them out, and thereby interject a new source of errors when this is done inadequately. In contrast, the envelopes were sent to the nursing units in disposable plastic bags.

Other advantages of the envelopes (e.g., over carts) included the fact that each was independent and could be completely separated for team or primary care nursing or for the giving of a single dose, and they were not dependent on the label on the cart drawer for patient identification. They could be used by the nurse to return an unused unit dose intact, recording the reason on the front. The empty envelope was used as a reminder for charting by the nurse.

Overall, the work of the nurse related to medications was greatly simplified in two ways: much of it was transferred to the pharmacy, and the remainder was simplified to the point that only the ability to read English and compare text (without having to "understand" it) was necessary to identify that a unit dose had arrived and was to be given to specified patient.

The effect of having the nurse transfer work such as dose preparation to the pharmacy was to centralize and concentrate it in one place. There the work involved was broken down into elements and the basic tasks restructured. Some tasks were assigned to machines, whereas the remainder were analyzed to determine the optimal utilization of personnel and staffing. As a result, some tasks were assigned to specialists (pharmacist, as opposed to a nurse), but this job analysis and restructuring also made it possible to assign some of the tasks formerly performed by the nurse to lower level (and less experienced) personnel. As a result, the sorting of orders to determine the doses due, for example, could then be assigned to workers instead of professionals; likewise, "pickers" could be used to "fill" the unit dose envelopes, since the description of the drug called for on the dispensing envelope matched the label on the correct unit dose—word for word and letter for letter.

The system provided, as a by-product, dose-by-dose inventory control (including narcotics), charging, and drug use data for both financial and patient care audits.

On evaluation, this system in operation resulted in a low rate of errors—1.9%, excluding wrong time errors. It also demonstrated the ability to save nursing time and see 57% of the time saved transferred to desirable activities (e.g., bedside care). Likewise, the utilization of the pharmacists time was improved.

This model system is still useful today, in that many current systems have yet to offer all of the features demonstrated, for reasons to be discussed.

As a model for the drug distribution system of the future, capable of full integration with modern clinical services, the following four features demonstrated by the most advanced systems today must be added:

1. Use of the latest data processing (e.g., computer and telecommunications) equipment

2. Automated charting (e.g., by having the nurse bar code read the dispensing envelope, the unit dose therein, and the patient identification band at the bedside, both as a final check and for automated charting)

3. Decentralization of the order editing function as an alternative where remote terminals are available and used by mobile pharmacist teams

4. Decentralization of the extemporaneous preparations (including IV admixtures) function to some degree (e.g., two separate locations in a 600-bed hospital) as an alternative when the nature and distribution of the workload and the layout of the hospital dictate

DRUG DISTRIBUTION TODAY

The drug distribution systems used today are variations of three concepts: floor stock, patient prescription, and unit dose dispensing.

In a floor stock system, a bulk supply of each drug product is stored on the nursing station in advance of need, and the nurse is totally responsible for all aspects of unit dose production (preparation) as well as administration.

In the patient prescription system, all drugs are retained in the pharmacy until receipt of the physician's initial order, whereupon a multiple-dose supply is dispensed for a specified patient. The nurse remains responsible for most aspects of the preparation of the unit doses, but is given the additional DISCON information provided on the label (e.g., identifying this drug and dose form as among those authorized for this patient). Commonly a 3-5 day supply of medication is dispensed.

A unit dose system generally means a system in which all drugs are retained in the pharmacy until receipt of the physician's order and then dispensed in unit dose packages. The nurse is relieved of all responsibility for preparing and labeling the unit dose for administration.

The percentage of hospitals that reported systems other than unit dose in 1983 was 25-28.3%, according to the Lilly survey and the American Society of Hospital Pharmacist (ASHP) survey (1,36). The Lilly survey elaborated further to report that 13% of these were floor stock systems. The trend over time has favored unit dose systems according to these surveys, and in 1983 the percentage of hospitals claiming to have "complete" unit dose systems, defined as 90% or more unit doses, was 61.1%. Another 10.6% claimed "partial" systems, and 9.7% said they had administrators' permission to install one. The Lilly survey reported that the percentage of hospitals utilizing the floor stock method was also "up to a slightly greater degree" but gave no further details.

Unfortunately, the label "unit dose system" means different things to different people, and the use of an operational definition useful for obtaining valid results in mail surveys (such as those cited) to measure the true extent of unit dose dispensing is lacking. For example, fewer hospitals reported having IV admixture programs than unit dose systems, suggesting a distinction between the two that is inconsistent with the unit dose concept. A recent national study of 58 nursing homes and 10 small hospitals reported that the decision of the pharmacists regarding whether or not to call theirs a unit dose system was often based only on whether more than a 1-day supply of drugs is dispensed at one time and/or whether or not strip packaged tablets and capsules were dispensed (25). Because of this problem, one can only safely state that most hospitals "report" that they have a unit dose system, as the term has meaning for them.

Performance Standards

Currently there is only one national, legally recognized performance standard based on outcome measures for a drug distribution system. The Health Care Financing Administration (HCFA) has established a minimum quality standard of zero "significant" (as judged by the inspector) medication errors, and not more than 5% significant ones, as a condition for participation of long-term care facilities (LTCF) and non–Joint Commision on Accreditation of Hospitals (JCAH)–accredited hospitals in the Medicare and

Medicaid programs (37). These error rates are determined by direct observation, and the rates are calculated by dividing the number of doses in error by the number of doses administered and omitted. A national study funded by HCFA that used direct observation to develop this standard projected that a maximum allowable standard of 6% would find the majority of U.S. LTCFs and small hospitals out of compliance (24).

It would seem reasonable to expect that there will someday be a national performance standard for medication errors in all hospitals (including those now subject only to the JCAH accreditation standards) set near the lowest level that has actually been attained in practice and for which reliable methods of measurement are available. Until such standards are identified and updated regularly by some central source (as USP does for drug standards), such standards will have to be determined and set for each hospital (hospital system).

Non–Unit Dose Systems

Floor Stock

Floor stock systems in which a bulk supply of each drug product is maintained on the nursing unit in advance of need and the nurse prepares the doses for administration have obvious advantages. The lines of communication for drug orders are short (the pharmacist is excluded), decisions about orders and dose preparation are decentralized and can be made at the patient's bedside, and distribution from the pharmacy to the patient care areas can be done on a batch rather than a continuous basis. Historically, this did not work well because the unit dose preparation process demanded drug knowledge beyond that of the typical nurse, and the drug inventory management requirements exceeded the capabilities (and interest) of the nursing personnel managing the typical unit.

Today, floor stock systems exist primarily in military and government hospitals, where the demand for unit doses is so specialized and thereby limited in variety that systems with more elaborate controls are not believed to be as important.

Automated dispensing machines installed on the nursing unit to dispense single unit packages to the nurse represent a form of a floor stock system, as does the use of a medication cart stocked with single unit packages delivered and left on the nursing unit daily.

Patient Prescription Systems

Patient prescription systems are distinguished by the fact that all drugs are retained in the pharmacy until the order is received, and then a multiple-dose supply is dispensed to the nursing unit labeled for use by a specific patient. Many distribution systems claiming to be unit dose dispensing systems actually fall closer to this category when the doses sent are in single unit rather than unit dose packages and when multiple doses of different drugs (e.g., a 24-hour supply) are sent all at one time. The placing of each patient's doses in a drawer of a medicine cart or cassette with his or her name on it performs essentially the same control function as labeling a prescription with the patient's name.

Pharmacist Review of Original Order

One important feature of drug distribution systems that is, to a degree, independent of the type of system is having a pharmacist review the physician's original order rather than a transcription by the nurse before the first dose may be given. It may be surprising to learn that this feature, traditional in community practice, became common in hospital pharmacy relatively recently.

This feature is not commonly associated with floor stock systems in which the nurse responds to a new order by preparing the first dose from floor stock without involving the pharmacist, but with systems in which floor stock drugs are stored on the nursing unit in dispensing machines that the nurse can gain access to only after the pharmacist has reviewed the order and activated the dispenser.

Unit Dose Dispensing Systems

To describe and characterize unit dose systems today in all of their variations is more difficult then it may seem, for good reason.

Historically, the unit dose dispensing concept evolved out of a revolution in the way pharmacists viewed their responsibilities for the particular steps in the hospital drug distribution system. This revolution was to view the system as a whole rather then as a chain of independent subsystems, each presided over by a different profession (medicine, pharmacy, nursing). The unit dose concept represented the first comprehensive and unified concept of the hospital drug distribution system as a whole. This characterizing feature "broke the mold" for thinking about drug distribution problems, and pharmacists soon began looking at nursing medication records, for example, and the chart.

This historical perspective is important in understanding why so much confusion and so many variations still exist, as well as why the implementation of this innovation has taken so long. For the first time, because of the sudden availability of government research funds for health care delivery research (33,35), there was a great deal of research data on a topic (systems analysis) that most pharmacy practitioners were not educationally prepared to evaluate.

The result is that today's apparent consensus in favor of unit dose dispensing hides a great degree of confusion that remains concerning what the concept means and entails; the interpretation of the results of the studies evaluating the applications to date; and as a result, a greater variety in the systems implemented than one might expect, given the unparalleled amount of research funds expended in this one area of professional practice.

The common belief that the unit dose concept and the research relating to it is widely understood may partly explain why the researchers studying drug distribution systems encounter such a seeming disparity between what is said and written about unit dose dispensing systems vs what is observed in practice.

Degree of Centralization

It was originally anticipated that the principal issues to be addressed in deciding how the unit dose concept should be applied would include centralization and communication (7).

The systems in place today vary primarily with regard to the degree of centralization of the functions shown below:

1. The communications involved in controlling the distribution of unit doses
2. The production of unit doses
3. The mechanism for the storage and delivery of the unit doses

In the literature, all unit dose systems that feature the use of satellite pharmacies (substations) located in the patient care areas are labeled "decentralized systems," although only the storage and dispensing of unit dose packages may take place there. Only about 13% of all hospitals have one or more satellite pharmacies, and this percentage has been relatively stable in recent years (1).

Factors external to the pharmacy that play an important part in prompting consideration of the use of satellites, each serving a predetermined number of beds, are:

1. Hospital policy calling for the general decentralization of most hospital services (NOTE: This was the impetus for the original decentralized system and was opposed by the pharmacist.)
2. Inadequate materials handling systems (e.g., elevators, dumbwaiters, trayveyors, pneumatic tubes, automatic carts) unable to provide adequate response times if centralized
3. Multiple building facilities, where decentralized pharmacy management is desired

External factors that may preclude the use of satellites include:

1. Lack of available space in the patient care areas
2. Insufficient concentration of beds on specialized patient care units for efficiency (minimal requirement believed to be about 85 beds of the same medical type, e.g., surgery, for efficiency via specialization) (38)
3. Higher cost of operation unacceptable to administration

The reasons why those pharmacies who have a choice sometimes choose to utilize satellites include the following:

1. Improvement of communications with other professionals via person-to-person interaction
2. Shared use of space and personnel for performance of clinical activities such as chart review, rounds, etc
3. Specialization in combined pharmacy dispensing and clinical services to a technically demanding type of patient population concentrated in one location (e.g., pediatrics, surgery, intensive care)

The last factor cited may be the most common today. A trend toward decreased use of satellites in general hospitals is being offset by their increased use in specialized hospitals (1).

The reasons why most pharmacies that have a choice have chosen systems that do not utilize satellites and choose to centralize at least the production of the unit dose packages include:

1. Lowest setup and operating cost
2. Higher cost effectiveness.

A centralized system is considered the least expensive system for reaching minimal standards of performance quality, i.e., "getting into unit dose dispensing." Then, as performance standards are raised, the cost continues to be less than for a satellite serving the same number of beds when considering drug distribution alone, with clinical activities set aside for cost justification on their own merits (39).

Satellite systems are easier to characterize and distinguish than the systems in the remainder of U.S. hospitals (48%) claiming to have complete unit dose systems. However, the homogeneity of satellite systems is not as great as it might first appear. A few simply prepare doses the way the nurses did it under the floor stock systems. Most depend on the central pharmacy to perform some tasks centrally, particularly the production of unit doses, and in many successful systems, their storage and delivery at least daily.

An examination of the mechanisms used by current systems claiming to be centralized unit dose dispensing systems reveals that, in terms of frequency of deliveries, they fall far short of matching the true pattern of the demand for unit doses. Of those hospitals reporting at least a partial unit dose system, 89.5% made deliveries at 24-hour intervals, and 7.2% made deliveries less often (1). Only 2% made deliveries as often as twice a day. In a sense, these "centralized" systems appear to have centralized the production and dispensing (release by pharmacist) of unit dose packages but decentralized their storage and delivery.

A system labeled the "decentralized pharmacist system" originating in the late 1970s has the pharmacist come to the patient care unit each day with approximately 500 of the most used drug products stored in a master mobile medication cart. There he dispenses a 24-hour supply of unit doses for each patient in a cassette and the first dose for each new order (40,41).

The decentralized pharmacist also performs an additional task on the patient care unit, the review of nursing medication records, which distinguishes this approach with regard to the third way in which unit dose systems vary in degree of centralization—the responsibility for DISCON information.

The degree of centralization of the task of originating and issuing the communications for controlling the distribution of unit doses varies. Generally, the ideal model of all such DISCON information coming from only one source has been realized in relatively few systems, mostly where on-line computerization of all DISCON information has been achieved.

Oddly enough, many satellite systems, in which it would presumably be relatively easy for the nurse and pharmacist to share the same patient medication profile information, nevertheless persist in duplicating this work, having the nurse prepare for her work a medication administration record (MAR), which involves essentially the same information as the patient medication profile prepared by the pharmacist. Moreover, cross-checking the two for consistency is not always routine or even required, even though it is a decentralized pharmacist system.

The same failing is true for many unit dose systems, although not all. Some attempt to provide the nurse with her MAR information via paper strips that are sent up to be attached to the MAR when new orders are written and discarded when orders are discontinued.

The delay in progress toward the model system is thought to be due, in part, to the reluctance of the pharmacist to cross "turf lines" and "tell nurses how to keep their medication records," along with the reluctance of nurses to let them. The increasing trend toward the implementation of the computerized patient record will hopefully overcome this problem.

Involvement in Medication Administration

Once it was shown that the quality of the performance of drug distribution systems could be significantly improved by relieving the nurse of the responsibility of performing many of the steps (particularly preparation for administration) preceding drug administration, it was perhaps inevitable that the "same medicine" would be tried on the final step—the administration of the unit dose. The utilization of pharmacists to administer drugs has been considered (42), but has been generally discarded for all except IV and emergency team participation for several reasons, primarily the increased cost.

Nurses have long experimented with central drug therapy systems featuring a centralized team of nurses specializing in medication preparation and administration (incidentally setting the pattern for the IV teams of today) (43).

An approach that featured greater involvement of the pharmacist in both unit dose production and administration was the central drug therapy team made responsible to the pharmacy department. Here the preparation of unit doses was checked (though not prepared) by a pharmacist before their administration by the nursing team (44).

All such approaches calling for the use of functionally specialized nursing teams ran afoul of the primary care nursing movement among nurses, which opposed functional assignments in principle and wished to see each nurse assigned instead to serve relatively few patients (e.g., 5-6 patients). The nurse's role would be to integrate all of the therapies received by that patient, not limited to drug therapy alone. Today, functional assignments are still common in many short-term general hospitals (i.e., 40-50%) and predominant at others (45).

At Ohio State University, researchers attempted to overcome such objections as well as the cost of the use of nurse medication teams by creating medication administration technicians, who received in-service training by nurses, but whose unit dose preparation activities were checked and supervised in practice by pharmacists stationed on the wards.

This concept has grown slowly. The 1983 Lilly survey reported that "pharmacy-controlled drug administration" was practiced by only 6.7% of reporting hospitals (1). The major obstacle to this approach has been the view that drug administration per se requires patient assessment, teaching, monitoring (e.g., blood pressure, respiration, pulse), and the ability to integrate drug therapy with other concurrent therapies.

To address this obstacle the researchers at Ohio State University conducted a study that showed that in the actual practice of administering medications most nurses did not, in fact, exercise such skills for lack of time. A compromise was reached whereby the nurses retained responsibility for observing, recording, and reporting desired and undesired effects and initiating appropriate action. They also evaluated

the need for doses ordered "prn." It should be noted that this approach does not propose that the use of medication technicians will, in fact, provide the nursing skills needed but not currently delivered but that those skills now for the first time would be exercised by the nurses by virtue of the nursing time freed from medication administration (46).

Another possible reason why this approach has grown so slowly may include the reluctance of pharmacists to take on the supervision of the task of the administration of the drug, for which they are poorly educated and trained as compared, for example, to unit dose preparation (10). Also, nurses have opposed this move, although their opposition may decrease as the nursing profession continues to move to new roles and away from areas of practice where they have little independent authority, such as medication administration. Also, the nurse-practice acts of some states still require the administering individual be a licensed nurse.

The ever-increasing pressure for cost containment could make the use of medication technicians more attractive, particularly when used in simple (low-cost) systems; and there is new evidence that they do reduce error rates (47).

Degree of Computerization

One of the most important developments that differentiates drug distribution systems today is the degree to which computers are utilized.

The most important application of the computer lies in its use as the one source of all DISCON information following order entry. It begins by helping the pharmacist to edit the information—performing cross-checks for patient allergies and drug-drug–food-lab test interactions and checking dosages. It can then maintain and provide this information, updated and on line, to all who need it, when and where they need it. This single source can generate patient profiles for the pharmacist, the MAR for the nurse, the dispensing orders or "pick list" for the pharmacy technicians, all automatic stop order notices for the physicians, all charges, inventory adjustments, and all labels.

Computerized systems make it feasible and practical to implement dispensing envelopes. This provides the ultimate in control of the individual unit dose and the reduction of medication errors but is dependent on the availability of computerized machine processing to produce the envelopes.

Computerization, with its ability to do all of the tasks demonstrated in the model system, has the potential for as big an impact on reducing errors as the unit dose dispensing concept, if not more so. The recent advent of affordable computer systems can be expected to accelerate the pace at which true unit dose dispensing throughout the hospital becomes feasible.

Articulation with Clinical Services

During the development of modern clinical pharmacy services, the drug distribution function was used by pharmacists as a springboard for developing and demonstrating new clinical activities as they evolved. This was a logical "entree" and provided access to those parts of the drug therapy system bordering the drug distribution system, which were the initial sites of the clinical pharmacy movement. The desire to implement clinical pharmacy activities prior to the time they could be cost justified on their own merits resulted in systems in which the two functions were so intermingled that it was difficult to determine which benefits (and which costs) should be ascribed to each function. A new criterion was proposed for a drug distribution system—it should place the pharmacist in a position and location where he would have time "free" for clinical activities. As great emphasis was placed on this one criterion, others such as the quality and efficiency of performance in distributing the unit doses were sometimes ignored. For example, a distribution system that poorly matched the staffing to the workload and resulted in many hours of idle time could be praised for "making more time free for clinical pharmacy."

Once several of the clinical activities were studied and their cost/benefits established, it became possible to look at the drug distribution and clinical functions separately and to consider as a separate matter the most effective and efficient integration of the two. Where this has been done, such integration has appeared less attractive. It would appear, for example, that the peak demand for clinical activities does not coincide with slack demand for drug distribution activities as some had hoped, e.g., both experience peak workloads in responding to the writing of new orders (27). The logistics and economies of scale are sometimes strikingly different between the two—the distribution function, for example, involves work units that (1) include products as well as information, (2) are much greater in number, (3) are more predictable in occurrence, and (4) more regular in their handling requirements.

The advent of computerized medication records accessible anywhere in the hospital may be expected to further free the drug distribution and clinical functions to find the degree of integration and the degree of centralization—decentralization—optimum for each. Some hospitals have already found the latter to be substantially different, with highly decentralized clinical teams and a more centralized distribution system.

PROCEDURES

Order Processing

Order Input

Typically the physician's order is put into the hospital medication system by his writing it in longhand on an order sheet form, which is a permanent part of the patient's medical record. Physicians may input orders directly via video display terminal (VDT), for example, with a light pen. However, all orders should be transmitted first to a pharmacist for review and editing. Efforts to skip this step or have the computer attempt to perform it have had a long record of failure over the years.

Methods currently used for transmitting the physician's medication orders in the original form (i.e., not a manual transcription) include (1) self-copying order forms, (2) electromechanical methods, and (3) telematics (computer telecommunications). Although telematics is the method of choice, the multicopy order form is still the most widely used. Physicians typically write medication orders among

all other orders; therefore, adding "no carbon" copy paper under the original is the least expensive and least objectionable method (9,33).

Some have redesigned the physician's order form to separate medication orders from treatment orders in parallel columns. This makes it easier for pharmacy personnel to review the sheet (48). However, medication orders inadvertently written in the treatment section are more easily missed by the pharmacist, and other orders relevant to drug therapy, such as potentially interacting laboratory tests, may also be overlooked. An entirely separate medication order form for medications alone is not desirable, since pharmacists should have all orders written for the patient available for his review (9).

Computerized systems that allow physicians to input orders at the patient care unit should have security mechanisms to prevent unauthorized order entry. Also, some states may have laws requiring handwritten physician's orders.

Review and Editing

All medication orders should be reviewed and edited by a pharmacist before they are acted upon by a nurse. Until computerized systems are available, orders for stat doses will be the exception, but these should be verified in retrospect at the earliest time.

In editing, the pharmacist should rewrite the medication order completely to standardize all drug nomenclature, abbreviations, terminology, dosage measurement systems, and administration instructions. Incomplete orders should be completed; conflicts with existing orders should be resolved; and it should be ascertained that the order is fillable, i.e., that the unit dose called for is in the formulary and can be supplied from stock. If extemporaneous packaging of the dose is required, the division of the pharmacy performing that function should be alerted. Any questions should be resolved by contacting the physician as necessary so that the edited order will be complete, unambiguous, and able to be carried out by all those involved.

The edited order should include the generic name of the drug (following by trade name in parentheses if it will appear on the label of the unit dose dispensed); strength; dosage form; route of administration; dosage regimen including actual times of day that doses will be administered; the ordering physician; and, ideally, an index number unique to that order. Orders for IV solution, both with and without additives, plus blood products should also be included.

Medication Order File

All edited orders should be entered into the master order file for access at any place and any time by all who will use the order, including nurse and physician. The file for each individual patient should display all (and only) current orders on that patient and include the patient's full name, hospital identification number, age, sex, nursing unit, admission date, admitting physician, diagnosis(es), surgical procedure(s), allergies, and special diets.

Any changes or clarifications in an order should be noted in writing in the file, including the initials of the person obtaining the order clarification (48).

Nursing Use

The medication file should be used to generate and update the nurse's MAR. The MAR serves as the nurse's primary listing of medication orders current on each patient, replacing the older medication cards and Kardex. The nurse's MAR is ideally updated electronically, but manual methods involving the sending of replacement printouts or adhesive strips have been used (33).

Except when envelope systems are used, the nurse must take the MAR along with her so that she can document each dose as it is administered, refused, or omitted for good reason. This creates a problem for physicians seeking access to the MAR information. To solve this problem, duplicate MARs are sometimes created and placed in the patient's chart at the end of each day for physician access (49).

In unit dose envelope systems, the order appears on front of the envelope, eliminating the need for the nurse to take the MAR along. The used envelope is retained for charting, which may be done automatically by passing it over a bar code reader on the nursing station.

A way of charting in which envelopes are not used is for the nurse to enter the doses given into the VDT. The most advanced systems, such as the one at the University of Alabama Hospital, anticipate that the nurse will chart onto the VDT inquiring why if it is not done and automatically reporting any failure to do so to nursing administration.

In advanced electronic systems, the nurse is alerted to the time doses are due automatically by VDT display or signal light (27,33). In manual systems, this may be done by a clock strip inserted at the bottom of each MAR, with a plastic signal that the nurse advances to the time the next dose (of any order) is due (9).

Pharmacy Use

The medication order file serves the pharmacy (as it serves the nurse) by providing a patient medication profile. It is also used for generation of orders for distribution of all scheduled doses due at a given time (including prn orders when the first dose is sent in advance). This set of distribution orders (i.e., dose setup document or "pick list") is derived from the medication order file and produced automatically at each filling time in computerized systems. In manual systems, the patient's medication order file can serve as the distribution order also (50). Some systems use separate distribution order documents, but this introduces inefficiency and error.

It is essential that permanent records of all orders written and all doses dispensed during the patient's hospitalization be maintained. Therefore, all order modifications such as cancellations, orders to withhold medications for a surgical procedure, npo (nothing by mouth) orders, etc must all be recorded and, when these cease to be current, transferred to the inactive permanent file.

Distribution

Picking

The dispensing of regularly scheduled medications that are already available in single unit packages, where all that is required is the ability to compare the name of the single unit package called for on the order with its counterpart on the package label, is referred to as "picking." The term "picker," taken from the wholesale drug industry, denotes a nonpharmacist who performs the task of filling the cassette drawers or envelopes for orders. The error rate for such workers was shown to be approximately 1 in 6000. This rate was four times better than the combined efforts of the pharmacist and nurse in the same study (33). In an outpatient pharmacy, one study found no significant difference between the error rates of pharmacists and technicians (51).

The pickers receive their orders in the form of a pick list, generated by the computer on hard copy (52) or soft copy (53) just prior (1-2 hours) to the time of the regularly scheduled dose delivery. As the pick list is generated, the inventory is updated and the charges posted automatically. In manual systems, the charges are commonly generated from the pharmacy, although the MAR has also been used.

A mechanism for written communication between the pharmacy and nursing departments regarding the disposition of a unit dose (e.g., the reason why it was omitted), npo status, etc is often used. In envelope systems, this is simply a printed form on the back of the envelope, but for cart systems, a separate card is required. This reduces telephone interruptions (54) and is especially useful in centralized systems.

Most systems (and some state regulations) require that the work of the pickers must be checked by a pharmacist before their output is released. However, as noted previously, it has been demonstrated that under favorable conditions their error rate can be much lower than for other parts of the system. When the nurse's final check is to bar code read and compare the label on the unit dose sent vs the unit dose called for in the order, then the checking of pickers can surely be eliminated.

Automated dispensing machines to replace the picker (if not the pharmacist) have been under study for more than 20 years (55). However, a machine for picking unit doses has only recently become commercially available, and its practicality has yet to be established (56).

Dispensing

Those doses not schedulable, i.e., prn doses plus all those requiring extemporaneous packaging or compounding should be dispensed from a separate area (or satellite). The majority of such orders will be for IV solutions, which present so many special problems they are discussed separately in Chapter 34.

Also filled there are preop orders, stat orders, and orders for those drugs not stocked in emergency carts (e.g., cardiopulmonary resuscitation carts) or cabinets in the nursing areas. The emergency drug supplies on the nursing units should be limited to those for which access must be quicker than the response time of the pharmacy service. (Speed is not an advantage if the dose will be in error.) The Pharmacy and Therapeutics Committee should approve and periodically review such drugs. Emergency supplies should be checked by pharmacy personnel periodically to ensure that they are in date and up to predetermined levels (48,57). Emergency boxes should be sealed with nonresealable devices (e.g., disposable locks, plastic bands) and dated on the outside with the date of the earliest expiring drug in the box (57).

It is recommended that prn medications be retained in the pharmacy and such doses sent only on request by the nurse, physician, or clinical pharmacist. Although this tends to increase the work of the pharmacist, it reduces the workload in the picking area considerably, since relatively few (21%) prn doses ordered are actually administered (27,58). The stress on the pharmacist is increased, since this exposes him to the same unit dose demand being experienced by the nurse, but the result is fewer extraneous doses on the floor available to the nurse, which can prevent medication errors (26). Less satisfactory approaches currently in use include:

1. Treat prn orders as if they are called for regularly scheduled doses but place only the first dose in a special compartment of the patient drawer when cassettes are used.

2. Maintain a separate drawer for prn medications for each patient on the medication cart, which remains on the nursing unit and is replenished daily.

3. Place frequently used prn medications (e.g., analgesics, antacids) on floor stock in the nursing area.

4. In envelope systems, have the picker send up the first dose to be stored in a special compartment for each patient on the nursing unit.

The last three approaches listed above suffer from added inefficiency and opportunity for error when the unused doses must be returned to stock (5).

Standing Orders

Some hospitals still allow physicians to use a preprinted set of orders for routine procedures (e.g., postpartum). A copy should be sent to the pharmacy once the physician has signed such orders. These are maintained on file for review and activation by the pharmacist (never a picker) when an order to activate them is received.

Floor Stock Items

Where floor stock is maintained, it is usually divided into "free" and "charge" floor stock. "Free" stock items are those few items considered so inexpensive and safe that their distribution is not controlled by the pharmacy. For safety, internal floor stock medications should always be stored separately from external medications. "Charge" floor stock includes those medications considered safe for preparation and administration by the nurse but whose cost is great enough to warrant a separate charge. The nurse's reorder for the dose is usually used to post the charge. Automated dispensing machines have been used for floor stock (55). Under unit dose systems only a few such over-the-counter items, such as back lotion and mouthwash, are permitted as floor stock.

Controlled Drugs

It is legal to dispense all controlled drugs in the same manner as other medications, as long as proper security is maintained (59); and the dose-by-dose accounting feature of the most advanced unit dose systems makes this possible (33). In systems lacking this feature, a copy of the medi-

cation administration record can serve as documentation of controlled drug administration (60). Computerized records and proof of use sheets are also acceptable to the drug enforcement administration (61) (see Chapter 60).

Patient Admissions, Transfers, and Discharges

In any drug distribution system, it is essential that the pharmacy be continually informed of patient admissions, transfers, discharges, and surgery schedules. This information is required for the pharmacy to accurately distribute medication to the patient's current location in the hospital. Hospitals can have a poor record in keeping up with patient location, and therefore, patient location (e.g., bed number) should not be used for patient identification. The pharmacy should have on-line, real-time access to the hospital system for monitoring admission/transfer/discharge activity.

After-hour Coverage

Although 24-hour coverage of the pharmacy would seem to be essential, at this time only 19.3% have achieved it, according to the most recent ASHP survey (36). The ASHP has stated the principles under which drugs may be obtained when the pharmacy is closed (48), and the JCAH standards for pharmaceutical services states (57):

Only prepackaged drugs shall be removed from the pharmacy when a pharmacist is not available. These drugs shall be removed only by a designated registered nurse or a physician, and only in amounts sufficient for immediate needs. Such drugs should be kept in a separate cabinet, closet, or other designated area, and shall be properly labelled. A record of such withdrawal shall be made by the authorized individual removing such drugs and shall be verified by a pharmacist.

Self-Administration

For years physicians have ordered certain drugs (e.g., antacids) "left at the bedside" for self-administration by the patient. Repeated efforts to increase the amount of this activity have been stalled by concern for the legal position of the hospital in such cases. Recently there has been an increased interest in this area, prompted in part by the desire to teach the patient how to use his or her medications correctly upon discharge, and also by the proliferation of devices such as those for self-administered analgesics. The economics of prospective payment systems have greatly increased efforts to increase the patient's involvement in self-care, and some hospitals are offering self-care nursing units at a greatly reduced patient cost (60). This may be expected to stimulate the self-administration of medications even further and will likely create a market for new kinds of simple devices capable of administering unit doses to patients at their bedsides.

Automated Administration Devices

In the future, the percentage distribution of the various drugs by dosage forms used may be expected to change dramatically, with the percentage of tablets and capsules dropping to less than 40%. Taking their place will be drugs administered by transdermal patch, by implanted devices, and by the respiratory route, among others. Implanted pumps for administering digoxin or insulin will require monitoring and dosage adjustment. How pharmacists will service these devices, how unit doses of respiratory drugs will be dispensed, etc is not at all clear. A pharmacist with a biomedical engineering background may be a necessary addition to the pharmacy staff.

Materials Handling System

When the materials handling system is selected for the hospital, the needs of the pharmacy have often been underestimated. It should be pointed out that the pharmacy department transports more units of materials throughout the hospital than any other department when unit dose systems are involved. For regularly scheduled medications, a trayveyor connecting the pharmacy and the nursing units aligned in a vertical tower is ideal, and a dumbwaiter or rail-mounted automated conveyor system, although offering batch rather than continuous delivery, is a close second.

For the delivery of the first doses of new orders, including stat and one-time orders, a pneumatic tube system is ideal (27,33). Cart delivery systems are the slowest and have the serious disadvantage of having to be "designed around" the queue for elevators. Messenger systems can be faster than cart systems by using the stairs for descent but are still the most labor-intensive method of delivery. Both carts and messengers are slow, in large part, due to the fact that items to be delivered must await pickup as opposed to the instant access feature of the pneumatic tube and trayveyor. Automated cart systems involving vertical and horizontal conveyor systems, including computer monitored systems, have not been very successful to date but with improvements may prove to be so in the future. The efficiency of all systems is greatly improved when the recipient is automatically notified of the arrival of the needed material. For example, a dumbwaiter should have a kick-off feature that turns on a signal light at the nurses' station that cannot be turned off without going to the dumbwaiter.

All parts of the materials handling system must protect medication from pilferage. Personnel employed as messengers should be thoroughly screened, and all automatic delivery equipment must have an alternate delivery method in the event of breakdown. The system should never leave medications unattended and accessible to patients and visitors on the patient care units (48).

Packaging

Three levels of packaging are required for unit dose systems: (1) one-at-a-time packaging in the dispensing area, (2) extemporaneous packaging in either a special area or the production area, and (3) production packaging.

In a true unit dose system, the circumstances that may result in a called-for dose not being prepackaged at the moment it is needed to be dispensed include (1) a drug unstable in ready-to-use form that must be reconstituted at the last moment, (2) a special dosage (e.g., one on a declining dosage schedule) not expected to be used again, and (3) new unit doses for which there has been insufficient time

following the receipt of the order to have the doses prepared extemporaneously or on a batch basis by the production packaging program.

The goal of the pharmacist should be to provide a unit dose package comparable to that provided by the production packaging or extemporaneous packaging program. For this reason, the same containers (e.g., syringes) and labels should be used. Special small volume devices are available for one-at-a-time packaging of tablets and capsules as well as oral liquids and injections.

Some unit doses may be prepared extemporaneously or batch packaged solely to relabel the drug to reduce confusion and possible error (33) (see Chapter 37).

Sources of Forms

Various forms for use in unit dose systems are pictured by Summerfield (62) in *Order Forms, Charts and Records in Hospital Unit Dose Distribution Systems* compiled and disseminated by Roxanne Laboratories (63) in Abbott's *Unit Dose Implementation Manual-Appendix A* (64), and in Buchanan's *Discussion of Unit Dose Documentation* in the *Practice of Pharmacy* (65).

A recommended content and format for the labels for noncommercially available unit doses has been published by the ASHP (66).

PROBLEMS OF CURRENT UNIT DOSE SYSTEMS

Some of the problems encountered with current systems relate simply to the adequacy of coverage. For example, 24-hour pharmacy service is offered by only about 19% of all hospitals today (1,36). Also, some systems exclude controlled drugs and IV drugs, and the special care areas (operating room, recovery) are seldom included. Such problems are important but are also readily apparent. Those less apparent and involving the unit dose concept itself are the focus of this section.

Doses Dispensed Before They Are Needed

Frequency of Scheduled Deliveries

As anticipated in the original article that gave unit dose its name, the major problems with such systems revolve around interhospital communications and transportation (7). This was reasonable to predict for a system that proposes to dispense all unit doses at the time they are due, when considering that the average hospital patient receives about 9-10 doses per day and that these must be given around the clock, 7 days a week (Fig. 32.2).

How do they do it? The answer is, most do not. The model system delivered unit doses 14 times per day to ensure that the next dose of any order never arrived on the nursing unit ahead of the time that the previous dose should have already been given or returned. However, according to the Lilly survey for 1983, only 2% of all unit dose hospitals delivered unit doses as frequently as twice a day. The vast majority, 89.5%, issued medications at 24-hour intervals (1), presumably because in doing so they complied with the

ASHP statement on unit dose drug distribution which states "for most medications not more than a 24 hour supply of doses is delivered to or available at the patient care area at any time" (67).

This statement was perhaps useful for its place and time in setting an achievable goal for hospital systems used to the pharmacy dispensing a 5-7 day supply. Now, however, there is additional evidence to support the hypothesis that the frequency of dose delivery (exchange) and the medication error rate are inversely related. In a 4-year study in a 622-bed not-for-profit hospital, the effects of poor pharmacy response time on medication error rates were described as follows (26):

[Because deliveries occurred only twice daily] . . . there were a great number of adjustment doses sent to the floor for placement in the cart by the nurse. These swelled the already heavy traffic of interim (new order) doses and stat orders, all queuing for transportation . . . to the nursing units.

A new nurse soon learned that response time was poor (e.g., "it takes a long time to get drugs from the pharmacy"). When a nurse found that the dose she needed was missing from cart . . . (for example due to the failure of an adjustment dose to arrive) . . . she was confronted by several unsatisfactory options including (1) ordering a replacement dose from the pharmacy with the expectation that *it* would likely *not* arrive in time for her to give it before going home, or (2) using the dose sent up for a later time, conveniently at hand in the patient's drawer. If she elected the first option, the replacement dose she ordered might arrive after her shift and be given to another patient in error (as was observed). If she elected the second option, the dose she used would be missing when the next nurse needed it, and an omission error might occur (as was observed).

The reports of the observer witnessing the administration of unit doses to the patients included many examples such as these two (26):

Isordil had been ordered as 10 mg, sublingual, q 6 h. When passing the noon medications, the nurse accidentally dropped one of the Isordil tablets on the floor. To replace it, she reached in the drawer, and took the dose *already there for the next time,* which in the current system had to be sent along with the first dose since there are only two cart deliveries per day. She did not order a replacement. The evening shift nurse, *not finding her dose in the cart at the time it was due,* omitted it.

An Atromid-S omission was similar. In that case the patient did not take the tablet, and instead left it on his breakfast tray where the nurse spotted it. Since that dose went into the garbage *she took the next dose (sent in advance)* out of his drawer in the cart and gave him that one. As a result, the evening nurse *found his drawer empty.* She remarked to the observer that this had happened the night before. She did fill out a slip, but the dose was never given.

It is probably not entirely a coincidence that the problem of "missing doses," meaning a dose the nurse expected from the pharmacy but said she did not receive, became prominent in the literature when the pace of unit dose implementation accelerated after the ASHP statement (requiring only one delivery per 24 hours) appeared in 1975 (68-73).

Procedures for "On Call" Deliveries (prns, IVs)

A similar situation may exist with regard to prn doses. In the model system, no doses were sent to the patient care areas in advance of need—all were dispatched only on call to a pharmacist and only after the existence of the proper order was verified. Yet most systems in existence today send the first dose of every prn order up in advance, despite the fact that 79-89% may never be administered, and represent not only wasted effort but also an increased opportunity for error (27,58).

What is the answer? There are a variety of developments on the horizon that promise relief. It seems reasonable to expect that the ASHP Statement on Drug Distribution Systems will be updated to call for more frequent deliveries per 24-hour period, probably 4-6 per day. Compliance will not be easy, and to do so using today's methods may increase costs. However, computerization will permit hospitals to switch to the envelope system, which is free of the need for carts, along with their competition for elevator space and the duplication of effort when they must be returned for cleaning and filling.

Automation may offer an entirely different approach, possibly negating the need for deliveries more frequent than just those needed to respond to orders changed or canceled that day. An automated bedside dispensing machine recently tested has been shown capable of reducing wrong time and omission errors by virtue of its ability to retain and keep each unit dose out of the hands of the nurse until the time it is due and then call her to come get it at that time (26). Another development on the horizon is a portable bar code reader, which the nurse would be required to use at the time of administration to read the patient's wrist band and then compare it with the unit dose described on the unit dose package she plans to adminster, both for identification of the patient and for authorization to proceed, transmitted from the central computer containing the current master order file on-line for all patients. With such controls, the effect of frequency of delivery might be significantly reduced as a source of error (although too-infrequent deliveries would be a source of delay).

Doses Not Dispensed in Unit Dose Packages

Another inadequacy of current systems is the extent to which they fall short of the goal of dispensing all doses in true unit dose packages. The extent to which current systems actually dispense all doses in true unit dose form has not been measured, but it is generally recognized that few if any have reached 100% in this respect. Typically, the first dose forms to be packaged for unit dose dispensing are oral tablets and capsules. However, the dose forms most likely to be involved in errors are oral liquids and injectables, in particular those for pediatric patients. Generally speaking, the dosage forms that are more difficult for the pharmacist to measure and package, e.g., injectables, ointments, eyedrops, and oral liquids, are the ones that give nurses the greatest problems (5).

In a recent study of a supposedly modern unit dose system, with adequate funding and staffing, 33% of the unit doses involved in the errors detected via the direct observation method had not been dispensed in unit packages. The notes of the observer included the following (74):

A wrong dose error involved the nurse's failure to apply a full one inch ribbon of Nitropaste as ordered. *It was not dispensed in unit dose form,* so the nurse had to measure out the dose. She gave only about ½ inch. [For another patient] Synthroid 150 mcg. daily was ordered. The pharmacy sent two tablets, one 100 mcg. and 50 mcg., but *not packaged together* (or attached packages) *as the unit dose concept requires.* The nurse tried to give time only one of these tablets but the patient told her "that isn't enough." [She then found the other tablet and gave it.]

One category of drug products too often excluded from unit dose packaging are nonprescription legend drugs, yet in this same study over one third of all errors detected (excluding wrong time) under the *improved* version of the system involved such nonprescription drugs. The observer had reported:

One evening, when the 10 P.M. medications were poured, though the order said Benyline Expectorant 2 drams—that is, 10 ml.— the nurse poured out 30 ml. The *pharmacy had sent a multiple dose container* which allowed this overdose to happen. Later, this patient was heard to tell the nurse she had given him "way too much."

All DISCON Information Not Controlled by One Source (Pharmacy) Duplication: Profile and MAR

Another shortcoming of existing unit dose systems is the extent to which they fail to provide a single source of DISCON information for pharmacists, nurses, and physicians. In one 622-bed hospital, such activity was costing the hospital $100,949 annually on the nursing unit and $60,466 annually in the pharmacy (28). The observer's report included the following (26):

[The patient's] physician ordered Tranxene 1 p.o., q.i.d. The order was incomplete, since no strength was specified, and also the drug was non-formulary. The pharmacy personnel *did not attempt to get the problems with the order corrected and then send a revised version to the nurse.* Instead, a pharmacist called the floor and left word that the order could not be filled. By the time this was relayed to the physician and a new order was entered in the chart, three days had elapsed. The patient was discharged the following day, and the first dose still had not yet arrived.

COST

General Effect of Drug Distribution on Costs

The total (system) cost of a hospital drug distribution system has never been studied and reported. Most hospital administrators do not know what the cost of their system is, and many may not even be familiar with the concept of a drug distribution system stretching across the various departments whose individual budgets are the customary focus of the budgeting and cost control processes.

It is clear that for the pharmacy department the labor invested in the drug distribution function is the most important cost to the department by a wide margin. The major portion of all pharmacist and technician time is spent in drug distribution (including IV admixture preparation) regardless of hospital size or profile. As noted earlier, in general hospitals with more than 200 beds, pharmacists spend about 74% of their time in dispensing, 16% in management tasks, and about 10% in clinical practice. In com-

parable specialized facilities, pharmacists spend 71% of their time in drug distribution and 16% and 13% in the other two categories, respectively. Generally, over 9 out of every 10 hours of technician time are devoted to the drug distribution function and, in specialized hospitals, practically all (1).

The most comprehensive study of the cost of drug distribution in hospitals to date was that conducted by the U.S. General Accounting Office (GAO). The GAO collected cost data on drug distribution systems in 30 hospitals, ranging from 75 to 500 beds, and whose pharmacies dispensed between 33,000 and 860,000 "prescriptions" per year. Nineteen of the hospitals operated traditional systems (floor stock, individual prescription, or combination), whereas the remainder operated unit dose systems. A comparison limited to personnel and medication costs led to the conclusion that the unit dose systems had lower life-cycle costs than a conventional system at higher annual prescription ranges, although this was reversed at the lowest ranges (Fig. 32.5).

The study also concluded that "the life-cycle savings are attributable, to a large extent, to a reduction in nursing time for administering medications." In the cost analysis, the GAO applied a 40% reduction in nursing time related to medication-related activities to determine the nursing cost of these activities for the unit dose system. The 40% was selected based on a literature review.

In terms of staffing, it was assumed that compared to floor stock systems, the unit dose systems required 1½ times the number of pharmacists and twice the number of technicians.

For a hypothetical 259-bed reference hospital, unit dose was projected to require the addition of two pharmacists and two technicians, but saving the equivalent of eight nurses, for a net savings of $1,060,000 over a 25-year life cycle (75).

The GAO study was important not only for its early independent assessment of the unit dose system concept by a nationally respected organization external to hospitals, but also for its approach, which acknowledged the importance of studying drug distribution as a system crossing several departments (28), in particular both pharmacy and nursing.

Unfortunately, too many hospital administrators have failed to pay attention. In 1975, Cameron and Vaughan (76) observed that despite the GAO study only 28% of all hospitals had converted to unit dose at that time. They believed the reason was that hospitals implementing unit dose systems were experiencing an increase in total cost (as opposed to the decrease they expected) on the order of $100,000 annually in a 350-bed community hospital. They traced the problem to the failure of administrators to properly manage the implementation process and insist on the budgetary reduction in the nursing department to reflect the nursing time saved and (necessary) to offset the increase in the pharmacy department.

In summary, the most important principle in evaluating the total cost of drug distribution is that the focus should include as much of the entire system as possible, because savings in one component may be more than offset by increased costs in the other, and vice versa. As the GAO study suggests, it is entirely possible to decrease the total cost of the drug distribution system simultaneous with an increase

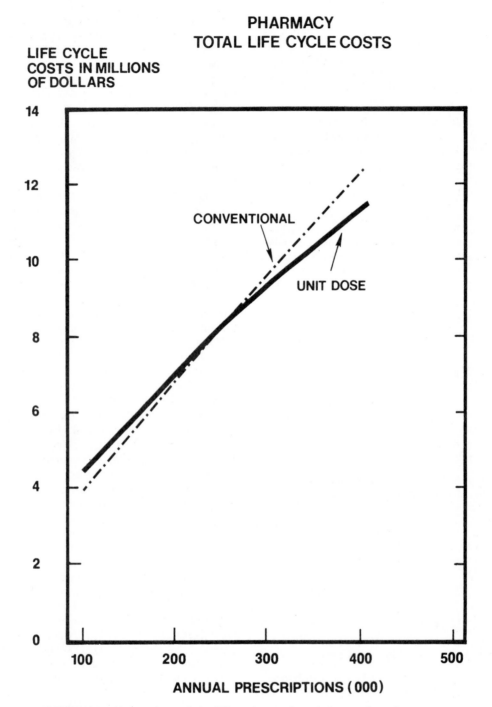

FIGURE 32.5 Comparative analysis of life-cycle costs for unit dose vs alternative systems.

in the size of the pharmacy budget when this increase is more than offset by savings in the substantial cost of medication preparation and administration. Because the cost of the latter is not regularly evaluated and reviewed, the uninformed administrator may falsely confuse the cost of operating the pharmacy with the cost of the total drug distribution system. This same mistake occurs in interinstitutional comparisons of pharmacy budgets or personnel requirements that fail to include comparable cost data for the drug distribution system components outside the door of the pharmacy department.

External Factors Affecting Cost

Factors other than the design of the system that affect the total systems cost of maintaining a hospital drug distribution system include (1) mission of the hospital, (2) objectives for the system, (3) enforcement of performance standards, (4) bed size, (5) physical layout of hospital, (6) policies on utilization of personnel, and (7) automation.

Mission

The mission of the hospital determines the patient mix (predominant diagnoses, severity of illness, acuity of care), which in turn affects the demand for drug distribution. For example, a study at Johns Hopkins Hospital showed that the cost per unit dose administered was approximately 50% greater in pediatric medicine compared to adult medicine, because more nursing time is required to administer each dose to pediatric patients and more extemporaneously prepared unit dose drugs are used by them (77). A similar study conducted by Schnell (78) produced the figure of 80%.

Objectives for the System

The objectives established for the drug distribution system can make a difference, for example, when they are reflected in the level of performance standards set. If a medication error rate standard as low as 2-3% of "all opportunities for error" is set, then the frequency of deliveries to the nurse should be much more frequent than once a day, and the percent of doses packaged in unit dose package form will have to be higher than the percent currently available from the manufacturer in this form—necessitating a more elaborate packaging operation. Will there be the centralized editing of all orders for both pharmacist and nurses? Will critical care areas receive special services? What will be the response time required for stat orders, now orders, and new orders?

Enforcement of Performance Standards

The establishment of performance standards will have little impact if deviations are not detected and enforced. Elaborate quality assurance systems based on process measures can be expensive, and more efficient systems based on outcome measures are being developed. A control system that effectively detects deviations without follow-up action to correct them is an economic waste (74).

Bed Size

The cost of drug distribution increases with the number of beds served, although the relationship is not direct. As might be expected, once a certain bed size (or prescription volume) is reached, the rate of growth in costs often slows as economies of scale set in.

Physical Layout of Hospital

The physical layout of the hospital is important, particularly regarding the materials handling challenges presented. Transportation times between the nursing stations and the pharmacy can significantly affect the cost of pharmacy operations, particularly with unit dose systems where deliveries are many times more frequent. The layout can determine whether pharmacy satellites are recommended, or even feasible.

Policies on Utilization of Personnel

Policies on the utilization of personnel can greatly affect cost, for example, where the use of pharmacy technicians is severely restricted or prohibited.

Automation

Automation is expected to increase efficiency by replacing personnel with automated systems. The more sophisticated and labor-intensive systems may expect to see greater benefits. Automated equipment currently in use includes packaging machines, dispensing machines, automated materials handling systems, and most important, computer applications (e.g., replacing paperwork, calculating staffing assignments, etc) (see Chapter 18).

Choice of System: Unit Dose vs Others

Total Systems Cost

In terms of total systems cost, the comprehensive GAO study made it clear that unit dose systems (of the centralized type studied) have a lower total cost than the combination floor stock and individual patient prescription system in all hospitals except those smaller than 250 beds filling under 250,000 medication orders per year. It should be noted that the GAO study assumed 24-hour service for unit dose dispensing in all bed sizes and did not include savings from reduced drug losses and more accurate billing (75). Subsequent studies have provided evidence that unit dose systems reduce costs in small (79) and medium (80,81) as well large hospitals (82).

Nursing Labor

The primary source of savings under unit dose systems is in nursing personnel labor. This seems reasonable to expect, since all of the activities of preparation for administration in addition to some administration activities and drug transportation are transferred from nursing to pharmacy in a unit dose system.

Unit dose does save nursing time. This has been demonstrated in 14 different studies (7,23,31,33,35,46,83-90). It is difficult to say exactly how much time, because the studies were affected by the properties of the hospital, the type of unit dose system, and the study design. It apppears safe to conclude that under the traditional combination system one third of a nurse's time is spent in medication-related activities, and this is roughly halved by unit dose; this "savings" represents one sixth of the total time or 16% (62).

Black and Upham (91) calculated that under a unit dose system nurses spent an average of 1.4 minutes less on each medication dose.

How the nursing time "saved" is reallocated must be considered, since it may not always be possible to reduce nurse staffing as a trade-off for the increased pharmacy staffing necessary to implement a unit dose system (81). The time saved on one nursing shift per nursing unit is usually not enough to free a full-time equivalent (FTE). If the time saved cannot be used for nursing staff reductions, or for compensation where nursing positions have gone unfilled and these positions can be transferred to the pharmacy, then the total cost might not be reduced. However, the evaluation of the model system showed that 57% of the nursing time saved was transferred into desirable activities such as bedside nursing, administration of drugs, and division management. The net effect of the unit dose system was to raise the percent of total nursing time spent in bedside nursing from 23.3-28.3%; the time spent in administration of drugs from 4.5-5.9% (the system provided ''nurses' package inserts'' to read before administering drugs); and the time spent in division management from 15.8-17.0% (33). Schnell's study of nursing activities in four hospitals before and after unit dose was implemented concluded that the time freed from medication activities was transferred to personal activities or direct patient care (23).

Other studies of systems that differed more from the model system were not as successful in ''capturing'' the savings to either reduce nursing personnel or increase patient care (86).

The direct approach to ensuring that saved nursing time is translated into a reduced overall cost (or increased value) is to accompany the conversion to unit dose with a decrease in nursing staff. If a nursing shortage exists, then an alternative is to delete the appropriate number of unfilled positions from the nursing budget at the time of conversion. A third approach is to restructure the job of the individual nurse in terms of job expectations, goals, and functions to achieve a qualitative improvement in nursing care at some extra cost to the drug distribution system as a whole (92).

Pharmacy Labor

The 1983 Lilly survey noted that unit dose and IV admixture services have had a definite impact on pharmacist and technician workloads, resulting in increased hours being worked in hospitals of every size, regardless of profile. Figures available for general hospitals from 50-300 beds revealed that the total hours per week worked by the pharmacist was on the order of two thirds more with unit dose and IV admixture systems than without (1).

Inventory Losses

Another basis for comparisons of unit dose with other types of drug distribution systems is with regard to their effect on materials cost. Specifically, the GAO found that drug losses due to waste and pilferage in hospitals using traditional distribution systems ranged from 25-50% compared to 9-12% for unit dose systems (93). The evaluation of the model system had found that under the control system drug losses were occurring from floor stock at the rate of 5½ times the average inventory ($2756 in 1964 dollars) maintained there (33).

Martinelli and Wurdack (94) showed that medication losses in their unit dose system were 75% less than in traditional systems.

An obvious reason for expecting reduced losses from floor stock under unit dose systems is the fact that they significantly reduce or practically eliminate the need for it, thus eliminating its availability for pilferage, deterioration, and waste. The fact that all doses are accounted for is a deterrent to pilferage. Waste is reduced when the preparation for administration is done in a centralized supervised place by those best equipped and qualified to do it (11). Otherwise, remaining portions of multiple dose injectables and oral liquids cannot legally be reissued, for example. The control of admixture waste through pharmacist monitoring can re-

sult in a reduction of admixture wasted from 4% down to 1.8% per year (95).

Inventory Control, Accounting, and Charging

Unit dose systems inherently offer greater accuracy in inventory control, cost accounting, and charging by virtue of the fact that the unit dose packages each patient receives come in complete, easily identifiable labeled units from a single centralized source—the pharmacy—as opposed to the preparation of such units extemporaneously by each nurse on each shift at each nurses' station. It is with the unit dose preparation process that nonpharmacists, e.g., accounting personnel, encounter the greatest difficulty in tracking physical inventory and identifying cost. Such personnel can track the ingredients that input the process, but have difficulty in calculating the theoretical output needed to look for shrinkage and losses. For this reason, accounting and charging systems that rely on nonprofessional personnel to identify the unit of drug administered, form the nurses' charting, for example, have proved inaccurate because such personnel have difficulty identifying the exact amount of drug administered. When the identification of the inventory unit to be dispensed is performed by the pharmacist as a by-product of the dispensing process, more accurate accounting becomes both achievable and inexpensive.

Black and Upham (91) showed that their unit dose system produced an 11.8% improvement in charting accuracy, which resulted in a savings of $0.68 per patient day from losses due to mischarges, pilferage, and waste. Unit dose charging accuracy saved $43,000 per year in the GAO reference hospital revenues (75).

Adaptability to Automation and Computers

The standardization and uniform labeling of all inventory units brought by the unit dose concept to all aspects of drug distribution, along with the concentration of repetitive tasks (e.g., dose preparation) and paperwork (e.g., MAR) in one place, makes unit dose systems ready targets for automation (33).

Intangibles

The effect of unit dose systems on liability can in turn affect costs. Claims based on medication errors are the most difficult for a hospital to defend, and so until all hospitals have unit dose systems, those without them will be in greater jeopardy. On the other hand, unit dose systems make claims of all kinds easier for the claimant to document.

When the burden and liability for dose preparation is shifted from the nurse to the pharmacist, his personal liability is increased but then offset by the overall total reduction in errors reaching the patient, provided this system achieves the error reduction intended. For this reason, the greatest legal risk to the employee pharmacist may come from employment of an ineffective unit dose system (33).

Job satisfaction has been found to be generally superior in unit dose systems, particularly for nurses (33,96). This may be of special importance in times of nurse shortages. A unit dose system also improves the hospital's ability to attract and retain highly qualified and motivated pharmacy personnel, whereas the additional workload and responsibilities may make those less qualified and less motivated less satisfied.

Summary

Comparison of Total Costs. It is possible to summarize the foregoing discussion with this statement: in almost all major studies comparing costs in a true dose system with costs of alternative systems representing a wide range of hospital types, sizes, physical layouts, and degree of implementation, the cost per dose to the hospital operating under a unit dose system was less. Only in the smaller hospitals (e.g., less than 300 beds) is the issue somewhat unclear.

Comparison of Types of Unit Dose Dispensing Systems. Generally speaking, decentralized distribution systems (via satellite pharmacies) are more expensive than centralized systems. This is because of the loss of economies of scale, poor utilization of personnel due to inflexibility in staffing, duplication of inventories, extra space and equipment costs, and poor intrapharmacy communication and control (97).

The physical layout of the hospital is possibly the only factor that can (on occasion) "swing the balance" of comparative costs to favor decentralization, such as when patients are grouped in different buildings and transportation systems are extremely limited. It is probably impossible to surpass the efficiency of the centralized approach when, for example, all nursing units are aligned vertically above the pharmacy and served by an automated trayveyor and pneumatic tube.

It is more difficult than is commonly appreciated to draw conclusions about the effect of the relative degree of centralization on the total cost of drug distribution, because in most studies of decentralized systems, the effects of the drug distribution function are confounded with those of the clinical function, making it difficult to separate the effects of the two. Most decentralized systems have been advocated not for their efficiency in drug distribution but rather to serve as a platform for the development of the clinical functions (see Chapter 54). In fact, it has even been argued that the inefficiencies of decentralized systems of distribution are a virtue in that the pharmacists are utilized so poorly that they have (otherwise unusable) time "free" for clinical activities.

As the pressures for cost containment have mounted, many decentralized systems have recentralized such functions as packaging and cart/cassette filling, leaving only the production of first, stat, and preop doses to be prepared on the satellite. (IV solutions are considered in Chapter 34.)

Studies of the effect of the degree of centralization on the cost of drug distribution function, both separate from and combined with various clinical functions, are sorely needed.

IMPLEMENTATION

The first step in implementing a drug distribution system is to read about them. Three recommended references are *The Unit Dose Primer* by Summerfield (62), *Source Book* on *Unit Dose Distribution Systems* (98), and *Planning and Preparation of Proposals for New Hospital Pharmacy Programs and Services* by McAllister and Lindley (99). The reader is urged to read carefully and critically, as many more system configurations and components have been recommended exuberantly than have been evaluated objectively for effectiveness. For example, the number of systems configurations evaluated by the observation method for their effect on medication errors is relatively few.

Proposing and Gaining Acceptance

The particular difficulty of proposing and gaining acceptance for a drug distribution system lies in the fact that this hospital-wide system crosses many departments and professions. It crosses the "professional turf" of the nurse, the physician, accounting, materials management, and computer services.

Summerfield (62) warns that the implementation process requires immense professional and personal commitment, during which time the director will have to use a range of personal and managerial skills: planning, justifying, proposing, persuading, educating, compromising, speaking, writing, meeting, and waiting. The interval between the date of the formal proposal and the day the last bid is placed on the system can span several years (63).

Innovations

An effort to gain acceptance for a unit dose system may be expected to encounter special difficulties due to the fact that this innovation (particularly those systems closest to the original concepts) is still moving through the normal five-step process of awareness, interest, evaluation, trial, and adoption (or demise). The theory of innovations teaches that this process may last from 10-20 years. An important requirement for acceptance is a perceived need (100), which may be totally lacking when hospital personnel refuse to accept the scope and/or significance of the medication error problem. Where this is true, a study of medication errors may be necessary to help identify the problem to which the new system is the solution. Bucceri and Baker (101) described a management model in which the pharmacist acts as the change agent and enlists opinion leaders in nursing to successfully convince their staff a unit dose system is preferable. However, Ketchum (100) found that the pharmacists themselves were the principal stumbling block in gaining acceptance for unit dose systems in hospitals, and so must be included as among those to be "won over" (100).

In planning to gain acceptance by nurses and pharmacists, it is useful to know how they differ in the criteria they use to evaluate a drug distribution system. For example, in one in-depth study, both accuracy and speed (in terms of saving time) top the list of 65 different criteria used by nurses. Of the 38 criteria used by pharmacists, "the acceptance of the system by others," such as the nurses and physicians, shared the top of the list with "speed of operation." Pharmacists apparently share a particular concern regarding how the system will be perceived by others. This suggests that it may be critical to convince the pharmacists in advance that the nurses and physicians will like the system to gain the pharmacists' acceptance. Ketchum (100) found that in the majority of hospitals where unit dose was considered but then abandoned, the negative attitude of the pharmacists was crucial (104).

On the Need for a Study

Studies may or may not be necessary to support a proposal to implement major changes in the drug distribution system. Certainly, it should not be necessary to reevaluate the unit dose concept, for example, but rather simply cite the GAO study (75), the JCAH standards (57), the ASHP statement on unit dose drug distribution systems (67), the current percent of hospitals having unit dose systems (36), the new HCFA conditions for participation in Medicare/Medicaid (37), and several similar hospitals that have installed systems similar to that contemplated.

The kind of study that usually is necessary is that which collects baseline data to estimate the resources required to implement and operate the system, and to show, through comparison with post implementation data, that the system has accomplished its goals. Data examined should include that showing the demand for unit doses as depicted in Figure 32.2. If this data is obtained from the nurses' charting, it may need to be corrected for charting errors (15). Charting can also serve as a source of information on the different dosage forms and strengths administered with estimates of frequency.

The cost of syringes, medicine, and other medication preparation supplies can be calculated from this same data to determine additional cost to the pharmacy and savings to the nursing department. The amount of nursing time to be saved and the amount of pharmacy time required (FTEs) should be calculated based on the estimating procedures presented in Chapter 9. (The use of ''standard'' estimates of the amount of nursing time saved based on studies conducted on different systems 15 years ago as recommended by some authors is not justified unless the systems and the hospitals in which they are installed are very similar to those where the original studies were conducted, which is highly unlikely.)

An additional reason for a pilot study conducted by an independent planning group or outside source is to evaluate the system design proposed to see if it really will produce the expected results (e.g., reduced medication error rate) in this hospital. For example, the affect on medication errors should be evaluated by direct observation of the doses as they are administered to the patients. Otherwise, the hospital may not get what it paid for (26,27,74).

In designing a medication system it is important to note the factors that have been found to be associated with error rates:

1. Work shift. Errors are more frequent on the day and evening shifts, when 75-80% of all doses are given. Wrong time errors tend to be more frequent on the day shift, when the interruptions for special treatments, visitors, etc, are more frequent.

2. Medical service. Pediatrics experiences more wrong dose errors as might be expected, whereas obstetrics-gynecology has more unordered drug errors.

3. The dosage forms. Those more likely to be involved in errors are not tablets and capsules, but rather (1) oral liquids, (2) intramuscular injections, and (3) suppositories.

4. Medication workload of the nurse.

5. Number of different orders in effect for same patient.

6. Nurses prone to these specific error types: (1) wrong dose and (2) omission.

7. Extent of measurement and calculations required.

8. Confusing drug nomenclature.

9. Automatic stop orders.

A system that is designed to focus on these factors should be the most effective in reducing errors.

At the minimum, a pilot study demonstrating the accomplishments of the goals of the proposed system on one nursing station is generally recommended to build acceptance for the system and ''work out the bugs'' before going hospital-wide.

Mapping Acceptance

In planning for acceptance, it is crucial to realize that the foci must be on reality as perceived by the significant audience. If the innovation offers a solution to a set of problems that are not perceived as problems by the nurses and physicians, for example, it is more likely to fail.

The term ''mapping acceptance'' was used to describe a program for achieving acceptance of a major systems change in one hospital. In-depth, 1-hour interviews were conducted with each of 18 key personnel in the administration (e.g., administrator), on the medical staff (e.g., chief of staff, chairman of each service, house staff), in nursing (e.g., director, supervisors), and in the pharmacy (e.g., supervisors, staff) to identify their perceptions of not only the key problems but the system objectives and performance standards they expected the new system to meet. All were also asked to express any strong feelings they had about a list of ''possible changes in the system.'' The results revealed a surprising degree of agreement on a few key problems, which made the planning of communications for ''selling the innovation'' much easier (26).

The Proposal

The elements of the successful proposal are listed below:
1. The problem the innovation is designed to solve
2. Brief description of how it works
3. Rationale for believing it can solve the problem (literature review, success in comparable institutions)
4. Evidence that it will work here (e.g., pilot study results)
5. Cost justification
6. ''Testimonials'' of key hospital personnel
7. Questions and answers, anticipating controversial issues

It is important to note that although the proposal is written for the administrator, he will likely have it reviewed by others, including nurses and physicians. The proposal must be well organized and well written, as the readers will use the quality of the proposal as an indicator of the knowledge, skills, and good judgment of the pharmacy director, and hence the quality and success potential of the system (62).

The wording should be in "the plain language of the institution regarding this problem area," which may be learned while mapping acceptance problems as described previously.

The rationale should include a literature search covering not only pharmacy but also prominent nursing, medical, and hospital administration journals and, ideally, an objective source from a field such as industrial engineering or accounting. (For unit dose systems, the GAO report cited previously is ideal.) The "everyone else has it" approach provides powerful support, but only when followed by evidence that the system is workable and cost justified in "this" hospital at "this" time. Resource requirements must be carefully assessed and honestly stated. Acceptance of the initial proposal is more likely if implementation can be phased, with the option to discontinue if important milestones are not achieved as planned.

Although "testimonials of key hospital personnel" will not be the actual title of a section in the proposal, support of the influential members of the hospital staff is very helpful. Indications of support can be woven into the text by quotes from key individuals. (Only mildly positive support that includes negatives can nevertheless be particularly helpful as reflecting a balanced and objective appraisal.)

The concerns of the administrator will focus on financial aspects and politics, such as how the innovation will affect the hospital budget, the balance of power between the groups of persons who he feels are crucial for his support, and considerations of liability and public relations. For the administrator, the proposal must address the cost of implementing the system and long-range cost benefits. Nursing concerns will focus on patient care aspects at two levels. First they will be the ones most interested in operational details, since the system will greatly affect their job roles and responsibilities more than those of others. Nurses will also be the personnel most concerned about the effect on the patients, as they are the ones who are with them 24 hours a day, 7 days a week.

Both nurses and physicians may be as interested in the financial aspects of the effect of the innovation as the administrator but lack the educational background to understand the issues and explanations; therefore, illogical misconceptions may be a problem (e.g., underrating the cost of the time involved in preparation of the medication by the nurse). The questions and answers section of the proposal is ideal for speaking to these issues without offending the readers. Medical staff personnel, in particular, have a tendency to consider themselves "experts on everything," and so it is a mistake to assume that communications with them can be "compartmentalized" to address only those topics for which they are educationally prepared (33). All parts of the proposal should be written with this in mind. The self-interest of all personnel affected by the system cannot be ignored and can also be addressed in this section, answering such questions as, Will there by any cuts in staff? to state a commitment to reduction by attrition.

When presenting study results, keep in mind that administrators focus first on understanding the results, and then on why it is reasonable to expect such results from implementation of the innovation. Other material such as the many details of the methodology (of which the author may be justly proud) should be reserved for the appendix to minimize "the noise" in this communication which might otherwise hinder the administrator from finding what he is seeking.

An excellent source of information concerning effective methods of selling, planning, and presenting a program proposal is available from McAllister and Lindley (99).

Every effort should be made to reduce the complexity and improve the clarity of the proposal. An easily understood proposal stands a greater chance of being adopted (102).

Cost Justification

As discussed previously, justifying the cost effectiveness of a drug distribution system is particularly complex because major cost elements are located in two traditionally separate budgets (nursing and pharmacy). For example, it may be clear that a true unit dose system will save nursing time; however, to justify a higher pharmacy budget, this time savings must be reflected in either a proposed decrease in the total cost of nursing care or in an increase in the quality of patient care justifying a net increase in the overall budget for the hospital. (Studies performed to compare the percent of nursing time spent on medication-related activities under traditional and unit dose systems are summarized in a table by Summerfield) (62). Arguments that true unit dose systems can be achieved without raising either total hospital cost or the pharmacy budget are unconvincing. Therefore, the pharmacist proponent must persuade the hospital administrator to either transfer funds from the nursing budget to the pharmacy budget or accept an increase in hospital costs while letting nursing keep the added time gained.

Historically, this has been a difficult political problem. Not every administrator has had the courage to put hospital cost containment foremost at the risk of offending his largest labor force (nurses). During periods of nursing shortage, the administrator's dilemma is somewhat relieved in that the money from the nursing budget can come from unfilled positions representing funds that could not be used by nursing anyway. A similar problem is presented in states where certificate of need boards restrict the number of hospital employees (103). Cost justifications must make clear how nursing will be affected and stress the net effect on patient care and total costs. Nevertheless, when the proposal is perceived by nursing as an encroachment of authority and empire building, implementation will be difficult in hospitals whose administrator lacks the courage to take on this battle in the interest of cost containment.

Planning

A plan for implementing a unit dose system must consider (1) planning committee, (2) personnel, (3) equipment, (4) facilities needed, (5) policies and procedures, (6) orientation and training, (7) schedule and sequencing the implementation, and (8) establishing quality assurance.

Planning Committee

Most authors recommend that a planning committee be established. The goals of such a planning committee are presented by Summerfield (62). The extent to which a committee participates in the implementation may differ, but the importance of having a multidisciplinary committee including representatives from pharmacy, nursing, administration, the medical staff, and financial services is undisputed. An industrial engineer is a valuable addition if available. The committee should be small, e.g., no more than eight or ten members. It is preferable (though not essential) for the chairman to be a pharmacist, whether he is the director of pharmacy (who may be more experienced and skilled at conducting meetings) or an associate (who will have more time). If the committee is allowed to "assume a life of its own" as a body somewhat removed and apart from the daily turf struggles of the competing departments, this may encourage objectivity and lend credibility to its actions.

It is clear that the planning committee should not be the Pharmacy and Therapeutics Committee, although the endorsement of (or at least avoidance of a negative position by) that committee is essential.

Personnel

Because of hospital to hospital variability and the wide variety of drug distribution systems within types, a fixed manpower requirement has been difficult to establish (104). Institution-specific variables are important. It is strongly recommended that directors of pharmacies develop their own staffing requirements with the measures described in Chapter 9. Several unique methods of scheduling personnel such as the 4-day week and the 7-day week have been tried for unit dose (105-109).

The use of supportive personnel or pharmacy technicians can be particularly tricky when their use is regulated by federal, state, and local laws that must be reviewed.

Equipment

The broad categories of equipment involved in drug distribution are (1) data processing and communications, (2) packaging, and (3) transportation and delivery. Sources of all of the equipment in these categories are given in Chapter 39. Only those items peculiar to drug distribution are mentioned here.

Data processing equipment needs are addressed thoroughly in Chapter 18. The primary need is to have all active medication orders "on line, in real-time" and accessible anywhere in the hospital that access is needed.

When implementing a unit dose system, a range of packaging and labeling equipment must be considered. A sequence of questions helpful in determining equipment needs is modified and presented here (33).

1. What are the percentages of total doses dispensed by dosage form (e.g., tablets and capsules, oral liquids, injectables, ointments, ophthalmics, etc)?

2. What percentage of all doses are not commercially available in unit dose packages? (See under "Definition").

3. Of the noncommercially available doses, how many different drugs and dosage strengths are represented?

4. Which ones should be prepackaged? Which ones should be prepared extemporaneously?

5. If doses are to be prepackaged, can contract acquisition be considered?

6. If prepackaged in house, should this be done in bulk or on call?

7. Based on the above, what criteria should be used in selecting the equipment for the in house packaging program contemplated?

An important reason for in-house packaging may be to avoid a commercial label, which is so confusing as to contribute to medication errors (33).

Medication carts and cassettes are often used with unit dose systems. The advent of primary care nursing, in which several nurses may be scheduled to give medications simultaneously, reduces the utility offered by a cart pushed room to room. When the purchase of several carts for one nursing station is viewed as extravagant, the solution has been to keep medications in one central location on the nursing unit (110). When carts with cassettes are used, only the cassettes are brought to the pharmacy for filling or are exchanged on the nursing station.

Carts and cassettes are unnecessary in medication envelope systems (19,33) and with the Friesen concept. In the latter, all patient supplies and records, including medications, are kept in or near the patient's room (111-113).

If unit dose carts are desired, the consideration for choosing carts is summarized in Abbott's *Unit Dose Implementation Manual* (64). For the decentralized pharmacist concept, the mobile master medication cart has special requirements that Superstine et al (114) have listed.

Facilities Needed

Since the hospital medication system reaches to almost all parts of the hospital and affects work activities, the design of the system to be installed necessarily has a major impact on the physical space, equipment, and furnishings needed. These are reviewed in Chapter 17.

Policies and Procedures

Policies and procedures need to be delineated in detail, recorded before implementation begins, and updated regularly. Buchanan's chapter on unit dose in the *Practice of Pharmacy* (65) includes a good discussion on procedural considerations and alternatives, as does Summerfield (62), in setting forth policies and procedures for unit dose systems. The preparation of a policy and procedure manual is discussed in Chapter 5.

Orientation and Training

After the initial set of operating procedures have been established, all future participants must be trained. It is particularly important in implementing a new system that all pharmacists, nurses, and physicians know not only how it is supposed to operate, but also why each task is performed and the program goals and performance standards of the system. This is important to enlist their aid in coping with the many unanticipated situations that are certain to occur.

Nurses are difficult to orient because such orientation

programs must cope with personnel spread across three shifts and 7 days of the week. Their interest in operational details is usually great, and both pharmacy staff and nursing staff represent "captive audiences" for orientation and training when these can be scheduled on "company time."

In the case of physicians, the times when they are in the hospital tend to be concentrated in periods that are few in number and easy to predict. Nevertheless, it can be difficult to get their attention unless the focus is on operational details related to saving them time and ensuring that their orders are carried out as they intend.

Scheduling and Sequencing the Implementation

If at all possible, it is preferable to set up temporarily two duplicate pharmacy operations following the conclusion of the pilot study. Then, implementation should proceed as fast as possible. It is essential to have experienced and knowledgeable nurses and pharmacists free from normal duties and designated "resource" persons to advise on each nursing unit for the initial day or two.

Establishing Quality Assurance

As soon as the drug distribution system has been installed, a quality assurance program should be established to pick up where any postimplementation studies have left off. How this may be done utilizing low-cost quality assurance system has to be described (74). The subject of quality assurance is addressed in Chapter 61.

REFERENCES

1. Deiner CH (ed): *Lilly Hospital Pharmacy Survey, 1983*, Indianapolis, Eli Lilly, 1983.
2. Anon: ASHP minimum standard for pharmacies in institutions. *Am J Hosp Pharm* 34:1346-1358, 1977.
3. Anon: APHA policy committee on professional affairs. *APharmacy Wkly* March 23, 1984, p 46.
4. McLeod DC: Philosophy of practice. In McLeod DC, Miller WA (eds): *Practice of Pharmacy.* Cincinnati, Harvey Whitney Books, 1981, p 1.
5. Barker KN, Heller WH, Kimbrough WW: *A Study of Medication Errors in a Hospital.* Fayetteville, University of Arkansas, 1966.
6. Frost and Sullivan: *Unit Dose Pharmaceuticals Market.* New York, Frost and Sullivan, 1979.
7. McConnell WE, Barker KN, Garrity LF: Centralized unit dose dispensing. *Am J Hosp Pharm* 18:531-541, 1963.
8. Schwartau N, Sturdavant M: A system of packaging and dispensing drugs in single doses. *Am J Hosp Pharm* 18:542-549, 1961.
9. Barker KN, Heller WM: The development of a centralized unit dose dispensing system. Part I. Description of the UAMC experimental system. *Am J Hosp Pharm* 20:568-579, 1963.
10. Barker KN, Heller WM: The development of a centralized unit dose dispensing system at UAMC. Part II. Why centralize the preparation of unit doses? *Am J Hosp Pharm* 20:612-613, 1963.
11. Barker KN, Heller WM: The development of a centralized unit dose dispensing system at UAMC. Part III. An editing center for physicians' medication orders. *Am J Hosp Pharm* 21:67-77, 1964.
12. Heller WM, Sheldon EC, Barker KN: The development of a centralized unit dose dispensing system for UAMC. Part IV. The roles and responsibilities of the pharmacist under the experimental system. *Am J Hosp Pharm* 21:231-237, 1964.
13. Barker KN, McConnell WM: The problems of detecting medication errors in hospitals. *Am J Hosp Pharm* 19:360, 1962.
14. Juran JM, Dingham RS: Service industries. In Juran JM (ed): *Quality Control Handbook,* ed 3. New York, McGraw-Hill, 1974.
15. Barker KN, Heller WM: The development of a centralized unit dose dispensing system for UAMC. Part VI. The pilot study—medication errors and drug losses. *Am J Hosp Pharm* 21:609-625, 1964.
16. Anon: Problem for physicians: Hospital medication errors. *JAMA* 195:31-32, 1966.
17. Barker KN: The effects of an experimental medication system on medication errors and costs. I. Introduction and errors study. *Am J Hosp Pharm* 26:324-333, 1969.
18. Hynniman CE, Conrad WF, Urch WA, et al: A comparison of medication errors under the University of Kentucky unit dose system and traditional drug distribution system in four hospitals. *Am J Hosp Pharm* 27:803-814, 1970.
19. Derewicz HJ, Zellers DD: The computer-based unit dose systems of the Johns Hopkins Hospital. *Am J Hosp Pharm* 30:206-212, 1973.
20. Brown WD, Blount CS, Harvey GD: Quality of pharmaceutical care in small hospitals. Report to the Missouri Regional Medical Program, Kansas City, MO, March 1976.
21. Hill PA, Wigmore HM: Measurement and control of drug administration incidents. *Lancet* 1:671-674, 1967.
22. Schnell BR, Anderson HA, Walter DE: *A Study of Unit Dose Drug Distribution in Four Canadian Hospitals, Final Report.* Saskatoon, College of Pharmacy, University of Saskatchewan, 1976.
23. Schnell BR: Study of unit dose distribution in four Canadian hospitals. *Can J Hosp Pharm* 29:85-90, 1976.
24. Barker KN, Mikeal RL, Pearson RE, et al: Medication errors in nursing homes and small hospitals. *Am J Hosp Pharm* 39:987-991, 1982.
25. Barker KN, Pearson RE, Hepler CD, et al: Effect of an automated bedside dispensing machine on medication errors. *Am J Hosp Pharm* 41:1352-1358, 1984.
26. Barker KN, Harris JA, Webster DB, et al: Consultant evaluation of a hospital medication system: Analysis of the existing system. *Am J Hosp Pharm* 41:2009-2016, 1984.
27. Barker KN, Harris JA, Webster DB, et al: Consultant evaluation of a hospital medication system: Synthesis of a new system. *Am J Hosp Pharm* 41:2016-2021, 1984.
28. Barker KN: Trends in drug distribution systems in hospitals. *Am J Hosp Pharm* 19:595, 1962.
29. Talley CR (ed): Aspirin for the nursing shortage headache: Upgraded pharmaceutical services. *Am J Hosp Pharm* 38:45, 1981.
30. Blumberg MS: Hospital automation: The needs and the prospects. *Hospitals* 35:34, 1961.
31. Barker KN, Brennan JJ, Heller WM: The development of a centralized unit dose dispensing system for UAMC. Part V. The pilot study—introduction and work measurement. *Am J Hosp Pharm* 21:412-423, 1964.
32. Barker KN, Smith M, Winters E: A study of the work of the pharmacist and the potential use of auxiliaries. *Am J Hosp Pharm* 29:35-53, 1972.
33. Barker K et al: *The Demonstration and Evaluation of an Experimental Medication System for the UAMC Hospital,* vol I. Fayetteville, Department of Editorial Services, University of Arkansas, 1967.
34. Kurtz A, Smith J: Three dimensional drug losses. *Hosp Top* 39:53-56, 1961.
35. Black HJ, Tester WW: Decentralized pharmacy operations utilizing the unit dose concept. Part I, *Am J Hosp Pharm* 21:344-350, 1964; Part II (with Greth PA), *Am J Hosp Pharm* 22:558-563, 1965; Part III, *Am J Hosp Pharm* 24:120-129, 1967.
36. Stolar MH: National survey of hospital pharmaceutical services 1982. *Am J Hosp Pharm* 40:963-969, 1983.
37. U.S. Department of Health, Education and Welfare: Section 3160; survey procedures for pharmaceutical service requirements in long-term care facilities. In *Transmittal No. 165, State Operations Manual for Provider Certification.* Washington DC, Health Care Financing Administration, Department of Health, Education and Welfare, 1984.
38. Barker KN: *Planning for Hospital Pharmacies.* HEW Publication No. FRA 74-4003, Rockville, MD; U.S. Department of Health, Education and Welfare, Health Resources Administration Health Care Facilities Service, 1974.
39. John GW, Burkhart VD, Lamy PP: Pharmacy personnel activities

and costs in decentralized unit dose drug distribution systems. *Am J Hosp Pharm* 33:38-43, 1976.

40. Jackson JC, Anderson RK, McGuire R: Decentralized pharmacist concept solves unit dose problems. *Hospitals* 52:107-110, April 1978.

41. Lipman AG, Blair JN, Hibbard FJ, et al: Decentralization of pharmaceutical services without satellite pharmacies. *Am J Hosp Pharm* 36:1513-1519, 1979.

42. Barker KN: On the administration of drugs—by pharmacists. *Hospitals* 38:106, April 1964.

43. Slonaker M: Administering drugs from a central drug room. *Am J Nursing* 62:108-110, 1962.

44. Beste DF: An integrated pharmacist-nurse approach to the unit dose concept. *Am J Hosp Pharm* 25:397-407, 1968.

45. Alexander VB, Barker KN: A national survey of pharmacy facilities. Part I. Introduction, space allocation. *Am J Hosp Pharm* (in press).

46. Latiolais CF, Berry CC, Lachner BJ, et al: A pharmacy coordinated unit dose dispensing and drug distribution system. *Am J Hosp Pharm* 27:886-910, 1970.

47. Jozefczyk KG, Schneider PJ, Pathak DS: *An Error Rate Study of Pharmacy Technician Administered Medications.* Columbus, College of Pharmacy, Ohio State University, 1984.

48. ASHP guidelines on hospitals drug distribution and control. *Am J Hosp Pharm* 37:1087-1103, 1980.

49. Corbet PD: Simplified records for a unit dose system. *Hospitals* 49:93-94, May 1975.

50. McLeod DC, Miller WA (eds): *Practice of Pharmacy.* Cincinnati, Harvey Whitney Books, 1981, p 412.

51. McGhan WF, Smith WE, Adams DW: *Med Care* 21:445-453, 1983.

52. Derewicz HJ, Simborg DW: The computer-based unit dose drug distribution system at Johns Hopkins Hospital: Second generation. *Hosp Pharm* 10:417-433, 1975.

53. Austin LH: Using a computer to run a modern hospital pharmacy. *Hosp Pharm* 14:74-80, 1979.

54. Beaman MA, Kotzan JA: Factors affecting medication-order processing time. *Am J Hosp Pharm* 39:1916-1919, 1982.

55. Manzelli TA: Utilization of the brewer system in the controlled distribution of medication within the hospital. *Am J Hosp Pharm* 18:560-566, 1961.

56. Anon: New pill-dispensing robot hikes pharmacy productivity. *Mod Healthcare* 14:122, 1984.

57. Tousignaut DR: Joint Commission on Accreditation of Hospitals' 1977 standards for pharmaceutical services. *Am J Hosp Pharm* 34:943-954, 1977.

58. Carroll RE, Gallina JN, Jeffrey LP: PRN drug utilization in a unit dose system. *Am J Hosp Pharm* 30:811-813, 1973.

59. ASHP guidelines for institutional use of controlled substances. *Am J Hosp Pharm* 31:582-588, 1974.

60. Anon: Room costs cut 25% by hospital. *Atlanta Constitution,* February 26, 1984.

61. Greenburg RB: Q/A—computer records for controlled substances. *Am J Hosp Pharm* 37:185, 1980.

62. Summerfield MR: *Unit Dose Primer.* Rockville, MD, American Society of Hospital Pharmacists, 1983.

63. *Order Forms, Charts and Records in Hospital Unit Dose Distribution Systems.* Columbus, OH, Roxane Laboratories, 1971.

64. Abbott Laboratories: *Unit Dose Implementation Manual.* North Chicago, IL, Miller and Fink, 1975.

65. Buchanan C: Unit dose drug distribution. In McLeod DC, Miller WA (eds): *The Practice of Pharmacy: Institutional and Ambulatory Pharmaceutical Services.* Cincinnati, Harvey Whitney Books, 1981, pp 403-427.

66. ASHP guidelines for single unit and unit dose packages of drugs. *Am J Hosp Pharm* 34:613-614, 1977.

67. ASHP statement on unit dose drug distribution. *Am J Hosp Pharm* 38:1214, 1981.

68. Pang F, Grant JA: Missing medications associated with centralized unit dose dispensing. *Am J Hosp Pharm* 32:1121-1123, 1975.

69. Cohen MR: Discrepancies in unit dose cart fills. *Hosp Pharm* 15:17-19, 1980.

70. Jarosinski PF: The importance of pharmacist surveillance in a unit dose drug distribution system. *Hosp Pharm* 13:491-500, 1978.

71. Tanner DJ: Patient profile medication administration records and cart exchange verification. *Hosp Pharm* 13:385-389, 1978.

72. Kitrenos JG, Gluc K, Stotter ML: Analysis of missing medication episodes in a unit dose system. *Hosp Pharm* 14:642-653, 1979.

73. Adelman DN: Reducing the number of missing doses with the aid of a computer system. *Hosp Pharm* 17:195-199, 1982.

74. Barker KN, Harris JA, Webster DB, et al: Consultant evaluation of a hospital medication system: Implementation and evaluation of the new system. *Am J Hosp Pharm* 41:2022-2029, 1984.

75. U.S. General Accounting Office: *Unit Dose Life Cycle Costs Analysis and Application to a Recently Constructed Health Care Facility. Study of Health Facilities Construction Costs.* A Report to the Congress by the United States General Accounting Office, 1972.

76. Cameron G, Vaughan RG: *Unit Dose: Cost/Benefit Dilemma for Hospital Pharmacies.* Chicago, Center for Hospital Management Engineering, American Hospital Association, 1979.

77. Arrington DM, Derewicz HJ, Lamy PP: Cost comparison of unit dose drug distribution for adult and pediatric medicine patients. *Am J Hosp Pharm* 31:578-581, 1974.

78. Schnell BR: A comparison of hospital drug distribution system costs on a pediatric and adult nursing ward. *Can J Hosp Pharm* 25:153-155, 1972.

79. Hendrix FL: The administrator of a small hospital looks at unit dose systems. *Hosp Form Mgt* 9:11-13, 1973.

80. Slater WE, Jacobsen R, Hripko JR, et al: Unit dose drops expenses. *Hospitals* 46:88-94, April 1972.

81. Minor MF: Justifying the cost of a unit dose system without reliance on savings for nursing. *Hosp Pharm* 10:94; 97-99, 1975.

82. Yorio D, Myers R, Chan L, Hutchinson RA, Wertheimer AI: Cost comparison of decentralized unit dose and traditional pharmacy services in a 600-bed community hospital. *Am J Hosp Pharm* 29:922-927, 1972.

83. Hynniman CE, Hyde GC, Parker PF: How costly is medication safety? *Hospitals* 45:73-85, September 1971.

84. Riley AN, Derewicz HJ, Lamy PP: Distributive costs of a computer-based unit dose drug distribution system. *Am J Hosp Pharm* 30:213-219, 1973.

85. Eberhardt RC: The effect of unit dose drug distribution on the allocation of nursing time in a neonatal intensive care unit. Thesis, Little Rock, University of Arkansas, 1982.

86. Slater WE, Hripko JR: The unit dose system in a private hospital. Part I. Implementation. *Am J Hosp Pharm* 25:408-417, 1968; Part II. Evaluation. *Am J Hosp Pharm* 25:641-648, 1968.

87. Blumberg MS: Packaging of hospital medication. *Am J Hosp Pharm* 19:270-273, 1962.

88. Fowler TJ, Spalding DW: Unit-dose or traditional system? *Hospitals* 44:154-160, August 1970.

89. Klotz R: Pediadose-pediatric unit dose dispensing. *Am J Hosp Pharm* 27:132-135, 1970.

90. Rosenberg JM, Peritore SP: Implications of a unit dose dispensing system in a community hospital. *Hosp Pharm* 8:35-39, 1973.

91. Black HJ, Upham R: Impact of unit dose pharmacy service on the time involvement of registered nurses with medication activities. Iowa City, The University of Iowa, 1971.

92. Anon: Unit dose system: The successful failure. *Hospitals* 47:138-146, July 1973.

93. U.S. General Accounting Office. *Potentially Dangerous Drugs Missing in VA Hospitals,* Washington, DC, 1975.

94. Martinelli BL, Wurdack PJ: Drug loss economics: Traditional drug distribution vs. unit dose. Presented at the Mid-Year Meeting of the American Society of Hospital Pharmacists, New Orleans, 1975.

95. Adachi WD, Endo AY, and Tanaka JY: Controlling admixture waste through pharmacist monitoring (letter). *Am J Hosp Pharm* 41:883, 1984.

96. Simon JR, LeMay RP, Tester WW: Attitudes of nurses, physicians and pharmacists toward a unit dose drug distribution system. *Am J Hosp Pharm* 25:239-247, 1968.

97. John GW: Pharmacy personnel activities and costs in decentralized and centralized unit dose drug distribution systems. *Am J Hosp Pharm* 33:38-43, 1976.

98. *Sourcebook on Unit Dose Distributing Systems.* Washington, DC, American Society of Hospital Pharmacists, 1978.

99. McAllister JC, Lindley CM: *Planning and Preparation of Proposals for New Hospital Pharmacy Programs and Services.* Chapel Hill, NC, Health Sciences Consortium, 1980.

100. Ketchum RM, Gibson JT, Freeman RA: Innovation diffusion in hospitals. Presented at the American Public Health Association Annual Meeting, Los Angeles, November 3, 1981.

101. Bucceri P, Baker JA: Management strategy for the diffusion on innovation: Unit dose drug distribution. _Am J Hosp Pharm_ 35:168-173, 1978.

102. Brief AP, Filley AC: Selling proposals for change. _Bus Horizons_ 19:22-25, April 1976.

103. Talley CR: Aspirin for the nursing shortage headache: Upgraded pharmaceutical services. _Am J Hosp Pharm_ 38:45, 1981.

104. Jeffrey LP, Gallina JN: Pharmacy staffing pattern for a unit dose medication distribution system. _Hosp Pharm_ 8:229-231, 1973.

105. Vogel DP: Four-day, 40-hour work week for pharmacy staff in unit dose drug distribution. _Hosp Pharm_ 9:258-268, 1974.

106. Gallina JN, Jeffrey LP: Personnel scheduling for unit dose. _Hosp Pharm_ 9:23, 1974.

107. Adelman D, Katz S: Four/three for staffing satellites. _Hospitals_ 48:68-70, December 1974.

108. Pang FJ: Seven days off, seven days on for total pharmacy service. _Hosp Pharm_ 9:21-22, 1974.

109. Hoffman RP: Expanding pharmaceutical services through efficient staff scheduling. _Hosp Pharm_ 14:192-200, 1979.

110. Lee HE: Effects of primary nursing on pharmaceutical services. _Am J Hosp Pharm_ 37:1093-1094, 1980.

111. Kay BG: Drug distribution in a Friesen concept hospital. _Hosp Pharm_ 8:366-375, 1973.

112. Lovett LT: Locked medication drawer at the patient's room—experience in one hospital. _Hosp Pharm_ 14:584-593, 1979.

113. Adams RW: Pharmacy services in a 240-bed Gordon Friesen-design hospital. _Hosp Pharm_ 14:594-606, 1979.

114. Superstine E, Lipman AG, Bair JN: Considerations in selecting a mobile master cart. _Am J Hosp Pharm_ 40:293-294, 1983.

CHAPTER 33

Administration of Medications

DICK R. GOURLEY, HENRY F. WEDEMEYER, and MICHAEL NORVELL

The administration of medications to the hospitalized patient is the result of the thoughts and actions of every department within the institution. From environmental services that prepares the patient room, to the admitting department that initially places the patient into the environment, to the nursing staff that cares for the patient, the medical staff that diagnoses and prescribes, and to the pharmacy that prepares the medication, all act to achieve the final result of actual administration of the drug to the patient. Also involved are the departments of clinical laboratories, pathology, radiology, and dietary. The implications are three. First, no single department or individual can perform the act of medication administration without prior preparation. Second, unless the correct medication is administered to the right patient at the right time, in the correct dose and form, the work of many clinicians has been wasted at the expense of the patient. Third, communication among all hospital staff involved in administering medications is essential but at times is the weakest link in the administration of medications to the hospitalized patient. This chapter will explore and discuss the implications to the hospital, the patient, and the individuals involved in the actual act of drug administration and some thoughts on the future of drug administration.

ENTERING, CHARTING, AND POSTING

The administration of any medication to a patient within the institution requires an order from a physician. Written medication orders are most commonly seen and least likely to result in misinterpretation; verbal medication orders are usually given when the physician is unable to come to the nursing unit until a later time. Both the registered nurse and pharmacist should be able to receive a verbal order from a physician and reduce it to writing in the medical record to be cosigned at a later time by the physician. There is also the standing order for routine procedures. Such orders are usually found on preprinted order forms and are specified for a certain period of time. A "one time only" order is usually administered at a specified time, and a "stat" order, one that is to be administered immediately, takes precedence over the regularly scheduled medications. The ordering of medications stat is sometimes abused, with the result that they soon become treated as any other routine order, making it difficult to respond to the true stat orders that are needed

immediately. Once the physician has initiated an order for a medication, he will usually "flag" a patient's chart to notify nursing personnel that there is a new order or change of orders. Someone, whether it be the nurse, ward clerk, or medication technician, must be assigned the responsibility of routinely checking for and initiating these orders. If responsibility is not given to someone, orders could go unfilled for a day or more, with the physician believing his orders are being carried out and the patient deprived of the proper care and treatment.

Once the medication order has been taken from the physician's order sheet, the transcribing of this order to the medication administration record must be done and a copy of the original order should be sent either to the pharmacist on the nursing unit, if there is one, or to the pharmacy so that the medications ordered can be prepared and dispensed and the order placed into the patient profile system of the pharmacy.

The information that should be placed on the medication administration record is:

1. The medication and dosage form to be administered. The dosage form is almost always important to the pharmacy, e.g., if the patient has a nasogastric tube and cannot swallow oral medication.

2. The proper dose of medication. This should be reviewed by the pharmacist before it is dispensed.

3. The route of administration.

4. The schedule of drug administration (time and frequency). It is to the advantage of the hospital staff to establish times for regularly scheduled doses. Some hospitals use military time in scheduling. This may reduce confusion when the time of day is not specified on a medication order. Some examples of dosing schedules used in hospitals are qd, 0900; hs, 2000; bid, 0900-1700 or 0900-2100; tid, 0900-1300-1700 or 0900-1500-2100; and qid, 0900-1300-1700-2100.

5. The patient's full name. No initials should be used, since two people with the same last name may be on the same nursing unit. If it should occur that two people with the same first and last name are on the same unit the designation John Smith "Heart" and John Smith "Liver," designating their medical problem, can be used to distinguish between them.

6. The patient's admission number, room number, and medical service.

7. Any special information (such as allergies, if patient is blind or deaf, or other special considerations).

8. The signature of the medication technician.

ADMINISTERING THE DRUG TO THE PATIENT

The individual administering the medication should remain at bedside until all the medication has been taken by the patient. Some patients may discard a medication if it is not palatable or if they suffer some adverse effects after taking the medication. If the patient refuses the medication, this must be reported to the nurse and pharmacist responsible for the patient and recorded in the medical record for the physician.

One advantage of a complete and effective unit dose dispensing system is that all doses are sent to the nursing unit in a ready-to-administer form, and all prepared doses have been checked by a pharmacist. The use of the medication technician works well in the unit dose system, particularly because only the doses ordered, in the proper dosage form, with only a sufficient supply (usually for 24 hours or less) are available to the medication technician. This reduces the possibility of administering too many doses or administering by the wrong route, errors which might occur more frequently if all dosage forms were available in large quantities for the technician to select.

Oral Medications

In the unit dose system, all oral medications are packaged so that there is no need for medicine cups to deliver the necessary doses. The medication technician selects from the patient's bin the doses needed for a specific time, and then takes them to the bedside. The patient is identified by his armband, and then solid oral medications are opened and placed in the patient's hand or the liquid medication containers are opened and handed to the patient to take. Some patients may require fruit juice, milk, or other liquid to take medications. These should be available on the drug dispensing cart taken into the patient's room.

Oral liquids and suspensions in unit dose packages are calculated to deliver the dose ordered. Also, oral syringes are calculated to deliver the dose ordered by compressing the plunger once. It is, therefore, unnecessary to flush the unit dose bottle, empty it into another container, or depress the plunger of an oral syringe more than once, since this could result in the delivery of an inaccurate dose.

Contraindications to oral administration are as follows: an unconscious patient; one who has difficulty swallowing, is vomiting, has had gastrointestinal problems or surgery; certain pediatric or geriatric patients; or an irrational patient.

Subcutaneous Injection Administration (SC, SQ, SubQ)

One of the three primary routes of parenteral administration, subcutaneous injection, is used for drugs that come as solutions or suspensions such as heparin or insulins. The main areas used for this type of parenteral administration are the thigh, abdomen, and upper arm. Patients who receive daily injections subcutaneously must rotate injection sites in order to reduce the chance of local irritation or damage. Usually a 23-gauge needle of ¾-inch length is selected and injected at a 45-60–degree angle with a quick dart-throwing action of the wrist (Fig. 33.1). The end of the syringe nearest the patient is then grasped and the syringe plunger drawn back to see if the needle has entered a blood vessel. If no blood appears in the syringe, the medication is injected. If blood does appear, then the needle should be withdrawn and another site selected several centimeters away. Before and after the injection is made, the injection site should be cleansed with a 70% alcohol or Iodophor sponge. At all times, before any medication is administered by any route, the patient should be identified by his armband, not the name on the bed or wall above the bed.

A new method of subcutaneous administration of medications involves the continuous infusion of drugs such as the delivery of insulin or narcotics via a programmable pump. The pump is filled with a 24-48–hour supply of medication, which is then administered over a predetermined amount of time and can be adjusted periodically by the patient.

Intramuscular Injection Administration (IM)

The injection of a drug intramuscularly requires more knowledge and practice than many of the other routes. This is not to suggest that it is more difficult to administer drugs by this route, but that more problems can result if administration is improper. The deltoid muscles of the arm and gluteal muscles of the buttocks are the usual sites for IM administration. Extreme care must be taken not to enter a blood vessel or damage a nerve when using this technique. After selecting the injection site and cleansing the skin, the needle is inserted by the dart technique through the skin at a 90-degree angle. The plunger of the syringe is pulled back to verify that a blood vessel has not been entered and if no blood enters the syringe the medication is injected and the needle removed quickly. Nerve damage can occur from placing an irritating drug too close to a nerve, so the selection of the injection site is important. The volume of drug to be injected is also important, since there will be some tissue tearing upon IM injection. Usually 3-4 ml is the recommended maximal volume. Larger volumes may be administered but usually not without pain and discomfort to the patient (Fig. 33.1).

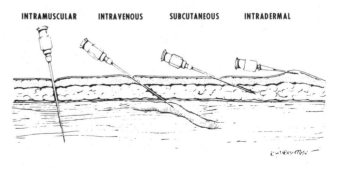

FIGURE 33.1 Injection techniques. (Reprinted by permission of Smith, Kline, and French Laboratories.)

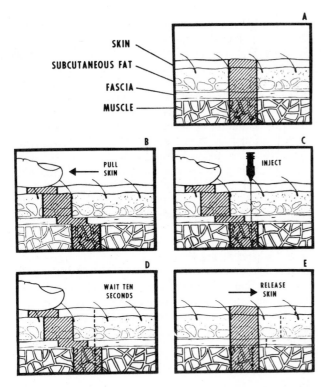

FIGURE 33.2 Z-track technique. (Reprinted by permission of Lakeside Laboratories.)

The Z-track method of IM injection, used to inject iron dextran, is accomplished by pulling the skin of the upper outer quadrant of the buttock firmly to one side and inserting the needle at a 90-degree angle, checking for blood, and then injecting. This method is used for drugs that are highly irritating or would stain the skin if they escaped into the surrounding tissue (Fig. 33.2).

Intradermal Injection Administration (ID)

The intradermal injection is used to inject antigens just below the dermal layer of the skin. This technique is used to check for circulating antibodies to the injected antigen and is used to test for such things as exposure to tuberculosis. Another application of intradermal testing is to test for anergy by injecting several antigens such as *Candida,* mumps, and tuberculin, which challenge the patient's immune system. The technique for intradermal injection is to cleanse the area with 70% alcohol or Iodophor, hold the skin taut, and insert the needle (usually 25-gauge, ¾ inch) bevel up, approximately ⅛ inch into the skin, at an angle almost parallel to the skin. The injection should raise a wheal or circumscribed elevation of the skin. The skin test is usually read at 24, 36, and 48 hours. A reddened area of induration of 5 mm or greater usually indicates a positive reaction or an intact immune system.

Intravenous Injection Administration (IV)

An IV injection provides the most rapid and complete absorption of a medication but is not without complications.

Thrombophlebitis, air emboli, speed shock, and injection of pathogens are a few of the adverse effects that must be avoided. Some of the indications for IV therapy are replacement of fluid and electrolytes, administration of antibiotics and drugs that may require a rapid high blood level, administration of drugs that are too irritating to be given intramuscularly or subcutaneously such as vincristine sulfate, parenteral nutrition, emergency situations such as cardiac arrest, and when no other route is available for the administration of medications.

Although the administration of medications by the IV route may be the responsibility of the registered nurse and not the medication technician, the technician should have an understanding of IV therapy and the drugs that are given intravenously, since it is usually the technician's responsibility to transcribe orders and interpret routes of administration from the physician's original order.

Before the administration of a medication intravenously, it is essential to check the medication, the dose, the fluid in which the drug is to be given, and the time for administration against the patient's chart. After checking these, all the necessary equipment such as alcohol or Iodophor sponge, needle, IV board, tape, and IV solution or admixture should be assembled. The patient should then be identified by his armband and the procedure explained to the patient to alleviate any apprehension. Venipuncture can then be performed with a needle or catheter, which should be checked after insertion to ensure proper placement in the vein and that it is adequately secured to the patient's arm. The patient should be advised not to adjust rates of flow of the solution and not to disturb the venipuncture site. Because of the many variables that affect the rate of flow of the solution (gravity, solution viscosity, temperature, possibly defective equipment), the rate of flow should be checked every hour or so depending on hospital policy. When the rate of flow is critical, such as in pediatric patients or patients receiving parenteral nutrition, an infusion pump may be needed to ensure the proper flow of solution into the patient.

When the patient is receiving IV drugs on an intermittent basis only, a heparin lock may be used. The system does not require a continuously running solution to keep the vein open but instead can be closed off and allow the patient more mobility between drug administrations. Before the drug is administered, the tubing is flushed with normal saline solution to remove any leftover drug, which may result in an incompatibility. The drug is then administered and is followed by another flush of normal saline solution. A small amount of heparin is then administered into the tubing to prevent the IV site from occluding.

Rectal Medication Administration

Rectal suppositories should be firm, not soft and may need to be moistened with a water-soluble lubricant for ease of insertion. The patient should be placed on his side with one leg extended and the other flexed prior to insertion. After removing the suppository from the foil wrapper, insert the suppository using a disposable glove, past the anal sphincter and hold the buttocks together, since the patient will have the urge to expel the suppository. Rectal ointments should be inserted well into the rectum with the applicator

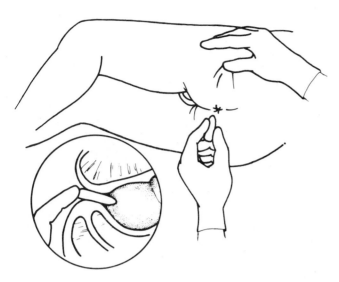

FIGURE 33.3   Rectal instillation technique.

or tube provided. The tube may need to be lubricated with petroleum jelly prior to insertion (Fig. 33.3).

Vaginal Medication Administration

For the administration of a vaginal cream or suppository, the patient should be instructed to lie on her back with her knees flexed and legs spread apart. The applicator provided should be moistened with a water-soluble lubricant or warmed water, if necessary, and with disposable gloves on both hands, the labia should be gently spread apart and the applicator gently inserted approximately 2-4 inches into the vagina or until resistance is felt. The plunger of the applicator should be depressed fully and then the applicator carefully removed. The applicator should be washed in warm soapy water after each application. Some points to remember are: (1) be sure the vaginal tablet has been removed from the foil wrapper, (2) check that the applicator is clean and the plunger moves freely before filling with cream or gel or adding the suppository; and (3) ensure that the patient is in a comfortable position and that privacy is ensured. No vaginal drugs should be administered to a pregnant woman without specific examination and orders from the patient's physician (Fig. 33.4).

Ophthalmic Drops and Ointment Instillation

Ophthalmic drops should be administered to the patient with his head tilted back and up. The skin below the eye just above the cheekbone should be pulled down and the fluid dropped into the lower conjunctival sac away from the tear ducts. The dropper tip should not touch the eye or lid to avoid contamination, and the fluid should be shaken well if it is a suspension before instillation. A thin line of ointment should be applied along the conjunctival surface of the lower lid with the same method used for an ophthalmic ointment. The patient should be instructed to close his eye for a short while to allow the medication to be dispersed throughout the eye. Be sure the tip of the ointment tube

does not touch the eye and the cap is replaced immediately (Fig. 33.5).

Instillation of Ear and Nose Medications

Ear drops are administered with the patient lying down and the affected ear facing up. After gently pulling the auricle of the ear up and back for an adult and down and back for a child, the drops should be instilled directly into the ear canal. Do not touch the ear canal with the dropper. The patient should remain lying down for several minutes, and if a cotton plug has been ordered, it should be placed at the opening of the ear canal, not down into it.

Nose drops should be administered to the patient with his head tilted back after he has cleared his nose by blowing. The patient should breathe through his mouth and the prescribed number of drops should be administered. The patient should keep his head tilted for several minutes. One should avoid touching the nostrils with the dropper. A nose spray is applied by squeezing the applicator bottle quickly and firmly into the nostrils once they have been cleared by blowing and with the head in an upright position (Figs. 33.6 and 33.7).

Topical Application of Medications

Before medications are applied topically, the affected area should be clean and any old medication removed. All topical medications should be applied in a thin layer and then covered with a sterile gauze or occlusive dressing. Rubber gloves should be used during the entire procedure. Ointment or creams may be applied with a tongue depressor or cotton-tipped swab; lotions, suspensions, and emulsions should be shaken well and then applied with a ball of cotton or applicator provided. Certain topical liquids should be measured with a medicine cup. Aerosol application should be applied in quick sprays after shaking the container well and having the patient cover his eyes, nose, and mouth. Do not breathe the aerosol spray.

APPLICATION OF TRANSDERMAL PRODUCTS

The transdermal system is a method of topically administering drugs such as nitroglycerin into the bloodstream for a sustained period of time. The system consists of a gel-like disc held in place by an adhesive bandage. The patient should be instructed to select an area of the skin that is free of hair, such as the upper arm, the inside of the forearm, or a hair-free portion of the chest. Areas with scar tissue, calluses, or areas that are irritated or damaged should be avoided. The skin should be clean and dry before application of the disc. The patient should be encouraged to change application areas each day (Fig. 33.8).

Sublingual Tablet Administration (SL)

Patients should be instructed to place the tablet under the tongue and leave it there until completely dissolved. The tablet should not be chewed or swallowed. Because of the nature of the drugs given sublingually and their ready dis-

Vaginal Suppository

HOW TO USE SUPPOSITORY INSERTER
1. Remove vaginal suppository from clear plastic package by peeling back protective foil closure. Moisten suppository in warm water for a second or two.

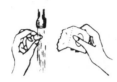

2. Pull out plunger (inner rod) of plastic inserter until it stops.

3. Place smaller, pointed end of suppository snugly into the open end of inserter.

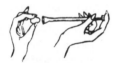

4. Grasp barrel (outer cylinder) of inserter at the bottom, with thumb and middle finger.

5. Lying on your back, push inserter into vagina as far as it will go comfortably without using force. With forefinger, depress plunger all the way down to insert suppository in vagina.

6. Carefully remove inserter from vagina, holding it by the barrel.

7. Wash inserter with warm, soapy water (do not boil). For easy cleaning, it may be disassembled by pulling plunger apart from barrel. Rinse and dry.

It is recommended that a pad be used to prevent staining of clothing.

Vaginal Ointment

FILLING THE APPLICATOR
1. Remove cap from tube. Screw applicator to tube.

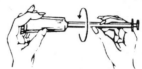

2. Pull out plunger (inner rod) of plastic inserter until it stops.

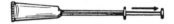

3. Hold tube with applicator pointing down. Squeeze tube, forcing contents into cylinder until it is full. Then remove applicator from tube.

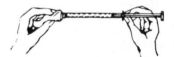

4. Hold filled applicator by cylinder and insert it into the vagina as far as it will go comfortably. Press plunger and deposit material. While keeping plunger depressed, remove the applicator from vagina.

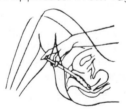

CARE OF THE APPLICATOR
After each use, take applicator and wash with soap and warm water. To take apart, hold cylinder of plunger and turn cap counterclockwise.
To reassemble, drop plunger back into cylinder as far as it will go. Place cap on end of plunger and turn clockwise until cap is tight.

FIGURE 33.4 Vaginal instillation technique. (Reprinted by permission from *US Pharmacist,* April 1977; original source: Merrell Laboratories.)

How to Instill Eye Drops in Your Own Eye

1. Remove cap from bottle.
2. Tilt head slightly back.
3. With index finger of free hand gently pull down lower lid.
4. Hold dropper pointed downward close to front of (but not touching) eye.
5. Instill prescribed number of drops into pocket between eye and lid.
6. Release eyelid, close eyes, and roll eyes slowly in a circular manner.
7. Replace and tighten cap.

How to Instill Eye Ointment in Your Own Eye

1. Remove cap from tube.
2. Stand in front of mirror and tilt head forward slightly.
3. With index finger of free hand gently pull down lower eyelid.
4. Hold tube in front of and parallel to eye.
5. By squeezing tube, apply a thin ribbon of ointment along inside surface of lower lid, taking care to avoid touching eye with tube.
6. Replace and tighten cap on tube.

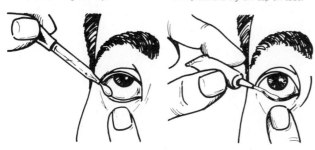

FIGURE 33.5 Ophthalmic administration. (Reprinted by permission from Strauss, Steven: *Your Prescription and You, A Pharmacy Handbook for Consumers,* ed 2. 1977.)

solution in moisture, the tablets should be stored in a cool, dry place and discarded if their potency is questionable.

CHARTING AND POSTING

In order to avoid errors and ensure proper administration of medications, proper and timely charting and posting of medications administered are essential. The most effective system is to post the medication at the time it is administered. It is also important to post medications not given and the reason for omitting dosage, such as the patient was in radiology or refused the medication. The charting and posting of medications is often the only form of communication for the nursing and the medical staff.

PREOPERATIVE AND POSTOPERATIVE CARE

Medications administered prior to surgery (preop) include both regularly scheduled medications and special preop medications such as atropine and meperidine. Once a patient has gone to surgery, new orders are necessary to resume preop medications or to order new medications, depending on the patient's status. Intravenous fluids with electrolytes and hyperalimentation solutions sometimes accompany the patient to surgery in the operating room, i.e., solutions with electrolytes should be administered by operating room personnel. If the hyperalimentation solution must go to the operating room with the patient, it is essential that enough solution be sent to last throughout the procedure and that surgery personnel be instructed that the hyperalimentation line should not be used for drawing blood or administering drugs.

□ 1. Tilt head to side with infected ear up.

□ 2. Without touching dropper to ear, gently squeeze dropper so medication will enter ear canal.

□ 3. Pull ear back, enabling drops to go down into ear canal.

□ 4. Hold head in tilted position for 10-15 seconds, gently using finger to push skin in front of canal (see arrow) to help spread the medication.

□ 5. Replace dropper in bottle.

□ 6. Use eardrops as directed until your doctor tells you to discontinue use.

*Shake well before using if suspension formula is prescribed.

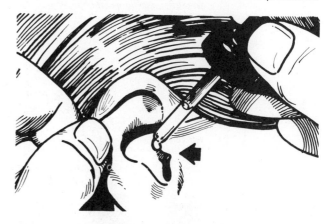

FIGURE 33.6 Ear instillation technique. (Reprinted by permission from Burroughs Wellcome Co.)

Nose Drops

Blow your nose before you use the drops. Lie down, and tilt your head slightly backward. Now place the medication in your nostril(s). Remain lying down for about 1-2 minutes so the medication will be absorbed.

Before replacing the dropper in the bottle, you should rinse the dropper with water after each use to prevent contaminating the drops.

Nose Spray

Blow your nose before you use the spray. Hold your head straight up and insert the tip of the nozzle (nosepiece) into the nostril. Squeeze the container firmly and quickly to apply each spray of medication

Rinse the tip of the nozzle with water or wipe it clean with a tissue after each use to prevent contamination.

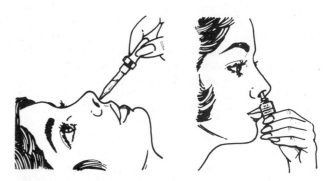

FIGURE 33.7 Nose instillation technique. (Reprinted by permission from Strauss, Steven: *Your Prescription and You, A Pharmacy Handbook for Consumers,* ed 2. 1977.)

How to use

Transderm®-Nitro
nitroglycerin
Transdermal Therapeutic System

The usual starting dose is one Transderm-Nitro 5 system. The dose may vary, however, depending on your individual response to the system. For instance, your doctor may decide to increase or decrease the size of the system, or prescribe a combination of systems, to suit your particular needs.

Where to place Transderm-Nitro

Select any area of skin on the body, **EXCEPT** the extremities below the knee or elbow. The chest is the preferred site, but the back is an excellent alternative because it is usually free of hair, skin folds, and excessive muscular movement. The area should be clean, dry, and hairless. If hair is likely to interfere with system adhesion or removal, clip the hair prior to applying the system. Do not shave. Take care to avoid areas with cuts or irritations. Do **NOT** apply the system immediately after showering or bathing. It is best to wait until you are certain the skin is completely dry.

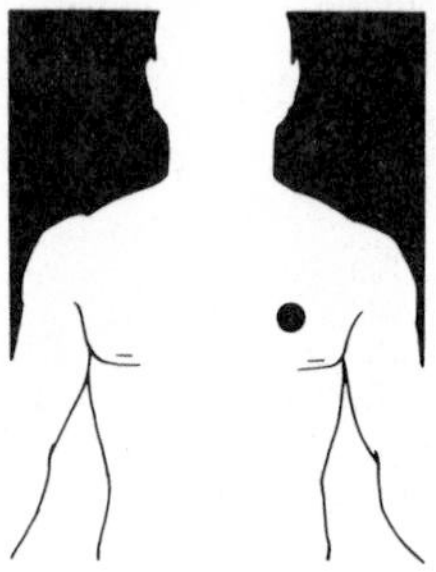

How to apply Transderm-Nitro

1. Open the package containing the system by tearing at the indicated indentations; then remove the system from the package (*Figure A*).

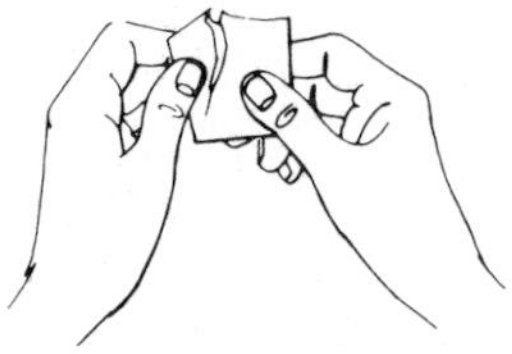

Figure A

2. Carefully pick up the system lengthwise with the tab up (*Figure B*)

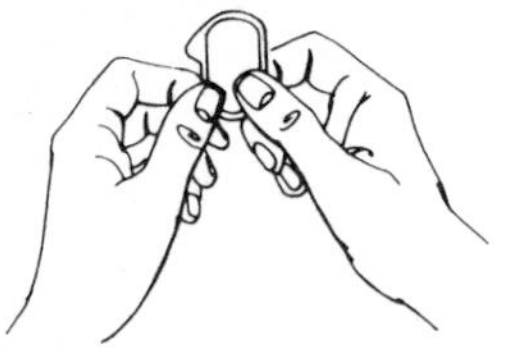

Figure B

3. With your thumbs, begin to remove the protective backing from the system at the tab (*Figure C*). Do not touch the inside of the exposed system, because the adhesive covers the entire surface.

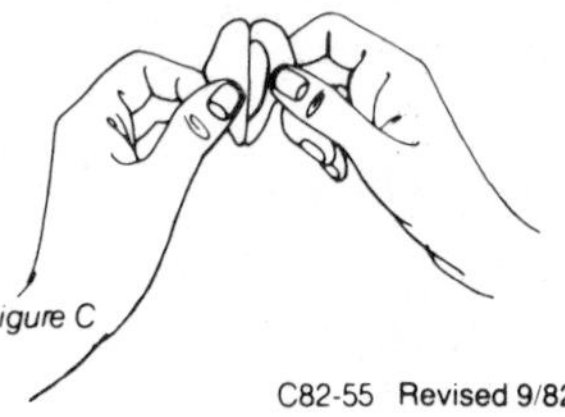

Figure C

C82-55   Revised 9/82   665934

FIGURE 33.8   Transdermal administration. (Reprinted by permission of CIBA Pharmaceutical Company.)

TRANSFERRING AND DISCHARGING THE PATIENT

Whenever a patient is transferred, it is essential that the receiving nursing unit or institution have an up-to-date medical record. For this reason, communication to the medication technician that a patient is being transferred is important so that all administered medications can be charted and posted in the medical record before the patient is transferred. The same holds true for the patient being discharged. Since the physician must make a discharge summary in the medical record, it is important that he be aware of medications administered or refused. At this time, he will also write discharge prescriptions. The pharmacist will need to know if there are any special medication needs, drug interactions, or other problems, in order to provide effective discharge counseling to the patient. Discharge orders should also include instructions for any medications brought into the hospital or medication that the patient was taking at home but did not bring into the institution. Information on prehospital medications is obtained from the medication history taken by the pharmacist at the time of the patient's admission and should be available in the medical record.

CHARGING FOR SERVICES

The most effective method of charging patients for medications administered is from the administration record. This avoids the need to credit for items not given and charges the patient only for what he has received. The amount the patient is billed depends on the charging structure for other hospital services, or medication administration fees may all be included in the medication charge. No matter what the charging system may be, the price of the drug alone should be readily identifiable for the purposes of budgeting, patient information, and third-party reimbursement. With the expansion of clinical pharmacy services, separation of reimbursement for these services from the cost of the drug product should be considered by both the administration of the institution and third-party payers.

4. Continue to remove the backing *slowly* along the length of the system allowing the system to rest on the outside of your fingers *(Figure D)*

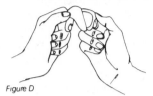

Figure D

5. Place the exposed, adhesive side of the system on the chosen skin site. It is extremely important to *press firmly* in place with the palm of your hand, and maintain the pressure for *10-15 seconds (Figure E)*.

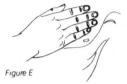

Figure E

6. Circle the outside edge of the system with one or two fingers *(Figure F)*. This, along with step 5, will insure optimum adhesion. Once the system is in place, *do not* test the adhesion by pulling on it. For your information, the adhesive in the Transderm-Nitro system will not feel as sticky as that on an adhesive bandage.

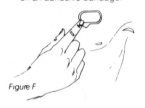

Figure F

7. Remove and discard the system after 24 hours. Dispose of the system by conventional means, such as in a trash container. Place a new system on a different skin site, following steps 1-6.

Please note:

Contact with water, as in bathing, swimming, or showering will not affect the system. In the unlikely event that a system falls off, discard it and put a new one on a different skin site.

Precautions:

The most common side effect that is encountered is transient headaches. These often decrease as therapy is continued, but may require treatment with a mild analgesic. Although uncommon, faintness, flushing, and dizziness may occur, especially when suddenly rising from the recumbent (lying horizontal) position. If these latter symptoms do occur, the system should be removed from the skin and your physician should be notified. For changes in dosage and frequency of application, consult your physician.

Keep these systems and all drugs out of the reach of children.

DO NOT STORE ABOVE 86°F (30°C).

Dist. by:
CIBA Pharmaceutical Company
Division of CIBA-GEIGY Corporation
Summit, New Jersey 07901

C I B A

Printed in U S A   C82-55 **Revised** 9/82 665934

FIGURE 33.8, cont'd

SELF-ADMINISTRATION OF DRUGS

The administration of medication to patients in the institution has evolved from the nurse administering the medication in a total floor stock system to a highly sophisticated unit dose dispensing system. Yet, most patients still go home on medications that are unfamiliar to them and do not know or understand the side effects. They may also be unsure of how to take the medication properly. Some pharmacy departments have initiated programs that will increase patient compliance once he leaves the institution, i.e., self-medication programs that involve the physician, nurse, pharmacist, and patient. Medications that are tailored for such programs include chronic drug administration such as digitalis, diuretics, and antiarrhythmics; medications that the patient will be taking for long periods of time, even life; or those drugs that have a narrow range of toxicity. In addition, patients may be allowed to administer drugs intravenously, such as antibiotics, narcotics, and total parenteral nutrition.

It is the role of the nurse and pharmacist in consultation with the physician to decide whether a particular patient should be placed on self-medication. The patient's condition, attitude, and ability to self-medicate will be factors in selection for self-medication. The process of selection is important because institutional and professional liability may increase when a patient is placed on self-medication, especially if patient instruction and monitoring are inadequate. At least one member of the family should also receive instructions. This will reinforce any instructions once the patient leaves the institution.

The patient should be instructed on what the medication is for, its action, side effects, storage conditions, and proper preparation and equipment that may be necessary. Before discharge, the patient should demonstrate and explain his ability to do all that has been taught before self-medication is begun. Along with all instructions, the patient should be given an instruction sheet to keep and take home. All information should be recorded in the patient's medical record. During the entire course of self-medication in the institution, the pharmacist and nurse closely monitor the patient, and the medication technician can be a valuable aid in this daily, routine monitoring and can relay questions the patient may ask to the proper professional.

If necessary, referral to a health care agency for assistance should be initiated as soon as possible in order to avoid complications at the time of discharge. When the patient is ready for discharge the pharmacist can help ensure compliance and further patient eduction by contacting the patient's community pharmacist, with the patient's consent, and inform him of the patient's condition and medications on discharge. The development of a close relationship between the hospital pharmacist and the community pharmacist is essential if one is to bridge the gap between the patient's hospitalization and home care.

IMPLICATIONS FOR THE COMMUNITY PRACTITIONER

The administration of medications to the patient, whether it be through health care personnel or self-medication, is no longer restricted to the institutional setting.

The ever-increasing pressures from government, consumers, and third-party payers to reduce the costs of health care have brought about the removal of some patients from the institutional environment into their home for hyperalimentation, home dialysis, and chemotherapy for the cancer patient. This affords the community practitioner a real opportunity to change his role from the merchandiser of a product to a professional practitioner and transform the community drugstore into a community health center. Similar relationships should be maintained with the outpatient pharmacy, if one exists, in the institution.

Evidence of this trend is provided by the surge of patient profiles and new laws requiring the pharmacist to counsel each patient receiving a drug in his pharmacy. Beyond this, however, is the expanded role of preparation and dispensing of hyperalimentation solutions, consultation and dispensing of factor VIII, injectable pain medication and cancer chemotherapy, and an active role as drug information consultant to the private practicing physician. Through development of a pharmacist-nurse team within the community setting, all immunizations could be administered to adult and pediatric patients, and home health care services such as appliances and proper use of over-the-counter products could be provided. Ultimately this community pharmacy setting could become the initial step in admitting the patient into the health care system. To bring this about will require the support of the professional organizations, college of pharmacy, institutional setting, and most important, the pharmacy practitioner.

NURSING CONSIDERATIONS

Traditionally the function of medication administration has been assumed by the nursing staff (usually by registered nurses). With the proliferation of specialty and supportive personnel in all of the health professions and the realization that medication administration is primarily a technical function, the task of administering medications in some hospitals has been delegated to effectively trained technical personnel. For example, the University of Nebraska Medical Cen-

ter employs licensed practical nurses, and the Ohio State University Hospitals employ pharmacy technicians to administer all medications except those given intravenously.

It might be considered foolish for the department to give up this traditional role, one that is still taught in nursing schools. When not involved in administering medications, the registered nurse is free to become more involved in direct patient care, primary nursing care, and more patient education. The nurse who is asked to give up this function may ask ''What will my role be and what will I be asked to give up next if I no longer administer medications?'' The nurse soon finds that the time saved is used to formulate patient care plans, to provide patient nursing care needs, patient and family teaching, and to coordinate all the other disciplines involved in the care, rehabilitation, discharge, and referral of the patient.

PHARMACY CONSIDERATIONS

If one accepts the premise that the total control of medications within the institution is the responsibility of the pharmacy department, then this control extends to the control of drug administration. Unless the medication is administered properly, such tasks as purchasing and rational product selection are wasted efforts.

Shifting the responsibility for the administration of medications to the pharmacy has far-reaching consequences. It requires that pharmacists be on the nursing unit, have a thorough knowledge of how to administer drugs, be educated and aware of the sociologic and psychologic needs of the patient, be willing to expand pharmacy hours of operation to evenings, nights, and weekends, and to develop a team concept on the nursing unit. This does not imply that the pharmacist should become the medication technician, for this would only be a shift of responsibility from one professional to another. The function of medication administration, however, may be delegated to pharmacy-trained and supervised clerks and technicians.

One of the concerns facing the pharmacist is the proper scheduling of medications when he has the knowledge of a particular drug's half-life, interaction with food, or fluctuation in pharmacologic action (e.g., biorhythms). The pharmacist must consider scheduling in the context of such factors as scheduled meal times, tests or procedures, and sleep.

LEGAL AND POLICY CONSIDERATIONS

The recognition that drug administration does not necessarily have to be performed by a registered nurse but rather by a trained technician has several legal implications. Some states and hospitals require that administration of medications be performed by a licensed individual. These regulations limit the ability of the hospital to be innovative and to better utilize professional and nonprofessional health care personnel, and also contribute to the high cost of health care.

Due to the numerous levels of personnel, frequent turnover, and the rotation of working shifts, written policies and procedures are necessary in order to have consistency in drug administration and to avoid errors due to poor communication.

It is important to ensure that the policies and procedures are written to create an effective system that reduces medication errors and not solely for regulation or self-protection. Some of the specific legal considerations of the medication technician are (1) knowing the drug and proper route of administration; (2) verifying any order that is unclear or questionable; (3) being sure that all orders are taken off the physician order sheet and all transcribing done correctly; (4) seeing that all prn doses are checked by the nurse in charge of the patient; (5) ensuring that the patient is always identified before a drug is administered; (6) checking that drugs are administered or discontinued at their proper time; and (7) having the proper attitude and realization of the moral responsibility to the patient.

ADMINISTRATIVE CONSIDERATIONS

If the task of drug administration is delegated to someone other than a registered nurse, a training program that involves both the registered nurse and registered pharmacist should be established. The act of administration of medications should also be under the supervision of both.The review of new orders, scheduling of doses, answering of drug information questions, and monitoring of therapy and adverse drug reactions are the responsibility of the pharmacist. The registered nurse is responsible for knowing the medication and its effects, reporting any adverse effects, and evaluating the need for a prn dose. Both should be involved in the education of the patient and the family concerning the patient's medications. Of utmost importance is teamwork and effective communication between the pharmacy and nursing staff.

IMPACT ON DRUG DISTRIBUTION SYSTEMS

The objective of drug distribution and drug administration is to provide for the safe and accurate use of drugs at all stages of the drug use system. In traditional systems where the nurse is responsible for dispensing, setting up, and administering all medications to patients, there is the greatest misuse of the nurse's talent and training. Such a system also opens avenues for medication errors.

The unit dose distribution system has been shown to be the most effective distribution system in terms of reduction of medication errors, savings in nursing time, and reduction in drug costs to the hosptial. If one adds to this the transfer of responsibility of medication administration to a trained technician under the supervision of the registered nurse and pharmacist, the result is more effective use of health care personnel, greater involvement of the nurse in direct patient care, and expansion of the pharmacist's role in the use of medications within the institution. The overall effect should be a system that is more responsive to the needs of the patient at a more reasonable cost.

QUALITIES AND RESPONSIBILITIES OF THE MEDICATION TECHNICIAN

Almost every area that is involved in the delivery of health care makes use of nonprofessional supportive personnel. This has come about because of the ever-increasing cost of health care, the greater demand for quality health care, and the recognition that many of the tasks performed in the past by professionals are of a technical nature and can easily, and sometimes more effectively, be performed by a trained technician.

The selection of individuals to perform the task of medication administration requires the initial input of both nursing and pharmacy. When selecting medication technicians, the following attributes and requirements should be looked for:

1. The proper attitude toward the job and patient
2. The ability to communicate to patients
3. The ability to work with the many levels of hospital staff and on the various shifts within the institution
4. Successful completion of a training course in medication administration that has been approved by the institution
5. Licensure as a licensed practical or vocation nurse if required by law

Functions to be performed include:

1. Observe and report any significant changes in the patient's condition or reactions to the appropriate nurse and pharmacist
2. Maintain any records related to drugs for patients being admitted, transferred, or discharged
3. Ensure the proper storage of drugs on the nursing unit (e.g., refrigerated items)
4. Keep sufficient inventory of supplies necessary for the administration of medications
5. Keep the medication area clean and organized
6. Administer the medications as dictated by patient profiles

The initial training of medication technicians should be outside the institution in a qualified school of pharmacy or nursing, technical school, or community college. The institution should not have to sacrifice patient care and professional time in order to give this basic background training. The development of the intitial training program should involve the professional nurse and pharmacist who practices within the institution, and there should be a time period of practical experience and demonstration of competency within the institution. The training programs should teach the medication technician the following:

1. Responsibility and relationship to the patient, physician, professional nurse, and pharmacist
2. Administration of medications by all routes
3. All recording and transcription in the necessary records
4. Policies and procedures of the institution and state and federal laws regulating the administration of medications
5. Responsibilities in intravenous therapy, if any
6. Dosage forms, route of administration, drug actions, side effects, and factors that influence drug action and absorption in a general way
7. Organization and layout of the institution
8. Medical abbreviations, terms, and procedures related to their jobs
9. Metric system of weights and measures
10. Proper procedure of physically handling the patient and isolation procedures

ADDITIONAL READING

Anon: A guide to correct use of dosage forms. *US Pharm* 51-54, April 1977.

Anon: *Report to the Congress. Study of Health Facilities Construction Costs B-164031(3)*.

Benya TJ: Responsibility for transcription of medication orders. *Drug Intell* 3:37, 1969.

Blackburn GL, et al: Nutritional assessment of the hospitalized patient. *JPEN* 1:11-22, 1977.

Fudge RP, Latiolais CJ: Blue Cross pays for clinical pharmacist services in training hemophiliacs for home care self-therapy. *Pharm Times* 36-41, January 1976.

Fudge RP, Vlasses PH: Third-party reimbursement for pharmacist instruction about antihemophilic factor. *Am J Hosp Pharm* 34:831-834, 1977.

Gregorich MR: Problems and concerns—a nurse. *Am J Hosp Pharm* 28:879-882, 1971.

Ivey M, Reilla M, Mueller W, et al: Long-term parenteral nutrition in the home. *Am J Hosp Pharm* 32:1032-1036, 1975.

Johnson WJ, Hathaway DJ, et al: Hemodialysis—comparison of treatment in the medical center community hospital, and home. *Arch Intern Med* 125:462-467, 1970.

Lachner BJ: Administrative implications. *Am J Hosp Pharm* 27:899-901, 1970.

Latiolais CJ: A pharmacy coordinated unit dose dispensing and drug administration system—philosophy, objectives and pharmaceutical implications. *Am J Hosp Pharm* 27:886-889, 1970.

Lucarotte RL, Prisco HM, Hafner PE, Shoup LK: Pharmacist-coordinated self-administration medication program on an obstetrical service. *Am J Hosp Pharm* 30:1147-1150, 1973.

Meakins JL, et al: Delayed hypersensitivity: Indicator of acquired failure of host defenses in sepsis and trauma. *Ann Surg* 186:241-250, 1977.

Myers LC: *Clinical Pharmacy Practice—Medication Administration*. Philadelphia, Lea & Febiger, 1972, pp 261-281.

Nold EG, Pathak DS: Third-party reimbursement for clinical pharmacy services: Philosophy and practice. *Am J Hosp Pharm* 34:823-826, 1977.

Shoup LK: Recruitment, selection and training of pharmacy technicians. *Am J Hosp Pharm* 27:907-910, 1970.

CHAPTER 34

Intravenous Admixture Systems

NEAL W. SCHWARTAU and W. ALAN WOODWARD

Of considerable importance in hospital pharmacy distribution systems are the preparation and distribution of medications for IV use. Although differences in magnitude may exist among hospitals, it appears that IV fluids with or without added medications are among the most commonly prescribed medications in the United States (1). Since IV admixture systems were reported in the literature a number of years ago, their development has progressed rapidly; such systems are currently operating in a considerable number of hospitals in the United States (2-17).

The development and management of an IV admixture system are essential parts of pharmacy services and require a considerable amount of dedication, perhaps even specialization. It should be emphasized that IV admixture systems are faced with many dynamic changes caused by technologic advances, regulatory changes, and product changes. It is therefore important to assess the admixture system on an ongoing basis and be aware of the advances in the literature to determine if the system and products that are presently being used are meeting the needs of the practice setting. The study of many of the chapters in this book is fundamentally important to provide a base for an optimal IV admixture system. A review of both past and ongoing literature will also be helpful in identifying important concepts for the system (18-20).

THE LITERATURE

One factor that seems to be considered basic or is an elemental characteristic of an IV therapy service is that of policies and procedures. Wuest (21-23) has shown that an ongoing management program can determine the needs of patients, help to establish objectives to meet these needs, and elaborate on the tasks required to meet the objectives. In these three articles, Wuest presented 30 policies and procedures that outline in detail the scope and objectives, purposes, and equipment that are needed to develop an IV therapy service. Pulliam and Upton (24) described a cooperative effort between the Pharmacy Committee and Nursing Practice Committee in defining the responsibilities and activities of a sepcialized team of nurses for administration of large-volume parenterals. Guidelines were established, and approval was received from the hospital's Medical Board prior to the establishment of a pharmacy-coordinated IV therapy program.

Another factor to be considered is personnel. Avis et al (25) emphasized the importance of developing a master procedural manual to provide a source of instruction and training for new personnel. Shoup (26) reported that a certain amount of personnel training should be the responsibility of undergraduate educators. The author stated that the college curriculum should include the proper procedures involved in preparing IV admixtures in training future hospital pharmacists. The students should possess a background knowledge of IV solution "systems" available from pharmaceutical manufacturers and should be familiar with various aseptic techniques involved in preparing IV admixtures.

Durgin (11), as well as Ravin et al (27), discussed the utilization of technical personnel in various aspects of an IV therapy service, in particular, the IV admixture system. The importance of technical personnel to these aspects of service should be emphasized (28,29).

Another aspect of personnel is the staffing of an IV admixture service. Meisler and Skolaut (30) reported that, in order to determine the personnel requirements for an IV admixture service, the following information should be obtained: how many IV units containing additives are utilized over a 24-hour period, what times of the day and by whom are they being compounded; when are orders changed, when do new orders become effective, what are the peak workload hours of the day, and when are infusions started? Many variables determine staff needs, and caution is warranted in extrapolating data from one study to an institution (31,32). It is more reasonable to attempt a time study and determine the in-house variables to assist in staffing determinations.

The results of a questionnaire developed by Ravin (33), revealed that the workload in providing an IV admixture service seemed to depend to a significant extent on how intermittent therapy was handled in the hospital. He suggested that further assistance regarding workload can be obtained by a survey of physicians' orders in the hospital. He suggested that information such as the number of medication doses prescribed to be administered via intermittent IV therapy and the number of large-volume parenterals prescribed with medication additions and their respective frequencies would also be helpful in determining workload. According to Ravin, once the projected workload is established, the staffing needs can be determined. The article also contained tables depicting the IV admixture staffing patterns in 20 of the hospitals that responded to the questionnaire. Loeb et al (34) and Lee (35) have commented on a new aspect of packaging premixed IV admixtures that offers the advantages of preparation-time savings and quality assurance. The extent of utilization of premixed admixtures and the handling of these within an admixture system will greatly affect the variance of staffing patterns among similar institutions.

Professional and legal reasons for the pharmacist's interest and concern regarding the preparation of large-volume IV solutions have also been elaborated. Ravin (36) stated that one of the professional reasons is a consideration of the mainstream function of pharmacy, i.e., the provision of pharmaceutical services as an integral part of the total patient care concept. Patterson (37) made reference to the legal considerations when he commented that the pharmacist may receive prescription orders calling for the use of Food and Drug Administration–approved drugs to prepare nonapproved dosage forms. Such an extemporaneous prescription for a single patient can be legally dispensed by the pharmacist, but at the same time the pharmacist may be responsible for knowing whether or not the nonapproved dosage form is safe.

Provisions of service within individual hospitals have been described by numerous authors. Skolaut (38) discussed the benefits of a centralized IV admixture service and how the patient eventually benefits. Ravin and Holysko (3) described a centralized pharmacy admixture service and also, among other things, the concept of an "IV call card" to alert the pharmacy to the delivery time of the next parenteral solution. Durgin (11) discussed 13 policies and procedures that described an admixture service. Brown (6) gave a stepwise outline of procedures that a hospital might follow in handling IV drug orders by the admixture service. Meisler and Skolaut (30) described a centralized admixture service and gave a breakdown of the type and frequency of additive used. Miller et al (39) conducted a time-and-motion study in an IV admixture service in order to examine the four major types of IV administration systems and the time involved in transferring various forms of additives (vials, ampules, etc) into each of the four systems. Wuest (21–23,40,41) and Ravin et al (27) described an IV admixture service and its procedures, facilities, and equipment.

Paolon (43) described the use of an IV therapy team of nurses responsible to pharmacy that resulted in better control of IV infusions and in the utilization of administration sets. Fewer mechanical problems with the IV system and more prompt reporting of adverse drug reactions were also described as benefits. Guidelines were given for the implementation of this IV therapy team. In another article, Paoloni (42) described the monitoring of IV solutions throughout the hospital by a team of highly trained and specially qualified personnel coordinated by pharmacy.

Wuest (41) presented an excellent discussion of an IV therapy team approach. The team consisted of a registered nurse, a licensed practical nurse, and an IV therapist. The IV therapy policies and procedures such as venipuncture procedure, procedures for inserting catheters, administration of parenteral fluids, preparation of IV fluids requiring additives, stat IV orders, and removal of air from tubing were described in detail.

Economic consideration of IV therapy, in partibular the admixture service, has been briefly mentioned by several authors. Skolaut (38) discussed the economics of centralized facilities in general. He commented that IV admixtures for the hospital could be provided much more economically if compounded on a production basis from a centralized area; other economic considerations were also discussed. Avis et al (25) discussed the cost factor and its importance in the preparation of injectables. Miller et al (39) discussed in some detail the economics of the four major types of IV administration systems ("closed systems" with air vent plastic bag system, etc) and the economic feasibility of the various types of additive containers (vials, ampules, etc) with each system. They concluded that the total compounding cost (per annum) of a centralized parenteral admixture service with each of the IV systems was most dependent on the type of medication additions used within an institution. Therefore, one IV system may be the most economical in one institution, whereas it is more expensive in another. Ravin (44) listed the expenditures for several pieces of equipment and types of materials that are needed to maintain an IV admixture service.

Of particular importance to the reader is an article entitled "Recommended Methods for Compounding Intravenous Admixtures in Hospitals" (45). "The purpose of this paper is to recommend procedures, facilities, and equipment needed for the safe and effective compounding (i.e., preparation for administration) of large-volume parenterals with additives in hospital (45)." This article should be mandatory study for any pharmacist who is or will be compounding IV admixtures. The surveillance and reporting of problems and recommendations for solving problems (46) with large-volume parenterals should also receive careful study.

A review of the indications for use, their potential hazards, and a description of the types of fluids administered can be found in an article by Lawson and Henry (48).

RATIONALE

The primary responsibility of a hospital is to mobilize and organize professional skills to provide the patient with the best possible care and treatment. When that treatment is IV therapy, the skills required in compounding IV fluid-drug admixtures as well as the knowledge to monitor their proper therapeutic use are possessed only by the pharmacist (49). Although the compounding function associated with oral dosage forms has to a large extent been assumed by the pharmaceutical manufacturer, experience has shown that 60-75% of all IV prescriptions require compounding. Studies have indicated that 5-10% of IV fluid-drug admixtures prepared by nurses on the nursing units were incompatible (50). Other studies have shown that the contamination rate for IV fluids prepared in the relatively contaminated atmosphere of a nursing unit is much higher than those prepared in the controlled environment of a laminar flow hood (11,51,52). A third reason for the establishment of a pharmacy-based IV admixture system in larger hospitals is that the total personnel time required to prepare admixtures in a pharmacy is less than the time required to prepare the same number of fluids on the nursing units (14).

Numerous articles have argued in support of the provision of IV admixture programs that are coordinated by pharmacy.

The basic support for this contention is that the hospital pharmacist, with appropriate training, should be in the position to prepare sterile admixtures (26). Grabowski (54) commented that, because of the pharmacist's knowledge of compounding and identifying incompatibilities, he is appropriately trained to assume this responsibility. Francke (55) supported Grabowski's statement and emphasized that the pharmacist is trained in pharmaceutical calculation, and that calculations are one of the greatest sources of error. Bogash (56), in a general way, cited the shortcomings of nurse's training relative to pharmaceutical compounding such as IV admixtures.

The Joint Commission on the Accreditation of Hospitals has recognized the importance of properly prepared admixtures to patient care in its accreditation standards. In the interpretation of Standard III, the statement is made that "the director of pharmaceutical service should be responsible for the admixture of parenteral products, when feasible" (57).

DEVELOPMENT OF SPECIFICATIONS

The development of a system to provide safe and effective IV fluid-drug admixtures requires a multidisciplinary approach. Such a system should be considered as a total hospital system and should be developed with the combined expertise of all personnel involved with IV therapy. A committee should be established with the guidance of hospital administration to evaluate present procedures and make recommendations for the type of system to be established. This committee should represent several departments of the hospital, including pharmacy, medical staff, nursing, business office, purchasing, and any other department of the institution that is involved in the purchase, administration, or preparation of or reimbursement for IV therapy. In order to develop specifications, each department should look at the following factors as they relate to their particular department:

1. The size of the hospital, type of patients, and number of IV fluids and medications administered. A critical point for some institutions will be dependent on the number of admixtures to determine if 24-hour admixture service is necessary, or if procedures need to be developed to ensure quality in the event the admixture is prepared on the nursing unit. It may be possible in some situations to prepare admixtures in advance and refrigerate them on the nursing unit or even purchase many of the most recently available admixtures in premixed forms, such as theophylline, lidocaine, and fluids with premixed amounts of potassium chloride. The necessity of a multidepartmental approach will be noticeable when the determinations of cost effectiveness of such premixed products must be determined.

2. The present procedures for insertion of IV catheters and their maintenance should be examined and, when needed, recommendations for improvements should be made. For example, an IV team may be desirable in which specially trained nurses are responsible for IV catheter insertion, initiating the administration of the fluids, and maintenance of catheter insertion site. The staff nurses are then responsible for controlling flow rate; other problems are handled by the IV team (9).

3. Does the hospital have a physicians' order system in which the pharmacist receives a direct copy of the physician's order? Does this system get the order to the pharmacist in a timely manner, or can it be changed to do so? (This feature is essential for safe and efficient IV admixture systems; if pharmacy receives the order after considerable delay, time does not permit appropriate therapeutic interventions.)

4. The type of physical distribution system within the institution and the dependability of such system. A hospital with a dumbwaiter or conveyor has an easier task than those which must depend on messengers.

5. Charting of IV fluids and drugs should be considered. Many charting systems were devised when IV fluid numbers were a fraction of those in use today. This is an excellent time to review the chart and redesign and update if indicated. (At present, one of the areas that is a problem for many institutions is the charting of total parenteral nutrition solutions and the number of additives. Although many systems can accomplish the task, the majority of these systems still require a large amount of space in the chart.)

6. The method of charging for IV fluids and drugs should be examined. A system must be devised so the patient will be billed for IV fluids and medications that are administered. Experience within the institution is showing an increasing number of third-party audits to determine the accuracy of the current billing systems. Steps to allow the billing process to be easily traced can save considerable amounts of time in participating in these audits that tend to be labor intensive without further financial benefit.

7. The types of IV pumps, monitors, infusion sets, containers, and any other device related to IV therapy should be assessed. It is important to note that the expense and utilization of these ancillary products may equal or exceed the cost of the medications themselves, and all practitioners should keep this in mind when considering a "new unique device." Specifications and recommendations for purchase may have to be made (58-60).

DESIGN OF THE SYSTEM

When the committee has considered all factors and determined the basic specifications for the system, the pharmacist can then design a system to meet the requirements of the institution. Since there are many systems currently in operation, it may be possible to establish one patterned after another hospital. However, modifications should be made to satisfy the institution's unique requirements.

In designing a system, the pharmacist will have to consider typical order flow, existing IV admixture systems, stability and compatibility information, types of IV fluid containers, compounding procedures, and infusion pumps and flow rate monitoring devices. Each of these will be discussed separately.

TYPICAL ORDER FLOW

In order to develop an admixture service, it is important to understand the order flow within an institution from the physician's order to the point of administration of the fluid:

1. The initial step in IV therapy starts when a physician writes an order for a specific fluid, additive(s), and rate of

administration. The nurse or ward secretary transcribes this order into a kardex or similar medication chart. (If a secretary transcribes the order, a nurse or pharmacist must check the transcription.) It is essential for pharmacy to receive the original order or direct copy. A transcribed order offers opportunity for error and should be avoided if possible.

2. The order is transmitted to the pharmacy by courier, pneumatic tube, or telephone if a stat dose is needed.

3. Therapeutic, chemical, and physical compatibility of an admixture may be achieved through systematic monitoring of a patient profile and available information on compatibility. Sources of compatibility information include, but are not limited to, current literature, IV compatibility publications, package inserts, manufacturer's correspondence, and charts.

4. If the IV admixture has met the requirements of compatibility, a label is prepared and checked against the original order for accuracy. A desirable label should contain the following minimal information: patient's name, patient's location, base fluid, additives and amount of each, time and date of preparation and expiration, and initials of person preparing the admixture.

Some institutions also include the rate of administration in milliliters per hour and/or drops per minute. Additional information may be added in the case of special requirements or precautions. Specific recommendations for labeling have been given by the National Coordinating Committee on Large Volume Parenterals (60).

5. Preparation of the IV admixture is accomplished by the use of a laminar flow hood free from the hazard of airborne contaminants. Prefiltered air delivered under pressure passes in a uniform manner through the high efficiency particulate air (HEPA) filter that removes 99.97% of all particles as small as 0.3 μm including airborne bacteria (7,11). A training manual (61) may be required for admixture personnel or students who are endeavoring to learn appropriate techniques and procedures associated with IV fluids, admixtures, and sterile products (62).

6. After the admixture is prepared, the final product is visually inspected for particulate matter, precipitates, or haziness and is stored in the pharmacy or dispensed to the nursing unit for administration or storage.

7. Prior to administration the nurse makes a final check for correctness and makes another visual inspection. If everything is in order, the fluid may be administered.

EXISTING IV ADMIXTURE SYSTEMS

When a pharmacy implements an admixture service, a system must be developed to handle the distribution of the end products of the admixture. Depending on the desires of the institution and the delivery system available, some decisions will have to be made on the extent of service and the inherent benefits of each system. Institutions that presently have an admixture service will commonly floor stock any fluid that does not have an additive. However, some institutions will provide all IV solutions, piggyback, and/or syringes of intermittent medications. In order to give a starting point of options, two systems will be abstracted to provide basic information and ideas for the development of a system within a given institution.

One type of IV admixture service has been described in a publication by the Ohio State University Hospitals and is distributed by Travenol Laboratories (17). All IV fluids without additives are floor stocked; those requiring an additive are prepared in the pharmacy and are sent to the nursing station according to the time needed. When the first IV fluid with an additive has been infused, the pharmacy will automatically send the next fluid based on the flow rate and volume of the solution. Nursing responsibility involves notifying the pharmacy if a fluid is either ahead of or behind schedule. Orders are filed in the pharmacy according to the need time of the next IV fluid. A computer-assisted IV admixture program developed at Methodist Hospital by Thompson incorporates a nursing and pharmacy profile that is printed on the nursing unit and is accessible in pharmacy via CRT or in printed formal identical to the nursing profile. Several features include (1) admission, discharge, and transfer capability, (2) patient billing, (3) label production for continuous and intermittent infusions, (4) drug interaction detection, (5) incompatibility screening, (6) intermittent and continuous fluid scheduling, and (7) data sheets for production lists of bulk-manufactured intermittent medications and workload statistics. Some items that will be refined and developed for the future expansion of the system will include (1) drug utilization review data, (2) infection control statistics that can be compared with laboratory data for antibiotic utilization review, and (3) inventory control and purchasing information.

In the present system, patient prescriptions are entered into the computer and scheduled according to patient needs. Nursing communicates changes to the pharmacy and the pharmacist updates the nursing profile and sends appropriate fluids and medications according to physician's orders on file. Whenever a profile is updated, a new version is printed on the nursing unit. By this team effort and cross-check, the staff is able to monitor the accuracy of nursing in providing the prescribed therapy. It has been the experience in the authors' institution that a key to the success of the program has been the profile created by pharmacy, used by nursing, and updated cooperatively. A document that is identical in each department eliminates the need of separate documents that often do not agree.

The author would like to caution practitioners against purchasing a "ready to go" system unless the ability to adapt the system to meet institutional differences is adequately demonstrated by the vendor. Questions of response time, number of operators, ability to expand the data base, ease of changing price information, formats of labels, and profiles are some of the problems that may be encountered. A complete document of specifications for an institution should be developed and compared to a system before a rational decision on purchase can be made. In some instances, it may be more practical to develop a system in-house or through an independent contractor (63).

An additional aspect of any system that develops is the need to establish policies and procedures that will allow continuity of therapy and a systematic approach to specific situations. For certain situations or specific medications, it may be prudent to develop an in-house protocol for the policy and procedure to ensure consistency and reduce the possibility of error.

STABILITY AND COMPATIBILITY

Stability and compatibility problems often have a significant impact on admixture policies and procedures as well as the type of delivery system used within an institution.

Drug stability in IV solutions is affected by storage temperature, type of IV fluid, exposure to light, and a drug's rate of decomposition at a certain pH (64). When IV admixtures are prepared in a pharmacy-based admixture service, they must be prepared in advance of scheduled times in order to control workload, to accommodate pharmacy hours, to allow time for distribution, and for other reasons unique to an institution. In the event a drug is ordered that is not sufficiently stable to be prepared and delivered in advance, the components must be provided along with instructions for extemporaneous compounding (65).

Intravenous drug compatibility problems occur many times as a result of an institution's particular IV administration system and sets. For example, many drug combinations are incompatible if mixed in one large-volume parenteral and administered over an extended time period. However, the same drugs are compatible when administered in separate fluids or in the same fluid over a short period of time (i.e., piggyback). A complete understanding of IV sets, volume control devices, piggyback systems, and unique problems with specific drug-drug combinations is essential for a pharmacist to decide what type of administration system is safest and most effective for a particular drug-fluid combination (66). Piggyback administration sets have been evaluated in a study by Raisch et al (67).

When a pharmacist is developing compatibility profiles and administration procedures for individual drugs, he will find conflicting data, a shortage of the desired information, and in some cases extensive lists of incompatibilities without explanation. A pharmacist must analyze the available data and make judgments on the information he feels is from a reliable source.

TYPES OF FLUID CONTAINERS AND EFFECTS ON TECHNIQUES

Most institutions that are starting an admixture service already have one type of IV fluid container, either glass bottles or plastic bags. In the development stages of an admixture service, it is important to determine how well the present fluid containers will work with the proposed delivery system. Special considerations should be given to space requirements on the nursing unit and in the pharmacy. If an institution is going to be involved in a total parenteral nutrition program, this should be integrated into the system. See Chapter 36 for a discussion of total parenteral nutrition.

Currently three systems are available for the preparation of antibiotics and other drugs that are administered intermittently. These will be referred to as "piggyback" systems.

Small-volume bags and partial-fill IV bottles can be used in the preparation of piggybacks by adding the reconstituted drug to the solution in the same manner used for large-volume parenterals. The advantage of this method is dosage flexibility and the ability to choose the desired type and quantity of fluid for each dose. A disadvantage is time needed for preparation.

A second method utilizes bottles that are prefilled with predetermined dosages of antibiotics that require only reconstitution in the bottle that subsequently serves as the piggyback bottle, thereby eliminating several steps in preparation. The disadvantage of this type of product is the loss of dosage flexibility unless additional antibiotic is added and the need for a separate system for those antibiotics not available in this type of container.

Another method available is the use of an in-line graduated cylinder to which medications can be added directly to a small volume of the patient's present IV fluid. The only advantage of this type of system is its ability to help minimize the amount of fluid. The disadvantages of this system range from addition of a drug to a potentially incompatible fluid to all the problems associated with airborne contamination.

An alternative to the piggyback/calibrated drip chamber administration is the mini-infusor system. A small battery-operated pump that holds a syringe containing the medication is used to deliver the dose through microbore tubing over a specified time. This system may have some advantages over the piggyback systems when IV fluids, minibag cost, and fluid restriction are being considered; however, it will be important to see how this system will fit into the total admixture program. An intermittent system that is under investigation uses a mini-infusor pump and manufacturer's vial to hold the medication prior to administration. In an unpublished work, the author points out the advantages of decreasing the cost of therapy by innovative methods such as hanging the entire dose for one day and keeping the number of devices used in preparation and administration to an absolute minimum. At this time, the state of art in the pharmaceutical industry is not geared to packaging that would allow this system to be feasible.

COMPOUNDING CONSIDERATIONS

In a hospital where the number of doses of antibiotics is low, all doses can be extemporaneously prepared. However, when the volume is great enough, it is practical to reconstitute a larger number of doses based on anticipated usage in relationship to the stability of the reconstituted antibiotic. Significant time and cost savings are possible when this method is utilized.

If an institution decides to implement a program for "bulk reconstitution" of antibiotics, it will be useful to develop the system in conjunction with the medical staff and have the pharmacy decide on the appropriate diluent for all antibiotics, leaving the option for change up to the physician in necessary situations. If pharmacy determines the standards, it will be easier to achieve larger numbers of the same diluent and dose. An additional advantage of having standard concentrations, is the ability to reuse antibiotics that were not administered, provided that they have been handled properly and have not exceeded the expiration date.

A related but different concept of mass production is seen with the availability of multidose admixture vials that contain several doses of commonly used additives such as aminophyllin, potassium chloride, and calcium gluconate. These products were developed as a response to several institutions' high use of these additives, and in some instances, these institutions were making their own solutions. As with all other systems and products, the pharmacist should be aware of the product and decide how and if it would be feasible and desirable for the institution.

An extremely important consideration in compounding is the use of aseptic technique. The contamination of IV fluids is well documented in the literature (68-71). Cortopassi and Kikugawa (72) evaluated antiseptics that may be used in preparing IV admixtures. In addition to American Society of Hospital Pharmacists' institutes on IV admixture services, a training manual is available that can assist in providing the fundamentals (61).

CHEMOTHERAPY COMPOUNDING CONSIDERATIONS

Pharmacy-based cancer chemotherapy preparation is becoming common in all institutions and will probably continue to grow in the forthcoming years. Chemotherapeutic agents represent a unique problem for institutions because of their toxicity and special considerations for handling and disposal. All institutions are encouraged to develop a system that will prevent the problems cited in the literature—a patient receiving a duplicate or wrong dose and other iatrogenic problems. Because of the dynamics of chemotherapy, it is important to read the current literature to ensure that the policy a hospital is using is appropriate to the state of the art in chemotherapy handling and administration.

The considerations in compounding chemotherapeutic agents adds a new dimension to IV admixture systems because, in addition to sterility of preparation, there is the added necessity of environmental protection and operator protection (73-76).(For a further discussion of chemotherapy, see Chapter 51.) Before any admixture system starts making chemotherapeutic agents, it will be necessary to investigate setup costs of equipment, space, and additional staffing if necessary. It has been the authors' experience that staffing data cannot be extrapolated from routine admixture services because the amount of time that is necessary for preparation of chemotherapeutic agents and the records that are normally inherent to these programs are extremely time consuming.

INFUSION PUMPS AND FLOW RATE MONITORING DEVICES

An integral part of any admixture program is the method by which fluids are administered to a patient. An accurate IV infusion rate may be difficult to maintain without the use of some type of monitoring device. Many hospitals without admixture services already use some type of monitor within certain areas of the hospital. Advances in infusion control systems are occurring continually; therefore, periodic reevaluation of an institution's infusion control procedures is warranted. A report on IV infusion pumps by Turco (77) is important reading for the uninformed or the person who desires to compare various types of pumps.

Most of the problems associated with the accuracy of IV infusion rates are caused by physical phenomena. Such physical phenomena include the viscosity, specific gravity, and surface tension of the fluid; the elasticity of the IV

tubing; the patient's venous pressure; and pressure within the fluid container itself. The manual clamp is not an accurate method of setting the flow rate, but its performance has been considered acceptable by the majority of practitioners. With respect to a manual clamp, it was found in one study that 17 corrections were necessary in order to maintain an acceptable accuracy within an 8-hour period (59). This time factor may be important in considering the cost of the proposed monitor or pump.

Some of the factors to consider in the purchase of infusion rate controllers are (1) cost of the unit, (2) cost of the tubing that must be used with the unit, (3) cost-benefit ratio for patient care, (4) maintenance requirements, and (5) ease of operation.

CONCLUSION

The addition of medications to parenteral solutions involves many important aspects such as stability, sterility, incompatibility, solubility, and proper labeling. It has been demonstrated that pharmacy-based admixture systems are cost effective and beneficial to patient care (50). However, the development of an admixture service is a delicate process that must be evaluated on a continual basis to meet changing needs and to improve present methods. Because institutions differ greatly in physical layouts, staffing requirements, and patient population, careful analysis of the present system is an important task in the development of a system. A review of the literature with an institution's needs in mind will yield much on systems that are presently in operation. Hospitals that have admixture services are excellent sources of information to help solve problems with a given system and provide ideas on what does not work for them as well as what does. Manufacturers of parenteral products may be of assistance in deciding what type of products and system will work in a particular institution. However, the most important factor in admixture service is instituting a system that provides the best IV therapy for the patient.

REFERENCES

1. Miller RR: Drug surveillance utilizing epidemiologic methods: A report from the Boston Collaborative Drug Surveillance Program. *Am J Hosp Pharm* 30:584-592, 1973.
2. Schawartau N, Sturdavant M: A system of packaging and dispensing drugs in single doses. *Am J Hosp Pharm* 18:542, 1961.
3. Ravin RI, Holyske M: A pharmacy centralized intravenous additive service. *Am J Hosp Pharm* 12:267, 1965.
4. Barker KM, Heller WM: The development of a centralized unit-dose dispensing system. *Am J Hosp Pharm* 20:568, 1963.
5. Allison E: An IV additive service in the pharmacy. *Hosp Pharm* 1:30, 1966.
6. Brown RG: IV additive program belongs in the pharmacy. *Hospitals* 43:92, 1969.
7. Paoloni CU: Procedures for handling intravenous additives: The nursing team approach. *Hosp Mgt* 108:12, 1969.
8. Pang FI: Transition to centralized IV additive service in a private hospital. *Hosp Pharm* 5:18, 1970.
9. Pulliam CC: Upton JH: Pharmacy coordinated intravenous admixture and administration service. *Am J Hosp Pharm* 28:92, 1971.
10. Sauve F: Pharmacist and a nutritional intravenous therapy program. *Am J Hosp Pharm* 28:106, 1971.
11. Durgin JM: Developing policies and procedures for an IV additive service. *Hosp Top* 48:47, 1970.

12. Francke GN, St. Clair H: IV additive services at Cincinnati Veterans Administration Hospital. *Drug Intell Clin Pharm* 5:377, 1971.
13. Schwartau NW, Schwerman EA Jr, Thompson CO, Hauff K: Comprehensive intravenous admixture system. *Am J Hosp Pharm* 30:607, 1973.
14. McLemore RA: IV additive service. *Hospitals* 45:96, 1971.
15. Bogash RC: Parenteral additive programs. *Hosp Formul Mgt* 2:98, 1967.
16. Ragland JG, Kroll KR: Pharmacists and nurses benefit from an IV additive program. *Hospitals* 42:136, 1968.
17. Godwin HN, Latiolais CJ: Developing a parenteral admixture service in a teaching hospital. Distributed by Travenol Laboratories.
18. Special Features. *Am J Hosp Pharm* 40:1920-1944, 1983.
19. Fink JL: Pharmcists as a liability reducing factor. *Am J Hosp Pharm* 39:1544-1546, 1982.
20. Proctor PA: Legal liability of a hospital for its pharmacy. *Hosp Mater Mgt Q* 4:60-63, August 1982.
21. Wuest JR: Initiating an IV additive service, 3. Development of policies and procedures. *Drug Intell Clin Pharm* 4:183-189, 1970.
22. Wuest JR: Initiating an IV additive service. 4. Development of policies and procedures. *Drug Intell Clin Pharm* 4:213-216, 1970.
23. Wuest JR: Initiating an IV additive service, 5. Development of policies and procedures. *Drug Intell Clin Pharm* 4:279-282, 1970.
24. Pulliam CC, Upton JH: A pharmacy coordinated intravenous admixture and administration service. *Am J Hosp Pharm* 28:92-101, 1971.
25. Avis KE, Carlin HS, Flack HL: Preparation of injectables—philosophy and master procedures. *Am J Hosp Pharm* 18:223-233, 1961.
26. Shoup LK: Instructions in preparing intravenous admixtures. *Am J Pharm Ed* 32:311-315, 1968.
27. Ravin RL, Gilbert JR, Comiskey JA: Two-year appraisal of a centralized IV additive service. *Hospitals* 41:88, 1967.
28. ASHP outcome competencies for institutional pharmacy technician training programs (with training guidelines). *Am J Hosp Pharm* 39:317-320, 1982.
29. Smith TP, Adams RC, Brewer CD: Supportive personnel training program based at a technical college. *Am J Hosp Pharm* 39:443-446, 1982.
30. Meisler JM, Skolaut MW: Extemporaneous sterile compounding of intravenous additives. *Am J Hosp Pharm* 23:557-563, 1966.
31. Hunt ML Jr, Tuck BA, Adams C: System to measure the use of Pharmacy Personnel. *Am J Hosp Pharm* 39:82-85, 1982.
32. Sebastian G, Thielke TS: Work analysis of an admixutre service. *Am J Hosp Pharm* 40:2149-2153, 1983.
33. Ravin RL: Steps in a parenteral admixture program. *Drug Intell Clin Pharm* 4:41-43, 1970.
34. Loeb AJ, Fishman DA, Kochis TR: Premixed intravenous admixtures: A critical challenge for hospital pharmacy. *Am J Hosp Pharm* :1041, 1983.
35. Lee HE: Premixed admixtures: A positive development for hospital pharmacy. *Am J Hosp Pharm* 40:1043-1044, 1983.
36. Ravin RL: Steps in starting an IV additive program. I. The reasons to begin. *Drug Intell Clin Pharm* 4:13-14, 1970.
37. Patterson FT: Dispensing for HDA nonapproved uses. *J Am Pharm Assoc* NS8:422, 1968.
38. Skolaut MW: Long-term benefits of a centralized IV additive service. *Am J Hosp Pharm* 25:536-537, 1968.
39. Miller WA, Smith GL, Latiolais CJ: Compounding costs and contamination rates of intravenous admixtures. *Drug Intell Clin Pharm* 5:51-60, 1971.
40. Wuest JR: Initiating an IV additive service, 4. Development of policies and procedures. *Drug Intell Clin Pharm* 4:213-216, 1970.
41. Wuest JR: Initiating an IV additive service, 5. Development of policies and procedures. *Drug Intell Clin Pharm* 4:279-282, 1970.
42. Paoloni CJ: Guidelines for administration of intravenous additives by nurses on the intravenous therapy team. *Hosp Mgt* 108:46, 1969.
43. Paoloni CJ: Procedures for handling intravenous additives. The nursing team approach. *Hosp Mgt* 108:12-22, 1969.
44. Ravin RL: Steps in starting an IV, additive program: Equipment and facilities required. *Drug Intell Clin Pharm* 4:97-99, 1970.
45. National Coordinating Committee on Large Volume Parenterals: Recommended methods for compounding intravenous admixtures in hospitals. *Am J Hosp Pharm* 32:261-270, 1975.
46. National Coordinating Committee on Large Volume Parenterals: Rec-
47. National Coordinating Committee on Large Volume Parenterals: Recommendations to pharmacists for solving problems with large-volume parenterals. *Am J Hosp Pharm* 33:231-236, 1976.
48. Lawson DH, Henry DA: Drug therapy reviews: Intravenous fluid therapy. *Am J Hosp Pharm* 34:1332-1338, 1977.
49. Heller WM: Should the pharmacist assume additional responsibilities for Medication preparation. *Am J Hosp Pharm* 18:521, 1961.
50. Thur MP, Miller WA, Latiolais CJ: Medication errors in a nurse-controlled parenteral admixture program. *Am J Hosp Pharm* 14:22, 1971.
51. Lamy PP, Kitler ME: Laminar flow: A method for contamination control. *J Mod Pharm* 14:22, 1971.
52. Morgan E, Fincher JH, Sadik F, Mikeal RL: Evaluation of laminar air flow and nursing station environments for the preparation of intravenous admixtures. *Am J Hosp Pharm* 29:1020, 1972.
53. Cooper CR: IV additive program: Survey of past experience. *Hospitals* 47:74, 1973.
54. Grabowski ZR: Intravenous additive services in hospital pharmacies. *Hosp Pharm* 2:14-18, 1967.
55. Francke DE: Preparation of parenteral admixtures—nursing or pharmacy functions? *Am J Hosp Pharm* 22:179, 1965.
56. Bogash RG: Parenteral additive programs. *Hosp Formul Mgt* 2:98, 1967.
57. Joint Commission on Accreditation of Hospitals. *Accreditation manual for hospitals*. Chicago, 1976, JCAH.
58. Coggin S: Device regulates the flow of IV solutions for critical patients. *Mod Hosp* 121:92, 1973.
59. Apelgren SA, Schwerman EA Jr: Maintaining a constant parenteral infusion rate. (Unpublished paper.)
60. National Coordinating Committee on Large Volume Parenterals: Recommendations for the labeling of large volume parenterals. *Am J Hosp Pharm* 35:49-51, 1978.
61. Hunt ML Jr, Latiolais CJ: *Training Manual for Central Intravenous Admixture Personnel*. Deerfield, IL, Travenol, 1972.
62. Turco S, King RE: *Sterile Dosage Forms*. Philadelphia, Lea & Febiger, 1974.
63. Nold EG: Computerization needs assessment. *Am J Hosp Pharm* 39:302-306, 1982.
64. Barrett CW: Drug stability and safety. *Pharm J* 206:267, 1971.
65. Jacobs J: Drug stability and compatibility in injections and intravenous infusion. *Pharm J* 205:437, 1970.
66. Grayson JG: Incompatibilities of multiple additives to intravenous infusion solutions. *Pharm J* 206:64, 1971.
67. Raisch DW, Johnson KT, Roth C: Evaluation of piggyback administration sets. *Am J Hosp Pharm* 34:1315-1323, 1977.
68. Arnold TR, Hepler CD: Bacterial contamination of intravenous fluids opened in unsterile air. *Am J Hosp Pharm* 28:614-619, 1971.
69. Deeb EM, Natsios GA: Contamination of intravenous fluids and bacterial and fungi during preparation and admininstration. *Am J Hosp Pharm* 28:764-767, 1971.
70. Hansen JD, Hepler CD: Contamination if intravenous solutions by airborne microbes. *Am J Hosp Pharm* 30:326-331, 1973.
71. Letcher KI, Thrupp LD, Schapiro DJ, et al: In-use contamination of intravenous solutions in flexible plastic containers. *Am J Hosp Pharm* 29:673-677, 1972.
72. Cortopassi RF, Kikugawa CA: Evaluation of antiseptics in the preparation of intravenous admixtures. *Am J Hosp Pharm* 34:1193-1196, 1977.
73. Auis KE, Leuchuk JW: Special considerations in the use of vertical laminar-flow workbenches. *Am J Hosp Pharm* 41:81-87, 1984.
74. LeRoy ML, Roberts MJ, Theisen JA: Procedures for handling of antineoplastic injections in comprehensive cancer centers. *Am J Hosp Pharm* 40:601-603, 1983.
75. Anderson RW, Puckett WH, Dana WJ, Nguyen TV, Theiss JC: Risk of handling injectable antineoplastic agents. *Am J Hosp Pharm* 39:1881-1887, 1982.
76. Hamilton CW: Risk to personnel admixing cancer chemotherapy. *US Pharm* 7:H1-H2, H4, H6-H8, 1982.
77. Turco SJ: Pressure for precision, a progress report on IV infusion pumps. *Am J Intraven Ther* 4:13, 16-21, 46, 48, 1977.

CHAPTER 35

Incompatibilities of Parenteral Admixtures

JAMES C. KING

The importance of parenteral dosage forms as pharmaceutical products is underscored by data indicating that, in 1964, the total U.S. expenditure for large-volume parenterals (LVPs) was $49 million. Fifteen years later, in 1979, this figure had risen to $400 million. With the increased use of parenteral nutrition products, it is expected that over $3 million will be spent on those products alone in 1985. Currently, about two thirds of our hospitals have at least a partial IV additive service to handle the nearly 300 million LVPs that are administered each year (1). Because at least half of those will contain at least one additive, it is important that those who prescribe, prepare, and administer LVPs know their compatibility and stability characteristics. It is too costly to prepare mixtures that cannot be administered because of the manifestations of incompatibility or which lose their potency before administration can be accomplished. The hazards of injecting carelessly prepared therapeutic agents speak for themselves. The standard of the Joint Commission on Accreditation of Hospitals noted that the hospital pharmacy should be responsible for the admixture of parenteral drugs when feasible. The National Coordinating Committee on Large Volume Parenterals has set forth recommended methods for compounding IV admixtures in hospitals.

A number of advantages are gained by the pharmacy's performing the compounding of extemporaneous parenteral mixtures. Pharmacists are the best trained in calculating doses, concentrations, and rates for administration, thereby helping to ensure that the patient receives the proper amounts of drug per unit of time. As the health care professional with the greatest background in chemistry, the pharmacist is the most qualified to predict chemical reactions that might occur with admixtures. Therefore, the number of incompatible combinations prepared should be greatly reduced. Also, because the atmosphere in the pharmacy is generally bacteriologically cleaner than in other sections of the hospital, where infected patients contribute to air contamination, preparation of the admixtures in the pharmacy is usually associated with a reduced incidence of solution contamination. The installation of laminar airflow hoods and facilities for inspecting finished solutions for particulate matter contamination contribute to the production of cleaner products.

Although this chapter will address itself primarily to the problems of incompatibilities in IV infusion admixtures, much of the information can be extrapolated to other parenteral mixtures such as those administered by IM injection. The principal differences are that those mixtures prepared for IM injection or for IV push usually contain higher concentrations of the therapeutic agents and are generally in contact with each other in the administration device for a shorter period of time. Because of the greater concentration, the potential for incompatibility is increased, but because of the shorter duration of contact, the potential for incompatibility may be simultaneously decreased.

It has been recognized that many hospitals today have pharmacy-operated centralized IV additive services, but many institutions may still place this responsibility on the nursing staff. In any case, if the pharmacy does not operate on a 24-hour basis, the nursing staff will still have some responsibility for determining the compatibility of admixtures. Additionally, because of turnaround time, even hospitals that have full-service IV additive activities may not prepare mixtures for the intensive care unit, where changes in orders occur very rapidly. It is therefore important to develop effective in-service education programs to assist the nursing staff in the absence of the pharmacist.

As will be pointed out later in this discussion, one of the techniques for avoiding compatibility problems is simply to avoid mixing drugs. This solution, however, is not always acceptable. If a patient has one IV drug running and requires a second drug, it is certainly less traumatic to him if a second venipuncture can be avoided. Also, if multiple IV solutions are being used simply for the purpose of avoiding admixtures, the volume of fluids that may be tolerated by the patient could be exceeded. Therefore, basically, the reasons for mixing multiple therapeutic agents relate to comfort of the patient and the avoidance of other problems. The responsibilities of those who prepare parenterals include the furnishing of a dosage form that is sterile, efficacious, and free of extraneous material. This means that the drugs added to it must be added by aseptic technique, that they must be compatible with each other, that potency has not been lost by mishandling, and that the drugs are administered in the proper dose and at the proper rate.

NATURE OF INCOMPATIBILITIES

For convenience, incompatibilities of parenteral admixtures are frequently referred to as physical incompatibilities and chemical incompatibilities. While in a strict sense all incompatibilities are really chemical incompatibilities has become useful in discussing the types of changes that might occur. Within the context of the present discussion, physical incompatibilities refer to those changes that are manifested by a change in color, precipitation, or evolution of a gas. On the other hand, chemical incompatibilities will be those in which there is no visible evidence of change but perhaps a loss in potency, or other evidence that there has been an alteration in the molecular structure of the drugs. Newton has reviewed the kinds of physical and chemical reactions that might occur. Therapeutic incompatibilities are outside the scope of this chapter and the reader is referred to Chapter 28 for that discussion.

After evaluating a mixture for its physical or chemical compatibilities, the true test would be the evaluation of therapeutic efficacy. To do this is tantamount to performing clinical studies on all of the combinations that might be prescribed; this is not feasible. The number of permutations of combinations of parenteral drugs is endless, considering dosage and concentration, temperature, interactions with administration devices, differences in formulations and other factors that come into play. Therefore, in the practical clinical situation, one must assemble what is known about a drug and what is known about similar therapeutic agents and extrapolate these data into the formation of the final decision.

CONTRIBUTING FACTORS

In addition to the therapeutic agent itself, there are a host of other factors that intermingle in the establishment of the final compatibility profile. In some instances incompatibility may be the fault of an adjuvant used by the manufacturer in stabilizing his brand of a particular drug. These adjuvants include the preservatives, stabilizers, or perhaps solubilizers that are a part of the marketed formulation. The pH of the basic infusion fluid, as well as the agents added to it, also have a very marked effect on the final compatibility. The official compendia permit rather wide ranges of pH in the standard infusion fluids; however, it may be useful to remember that fluids such as 5% dextrose in water, although having an acid pH, are really not very acidic. They have essentially no buffer capacity, and therefore, the addition of another therapeutic agent will have a marked effect on the resulting pH. It is the effect of the pH conferred by the first additive that will have the greatest effect on the compatibility of a second additive from the standpoint of the pH. The infusion fluid contributes to the final compatibility in other ways. For example, they may contain certain ions such as calcium, which would be incompatible with specific other additives. The bisulfite stabilizer in some basic total parenteral nutrition (TPN) mixtures can decompose certain of the vitamins that are frequently added to those mixtures (3).

The concentration of the additives is also very important in establishing whether a mixture should be rated as being compatible. In the majority of cases, if the concentrations of additives are increased, the likelihood of incompatibility is increased. There are, however, exceptions to this rule. For example, thiopental sodium has been noted to be incompatible in Normosol R at a concentration of 1 g/liter, although at a concentration of 2 g/liter, the mixture appears acceptable (4). The matter of concentration also comes into a discussion of the physical design of the containers in this chapter.

It is obvious that the time of contact is important in the loss of potency of certain groups of drugs. When preparing IV infusions, one must keep in mind that some time may elapse before the infusion is begun and that perhaps 8 hours will be required for the administration to be completed once it has begun. Therefore, it is not unusual for 12 hours or more to elapse between the time the mixture is made and the time when the final portions have gone into the patient. If a drug loses potency rapidly, it is easy to see that the final portions of the solution may have diminished therapeutic effect. For this reason, and perhaps even more for the possibility of accidental contamination, good pharmaceutical practice dictates that extemporaneous parenteral mixtures be administered within 24 hours of their preparation. This practice is not intended to apply to mixtures that are mass produced for freezing to be thawed for administration at some future date.

The temperature at which mixtures are maintained may also affect potency by the time of administration. As a group, antibiotics can be expected to deteriorate unless underrefrigerated; some antibiotics, however, are reasonably stable at room temperature. In no case should IV mixtures be subjected to elevated temperatures. Carts holding the products after admixture should not be left near windows where direct sunlight falls on the containers, nor should solutions be hung where direct sunlight through the window of the patient's room can fall on them.

The order of mixing will occasionally have some effect on compatibility, especially with respect to the concentrations that will be tolerated. This is sometimes of importance in the preparation of TPN mixtures to which calcium salts must be added. If the calcium is added last, the solution will tolerate higher concentrations of the calcium salt than when it is put into the mixture as the first additive. In order to avoid incompatibilities due to high concentrations, the mixtures should be agitated after the addition of each drug (5).

Finally, the materials from which containers are fabricated may be a source of incompatibility. This consideration often extends to administration sets and devices such as syringes and infusion pumps. This area of concern will be expanded upon in the pages that follow.

SOLVING THE PROBLEMS

Testing all variations of the many contributory factors presents an impossible task. There is no practical way by which all of the drugs from each of the various manufacturers can be tested in all concentrations, in all infusion fluids, under all of the various environmental conditions.

Therefore, the pharmacist is obliged to work with those situations that are most commonly encountered with respect to concentration, infusion fluid, etc. A number of incompatibility charts have been published by various manufacturers from time to time. These are helpful but certainly do not cover all of the possibilities. In recent years, two major compilations of incompatibility data have been assembled (6,7). These attempt to pull together all of the information available from the various manufacturers, the professional literature, and other sources so that the information is available in a single volume. These compilations are most useful if one remembers that they are intended to be used as guides and that the data should not be construed as absolute. Some of the reasons why these should not be viewed as hard and fast data is that many of the sources used in preparing them did not furnish a great deal of data on the methodology by which the determinations were made. Also the variabilities of concentration and the other contributing factors noted above cannot be covered in any single work.

When using compatibility charts, compilations, or journal literature, one must bear in mind that the absence of precipitation or color changes does not constitute full compatibility. Other parameters by which compatibility may be measured include microbiologic assay, spectrophototometric studies, iodometric techniques, chromotography, and various methods of measuring particulate matter. The apparent compatibility substantiated by any of these methods, again, does not guarantee full compatibility. Clearance of an admixture by any of these techniques simply eliminates another reason why that mixture should not be prepared. Assuming an admixture has not been judged incompatible by any of the methods used, and hopefully there will be several, about all one can say with certainty is that there appears to be no reason why the combination in question should not be prepared.

There are some "rules of thumb" that may be useful in estimating whether a given mixture should be prepared. Probably the most common cause for an incompatibility is a simple acid-base reaction. Therefore, if one is asked to prepare a mixture containing a drug that is the sodium salt of a weak acid and the hydrochloride salt of a weak base, he should be alert to the possibility of an interaction leading perhaps to precipitation. One should also be cautious of those mixtures in which di- or trivalent ions are involved. Calcium salts are especially likely to be bothersome. Many of the so-called balanced solutions contain some levels of calcium and/or magnesium ion. It is easy to forget the precise content of these balanced solutions and to overlook that possibility. Finally, the relative instability of certain drugs can be predicted by the form in which they are marketed. That is, if a drug is marketed as a lyophilized powder as contrasted to an aqueous solution, that particular drug is probably somewhat unstable after reconstitution and mixing within an infusion fluid.

It is fortunate that potassium chloride is the most common additive in IV solutions. It is a neutral salt comprised of monovalent ions and as such is not likely to produce compatibility problems. Therefore, if a drug is compatible with sodium chloride or in normal saline solution, it will very likely be compatible with potassium chloride.

ADDITIONAL CONSIDERATIONS

In recent years, it has become common practice to use final filters on many of the IV solutions administered to hospital patients. This practice is intended to reduce vascular irritation by eliminating, insofar as possible, particulate matter from entering the veins. Final filters are never to be used as a substitute for sterile technique; nor should final filters be used as a method for overcoming an incompatibility. To place a final filter on an administration set to filter out a precipitate that has formed is sheer folly. Certain drugs, e.g., amphotericin B, may be removed by the filter. Also, the reader is reminded that emulsions cannot be administered through membrane filters.

Hospital pharmacists had just begun to collect data on the compatibility of IV admixtures in the traditional glass container when plastic containers for IV fluids made their appearance on the market. The data that were generated for the systems in the glass container may not always be applicable to those in the plastic container. Certain drugs such as insulin may be adsorbed by both glass and plastic, reducing the quantity that is received by the patient substantially. Other drugs also have a propensity for being adsorbed by plastic containers and sets; the degree varies with the individual drug and plastic polymer. In one study, 67% of the vitamin A put into a polyvinyl chloride (PVC) container was sorbed by the plastic. Lesser amounts of warfarin and methohexital sodium were also sorbed (8).

The variability of sorption characteristics is nicely illustrated by observations of diazepam in a variety of conditions. There can be significant loss of diazepam potency when dilutions of it are stored in PVC containers but not when stored in glass bottles (9). However, even if glass bottles are used for the solutions, there can be sorption of the drug by the PVC tubing of the administration set (10) or some plastic burette chambers (e.g., Soluset or Buretrol) (11). Polyolefin semirigid containers (Accumed) seem to be acceptable alternatives to glass containers (12). Finally, some quantities of diazepam are sorbed by plastic infusion sets made of cellulose propionate and PVC tubing; substantial quantities were sorbed by a simulated infusion pump system made of glass syringe and Silastic tubing. The sorption was not significant when polyethylene tubing was used (13). As new types of plastic containers and administration sets are developed by the manufacturers, the compatibility characteristics of those polymers with the more than 200 parenteral drugs that might be added will have to be determined anew.

In preparing mixtures for parenteral administration, the pharmacist must be conscious of which route of administration is appropriate for each particular agent. There are some that may be administered only intravenously, some only intramuscularly, and others that may be administered by either route. This makes it possible in some cases to avoid an incompatibility. Should two drugs be contraindicated in the same solution but be required by the patient, one may prepare one of them for administration by the IV route and suggest that the other be given by IM injection. This presumes that therapeutic incompatibility does not exist.

In recent years, it has become practice in some of the

large hospitals that handle many units of IV mixtures daily to prepare large numbers of common combinations and to freeze them for thawing just prior to administration. When doing this, the IV additive service must determine the advisability of freezing a particular agent lest it lose its potency. For example, ampicillin sodium has been shown to decompose faster when frozen than when kept under ordinary refrigeration. A principal hazard in the preparation of large numbers of units for freezing is that if an error is made, a large number of units will be lost, or there may be a large number of therapeutic misadventures before the error is discovered. Also, should there be a change in protocols in the institution, a great financial loss could be incurred by having a large stock of mixtures that are no longer in use. A concern that is related to the practice of freezing admixtures is the use of microwave ovens for thawing them quickly. It seems that the greatest concern, presently, is whether the microwaves will decompose the active drugs or whether they may have some adverse effect on the containers (especially plastics) that will then affect the quality of the parenteral mixture. To date, there have not been any major reports that microwave ovens deteriorate any particular drugs or affect plastic containers of parenterals adversely. The only major problem area seems to be the uniformity of thawing, i.e., "cold" and "hot" spots in the oven that could produce spots of decomposition.

EXAMPLES OF COMPATIBILITY PROBLEMS

Although it is impossible to present complete data on any drug in this discussion, some comments on certain of the most commonly used agents may be helpful.

The optimal pH range for the stability of aminophylline is above pH 8.0. Crystals of theophylline will deposit below pH 8.0 but probably not unless the concentration is over 40 mg/mg. Therefore, this incompatibility is more apt to occur if admixtures of aminophylline are made in syringes or small volumes of fluids than if components are added separately to large-volume IV fluids. The high pH of aminophylline may create stability problems with a number of antibiotics and other alkaline-labile compounds.

Ampicillin sodium is a rather unstable antibiotic. It appears to be most stable if mixed with normal saline solution or certain electrolyte solutions such as Isolyte M or Isolyte P. In dextrose-containing fluids or Ringer's lactated injection, its potency drops rapidly. It is good practice to prepare solutions of ampicillin just before use and to avoid using fluids containing dextrose. If short-term storage is unavoidable, refrigeration will prolong potency; however, freezing is to be avoided.

No guaranteed successful method for preparing infusions of phenytoin (Dilantin) has been developed. All investigators report immediate precipitation if one attempts to dilute the drug with dextrose and the various Ringer's mixtures. Phenytoin is insoluble in aqueous infusion fluids and should be diluted only by the diluent provided by the manufacturer. One report suggests that when direct IV injection is not practical, a dilution with not more than 50 ml saline solution may be stable enough to be infused in not more than than 1 hour (14). However, it does seem that small microcrystals

of Dilantin may be found if the solutions made with saline solutions are examined microscopically.

Rather recently, it has been reported that two European phenytoin products are less likely to produce crystallization than Dilantin. If those formulations (phenhydan and phenytoin concentrate) become available in the United States, there may be less problem in preparing infusions of phenytoin (15). Until then, slow IV push is the only approved way to administer Dilantin injection and its addition to IV infusions is not recommended because of lack of solubility and resultant precipitation.

In addition to its lack of solubility, one should remember that Dilantin is alkaline.

Like phenytoin, diazepam is a poorly soluble drug in water, and if it is mixed with only a small volume of aqueous solution, precipitation is usually seen immediately. However, if additional amounts of aqueous solutions are added, the precipitate will dissolve. Originally, the manufacturer warned against the dilution of diazepam with other solutions or drugs. The product information now states that if it is not feasible to administer diazepam directly intravenously, it may be injected slowly through the infusion tubing as close as possible to the vein insertion. Literature reports indicate that dilutions of 1:50 or 1:100 of the drug in 5% dextrose injection, normal saline solution, Ringer's solution or Ringer's lactated injection are soluble and stable for up to 24 hours (16-17).

Metaraminol bitartrate (Aramine) is an example of an acidic drug. Its acidity may be deleterious to acid-labile additives such as certain antibiotics and hydrocortisone sodium succinate. Hydrocortisone sodium succinate may hydrolyze to a significant extent when combined with acidic agents. Extensive experiments on combinations of metaraminol bitartrate with hydrocortisone sodium succinate or methylprednisolone sodium succinate in normal saline solution or D5W solution have given such inconsistent results that it is recommended that such combinations not be mixed. Cimetidine hydrochloride injection is also acidic and can be expected to produce precipitates when mixed with many of the cephalosporin antibiotics, penicillin, aminophylline, barbiturates, and other alkaline medications.

As a final example, because of its importance and widespread use, nitroglycerin injection should be included. Large quantities of nitroglycerin in 5% dextrose injection or in normal saline solution were lost when the solutions were stored in PVC containers (18-20). One of those studies also reports that when Silastic tubing was used in bulk processing of nitroglycerin solutions, as much as 15% of the nitroglycerin activity was adsorbed onto the tubing. Still another report indicates that, in polyolefin or glass containers, solutions of 50 μg/ml nitroglycerin in D5W and in normal saline solution retained satisfactory potency at 4°, 25°, and 40° C for 48 hours, whereas large and rapid losses of potency were observed in PVC containers under the same test conditions (21). An additional study reported no change in the concentration of nitroglycerin in glass or polypropylene syringes for 5 hours. However, solutions in cellulose propionate (Buretrol) lost approximately 40% potency in 2 hours; PVC tubing increased the adsorptive effect to about 70%. An immediate loss of 80% was observed when solutions were placed in Viaflex bags. The uptake of nitroglycerin by PVC tubing and catheters (e.g., Swan-Ganz) ranged from 65-75% in less than 1 hour (22). In summary, cellulose propionate, PVC, and siliconized rubber have an adsorptive capacity for nitroglycerin; glass, polypropylene, and polyethylene do not appear to sorb nitroglycerin significantly. As compared with the erratic sorption by conventional sets, the Tridilset appears to lack sorptive capacity for nitroglycerin (23).

Significant quantities of chlorpromazine, promethazine, promazine, thiopental, and trifluoperazine were found to be sorbed by plastic infusion sets made of cellulose propionate and PVC tubing. Only small quantities of those drugs were sorbed if polyethylene tubing were used. It is also important to be aware that BCNU (carmustine) and bleomycin show rapid loss of potency when solutions of them are prepared in PVC containers (24).

Still other drugs have been shown to lose potency in plastic containers, but there does not seem to be a pattern to allow generalization. Therefore, when in doubt, compatibility tables should be consulted (6,7).

AVOIDING SOME POTENTIAL PROBLEMS

Of course the simplest way of avoiding imcompatibilities is simply not to mix multiple therapeutic agents. Several techniques may provide acceptable alternatives. If two agents that are incompatible are required for an individual patient, the technique of separate routes of administration may be considered. If the IM and IV routes cannot both be used, one may then consider setting up two IV infusions. However, because the problem of exceeding volume limitations may be encountered by this alternative, one should then look into the possibility of using a secondary administration to give the second drug through a small volume infusion using the piggyback technique. If this is done, it may be advisable to rinse the tubing through which the infusion is to be run, lest residual solution in the line create a problem with the secondary. This is mandatory in the instance in which the incompatibility is manifested by development of a precipitate. It is, however, not so critical if the incompatibility involves a potency loss that would be encountered over a period exceeding 1 hour or longer. Several studies on compatibility profiles of mixtures using this technique have been published, but the data are still limited. As a final alternative, one can consider giving one of the drugs in one of the bottles of infusion and the other in the second bottle scheduled for the day; i.e., to put them in alternate bottles.

EXTEMPORANEOUS INCOMPATIBILITY DETERMINATION

Because it is unlikely that any sort of compilation will cover all of the mixtures that might be prescribed, the hospital pharmacist should be able to make some basic compatibility determinations himself. The rules of thumb that have already been described are a good starting place. As a second step, he may prepare a mixture of the new combination and observe it for several hours before delivering it to the floor. Then he should advise the nursing personnel to continue watching the mixture for any unanticipated problem. In the case of antibiotics, he may enlist the assistance of the hospital laboratory to determine whether or not the antibiotic has had its potency affected by admixture. As a standard of comparison, the antibiotic in normal saline solution or sterile water for injection is probably the best available reference point.

When a new drug comes on the market, there are seldom any IV compatibility data available with it. However, clinicians will soon want to be mixing other drugs with the new product, and the advice of the pharmacist is sought in determining the advisability of this new combination. As an extemporaneous approach to providing information, it is suggested that the pharmacist compare the new drug with similar agents on which data are already available. For this, some generalizations about the stability with reference to pH, compatibility with divalent ions, and potency loss with respect to time and temperature might be made. At best, this is a "guesstimation," and such armchair chemistry may not hold up; however, in the absence of comprehensive studies it might provide the only data available.

If a pharmacist has completed some determinations on the compatibility of admixtures not previously reported, he should assume his professional responsibility in disseminating the information to others. The hospital pharmacy newsletter is an appropriate medium for disseminating the information within the hospital. However, the professional journals would provide a broader coverage; a letter to the editor may be all that is required. In addition, one of the compatibility compilations cited (6) has the mechanism whereby the observations can be given even broader distribution. It is through the sharing of experiences and information that the pharmacist's ability to serve as advisor and drug consultant is enhanced.

REFERENCES

1. Turco SJ: Clinical use of parenterals: Past, present, and future. *Parenterals* 1:1-3, 1983.
2. Newton DW: Physicochemical determinants of incompatibility and instability of drugs for injection and infusion. In Trissel LA: *Handbook on Injectable Drugs*, Bethesda, American Society of Hospital Pharmacists, 1983.
3. Rigamonti S: Stabilita della soluzioni iniettabili di vitamina B-1 in presenza di antiossidanti. *Boll Chim-Farm* 103:358-367, 1964.
4. *The Life-care flexible I.V. container, I.V. additive compatibility studies 97-3643-4.* North Chicago, IL, Abbott Laboratories, 1976.
5. Kobayashi NH, King JC: Compatibility of common additives in protein hydrolysate/dextrose solutions. *Am J Hosp Pharm* 34:589-594, 1977.
6. King JC: Guide to parenteral admixtures. In *Cutter Guide to Parenteral Admixtures*, 11701 Borman Dr, St Louis, MO, 1984.
7. Trissel LA: *Handbook of Injectable Drugs*, Bethesda, American Society of Hospital Pharmacists, 1983.
8. Moorhatch P, Chiou WL: Interactions between drugs and plastic intravenous fluid bags, part i: Sorption studies in 17 drugs. *Am J Hosp Pharm* 31:72-78, 1974.
9. Parker WA, Morris ME, Shearer CA: Incompatibility of diazepam injection in plastic intravenous bags. *Am J Hosp Pharm* 36:505-507, 1979.
10. MacKichan J, Duffner PK, Cohen MD: Adsorption of diazepam to plastic tubing *N Engl J Med* 301:332-333, 1979.
11. Parker WA, MacCara ME: Compatibility of diazepam with intravenous fluid containers and administration sets. *Am J Hosp Pharm* 37:496-500, 1980.
12. Mason NA, Cline S, Hyneck ML, et al: Factors affecting diazepam

infusion: Solubility, administration-set composition, and flow rate. *Am J Hosp Pharm* 38:1449-1454, 1981.

13. Kowaluk EA, Roberts MS, Polack AE: Interactions between drugs and intravenous delivery systems. *Am J Hosp Pharm* 39:460-467, 1982.

14. Carmichael RR, Mahoney CD, Jeffrey LP: Solubility and stability of phenytoin sodium when mixed with intravenous solutions. *Am J Hosp Pharm* 37:95-98, 1980.

15. Glacona N, Bauman JL, Siepler JK: Crystallization of three phenytoin preparations in intravenous fluids. *Am J Hosp Pharm* 35:630-634, 1982.

16. Morris ME: Compatibility and stability of diazepam injection following dilution with intravenous fluids. *Am J Hosp Pharm* 35:669-672, 1978.

17. Newton DW, Driscoll DF, Goudreau JL, et al: Solubility characteristics of diazepam in aqueous admixture solutions: Theory and practice. *Am J Hosp Pharm* 38:179-182, 1981.

18. Sturek JK, Sokoloski TD, Winsley WT, et al: Stability of nitroglycerin injection determined by gas chromatography. *Am J Hosp Pharm* 35:537-541, 1978.

19. Baaske DM, Amann AH, Wagenknecht DM, et al: Nitroglycerin compatibility with intravenous fluid filters, containers, and administration sets. *Am J Hosp Pharm* 37:201-205, 1980.

20. Boylan JC, Robison RL, Terrill PM: Stability of nitroglycerin solutions in viaflex plastic containers. *Am J Hosp Pharm* 35:1031, 1978.

21. Amann AH, Baaske DM, Wagenknecht: Plastic I.V. container for nitroglycerin. *Am J Hosp Pharm* 37:618, 1980.

22. Ingram JK, Miller JK: Plastic absorption adsorption of nitroglycerin solution. *Anesthesiology* 51-3S:S132, 1979.

23. Baaske DM, Amann AH, Karnatz NN, et al: Administration set suitable for use with intravenous nitroglycerin. *Am J Hosp Pharm* 39:121-122, 1982.

24. Benvenuto JA, Anderson RW, Kerkof K, et al: Stability and compatibility of antitumor agnets in glass and plastic containers. *Am J Hosp Pharm* 38:1914-1918, 1981.

CHAPTER 36

Enteral and Parenteral Nutrition

JAY M. MIRTALLO and MARY LOU EBBERT

Malnutrition has been recognized by clinicians, especially surgeons, to adversely affect the patient's hospital course. Maintenance of lean body mass and other nutritional parameters have been noted to be important to patient survival. These nutritional parameters, e.g., serum albumin and skin test responsiveness, have been shown to be predictive of postoperatuve morbidity and mortality (1). In recent years, the demonstration by Dudrick et al (2,3) of successful catheterization of the subclavian vein for IV provision of hypertonic nutrients and the achievement of normal growth and development of beagle puppies via IV nutrition solely created a major advance in the provision of nutrition to the hospitalized patient—total parenteral nutrition (TPN). Since then, the therapy has been refined for subsequent use in humans and included advances in TPN formulations and techniques for their delivery, which have resulted in the acceptance of TPN as an important therapeutic modality for certain clinical conditions. Also, this emphasis on nutrition support has led to the development of new products and techniques (such as specially designed enteral catheters, feedings, and surgical placement of enteric feeding tubes) for the provision of enteral nutrition.

TABLE 36.1 Nutrition Support Personnel Activities

Personnel	Activity
Nurse	Assist in catheter insertion
	Catheter care
	In-service education
	Liaison with department of nursing
	Home patient education
	Mechanical and metabolic monitoring of therapy
	Patient and family support
Pharmacist	Parenteral formulation design
	Metabolic monitoring of therapy
	Availability of IV nutrients
	Ensure proper preparation and delivery of TPN solutions
	Supply management and education of home patients
	Pharmacologic interventions with nutrition support
Dietitian	Enteral formulation design
	Nutritional assessment
	Determine nutrient needs
	Estimate oral caloric intake
	Home patient instruction
	Ensure proper preparation and delivery of enteral feeding products
	Availability of special enteral nutrition products

These advances in nutritional therapy were not without complication, but it was soon discovered that key support personnel working as a team could minimize therapy-related problems (4). Significant activities for the pharmacist, nurse, and dietitian in nutrition support services were identified (Table 36.1). Initially, the hospital pharmacy and the pharmacist were instrumental in ensuing sterile, pyrogen-free, stable, and compatible solutions. From this initial involvement, pharmacists have assumed important roles in the delivery and use of parenteral and enteral nutrition. It is the purpose of this chapter to provide an overview of nutrition support of the hospitalized patient so as to yield a fundamental knowledge base for a novice to become involved with this therapy or to provide a reference for the experienced clinician. Specific topics that will be addressed include nutritional assessment, requirements, and formulation design in addition to therapeutic complications, monitoring parameters, special considerations in organ failure, and enteral nutrition therapy.

CONSEQUENCES OF MALNUTRITION

Protein-calorie malnutrition (PCM) is estimated to affect one fourth to one half of medical and surgical patients who require hospitalization for 2 weeks or more. During the hospital course, PCM may develop further while patients are maintained on restricted diets for tests or as a result of altered metabolism created by the underlying disease. These patients with PCM may be more likely to have delayed wound healing, susceptibility to infection, and prolonged hospitalization (5).

As the patient is starved, the hormonal balance of the body is altered such that endogenous stores of nutrients are mobilized and utilized for energy and substrate synthesis. The first body compartment to be affected by inadequate nutrition is that which contains the skeletal, cardiac, and smooth muscle. Following glycogen depletion, these tissues are the first to be utilized for energy. Skeletal atrophy is enhanced by the immobilization that often accompanies disease. Cardiac muscle was once thought to be spared during starvation. Now it is known that the myocardium is wasted and electical activity is diminished as malnutrition progresses (6).

Body levels of visceral proteins (albumin, transferrin, prealbumin) become depressed along with losses in lean body mass. Therefore, many intracellular activities become impaired as a result of transport protein depletion. Coupled with this is a depressed immune system cuased by impaired synthesis and function of antibodies, lymphocytes, and complement and acute phase proteins. Concurrent malnutrition and infection can be potentially devastating, since infectious processes augment a hormonal stress response that promotes an accelerated rate of protein wasting.

Surgical and trauma patients rely on intact immune defense mechanism for recovery. They are additionally dependent on wound healing processes. Depressed tissue synthesis leads to depressed granulation tissue formation with a prolonged recovery and hospital stay. Malnutrition in this setting could significantly increase morbidity and mortality.

Organ systems may fail as malnutrition progresses. In addition to the cardiac failure alluded to above, the lungs are also subject to deteriorization. The lungs fail as the intercostal muscles atrophy and as surfactant synthesis is impaired. The intestinal tissue is not spared either. Even though the gastrointestinal tract and its associated organs are the organs responsible for maintaining nutritional status, even a previously healthy bowel can become afunctional. A starved gastrointestinal tract may not accept food readily in order to facilitate nutritional repletion. Malnutrition causes villi to flatten and fuse; it causes microvilli to disappear, thereby functionally decreasing gastrointestinal surface area required for optimum absorption of nutrients. Additionally, bowel tissue becomes edematous due to low circulating albumin levels (6). Finally, the entire gastrointestinal tract becomes totally unable to digest and absorb nutrients when this occurs, and only parenteral nutrition can generate a repleted nutritional state.

Failure to meet maintenance energy and protein requirements affects all body tissues and functions. This fact illustrates the importance of nutritional support for all individuals. A proposed relationship of lean body mass depletion and associated morbidity and mortality is presented in Table 36.2 (5,6).

Clinically, a semistarved individual presents with generalized weakness, is unable to sustain even minimal physical activity, complains of coldness especially in the extremities, is anxious, and has aches in the ribs, sternum, pelvis, and lower extremities. Sexually, women may become amenorrheic and men may be impotent. On physical examination, the person appears pale with temporal wasting

and is cyanotic in the extremities. With advanced PCM, edema is common, especially in the feet and legs; the skin has a parchment appearance and looks prematurely aged. The hair is brittle and easily "pluckable," and the body temperature, pulse, and blood pressure are often subnormal. Finally, the mass and functional capacity of skeletal muscle, the heart, and visceral organs decline.

The causes of malnutrition vary and are briefly summarized in Table 36.3.

NUTRITIONAL ASSESSMENT

The first step in nutritional therapy should be completion of a nutritional assessment, since it determines present nutritional status and can help identify treatment objectives. An adequate nutritional assessment includes a complete nutritional history, anthropometric measurements, and several biochemical assessments, since no single parameter can fully evaluate nutritional condition.

Nutritional History

The nutritional history can be obtained largely by conversing with the patient. Weight loss or gain should be recorded as "change per unit time." Acute weight fluxes are always more serious than chronic ones. Any recent surgery or trauma, especially to the gastrointestinal tract, should be evaluated to help assess its functionality. Abnormal dietary habits or social history may prove helpful in planning long-term nutritional goals. In short, the nutritional history forms the backbone of the overall nutritional plan.

Anthropometric Measurements

Anthropometric measurements provide objective values that compare the patients fat and muscle stores to the norm. Fat resources are evaluated by taking the triceps skinfold and subscapular skinfold measurements and comparing them to standardized tables. Presence of edema or subcutaneous emphysema will falsely elevate the readings as will IV fluid administration. A second shortcoming to these assessments is the variability induced by different individuals performing the measurements.

Somatic protein mass is measured by three weight comparisons, midarm circumference, and midarm muscle area. The percent ideal body weight and current weight as a percentage of usual weight can be interpreted according to

TABLE 36.2 Proposed Relationship of Lean Body Mass Depletion and Patient Morbidity and Mortality

Lean Body Mass Depletion (%)	Metabolic Consequence
10	Growth retardation (child), decreased muscle mass: skeletal, cardiac, smooth
15	Anemia, decreased visceral proteins
20	Impaired immune response, complement, antibodies, acute phase proteins
25	Impaired wound healing, response to trauma, impaired organ function, gut, liver, heart
28-30	Impaired adaptation, urinary tract infection, bed sores
>30	Nitrogen death

TABLE 36.3 Causes of Malnutrition

Causes	Etiology
Anorexia, altered intake	Psychologic (anorexia nervosa, severe depression), medications, dietary restrictions
Increased nutrient loss	Emesis, enteric suction, fistula, gastrointestinal malabsorption
Hypermetabolism	Severe injury or burns
Altered metabolism	Cancer, advanced cardiac or pulmonary insufficiency, renal or hepatic failure

TABLE 36.4   Degree of Protein Calorie Malnutrition

	Mild	*Moderate*	*Severe*
Percent ideal body weight	80-90%	70%-80%	<70%
Percent usual weight	85-95%	75%-84%	<75%
Recent weight change	1 week	1-2%	>2%
	1 month	5%	>5%
	3 months	7.5%	>7.5%
	6 months	10%	>10%

previously published tables (7). Recent weight change is calculated by the formula

$$\frac{\text{Usual weight} - \text{Current weight}}{\text{Usual weight}} \times 100(\%)$$

Changes can be interpreted according to the information provided in Table 36.4. It should be kept in mind that weight comparisons cannot appropriately reveal nutritional status when isolated from other anthropometric parameters. Weight should be used solely as a guide for interpretation of other anthropometric measurements. Midarm muscle circumference and midarm muscle area should be determined at the same location as the triceps skinfold. These measurements assume that the arm and arm muscle are circular and that the bone area may be disregarded. These assumptions plus measurement variability contribute to singularly uninterpretable results. Again, all other anthropometric measurements must be available for relative comparison before conclusions can be drawn from them.

Biochemical Measurements

Biochemical measures are available to determine visceral protein mass and immunocompetence. Visceral proteins can be measured by direct assay of albumin, transferrin, total iron binding capacity (TIBC), prealbumin and retinal binding protein. Albumin has a long half-life and large body stores, making its levels inappropriate for assessment of acute nutritional changes. Additionally, albumin levels can be increased with administration of blood products, especially exogenous albumin. Transferrin or TIBC measurements are more appropriate to illustrate short-term nutritional changes, since the transport proteins measured by these tests have relatively limited body pools as well as short half-lives. Both TIBC and transferrin can detect nutritional changes within 1 week. Prealbumin and retinal binding protein have short half-lives of 2 days and 10 hours, respectively. They are, however, very sensitive to the influences of stress and are therefore of little clinical importance.

Immunocompetence is assessed by total lymphocyte counts and delayed cutaneous hypersensitivity to a skin test battery. The total lymphocyte count measures both cellular and humoral immunity since 25% of lymphocytes are B cells. Lymphocyte counts have been correlated to hypoalbuminemia and are therefore thought to be related to protein deficiency. However, a total lymphocyte count less than 2000 cells/mm³ indicates the need for additional nutritional

workup since lymphocytopenia may be caused by surgery, stress of injury, radiation therapy, or chemotherapy.

Impaired cell mediated immunity as measured by skin test antigen recall has been associated with increased risk of morbidity in all hospitalized patients. Complete unreactivity (anergy) alone is considered to indicate a significant risk factor for mortality in the elderly, a poor prognosis in a variety of malignant diseases, and an increased risk of sepsis in surgical patients. As with the total lymphocyte count, skin antigen sensitivity can be blunted by high levels of stress.

In conclusion, a nutritional assessment yields a composite picture of a patient's nutritional status. By evaluating nutritional history, anthropometrics, and biochemical indices, a plan can be derived for appropriate nutritional therapy.

NUTRITIONAL REQUIREMENTS

The seven basic nutrients required by the human body are given in Table 36.5. The source and some specific comments regarding each individual nutrient are included. The requirements for nutrients have been well defined in health with the minimum daily requirements (MDR) and recommended daily allowances (RDA) updated by the World Health Organization. These are quantities of nutrients required in the diet to prevent deficiency syndromes. The question arises as to what alterations in requirements results as it relates to quantities and relative proportions of nutrients in the diet result from human disease. Often an accurate assessment of these nutrients is not available for the hospitalized patient, thereby highlighting the importance of recognizing that the average requirements that will be discussed in this section are, at best, estimates that require careful monitoring for efficacy and complications. Often the patient's clinical condition, presence of altered nutritional status, and the primary therapy for the underlying disease alter the patient's requirement for and tolerance to nutrition intervention. In these instances, individualized nutrient therapy is recommended. With these concepts in mind the nutritional requirements of the hospitalized patient will be discussed and an attempt will be made to identify specific concerns where aberrations from the norm may be common.

Calories

The human body can draw energy from carbohydrates, fat, protein, and alcohol. Generally, the majority of calories are taken in as carbohydrate and fat; 40% of total calorie intake each, with protein providing from 15-20% of total calories per day. Generally, caloric requirements of the hospitalized patient are based on the recommendation of Long et al (8). These include an estimate of basal energy expenditure (BEE) using the Harris-Benedict equation (Table 36.6) (9). The caloric requirement (CR) is then approximated by consideration of injury and activity by the following relationship (8).

$$\text{CR} = \text{BE} \times \text{Activity factor} \times \text{Injury factor} \quad \text{(1)}$$

Activity Factor	*Use*	*Injury Factor*	*Use*
Confined to bed	1.2	Minor operation	1.20
Out of bed	1.3	Skeletal trauma	1.35
		Major spesis	1.60
		Severe thermal burn	2.10

TABLE 36.5 Essential Human Nutrients for IV Diets

Nutrient	Source	Comments
Carbohydrate	Dextrose	Caloric source, 3.4 kcal/g as hydrous form, 4.0 kcal/g as anhydrous form, nitrogen-sparing effect, inexpensive
Fat	IV fat emulsion, 10%, 20%	Caloric source, 9.0 kcal/g; 1.1 and 2.0 kcal/ml as 10% and 20% IV fat emulsion, respectively; provides essential fatty acids, some calories from IV formulation provided from glycerol, no nitrogen-sparing effect, relatively expensive
Protein	IV amino acid solutions	Provide substrate for tissue synthesis and repair, provides calories, 4.0 kcal/g; special formulations designed for specific clinical conditions available
Electrolytes	Various	Includes Na, K, Cl, acetate, Mg, phosphorus, calcium; some manufacturers have developed standard formulations of these chemicals for use in preparation of TPN solutions
Vitamins	Various	Recent recommendations by the American Medical Association National Advisory Group have resulted in redesign of parenteral vitamin products; note that availability of individual parenteral vitamins is required to treat deficiency states.
Trace elements	Various	Includes Zn, Cu, Cr, Mn; availability of Se, Mb followed
Water		Usual fluid requirements in range of 1.5 liter/m² unless restriction for disease required

Determinations by this method usually provide a CR in the range of 2000-2500 kcal/day. It is important to note that calorie needs vary depending on patient activity, severity of illness, age, and the presence or absence of malnutrition. In some conditions, BEE is not an accurate measure of actual resting energy expenditure (9).

Basically carbohydrate and fat provide the majority of calories in the diet. For TPN, dextrose has emerged as the major source of carbohydrates, although nondextrose carbohydrates such as fructose and sorbitol have been evaluated (10). Although the nondextrose carbohydrates may have some advantages over dextrose, the disadvantages related to phosphate depletion for fructose, for example, have limited their use. Hydrous dextrose providing 3.4 kcal/g yields 850 and 1190 kcal/liter of TPN for 25% and 35% final dextrose concentrations solutions, respectively.

Intravenous fats are available as either safflower or soybean oil emulsions containing an egg yolk phosphatide as an emulsifier and glycerol to provide tonicity. These solutions may be administered by peripheral vein. When used as a calorie source, the total dose should not exceed 60% of total calories per day. Although use as a calorie source is more common due to reported complications from carbohydrate infusions (11) and reduced product cost over recent years. IV fats are used primarily to prevent the development of an essential fatty acid (EFA) deficiency. This complication may be successfully prevented by the administration of 4% of total calories as the EFA, linolenic and linoleic acids. The content of these fatty acids in IV formulations vary depending upon the oil used in formulating the product such that soybean oil provides a total EFA content of 62% from both linolenic and linoleic acid and safflower oil yields 71% total EFA as linoleic acid only. Both products have been shown to be effective caloric substrates and to prevent the clinical and biochemical signs of EFA deficiency. The dose of IV fats to prevent EFA deficiency can be provided as 500 ml of a 10% solution twice weekly, but it appears that an appropriate interval between infusion days be maintained in order to prevent abnormalities in biochemical indicators of EFA deficiency (12).

Protein

Protein is the most important human nutrient required for tissue synthesis, repair, transport of body nutrients and waste, and maintenance of immune function. For this purpose, it is desired that the protein administered be preferentially used for these processes and not as energy. This results in the recommendation that sufficient nonprotein calories be provided so as to support efficient body protein use. The recommended calorie:nitrogen ratio for IV diets is in the range of 120-150:1 with adjustment for the critically ill patient to 80-100:1. For the hospitalized patient, protein of high biologic value (high in content of essential amino acids) as provided by the commercially available amino acid products is recommended. Requirements based on body weight yield an MDR of 0.3-0.4 g/kg/day, an RDA of 0.8 g/kg/day, and recommended doses for hospitalized patients of 1.0-1.5 g/kg/day. As the illness becomes more critical, protein dosages in the range of 2.5-3.0 g/kg/day have been recommended. It should be noted though that efficiency of protein synthesis is not only affected by the amount of amino acids but also by the relative balance of the amino acids at the site of protein synthesis. Therefore, excess as well as lack of specific amino acids may impair protein synthesis.

Usually, determination of caloric needs and provision of commercially available amino acid solutions in combination with dextrose in quantities sufficient to meet these needs will also provide adequate protein doses and calorie:nitrogen ratios for successful nutrition support (13).

Electrolytes, Trace Elements, and Vitamins

These nutrients are required for proper enzymatic and energy conserving or expending reactions within the body. Also, various nutrients are incorporated in cellular constit-

TABLE 36.6 Harris-Benedict Equation for Prediction of Basal Energy Expenditure (BEE)[a]

$$BEE = 66.47 + 13.75W + 5.0H - 6.76A \text{ males}$$
$$BEE = 655.10 + 9.56W + 1.85H - 4.68A \text{ females}$$
Where: W = weight in kg
H = height in cm
A = age in years

[a]Reprinted by permission from Long CL, Schaffel N, Greger JW, et al: Metabolic response to injury and illness: Estimation of energy and protein needs from indirect calorimetry and nitrogen balances. *J Parenter Enter Nutr* 3:452-456, 1979.

TABLE 36.7 Requirements for Daily IV Electrolytes and Trace Elements

Nutrient	Daily Requirement
Sodium	70-100 mEq
Potassium	100-120 mEq
Magnesium	8-16 mEq
Calcium	3-8 mEq
Chloride	105-120 mEq
Phosphate	30-45 mmol
Acetate	20-40 mEq
Zinc	2-4 mg
Copper	0.5-1.5 mg
Chromium	20 mg
Manganese	1-3 mg
Selenium	—
Iron	1-2 mg[a]

[a]Based on normal daily losses. Supplementation not recommended by these authors unless a deficiency has been clearly documented.

uents as the patient becomes anabolic. Daily requirements for electrolytes and trace elements are listed in Table 36.7. The electrolyte requirements are based on anabolic requirements and consideration for normal renal excretion. At the minimum though, Rudman et al (14) found that an optimal ratio of electrolytes per gram of nitrogen administered that promotes appropriate lean body mass repletion are phosphorus, 0.8 g; potassium, 3 mEq; sodium, 3.9 mEq; chloride, 2.5 mEq; and calcium, 1.2 mEq. Supplemental electrolytes are required when extraneous fluid losses occur from fistulas and/or ostomies.

The doses of trace elements may also be altered when extraneous fluid losses are present and result in recommending supplemental parenteral zinc (1 mg/ml) for small bowel fluid of 4 ml/liter of loss and for stool or ileostomy loss of 6 ml/liter. Also, an additional 3 ml/day of zinc is recommended for the critically ill patient. Recent interest in selenium has emerged as a result of a reported case of deficiency (15). Also, selenium requirements may be in-

creased when more calories are provided as fat in order to support appropriate activity of glutathione peroxidase.

Vitamins are dosed according to the recommendation of the American Medical Association National Advisory Group suggestions (Table 36.8) (16). Supplemental vitamins may be required in the critically ill, particularly in relation to collagen synthesis and wound repair—vitamin C or maintenance of peroxidase activity—vitamin E. Previous deficiency states and some organ failure also will alter the appropriate dose of vitamins.

TOTAL PARENTERAL NUTRITION

Indications

Total parenteral nutrition is a treatment modality that should only be employed when enteral nutrition is not plausible. Examples of such situations can be found in Table 36.9. Notice that each indication for that parenteral nutrition is a relative contraindication to enteral therapy. The enteral route is always preferred, since it preserves gastrointestinal mucosal integrity better, carries less infectious risk, and is more cost effective than the parenteral route.

Formulation Design

As its name implies, TPN must supply all necessary nutrients for synthesis of lean body mass, wound healing, and maintenance of immune function. Therefore, macronutrients and micronutrients are necessarily contained in each TPN regimen. Only the macronutrients including protein, carbohydrate, and fat, will be considered in this section.

Protein

Protein hydrolysate solutions that were utilized in the early days of parenteral nutrition have now been replaced with synthetic crystalline amino acid products. The newly developed formulations have the advantages of being as-

TABLE 36.8 Suggested Formulations for Children Age 11 Years and Above and Adults[a] (Results Do Not Include Requirements for Pregnancy or Lactation)

Vitamins	RDA Adult Range	Multivitamin Formulation for IV Use	Water-soluble Vitamin Formulation for IM Use
A, IU	4,000-5,000[b]	3,300	
D, IU	400	200	
E, IU	12-15	10.0	
Ascorbic acid, mg	45	100.0	100.0
Folacin, μg	400	400.0	400.0
Niacin, mg	12-20	40.0	40.0
Riboflavin, mg	1.1-1.8	3.6	3.6
Thiamin, mg	1.0-1.5	3.0	3.0
B6 (pyridoxine), mg	1.6-2.0	4.0	4.0
B12 (cyanocobalamin), μg	3	5.0	5.0
Pantothenic acid, mg	5-10[c]	15.0	15.0
Biotin, μg	150-300[c]	60.0	60.0

[a]Reprinted from American Medical Association National Advisory Group: Recommendations for Parenteral Vitamin Formulations; adapted from Multivitamin preparations for parenteral use. A statement by the nutrition advisory group. AMA Department of Foods and Nutrition, 1975. *J Parenter Enter Nutr* 3:258-262, 1979.
[b]Assumes 50% intake as carotene, which is less available than vitamin A.
[c]RDA not established, amount considered adequate in usual dietary intake.

TABLE 36.9 Indications for Parenteral Nutrition

Failure of or inadequate enteral nutrition
    Short bowel syndrome
    Moderate malabsorption
    Major burns
    Long bone fractures
Enteral nutrition should be avoided
    Enterocutaneous fistulas
    Severe pancreatitis
    Acute inflammatory bowel disease
    Gastrointestinal destruction
    Paralytic ileus
    Short bowel syndrome
    Severe malabsorption
Enteral nutrition is hazardous
    Geriatric patient
    Comatose patient

sociated with a low incidence of metabolic acidosis (commonly reported with early therapies) and being of known composition. All general use crystalline amino acid preparations appear to have clinically equivalent amino acid profiles. Generally, 16% of protein is nitrogen, but this conversion varies with the commercial source of amino acids. Available concentrations of parenteral amino acids ranges from 3-10%, thereby allowing protein dose individualization.

Some products are formulated with maintenance electrolytes that must be considered in calculating the total electrolyte dose of each TPN formulation. Complete comparative lists of electrolyte content, amino acid profile, and amino acid concentration may be found by consulting other reference sources (17).

Some research has indicated specific amino acids may be important in certain disease states. So far specialized nu-

tritional products have been designed for hepatic disease, renal disease, and high stress, but clinical superiority of these products remains to be proved. Relative comparisons of the amino acid content of the available specialty products can be found in Table 36.10.

Carbohydrate

Dextrose is the most widely utilized carbohydrate in parenteral nitrition because of its low cost, availability, and proven utility. As with crystalline amino acid products, dextrose is available in a wide variety of concentrations to allow formulation individualization. A relatively new carbohydrate source is glycerol. It yields the same kcal/g as dextrose but has the advantage of not stimulating insulin release. Currently glycerol is only used in a 3% concentration for peripheral alimentation uses.

Fat

Parenteral fat must be administered as a lipid emulsion. Presently, products are available in 10% or 20% concentrations that yield 1.1 kcal/ml or 2.0 kcal/ml, respectively. Fat emulsions are used to deliver essential fatty acids and to replace carbohydrate calories in patients who are dextrose intolerant or who have a high degree of respiratory compromise. The three available fat emulsion brands are considered to be clinically equivalent, despite slight difference in their concentration (Table 36.11).

Crystalline amino acids and dextrose compose the base solution from which most TPN formulations are derived. By varying each components dose and perhaps by adding fat, a combination can be designed to meet each patient's nutritional needs that is well tolerated. Sample base solu-

TABLE 36.10 Parenteral Amino Acid Products for Special Clinical Conditions

Disorder	Amino Acid Product	Manufacturer	Specific Amino Acid Content Alteration
Hepatic failure	Hepatamine	McGaw	Increased branched-chain amino acids, decreased aromatic amino acids
Renal failure	Nephramine	McGaw	Only essential amino acids plus histidine and cysteine
	Aminosyn RF	Abbott	Only essential amino acids plus histidine and cysteine
	Renamin	Travenol	Essential and nonessential amino acids with an increased proportion of essential amino acids to 60% of total amount
High-stress trauma	Branch Amin	Travenol	4% branched-chain amino acids

TABLE 36.11 Commercially Available IV Fat Emulsions

Product	Source	Available Concentrations	Fatty Acid Source	Content
Liposyn	Abbott	10%, 20%	Safflower oil	Linoleic acid, 77% Linolenic acid, 0.1% Others, 23%
Intralipid	Cutter	10%, 20%	Soybean oil	Linoleic acid, 50-54% Linolenic acid, 8.5% Others, 35%
Travamulsion	Travenol	10%	Soybean oil	Linoleic acid, 54% Linolenic acid, 6% Others, 38%

TABLE 36.12 Suggested Parenteral Formulation Designs for Hospitalized Patients

Parenteral Nutrient		Amino Acids		Combined Nutrient Volume (liter)	Content/liter of Final Solution		Suggested Use
Dextrose					Nitrogen (g)	Calories (kcal)	
(g)	(kcal)	(g)	(kcal)				
250	850	42.5	170	1.0	7.15	1020	Standard TPN or hepatic failure
350	1190	42.5	170	1.0	7.15	1360	Hepatic failure or renal failure with or without dialysis
350	1190	21.3	85	1.0	3.58	1280	Renal disease, hepatic disease
467	1485	28.4	114	0.75	4.77	1600	Renal disease
250	850	21.3	85	1.0	3.58	940	Renal disease, protein intolerance
333	1133	28.4	114	0.75	4.77	1250	Renal disease, fluid intolerance
467	1486	20.0	80	0.75	3.36	1560	Acute, oliguric renal failure
250	850	27.5	110	1.0	4.63	960	Acute, nonoliguric renal failure
350	1190	27.5	110	1.0	4.63	1300	Acute, nonoliguric renal failure
233	793	56.7	227	0.75	9.52	1020	Severe stress, extraneous protein output i.e., burns, fistula, renal disease, pulmonary compromise, diabetes[a]

[a]Formulated to concentrate protein content and reduce carbohydrate calories and providing the remainder of total calories as parenteral fat.

tions with suggested speciality uses can be found in Table 36.12.

Compatibility, Stability, and Sterility

Crystalline amino acids are chemically stable when mixed with dextrose for at least 30 days at a time. Standard maintenance electrolytes do not affect this stability and are compatible with the base solutions. Inorganic phosphate, magnesium, and calcium, though, may precipitate when supranormal concentrations are required. Complete compatibility and stability characteristics for TPN solutions have been delineated by several authors (18-20); the reader is encouraged to consult these sources.

Recent trends have advocated the admixing of drugs with TPN. Reasonable compatibility and stability characteristics have been found for hydrochloric acid (21), cimetidine (22), aminophylline (23), and several antibiotics (24-26). Even though combining nutritional therapy with pharmacologic therapies has been proved chemically feasible, one must be sure that both therapeutic and nutritional goals can be met simultaneously before such combinations become routine.

Another nutritional nuance is that of combining crystalline amino acids, dextrose, and fat emulsions in one final container chemical stability of this nutrient mix, but the stability may be affected by large quantities of divalent cations, the presence of a low pH, and extreme temperatures (27).

Since TPN provides a complete mix of nutrients, it was believed to have been supportive of microbial and fungal growth if inadvertently contaminated during preparation and administration. Indeed, this was reported with TPN solutions with protein hydrolysates as the amino acid source (28). Further work showed inhibition of bacterial growth in TPN solutions with synthetic amino acids as the protein source and survival and proliferation of fungal species; however, this growth rate was retarded as compared to the protein hydrolysate TPN solutions (29). Therefore, current TPN solutions may only support fungal growth. In contrast, fat emulsions support the multiplication of various bacterial and fungal species (30). To ensure compatibility, stability, and sterility of TPN solutions, preparation should be in an asep-

tic manner under laminar flow and under the direct supervision of a qualified pharmacist who is well versed in the chemical nature of the individual TPN ingredients and the overall capability of the final solution to support and promote microbial and/or fungal growth.

COMPLICATIONS

Metabolic and mechanical complications of TPN have been frequently reported but, as mentioned previously, have been minimized by the provision of therapy by a team of individuals specializing in this practice area.

Mechanical Complications

Mechanical complications involving TPN relate to catheter placement problems such as pneumothorax, hydrothorax, or subclavian artery cannulization. Malposition of the catheter is noted when the tip of the catheter is located in any place other than the superior vena cava. The most frequent complications of subclavian catheters, though, are infection and thrombosis. Reported rates of subclavian catheter infection range from 6-27% and vary considerably, dependent on the author's definition of suspected or confirmed catheter sepsis. *Candida* species have been reported as the predominant offender in cases of catheter sepsis; however, it has been our observation that *Staphylococcus epidermidis* contamination of catheters is becoming a common offending agent. The etiology of infection may be due to poor aseptic technique in catheter insertion or care, catheter seeding from an alternate site, or contaminated TPN infusate. Generally the current TPN solutions that contain amino acids solely are poor supporters of microbial growth; only *Candida* species are capable of survival but have only minimal capabilities to proliferate in solution. Still it is recommended that preparation of these solutions be done by qualified individuals under laminar flow aseptic areas in the hospital pharmacy. Also, it is recommended that policies and procedures for subclavian catheter care be adhered to strictly. These guidelines are completely summarized in the section of the first edition of this text (31).

Thrombosis of the subclavian vein and the major vessels

TABLE 36.13   Common Electrolyte and Metabolic Abnormalities Occurring in TPN Patients

Disorder	Etiology	Treatment
Hyponatremia	Fluid excess, sodium depletion	Fluid restriction, sodium replacement
Hyperkalemia	Acidosis, renal failure	Correct acidosis, potassium restriction
Hypokalemia	Inadequate intake, extraneous fluid loss, alkalosis	Include in TPN formulation, replace losses, correct alkalosis
Hyperchloremia	Excess cationic amino acid,[a] bicarbonate losses, chloride excess	Verify amino acid content of commercial product, replace losses, use acetate salts
Hypochloremia	Inadequate replacement of gastric loss	Administer chloride
Hypermagnesemia	Renal failure, antacids	Restrict intake, stop antacids
Hypomagnesemia	Gastrointestinal fluid losses	Replace losses
Hyperphosphatemia	Renal failure	Restrict intake
Hypophosphatemia	Inadequate intake, antacids, alkalosis, alcohol ingestion, diabetic ketoacidosis	Provide phosphate, stop antacids, correct underlying disorder
Acidosis	Bicarbonate loss	Control excess loss and replace deficit
	Excess acid	Eliminate source of acid
Alkalosis	Inadequate gastric loss replacement, hyperventilation	Replace acid deficit and continued losses, control underlying disorder
Hyperglycemia	Stress	Control underlying disease
	Excess glucose administration	Insulin or restrict glucose
	Aberrant TPN infusion rate	Use infusion pumps for delivery, never exceed ordered rate of infusion
Hypoglycemia	Sudden cessation of TPN infusion, excess insulin	Taper rate of TPN infusion over 2-6 hours
		Restrict exogenous insulin administration
Hepatic enzyme elevation	Possible hepatoxicity due to amino acid imbalance, excessive glycogen, and/or fat deposition in liver	Reduce rate of infusion and carbohydrate intake and discontinue TPN if necessary

[a]Commercial formulations of amino acids have been reformulated to include these amino acids as acetate salts, thereby minimizing net acid production from protein synthesis.

leading to the right atrium of the heart is reported in 1-4% of patients receiving TPN. However, subclinical evidence of thrombosis has been observed in as many as 30% of patients (32). This particular patient population is more prone to thrombosis, since local trauma or irritation to the vein from the presence of a stiff catheter or infection and/or the presence of a hypercoagulable state from their underlying disease. Symptoms of subclavian vein thrombosis include the following: pain, swelling, and the development of collateral venous circulation in the arm, neck, and chest; the presence of a palpable venous cord; and the presence of fever of unknown etiology.

Metabolic and Electrolyte Abnormalities

Metabolic and electrolyte abnormalities occur commonly and may or may not be related to the nutrition therapy but are managed in some instances by content manipulation of the TPN formula. The occurrence of these disorders is frequent (33) in the patient requiring nutrition support and requires careful assessment of the cause of the disorder in order for adequate correction of the problem. Table 36.13 lists the common electrolyte and metabolic problems that occur frequently in TPN patients and provides the usual etiologies and appropriate treatments.

Patient Monitoring

Protocols for patient monitoring of TPN patients are designed to provide data necessary to recognize therapeutic efficacy or complications of treatment. Nutritional efficacy may be determined from estimates of nitrogen balance, assurance of weight maintenance (it is usually not possible to achieve appropriate weight gain until after successful treatment of the underlying disease), and improvements in vis-

ceral protein status. Accordingly, nitrogen balance (NB) is calculated by the following formula (34):

$$NB = NI - (UUN + F) \qquad (2)$$

where NB = nitrogen balance, g/day; NI = nitrogen intake, g/day; UUN = 24-hour urine urea nitrogen excretion, g/day; and F = factor to consider daily insensible nitrogen losses such that UUN <5.0, F = 3.0, UUN = 5-10, F = 3.5, UUN >10, F = 4.

Transferrin (Tf) is a visceral protein that, because of its relatively short half-life (8 days), may respond to nutrition intervention. However, this value is also affected by the patient's iron status and is markedly depressed during periods of stress. The TIBC is a functional measure of Tf that is also useful in determining iron status of the patient.

Laboratory values and physical patient parameters are used to evaluate balance for maintenance of acid-base and fluid-electrolyte status and septic or hemodynamic complications of therapy. A suggested patient monitoring protocol is provided in Table 36.14. Prior to the institution of TPN therapy, baseline data should be obtained and include all of the data listed in Table 36.14. Other data such as patient history, including both medical and surgical problems and especially the current status of critical organ functions, are very useful. At the start of therapy, evaluation of these data can provide a complete assessment of the patient and be predictive of specific problem areas that may arise from nutrition intervention such that priorities for monitoring may be determined. The key to adequate monitoring is to establish a protocol such that possible complications of therapy can be detected early and prevented. Also, with the change in current federal reimbursement schemes, scrutiny should be used in establishing a monitoring protocol such that optimal therapy be assured but costs of monitoring minimized. This may best be accomplished via a nutrition support ser-

TABLE 36.14 Suggested Patient Monitoring Data

	At Initiation of Therapy or in an Unstable Patient	Patient Stabilized
Blood determinations		
Na^+	Daily	72 hours
K^+	Daily	72 hours
Cl^-	Daily	72 hours
$CO_{2=}$	Daily	72 hours
CA^{+2}	48 hours	96 hours
$PO_{4=}$	48 hours	96 hours
Mg^{+2}	48 hours	96 hours
Blood urea nitrogen	48 hours	96 hours
Creatinine	48 hours	96 hours
Total protein	48 hours	Weekly
Albumin	48 hours	Weekly
Hemoglobin	96 hours	Weekly
Hematocrit	96 hours	Weekly
Prothrombin time	Weekly	Biweekly
FBS	Daily	72 hours
Urine determinations		
Glucose	4-6 hours	12 hours
Acetone	4-6 hours	12 hours
Specific gravity	12 hours	Daily
Patient data		
Blood pressure	4-6 hours	Each shift
Pulse	4-6 hours	Each shift
Temperature	4-6 hours	Each shift
Respirations	4-6 hours	Each shift
Input-output	Daily	Daily
Weight	Daily	Twice weekly

vice having a specialized interest and experience in this treatment area.

Special Considerations in Organ Failure

Organ failure impairs the body's ability to metabolize and excrete nutrient substrate. The requirements for nutrients may be altered or similar to those of hospitalized patients with normal organ function. Important to patients with organ failure is adequate provision of nutrients without worsening symptoms or severity of the underlying disorder. To ensure safe and effective nutrition support, these patients require more careful monitoring and, in some cases, modified quantities of nutrients. When nutrient intake is restricted, the patient may be predisposed to the development of malnutrition with its inherent complications. Current approaches to nutrition support in organ failure, especially renal failure, is to provide nutrients in increasing quantities according to the patient's tolerance with careful attention to avoiding excess nutrient administration. Monitoring protocols include parameters to determine tolerance and efficacy.

This section will deal with special considerations in nutrition support in renal, liver, cardiac, and/or pulmonary failure. In addition, special consideration will be given to the patient with enterocutaneous fistula(s) or severe extraneous fluid losses. Unfortunately, these disorders seldom occur independent of each other with more than one disorder commonly occurring in an individual patient. The difficulty arises when combining principles of a specific organ dysfunction at the same time another organ is failing.

Renal Failure. Renal failure is a broad classification for a variety of disorders associated with the urinary tract. In effect, there is an impairment in the body's ability to excrete water and nonmetabolized solute provided by the diet in addition to the end products of nitrogen metabolism. Aberrations in synthesis and metabolism of amino acids and protein probably occur as a result of impairment caused by the buildup or accumulation of waste products of the body. Generally, protein restriction to a dose of 0.4-0.5 g/kg/day is required with the glomerular filtration rate <20 ml/min, providing protein of high biologic value (high in content of essential amino acids). For dialysis patients, the protein dose may be liberalized (1.0-1.2 g/kg/day) to offset losses in the dialysate. Parameters to monitor for adequate protein dosage are urea accumulation rate, nitrogen balance (equation 3), and visceral protein status (35).

$$NB = NI - Up \tag{3}$$

where NB = nitrogen balance, NI = nitrogen intake (g/day), Up = Urea production (accumulation) rate (g/day)

$$Up = UUN - \frac{[(W_i)\,(BUN_i) - (W_f\,(BUN_f)]}{1000} \times 2.73$$

where UUN = urine urea nitrogen (g/day), W_i, BUN_i = patient weight (lb) and BUN (mg/dl) upon initiation of the 24-hour urine collection, and W_f, BUN_f are those values measured upon completion of the 24-hour collection period.

Measures of plasma and muscle amino acids have provided inconclusive evidence of the therapeutic usefulness of special amino acid formulations in renal failure (36). Also, the expense of these measures prohibits the usefulness of these results in general practice. Sargent et al (37) uses urea mass balance and kinetics to estimate protein requirements in renal failure and the acutely ill. This is based on the premise that urea production is related to nitrogen intake (Fig. 36.1) and the catabolic status of the patient (38). On any given dose of protein, the urea excretion rate (mg/min) will increase accordingly until an equilibrium is reached with regard to urea produced and renal urea excretion. The urea excretion rate (G) is predictive of a protein catabolic rate (PCR) in grams per day such that

$$PCR = 9.35\,G \pm 11.04$$

TABLE 36.15 Laboratory Monitoring of TPN[a]

	Initial	Steady-state
Glucose	Every 6 hours	Every 12-24 hours
Electrolytes (Na, K, Cl, CO_2)	Daily	Thrice weekly
Calcium	Twice weekly	Weekly
Magnesium	Twice weekly	Weekly
Phosphorus	Every other day	Twice weekly
Osmolality	Daily	Twice weekly
BUN, creatinine[b]	Daily	Every other day
TIBC	Weekly	Weekly
Urine creatinine, BUN	Twice weekly	Twice weekly

[a]Reprinted by permission from Mirtallo JM, Fabri PJ: Nutritional support of the renal patient. *Hosp Formul* 17:1186-1192, 1982.
[b]Dialysis patients: obtain pre- and postdialysis levels.

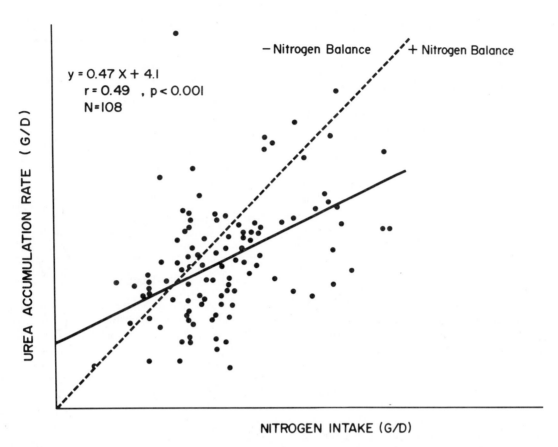

FIGURE 36.1 Linear plot (solid line) of urea accumulation rate in grams per day vs nitrogen intake in grams per day. The dashed line represents nitrogen equilibrium as calculated by equation 1. Least squares regression line is $y = 0.47 \times \pm 4.1$, $r = 0.49$, $P < 0.001$.

According to mass balance principles, nitrogen equilibrium is achieved when protein intake (g/day) equals the PCR (g/day). A problem exists in extrapolating this data to these patients since many factors are usually present that alter urea disposition in the body. A correlation with positive nitrogen balance and improvements in measures of visceral protein status (TIBC) has been observed by our group (38). Table 36.15 provides parameters to monitor nutrition support in renal failure. Impaired excretion of electrolytes, glucose, and other solutes is present. However, depletion of electrolytes may occur when the patient becomes anabolic, since tissue synthesis causes an intracellular shift of ions such as potassium, phosphate, and magnesium. In addition, impaired acid and alkali regulation occurs, causing complex acid base imbalances that may require arterial blood gas monitoring for accurate assessment of the underlying disorder.

Hepatic Failure. Most reactions of intermediary metabolism occur in the liver, and any dysfunction could significantly alter nutrition support. In effect, abnormalities in plasma amino acids have been reported that correlate with the development of encephalopathy (39). This imbalance relates to an increase in the ratio of aromatic to branched-chain amino acids in the plasma. Improvements in encephalopathic symptoms have occurred when an amino acid solution high in branched-chain amino acid content is infused (40). However, many factors contribute to hepatic encephalopathy, i.e., ammonia, amino acid imbalances, short-chain fatty acids, electrolyte imbalances, and acid-base abnormalities. The excessive cost of the branched-chain amino acid–enriched formula and the variable reported effects on morbidity and mortality are factors related to the use of this product, with some recommending its use only when failure of standard nutrition support is determined. Parameters to monitor include daily evaluation of mental status via patient signature, serial ammonia levels, and nitrogen intake vs urea accumulation rate. Also, clotting parameters may be useful in determining severity of the underlying disorder. In the presence of ascites, body fluid tonicity and sodium balance are impaired and may require sodium as well as fluid restriction.

Cardiac Failure. Malnutrition produces a loss of cardiac contractility and sarcoplasmic proteins. Reduction in cardiac function (cardiac output, stroke volume) occurs as cardiac mass decreases. Bradycardia and hypotension allows the heart to function at a reduced oxygen need, thereby delaying heart failure (41). Since replacement of myocardial contractile proteins occurs gradually during refeeding, over-zealous feeding programs may exceed the heart's capacity to meet the increased metabolism of the patient (42). As a result, heart failure may be worsened or precipitated. As a general rule, fluid and sodium restriction are recommended. Advancement of nutrient doses should be gradual. Careful attention should be given to the heart (S_3 gallop), lungs

TABLE 36.16 Electrolyte Replacement for Extraneous Fluid Losses

Source	Major Electrolyte Lost	IV Replacement Solution
Gastric	Chloride, hydrogen	0.9% sodium chloride
Pancreatic	Sodium, bicarbonate	Lactated Ringer's solution with added bicarbonate
Bile	Sodium, chloride, bicarbonate	Lactated Ringer's solution
Small bowel	Sodium, chloride, bicarbonate	Lactated Ringer's solution
Diarrheal stools	Sodium, chloride, bicarbonate	Lactated Ringer's solution with added bicarbonate

TABLE 36.17 Indications for Enteral Nutrition Therapy

Patients who cannot eat normally
   Head and neck surgery
   Partial esophageal obstruction
   Semicomatose
Patients who cannot eat enough
   Preparation for GI tests
   Long bone fractures
   Multiple trauma
   Major burns
   Cancer
Patients who should not eat normal diets
   Mild to moderate pancreatitis
   Low-output fistulas
   Mild to moderate inflammatory bowel disease
Patients who will not eat
   Geriatrics
   Psychiatric patients

(rales), and peripheral tissue (edema). Hyperglycema is common in these patients, but, more acutely, abnormalities in electrolyte or trace elements may induce arrhythmias or further impair cardiac function. Since chronic diuretic use may lead to depletion of electrolytes, careful attention to potassium, chloride, magnesium, and phosphate levels is required.

Pulmonary Disease. Pulmonary function is moderated by neurologic, mechanical, and physiologic mechanisms. Undernutrition impairs pulmonary function via catabolism of respiratory muscles. Metabolically, refeeding may influence pulmonary function by increasing CO_2 production and respiratory quotient (43). If the lungs are not capable of increasing function (minute expiratory volume, respiratory rate), failure may ensue or the ability to wean the patient from a respirator will be impaired. The caloric source yielding the most CO_2 production and elevated respiratory quotient is carbohydrate. The use of fat as a caloric source allows for reduced quantities of dextrose to be administered and has been reported to be effective in assisting patients to be weaned from a respirator. It may also be proposed that overfeeding a patient, resulting in excess CO_2 production from lipogenesis, will also place further stress on the lungs. Commonly, metabolic carts for measurement of CO_2 production, respiratory quotient, and caloric expenditure are not available. Metabolic monitoring is therefore performed by measuring arterial blood gases, respiratory rate, and if the patient is on a respirator, minute expiratory volume. Serum CO_2 may also be useful in determining an acid-base abnormality that requires a diagnostic workup.

Gastrointestinal Fistulas

Fluid losses from fistulas result in significant depletion of fluid, electrolyte, trace element, and nitrogen stores in the body. Assessment of electrolyte content of these fluids may be accomplished; however, losses of other nutrients may go on without recognition. Severe derangement in fluid, electrolyte, and acid-base balance may occur. Further prolonged net negative nitrogen balance may persist as a result of trace element deficiency or unrecognized nitrogen loss. Careful assessment and replacement of this fluid is required for adequate nutrition support to be possible (Table 36.16).

ENTERAL NUTRITION

Enteral nutrition techniques are useful in most patients with patent, functioning gastrointestinal tracts. When compared to the parenteral route, enteral alimentation offers the advantages of maintaining structural and functional integrity of the small intestine, causing fewer side effects, and minimizing costs. This section will address several aspects of enteral nutrition, including patient selection, indications, contraindications, formula selection, monitoring parameters, and delivery systems.

Patient Selection

The patient selection process for enteral nutrition should always begin with a complete nutritional assessment as outlined in the "Nutritional Assessment" section. Candidates for enteral nutrition support can be divided into four basic categories involving several patient types. These categories and the patients included in each can be found in Table 36.17.

Contraindications

Contraindications to enteral nutrition therapy are largely composed of severe manifestations of the indications list and should be evaluated before initiation of therapy. For instance, a complete esophageal obstruction would prevent passage of a feeding tube. Comatose patients are at a high risk of aspiration and therefore should be fed parenterally, as should some elderly patients who have impaired gag reflexes, thereby predisposing to aspiration pneumonia. Further contraindications include the presence of an ileus, any abdominal distention, gastric residual volumes exceeding 150 ml, severe malabsorption syndromes, and large high-output fistulas.

Formula Selection

Enteral formula selection should involve consideration of viscosity, osmolality, lactose content, caloric density, and cost. A simple correlation to keep in mind is that usually as nutrient simplicity increases, so does osmolality and cost. The three main nutrient categories are protein, carbohydrate,

TABLE 36.18   Enteral Nutrient Complexity

| | Molecules | | |
Nutrient	Intact Entity	Partially Digested	Simple
Carbohydrate	Corn syrup solids Cornstarch Fruit, vegetable, cereal solids	Maltodextrans Lactose Sucrose Glucose Oligosaccharides	Glucose Galactose
Fat	Butterfat Corn oil Soy oil Safflower oil	Medium-chain triglycerides Monoglycerides Diglycerides	Fatty acids
Protein	Milk Eggs Meat	Sodium caseinate Calcium caseinate Soy protein isolate Dipeptides Tripeptides	Amino acids

and fat. Each of these is available as large intact, partially digested, or simple molecules. Table 36.18 lists examples of each nutrient group categorized by complexity.

All feeding formulas can be classified as either supplemental or tube formulations. Supplemental products are palatable enough to be taken by mouth but may also be given through a tube. Tube feeding formulas lack acceptable taste and smell. They must, therefore, be administered through a delivery system that bypasses the nose and tastebuds.

As with parenteral nutrition, disease-specific formulations have been developed for enteral use. Essential amino acid products for use in patients with renal failure have been marketed as well as high-proportion branched-chain formulas for patients with hepatic dysfunction or trauma. Since some of these products contain little or no supplemental vitamins or electrolytes, formula alterations may be necessary for some patients.

Complications, Management, and Monitoring

Tube feeding complications are of three types (Table 36.19). Aspiration, the most fearful of the mechanical complications, should be prevented, if possible, by only increasing the formula flow rate in the absence of gastric distention or nausea and maintaining the head elevation at 30 degrees.

Gastrointestinal side effects occur most frequently at the initiation of feeding. Cramping and distention are best managed by decreasing the flow rate and using lactose-free products. Vomiting and/or diarrhea can also be managed sometimes with rate reduction. Additionally, formula dilution may also be helpful. On occasion, antidiarrheal agents may become necessary but should only be used in the absence of a toxin-producing intestinal infection.

Metabolic side effects may be the most serious complications resulting from enteral nutrition therapy. Hypertonic dehydration occurs when a patient's overall fluid requirements are not met. Some calorically dense formulations contain only 60% free water. Diluting the formula or maintaining an IV electrolyte should correct the problem. Glucose intolerance can occur frequently, since many enteral products contain high carbohydrate loads. If not adequately

treated with insulin or flow rate reduction, fulminant hyperosmolar nonketotic coma could result. The most commonly experienced electrolyte abnormalities are hyponatremia, hyperkalemia, and hypophosphatemia. Electrolyte deficiencies can be managed with appropriate supplementations; however, hyperkalemia may require a formula change to a diluted calorically dense alternative.

Close patient monitoring is always beneficial and should follow a schedule similar to the guidelines suggested for parenteral nutrition.

Choice of Administration Route

The appropriate route for enteral nutrition administration should be chosen with each patient's anatomy and gastrointestinal functional capacity in mind. Oral supplements may be taken by mouth if the patient is capable and willing to cooperate. In uncooperative or incapable patients, a nasogastric or nasoduodenal tube should be considered for short-term use. Most available tubes are small bore, sift, and pliable. Such characteristics make them relatively comfortable and acceptable to patients. These tubes are utilized in conjunction with an enteral pump system that allows either continuous or intermittent fluid infusion.

For long-term treatment, a feeding gastrostomy or jejunostomy tube should be inserted surgically. Bolus feedings are given by the gastrostomy route that can only be used if

TABLE 36.19   Tube Feeding Complications

Mechanical	Aspiration pneumonia Mucosal erosions Tube lumen obstruction Tube displacement Nasopharyngeal irritation
Gastrointestinal	Cramping Diarrhea Distention Vomiting
Metabolic	Electrolyte imbalance Fluid overload (dilute formulas) Glucose intolerance Hypertonic dehydration

the patient has a normal gastric emptying capacity. Advantages of gastrostomy feedings are freedom from an infusion device and easier tube maintenance. Feeding jejunostomies, on the other hand, do require an enteral pump system to propel the formula through the small lumen of the catheter. Finally, the choice of enteral liquid feeding may depend on the routes of delivery.

Summary

Enteral nutrition support involves many considerations. Each prospective patient should be carefully analyzed to ensure that enteral feeding is indicated and that no contraindications exists. Next, the formula and delivery system must be chosen in accordance with the patient's nutritional history, functional qualities, and anatomic characteristics in mind. Monitoring should begin before therapy initiation and continue throughout the treatment period. For most patients, enteral nutrition support is not a permanent therapy. When used correctly, it can be an effective, efficient, and safe method of promoting patient recovery.

REFERENCES

1. Buzby GP, Mullen JL, Matthews OC, et al: Prognostic nutritional index in gastrointestinal surgery. *Am J Surg* 139:160-167, 1980.
2. Dudrick SJ, Groff DB, Wilmore DW: Long-term venous catheterization in infants. *Surg Gynecol Obstet* 129:805-809, 1969.
3. Dudrick SJ, Wilmore DW, Vars HM, Rhoads JE: Long term total parenteral nutrition with growth, development, and positive nitrogen balance. *Surgery* 64:134-142, 1968.
4. Nehme AE: Nutritional support of the hospitalized patient. The team concept. *JAMA* 243:1906-1908, 1980.
5. Heymsfield SB, Bethel RA, Ansby JD, et al: Enteral hyperalimentation: An alternative to central venous hyperalimentation. *Ann Intern Med* 90:63-71, 1979.
6. Steffie WP: Malnutrition in hospitalized patients. *JAMA* 244:2630-2635, 1980.
7. Blackburn GL, Bistrian BR, Maini BS, et al: Nutritional and metabolic assessment of the hospitalized patient. *J Parenter Enter Nutr* 1:11-22, 1977.
8. Long CL, Schaffel N, Gieger JW, et al: Metabolic response to injury and illness: Estimation of energy and protein needs from indirect calorimetry and nitrogen balance. *J Parenter Enter Nutr* 3:452-456, 1979.
9. Mirtallo JM, Joch L, Fabri PJ: Caloric requirements of patients receiving total parenteral nutrition. *Hosp Formul* 18:57-64, 1983.
10. Vanden Berghe G, Hers HG: Dangers of intravenous fructose and sorbitol. *Acta Pediatr Belg* 31:115-123, 1978.
11. Askanazi J, Rosenbaum SH, Hyman AI, et al: Respiratory changes induced by the large glucose loads of total parenteral nutrition. *JAMA* 243:1444-1447, 1980.
12. Bivins BA, Rapp RP, Record K, et al: Parenteral safflower oil emulsion (Liposyn 10%). Safety and effectiveness in treating or preventing essential fatty acid deficiency in surgical patients. *Ann Surg* 191:307-315, 1980.
13. Mirtallo JM, Fabri PJ, Radcliffe K, et al: Evaluation of nitrogen utilization in patients receiving total parenteral nutrition. *J Parenter Enter Nutr* 7:136-141, 1983.
14. Rudman D, Millikan WJ, Richardson TJ, et al: Elemental balances during intravenous hyperalimentation of underweight adult subject. *J Clin Invest* 55:94-104, 1975.
15. Johnson RA, Fallen JT, Maynard EP, et al: An occidental case of cardiomyopathy and selenium deficiency. *N Engl J Med* 304:1210-1212, 1981.
16. Multivitamin preparations for parenteral use. A statement by the nutrition advisory group. AMA Department of Foods and Nutrition, 1975. *J Parenter Enter Nutr* 3:258-262, 1979.
17. Parenteral Nutrition Therapy. In Alpers DH, Clouse RE, Henson WF (eds): *Manual of Nutritional Therapeutics*, ed 1. Boston, Little, Brown, 1983, pp 233-268.
18. Jurgens R, Henry RS, Welco A: Amino acid stability in a mixed parenteral nutrition solution. *Am J Hosp Pharm* 38:1358-1359, 1981.
19. Henry RS, Jurgens RW, Sturgeon R, et al: Compatibility of calcium chloride and calcium gluconate with sodium phosphate in a mixed TPN solution. *Am J Hosp Pharm* 37:673-674, 1980.
20. Kaminski MV, Harris DF, Collin CF, et al: Electrolyte compatibility in a synthetic amino acid hyperalimentation solution. *Am J Hosp Pharm* 31:244-246, 1974.
21. Mirtallo JM, Rogers KR, Johnson JA, et al: Stability of amino acids and the availability of acid in total parenteral nutrition solutions containing hydrochloric acid. *Am J Hosp Pharm* 38:1729-1731, 1981.
22. Tsallas G, Allen LC: Stability of cimetidine hydrochloride in parenteral nutrition solutions. *Am J Hosp Pharm* 39:484-485, 1982.
23. Niemiec PW: Vanderveen TW, Hohenwarter MW, et al: Stability of aminophylline injection in three parenteral nutrient solutions. *Am J Hosp Pharm* 40:428-432, 1983.
24. Scheentz DH, King JC: Compatibility and stability of electrolytes vitamins and antibiotics in combination with 8% amino acid solutions. *Am J Hosp Pharm* 35:33-44, 1978.
25. Athanikar N, Boyer B, Beamer R, et al: Visual compatibility of 30 additives with a parenteral nutrient solution. *Am J Hosp Pharm* 36:511-513, 1979.
26. Reid MD, Perry EB, Fennell SJ, et al: Antibiotic compatibility and stability in a parenteral nutrition solution. *Chemotherapy* 25:336-345, 1979.
27. Black C, Popovich NG: A study of intravenous emulsion compatibility. Effects of dextrose, amino acids, and selected electrolytes. *Drug Intell Clin Pharm* 15:182-193, 1981.
28. Deeb EN, Natsios GA. Contamination of intravenous fluids by bacteria and fungi during preparation and administration. *Am J Hosp Pharm* 28:765-767, 1971.
29. Goldmann DA, Martin WT, Worthington JW: Growth of bacteria and fungi in total parenteral nutrition solutions. *Am J Surg* 126:314-318, 1973.
30. Deitel M, Fuksa M, Kamirnsky VM, et al: Growth of microorganisms in soybean oil emulsion and clinical implications. *Internat Surg* 64:27-32, 1979.
31. Yost RL: Total parenteral nutrition. In Brown TR, Smith MC (eds): *Handbook of Institutional Pharmacy Practice*, ed 1. Baltimore, Williams and Wilkins, 1979, pp 295-301.
32. Fabri PJ, Mirtallo JM, Ruberg RL, et al: Incidence and prevention of thrombosis of the subclavian vein during total parenteral nutrition. *Surg Gynecol Obstet* 155:238-240, 1982.
33. Henry M, Mirtallo JM, Fabri PJ: Pretreatment laboratory abnormalities in patients receiving TPN. *Nutr Support Serv* 3:15-17, 1983.
34. Rutten P, Blackburn GL, Flatt JP, et al: Determination of optimal hyperalimentation infusion rate. *J Surg Res* 18:477-483, 1975.
35. Mirtallo JM, Fabri PJ: Nutritional support of the renal patient. *Hosp Formul* 17:1186-1192, 1982.
36. Furst P, Alvesstrand A, Bergstrom J: Effects of nutrition and catabolic stress on intracellular amino acid pools in uremia. *Am J Clin Nutr* 33:1387-1395, 1980.
37. Sargent J, Gotch F, Borah M, et al: Urea kinetics, a guide to nutritional management of renal failure. *Am J Clin Nutr* 31:1696-1702, 1978.
38. Mirtallo JM, Fabri PJ: Effect of nitrogen intake on urea appearance in patients receiving TPN and hemodialysis. *Drug Intell Clin Pharm* 17:434, 1983.
39. Fischer JE, Funovics JM, Aguirre A, et al: The role of plasma amino acids in hepatic encephalopathy. *Surgery* 78:276-290, 1975.
40. Fischer JE, Rosen HM, Ebeid AM, et al: The effect of normalization of plasma amino acids on hepatic encephalopathy in man. *Surgery* 80:77-91, 1976.
41. Heymsfield SB, Bethel RA, Ansby JD, et al: Cardiac abnormalities in cachectic patients before and during nutritional repletion. *Am Heart J* 95:584-594, 1979.
42. Weinsin RL, Krumdrick CL: Death resulting from overzealous total parenteral nutrition: The refeeding syndrome revisited. *Am J Clin Nutr* 34:393-399, 1980.
43. Askanazi J, Weissman C, Rosenbaum SH, et al: Nutrition and the respiratory system. *Crit Care Med* 10:163-172, 1982.

CHAPTER 37

Packaging Pharmaceuticals in Institutions

F. MAURIECE SMITH

Packaging pharmaceuticals has always been one of the functions of the profession. However, pharmacy practice has changed during the past few decades so that now this function consists primarily of repackaging a manufactured dosage form on receipt of a prescription. In institutions, however, greater efficiency has been achieved by repackaging the more commonly used (or "fast-moving") drugs into standard quantities prior to actually receiving orders. This anticipation of need, or "prepackaging," started with the packaging pharmacist preparing nursing unit stock and then progressed to the supplying of traditional patient dispensing programs. In many institutions, this activity presently supports unit dose drug distribution systems, although the other two types of packaging programs still exist.

It is the intent of this chapter to discuss the major considerations relating to packaging or repackaging sterile and nonsterile pharmaceuticals, in many cases irrespective of type of dispensing system served. These same considerations must be evaluated unless otherwise indicated, whether packaging a dosage form prepared in the institution or repackaging one purchased from a manufacturer. In fact, the term "repackaging" is often shortened to "packaging" in hospital jargon.

There are a number of published recommendations that must be considered by those who repackage pharmaceuticals. The USP (1) discourages the practice and states that the pharmacist may become responsible for its stability. It further declares that if it is necessary to repackage a drug, the manufacturer should be consulted concerning potential problems. The American Society of Hospital Pharmacists (ASHP) published guidelines to direct institutional pharmacists in repackaging oral solids and liquids (2) and to assist manufacturers and pharmacists in developing and producing unit dose and single unit packages (3). According to the latter, there are four basic functions that drug packages must fulfill: (1) identify their contents completely and precisely; (2) protect their contents from deleterious environmental effects; (3) protect their contents from deterioration due to handling; and (4) permit their contents to be used quickly, easily, and safely (3).

Predominantly two types of packages are found in insti-

tutions at the present time (Fig. 37.1). The first is a *unit-of-use* or *dispensing* package, commonly called a "prepack." This container, usually holding several doses, requires only the addition of a prescription label to render it suitable for dispensing. These are useful in traditional floor stock systems and for inpatient and outpatient dispensing. The second type is the *single-unit* package, containing one separate and distinct dosage form. Examples might be one tablet or capsule, one teaspoonful (5 ml) of liquid, one 10-mg (2-ml) syringe, etc. These are not the same as a unit or single-dose package, which contains a particular dose of a drug for a specific patient (3). Therefore, that patient's "unit dose" of two tablets may be dispensed by the pharmacist as two single-unit packages of one tablet each, joined together in some fashion. The USP, however, differentiates between the terms "unit dose" and "single-unit" containers, restricting use of the latter term to "articles intended for parenteral administration only" (4).

As previously mentioned, the concept of "prepackaging" is based on predicting future needs of the inpatient and/or outpatient dispensing areas and/or IV admixture service. On the other hand, packaging activities *not* fitting this description are those pharmaceuticals prepared on a day-to-day basis, such as IV admixtures, new dose sizes, etc, and are referred to as "extemporaneous" products.

From an administrative viewpoint, one of the primary reasons for packaging drugs before they are needed is efficiency. By preparing numerous doses at one time, the costs of repackaging are distributed among several doses. On the other hand, if only one or two doses are repackaged, they must bear the entire burden of all costs associated with this function. Therefore, by minimizing the number of drug doses packaged "extemporaneously" and maximizing the number that are "prepackaged" and kept in stock, the administrator is often able to cut costs. In a more efficient operation, daily workload can often be decreased somewhat or, at least, distributed better so packaging personnel can aid dispensing areas during busier times. Another advantage of prepackaging drugs is that it enables the pharmacist to apply batch concepts and principles. For example, if 100 tablets from a single manufacturer's lot are repackaged at

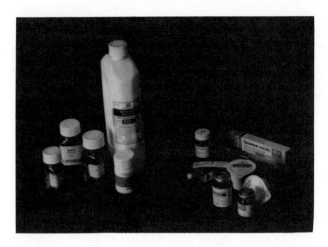

FIGURE 37.1 Two general types of packaging in institutional use, with unit-of-use packaging on the *left* and single unit packaging on the *right*.

one time by the same individual using a single method, those tablets are considered to be a "batch" or "lot" of that drug and are assigned a "lot" or "batch" number. Since all tablets are expected to share common characteristics, random samples can be removed from the batch and subjected to various quality control tests. The results of these tests are then projected to be the attributes of *each* batch unit. On the other hand, products packaged extemporaneously are considered to be individual units and cannot be treated as batches for testing purposes.

In order to enjoy these and other advantages of prepackaging, an institutional pharmacist must assume the same basic philosophy of his industrial counterpart, ". . . that no effort is too great to make the finished product as near perfect as possible" (5). From start to finish each step in repackaging a pharmaceutical dosage form must be taken with this goal in mind. The "quality" in quality control is built (or, in this case, packaged) into the final product, *not* tested into it!

ESTABLISHING A PACKAGING PROGRAM

The packaging operation at each institution is, of course, unique to its own needs, the most important of which is type of drug distribution system in use. Other considerations are costs, personnel, facilities, accreditation standards, and state and federal laws and regulations, etc.

Once an institution commits to establishing an in-house packaging program, a pharmacist should be assigned to supervise supportive personnel and coordinate the operation with dispensing and clinical activities. Besides possessing basic pharmaceutical knowledge and physical abilities, the individual must also be well trained in all techniques to be used, including quality control tests. Many institutions employ supportive personnel to perform the repetitive functions of packaging. They should wear clean clothing, have good sanitation and health habits, and be free of illness, lesions, etc (6). The supervisor pharmacist is responsible for their training as well as day-to-day monitoring of performance.

It is recommended that the packaging operation be isolated from other pharmacy activities and arranged to prevent contaminations and mix-ups (6). Access to the area should

be limited to packaging personnel only. Cleaning, maintenance, and proper operations are facilitated if the area is suitably constructed. The environment should be temperature- and humidity-controlled, if at all possible, to minimize degradation caused by heat and moisture. Both the packaging and storage areas should *not* exceed a relative humidity of 75% at 23° C (2). Also, if drugs with a high vapor pressure are packaged, they should be isolated from other stored products to minimize cross-contamination (2). Additional special considerations for a separate area in which to package sterile pharmaceuticals are well documented in the literature (7).

The packaging pharmacist supervisor must be aware of both the capabilities and limitations of the equipment in use as well as its correct operation and maintenance. Specifications should be gathered prior to purchase and must be updated regularly as required by new applications for that particular equipment. All equipment and systems should be operated and maintained in accordance with the manufacturer's instructions. "There should be valid justification and authorization by the supervisor for any deviation from those instructions on the part of the operator" (2).

Another important parameter to be considered at the time of equipment purchase is the type of containers or packaging materials to be used. Will the final packaged product meet compendial standards? According to *USP XX*, the container should not interact physically or chemically with the drug placed in it so as to alter the strength, quality, or purity of its contents beyond permissible limits (8). Also, where "tight" or "well-closed" containers are specified in individual monographs, the container must meet permeation standards (8). The packaging pharmacist supervisor should obtain data from the manufacturer on the characteristics of all containers and packaging materials used. Such information includes data on chemical composition, light transmission, and physical specifications. Specific information necessary for single-unit packaging materials, both sterile and nonsterile, will be discussed later. It is the supervisor's responsibility to see that all Food and Drug Administration (FDA) and USP requirements concerning types of packages required for specific drug products are followed!

The final, but by no means least important, consideration in developing a packaging program is the quality control function. The packaging pharmacist supervisor must know FDA regulations as well as compendial requirements and how they apply to his or her unique operation. Although chemical stability is only one facet of the quality control spectrum, it causes much concern. This is manifested in *USP XX* in at least seven ways, including monograph packaging and storage requirements as well as standards for repackaging and storage (9). It further explains that an expiration date determined by the manufacturer for a drug in a particular package may *not* be applicable if the product has been repackaged in a different container. Information relating to the repackaged product and its storage, expiration, etc should be gathered from the compendia and literature reports as well as the manufacturers' quality control laboratories. In the absence of in-house stability testing programs, pertinent facts gathered in this manner are the basis for establishing a packaging procedure and should be collected on a control sheet or card for each individual product (Fig. 37.2).

DEPARTMENT OF PHARMACY
PACKAGING DIVISION

Repackaging Worksheet

Name of Product_____   Auxiliary Label_____
Dosage Form_____   _____
Dosage Strength   Special Considerations (Storage, Stability, Packaging
   or Concentration_____   Materials, Delivery Volume, etc.)
Amount/Packaged Unit_____   _____
Container Type and Size_____   _____
Drug Code Number_____   _____

Item No.	Date	Manufacturer's			Pharmacy Exp. Date	Units Packaged	Pharmacy Control No.	Packaged By	Approved By:			Date Released
		Name	Lot Number	Exp. Date					Drug	Quan.	Label	
1												
2												
3												
4												
5												
6												
7												
8												
9												
10												
11												
12												
13												
14												
15												
16												
17												
18												

FIGURE 37.2 An example of a repackaging worksheet.

Control records of all packaging runs must be kept. These records should include the following information: (1) complete description of the product, i.e., name, strength, dosage form, route of administration, etc.; (2) the product's manufacturer or supplier; (3) control number; (4) the pharmacy's control number if different from the manufacturer's; (5) expiration dates of the original container and the repackaged product; (6) number of units packaged and the date; (7) initials of the operator and checker (if any); (8) a sample of the label and, if feasible, a sample of the finished package which should not be discarded until after the expiration date and which should be examined periodically for signs of deterioration; (9) description (including lot number) of the packaging materials and equipment used (2).

After outlining some of the general considerations of packaging system design, it can be seen readily that well-written policies and procedures are central to a drug packaging program. As previously stated, these should follow compendial and FDA requirements as well as ASHP guide-lines where appropriate. They should not stop at general procedures but should include specific directions for operation, maintenance, and cleanup within each system used and, via the control card, each product packaged. They should also include a means of accounting for all doses of drug as well as all containers and labels. A method for determining the expiration date assigned to each drug should be described. Of course, the same criteria should also apply to extemporaneous packaging. Creating and updating these procedures is the responsibility of the packaging pharmacist supervisor.

PACKAGING FOR TRADITIONAL DISPENSING

"Unit-of-use" is a term now used to describe the dispensing package, or "prepack," used in hospital pharmacies for many years. Historically, the advantage to this type of package was to have available, in advance, quantities of floor stock drugs frequently used in that institution. However, it became apparent that a pharmacist reviewing medication orders was preferable to the convenience factor. Therefore, dispensing systems were developed whereby patients received a 2-5 day supply of each medication after review of the order. Of course, the utility of prepackaged drugs became even more apparent for those frequently prescribed medications, and it was evident that much dispensing time and money could be saved (10). Additional advantages were discovered as labeling systems developed, such as providing a standard structure or format, including uniform pricing codes, etc. This improved the aesthetic appearance of the product, and the entire system streamlined the dispensing function.

A large selection of equipment is available for such repackaging needs as described above (see Chapter 39). The simplest devices are, of course, the counting trays and are available as either the standard tray used in prescription dispensing or the perforated trays that deliver a specific number of units (e.g., 100 tablets) through a chute into a bottle. Since these trays are inconvenient when packaging large quantities of a product, many institutions have been able to cost-justify the purchase of batch counting machines for use in drug prepackaging. Recently, several types of tabletop counting machines have become available. These were designed for routine prescription filling but can be used for small-to-medium lot sizes of prepackaged drugs without getting into the greater cost of batch counters. Several types of liquid filling apparatus are also available, ranging from small peristaltic pumps with one filling line to syringe-type units capable of filling a number of containers on a single stroke.

Labels for small and medium lot sizes can be easily prepared by magnetic tape or card typewriters, but these are not very efficient for larger batches. Pharmacies can purchase preprinted labels, typing or stamping lot numbers and expiration dates on them when needed. Frequently, the purchase of a label-printing machine can be justified by volume of use. In departments with computer time available, generating labels for either small or large batches is often more efficient than any of the methods above.

The expiration date assigned to prepackaged items is dependent on several factors. Containers meeting USP standards such as "tight" and "well-closed" are now stocked in all pharmacies for prescription dispensing and are preferred for drug prepackaging as well. *USP XX* describes a relatively simple test to determine moisture permeability of containers in which drugs are packaged, stored, and dispensed where monographs specified "tight" or "well-closed" containers (11). With the use of desiccant pellets in a specified number of containers, weight gain due to moisture is measured and related by formula to container volume. Information from the manufacturer should also be available. In addition, such things as the number of times the container is expected to be opened and the presence of desiccant capsules in the manufacturer's bottle must be considered in any expiration policy developed by a pharmacy for prepackaged bottles of drugs.

Some of the problems inherent in free floor stock systems, such as waste, errors, undetected expiration dates, contamination, and drug security and control are still present in individual patient prescription dispensing systems. Partially

used packages returned for credit are sometimes refilled to their original amount, and this is not always done with doses from the same batch. This leads to the distinct possibility that an individual tablet or capsule may have been exposed to the atmosphere or handled several times before it was actually consumed. Also, the drug product labeling does not remain with the dose until it is administered. However, some states have taken steps to correct these problems by regulating when and under what circumstances drugs may be returned to stock or reused.

In any case, these problems can be dealt with rather easily. Commercial availability of single-unit packages of commonly dispensed drugs has led to their use in traditional dispensing, even in the absence of a unit dose system. A common practice, for example, is to replace a 20-capsule prepackaged bottle of drug with a 20-capsule prepackaged plastic bag of single-unit doses. In the latter case, the integrity of each package is undisturbed, so the manufacturer's expiration date remains valid. Thus, drug labeling stays intact at the patient's bedside, and returned drugs are still in the manufacturer's package with the original expiration date, untouched and uncontaminated, making reissue a much easier and safer process (Fig. 37.3).

Zip-loc plastic bags are cheaper than bottles, but this cost savings is often nullified by the purchase of more expensive single-unit drug packages instead of bulk containers. Another disadvantage to this method is that automatic counters cannot be used. The comparative merit of these advantages and disadvantages will, of course, vary from institution to institution.

Unit-of-use prepackaging by pharmacies can be of benefit to outpatient dispensing areas as well. The principles, systems, and equipment already discussed can be easily adapted to various "fast-moving" drugs in an outpatient pharmacy. Tight containers with childproof caps are preferred, since their use diminishes concern about stability problems. However, a stock rotation procedure should be established, providing a means of removing packages from dispensing stock sufficiently in advance of their expiration dates so that those dispensed to a patient can be completely used up before expiring.

As with all other products, drugs prepackaged for use in outpatient dispensing areas should be adequately labeled, even if the label will be removed or covered up at the time of dispensing. These labels can provide added convenience if they are purchased with removable adhesive. Therefore, the label can be detached from the bottle and placed on the prescription itself, leaving a permanent record of the lot number, expiration date, and NDC number (for third-party billing) of the drug dispensed to the patient. Recording of this type of information is currently considered to be a good standard of practice and may be required on all prescriptions in the future.

The pharmaceutical industry has already made available many products in unit-of-use packages. These have (1) labels that detach, leaving only identification, lot number, and expiration information on the bottle; (2) childproof caps; and, sometimes, (3) peel-off labels suitable for attachment to the prescription. The cost of these packages is usually higher than bulk prices, but this can be offset somewhat by savings in time, labor, and bottle costs. Many institutions

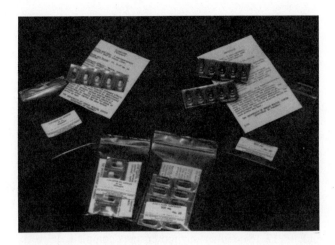

FIGURE 37.3 Unit-of-use package for individual inpatient prescriptions using single-unit drug packages.

are benefiting from the availability of these packages, and this industry trend should be encouraged.

PACKAGING FOR UNIT DOSE DISPENSING

As described earlier in this text (see Chapter 32), the advent of unit dose distribution systems was responsible for some rather significant changes in institutional pharmacy practice. Most important to the packaging area, medications are to be dispensed in as ready-to-administer form as possible, i.e., contained in single-unit packages (12). The pharmaceutical industry, realizing the marketing potential, has responded to this development with the introduction of numerous drugs in single-unit packages. Unfortunately, only a fraction of the doses used in hospitals are commercially available, so those committed to this type of distribution are forced to do their own repackaging from bulk containers, in spite of all recommendations to the contrary!

The need and extent of repackaging varies among institutions and their commitment to the unit dose concept. Ideally, all drugs administered to the patient by *any route* will be in single-unit form. However, not all of the drugs in an institution are used in sufficient quantities to justify prepackaging, i.e., their use cannot be anticipated. Thus, the first step in the development of a single-unit packaging program is to define a "standard inventory" for unit dose use separate from those items to be packaged on an extemporaneous basis only. At the same time, anticipated usage should be determined. This information is the groundwork for selecting the type of single-unit packaging to be used.

There are some other factors to consider in selecting types of single-unit packages to use. All containers and packaging materials must have the necessary physical characteristics to protect their contents from (as required) light, air, moisture, temperature, and handling. Furthermore, these materials should not deteriorate or adsorb, absorb, or otherwise deleteriously affect their contents during shelf-life (3). The shape and form of each type of container used should be such that the package will survive normal handling and be easy to open and use with little or no special training.

Based on the characteristics of the containers selected, the nature of each drug repackaged, and anticipated storage

conditions, the pharmacist must determine a suitable expiration date to place on the label of each unit. Fortunately, the FDA has issued a clarifying policy statement regarding expiration dating of unit dose repackaged drugs. Although their Current Good Manufacturing Practice (CGMP) regulations mandate that drug products bear expiration dates derived from tests conducted on samples stored in the same immediate container, the FDA will waive that requirement of repackagers of solid and liquid oral dosage forms in unit dose containers under the following conditions: (1) the unit dose container complies with the Class A or Class B standard described in *USP XX;* (2) the expiration date does *not* exceed 6 months; (3) the 6-month expiration period does *not* exceed 25% of the remaining time between the date of repackaging and expiration date on the original manufacturer's bulk container of the drug repackaged; and (4) the bulk container has not been previously opened (13). This policy does *not* apply to other dosage forms, other types of packages, antibiotics, or other drugs with documented stability problems, e.g., nitroglycerin and digoxin.

Oral Solids. Containers used for single-unit packaging of these products include heat– or Zip-loc–sealed plastic bags, paper-/adhesive-sealed cups, paper/foil heat-sealed plastic blister packs, and heat-sealed strip packages. These are available for use in manual, semiautomatic, and automatic filling systems, with the automated strip packers generally providing the greatest packaging rates. The complexity of use associated with each system roughly parallels the degree of automation. Many institutions have found that a combination of two systems, one for routine work and another for extemporaneous use, is desirable. The utility of each of these systems is determined by more than simple cost, efficiency, and convenience.

Package integrity, an important consideration, is directly related to stability but is quite variable among the different systems. The problem was studied by Reamer et al (14,15) in two reports on moisture permeation of various single-dose packaging materials. In the first study, significant problems regarding permeation were demonstrated in all systems tested (14). This and other data led the ASHP to recommend, in the absence of valid stability data, an arbitrary expiration date of not more than 60 days from the date of repackaging or as defined by FDA or USP (2). The second study described several new materials for repackaging, showing markedly improved permeation characteristics (15). Overall, however, quality of single-unit packaging materials varied greatly, probably due, in part, to the lack of compendial or industry standards. As a result of this study, standards and classification systems were proposed and eventually adopted in *USP XX* (11). In any case, pharmacists should also obtain detailed information on the characteristics of the materials to be used, especially since few institutions are equipped to perform routine stability testing of all solids. Necessary information includes chemical composition, light transmission, size, thickness, recommended sealing temperatures, and storage requirements. Class of package (A or B) obtainable is important information also, although it is *not* guaranteed because both heat and adhesive seals are also dependent on other variables, such as equipment and personnel performance and past storage conditions.

Specific packaging procedures vary from product to prod-

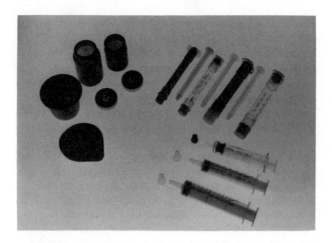

FIGURE 37.4 Examples of available liquid single-unit containers on the market today.

uct, depending on such factors as moisture and light sensitivity. The quality of the package seal is dependent on heat, pressure, wrinkles, and thickness of the materials involved. Variations in these factors should be recognized and adjustments made accordingly. Handling of drugs in the packaging process should be minimized, and each package should be inspected. Also, temperature and humidity in the storage area should be monitored and obvious problems avoided, such as a working still or labwasher in the area.

Oral Liquids. Containers available to repackage liquid doses include plastic or glass vials with aluminum caps, slit-top resealable glass vials, and plastic or aluminum cups with paper/foil tops (Fig. 37.4). These are generally used for standard size doses. For smaller doses, plastic or glass oral syringes that do not accept hypodermic needles are available. Both bottles and syringes are available with amber coloring to filter out UV light when such a precaution is indicated. Filling equipment commonly used includes simple graduated cylinders, hand-held syringes, various semiautomatic or "control" syringes and stopcock assemblies, and automatic syringe-type or peristaltic filling machines. Most of these are available with a choice of permanent or disposable features. The selection of a system depends somewhat on the ease of filling. Vials, cups, and breechfill oral syringes are easily adapted to manual, automatic, and semiautomatic filling, but front-fill oral syringes are not as versatile. A manual method for rapidly filling the latter type of syringes has been described (16).

Most of the stability characteristics of liquid dosage forms will be considered in the "Sterile Products" section of this chapter. However, two points specific to oral liquids need to be made. The large number of alcohol-containing formulations of oral liquids often creates problems when packaging in plastic containers, as the plastics generally permit a rather high level of vapor transmission. This can result in alcohol or other solvent loss, adversely affecting the formulation. Also, the tendency of a suspension to cake increases at the ratio of the height of a bottle to the area of its base decreases, a situation found in unit dose vials as opposed to standard prescription bottles. These and other factors usually dictate product-specific expiration policies for oral liquid doses. The importance of collecting stability

information from drug manufacturers and of performing in-house stability testing cannot be overemphasized. In the absence of such information, a relatively short, arbitrary expiration date must be assigned.

Other areas of quality assurance important in oral liquid dose filling include handling procedures. These dosage units are generally not intended to be sterile, but cleanliness in the operation is mandatory. Doses should be sealed as soon as possible after filling. Calculation of the overfill necessary to allow the delivery of the labeled contents of the package to the patient can become difficult where very small volumes are to be used. Some institutions prefer the use of oral syringes in these cases, whereas others have found that placing the exact dose in a larger vial with specific directions to dilute or rinse before use enables them to solve this problem (17,18). Either method ensures complete delivery of an accurate amount of drug without overdosing the patient.

Oral Powders. These dosage forms are generally packaged into open-top single-unit vials or cups as used for liquids. Antibiotic powders to be reconstituted for oral use are a convenience in this regard, avoiding the short, reconstituted expirations; but the liabilities of antibiotic stability after repackaging and problems of cross-contamination, etc must be carefully considered before repackaging is attempted. Other powders generally present less risk. Filling is most accurately done by weight, a time-consuming process; but, if the drug is granular and free-flowing so as not to pack significantly, a volume measurement can sometimes suffice. Directions for proper use or reconstitution should be included on the label of such items.

Suppositories. A packet of lubricant and an examining glove or finger cot, along with the suppository, are usually packaged in a small bag and labeled. This is of obvious convenience for nursing personnel. It is recommended that only foil-wrapped suppositories from manufacturers be used for this purpose.

Regardless of dosage form or type of packaging system used, all labeling must conform to state, federal, and compendial requirements. According to ASHP guidelines (3), the desired copy and format are as follows:

Nonproprietary name
Dosage form (if special or other than oral)
Strength
Strength of dose and total contents delivered
Special notes (such as storage conditions)
Expiration date
Control number

The rapid growth of and increased demand for single-unit packages has led to the emergence of custom repackaging companies (19). These companies offer various repackaging services to institutions and are worthy of consideration when contemplating a unit dose repackaging program.

PACKAGING STERILE DOSAGE FORMS

The packaging of sterile pharmaceuticals in an institutional setting is accomplished in a manner not too different from some of the nonsterile methods already discussed. The

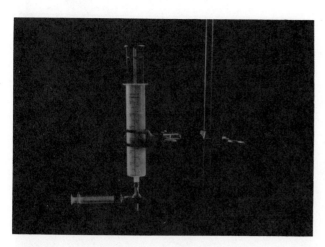

FIGURE 37.5 Stopcock filling method. Injection material is collected into large syringe that serves as a reservoir for filling smaller units.

TABLE 37.1 Types of Sterile Products Amenable to Prepackaging

Product Description	Used by	Examples
Antibiotics reconstituted and refrigerated or frozen	IV admixtures	Cefazolin Na, 10 g/50 ml (frozen)
		Polymyxin B sulfate, 50 mg/5 ml (refrigerated)
	Unit dose	Cefazolin Na syringes, 1 g/3 ml (frozen)
Repackaged large-volume parenteral solutions	IV admixtures	Hyperalimentation solutions (house formulas)
	Pediatrics	Plasma protein fraction, 30-ml vials (single use)
Injections repackaged into syringes	Unit dose	Gentamicin sulfate 70 mg/1.75 ml
		Heparin Na, 2500 units/0.25 ml
Repackaged respiratory therapy solutions	Unit dose	Isoetharine HCl, 1%
		Metaproterenol sulfate, 5%
Ophthalmics reconstituted and packaged	Unit dose Outpatient pharm.	Chloramphenicol, 0.5%
		Echothiophate iodide, 0.25%

equipment or apparatus for filling is often of the same general type, from large operations with automatic machine fillers to smaller ones with automatic or "control" syringe techniques. Both sterile and nonsterile packaging areas must also be very concerned about the stability of their repackaged formulations. Beyond this point, however, the concerns of each operation differ; for this reason, some larger institutions separate these packaging functions into a sterile products division and a drug packaging division. In smaller hospitals, aseptic packaging may be incorporated into the IV admixture workload and nonsterile packaging into the unit dose workload.

Before initiating an aseptic packaging program, many factors should be weighed before realistic goals can be set. The first thing to be considered is the question: "Is there a *need* to repackage sterile products?" The areas providing answers are, most likely, unit dose and IV admixtures. The pharmacist must determine how many different products could be packaged ahead of time and their anticipated volume of use. Table 37.1 outlines a variety of sterile products that might be prepackaged.

Once needs are established and verified, the personnel to operate such a program can then be identified. Besides possessing basic pharmaceutical skills, any person working in sterile products packaging must have also received intensive training in aseptic technique (20). Since one thoughtless act could jeopardize an entire batch of product, the fate of a sterile products packaging area should rest in the hands of efficient, responsible, well-trained individuals.

At this point, the pharmacist can begin to look more closely at specifics. Individual products, methods, equipment, containers, etc, must be studied and compared. Of course, the most important place of equipment, and probably the biggest investment, is the laminar airflow (LAF) hood in which the actual packaging is done. Methods of packaging have been discussed in many articles over the years and are quite varied. The manufacturers of sterile containers, such as syringes, often have packaging systems and equipment as part of their product line. Ancillary pharmaceutical supply houses also offer packaging aids and plans. Examples of methods in use include syringe-type filling machines, peri-

staltic pumps, spring-loaded automatic syringes, and various stopcock and transfer assemblies (Fig. 37.5).

Generally, from an economic efficiency standpoint, there is an advantage in selecting a system readily adaptable to any and all types of containers that might be filled. By following such a philosophy, the institutional pharmacist invests, in the long run, less money in equipment and less time in training personnel in several different methods.

Regardless of the system chosen, it is wise to test it under actual use conditions before implementation. For example, it might be decided to collect the contents of vials or ampules into a large evacuated container so the injection could be more easily repackaged into syringes with the use of a filling machine. Before production runs are instituted and the pharmacist commits heavily to that particular system, a pilot run should be made, using vials or ampules of sterile culture medium instead of product. Their contents are aseptically collected in the evacuated bottle, as mentioned, and this is attached to the filling machine. Disposable glass or plastic syringes are filled with this broth and then incubated to determine if this process can, indeed, produce a sterile product. A few of the syringes should be deliberately contaminated to prove this media would support growth if organisms are there. A more complete discussion of control measures to be used is treated later under "Sterility Testing."

Although there are many brands of sterile empty syringes on the market, made of either glass or plastic (Fig. 37.6), there are really only two basic approaches to filling them. The "front fill" method is designed for introduction of substances into the syringe barrel through the front opening, where the needle is attached prior to administration. The other concept employed is the "breech" or "open cartridge fill," which involves introducing the product through the plunger stopper or open end. In both cases, a sealing process generally follows immediately thereafter (Fig. 37.7 and 37.8).

Probably the only other major type of container to be filled is a vial with a rubber stopper closure requiring a vented needle to allow the escape of air as fluid is added.

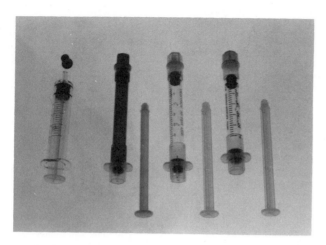

FIGURE 37.6 Some glass syringes available for packaging injections and respiratory therapy solutions.

Some institutions also fill into open-top containers, such as ophthalmic bottles, ampules, IV containers, irrigating bottles, etc. About the only requirement here might be a filling bell along with excellent technique.

When systems under consideration are reduced to a workable number, the next step is to weigh costs—not just the initial investment, but *total* operating costs over a period of time. Certainly the initial dollar output is significant, especially if an additional laminar flow hood must be purchased. But one must also examine closely the cost of syringes with each system, as well as the amount of personnel time required. Not all systems involve the same amount of time in setting up, filling, disassembling, and cleaning up. Some use entirely disposable parts, whereas others require cleaning, repackaging, and sterilizing. Another expense to be considered is that of storage space, storage containers, etc. Are there enough refrigerators, freezers, boxes, shelves, etc to store an adequate supply of each product?

When all other packaging system details are worked out, the pharmacist must then consider product specifics. To select a packaging system for injections, the nature of each injectable formulation must be known and the following factors considered: (1) solvent system requirements (2) light sensitivity, (3) oxygen sensitivity, (4) trace metal catalytic effects, and (5) pH range for stability (21). Packaging system parameters that must be regarded are the composition and moisture-vapor permeation properties of the containers; any special treatment of the final product, such as freezing or autoclaving; and the potential for physicochemical interaction of the formulation with container components (21). Therefore, as products to be packaged are identified, each must be thoroughly studied with respect to compendial monographs (when applicable) and manufacturer's data, mode of degradation, optimal storage conditions, projected time of expiration, and any other physicochemical information available. From a feasibility standpoint, probably the biggest factor is the expiration time. If it is too short, it may be difficult to rationalize packaging such an item because of the workload of other products and the time required to get quality control results back. As a general rule, it is best to consider packaging only products that are

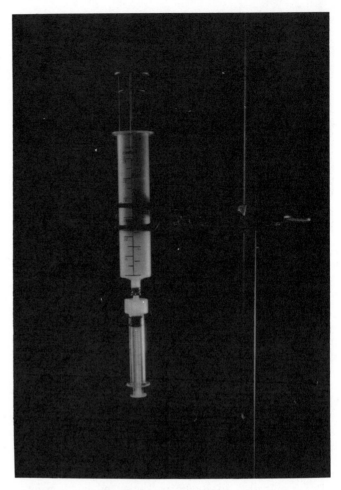

FIGURE 37.7 An example of the "front fill" method that uses a "syringe tip connector."

stable for at least 1 month, since it takes 1 week or more to get sterility test results back.

For each item packaged, a procedure must be written specifically describing methodology, equipment, etc as well as the quality control testing methods to be used. Generally, this is accomplished through the use of a worksheet that is carefully designed to include a permanent, written record of *all* phases of production and testing. Therefore, to meet this stringent criterion, the following information should be included: (1) name of product; (2) packaging control (or "lot") number; (3) ingredient(s) used, source manufacturer's name, expiration, lot number, and amount; (4) equipment needed; (5) procedure used; (6) size and type of container in which product is repackaged, source manufacturer's name and lot number, and number of containers used; (7) quantity in each unit packaged; (8) final number of units packaged; (9) expiration date; (10) quality control tests conducted, with space for recording results; (11) name of person packaging the product; (12) name of person checking it; and (13) spaces for describing any special considerations, stability data, literature references, and calculations. In some institutions, space is also provided on the worksheet to calculate packaging costs for each batch. (Fig. 37.9*A* and 37.9*B*).

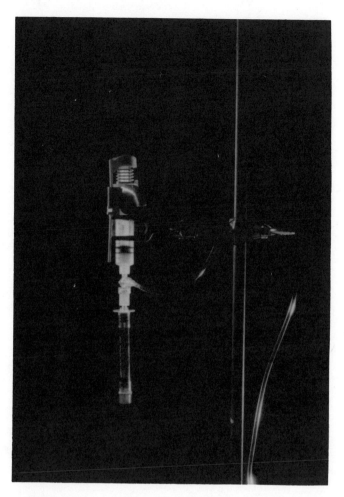

FIGURE 37.8 An example of the "breech fill" method that uses a "fluid dispensing system" and Hypod syringe.

As mentioned earlier, the ability to regard packaged items as a single batch is an advantage as well as a responsibility in quality control. Proven industrial concepts of batch analysis are scaled down and utilized. Random samples of repackaged injectables are subjected to sterility, stability, particle, and pyrogen testing. These are all required to comply with compendial standards outlined in individual drug monographs as well as in the general chapter on tests and assays (22).

Although compendial requirements for ophthalmic and respiratory therapy drugs (23) are not as stringent, most institutions use the same care in packaging these as they do injectables. Ophthalmics must be stable, sterile, and particle-free, with no pyrogen test required. The only criterion in USP monographs of respiratory therapy agents is stability. However, due to the nature of their use, it is best to package them aseptically and conduct sterility tests.

Looking at the four quality control objectives individually, the institutional pharmacist probably has the most difficulty with stability determination. Most places have neither the personnel, equipment, nor expertise to establish proper testing programs. Therefore, the alternative is to rely on published studies or data supplied by the manufacturer's quality control laboratory.

In no instance can it be rationalized that, if an injection is stable in the manufacturer's vial, it is also stable in a syringe. In removing the contents from vials or ampules and repackaging it in syringes, the injection is exposed to an entirely new and different set of conditions. Everything contacting the active drug must be considered in relationship to its final effect, from atmosphere to packaging components to formulation ingredients. Therefore, the influence of all components on the stability of the product and the effectiveness of a particular packaging system in preserving that product during prolonged storage must be evaluated under varying conditions of heat, light, and moisture. The substances most generally in contact with a product are glass, plastic, rubber, metals, and some sort of environmental layer (air, nitrogen, carbon dioxide, etc).

Glass has been the container material of choice for years because of its chemical resistance or "inertness." However, various analytical techniques have proved this to be a false assumption, with alkali release into some products causing problems. The USP (24) defines and describes four types of glass, and each individual injection monograph specifies the type to be used in packaging that particular product. Table 37.2 outlines this information. Notice that types I, II, and III may be used to package parenterals, depending on the nature of the injection formulation and time of sterilization. As a general rule, products with pH over 7.0 at any time during shelf life should be put in type I glass containers, whereas type II can be used for solutions of pH 7.0 or less. Either type II or III may be used to package sterile powders and oils and are preferable from an economic standpoint to type I. Therefore, when repackaging injections, it is necessary to know the glass composition and type for syringes being used and to determine its suitability for each different parenteral formulation.

Advancement in the field of polymer technology have enabled development of several types of plastic suitable for use in packaging and storing sterile pharmaceuticals. Different polymers, such as polyethylene or polypropylene, exhibit different characteristics that may be altered somewhat to meet packaging needs. A particular plastic may be obtained in different densities or with modifying additives to change its physicochemical properties. The six classes of plastic and their criteria are described in the USP (25). One can easily see why it is imperative to determine the stability of each product in contact with the specific plastic container in which it is packaged.

One property of plastic seemingly causes most of the problems attendant with its use. That, stated simply, is the permeation in both directions as shown:

Sterile solution = Plastic polymer

= Ambient environment

Also, additives can be leached from the plastic material into the sterile solution (26), or components of the sterile product can be attracted to the plastic or actually bound to a rearranged polymer structure. Some of the ways in which these factors affect a product packaged in a plastic container are listed in Table 37.3.

The final container component generally in contact with injections is rubber and, being a polymer also, it shares may of the problems of plastics. Its molding properties, con-

DEPARTMENT OF PHARMACY
STERILE PRODUCTS DIVISION

Repackaging Worksheet

Name of
Product:_____

Pharmacy
Control Number: S_____

Requested by:_____Packaged by:_____

Special considerations:

Use (IV, IM, ophth., etc.):

Literature reviewed:

Stability data:

Contents:	Amount Used:	Manufacturer's Name, Lot Number, & Expiration:	Filled By:	Checked By:
Container Size & Type:	Number Used:	Manufacturer's Name, Lot Number, & Expiration:	Filled By:	Checked By:
Other Materials:	Quantity:	Manufacturer's Name, Lot Number, & Expiration:		Checked By:

FIGURE 37.9A   An example of a repackaging worksheet (front) for sterile products.

formity characteristics, elasticity, and ability to "relax" and reseal after puncture dictates its use as closure material for all sizes and shapes of injection containers. As with plastic formulations, rubber packaging components are numerous and may include, in addition to the rubber polymer, accelerators, activators, fillers, plasticizers, and reinforcing agents (26). Lubricants from the molding process may also still be present on the surface; therefore, it can only be reiterated that the effect of the container on each drug formulation (and vice versa) must be determined before use.

Although it is generally not considered a packaging component, the atmospheric layer between the pharmaceutical and the container certainly can have a great influence on the stability of that product. Since many drugs break down as a result of oxidation reactions, their injectable forms are often packaged under nitrogen or, in some cases, carbon dioxide to retard this process and prolong shelf life. Their formulations might also include antioxidants, with or without chelating agents and buffers, to accomplish the same purpose. Often the pharmacist is not aware of these special precautions and does not suspect any stability problems. As a general rule, therefore, when repackaging an injection

Procedure for packaging:

Labeling & packaging data:

   Number of packaged units:_____   Sample & auxiliary labels:

   Quantity per unit:_____

   Delivery volume (if applicable):_____

   Expiration date:_____

   Labeled by:_____

Quality control data (attach results if separate report form):

   Clarity:_____

   Container check:_____

   Label check:_____

   Assay:_____

   Sterility test:_____

   Pyrogen test:_____

   Leaker test:_____

   Others:

_____

_____

Packaging costs:

   Contents: $_____

   Containers & labels: $_____

   Equipment, disposables, & Q.C.: $_____

   Labor

      Pharmacist_____hours @ $_____/hr: $_____

      Technician_____hours @ $_____/hr: $_____

   Total batch cost: $_____

   Cost per unit: $_____

Batch released by:_____Date:_____

                           Quality control pharmacist

FIGURE 37.9*B*   Back of repackaging worksheet.

containing a metasulfite, bisulfite, or sulfite salt, special precautions should be taken to avoid introducing oxygen and ititiating the auto-oxidative process.

Degradation can also occur when certain pharmaceutical formulations absorb radiant energy, bringing about oxidation-reduction reactions, polymerization, etc. The UV portion of the light spectrum, with its large energy level, is the primary offender in such photochemical reactions. Several variables, such as intensity and wavelength of light as well as container color, composition, etc, all have an effect on reaction rates (27). Therefore, dosage froms that are light-sensitive should be protected by using amber containers or some sort of light-resistant covering.

As a general rule, degradation rates may also be influenced by such factors as solution pH, presence of a catalyst, and storage temperature. Therefore, periodic determinations of solution pH made during product shelf life may provide the first clue that a batch stability problem exists. These values are recorded on the product worksheet; thus any significant changes or ''trends'' will be readily apparent. Storage temperatures should also be checked frequently, since many reactions are greatly accelerated by even a small

TABLE 37.2   A Description of Glass Types

Type	General Description	Use	Sterilization Requirements for Container
I	Highly resistant borosilicate glass	P	Before or after filling with solution
II	Treated soda lime glass	P	Should be sterilized before filling
III	Soda lime glass	P	Must be sterile before filling
NP	General purpose soda lime glass	NP	Not sterilized

P = parenteral; NP = nonparenteral.

TABLE 37.3   Effect of Plastic or Rubber Interacting with Injection Formulation

Physical Factor	Result	Possible Effect
Moisture-vapor transmission	1. Water leaves package	Loss of injection volume
		Increased concentration of solutes
	2. Water enters package	Powdered or lyophilized drugs could hydrolyze
	3. Air enters package	Catalyzes oxidation, hydrolysis, etc of solution
Sorption	Solution ingredients sorb to plastic	Loss of drug, antibacterial agents, etc from solution
		Container deformation
Leaching	Plastic formulation ingredients into sterile product	High levels of DEHP, etc
		Solution discolored, degraded, etc

increase. Some institutions have installed temperature-sensing devices that sound an alarm when the temperature in their refrigerator and/or freezer rises more than a few degrees.

To sum up the stability issue, specific potency information from one source or another must be obtained on each repackaged product *if at all possible*. However, if no information is available, meticulous attention to the factors discussed should enable a pharmacist to make a decision whether or not adequate stability might be expected on repackaging. If so, a short expiration period of 30-90 days is placed on the label (28). However, if this last method is used, the benefit to risk should be carefully calculated.

The other criteria for injections are much easier to examine. As a general rule, USP requirements must be observed and procedures followed as written unless it can be proved that another method is equal or superior to the official one.

Some institutional pharmacies rely entirely on their microbiology department to perform all batch sterility testing. The pharmacist merely sends his samples to the microbiologist for inoculation, incubation, and a final sterility test report. In other institutions, pharmacy personnel perform the inoculation phase. In either case, testing to determine the presence or absence of microorganisms is based on introduction of the contents of the correct number of samples into culture media as described in the compendia (29). For small injection volumes with no antibacterial substances in the formula, the direct inoculation method might be used. For large-volume parenterals and formulations with inhibitory materials present, a membrane filter method should be employed, thereby concentrating microorganisms on the filter surface and physically separating them from the injection solution. The filter is then placed in culture media or vice versa.

After inoculating the broth by one method or the other, the containers are incubated at prescribed temperatures for 1 week or more. At the end of this time period, they are then examined for turbidity, indicating microbiologic growth. Most often, the microbiology department conducts

the incubation and examination phases, as mentioned, reporting their findings to the sterile products pharmacist.

Knowledge of the statistical basis of sterility testing is helpful in recognizing the limitations of such a test (30). Therefore, it is best to design as many safeguards as possible into the testing procedure, such as the utilization of "control" tubes during the process. A "positive" control can be prepared by running a few drops of water into a tube of broth, testing its ability to promote growth. "Technique" control tubes require the operator to perform the sample procedure without product, i.e., going through the same direct inoculation or membrane test motions as done with the product. Other tubes included are the "broth" controls, which are simply unopened tubes of media that, obviously, should not grow anything. Additional tubes or plates might be opened in the LAF and serve as "hood" controls. If any of the control tubes fail to respond as expected, the results of that particular sterility test are suspect, and the USP procedure for retesting must be observed.

Performing the compendial test to detect the presence of pyrogens is a little more difficult than testing for microorganisms. Since it is a qualitative rabbit fever response test, most institutions do not have the animals or the facilities to conduct such examinations (31). Therefore, the alternative has long been to send batch samples to an independent laboratory, at considerable expense and delay, or release the product without benefit of pyrogen testing. Another option was developed in the early 1970s with the discovery of the limulus amebocyte lysate (LAL or "limulus") test (32). This is an in vitro bacterial endotoxin test involving inoculation of microgram quantities of test material into a small amount of lysate and observing for gel formation, indicating the presence of pyrogenic substances. There are some products that inhibit gelation, even in the presence of endotoxin, so a series of positive and negative control tests should be conducted before actually testing the product.

"Good pharmaceutical practice requires also that each final container of injection be subjected individually to a physical inspection, whenever the nature of the container permits, and that every container whose contents show evidence of contamination with visible foreign material be rejected'' (22). Visual inspection for clarity is usually done by swirling the solution under a good light in front of dark and light backgrounds, respectively. The limitation here, of course, is the visual acuity of each inspector. Automated particle counters and membrane filtration methods are more sensitive and accurate, but they are also expensive and usually destroy the samples.

Other quality control functions involve leaker testing ampules and certain types of syringes as well as final inspection of all repackaged products, their labels, and any accompanying information. The leaker test is designed to reveal physical flaws in containers that allow contaminants access from outside. Most weaknesses are readily detected through the use of a dye solution and pressure differentials (33).

Requirements for packaging, storing, and labeling injections, inhalants, and ophthalmics appear in the USP in both individual monographs as well as the general test section. It also devotes a special section to injections (22). As a general working rule, however, label information should include everything necessary for the safe and proper use of that particular product. Since it is often impossible to fit all this directly onto the label itself, a package insert can accompany the product.

CONCLUSION

Packaging pharmaceutical dosage forms should be undertaken only after all factors are carefully considered. Written procedures should be developed; specifications must be obtained for packaging materials and operating instructions for equipment; materials and equipment should be evaluated for moisture permeation by the USP test; relatively short expiration dates for all products should be established; and packages should be stored in low-humidity areas. The packaging pharmacist should become familiar with indicators of the characteristics of specific drug products, such as the use of light-resistant bottles by the manufacturer or the necessity of ''tight'' containers when the manufacturer includes desiccants in a bulk container. One should ''overpackage,'' i.e., use relatively impermeable materials even when the drug is relatively stable to moisture, and overwrap or store it in less permeable containers (34).

Such a carefully conceived plan will allow each product to meet all requirements, both official and departmental, and will include *total* quality control. The latter, obviously, must be a concern throughout the life of a product, from inception to administration. The ''quality'' from quality control must be *built* into each packaged unit, not tested into it as an afterthought. With this in mind, the quest for those ''perfect'' dosage forms should be much easier, and the institutional packaging personnel can take tremendous pride in a difficult job well done.

REFERENCES

1. The *United States Pharmacopeia*, 20th rev, and *The National Formulary*, ed 15. Rockville, MD, The United States Pharmacopeia Convention, 1980, p 1036.
2. American Society of Hospital Pharmacists: Guidelines for repackaging oral solids and liquids in single unit and unit dose packages. *Am J Hosp Pharm* 34:1355, 1977.
3. American Society of Hospital Pharmacists: Guidelines for single unit and unit dose packages of drugs. *Am J Hosp Pharm* 34:613-614, 1977.
4. *The United States Pharmacopeia, op. cit.,* p 8.
5. Avis KE: Sterile products. In Lachman L, Lieberman HA, Kanig JL (eds): *The Theory and Practice of Industrial Pharmacy*. Philadelphia, Lea & Febiger, 1970, p 603.
6. Food and Drug Administration, Department of Health and Human Services: *Code of federal regulations: Food and drugs—current good manufacturing practice for finished pharmaceuticals*. 21CFR 211.28-.45, April, 1983.
7. Avis KE: Parenteral preparations. In Osol A, (ed): *Remington's Pharmaceutical Sciences*. Easton, PA, Mack, 1980, pp 1471-1475.
8. *The United States Pharmacopeia: op. cit.,* pp 7-8.
9. *ibid,* p XI.
10. Campbell WH, Christensen DB, Johnson RE, et al: Identifying economic efficiencies resulting from a drug repackaging program. *Am J Hosp Pharm* 31:954-960, 1974.
11. The *United States Pharmacopeia, op. cit.,* pp 954-955.
12. American Society of Hospital Pharmacists: ASHP statement on unit dose drug distribution. *Am J Hosp Pharm* 32:835, 1975.
13. Food and Drug Administration, Department of Health and Human Services: *Compliance Policy Guidelines*. 7132b.11, October 1, 1980.
14. Reamer JT, Grady LT, Shangraw RF, et al: Moisture permeation of typical unit dose repackaging materials. *Am J Hosp Pharm*. 34:35-42, 1977.
15. Reamer JT, Grady LT: Moisture permeation of newer unit dose repackaging materials. *Am J Hosp Pharm*. 35:787-793, 1978.
16. White SJ, Miller PO, Godwin HN: Unit dose innovations. *Am J Hosp Pharm*. 32:814-817, 1975.
17. Minerath MI: Responses to request for suggestions on unit dose packaging of small-volume oral liquids. *Am J Hosp Pharm*. 33:880,885, 1976 (letter).
18. O'Donnell J: Responses to request for suggestions on unit dose packaging of small-volume oral liquids (letter). *Am J Hosp Pharm* 33:885, 1976.
19. Labreque J: Regional service center provides prepackaged medications. *Hospitals* 50:73-76, 1976.
20. Avis KE: *op. cit.,* p 1474.
21. Nedich RL: Selection of containers and closure systems for injectable products. *Am J Hosp Pharm* 40:1924-1927, 1983.
22. The *United States Pharmacopeia, op. cit.,* pp 861-863.
23. *ibid.,* pp 1026, 1027-1028.
24. *ibid.,* p 949.
25. *ibid.,* p 951.
26. Nedich RL: *op. cit.,* pp 1925-1926.
27. Lintner CJ: Stability of pharmaceutical products. In Osol A, (ed): *Remington's Pharmaceutical Sciences*. Easton, PA, Mack, 1980, p 1429.
28. Turco S, King RE: *Sterile Dosage Forms*. Philadelphia, Lea & Febiger, 1974, p 202.
29. *The United States Pharmacopeia, op. cit.,* pp 1039-1034.
30. Phillips GB, Miller WS: Sterilization. In Osol A (ed): *Remington's Pharmaceutical Sciences*. Easton, PA, Mack, 1980, pp 1400-1402.
31. *The United States Pharmacepeia, op. cit.,* pp 902-903.
32. *ibid,* pp 888-889.
33. Avis KE: *Parenteral, op. cit.,* p 1486.
34. Zellmer WA: Unit dose repackaging (editorial). *Am J Hosp Pharm* 34:27, 1977.

ADDITIONAL READING

Banker GS, Rhodes CT: Packaging of pharmaceuticals. In *Modern Pharmaceutics*. New York, Marcel Dekker, 1979.
Eudailey WA: Membrane filters and membrane-filtration processes for health care. *Am J Hosp Pharm* 40:1921-1923, 1983.
Frieben WR: Control of the aseptic processing environment. *Am J Hosp Pharm* 40:1928-1935, 1983.
Newton DW: Physicochemical determinants of incompatibility and instability of drugs for injection and infsuion. In Trissel LA (ed): *Handbook of Injectable Drugs*, ed. 3. Bethesda, American Society of Hospital Pharmacists, 1983, pp xi-xxi.
Trissel LA: *Handbook of Injectable Drugs*, ed. 3, Bethesda, American Society of Hospital Pharmacists, 1983.

CHAPTER 38

Quality Control and Standards

JAYANT A. PATEL

The intent of this chapter is to provide guidelines for all phases of quality control in the hospital pharmacy. However, implementation and modification of the acceptable standards described in the current Good Manufacturing Practice (GMP) (1) must be tailored to the needs and type of services offered by each hospital pharmacy. If a hospital engages in drug manufacturing, repackaging, reprocessing, or relabeling to supply its needs, it must follow GMP regulations as a guide to ensure that the drugs they manufacture, repackage, or relabel meet the standards of pharmaceutical integrity (identity, purity, strength, quality, safety).

Such self-regulating practice will make government regulatory activity unnecessary. However, when multiple institutions (hospitals, clinics, nursing homes, drugstores, etc) are involved jointly in manufacturing, repackaging, or relabeling, they fall under the Federal Food, Drug and Cosmetic Act and thus invite govermnent regulation (2).

The guidelines presented here are not necessarily applicable to large hospitals only. Certain functions of quality control can be integrated into the production unit provided there is no conflict in maintaining the integrity of the drug products processed. The criteria used to establish a separate quality control function depend upon the extent of the activities, number, and type of personnel involved.

The control laboratory may not be equipped with sophisticated instruments such as a gas chromatograph, high-performance liquid chromatograph, or atomic absorption analyzer in the formative years, and conventional methods of analysis such as simple titrations, refractive index, and melting point determinations can then be made. The growth of the control laboratory facilities can be extended to provide bacteriologic, toxicologic, and therapeutic monitoring of drugs and may be a source of new revenues to a pharmacy department as well as offer an avenue for professional growth to the hospital pharmacists.

Control of quality in the formulation, manufacture, and distribution of pharmaceutical, biological, and other medicinal products is the organized effort employed by a company to provide and maintain in the final product the desired feature, properties and characteristics of identity, purity, uniformity, potency, and stability within established levels so that all merchandise shall meet professional requirements, legal standards, and also such additional standards as the management of a firm may adopt (3).

The above is the principle adopted by the Pharmaceutical Manufacturers Association and is equally applicable to any institution, whether a drug manufacturer or hospital pharmacy. Whatever control system is devised, it must be adequate and effective in attaining its purposes.

Pharmaceutical production presents many problems and conditions that make it a complicated operation, especially when the quantity prepared is large. Quality control must be built into the manufacturing process itself; it is not something that can be added after the product is made. Quality control is an organized effort of all individuals directly or indirectly involved in the production, packaging, and distribution of quality medications that are safe, effective, and acceptable. Its ultimate success depends on the cooperation of all individuals.

In hospital pharmacies, quality control should encompass not only formulation, compounding, and dispensing but must also include packaging, purchasing, storage, and distribution of medication to the ultimate user, the patient.

AUTHORITY FOR QUALITY CONTROL

The total control of quality for drugs is a hospital-wide activity for all segments of a pharmacy department. However, the responsibility for auditing the control system and evaluating product quality is that of the quality control unit, sometimes referred to as "assay and control." In hospital pharmacies with separate assay and control capability, this unit is independent and responsible to the director and/or assistant director of pharmacy services. The assay and control or quality control unit may consist of a pharmacist supervisor and technicians, depending on the scope of service. The supervisor of the quality control unit should be assigned authority to approve, reject, or order the reprocessing of products or procedures.

CONTROL LABORATORY

An important prerequisite for efficient functioning of quality control, in addition to qualified personnel, is that it must have adequate facilities (space and equipment) (4), to perform all necessary analyses and to maintain records. Likewise, the production and packaging sections should have facilities adequate to produce quality pharmaceuticals in quantities sufficient to meet patient demand.

INTERRELATIONSHIP OF ASSAY AND CONTROL AND PRODUCTION SECTIONS

The responsibility of the production section is to produce quality products, and the responsibility of assay and control is to examine and approve the formulas and procedures by which products are produced and to approve all final products so that the goals of quality control, as previously outlined, may be attained. The production pharmacist may perform certain in-process control procedures such as pH determination, viscosity, specific gravity, tablet disintegration and hardness tests, etc.

Assay and control can be a potential source of irritation to the various production sections, and the reverse is also true, unless proper individuals are chosen and the purpose of the function of each is clearly delineated and understood by all. Each pharmacist should have the necessary scientific knowledge and skills and be cooperative in spirit and quality conscious. For example, one important area requiring cooperative efforts is the determination of production size batches in relation to the shelf life, stability, and rate of distribution.

RECORDS

A large amount of record keeping is necessary to monitor the different aspects of quality control and production that must be readily retrievable (5). Good maintenance and an adequate number of records are basic requirements of any well-designed quality control system. The dynamic growth of computer technology has made quality control record keeping much easier and readily retrievable. All necessary reports can be generated from the data stored. The increased use of computers in other areas of pharmacy makes access to such a system a reality.

GENERAL CONSIDERATIONS

The following discussion covers the general areas of quality control of pharmaceutical preparation and production in outline form. This has been exerpted from *General Principles of Control of Quality in the Drug Industry,* adopted by the Board of Directors of the Pharmaceutical Manufacturer's Association (3).

1. Buildings for manufacturing, testing, and storage operations are of adequate design, size, and construction to:
   a. Provide for proper receipt and storage of raw materials
   b. Allow proper segregation and identification of material during manufacturing and packaging
   c. Provide for ease in maintaining cleanliness and for avoiding contamination
   d. Provide suitable sampling facilities
   e. Provide adequate laboratory facilities
   f. Provide proper storage for final products
2. Equipment is:
   a. Properly located
   b. Adequate for the required operations
   c. Constructed to facilitate cleaning
   d. Properly maintained
3. Raw materials are controlled by:
   a. Establishment of suitable specifications
   b. Development of adequate test procedures
   c. Specific identification markings
   d. Proper storage conditions
   e. Adequate sampling
   f. Appropriate testing
   g. Requiring compliance with specifications
   h. Providing for quality control release
   i. Maintaining records and samples whenever appropriate
4. Manufacturing operations are controlled by:
   a. Use of suitable batch numbering system
   b. Preparation of formula or batch records
   c. Checking of ingredients (identity, weight, measure)
   d. Maintaining identity during processing
   e. Checking quality during processing
   f. Checking yield against theory
   g. Adequate sampling and testing
   h. Requiring compliance with specifications
   i. Maintaining appropriate records and samples
5. Packaging and finishing are controlled by:
   a. Establishment of specifications for packaging and packaging operations
   b. A formal procedure providing for the inspection and issuance of packaging materials including labels and labeling
   c. Providing for the proper disposition of unused labels and labeling
   d. Use of suitable batch, lot, or control numbers
   e. Maintaining identity of product before and during packaging
   f. Checking final yield against theoretical yield
   g. Sampling and checking for compliance with specifications
   h. Providing for release by quality control
   i. Maintaining appropriate records and samples
6. Finished stock quality is maintained by:
   a. Providing proper storage conditions
   b. Collection and review of stability data
   c. Investigating all significant complaints concerning quality of products
   d. Providing for the disposition of returned goods

Based on the above principles, the following quality control standards for drugs have been adopted at the University of Michigan Pharmacy Department (6). These standards may be modified depending on organizational pattern, available space and facilities, and scope and volume of preparations manufactured.

RAW MATERIALS

Specifications

To manufacture finished pharmaceuticals satisfactorily, superior raw materials are necessary. Thus, the control effort begins with the incoming materials, making it necessary to decide on the specifications (USP, BP, etc) to ensure materials of proper quality. This function is performed through the cooperative efforts of assay and control and purchasing. Many times the items specified will be for USP or ACS reagent grade materials, perhaps with certain modifications such as density, mesh size, freedom from pyrogens, viscosity (7). However, very definite specifications will become necessary for many materials that may be otherwise graded

TABLE 38.1 Raw Material Specifications: Pyridoxal Phosphate

Pyridoxal phosphate: $C_8H_{10}NO_6P$, mol wt 247.15. Pyridoxal phosphate contains not less than 99% of $C_8H_{10}NO_6P$.

Description: It is a light yellow crystalline powder.

Loss on drying: Dry at 105° C. It is not more than 1% of its weight.

Melting range: Class Ia 142-145° C decomposition.

Identification: The solution used for assay exhibits the same characteristics spectrum as the reference standard (in solution 0.1 N phosphoric acid).

Assay: Prepare a solution of the crystals to contain 20 µg/ml in 0.1 N phosphoric acid solution and compare with a solution of reference pyridoxal phosphate of the same strength using the 295 mµ wavelength on a UV spectrophotometer. The absorbance is 95-105% of the reference standard.

Drug Analysis Laboratory
University Hospital
JAP 10/1977

(Table 38.1). In such cases, one alternative method is the acceptance of the material based on the manufacturer's information on assay specifications, physical characteristics, and purity, with particular emphasis on heavy metal contents.

Receipt and Lot Number Assignment

A lot is a single batch of raw material that may be in one or more containers but is represented by a single manufacturer's control number. As each lot of incoming material from the supplier is received, the assay and control section is notified, and the lot is quarantined to prevent use until tested. Each manufacturer's lot is then reassigned a lot number from the crude stock inventory record by which the material is subsequently identified until it all has been used. The lot number is assigned by a consecutive number system

in order of receipt. This lot number must have distinguishing characteristics that will avoid confusion with any numbers already placed on the container by the supplier and is placed on a supplementary label that is attached to the container.

Crude Stock Inventory Record (Fig. 38.1)

This record is kept in a log book and provides the following information: (1) name of chemical, (2) chemical grade, (3) quantity received, (4) date received, (5) name of manufacturer, (6) manufacturer's lot or batch number, (7) lot number assignment and expiration date, (8) "approve for use" or rejected and signature of the analyst.

Identity and Purity

An examination for identification, purity, and assay of the raw material should be performed. If the material is USP, NF, or reagent grade, the minimum assay of the manufacturer is assumed. If it is not graded as mentioned above, an assay report should be obtained from the manufacturer, and a decision made whether the material meets the desired specifications; otherwise the minimum assay will be performed. However, assays are usually performed on certain labile chemicals such as calcium chloride (anhydrous) and magnesium sulfate, which readily gain or lose moisture.

Tests for Identity and Purity

Purity and identification can be tested by various methods. It is not usually necessary to perform all the official tests but only certain minimum chemical and physical tests sufficient to identify the material and ascertain its purity. For example, a mixed melting point or optical rotation determination may suffice for purity tests; a simple chemical-

Lot # (Pharmacy)	Name of Chemical	Grade	Date received	Mfg.	Lot# Exp.Date	Quantity received	remarks	Approval date
UM601	Sodium chloride, cryst.	USP	7-7-77	XYZ Chem.	000726 None	2X100lbs	Fiber drums	JAP 7-8-77
UM602	Alcohol 95%	USP	7-8-77	USChem	TI3366 none	1X54 Gal.	metal drum	7-8-77 AR
UM603	Dextrose,Anhydrous	USP	7-10-77	Starch Prod.	MBKX none	5X100 lbs.	Bags	PMJ 7-12-77
UM604								
UM605								
UM606								

FIGURE 38.1 Crude stock inventory record.

Name of Chemical: Dextrose, anhydrous U.S.P.

Pharmacy Lot #	Description	Identification	Solubility	Specific Rotation	Acidity	Color of solution	Heavy metals	soluble starch	Approval	Analyst date
UM603	passes	passes	passes	passes	passes	passes	0.0005 %	passes	approved	PMJ 7/12/77

FIGURE 38.2 Crude stock control record.

color reaction, characteristic odor, taste, or physical appearance could identify the drug. In fact, physical tests such as mixed melting points, refractive index, and optical rotation may be interpreted to indicate the purity and also to serve as an empirical check on the assay and identification. The infrared spectrometric assays are quite useful in characterization of various organic compounds.

Expiration Date

An expiration date has now become mandatory for all commercially available dosage forms, and this same number might be used as an upper limit on storage time if the commercial product is repackaged in the pharmacy. One must bear in mind, however, that conditions of storage or type of container into which the dosage form is transferred or stored may shorten the expiration date. Here, as in all cases of repackaging, one must remember that the repackager assumes part of any liability when repackaging a commercially available dosage form.

Expiration dates for extemporaneously compounded and in-house formulas are usually established by the formula committee (see below) and are based on stability date of ingredients, turnover time based on use rate, and any other significant information that might be gleaned from the literature. Many times, an expiration date must be empirically assigned.

Crude Stock Control Record

The examination is reported in the crude stock control record (Fig. 38.2). The system usually consists of a file of cards for each raw material and contains the lot number, information of identification and purity, signature of the analyst, approval for release, and the date released. The cards are filed alphabetically by the name of the raw material. There should be space available to enter the type of tests performed.

Approval for Use

No raw material can be used unless it has been approved for use by the assay and control section. If the raw material meets the specifications, a label is attached to the containers.

The label (Fig. 38.3) should contain the following information: (1) "approved for use," (2) date released by the assay and control section, (3) lot number, (4) signature of the analyst.

PHARMACEUTICAL PRODUCTION

Formula of the Product

Only approved manufacturing formulas and raw materials must be used. No additions, deletions, or modifications of the approved formula and procedure can be performed without the approval of the formula committee.

Formula Committee

This committee usually consists of at least three qualified pharmacists, including the supervisor of assay control. Its purpose is to establish formulas and procedures for all products produced in the pharmacy and to approve any revisions in these formulas or procedures.

Master Formula Card

The approved formula is entered on the master formula card (Fig. 38.4), which is kept on permanent file. The master form gives complete information and specifications

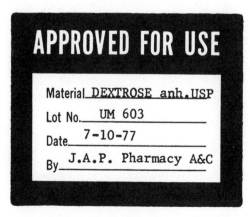

FIGURE 38.3 Product approval label.

PHARMACY DEPARTMENT

Master Formula Card

		Attach Label Here	

Product: Sterile Solution: Ethanol 8.66% v/v and   Batch No. 03238411EXP 3/24/84-5P.M.

Sodium Chloride 8.766% w/v (200 ml will yield 300 mMol of each)

	Lot No.	Ingredients	Amount	Weighed By	Checked By
1	UM-6011	Sodium Chloride USP	87.66 g	VB	EGC
2	UM-100/2	Absolute alcohol 100% USP	86.60 ml	VB	EGC
3	Abbott XYZ-Z	Water for injection qs	1000.0 ml	VB	EGC
4					
5					
6					
7					
8					

Directions for manufacture:

1. Mix well.

2. Pass through a 0.2 micron membrane filter.

3. Package into a 200 ml evacuated sterile bottle.

4. Inspect.

5. Label.

6. Send 2 samples to assay & control.

Amt. of EtOH for 300 mMol

EtOH M.W. 46.07
1 mMol = 46.07

$$\frac{300\ mMol}{x} = \frac{1\ mMol}{46.07}$$

x = 13821 mg or 13.821 g

Amt. EtOH in ml

(spec. gr.) d = 0.798 or 0.798 g/ml

$$\frac{13.821\ g}{x} = \frac{0.798\ g}{1\ ml}$$

x = 17.32 ml EtOH 100%

Final Strength of Solution

% of EtOH v/v

$$\frac{17.32\ ml}{200\ ml} = \frac{x}{100}$$

x = 8.66%

Packaging and Labeling

Containers Normally Required:

                                     1 × 125 ml

Theoretical Yield 5 × 200 ml   Actual Yield 4 × 200 ml   Reason for discrepancy, if any: Loss in filter, rinse.

Manufactured by V. Bernard   Time 1.5 hr   Control Action:

     Assistant S. Marchant   Time 2.0 hr   By JAP   Date 3/23/84

IN-PROCESS CONTROL DATA are to be recorded on the back of this sheet.

FIGURE 38.4 Master formula card.

on each formula: (1) name of ingredients and its chemical grade, (2) quantity of ingredients, (3) a space for the lot number and expiration date of ingredients, (4) spaces for the signatures of the persons doing the weighing and checking, (5) complete directions for preparation, (6) packaging instructions, (7) labeling instructions, (8) spaces for the signature of the preparer and helper, (9) time spent, (10) space for approval for release, (11) control number and expiration date of batch, (12) theoretical and actual yield, (13) storage instructions, (14) in-process control directions for the compounding pharmacist, such as tablet disintegration and weight variation tests and specific gravity, and (15) method of collection of samples for assay and control unit.

Nonestablished Formulas

New or nonestablished formulas should be reviewed and then established by the Formula Committee for use by the production section. A pilot study plan should be devised whereby trial batches can be analyzed for stability under accelerated storage-aging conditions and at various time intervals. If the results receive a satisfactory evaluation, the formula is released for production. Records of these studies are to be kept in a special log book on product development and research.

Manufacturing Process

The production pharmacist should notify the supervisor of assay and control of the products to be prepared that day in order to facilitate quick analysis of a batch if warranted before packaging or reprocessing.

Daily Production Log Book

The manufacturing section should keep a daily production log book, entering the following information: (1) name of product, (2) control number and expiration date, (3) batch quantity and number of packages, (4) date manufactured, (5) signature of the pharmacist in charge of operation, and (6) "approved for use" (to be entered upon decision of assay and control to approve or reject the batch).

Working Formula or Batch Card

When a preparation is to be manufactured, a duplicate of the master formula manufacturing card is made, and this copy serves as a worksheet, administrative control form, and production record.

In-Process Controls

Every effort must be made to ensure quality preparations. Although all compounding procedures require the skill and knowledge of the pharmacist, certain procedures require special attention. The production of sterile products or research tablet formulations require additional control measures.

Certain control and inspections should be made routinely by the pharmacist during the production of all types of products. He will enter the lot number of the approved raw material on the formula worksheet to identify the materials used. He will check the weights or volume of each ingredient to avoid error. The pharmacist will then perform certain pharmaceutical tests on selected products during production. These tests will be indicated on the formula card and will include such tests as pH, particulate matter, vacuum check of containers, tightness of the container caps, and package leakage. Any discrepancies of any nature should be investigated and explained satisfactorily before the process is continued.

PACKAGING AND LABELING

General Procedures of Packaging

The packaging operation should be carefully performed and supervised. It may be necessary to perform periodic mixing during the packaging operation to ensure uniformity of the product in each package, particularly during the packaging of suspensions or other preparations that have the tendency to settle out or stratify on standing.

Clean bottles should be used, all closures should be tight, and labels should be uniformly placed.

Approval before Packaging

The finished product must be checked and approved by assay and control before packaging (except the commercial products).

Specifications of Containers

All packaging materials such as bottles, vials, closures, and other related items should be used and examined with the same care that is given to raw materials. The packages are specified on the master formula card for each product.

Labeling on Stock Containers

Each product and its stock container should be labeled properly by including (1) the name of the products, (2) active ingredients and quantity of each, (3) control number and auxiliary labels if necessary, and (4) expiration date.

The type of label to be used and the information to be included on the label itself will be noted in the master formula card. If a proprietary name is used, the generic name should also appear on the label.

Control Number System

The control number consists of eight digits, designating the month, day, and year when the product was manufactured or packaged. The last two digits identify the unit involved and batch number (Fig. 38.5). By this system of control numbers one may (1) identify each production batch; (2) establish the history of the batch, source of each ingredient, record of tests made on each ingredient, as well as on the final product, identity of individuals responsible for each step in the manufacturing process, and quantity manufactured; and (3) provide a means of recalling the product if necessary.

```
        MONTH    DAY    YEAR    UNIT    BATCH NO.
         07      07      77      0          0


     Unit Identification Code
     0                Allergy laboratory
     1-2              Small volume sterile products
     3                Pre-packaging tablets and capsules
     4                Pre-packaging liquids
     5                Large volume parenterals
     6                Stain and reagents
     7-9              Bulk non-sterile compounding

  The first batch number for each unit begins with "0" e.g., first batch
  number, for Allergy laboratory will be control number 07077700,
  second batch 07077701 etc.
  Stains and reagent laboratory
     First control number will be 07077760
                       Second 07077761
                         Third 07077762
```

FIGURE 38.5   Control number system.

Quarantine Period

All manufactured products will be placed in quarantine until such time as they are approved or rejected by assay and control.

Samples for Assay

Properly selected random samples of the batch of finished product, clearly labeled, should be submitted to assay and control for all sterile products, all products for internal use, and for selected external products so designated. The number and size of samples and the method of their collection are dependent on the nature of the product. Information concerning collection of samples will be found on the master formula card. The master formula batch card copy will also accompany the samples.

CONTROL OF FINISHED PRODUCT

Control During the Manufacturing Process

The role of the production pharmacist in this activity has been discussed previously. It is the responsibility of assay and control to check the procedure and finished product and see that proper corrections, if necessary, are made before packaging. Assay and control will also check manufacturing procedures from time to time. The most frequent errors that occur are errors in weighing and measuring, wrong ingredients, and improper mixing.

Control Samples

The method of collection of samples has been discussed previously. These random samples will become the basis of analysis of the entire batch of the product manufactured.

A sample of the product should be retained for reference and periodically analyzed as a check on stability. It may be necessary to recall products that have lost potency more rapidly than anticipated or that, for some other reason, are no longer acceptable. Those products that have an expiration date should also be checked periodically. Such studies should be recorded in a log book on product development and research.

Methods of Analysis

Although the majority of the methods conform to the official techniques described in the *United States Pharmacopeia, National Formulary, British Pharmacopeia, Pharmacopeia Internationalis, Method of Analysis of the Association of Official Agricultural Chemists*, etc, other sophisticated techniques such as high-performance liquid chromatography or gas liquid chromatography, which may be more efficient and just as accurate, may be employed (7). All assay techniques used by the assay and control lab are written and documented and kept in a plastic-covered, loose-leaf binder.

Every type of product made must be subjected to careful, intelligent scrutiny and tests. Nothing should be overlooked or taken for granted.

Assay and Control Records

These records on the finished products consist of the following:

Daily Assay Log Book. The records of analyses of products routinely produced are kept in the log book. It includes the following information: (1) techniques (weighing, measurement, mathematical calculations, methods, other necessary data), (2) name of the product, (3) control number and expiration date, (4) date, (5) book and page number of the log book, and (6) signature of the analyst.

The pertinent data, as well as the book and page numbers, must be transferred to the product control report.

UNIVERSITY OF MICHIGAN HOSPITAL
PHARMACY DEPARTMENT

PRODUCT CONTROL CARD

STERILE SOLUTION: ETHANOL 8.66% v/v and
SODIUM CHLORIDE 8.766%, 200 ml

UM LOT No.	Date Recvd.	Exp. date	Control ref.	Sterility test	pH	Particulate matter	Ethanol % L.A.	Sodium Chloride	No. of Containers	Approval date
03238411	3/23/84	3/24/84	84-103	Membrane Filtration	6.8	None	99.8% GLC	98.0% USP	2	3/23/84

FIGURE 38.6 Product control record.

Product Control Report. This report contains the summary form of pertinent assay data of products routinely formulated (Fig. 38.6):

1. Name of the product
2. Control number and expiration date
3. Book and page numbers of the daily log book
4. Drug assayed for
5. Method of assay (USP, NF, IP, HPLC, GLC, etc)
6. Results of the assay
7. Other tests:
   a. pH
   b. Viscosity
   c. Tablet disintegration, hardness, and weight variation
   d. Specific gravity
   e. Sterility
   f. Pyrogen tests
   g. Alcohol determination
   h. Refractive index
   i. Others
8. Disposition of the product—whether accepted or rejected
9. Date released
10. Signature of the analyst

It is filed alphabetically according to the name of the product.

Log Book on Product Development and Research. This is a record of assays performed on investigational formulas and special products not routinely manufactured. All research data are also included.

Approval of Product for Use

If the results of the analysis meet the requirements of quality control, the product is approved and released from quarantine. The decision for release or rejection of the batch will be forwarded to the manufacturing section, which will record the decision in the daily manufacturing log. All rejected batches will either be corrected by dilution or fortification and submitted again for analysis or will be destroyed.

All approved batches will be designated by the "Approved For Use" label (Fig. 38.3), and this label is attached to all bulk stock containers. Then the stock containers and prepackaged dispensing unit sizes may be released.

PRODUCTION RECORDS

Production Records

The production data on all products will be entered on the record card whether approved for dispensing or rejected and recommended for destruction. The record is filed alphabetically by the name of the product and contains the following information: (1) name of the product, (2) control number and expiration date, (3) batch quantity, and (4) annual total batch quantity.

The batches that have been rejected and subsequently destroyed should be entered distinctively, such as by the use of red lettering.

Packaging Record of Formulated Products

It is recognized that some of the products formulated are packaged into (1) stock containers and subsequently pack-

aged into smaller dispensing units and/or (2) prepackaged into single units directly (8). To facilitate the maintenance of records, the production pharmacist should enter the pertinent packaging data on the packaging report.

Packaging Report

This report is sent by the production pharmacist to the supervisor of assay and control, who will check and approve the report and then submit it to inventory control for keeping the proper records in the package control records.

The package report includes (1) name of the product and strength or concentration, (2) control number and expiration date, (3) quantity packaged, (4) size of package, (5) type of containers used, (6) number of packages, (7) time spent and by whom, (8) label used, and (9) approved by assay and control.

Packaging and Extemporaneous Compounding Record

This record provides the following information (Fig. 38.7): (1) name of the product, strength or concentration, or formulation, (2) manufacturer, (3) control number and expiration date, (4) quantity packaged, (5) size and type of container, (6) the product label and auxiliary labels, (7) stability, (8) description of the product, (9) filled by, and (10) approved by.

Reconstitution of Medications

Reconstitution and packaging of oral or parenteral antibiotics for single-unit package must be segregated in order to avoid cross-contamination into other products (8), preferably using separate rooms and laminar flow hoods. Control records must be maintained, as described previously for other drugs.

Quality Control of IV Additive Service

A hospital pharmacy IV admixture service may involve the use of varying numbers of pharmacists and technicians. In addition to the pharmacist's concern for physical, chemical, or therapeutic incompatibility of ingredients, these solutions must be monitored for possible in-process microbial contamination. This microbial contamination of the compounded IV fluids may result from faulty compounding technique or malfunction of equipment, such as a perforated HEPA filter in the laminar flow hood or contaminated vacuum lines or syringes (9,10). Sterility test monitoring of this compounding laboratory on a daily basis must be implemented. Proper performance of the laminar flow hood must be routinely checked for breaks in the HEPA filters, either by environmental health specialists or qualified maintenance personnel. A suitable method for surveillance of bacterial comtamination must be enforced rigorously. The membrane filtration technique has been found to be accurate (11). The identification of the positive cultures can be performed by the microbiology laboratory of the hospital.

Tabulation of test results and identification of positive cultures are essential information for the Hospital Infections

UNIVERSITY HOSPITAL PHARMACY
ANN ARBOR, MICHIGAN   LABEL SAMPLE

PACKAGING AND
EXTEMPORANEOUS COMPOUNDING RECORD

Name of Drug _____   Formulation:

Dosage Strength or Conc. _____

Stability _____

Size & Type of Container _____

Quantity per Unit _____

Auxiliary Labels _____

Date	Ingredients Used	Mfr.	Mfr. Lot. No.	Exp. Date	No. of Units	Pharmacy Control No.	Pkg. By	Appr. By

FIGURE 38.7 Packaging and extemporaneous compounding record.

Committee in assessing possible origin of any extraordinary hospital infections.

Investigational New Drug Application and Double-Blind Studies

Assay and control also provides pertinent quality control information to the medical staff in preparation of the required investigational new drug application for the sections on formulations, assay, packaging, and stability (12).

Maintenance of records for double-blind studies may be coordinated by assay and control with other involved units.

Therapeutic Monitoring and Toxicology

As an outgrowth of assay and control in the institutional pharmacy practice, therapeutic monitoring of drugs can be considered quality control of the drug dosage administration process. This assumption is a reality as demonstrated by Curtis et al (13). The therapeutic monitoring service is not only a valuable aid to inpatient treatment and convalescence, but also to outpatient counseling and therapy.

REFERENCES

1. Current good manufacturing practice in manufacture processing, packaging and holding. *Fed Reg* Part 133, 28 FR 6385, June 20, 1963.
2. Byers TE: FDA regulations and unit of use packaging. *FDA Handbook of Total Drug Quality.* FDA Publication No. 64, Rockville, MD, U.S. Department of Health, Education and Welfare, July 1971, pp 62-67.
3. *General Principles of Total Control of Quality in the Drug Industry.* Washington, DC, Pharmaceutical Manufacturers Association, May 3, 1961.
4. Chafetz L: Considerations in equipping a hospital pharmacy control laboratory. *Am J Hosp Pharm* 22:573-577, 1965.
5. Benya TJ: Records—a control device in production. *Am J Hosp Pharm* 23:385-395, 1966.
6. *Procedure Manual Quality Control Drugs.* Ann Arbor, The University of Michigan Medical Center, Pharmacy Department.
7. Feldman EG: The relationship of control procedures to drug standards. *Am J Hosp Pharm* 21:388-396, 1964.
8. Patel JA, Curtis EG, Phillips GL: Quality control guidelines for single unit packaging of parenterals in hospital pharmacy. *Am J Hosp Pharm* 29:947-951, 1972.
9. Arnold TR, Helper CD: Bacterial contamination of intravenous fluids opened in unsterile air. *Am J Hosp Pharm* 28:614-623, 1971.
10. Deeb EN, Natsios GA: Contamination of intravenous fluids by bacteria and fungi during preparation and administration. *Am J Hosp Pharm* 28:764-767, 1971.
11. Miller CM, Furtado D, et al: Evaluation of three methods for detecting low-level bacterial contamination in intravenous solutions. *Am J Hosp Pharm* 39:1302-1305, 1982.
12. Patel JA: Chemical control information on investigational new drug application (IND). *Am J Hosp Pharm* 26:178-179, 1969.
13. Curtis EG, Patel JA: Pharmacy based analytical toxicology service. *Am J Hosp Pharm* 32:685-693, 1975.

CHAPTER 39

Hospital Pharmacy
Equipment and Supplies

THOMAS R. BROWN

The opportunity to purchase new equipment and supplies for hospital pharmacy use is usually an exciting experience, especially when the purchase will improve professional capability. However, the procurement process can lead to anxiety and frustration when the process becomes tedious and time consuming, and the results are unsatisfactory. In order to initiate a new patient care system, or plan, renovate, or remodel a facility or similar project, this procurement process plays an important role.

The procurement process for equipment and supplies requires an organized effort that will minimize the likelihood of problems and increase the potential for success. The process begins with a decision concerning what is to be purchased and then, more specifically, what features or characteristics are required to fulfill the need. Obviously, the type of item to be purchased dictates the degree of specifications required. The purchasing procedures in any given institution may well define the procurement process at this point, but surveillance to expedite purchases may be required.

The more important components of the process of purchasing seem to involve the early considerations in the selection process and involve a number of considerations. Although many are self-evident, they are certainly important and deserve reasonably exhaustive consideration.

EQUIPMENT CONSIDERATIONS

Before purchasing an item of equipment, a thorough investigation of motives, needs, and practical matters regarding the equipment is essential. A thought process that is not reasonably exhaustive may lead to a purchase that is disappointing at best. Consider the following items and questions in developing the logic for the purchase of equipment:

1. Functionality. Is the item what the department needs? Will it improve the service? Will it be a dteriment to the service? What functions will it serve? Will the item perform the functions in a ''hospital-specific'' way?
2. Personnel. Does the pharmacy currently have personnel who can operate the equipment? If it involves a totally new environment, can current personnel adjust to a new way of working? Can the current facility manage the new equipment as well as personnel? Many other questions regarding personnel may be important locally.
3. Cost. Is the equipment worth the expense? Can the cost be recovered? Will the equipment generate new revenue? Is the expense unavoidable? Is the item comparatively reasonable in cost? Cost is a factor that must be weighed carefully, particularly relative to the quality of the item considered for purchase.
4. Maintenance. Is the item difficult to service, clean, repair, etc? Are repair facilities available? Are service agreements available, and, if so, what is the cost? Can the item be repaired in house? Are maintenance manuals available (also repair manuals)? What about backup support if repair takes a long period of time? Are repair parts easy to obtain, and are they expensive? Is telephone assistance available for repair? Many others.
5. Ease of use. Are instruction manuals provided? Are they understandable? What about setup and demonstration after purchase? Are there special courses for users? Is there telephone assistance available for problems with use? Many others.
6. Portability. Will the equipment need to be moved? Can it be moved? Is the equipment flexible enough to meet changing needs or new facilities? Will alterations be needed if the equipment is moved?
7. Lease vs purchase. Is the equipment a short- or long-term need? What are the advantages of leasing? Is a service agreement included with leasing? Is it possible to lease now with a purchase option? There are many things to consider that may save money and headaches.
8. Aesthetics. Be sure to consider color, size, shape, placement, etc, in order to maintain or improve a pleasant workplace. Although often overlooked, it may be possible to obtain the needed equipment with all desired functions and aesthetics with little additional investment.

9. Shared equipment. Can a piece of equipment be shared with another department? Is it desirable to share the item?

10. Reliability. Is the manufacturer reputable? Are expendable supplies required that create a dependency on a single source in order to operate the equipment? Will supplies be reasonably available? Consider alternate sources.

11. State-of-art. Is this item last year's model? Will the next version (if forseeable) make the current model obsolete? Can state-of-the-art be updated and maintained? Will the purchased model have to be replaced to keep up-to-date?

12. Special requirements. Does the equipment require special alterations to the building or will it fit nicely into available space? What about requirements for water, electricity, light, etc? Will it fit through the door? What about special temperature requirements? Many other factors must be considered.

These are but a few considerations that must be given careful, early attention when deciding to purchase an item. There are many that must be considered locally—do not overlook them.

SCOPE AND LIMITATIONS

The starting point for this compilation of suppliers of equipment and supplies was the first edition of this text. The scope of the compilation is limited to those types of equipment and supplies the hospital pharmacist would need in planning a new facility or planning the expansion or remodeling of an existing one. It was outside the scope of this compilation to include drug or drug-related products, equipment required for the large-scale manufacture of injections, tablets, capsules, liquids, etc, or to include commonly used articles that can be obtained locally by hospital pharmacists, such as common office equipment and supplies, carpets, typewriters, etc.

The section headings below indicate the type of equipment and supplies that can be found within. The "Miscellaneous Equipment and Supplies" section encompasses a wide variety of items that could not be placed in one of the other nine sections but did deserve to be included in the compilation. Because of the dynamics of the industries that support pharmacy practice, particularly those dealing with equipment and supplies, it is virtually impossible to guarantee that an individual supplier still offers specific equipment and/or supplies.

ADMINISTRATIVE FURNISHINGS AND FILING EQUIPMENT AND SUPPLIES

Acme Visible Records, Inc. Crozet, VA 22932	Automated and manual card filing and retrieval system; trays for hinged cards (or card books)
Avery Label Co. 777 E. Foothill Blvd. Azusa, CA 91702	Office labels and aids
Blickman Casework and Design Corp. Weehawken, NJ 07087	Pharmacy casework
Browne-Morse Co. 110 E. Broadway Muskegon, MI 49443	Office furniture and accessories; bookcases, side files; filing cabinets
Cresco Systems 563 Alder St. Fall River, MA 02722	Narcotic and controlled drugs inventory control record system
A.B. Dick (local representative)	Photocopying and duplicating equipment
Drug Package, Inc. O'Fallon, MO 63366	Record filing system
Equipto 225 S. Highland Ave. Aurora, IL 60507	General office furniture
Fisher Scientific Co. 203 Fisher Bldg. Pittsburgh, PA 15219	Office furniture; filing cabinets
Globe-Weis System Co. P.O. Box 398 Wauseon, OH 43567	Filing and general office equipment and supplies
Grant Rapids Sectional Equipment Co. P.O. Box 6306 Grand Rapids, MI 49506	Office furniture and accessories
Hauserman, Inc. 5711 Grant Ave. Cleveland, OH 44105	Modular office furniture
IBM Corporation (local representative)	Photocopiers
Kewaunee Manufacturing Co. P.O. Box 5400 Statesville, NC 28677	Metal filing cabinets
Kole Enterprises P.O. Box 33152 Miami, FL 33152	Pull drawer files, metal filing cabinets; office furniture and accessories
Lyon Metal Products, Inc. 1933 Montgomery St. Aurora, IL 60507	Desk and counter filing cabinets; office desks and accessories; book cases
Herman Miller, Inc. Zeeland, MI 49464	Office furniture and accessories
Modern Office Devices, Inc. 731 Hempstead Turnpike Franklin Square, NY 11010	Prescription files; numbering machines
Myrtle Desk Co. P.O. Box 1750 High Point, NC 27261	Office furniture
Owens-Corning Fiberglas Corp. (local representative)	Office acoustical equipment (partitions)
Randomatic Data Systems, Inc. 216 Robbins Ave. Trenton, NJ 08638	Automated filing systems
Remington Rand (local representative)	Manual index filing system; filing cabinets; automatic filing systems
Rockaway Metal Products Corp. 175 Roger Ave. Inwood, Long Island, NY 11696	Modular work stations; office furniture; movable partitions
Roto Photo Co., Inc. 2835 N. Western Ave. Chicago, IL 60618	Multipurpose filing system
Sherwood Medical Inc. 1831 Olive St. St. Louis, MO 63103	Revolving filing equipment
Steelcase, Inc. 1120 36th Street, SE Grand Rapids, MI 49501	Modular office furniture and filing systems

Wang Laboratories Inc. Tewksbury, MA 01876	Automated typing systems
Westinghouse Electric Corp. Architectural Systems Div. 4300 36th St. SE Grand Rapids, MI 49508	Office furniture; movable partition systems, storage systems
Wheeldex, Inc. P.O. Box 2028 Cedar Rapids, Iowa 52406	Manual and mechanized filing equipment; rotary files
Xerox Corporation (local representative)	Photo copiers and printers

COMMUNICATION EQUIPMENT

Alden Electronic and Impulse Recording Equipment Co., Inc. Westboro, MA 01581	Facsimile communications systems
American District Telegraph Co. 1 World Trade Center Suite 9200 New York, NY 10048	Security alarm systems
Bell System Data Communication Service (local representative)	Two-way communications system; data transmitting systems; teletype equipment
Dictaphone Corporation (local representative)	Communications equipment; dictation systems
Dukane Corporation Communication Systems Div. 2900 Dukane Drive St. Charles, IL 60174	Nurse/patient communication systems; intercom systems; sound systems
Executone Inc. 29-10 Thomson Ave. Long Island City, NY 11101	Communication systems; intercoms; alarm systems; paging systems
General Electric Co. Data Communication Products Dept. Waynesboro, VA 22980	Communication systems
Magnavox Co. (local representative)	Facsimile copying and transmitting equipment
Motorola Communications and Electronic Inc. (local representative)	Communication systems; music systems; public address paging systems
Picker Briggs Corp. 4135 W. 150th St. Cleveland, OH 44135	Audio and visual hospital communication systems
RCA Service Company (local representative)	Communication systems; entertainment systems; visual nurse call systems
Telautograph Corporation 8700 Bellanca Ave. Los Angeles, CA 90045	Telewriter systems; medication order communication systems
Talos Systems, Inc. 7419 E. Helm Drive Scottsdale, AZ 85260	Voice/graphic communications systems
Victor Graphic Systems 95F Hoffman Lane S. Central Islip, NY 11722	Automated handwriting communications systems (facsimile transmitting equipment)
Xerox Corp. (local representative)	Facsimile communications systems

COMPUTER SYSTEMS

The following vendors should be contacted regarding hardware and software:

Advanced Concepts & Programs for Institutions, Ltd. (ACPI)
1 Old Country Raod
Carle Place, NY 11514

American Druggist Blue Book
Data Center
875 Mahler Road, Suite 200
Burlingame, CA 94010

AMI Professional Hospital Services
12960 Coral Tree Place
Los Angeles, CA 90066

Apothetech
23800 Hawthorne Blvd.
Torrance, CA 98505

ARC Data Systems, Inc.
185 Cross St.
Fort Lee, NJ 07024

Autoscript, Inc.
11 Mountain Ave.
Bloomfield, CT 06002

BAC-Data Medical Information Systems, Inc.
Campus Road
Totawa, NJ 07512

Bard MedSystems Division
87 Concord St.
North Reading, MA 01864

BDM Information Systems, Ltd.
3032 Louise St.
Saskatoon, Saskatchewan
Canada S7J 3L8

Burroughs Hospital Information Systems (BHIS)
Burroughs Corporation
Health Care Services
2101 East Rexford Road,
Suite 203
Charlotte, NC 28215

Cedar Systems, Ltd.
1224 West Main St., 6th Floor
Charlottesville, VA 22903-2864

Comco Tec
825 North Cass Ave., Suite 104
Westmont, IL 60559

Commercial Computer Services, Inc.
3000 Dundee Road, Suite 402
Northbrook, IL 60062

Compucare, Inc.
8200 Greensboro Drive, Suite 800
McLean, VA 22102

Computer Synergy, Inc.
2201 Broadway, Suite 401
Oakland, CA 94612

Continental Healthcare Systems
8900 Indian Creek Parkway
Bldg. 6, Suite 550
Overland Park, KS 66210

Data Med, Inc.
155 26th Ave., Southeast
Minneapolis, MN 55414

Datacare, Inc.
2602 Franklin Road, Southwest
Roanoke, VA 24014

Dataform Systems, Inc.
5543 East Blvd., Northwest
Canton, OH 44718

Datamedix
Route 1
Sharon, MA 02067

Datastat
National Data Corporation (NDC)
1 NDC Plaza
Atlanta, GA 30329

DCC-PHARM
Dynamic Control Corporation
1311 South Semoran Blvd.
Winter Park, FL 32792

Digimedics Incorporated
501 Cedar St.
Santa Cruz, CA 95060

DIMES, Inc.
71 Elton Ave.
Watertown, MA 02172

DOSE Pharmacy Systems
1645 Dorchester Ave.
Plano, TX 75075

Doxsis Systems
6335 Southeast 82nd Ave.
Portland, OR 97266

Electronic Data Systems Corporation (EDS)
7171 Forest Lane
Dallas, TX 75230

Enterprise Systems, Inc.
233 Waukegan Road, Suite 100 East
Bannockburn, IL 60015

Erudite Systems
Weirton, WV 26062

Filetti, Inc.
241 Frontage Road, Suite 46
Burr Ridge, IL 60521

Florida Hospital Systems
2626 West Oakland Park Blvd.
Suite 110
Fort Lauderdale, FL 33311

Gamma Systems Services
1027 5th Ave.North, Suite A
St. Petersburg, FL 33705

General Computer Corporation
2045 Midway Drive, P.O. Box 304
Twinsburg, OH 44087

Health Care Log
Health Care Logistics, Inc.
934 South Washington, P.O. Box 25
Circleville, OH 43113

Health Information Systems, Inc.
4522 Fort Hamilton Parkway
Brooklyn, NY 11219

Honeywell Information Systems
200 Smith St.
Waltham, MA 02154

Hospital Computer Systems, Inc.
Professional Plaza
Colts Neck, NJ 07222

Hospital Data Center of Virginia, Inc.
962 Norfolk Square
Norfolk, VA 23502

Hugh Cort Computers
4 Office Park Circle, Suite 108
Birmingham, AL 35253

IBM Patient Care System
400 Paron's Pond Drive
Franklin Lakes, NJ 07417

Intermountain Health Care
Management Systems Division
36 South State
Salt Lake City, UT 84111

KIYO Systems
13722 Golden West St.
P.O. Box 330
Westminster, CA 92683

Laurel Mountain Software
1318 Route 271 South
Ligonier, PA 15658

Lenco Laboratories, Inc.
P.O. Box 862
Lynbrook, NY 11563

MacBick
Bard MedSystems Division
558 Central Ave.
Murray Hill, NJ 07974

MAI Application Software
Corporation
18010 Skypark Circle, Suite 100
Irvine, CA 92708

Mastercare Pharmacy Systems
3801 Gaston Ave., Suite 301
Dallas, TX 75246

Mavis Computer Systems
11257 Coloma Road
Rancho Cordova, CA 95670

McDonnell Douglas Health
Services (MCAUTO)
5575 Campus Parkway
Hazelwood, MO 63042

Medical Cybernetics, Inc.
133 South Main St.
Salisbury, NC 28144

Medical Engineering, Inc. (MEI)
2675 Winkler Ave., Suite 108
Fort Myers, FL 33901

Medical Information Technology,
Inc. (MEDITECH)
255 Bent St.
Cambridge, MA 02141

Medical Scientific International
Corporation
5640 Nicholson Lane, Suite 111
Rockville, MD 20852

Medication Services, Inc. (MSI)
714 C St., Suite 2
San Rafael, CA 94901

Mediflex Systems Corporation
990 Grove St.
Evanston, IL 60201

Medi-Span, Inc.
P.O. Box 459
110 North 9th St.
Zionsville, IN 46077-0459

Medlab, Div. of Control Data
Corporation
P.O. Box O (HQVOO3)
Minneapolis, MN 55440

Medpro Pharmacy System
HBO and Company
301 Perimeter Center North
Atlanta, GA 30346

Medso Pharmacy System
Medso Incorporated
4144 Crossgate Drive
Cincinnati, OH 45236

Mini-Pharm
Interactive Business Systems, Inc.
20 West Kaley St.
Orlando, FL 32806

National Data Communications,
Inc. (NADACOM)
5440 Harvest Field, Suite 150
Dallas, TX 75230

NCR Corporation
Medical Systems Marketing
1700 South Patterson
Dayton, OH 45479

1 Up Pharmacy Software
(formerly AIDS Pharmacy
Systems)
1330 West 139th St.
Gardena, CA 90247

Patient Management Application
Systems, Div. of Compucare
PCI Systems, Inc.
1527 Madison Raod
Cincinnati, OH 45206

Pharmacy Computer Services, Inc.
208 Northwest 6th, Suite 2
Grants Pass, OR 97526

Pharmacy Systems Design
5711 Schaefer
Dearborn, MI 48126

Pharmcom
2301 Ave. J
Arlington, TX 76011

Pharmserv
3 PM, Inc.
30881 Schoolcraft
Livonia, MI 48150

Plus/7 Pharmacy System
Pentamation Enterprises, Inc.
10 Loveton Circle
Sparkes, MD 21152

PREP (Patient Records Electronically Prepared)
HPI Health Care Services, Inc.
10960 Wilshire Blvd., Suite 2000
Los Angeles, CA 90024

Professional Drug Systems, Inc.
2320 Schuetz Road
St. Louis, MO 63141

PRX Systems
Western States Pharmacy
Consultants, Ltd.
5797 Central Ave.
Boulder, CO 80301

Realtime Network Applications,
Inc. (RNA)
716 East Main St., P.O. Box 26249
Dayton, OH 45426

Script Control
James W. Daly, Inc.
66 Broadway, Route 1
Lynnfield, MA 01940

Shared Medical Systems (SMS)
51 Valley Stream Parkway
Malvern, PA 19355

Signature Software Systems, Inc.
5601 Stouder Place, Northwest
Pickerington, OH 43147

SOFCOR
2202 14th St.
Meridian, MS 39301

Software Consulting Services
Ben Franklin Technology Center—
125
Lehigh University
Bethlehem, PA 18015

Space Age Computer Systems,
Inc.
4400 Jenifer St., Northwest, Suite
200
Washington, DC 20015

Systems Associates, Inc. (SAINT)
412 East Blvd., P.O. Box 36305
Charlotte, NC 28236

TBL
720 South Kimball
Southlake, TX 76092

Technicon Data Systems, Inc.
1011 East Touhy Ave., Suite 555
Des Plaines, IL 60018

Travenol Laboratories, Inc.
1 Baxter Parkway
Deerfield, IL 60015

Wang Laboratories
Lowell, MA 01853

Whittaker-Medicus
990 Grove St.
Evanston, IL 60201

EQUIPMENT AND SUPPLIES FOR MEDICATIONS AND MATERIALS HANDLING

Akro-Mills, Div. of Myers Ind.
P.O. Box 989
Akron, OH 44309 — Medication cabinets and carts

American Sterilizer Co.
2425 W. 23rd St.
Erie, PA 16512 — Automated materials and distribution equipment; medication carts

Artromick International Co.
2008 Zettler Road
Columbus, OH 43232 — Medication carts

Automatic Tube Co.
17 Paul Drive
San Rafael, CA 94903 — Pneumatic tube systems

J.L. Baldwin Conveyor Co.
2726-32 N. Ashland Ave.
Chicago, IL 60614 — Materials handling conveyors

Bard MedSystems, Div. of C.R.
Bard, Inc.
558 Central Ave.
Murray Hill, NJ 07974 — Medication carts; mobile satellites

Bay Products, Div. of American
Metal Works, Inc.
8701 Torresdale Ave.
Philadelphia, PA 19136 — Mobile cabinets and multipurpose carts

Becton-Dickinson
Medication Delivery Systems
Rutherford, NJ 07070 — Medication carts; medication drawer transfer carts

Blickman Health Industries, Inc.
20-21 Wagnaraw Road
Fair Lawn, NJ 07410 — Medication carts

John Bunn Corp.
1716 Main St.
Buffalo, NY 14209 — Plastic medication trays, racks and holders; medication carts

Castle Company, Div. of Sybron
Corp.
Rochester, NY 14623 — Automated rail systems for transporting materials

Columbus McKinnon Corp, Conveyor Div.
Tonawanda, NY 14150 — Automatic cart transportation systems

Contempra Furniture Div., Fisher
Scientific Corp.
1410 Wayne Ave.
Indiana, PA 15701 — Utility carts; movable lab carts and tables

Diebold Inc., Lamson Div.
Lamson St.
Syracuse, NY 13201 — Computerized air tube (pneumatic) systems

Drustar, Inc. A Johnson & Johnson Co. Brookham Drive Grove City, OH 43132	Medication delivery systems
Dynalab Corporation Box 112 Rochester, NY 14601	Multipurpose carts; tote boxes; dollies, carrying baskets, mobile benches
Equipto 225 S. Aurora Ave. Aurora, IL 60507	Multipurpose carts, mobile bench cabinets
General Equipment Manufacturers (SystaModule Div.) P.O. Box 1059 Jackson, MS 39205	Multipurpose carts and tables
Grand Rapids Sectional Equip. P.O. Box 6306 Grand Rapids, MI 49506	Narcotic carts
Health Care Logistics, Inc. P.O. Box 25 Circleville, OH 43113	Utility carts & bins
Healthmark Industries Co. 17006 Mack Ave. Grosse Pointe, MI 48224	Plastic tote trays and boxes
Hollywood Plastics, Inc. 4560 Worth St. Los Angeles, CA 90063	Carrying trays
Kewaunee Scientific Equipment P.O. Box 5400 Statesville, NC 28677	Utility tables; carts
Kole Enterprises P.O. Box 520152 Miami, FL 33152	Transportation trucks and utility carts; carrying trays; general accessories
Labconco Corp. 8811 Prospect Kansas City, MO 64132	Multipurpose lab carts; portable tables and benches
Lakeside Manufacturing, Inc. 1977 S. Allis St. Milwaukee, WI 53207	Multipurpose carts, trucks, and accessories; medication carts; dollies
Lamson Division Syracuse, NY 13201	Pneumatic tube systems
Lewis Systems 426 Montgomery St. Watertown, WI 53094	Plastic bins and boxes; movable racks for bin storage and transport
Foremost-McKesson, Inc. Crocker Plaza One Post St. San Francisco, CA 94104	Medication carts and trays
Herman Miller, Inc. Zeeland, MI 49464	Utility carts; multipurpose carts; carrying trays; delivery carts
Lionville Systems, Inc. Lionville, PA 19353	Decentralized Pharmacy
Modern Metals Industries, Inc. P.O. Box 888 El Segundo, CA 90245	Medication and cassette transfer carts
Monarch Metal Products, Inc. New Windsor, NY 12250	Medication carts
Nestier Div., Midland-Ross Corp. 10605 Chester Road Cincinnati, OH 45215	Modular distribution container systems
Parke-Davis 208 Welsh Pool Rd. Lionville, PA 19353	Medication carts
Powers Regulator Co. 10825 E. 47th Ave. Denver, CO 80239	Pneumatic tube systems

Rapistan, Inc. Grand Rapids, MI 49505	Materials handling conveyor systems; automatic cart transport systems
Sherwood Medical Ind., Inc. 1831 Olive St. St. Louis, MO 63103	Medication carts; supply trucks; utility carts
Standard Conveyor Co. North St. Paul, MN 55109	Pneumatic tube systems; automatic vertical conveyor systems
Thymer Industries 392 7th Ave. Newark, NJ 07107	Medication carts; emergency carts
Trans-Aid Corp. 1609 E. Del Amo Blvd. Carson, CA 90746	Medication carts
Waterloo Industries Waterloo, IA 50704	Medication carts; utility carts; emergency carts; plastic trays and accessories
Wayne-Ferrell Co. P.O. Box 2201 Iowa City, IA 52240	Unit dose drug distribution materials handling equipment
The Paul O. Young Co. Line Lexington, PA 18932	Multipurpose carts; dolly trucks; casters and wheels

EQUIPMENT AND SUPPLIES FOR PACKAGING ORAL SOLIDS, ORAL LIQUIDS, INJECTABLES, AND MISCELLANEOUS DRUG PRODUCTS

Agnew-Higgins Garden Grove, CA 92642	Laminar air flow hoods
Air Control, Inc. 1448 Countyline Huntington Valley, PA 19006	Laminar airflow hoods
American Sterilizer Co. 2425 W. 23rd St. Erie, PA 16512	Laminar airflow hoods
Americare, Inc. 3030 Quigley Rd. Cleveland, OH 44113	Oral solid unit dose packaging and labeling machine; oral liquid unit dose packaging and labeling machine; small-volume syringe or vial filling apparatus
Apex Medical Supply, Inc. 9701 Penn Ave. South Bloomington, MN 55431	Oral medication syringes
Arenco Machine Co., Inc. 500 Hollister Road Teterboro, NJ 07608	Oral solid and oral liquid (industrial) packaging machines
Arvey Corp., Lamcote Div. 3500 N. Kimbal Ave. Chicago, IL 60618	Unit dose packaging
The Associated Bag Co. 160 South 2nd St. Milwaukee, WI 53204	Reusable plastic bags
Atmos-tech Ind. 204 Pinebrook Road Eatontown, NJ 07724	Laminar airflow hoods
Automated Prescription Systems, Inc. P.O. Box 686 Pineville, LA 71360	Automatic drug counting machines
The Baker Company, Inc. Sanford Airport Sanford, ME 04073	Laminar airflow hoods
Baxa Laboratories, Inc. Skokie, IL 60076	Oral liquid dispensers
Baxter Laboratories, Div. of Travenol Lab., Inc. Morton Grove, IL 60053	Needles and ancillary supplies; laminar airflow hoods

Becton-Dickinson
Medication Delivery Systems
Rutherford, NJ 07070 — Oral solid packaging equipment liquid packaging equipment; glass vials and caps; cappers; crimpers syringes and needles; laminar airflow hoods, syringe filling stands, Cornwall pipetting outfits

Bel-Art Products
Pequannock, NJ 07440 — Portable laminar airflow work stations; plastic containers for packaging

Bio-Logic Controls
P.O. Box 806-T
Eatontown, NJ 07727 — Sterile air clean work station

Brockway Glass Co., Inc.
Brockway, PA 15824 — Dispensing containers

Burron Products, Inc.
824 12th Ave.
Bethlehem, PA 18018 — Syringes and needles; syringe and needle dispensers; IV equipment

Celluplastics, Inc.
McCullough Ave.
Brockway, PA 15824 — Prescriptionware vials; safety closures

Chemical and Pharmaceutical Ind. Co., Inc.
260 W. Broadway
New York, NY 10013 — Oral solid packaging equipment liquid filling equipment

Contamination Control Labs. Inc.
P.O. Box 867
Lansdale, PA 19446 — Laminar airflow hoods; IV container inspection station

Contempra Furniture Div., Fisher Scientific Corp.
1410 Wayne Ave.
Indiana, PA 15701 — Sterile extemporaneous preparation module (with laminar airflow hood)

Continental Plastics of Oklahoma, Inc.
3421 N. Lincoln Blvd.
Oklahoma City, OK 73105 — Dispensing containers

Coordinated Systems Corp.
7300 Industrial Park
Pennsauken, NJ 08110 — IV dispensing system

Cozzoli Machine Co.
401 E. 3rd St.
Plainfield, NJ 07060 — Liquid filler and capper; ampule sealer, laminar airflow hood

Creative Packaging Co.,
Div. of Eli Lilly and Co.
4411 Hollins Road, NE
Roanoke VA 24012 — Multipurpose containers for packaging

Crompton and Knowles Corp.
345 Park Ave.
New York, NY 10022 — Strip packaging machines

Cutter Laboratories
Berkeley, CA 94710 — Needles and ancillary supplies

Drug Package Inc.
O'Fallon, MO 63366 — Oral solid medication dispensers

Drustar, Inc., A Johnson & Johnson Co.
Brookham Dr.
Grove City, OH 43123 — Packaging trays and cups with labeling systems

Dynalab Corporation
Box 112
Rochester, NY 14601 — Multipurpose plastic vials and bottles; prescription containers; (serum) vials for injectables

Emblem Medic Industries
30355 Umatilla
Englewood, CO 80110 — Unit dose printing and packaging apparatus and supplies

Emblem Tape and Label Co.
1420 Blake St.
Denver, CO 80202 — System for packaging unit dose oral solid items

E.S. Medical Products
P.O. Box 1043
Melville, NY 11746 — Unit dose oral solid packaging systems

Ferno Forge
Industrial Way
Wilmington, MA 01887 — IV preparation stations with laminar airflow hoods

L.C. Gess, Inc.
5235 Tractor Rd.
Toledo, OH 43612 — Oral solid and liquid unit dose packaging machines

Health Care Logistics, Inc.
P.O. Box 25
Circleville, OH 43113 — Oral solid and liquid packaging systems

H. Hutson
P.O. Box 1415
Denver, CO 80201 — Bottle and jar openers

I.T.L. Industries, Inc.
Box 877
Newark, OH 43055 — Vials and automatic pill counter

Jelco Laboratories
Raritan, NJ 08869 — Needles and syringes; needle cutter container

Walter H. Jelly and Co., Inc.
2822 Birch St.
Franklin Park, Il 60131 — Cellulose seals for packaging

Kapak Industries, Inc.
9809 Logan Ave.
S. Bloomington, MN 55431 — Plastic bags; electric bag sealers

KCL Corporation
Shelbyville, IN 46176 — Reclosable polyethylene bags

Kerr Glass Mnaufacturing Corp.
Lancaster, PA 17604 — Dispensing containers

Labconco Corp.
8811 Prospect
Kansas City, MO 64132 — Laminar airflow hoods

Lakso Company, Inc.
Box 442
Fitchburg, MA 01420 — Oral solid strip packaging machines; counting and prepackaging equipment

Laminar Flow, Inc.
739 E. Elm St.
Conshohocken, PA 19428 — Laminar airflow hoods

Kirby Lester, Inc.
P.O. Box 43
Riverside, CT 06878 — Automated tablet counters

Lunaire Environmental, Inc.
4 Quality St., Box 3246
Williamsport, PA 11701 — Sterile air safety cabinet

Lynn Peavy Co.
Box 5555
15551 W. 190th St.
Lenexa, KS 66219 — Zip-lip plastic bags

M & M Plastics, Inc.
4120 S. Creek Road
Chattanooga, TN 37406 — Reversible cap (child-resistant, conventional) dispensing containers

Manostat
519 Eighth Ave.
New York, NY 10018 — Syringe type pipetting-liquid filling apparatus

Medical Packaging Inc.
1800 Lark Lane
Cherry Hill, NJ 08003 — Strip packaging and labeling equipment

Med-A-Safe Co., Div. of ITL, Ind., Inc.
Box 877
Newark, OH 43055 — Automatic tablet/capsule counter

Medi-Dose, Inc.
1671 Loretta Ave.
Feasterville, PA 19047 — Oral solid unit packaging

Medipak, Inc.
Box 201
1009 West Ash
Springfield, IL 62705 — Amber plastic bags; bag sealers

Mediset
Drug Intelligence, Inc.
Dept. AD-31
Hamilton, IL 62341

Packaging and monitoring system for self-administration of medication

McGaw Laboratories
2525 McGaw Ave. (Irvine)
P.O. Box 11887
Santa Ana, CA 92711

Laminar airflow hoods

Millipore Filter Corp.
Bedford, MA 01730

Sterile packaging equipment

MPL Solo Pak Division
1820 W. Roscoe St.
Chicago, IL 60657

Liquid filling apparatus; needles and syringes; nebulizer injectors; and liquid syringes

National Instrument Co., Inc.
4119-27 Fordleigh Rd.
Baltimore, MD 21215

Syringe filling apparatus; oral liquid filling apparatus; capsule filler; bottle cappers

Owens-Illinois
Toledo, OH 43601

Empty sterile vials for injectables; vial filling, capping and labeling equipment; glass syringes, rubber tips, and plunger rods, syringe filling, equipment; all types of prescriptionware containers; unit dose vials for oral liquids; plastic hinged containers; aluminum caps; strip packaging materials

NuAire, Inc.
2100 Fernbrook Lane
Plymouth, MN 55441

Laminar air and safety hoods

Parke-Davis
208 Welsh Pool Rd.
Lionville, PA 19353

Oral solids unit dose packaging equipment and accessories; laminar air flow hoods

Pennsylvania Glass Products Co.
430 N. Craig
Pittsburgh, PA 15213

Dispensing containers

Pharmaseal
Glendale, CA 91201

Packaging aids for unit dose and IV programs

Phenix Box and Label Co.
4120 Pennsylvania Ave.
Kansas City, MO 64111

Dispensing containers

Popper and Sons, Inc.
300 Denton Ave.
New Hyde Park, NY 11040

Needles and glass syringes

Production Equipment Inc.
17 Legion Place
Box 236
Rochelle Park, NJ 07662

Oral solid counting machines; oral liquid filling machines; oral solid prepackaging equipment

Pure Aire Corp.
15544 Cabrito Road
Van Nuys, CA 91406

Laminar airflow hoods

Raytron Corp.
5235 Tractor Rd.
Toledo, OH 43612

Laminar airflow hoods with built-in syringe filter and labeler; strip packaging machines; liquid filling machines; vial filler-capper-labeler apparatus; syringe filler and labeler

Regional Service Center, Inc.
260 New Boston Park
Woburn, MA 01810

Single-unit packaging

Remind-A-Pac, Inc.
Southfield, MI 48075

Drug packaging system (outpatient)

R$_x$ Count Corp.
14129 Chadron Ave.
Hawthorn, CA 90250

Oral solid prepackaging machines

Shaw-Clayton Plastics, Inc.
123 Carlos Dr.
San Rafael, CA 94903

Hinged-lid plastic containers

Sherwood Medical Industries
1831 Olive St.
St. Louis, MO 63103

Syringe filling equipment; syringes, needles, cartridges, plungers and other accessories; syringes for oral medications; laminar airflow hoods to accommodate syringe filling apparatus

SystaModule Div., General Equipment Manufacturers
P.O. Box 1059
Jackson, MS 39205

Sterile extemporaneous preparation module (with laminar airflow hood)

Temco Pre-Pac
P.O. Box 3881
1209 Grand Central Ave.
Glendale, CA 91201

Packaging system for unit dose

Henry Troemner, Inc.
6825 Greenway Ave.
Philadelphia, PA 19142

Laminar airflow hoods

U.D.M. Packaging
2005 Mt. Vernon Ave.
Pomona, CA 91768

Oral solid unit dose package machine

U.S. Bottlers Machinery Corp.
4015 N. Rockwell
Chicago, IL 60618

Semiautomated liquid filling equipment

VECO International
15565 Northland Drive
Southfield, MI 48075

Laminar flow hoods; IV inspection system

Wayne-Ferrell Co.
P.O. Box 2201
Iowa City, IA 52240

Unit dose drug distribution packaging equipment and supplies

Wheaton Medi-Systems
1000 N. 10th St.
Millville, NJ 08332

Vials for oral liquids; dispensing containers; dispensers for filling single-dose containers

Wrap-Aid Machine Co., Inc.
189 Sargeant Ave.
Clifton, NJ 07103

Oral solid strip packaging equipment and accessories

EQUIPMENT AND SUPPLIES FOR PRINTING AND LABELING

Avery Label Co.
777 E. Foothill Blvd.
Azusa, CA 91702

Label printing machines and labels; wrap-around labeling systems

Briggs Corp.
Des Moines, IA 50306

Multipurpose labels

Drug Package Inc.
O'Fallon, MO 63366

Pressure-sensitive labels; manual numbering machines; counter label holders and label accessories

Drustar, Inc., A Johnson & Johnson Co.
Brookham Dr.
Grove City, OH 43123

Medication cups and labels; label printers

Dymo Visual Systems, Inc.
P.O. Box 1568
Augusta, GA 30903

Electric and manual tape label makers accessories

Emblem-Medic Industries
3035 S. Umatilla
Englewood, CO 80110

Labels and label printers

Emblem Tape and Label Co.
1420 Blake St.
Denver, CO 80202

Unit dose oral solid packaging and labeling system

The Engle Press
P.O. Box 187
Pitman, NJ 08071

Roll prescription labels

E.S. Medical Products
P.O. Box 1043
Melville, NY 11746

Oral solid unit dose label printer

Howard Sales Inc.
3210 Belt Line Road
Dallas, TX 75234
| Labeling/marking systems for pressure sensitive labels

Labelon Corp.
10 Chapin St.
Canadaigua, NY 14424
| Marking/copying products; preprinted tapes; labels; rubber stamp kits; xerographic toners; thermal copy paper

Mayfield Printing Co.
Mayfield, KY 42006
| Prescription labels

Medi-Dose, Inc.
1671 Loretta Ave.
Feasterville, PA 19047
| Labels

Medipak, Inc.
1009 W. Ash
P.O. Box 201
Springfield, IL 62705
| Pressure-sensitive preprinted labels

Modern Office Devices, Inc.
731 Hempstead Turnpike
Franklin Square, NY 11010
| Preprinted pressure-sensitive labels; manual labeling equipment

Monarch Marking Systems Co.
P.O. Box 1201
Dayton, OH 45401
| Label printing machines

Owens-Illinois
Toledo, OH 43601
| Bottle and vial labeler; labels and accessories

Parke-Davis & Company
208 Welsh Pool Road
Lionville, PA 19353
| Labeling equipment and accessories

Phenix Box and Label Co.
4120 Pennsylvania Ave.
Kansas City, MO 64111
| Accessory labels; self-adhesive and removable labels

Professional Tape Co., Inc.
144 Tower Drive
Burr Ridge
Hinsdale, IL 60521
| Labels and labeling equipment; label dispensers; tape and tape dispensers; IV infusion rate labels.

Raytron Corp.
Toledo, OH 43612
| Automatic bottle or vial labelers

Shamrock Scientific Specialty Systems Inc.
34 Davis Drive
Bellwood, IL 60104
| Labels and label dispensers

Saxon Adhesive Products, Inc.
880 Garfield Ave.
Jersey City, NJ 07305
| Labels

Soabar Co.
7722 Dungen Road
Philadelphia, PA 19111
| Marking and label printing machines; labels

Sohn Manufacturing Inc.
Elk Hart Lake, WI 53020
| Label printing machines, labels and supplies

United Ad Label Co. Inc.
12115 S. Shoemaker Ave.
Box 2165
Whittier, CA 90610
| Pharmacy labeling systems

Weber Marking Systems Inc.
711 Algonquin Road
Arlington Heights, IL 60005
| Automatic label makers (printers)

MICROFILM READERS, PRINTERS, AND SUPPLIES

Acme Visible Records, Inc.
Crozet, VA 22932
| Microfilm readers and copiers

Alden Electronic and Impulse Recording Equipment Co. Inc.
119 N. Main St.
Brockton, MA 02401
| Microfilm readers and copiers

Avery Label Co.
777 E. Foothill Blvd.
Azusa, CA 91702
| Microfiche jackets and labels

Bell & Howell Co.
(local representative)
| Microfilm readers and copiers

Datagraphix, Inc.
P.O. Box 82449
San Diego, CA 92138
| Microfilm readers and printers; film processors and duplicators; microfilm viewers and accessories

Drug Package, Inc.
O'Fallon, MO 63366
| Microfilm camera and viewer; microfilm supplies

Kukane Corp., Audio Visual Div.
2900 Dukane Drive
St. Charles, IL 60174
| Microfilm readers

Eastman Kodak Co.
(local representative)
| Microfilm readers and copiers; portable microfilmers; microfilm files

Emergency Medical Data Service
P.O. Box 6730
San Francisco, CA 94101
| Microfilm data systems

Alan Gordan Enterprises, Inc.,
Microfilm Div.
5362 N. Cahuenga Blvd.
North Hollywood, CA 91601
| Microfilm readers and printers

Kleer-Vu, Microfilm Div.
666 Third Ave.
New York, NY 10017
| Microfilm readers

Minnesota Mining and Manufacturing and Co. (3M), Microfilm Products Div.
Saint Paul, MN 55101
| Microfilm readers and printers

NCR Corp.
Valleywood DPC
3100 Valleywood Dr.
Dayton, OH 45429
| Microfilm readers and copiers; automatic microfiche enlarger printer; processing services

Philips Roxane Labs, Inc.
330 Oak St.
Columbus, OH 43216
| Labeling equipment and supplies

Remington Rand, Systems
(local representatives)
| Microfilm readers and copiers

Xerox Corp.
(local representative)
| Microfilm printers

PHARMACY AND MEDICAL RECORDS FORMS

Acme Visible Records, Inc.
Crozet, VA 22932
| Pharmacy, nursing, etc. forms; patient profile records

Business Controls Corp.
P.O. Box 3287
Tulsa, OK 74101
| Inventory control forms; physician order forms; patient profile forms

Cresco Systems
563 Alden St.
Fall River, MA 02722
| Controlled drug forms; medication order forms

Diebold Inc.
Canton, OH 44702
| Patient profile forms; pharmacy and medical records forms

Drug Package, Inc.
O'Fallon, MO 63366
| Family records; prescription files

Drustar Inc., A Johnson & Johnson Co.
Brookham Dr.
Grove City, OH 43123
| Pharmacy and nursing records; medication order forms

Modern Office Devices, Inc.
731 Hempstead Turnpike
Franklin Square, NY 11010
| Pharmacy and medical records forms

Parke-Davis
208 Welsh Pool Road
Lionville, PA 19353
| Pharmacy and nursing records; physician order forms; patient profile forms

Phenix Box and Label Co.
4120 Pennsylvania Ave.
Kansas City, MO 64111
| Patient profile cards; prescription records and files

Physician's Record Co.
3000 S. Ridgeland Ave.
Berwyn, IL 60402

Pharmacy and medical record forms

Randomatic Data Systems, Inc.
216 Robbins Ave.
Trenton, NJ 08618

Pharmacy and medical records forms; patient profile forms

Reynolds and Reynolds Co.
Dayton, OH 45401

Hospital records and forms; business and accounting forms; inventory control record forms

Trans-Aid Corp.
1609 E. Del Amo Blvd.
Carson, CA 90746

Pharmacy and medical records forms

STORAGE FACILITIES AND REFRIGERATORS

Acme Visible, Inc.
Crozet, VA 22932

Metal storage cabinets

Akro-Mils, Div. of Myers Industries
P.O. Box 989 TR
Akron, OH 44309

Plastic bins; modular drug storage cabinets; dividers; drawer boxes; storage cabinets on rotary base

American Sterilizer Co.
2424 23rd St.
Erie, PA 16512

Built-in and freestanding cabinets and casework; medication stations

Automated Prescription Systems, Inc.
P.O. Box 686
Pineville, LA 71360

Oral solid storage and automated counting-dispensing units

Bally Case and Cooler Inc.
Bally, PA 19503

Walk-in coolers, freezers, refrigerators

Bay Products
701 Torresdale Ave.
Philadelphia, PA 19136

Modular work benches; storage facilities; cabinets and bins; stacking boxes

Blickman Casework and Design Corp.
530 Gregory Ave.
Weehauken, NJ 07087

Built-in and freestanding cabinets and casework; drug and narcotic cabinets

Brown-Morse Co.
110 E. Broadway
Muskegon, MI 49443

General casework cabinets and benches

Columbus Show Case Co.
Columbus, OH 43212

General casework showcases

Contempra Furniture Div., Fisher Scientific Corp.
1410 Wayne Ave.
Indiana, PA 15701

General pharmacy casework; narcotic storage units; modular, freestanding self-contained storage facilities; unit dose dispensing; IV admixture preparation

Diebold Inc.
Canton, OH 44702

Automated drug storage and retrieval systems (or power files)

Drustar Unit Dose System, Inc.
1385 Brookham Drive
Grove City, OH 43123

Storage tables for unit dose items

Dynalab Corp.
Box 112
Rochester, NY 14601

Plastic storage boxes; stacking trays

Equipto
225 S. Highland Ave.
Aurora, IL 60507

Metal storage units; general casework; tables; bulk storage units

Ferno Forge
Industrial Way
Wilmington, MA 01887

Modication preparation stations; IV preparation stations; storage units; refrigerators/freezers

Foremost-McKesson, Inc.
Crocket Plaza
One Post St.
San Francisco, CA 94104

Unit dose systems; storage units and general casework

Gem Refrigerator Co.
650 E. Erie Ave.
Philadelphia, PA 19134

Refrigerators

General Equipment Manufacturers, SystaModule Div.
P.O. Box 1059
Jackson, MS 39205

General pharmacy casework; storage units; cabinets; dispensing units; narcotic storage units

Geneva Industry Inc.
Geneva, IL 60134

General casework wall and base cabinets; workbenches; undercounter refrigerators

Grand Rapids Sectional Equipment Co.
P.O. Box 6306
Grand Rapids, MI 49506

General wood casework; narcotic storage units; multipurpose storage units

Hamilton Manufacturing Co.
Two Rivers, WI 54241

General casework storage units

Hollywood Plastics, Inc.
4560 Worth St.
Los Angeles, CA 90063

Storage trays

Jewett Refrigerator Co. Inc.
2 Letchworth St.
Buffalo, NY 14213

Refrigerators; freezers

Kelmore, Inc.
599 Springfield Ave.
Newark, NJ 07103

Upright refrigerators/freezers; undercounter refrigerators; chest-type freezers; explosion-proof refrigerators

Kelvinator Commercial Products, Inc.
621 Quay St.
Manitowac, WI 54220

Refrigerators, freezers

Kewaunee Manufacturing Co.
P.O. Box 5400
Statesville, NC 28677

General casework

Kole Enterprises
P.O. Box 520152
Miami, FL 33152

Cardboard storage bins; metal storage shelves; storage boxes; stacking cabinets; safes, refrigerators

Lab Line Instruments, Inc.
Lab Line Plaza
Melrose Park, IL 60160

Laboratory casework; storage units; walk-in refrigerators; freezers

Lewis Systems
426 Montgomery St.
Watertown, WI 53094

Plastic bins and storage racks

Lundia Myers Industries, Inc.
Decatur, IL 62525

Movable shelving and storage facilities

Medipak, Inc.
P.O. Box 201
1009 West Ash
Springfield, IL 62705

Storage bins

Metropolitan Wire Goods Co.
Wilkes-Barre, PA 18705

Wire and metal shelving; movable storage units

Herman Miller, Inc.
Zeeland, MI 49464

Modular storage equipment; dispensing facilities; modular casework

Nor-Lake Inc.
Second and Elm
Hudson, WI 54016

Biologic and undercounter refrigerators; walk-in coolers; freezers

Parke-Davis Co.
208 Welsh Pool Road
Lionville, PA 19353

Drug dispensing stations; unit dose bins and storage units; general casework

Precision Scientific Co.
3737 W. Cortlant St.
Chicago, IL 60647

Refrigerators

Puffer-Hubbard Refrigerator Div.
E. Jackson St.
Grand Haven, MI 49417

Refrigerator, freezers

Remington Rand Systems
(local representatives)

Power files for mechanized drug storage and retrieval; metal filing and storage cabinets

Saginaw Industries Co.
Saginaw, MI 48605

General pharmacy casework; storage units

The C. Schmidt Company 11400 Grooms Road Cincinnati, OH 45242	Walk-in and biologic refrigerators; freezers
Shaw-Clayton Plastics, Inc. 123 Carlos Drive San Rafael, CA 94903	Hinged-lid plastic drug containers
Sherwood Medical Inc. 1831 Olive St. St. Louis MO 63103	Built-in and freestanding cabinets and casework; drug and narcotic cabinets
St. Charles Manufacturing Co. St. Charles, IL 60174	Built-in and freestanding cabinets and casework; drug and narcotic cabinets; refrigerators
R.C. Smith Co. 801 E. 79th St. Minneapolis, MN 55420	Modular casework systems
SystaModule Div., General Equipment Manufacturers P.O. Box 1059 Jackson, MS 39205	Modular, freestanding, self-contained storage facilities for outpatient dispensing, unit dose dispensing, IV admixture preparations and traditional inpatient dispensing; storage bins and boxes
Thymer Industries 392 7th Ave. Newark, NJ 07107	Medication carts; emergency carts
Watson Manufacturing Co., Inc. Jamestown, NY 14701	General pharmacy casework; storage units; cabinets; dispensing units; storage trays; narcotic cabinets

ENTERAL AND PARENTERAL INFUSION PUMPS

Abbott Laboratories Abbott Park North Chicago, IL 60064	Volumetric pumps and controllers
American McGaw Div. American Hospital Supply Corp. P.O. Box 1187 Santa Ana, CA 92711	Volumetric pumps
Anatros Corporation 1922 Junction Ave. San Jose, CA 95131	IV controllers
AVI, Inc. 1118 Red Fox Road St. Paul, MN 55112	IV variable pressure pumps
Bard Med Systems Div., C.R. Bard Inc. 87 Concord St. North Reading, MA 01864	Syringe pumps
Biosearch Med. Products 35 Industrial Parkway Somerville, NJ 08876	Enteral nutrition pumps
Centaur Sciences Inc. 180 Harvard Ave. Stamford, CT 06902	IV controllers
Chesebrough-Ponds Inc. 33 Benedict Place Greenwich, CT 06830	Enteral nutrition pumps
Cormed Inc. 591 Mahar St. P.O. Box 470 Medina, NY 14103	Mobile infusion pumps
Critikon, Inc. 1410 N. West Shore Blvd. Tampa, FL 33607	Volumetric pumps
Cutter Medical Berkeley, CA 94710	IV controllers

Diatek, Inc. 3910 Sorrento Valley Blvd. San Diego, CA 92121	Volumetric pumps
DNA Medical Inc. 3385 West 1820 South Salt Lake City, UT 84104	IV controllers
IMED Corporation 9925 Carroll Canyon Road San Diego, CA 92131	Volumetric pumps controllers
IMS 311 Rt. 46 West Fairfield, NJ 07006	Volumetric pumps
Infusaid Corp. 1400 Providence Highway Norwood, MA 02060	Implantable pumps
IVAC Corporation P.O. Box 2385 La Jolla, CA 82038	Volumetric/pressure pumps IV controllers; enteral pumps
Omni Flow 4 Henshaw St. Woburn, MA 01801	Volumetric pumps
Pacesetter Systems Inc. 12884 Bradley Ave. Sylmar, CA 91345	Mobile infusion pumps
Quest Medical Inc. 3312 Wiley Post Road Carrolton, TX 75006	IV controllers
Ross Labs Columbus, OH 43216	Enteral nutrition pumps
Sage Instruments Orion Research Inc. 380 Putnam Ave. Cambridge, MA 02139	Volumetric pumps
Sigmamotor, Inc. 14 Elizabeth St. Middleport, NY 14105	Volumetric/pressure pumps
Travenol Lab, Inc. Nutrition and Flow Control Div. 1 Baxter Parkway Deerfield, IL 60015	Volumetric pumps/controllers
Valleylab 5920 Longbow Drive P.O. Box 9015 Boulder, CO 80301	Volumetric pumps

MISCELLANEOUS EQUIPMENT AND SUPPLIES

Alsop Engineering Corp. Milldale, CT 06467	Stainless steel tanks; mixers, filters and filtering apparatus
Alza Corp 950 Page Mill Road Palo Alto, CA 94304	Liquid infusion system
American Sterilizer Co. 2425 W. 23rd St. Erie, PA 16512	Distillation apparatus
Barnstead Co., Div. of Sybron Corp. 225 Rivermoor St. Boston, MA 02132	Purification systems
Baxter Laboratories, Div. of Travenol Laboratories Inc. Morton Grove, IL 60053	In-line filters for IV infusions
Bel-Art Products Pequannock, NJ 07440	Magnetic stirrers; pharmaceutical glassware
Brown-Morse Co. 110 E. Broadway Muskegon, MI 49443	General laboratory casework and fixtures

Chemical and Pharmaceutical Ind. Co., Inc.
260 W. Broadway
New York, NY 10013

Ointment mills, mixers and blenders; manual tube filling machines; small-scale manufacturing equipment; quality control equipment

Corning Glass Works
Corning, NY 14830

Water demineralizer unit; laboratory glassware

Cox Instrument Div.
15300 Fullerton Ave.
Detroit, MI 48227

Membrane filters and apparatus

Cutter Laboratories, Inc.
Berkeley, CA 94710

In-line filters for IV infusions

Dynalab Corporation
Box 112
Rochester, NY 14601

Pharmaceutical glassware; prescription balances; stirring plates, hot plates

EM Laboratories, Inc.
500 Executive Blvd.
Elmsford, NY 10523

Ph indicator systems

Ertel Engineering Co.
8-14 N. Front St.
Kingston, NJ 12401

Filtration apparatus; mixing tanks

Extracorporeal Medical Specialties Inc.
Ross and Royal Roads
King of Prussia, PA 19406

IV in-line final filters

Gelman Instrument Co.
600 S. Wagner Road
Ann Arbor, MI 48106

Membrane filters and filtering apparatus; prefilters

General Equipment Manufacturers, SystaModule Div.
P.O. Box 1059
Jackson, MS 39205

General pharmacy casework and fixtures

Geneva Industry Inc.
Geneva, IL 60134

General laboratory casework and fixtures

Grand Rapids Sectional Equipment Co.
P.O. Box 6306
Grand Rapids, MI 49506

General pharmacy casework and fixtures

High Efficiency Filter Corp.
P.O. Box 995
Eatontown, NJ 07724

Contamination control equipment and accessories; HEPA filters

Kerr Glass Manufacturing Corp.
Lancaster, PA 17604

Laboratory glassware

Kewaunee Manufacturing Co.
P.O. Box 5400
Statesville, NC 28677

General laboratory casework and fixtures

Lab-Line Instruments, Inc.
Lab-Line Plaza
Melrose Park, IL 60160

Stirring equipment; sterilizers; general laboratory casework

Johns-Manville
P.O. Box 5108
Denver, CO 80217

Filter products and systems

Manostat
519 Eighth Ave.
New York, NY 10018

Peristaltic pumps and pump dispensers; electric laboratory stirrers

Market Forge Co.
Everett, MA 02149

Sterilizers

McGaw Laboratories
2525 McGaw Ave. (Irvine)
P.O. Box 11887
Santa Ana, CA 92711

In-line final filters

Herman Miller Inc.
Grand Rapids, MI 49464

Physical facilities for drug storage, distribution and dispensing

Millipore Corporation
Bedford, MA 01730

Filtration apparatus

RC. Musson Rubber Co.
P.O. Box 7038
1320 East Archwood
Akron, OH 44306

Antifatigue floor mats

Nucleopore Corp.
7035 Commerce Circle
Pleasanton CA 94566

Membrane filter apparatus

Omnimed, Inc.
Cooper St. and Rt. 130
Burlington, NJ 08016

Emergency drug kit

Pall Biomedical Products Corp.
Glen Cove, NY 11542

IV final filter

Parke-Davis
208 Welsh Pool Rd.
Lionville, PA 19353

Unit dose drug distribution system and facilities

Phenix Box and Label Co.
4120 Pennsylvania Ave.
Kansas City, MO 64111

Pharmaceutical glassware; prescription balances

Saginaw Industries
Saginaw, MI 48605

General pharmacy casework

Sargent-Welch Scientific Co.
7300 North Linder Ave.
Skokie, IL 60076

Quality control equipment; laboratory glassware

Seitz Filters
P.O. Box 538
Milldale, CT 06467

Filters and filter equipment

Sherwood Medical Industries
1831 Olive St.
St. Louis, MO 63103

Medication preparation stations; filtered aspiration needles

Spectrex Co.
3594 Haven Ave.
Redwood City, CA 94063

Particle counter and identifier

Star Tank and Filter Corp.
875 Edgewater Road
Bronx, NY 10474

Filter units

St. Charles Manufacturing Co.
St. Charles, IL 60174

General pharmacy casework and fixtures; medication preparation stations

Toledo Scale
Toledo, OH 43612

Portable all-purpose scales and balances

Torsion Balance Co.
Clifton, NJ 07013

Prescription balances and accessories

Watson Manufacturing Co., Inc.
Jamestown, NY 14701

Medication preparation stations; general pharmacy casework and fixtures

Wheaton Medi-Systems
1000 North 10th St.
Millville, NJ 08332

Automatic waterstill

Research

CONDUCT OF AND PARTICIPATION IN RESEARCH

The institutional pharmacist must be prepared to participate in clinical research originated by the medical staff and to conduct pharmaceutical research or initiate research himself. In doing so, he may act as the principal or co-principal investigator or he may use the resources of the department to support a particular research study. The pharmacist must be able to establish a data base, either for the drugs being used or the patients participating in the study. Equally important, he must have the ability to collect appropriate data, interpret them, apply the conclusions drawn from the data, and transmit the results in an adequate manner.

An educational background with appropriate orientation and training in research methodology, including criteria for and structure of a research report, is mandatory.

CHAPTER 40

Philosophy and Design of Research

THOMAS R. SHARPE

The institutional pharmacy practitioner is constantly involved in research, either directly or indirectly, as a part of professional life. The pharmacist is indirectly involved as a "consumer of research." As a consumer, the pharmacist must critically evaluate the pharmacy and medical literature to make informed decisions affecting everyday pharmacy practice and to advise patients and health professionals concerning appropriate drug use.

The pharmacist is often directly involved in research as well. This may involve participation in research to establish fundamental knowledge concerning drug activity of investigational new drugs. The pharmacist may also be conducting research to evaluate the effect of alternative decisions regarding delivery of pharmaceutical services.

Whatever the extent of this involvement, either as consumer or researcher, to act most effectively the practitioner must have an understanding of the principles of research design and statistics. This chapter addresses the first of these needs: research design.

IN SEARCH OF CAUSE

Evidence and Causal Analysis

The major goal of scientific research is to establish causal laws that enable us to predict and explain scientific phenomena. More often a given research project has the explanation of relationships among the variables selected for study as its somewhat less lofty aim. In either case, the aim is to establish knowledge based on reliable and valid information and facts.

Many methods exist for establishing this knowledge. Charles Pierce has identified four general ways or methods of knowing (1):

1. *Method of tenacity.* People hold firmly to the "truth" because they know it is the truth. If it were not the truth they would not hold firmly to it. Repetition of "facts" makes them truth, and they may even infer "new" truths from these false propositions.

2. *Method of authority.* If an idea has the weight of public sanction and tradition behind it, it is "truth." If the Bible or noted scientist says it, it is so.

3. *Method of priori.* "Truth" is established if the idea agrees with "reason" or the way things "should be." This is also sometimes referred to as the *method of intuition.*

4. *Method of science.* The "truth" of a proposition is determined by *objective empiricism.* It is *objective* because it is without investigator bias; it is *empirical* because it is based on observation and experimentation.

Each of these methods is based on assumptions. The *method of tenacity* assumes all persons know truth—hardly a tenable assumption. The *method of authority* assumes that some people know truth. The problem here is in objectively determining who knows truth and who does not. The *method of a priori* assumes that people can find truth without empirical evidence (observation). The problem with this method is that two persons using rational processes may reach different "truths" or conclusions, both of which agree with reason. Which conclusion is correct?

Because each of these methods can lead to false conclusions, scientists found it necessary to develop their own criteria for establishing knowledge—the *method of science.* This method assumes that truth can be found only with empirical evidence.* The scientific method is the focus of our discussion of research design.

The Stimulus-Response Model

All experimental designs have as an underlying assumption some variation of the stimulus-response (S-R) model, which, in turn, is based on the assumptions of the scientific method. This model can be illustrated as follows:

$$S \rightarrow R$$

According to this model, a stimulus treatment (S) when applied to a treatment subject elicits some direct and measurable response (R). The treatment may be administration of an experimental psychotropic drug or an intervention program to provide the patient with information concerning the importance of consuming an entire course of antibiotic therapy. In the first example, the response might be a change in pupil size or some objective measure of mood elevation. In the latter example, the response might be an increase in patient compliance. A variation of the S-R model is the model in which some intervening mechanism takes place

---

*The *method of science* has additional assumptions known as the postulates of science. Space limitations do not permit a full discussion of these postulates. Instead, the reader is referred to Brown CW, Edwin EG: *Scientific Method in Psychology.* New York, McGraw-Hill, 1955, pp 15-34.

within the organism (person, rabbit, rat, etc) prior to the response. The model is illustrated below:

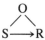

According to this model, a stimulus treatment when applied to a treatment subject elicits a measurable response that is first mediated by some intervening mechanism. Regardless of which model is applied, the adequacy of the research design will determine whether the investigator can make the crucial step from *association* (correlation between S and R) to *causation*.

Establishing Causality

There are three generally accepted scientific criteria for establishing causality in the S-R model. These include the following:

1. *Association*. If two or more variables are not associated (i.e., correlated, related), one cannot possibly cause the other.

2. *Time priority*. To establish cause, the independent variable (stimulus variable) must occur first or change prior to the dependent variable (response variable).

3. *Nonspurious relationship*. A nonspurious relationship is defined as an association between two variables that cannot be explained by a third variable. Rival hypotheses concerning the relationship are eliminated. If the effects of all relevant variables are eliminated and the relationship between the independent and dependent variables is maintained, then the relationship is nonspurious.

Association. Two characteristics of an association strengthen the conclusion that one variable is the cause of the other. Although not a sufficient condition for establishing causation, the greater the *magnitude* of the relationship between two variables, the more confidence one has that the association is truly causal. High magnitude alone, however, is not a sufficient condition for an interpretation of causality.

A second characteristic of an association that increases the plausibility of a causal interpretation is *consistency*. If the relationship persists under a variety of conditions, confidence in the causal nature of the relationship is increased. For example, one argument supporting the proposition that smoking causes cancer is that this relationship has been found in (1) prospective as well as retrospective studies, (2) studies of animals as well as humans, (3) studies in different localities, (4) studies among different ethnic and racial groups and among males as well as females, and (5) studies conducted from one time period to another.

Magnitude and consistency of an association should be treated only as a guide in assessing causality, however. A true causal association, for example, may exist when two variables are just barely related, because there may be several factors producing an event. All the factors may be important because they combine their small influences to cause the event. For example, possible causal factors in an individual's decisions to join a professional pharmacy organization may include leadership ability, power seeking, professionalism, self-esteem, and attempting to establish business contacts. All of these factors (and others) may be necessary to explain organization membership.

The consistency of association should also be considered cautiously. All causal relationships apply only under certain circumstances. Consequently, if results are not consistent, it may be that the causal relationship is valid only in certain situations. Conversely, even if consistency of the relationship exists, this is a necessary *but not sufficient* condition to establish causality.

Time Priority. This assumption is based on the fact that an event in the future cannot determine an event in the past or present. However, there are many relationships where time priority is difficult to determine. For example, an equally plausible explanation of our previous example of organizational membership might be that those who join professional organizations become more interested in professionalism, power, business contacts, etc. (Which came first, the chicken or the egg?) Without knowledge concerning time priority, we are limited to making conclusions only with respect to association (correlation) among the variables of concern. Causal relationships cannot be determined.

Spurious Relationship. Controlling for all relevant variables is the basic problem that must be addressed when trying to determine whether the interpretation of a relation is spurious. Assuming that the effects of all relevant variables have been eliminated, we can more confidently interpret the relation as causal and not due to other factors.

Even if we have controlled for all variables that we consider relevant, the possibility still exists that some variable we have not considered is acting in the phenomenon. If it can be shown, for example, that certain genetic factors predispose a person to smoking and also determine who will develop lung cancer, then it would be spurious to interpret the relation between smoking and cancer as causal. Only in experiments which randomly assign individuals to treatment and control groups can we be sure that we have controlled for all other factors, both known and unknown.

Thus only when all three conditions of association, time priority, and nonspurious relationship exist can we draw conclusions concerning causal relationships. The measurement of magnitude of association is determined through appropriate application of statistical procedures.* It is in the realm of research design that the questions of time priority and nonspurious relationships are directly addressed.

CHARACTERISTICS OF EXPERIMENTAL DESIGNS

The application of the research model to experimental research is presented in Figure 40.1. This model depicts the activity flow of the research act, including definition of the population, selection of a representative sample for study, random assignment of the sample to experimental and control groups, administration of the experimental treatment to one group and no treatment (placebo) to the other, comparison of resulting differences between the two groups, and, finally, interpretation of differences found. Actually

---

*The reader is referred to Chapter 42 for an excellent practical discussion of statistics.

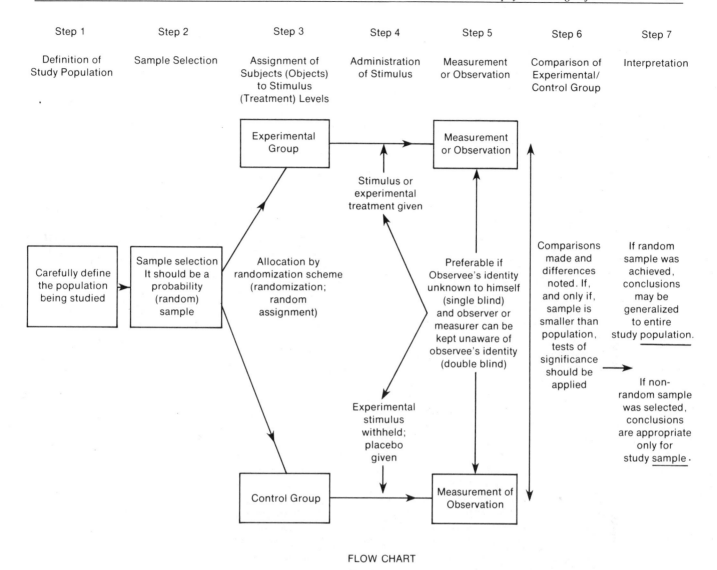

Step 1	Step 2	Step 3	Step 4	Step 5	Step 6	Step 7
Definition of Study Population	Sample Selection	Assignment of Subjects (Objects) to Stimulus (Treatment) Levels	Administration of Stimulus	Measurement or Observation	Comparison of Experimental/ Control Group	Interpretation

FLOW CHART

FIGURE 40.1 Implementation of an experimental design. This flow chart illustrates optimum principles and sequence to be followed in conducting a valid experimental design. (Adapted by permission from Greenberg, B.G., Mattison, B.F.: The whys and wherefores of program evaluation. Can. J. Public Health, 46:298, 1955.)

there are several forms of experimental designs. The selection of the best design will depend on the nature and limitations of the specific research situation. Before examining these variations, however, it would be helpful to examine the characteristics which are universal to true experimental designs.

Suchman (2) outlined three main conditions of the experimental method. These include (1) sampling equivalent experimental and control groups; (2) isolation and control of the stimulus; and (3) definition and measurement of response.

Sampling Equivalent Experimental and Control Groups

The problems of selecting subjects for research projects may be discussed under three headings: (1) defining the population universe for study; (2) selecting the specific samples to be included in the study; and (3) dividing the sample into equivalent experimental and control groups.

Defining the Study Population. The definition of the population to be studied will largely depend on how the results of the study are to be applied. The crucial question is, "To which groups am I going to generalize the results of my study?"

Probably the most common error in this regard is defining the population too broadly. The population should not be defined as greater than the group from which the research can and does randomly sample. For example, a study conducted among patients admitted during a 3-month period to a single service of a given hospital should not define its population as (nor later generalize findings to) "patients admitted to hospitals."

Sample Selection. Scientists seldom study a total population. Many populations are impossible or impractical to study directly because the researcher lacks accessibility, sufficient time, or the financial resources to collect data on such a large number of study units. Therefore, data are usually gathered on only a part, or *sample*, of the population. The researchers then try to specify conclusions concerning the population based on knowledge derived from studying relationships in the sample.

The size of the sample to be selected will depend a great deal upon the anticipated degree of effect—the greater the degree, the smaller the sample required. Additionally, the more population subgroupings and the more variables introduced simultaneously, the larger will be the sample required. Statistical procedures are available to aid the researcher in choosing an adequate sample size to fit the needs of the particular study situation.

Random sampling is a method of drawing a sample (e.g., using a table of random numbers) of the population such that every member of the population has an equal chance of being selected. Thus, a random sample is representative of the population from which it was drawn; no bias exists with regard to the characteristics of the sample selected. If 70% of our population is made up of females, for example, we can expect our sample, because we selected it randomly, to contain the same proportion of women.

Stratified random sampling is a refinement of the simple random sampling discussed above. This procedure first divides the population into strata. Strata might consist of age groups, men and women, caucasians and noncaucasians, etc. Random samples are drawn from each of these strata in proportion to their presence in the population. For example, if 12% of the total population is age 25-35 years, then 12% of the total sample would be drawn from this age stratum. Stratified random sampling is especially useful when the investigator has some basis for expecting that the strata are related to the phenomenon being studied and/or when the investigator wishes to ensure that very small strata are not excluded from the sample.

Several forms of nonrandom sampling are also used. These include:

1. Convenience sampling. Selection is based solely on the convenience to the investigation of obtaining the sample. An example would be all patients in a given hospital ward, or students in an undergraduate pharmacy class.

2. Quota sampling. The population is divided into groups according to selected characteristics which are considered important to the study. A percentage (quota) of individuals is then selected from each category.

3. Interval sampling. Individuals are selected in a periodic sequence. An example would be every person entering the hospital on Mondays.

4. Judgment sampling. Selection is based on the investigator's judgment alone that the members of the sample are representative of the population. A psychiatrist selecting a few "typical" manic depressives is an example of this method.

5. Systematic sampling. Selection is accomplished by choosing every *n*th person from a population. This is a common procedure when a list of all persons in the population is available. An example of this method is the selection of a 10% sample of American Society of Hospital Pharmacists (ASHP) members by selecting the first name

randomly, and every tenth name thereafter from the ASHP roster of members. In most instances, this method is equivalent to true random sampling.

Regardless of the specific sampling procedure used, it cannot be emphasized enough that without some form of random sampling no conclusions can be inferred concerning relationships in the population. If the researcher does not sample randomly, he must be satisfied with conclusions concerning relationships only in the sample.

Random Assignment to Experimental and Control Groups. In the behavioral sciences, the bedrock essential for any true experimental design is the random assignment of subjects to treatment conditions. The design may entail only one independent variable, such as (1) presence or absence of a particular type of patient instruction or (2) different levels of a particular drug administered to depressive patients. In practice, the number of levels of an independent variable range from two (usually a comparison of a treatment condition with a control condition) up to eight or more. The design, alternatively, may entail several independent variables rather than only one. However simple or complex the design, the essence of the true experimental design is that the available pool of subjects is randomly sorted into the various groups. The only restriction usually employed in this regard is that an equal (or nearly equal) number of people be placed into each group.

The beauty of randomly assigning subjects to groups of an experimental design is that the procedure *absolutely guarantees* that, prior to participation in the experiment, subjects on the average will not differ with respect to any characteristic more than could be expected by chance alone. By "chance alone" is meant the probability distributions associated with the random sorting of subjects into treatment groups. Thus, the subjects in an investigation of methods of training patients to monitor their diabetes condition would vary in terms of height, intelligence, social class, personality characteristics, and many other human traits before being introduced to experimental treatments. After being randomly allocated to groups of the design, subjects would still vary within groups with respect to all such human traits; and the sheer act of randomly allocating subjects would lead to a predictable amount of variation in average values of these traits across the groups of the experimental design. However, the randomization process would ensure that there were no systematic influences tending to make the average value of any extraneous variable higher in one group than in another.

Isolation and Control of the Stimulus

Careful formulation, isolation, and manipulation of the stimulus (independent) variable are crucial to the experimental design.

Careful formulation and definition of the stimulus are important to increasing reliability of study measurements. When the stimulus is administered, it is important that each member in the experimental group receives exactly the same treatment. This careful stimulus specification is important both to the immediate study situation and for those who may wish to replicate the investigation at their own institutions.

Statements such as "an education program was administered'' or ''50 patients in the experimental group received intensive counseling'' are unacceptable. The specific content, including message, medium, and situational environment (among others) must be clearly delineated concerning the ''education program'' and ''intensive counseling.'' Stimulus variables should be defined in measurable terms.

Isolation of the treatment stimulus is also extremely important. Introduction of extraneous stimuli can confound the effects resulting from the stimulus treatment. That is, the effects of the extraneous stimuli cannot be separated from the experimental stimulus, whose effects the investigator intends to isolate for study. Care should also be exercised to isolate experimental from control subjects. ''Cross-contamination'' between these two groups is a problem which often goes unrecognized.

Definition and Measurement of Response

Precision in operationally defining response (dependent) variables is just as important as careful specification of the stimulus treatment. As with the latter, the dependent variables should be operationally defined in measurable terms. As such, they should be characterized as reliable and valid. Let us examine reliability and validity more carefully.

RELIABILITY AND VALIDITY

Reliability

In the simplest sense, reliability is consistency. The reliability of a measure refers to the degree to which the measure produces consistent results upon repeated application. In other words, reliability is the relative absence of random, or unsystematic, errors of measurement. This reliability can be classified into four types:

1. *Congruency.* The extent to which several indicators measure the same thing

2. *Precision.* The extent to which an indicator is consistent for a single observer

3. *Objectivity.* The extent to which the same instrument is consistent for two or more observers

4. *Constancy.* The extent to which the object being measured does not fluctuate

Suchman (3) outlines five sources of unreliability in experiments. The major sources of this unsystematic variation in experiments are:

1. *Subject reliability.* The subject's mood, motivation, fatigue, etc may momentarily affect his physical and mental health and attitudes and behaviors. When such factors are of a transient nature, they may produce unsystematic changes in subject responses.

2. *Observer reliability.* The same personal factors will also affect the way in which an observer makes measurements. These observer factors will not only tend to affect the subject's reactions, but also the observer's interpretation of the subject's responses.

3. *Situational reliability.* The conditions under which the measurement is made may produce changes in results which do not reflect ''true'' changes in the population being studied. If the variation in the experimental situation is random, then these situational factors will produce unsystematic responses which produce unreliable results.

4. *Instrument reliability.* All of the aforementioned factors will combine to produce an evaluative instrument of low reliability. However, certain specific aspects of the instrument itself may also affect its reliability. Poorly worded questions in an interview, for example, especially those which are ambiguous or ''double-barreled,'' may lead to random variation in responses.

5. *Processing reliability.* Simple coding or mechanical errors, when they occur at random or in an unsystematic manner, may also lead to a lack of reliability.

Since all measurement contains some error, the problem for the researcher is to reduce this random error such that it does not interfere with the valid use of the measurement instrument. Reliability can best be controlled by careful attention to factors that permit large chance errors to enter into the experiment. Such unreliability often results from carelessness and inadequate precautions against unsystematic error.

Validity

Validity refers to the degree to which a measure or procedure succeeds in doing what it purports to do. It answers the question: Are we indeed measuring what we say we are measuring?

In contrast to reliability, which is a measure of random error, validity reflects those errors which are systematic. Therefore, errors of validity represent some form of bias which slants the results in a particular direction rather than at random. Thus, the factors which affect validity may be incorrectly interpreted as causal.

Fundamental to an understanding of validity is the distinction between internal and external validity. *Internal validity* is the basic minimum without which any experiment is uninterpretable: Did in fact the experimental treatments make a difference in this specific experimental instance? *External validity* asks the question of generalizability: To what populations, settings, treatment variables, and measurement variables can this effect be generalized?

Campbell and Stanley (4) identified eight classes of extraneous factors, which, if not controlled in the experimental design, might produce effects confounded with the effect of the experimental stimulus. These threats to internal validity represent the effects of:

1. *History:* Events, other than the experimental treatment, occurring between pre-test and post-test and thus providing alternate explanations of effects

2. *Maturation:* Processes within the respondents or observed social units producing changes as a function of the passage of time per se, such as growth, fatigue, secular trends

3. *Testing:* The effect of taking a test upon the scores of a second testing

4. *Instrumentation:* In which changes in the calibration of a measuring instrument or changes in the observers or scores used may produce changes in the obtained measurements

5. *Regression artifacts:* Pseudo-shifts occurring when persons or treatment units have been selected upon the basis of their extreme scores

6. *Selection:* Biases resulting from differential recruit-

ment of comparison groups, producing different mean levels on the measure of effects

7. *Experimental mortality:* The differential loss of respondents from comparison groups

8. *Selection-maturation interaction:* Selection of biases resulting in differential rates of "maturation" or autonomous change.

Four factors that jeopardize external validity, or representativeness, were also outlined:

9. *Interaction effects of testing:* The effect of a pretest in increasing or decreasing the respondent's sensitivity or responsiveness to the experimental variable, thus making the results obtained for a pretested population unrepresentative of the effects of the experimental variable for the unpretested universe from which the experimental respondents were selected

10. *Interaction of selection and experimental treatment:* Unrepresentative responsiveness of the treated population

11. *Reactive effects of experimental arrangements:* "Artificiality"; conditions making the experimental setting atypical of conditions of regular application of the treatment: "Hawthorne effects"

12. *Multiple-treatment interference:* Where multiple treatments are jointly applied; effects atypical of the separate application of the treatments

CLASSIFICATION OF RESEARCH DESIGNS

Campbell and Stanley (5) classified some 15-20 common experimental and quasi-experimental designs and evaluated them according to their typology of threats to internal and external validity. Several of these designs are discussed below, with particular emphasis on *internal* validity.

In the graphic presentation of these designs an X represents the exposure of a group to the experimental treatment, and O refers to the process of observation or measurement. Xs and Os in a given row are applied to the same specific persons. The left-to-right dimension indicates temporal order, and Xs and Os vertical to one another are simultaneous. An R indicates random assignment to experimental and control groups. Finally, rows which are not separated by dashes represent comparison groups equated by randomization, while those separated by such a line represent comparison groups not equated by random assignment.

Preexperimental Designs

Design 1: The One-Shot Case Study

$$O_1 \quad X \quad O_2$$

Example†: Eight cases of thrombosis (including one death) in patients treated with the antipsoriatic agent azaribine were reported during the first year of marketing, during which time an estimated 500-1000 patients were treated with the drug. The severity of the adverse reactions led to an FDA request on August 12, 1976, that

---

†All examples are hypothetical, unless otherwise indicated.
‡In this case, however, the FDA was wise in removing the stimulus (azaribine) from the market. This design does not allow us to determine whether the observations resulted from the stimulus, but it also does not allow us to determine they did not. The risk was simply too great to continue to allow the manufacturer to market the drug.

the manufacturer withdraw the drug from the market. (Source: *FDA Drug Bulletin,* August-October 1976.)

In this design, observations are made only after the treatment has been administered. This is the simplest form of research design and the most frequently used in pharmacy and medicine. Unfortunately, it is also the weakest form of design. Since there are no baseline measurements or control groups in the study, there is no way to evaluate whether the observations were a result of the stimulus.‡

The popularity of this design derives primarily from its simplicity and ease, but it leads to results which are primarily "testimonials" concerning the effect of the stimulus variable. (In research, as well as other endeavors, there is no such thing as a free lunch.) Primary sources of invalidity from this design include history, maturation, selection, and mortality.

Design 2: The One-Group, Pre-Test, Post-Test Design

$$O_1 \quad X \quad O_2$$

Example: A study to determine the analgesic activity of AX-735, an investigational new drug, was conducted among a sample of 50 patients in a hospital general medicine service. Patient reports of pain after administering a pinprick to the right forearm served as the measure of pain threshold (PT). PT was measured, a 200-mg oral capsule of AX-735 was then administered to all patients in the sample, and the PT measured again 4 hours after medication. A significantly lowered PT was found after medication, which the researchers attributed to AX-735 analgesic activity.

This design introduces a baseline measure before the stimulus is administered, followed by measure after the stimulus has been given. The design is an improvement over the previous one, because it allows the researcher to objectively measure change. However, *it does not allow the researcher to attribute this change to the stimulus which was administered.*

Five main threats (i.e., sources of plausible rival hypotheses) to internal validity plague this design. They include the following:

1. *History.* Other extraneous events may occur simultaneously with the experimental stimulus which influence the effect being measured.

2. *Maturation.* The effect may be due to "unstimulated" change as a result of time alone; i.e., some people improve with or without exposure to the stimulus.

3. *Testing.* The "before" measure itself may constitute a stimulus, regardless of the experimental stimulus itself.

4. *Instrumentation.* The "after" measure may reflect time changes in measurement due to fatigue or instrument unreliability.

5. *Statistical regression.* Unreliability may produce statistical regression with shifting values toward the mean.

Design 3: The Static Group Comparison

$$\frac{X \quad O_1}{O_2}$$

Example: A study to determine the analgesic activity of AX-735, an investigational new drug, was conducted among a sample of 50 patients in a hospital general medicine service. Patient reports of pain after administration of a pinprick to the right forearm served as the measure of pain threshold (PT). Twenty-five patients on one floor of the service were administered a 200-mg oral dose of AX-735, and the PT measured 4 hours later. Twenty-five patients on the other floor were administered an inert (placebo) oral capsule, and the PT measured 4 hours later. A significantly lower PT was found in the AX-735 group compared to the placebo group, which the researchers attributed to AX-735 analgesic activity.

This design represents the basic logic behind much epidemiologic research, where two groups with varying frequency of a disease condition are compared and differences between the two are viewed as possible causes of the disease. As in the previous two examples, however, the conclusions of the investigators are unwarranted.

The static group comparison merely gives the appearance of providing a control group. While it does effectively control for problems concerning history, testing, instrumentation, and regression, two main sources of rival hypotheses (threats to internal validity) still remain: selection and mortality.

1. *Selection.* If O_1 and O_2 differ, this difference could well be due to differential recruitment of persons making up the groups; the groups might have differed anyway, without the occurrence of X.

2. *Mortality.* Differences in O_1 and O_2 may be due to differential dropout of persons from the groups. Thus even if the two groups had once been equivalent, they might differ now because of the selective dropout of persons from one of the groups.

True Experimental Designs

With this group of designs we finally come to the classic experimental design illustrated in Figure 40.1. These designs allow the researcher both to objectively measure change and to attribute this change (if it exists) to the experimental stimuli.

Design 4: The Pre-Test, Post-Test Control Group Design

$$R\ O_1\quad X\quad O_2$$
$$R\ O_3\quad\quad\ O_4$$

Example 1. One hundred pharmacists who attended a weekly continuing education seminar were randomly assigned to experimental and control groups which met in different buildings. During week 1 a knowledge test concerning drug therapy for diabetes mellitus was administered to both groups. During the session of week 5 the experimental group was shown a commercially available film concerning diabetes mellitus drug therapy, while the control group was shown a film on a different subject. During week 12 both groups were readministered the knowledge test. Mean improvement score for the experimental group ($O_2 - O_1$) was significantly ($P < 0.05$) greater than for the control ($O_4 - O_3$). The investigators attributed the difference in knowledge to the film stimulus.

Design 4 is the most frequently used of the three truly experimental designs. This design uses two equivalent groups which are as alike as possible before the stimulus is administered. Equivalence is obtained by random assignment to experimental and control groups. A "before" measure is made to determine the baseline from which change is to be evaluated. The experimental group is exposed to the experimental treatment, and the control group receives no treatment or a placebo. An "after" measure is then obtained for both the experimental and control group. If we let $d_{expt} = O_2 - O_1$ and $d_{cont} = O_4 - O_3$, then if d_{expt} differs significantly from d_{cont} (after applying the appropriate statistical test), the researcher can attribute that difference to the experimental treatment.

All threats to internal validity are controlled with this design. History is controlled because extraneous variables occurring between the pre-test and post-test which might have produced an $O_1 - O_2$ difference would also produce an $O_3 - O_4$ difference. Similarly, rival hypotheses concerning maturation, instrumentation, and testing are ruled out. Selection is ruled out as an explanation of difference, since random assignment of treatment groups has assured group equality (this can be verified by testing for differences between O_2 and O_3). Mortality can be evaluated as a rival explanation by examining to see if differential dropout rates exist between the experimental and control groups.

Example 2. The anxiolytic effects of alprazolam were evaluated in a double-blind randomized comparison with diazepam and placebo in 46 outpatients suffering from anxiety of moderate to severe intensity. Patients were randomly allocated identical capsules containing alprazolam, 0.5 mg, diazepam, 5 mg, or placebo over a 28-day period. Initial dosage was 1 cap tid and after day 4 could be modified (increased or decreased), within established parameters, according to response. Anxiety was assessed using the Hamilton Anxiety Rating Scale (HARS). The scale was completed before the start of medication and at the end of weeks 1, 2, and 4. Average (mean) improvement scores on the HARS were 54.7% ($P < 0.001$), 41.3% ($P < 0.01$), and 28.9% ($P < 0.05$) for alprazolam, diazepam, and placebo, respectively, but differences between groups did not reach statistical significance. Based on these results and similar results using other measures, the investigators concluded that the results confirm that alprazolam is effective in the treatment of anxiety symptoms. (Adapted from Davison K et al: A double blind comparison of alprazolam, diazepam, and placebo in the treatment of anxious out-patients. *Psychopharmacology* 80:308-310, 1983.)

It is not sufficient merely to select an appropriate research design, however. Example 2 depicts a study using an appropriate experimental design, but the investigators have drawn inappropriate conclusions from their own statistical analysis. For both experimental groups (alprazolam and diazepam), significant differences were found in mean HARS scores when comparing post-test to pre-test (O_2 vs O_1) scores. But significant differences were also found when comparing the control post-test and pre-test scores (O_4 vs O_3). More important, no significant differences were found between the placebo group post-test scores (O_4) and the experimental group post-test scores (O_2). Thus, although significant changes in anxiety level were found in the experimental groups, these changes were no greater (or no less) than changes found in the control group. Other studies no doubt appropriately document the therapeutic effectiveness of alprazolam (and diazepam); this study, however, does not.

Design 5: The Post-Test Only, Control Group Design

$$R \quad X \quad O_1$$
$$R \qquad O_2$$

Example: A double-blind randomized trial was conducted to determine the effect of dietary sodium (Na) on systolic blood pressure (SBP) in healthy newborn infants. Infants (n = 476) were randomly assigned to a low-Na (experimental) or normal-Na (control) diet starting immediately after birth. Subjects received experimental or control diets (formula milk and solid foods) free of charge for 6 months. Careful monitoring of breast feeding and deviations from supplied diets was conducted; Na excretion was determined via periodic casual urine samples taken to verify differences in Na intake by the two groups. Average Na intake of the control group was almost three times greater than the low-Na experimental group. SBP was significantly lower (2.1 mm Hg) at week 25 for the experimental group. The investigators attributed the difference in SBP to the experimental low-Na diet. (Adapted from Hofman A et al: A randomized trial of sodium intake and blood pressure in newborn infants. *JAMA* 250:370-373, 1983.)

The pre-test is a concept "dear to the hearts" of researchers, especially in the social sciences. Actually, however, it is not essential to true experimental designs. Design 5 is similar to the previous design, except that pre-test observations are not conducted.

The rationale behind this simplification of design 4 is that randomization can suffice without the pre-test to ensure equivalence of experimental and control groups prior to administering the study treatment. The most adequate all-purpose means to ensure initial equivalence of groups is randomization.

Simply stated, this design controls for all the threats to internal validity that the previous design does, but without actually measuring them. This design considers the measurement of these controls to be an academic question. (Perhaps, after all, there is such a thing as a free lunch, or at least a cheaper one.)

Design 6: The Solomon Four-Group Design

$$\begin{array}{l} R \; O_1 \quad X \quad O_2 \\ R \; O_3 \qquad O_4 \end{array} \right\} \text{This part is design 4}$$

$$\begin{array}{l} R \qquad X \quad O_5 \\ R \qquad\qquad O_6 \end{array} \right\} \text{This part is design 5}$$

This design controls and measures both the experimental effect and the possible interaction effects of the measuring process itself. The contribution of this design, then, is that it allows the researcher to determine whether the pre-test itself acted as a stimulus in the experiment. Often a pre-test will "sensitize" the study subjects to the phenomenon which the researcher is investigating. Evidence for this interaction between testing and X exists if O_2 differs significantly from O_5 and/or O_4 differs significantly from O_6 (note that the only difference with respect to the two groups within each of these pairs is whether a pre-test administered).

Quasi-Experimental Designs

Often the realities of conducting research "in the real world" prevent the researcher from gaining full control over sample selection, randomization, and scheduling experimental stimuli. In these situations, a truly experimental design is not possible. For these situations, Campbell and Stanley suggest some 10 to 15 alternative quasi-experimental designs. Three examples include:

Design 7: The Time Series Experiment

$$O_1 \; O_2 \; O_3 \; O_4 \quad X \quad O_5 \; O_6 \; O_7 \; O_8$$

Design 8: The Equivalent Time-Samples Design

$$X_1O \; X_oO \; X_1O \; X_oO$$

Design 9: Nonequivalent Control Group Design

$$\frac{O_1 \quad X \quad O_2}{O_2 \qquad O_4}$$

These designs differ from the true experimental designs in that the former do not *control* for threats to internal validity (rival hypotheses), but to a greater or lesser degree (depending on the specific design) they do allow the researcher to determine whether a given rival hypothesis can be ruled out through circumstantial evidence. Thus quasi-experimental designs are sufficiently probing to warrant their use under limited circumstances, but they should never be employed when the more valid true experimental designs are possible and practical.

CONCLUSION

A research design designates the logical manner in which individuals or other units are compared and analyzed. This design and the appropriately selected and applied statistical procedures serve as the basis for making interpretations from the data. The purpose of the design is to ensure a comparison that is not subject to alternative interpretations. While statistics allow us to make correct judgments concerning whether significant differences exist between two (or more) groups or whether two (or more) groups are significantly associated with respect to some variable, statistics alone do not allow us to make cause-and-effect statements about these relationships. Only when the statistics are applied within the framework of an appropriately selected and properly implemented research design can such causal statements be justified.

This discussion has sought to provide an understanding of the principles underlying effective design of research which must be practical in dealing with the "real world." Below are some practical guidelines which are derived from those principles. By following these guidelines, the researcher can avoid the common pitfalls of conducting research in the clinical or social setting.

1. Carefully define the study population. An imprecisely defined population prevents the researcher from drawing a random sample (if you do not know what the population is, how can you assure that each member has an equal probability of being selected). This imprecision also leads to

ambiguity concerning to whom generalizations can be extended.

2. Sample randomly from your population whenever possible. If you cannot sample randomly, don't extend your conclusions further than to the sample you have selected.

3. Randomly assign your subjects to experimental and control groups. This is the bedrock essential for any true experimental design and is essential if conclusions concerning casual relationships are to be made.

4. Carefully define all variables and the conditions of the experiment. Independent and dependent variables should be operationally defined in measurable terms. Careful variable specification is the foundation for reliable measurement.

5. Carefully isolate the experimental and control conditions. The objective is to assure that the *only* difference between the experimental and control groups is the presence or absence of the stimulus. Extraneous stimuli and/or "cross-contamination" of experimental and control groups ruins the validity of the study.

6. Carefully develop your measurement instrument and be certain to pretest it. Whether the measurement instrument is a mercury sphygmomonometer or an attitude scale, it should be carefully pretested to ensure its reliability.

7. Carefully train your observers in the proper use of your measurement instrument. This will help reduce unreliable measurement and observer bias.

8. Observe unobtrusively if possible. Subjects who do not know they are being tested are more likely to produce valid (unbiased) responses.

9. Conduct the investigation under double-blind conditions if possible and practical. Both observer and subject bias are controlled using this procedure.

10. Choose an *appropriate* statistic for making comparisons. Improper use of statistics is a common source of incorrect conclusions.

11. Never use a quasi-experimental design if a true experimental design can be used in your particular research situation. If you must use a quasi-experimental design, choose the one which controls the greatest number of validity threats which are applicable to your study.

12. Don't "step outside" of your data. Be careful that conclusions are firmly supported by your data, statistics, and research design. Intuition, opinions, editorial comment, and even "wild guesses" are acceptable, but only if clearly labeled as such.

REFERENCES

1. Buchler J (ed): *Philosophical Writings of Pierce.* New York, Dover, 1955, pp 5-23.
2. Suchman EA: *Evaluative Research.* New York, Russell Sage Foundation, 1967, pp 102-111.
3. *ibid.*, pp 118-120.
4. Campbell DT, Stanley JC: *Experimental and Quasi-Experimental Designs for Research.* Chicago, Rand McNally, 1963, pp 5-6.
5. *ibid.*, pp 6-76.

SUGGESTED READING

Babbie ER: *The Practice of Social Research,* ed 2. Belmont, Calif, Wadsworth, 1979.
Brown CW, Ghiselli EW: *Scientific Method in Psychology.* New York, McGraw-Hill, 1955.
Campbell DT, Stanley JC: *Experimental and Quasi-Experimental Designs for Research.* Chicago, Rand McNally, 1963.
Cook TD, Campbell DT: *Quasi-Experimentation: Design and Analysis Issues for Field Settings.* Chicago, Rand McNally, 1979.
Kerlinger FN: *Foundations of Behavioral Research,* ed 2. New York, Holt, Rinehart & Winston, 1973.
Labovitz S, Hagedorn R: *Introduction to Social Research,* ed 3. New York, McGraw-Hill, 1981.
Simon JL: *Basic Research Methods in Social Science,* ed 2. New York, Random House, 1978.
Suchman EA: *Evaluative Research.* New York, Russell Sage Foundation, 1973.

CHAPTER 41

Evaluation*

ALAN B. McKAY and DAVID A. KNAPP

Pharmacists have had to cope with enormous changes and growing complexity in health care during the past decade. New classes of potent therapeutic agents, innovative drug delivery systems, and increased societal demands for safer methods of drug testing and surveillance have dictated an expanded role for the pharmacist in health care.

The health care delivery system has also grown more complicated and more challenging as pharmacists increasingly find that they must practice their profession within the framework of a complex organization such as a hospital, a health maintenance organization, a preferred provider organization, or a corporate chain. Their compensation is often dictated by private insurance plans or public assistance programs. Rapid technologic change, e.g., automated patient records and electronic data transfer, also plays a significant role in altering the traditional practice environment of pharmacy.

Pharmacy has responded to these changes by modifying its educational programs and emphasizing the clinical components of practice in all settings. Pharmacists have adopted many new roles and have developed innovative programs aimed at providing high-quality pharmacy services in an economic and cost-effective manner.

This climate of change includes a constant call for evaluation. Program evaluation will be the key to validating and justifying the existence of successful programs and modifying or eliminating unsuccessful ones. The need to document the efficiency and effectiveness of both existing and innovative pharmacy programs requires pharmacists to become actively involved in program evaluation. Whether the pharmacist is directly responsible for program evaluation or has operational responsibility for the program being evaluated, familiarity with the concepts and methods of program evaluation is essential.

Evaluation itself is a simple concept to understand. We all evaluate things everyday. Every time persons make decisions, i.e., choose among alternatives, they engage in evaluation, even though most of the time this evaluation is implicit rather than explicit. While most evaluation is informal, it helps to provide insight into the possible short-term solutions to specific problems. An informal process is usually sufficient for most of the day-to-day decisions that pharmacy managers make.

However, from time to time, a practitioner may be called upon to more formally evaluate the ongoing activities of a program. The effectiveness and efficiency of the activities are often the major concerns, and immediate evaluation is needed to facilitate decisions that must be made rapidly. The emphasis is on a rapid but thorough assessment of the internal workings of the program in question. Such an assessment requires a more deliberate and complex process.

This chapter is concerned primarily with the more formal type of assessment—the use of evaluative research techniques based upon the scientific method. Program evaluation, as discussed in this chapter, is a rigorous attempt to assess the degree to which a program meets its objectives. The techniques of the scientific method utilized in evaluative research contribute to a decision process that is accurate and objective. Such an approach requires more resources than informal evaluations, but provides three advantages not found in less stringent methods:

1. It is applicable to evaluating programs where the outcomes are complex, hard to observe, or made up of many elements interacting in diverse ways.

2. It provides substantiation for decisions that are crucial or expensive.

3. It provides evidence that may be needed to convince skeptics of the validity of the conclusions of the evaluation.

Evaluative research is often initiated as a response to a problem in an existing program. Although this is a valid use of the process, since it initiates inquiry into situations where help is needed, the situation has two drawbacks: first, it is technically difficult to begin evaluation after a program is operating; and second, each evaluation often takes place in a crisis atmosphere as opposed to the routine inclusion of an evaluative component at the onset of new programs or demonstrations. For optimum results, evaluation must be built in from the planning stage rather than being tacked on later.

Advance planning requires program personnel and researchers to work together from the outset; the researcher must recognize the administrative constraints upon the design and measures, while the administrator must recognize the need for as controlled a situation as possible. Implicit in the relationship is an understanding that, for maximum payoff, the results of the evaluation must be useful to the

---

*An earlier version of this chapter was adapted from *Evaluating Pharmacists and Their Activities*. Washington, DC, American Society of Hospital Pharmacists, 1973.

administrator for purposes of improving the program as it moves toward predetermined objectives.

A FRAMEWORK FOR EVALUATIVE RESEARCH

It must be possible, theoretically, to describe in sufficient detail how a program should work so that specific techniques may be devised to measure the degree to which the program does work. Thus, the underlying framework of the program also provides the framework for the evaluative research (Table 41.1). The framework usually includes a general goal which sets the direction of the project. The specific objectives of the program spell out the end results desired. Each specific objective subsumes one or more intermediate or sub-objectives, each of which must be accomplished before the overall program objectives can be reached. Each sub-objective requires planning and implementing specified activities that, in turn, require the allocation of resources. The program framework must be elucidated in sufficient detail to permit the program evaluator to decide what specifically to evaluate and how to structure the evaluation measures. The operational definition of the framework of evaluation is easier to do before a program begins, which reinforces the notion that the evaluation team should be involved in planning from the outset of the program. By working together, the evaluation personnel can better understand the rationale behind the goals, objectives, and sub-objectives, while the program planners can be helped to clarify their thinking by the evaluators' insistence on precise operational definitions.

As a crucial basis for effective decision making, evaluative research may provide data and feedback on a program during its development and operation. Such *formative* evaluation can be of great significance to program personnel by helping them maximize the success of the program. Preliminary information from formative evaluation can be utilized to change the program in order to improve its ultimate impact.

Summative evaluation is concerned with the assessment of impact once the program is fully developed and is operational. This type of evaluation consists of determining:

1. How the program was implemented
2. The success of the program in meeting its objectives
3. The effect of the program on the social environment
4. And why the desired effects did or did not occur

TABLE 41.1 A Framework for Evaluative Research

I. Identification of program goals including specific measurable objectives and operational definitions

II. Identification and analysis of problems with which the program must cope

III. Description and standardization of the program activity to be observed

IV. Measurement of the degree of change that takes place in the program activity

V. Attribution of observed changes to the program activity or some other cause

VI. Determination of the desirability of the program effect (e.g., were the program goals achieved and, if so, to what extent?)

Summative evaluation is usually more powerful methodologically and focuses on the long-term outcomes of a program.

Determination of Objectives

Since overall program plans seldom spell out objectives in enough detail to meet the needs of evaluators, the development of a clearly stated set of objectives is the first task in evaluative research. Three levels of objectives are involved: the ultimate objective, stated in general long-range terms (e.g., to improve health), the program objective or immediate goal of the program in question (e.g., to reduce adverse drug reactions in a hospital to a given level), and the sub-objectives, those specific goals which must be met en route to meeting the program objective (e.g., reaching a point where all patients on a given hospital floor are monitored constantly for adverse drug reactions).

To cite another example, an investigator may wish to evaluate the effectiveness of a drug information center in the hospital. The ultimate objective might be the elimination of irrational prescribing in the hospital; the program objective might be the provision of accurate and appropriate drug information to all members of the hospital staff; and a sub-objective might be the assurance that all physicians in the hospital are aware of the existence of the drug information center.

The specification of an adequate number of sequential sub-objectives permits the investigator to devise measures of effectiveness at several points along the line toward the program objective. Measuring progress toward specific sub-objectives is easier than more global assessments and also permits pinpointing problem areas if there is an overall lack of program effectiveness. Viewed in this respect, the importance of clearly linking sub-objectives with the overall program objective is essential.

Determination of Activities and Resources

To avoid confusion in the evaluation process, care must be taken to clearly differentiate objectives and activities. Activity is work performed; objectives are states to be reached. The classic analogy is that of a bird flying: flapping its wings is the activity; its destination is the objective (1).

Spelling out activities in detail makes the evaluator more conscious of what is being measured. A frequent weakness of evaluative studies in the drug area is that activities are measured, rather than the attainment of objectives or sub-objectives. For example, studies of the pharmacist's role in providing drug information may concentrate on determining the number of requests for information received by pharmacists, rather than upon the effect of the information on the behavior of the recipient. Measuring the number of requests is often important and provides needed data, but evaluators sometimes assume that an activity measure reflects accomplishment of a program objective, which it usually does not. By specifying clearly the differences between activities and objectives, problems of this sort can be minimized.

Activities and sub-objectives are linked by a series of

assumptions that may be tested as hypotheses as the evaluation progresses. As each small link between activity and sub-objective is proved or disproved, the overall evaluation of the program is strengthened. Such specificity permits careful pinpointing of difficulties uncovered during the evaluative process.

It is important to identify the resources invested in each set of program activities. This permits the determination of whether the resources were used as planned and whether their use was efficient. If failure to reach the program objectives were due to the unavailability of resources, such a problem can be identified.

Measurement

The next step in evaluative research is to measure the degree to which a program attains its objectives. This involves choice (and often development) of measurement techniques and decisions regarding when and how to measure. Only a brief treatment of measurement can be attempted here. For details, one of the many standard references in the area, such as Cronbach (2) and Rossi et al (3), should be consulted.

It is often useful and sometimes essential to collaborate with experts from the social sciences and statistics at this stage in evaluation. Such specialists can assist in the choice of appropriate measures since, in many cases, specific instruments for measuring desired characteristics are available in the literature. For example, numerous well-constructed personality tests may be found to measure traits such as hypochondriasis, dogmatism, and anxiety. Some attitude scales specifically related to pharmacists and drug use may also be found in the literature, but data on reliability and validity should be carefully examined before they are used.

If specific measuring instruments cannot be found, the literature will often provide general techniques which can be adapted easily to specific needs. The semantic differential, for example, has been successfully used to measure respondents' connotational definitions of terms related to pharmacy (4). Established and well-accepted methods for devising attitude scales can be readily applied to attitude measurement problems in pharmacy.

Of course, not all evaluative research requires attitude measurement. The evaluation of the quality of health care, for example, involves the development of criteria of good care coupled with specific measures of each criterion. Table 41.2 illustrates the criteria, measures, and standards developed by King in order to evaluate the quality of pharma-

TABLE 41.2   Criteria, Measurement Process, and Standards for Quality[a]

Function	Criteria	Measurement Process	Standards
Dispensing	Completeness	Random sample of filled prescriptions	All labels in sample must contain prescription number, name of patient, prescriber, date, directions for use, expiration date (when applicable), and pharmacist's initials
	Accuracy	Random sample of filled prescriptions	Correct drug, form, and strength; correct count and name of drug on label of all filled prescriptions in sample
	Degree of legal compliance	Random sample of filled prescriptions for scheduled drugs	Entire sample must conform 100% to state in which evaluation occurs and federal regulations
	Degree of administrative compliance	Retrospective review of filled prescriptions	At least 90% of sample should be filled in accordance with program policies
Delivery	Responsibleness	Random sample of patients is called to verify receipt and/or that medication was left in a safe place	95% of patients called verify receipt of medication
Patient counseling	Completeness	Direct observation using a work sampling technique	Each verbal communication to counsel a patient on drug usage should include explanation of directions, explanation of special precautions, requests for verbal feedback
	Accuracy	Direct observation using a work sampling technique	All directions and precautions given to patient should be correct (i.e., according to acceptable reference standards)
	Utility	Immediate interview of patient	Information given to the patient is perceived as useful in at least 75% of interviews
Maintaining patient profiles	Completeness	Random sample of patient profiles	Profile cards used allow collection of following data: patient name, address, telephone number, and birthdate; previous drug allergies, idiosyncratic reaction, and/or other untoward drug effects; patient diseases/condition; previous ineffective therapy; prescription number; date of service; drug product name/manufacturer; dosage form, strength, and quantity dispensed; prescriber's name; and identification of dispensing pharmacist
			Each profile in sample contains all drugs given to patient (excluding injections and immunizations only if the service does not have access to medical records)
	Accuracy	Comparison of a random sample of filled prescriptions (or patient charts) with profiles	All entries in all profiles in the sample correspond to information on prescriptions in the patient's medical chart
	Utility	Random sample of patient profiles	At least one notation on one profile consisting of date and statement of therapeutic problem
	Use	Direct observation	Profile is reviewed before prescription is filled

[a]Reprinted by permission from King RC: Evaluating pharmaceutical service in community health centers. *Contemp Pharm Pract* 2:35, 1979.

ceutical services in community health centers. If appropriate measures cannot be found in the literature, the investigator will have to prepare his own. Unfortunately, this practice often results in one of the major weaknesses found in the evaluation of the pharmacist's role or drug-related systems. All too often, measuring instruments are drawn up hastily and administered without proper attention to potential ambiguities, bias, and other hazards. Proper development demands expert guidance (or at least the use of appropriate references), attention to detail, and ample time to allow for pre-testing under field conditions prior to the actual evaluation.

Because of restraints of time or resources, it may not always be possible to develop measures for all sub-objectives. In these cases, the investigator is forced to rely on a more limited set of measures. Evaluative research often suffers from this sort of problem since resources allocated to the measurement process are sometimes inadequate. This is yet another reason why evaluative research should be built into a program at the beginning so that adequate time and resources can be made available.

The timing of the measurements will be determined by the timing of the objectives and the sub-objectives. As stated previously, the most thorough approach to evaluation is to devise measures of the attainment of each of the separate sub-objectives so that a progression of information about each step toward the program objective is created. Thus, evaluative measurements would begin to be made from the outset of the program. Evaluative research is a continuous process; measurement of results cannot be put off until the end.

Determining Effectiveness

In conducting evaluative research, the investigator is not only seeking to determine the extent to which program objectives are met, but to find out how much of the success of the program is attributable to the activities performed. In other words, some means is necessary to separate out the specific effects of the program from progress toward the objectives which would have occurred in the absence of the program. Thus, a major concern of those conducting evaluative research is the design and implementation of well-controlled experiments in the real world. Experimental design is discussed in Chapter 40, and readers are referred to Flay and Best (5), who have identified 13 research design problems associated with evaluation.

Three additional considerations deserve attention when discussing how to determine effectiveness: (1) obtaining an appropriate sample, (2) isolating the variables which are to be measured, and (3) defining criteria for use in interpreting results.

The sample chosen for evaluative research must be a part of the target population to which it is desired to generalize. In this respect, it should be noted that much experimentation with roles of the pharmacist and with drug-related systems takes place in large teaching hospitals which are unrepresentative of care settings in general. In this regard, demonstration of new roles or systems may be classified as one of two types: (1) demonstration of feasibility, in which the object is, for example, to see if a pharmacist is capable of performing a new role, given an ideal situation, and (2) demonstrations of potential, in which the object is to illustrate that the new role can readily be implemented in existing settings without a major increase in required resources. Pharmacy has seen far more of the former type of projects than the latter!

Isolating the variables to be measured in an evaluation project is obviously important in order to know precisely what is being evaluated; thus, the priority of specifying in detail each activity and sub-objective for purposes of proper analysis. With regard to the evaluation of demonstration projects, it is vital to separate the effects of the program from the effects of the staff. Since demonstration project directors make special efforts to select staff who are extremely well qualified and motivated, it is difficult to generalize to applications using less outstanding staff members.

Finally, criteria must be defined for the judgment of the results obtained from the evaluation. Criteria represent the investigator's value judgments about desired outcomes. For a theoretical discussion of criteria in the context of drug prescribing review, see Knapp et al (6). For a more general (and exhaustive) treatment of criteria for the quality of health care, see Donabedian (7).

Reliability and Validity

Attention to reliability and validity is as important in evaluative research as it is to any other type of research. Reliability is the extent to which a technique consistently measures whatever it measures regardless of the investigator or the situation. For example, a wooden ruler with clear markings will provide reliable linear measurements no matter who uses it.

Validity is the extent to which a technique measures what it is intended to measure. For the above ruler to be valid as well as reliable, its markings must be consistent with accepted standards of length (i.e., inches, centimeters). Reliability is a necessary prerequisite of validity.

These concepts are discussed generally in Chapter 40 and more specifically with regard to evaluation by Suchman (8).

APPROACHES AND TECHNIQUES

This section will deal in a general way with the issues of what is to be assessed and what techniques are available for use in the assessment process. Several approaches to the first issue, drawn primarily from classifications suggested by Donabedian (9) and Suchman (10), are provided. Donabedian proposes that quality of care can be measured by assessing structure, process, and outcomes of care, and it seems that this framework can be readily applied to most evaluative research situations. To these classifications Suchman would add assessment of efficiency and of the adequacy or impact of the program or activity. Each of these approaches is discussed in this section along with illustrations from the substantive areas of drug-related systems and the role of the pharmacist. Several examples of assessment techniques also are included. The techniques discussed are intended only to be exemplary and are not presented as methods of choice. Any scientifically based research technique could be used in evaluative research where appropriate.

Structure

Structure concerns the resources available to the program under evaluation and the setting in which it takes place. It includes the facilities, equipment, and supplies provided; the number, type, and quality of personnel employed; the administrative systems of record keeping and retrieval; financial strength; interrelationships with other relevant units; organizational support; and the like. Structure usually involves persons and things which are directly observable and easily measurable and, as such, is frequently one of the first things evaluated. The relationship of structure to process and outcome is often hazy, however, and structure evaluation alone is apt to be insufficient. Owning a computer, for example, does not mean it is being used properly or at all.

It is important, however, to evaluate structure along with other elements of the program. Structural instrumentalities are usually prerequisite to program activities, and therefore, their absence can be a good measure of an inadequate program. If a pharmacy is evaluated with regard to its ability to monitor drug therapy in its patients, the absence of an adequate system of patient drug records would be an accurate index of quality (unless the pharmacist had few patients and an excellent memory!).

Many examples of structural assessment can be found in the pharmacy field. Minimum standards for practice set by state laws and board regulation often are primarily of a structural nature: minimum floor space requirements for the prescription department, presence of basic compounding equipment and reference books, and presence of a licensed pharmacist at all times. In a similar vein, a large component of the accreditation requirements of pharmacy schools relates to structural variables, such as the number and training of faculty in each department, physical facilities, and organizational autonomy of the school in curriculum matters. Of recent importance are the existence and availability of facilities and equipment for clinical training and for hands-on experience with computers.

The usual technique for evaluating structure is simply description, based upon reports or direct observation by the investigators. Most structural elements are apparent and readily measurable. The mere presence of such elements, while necessary, is not sufficient, however; more important is the manner in which they are used. This leads to consideration of the evaluation of process.

Process

Most evaluative research involves the assessment of the process of care in some respect, on the one hand because structure, although easily measured, is an inadequate predictor of a successful program, and on the other hand because outcome, although the ultimate validator, is difficult to define and measure. Process means different things to different authorities in the evaluation field, but three aspects stand out as worthy of consideration: (1) the amount and kinds of activities performed, (2) the quality and appropriateness of these activities, and (3) the meaning of these activities to relevant groups.

Amounts and Kinds of Activities. The most frequently encountered form of process evaluation asks simply: "Who does how much of what?" Recalling the analogy of the flying bird, the data called for would be the number of times it flapped its wings; if required, further detail would call for the number of flaps per wing. This kind of data is usually easy to obtain, since it is often collected for administrative purposes anyway. Examples in pharmacy are such indices of activities as the number and type of prescriptions dispensed per day per pharmacy and the number and type of drug information consultations provided to physicians and patients in a given time period. Quantity measures such as workload and productivity can be indexed for comparison across programs (11).

Quality and Appropriateness of Activities. A step up in complexity is the assessment of the effectiveness of performed activities, both in terms of some criteria of quality and with regard to appropriateness to the specific situation. Again referring to hospital drug information centers, many collect much more information than just the number and type of requests received. Some classify requests by type of requestor, note the source of information consulted, and even ask the requestor for an evaluation of the usefulness of the information provided. While this additional material is useful in the evaluation process, other data would be important also, such as the quality of the center's response: its completeness, understandability, relevance, succinctness, etc. If outcome measures are to be employed using changes in the health status of patients as criteria, it is essential to establish that information provided by the center is appropriate and of high quality. Unfortunately, this type of measure is usually lacking in evaluations of drug information centers; more frequently, information disseminated is assumed to be correct.

Outcomes

Since drug use and the practice of pharmacy are components of medical care, the ultimate criterion of their successful application would be a positive change in the health status of patients treated. The problem is that medical care is often an all-or-nothing proposition, and it is extremely difficult to establish the contribution of any particular component to patient outcomes. Sometimes the effects of medical care cannot be fully evaluated for weeks, months, or even years after treatment, time spans which are not very useful for evaluative research purposes.

Of course, outcomes may be defined in various ways, and they need not always be ultimate patient outcomes. For example, the achievement of a sub-objective can sometimes serve satisfactorily as an outcome measure. Since activities and sub-objectives are continually linked in sequence as the program proceeds toward the major objective, attainment of such sub-objective may be viewed as an intermediate outcome. Thus, the line between process evaluation and outcome evaluation is easily blurred in actual practice.

For example, determining appropriate outcome measures for the effectiveness of pharmacists in practice depends upon a clear definition of the extent of their role. If the role definition includes partial responsibility for determining drug therapy and requires pharmacists to monitor this therapy, outcome measures should assess the effects of therapy on the patient. On the other hand, if the pharmacist's role is limited to accurately dispensing prescribed drugs, the outcome measure might consist of an evaluation of dispensed prescriptions as they are obtained from the pharmacy.

A possible technique to evaluate the effectiveness of pharmacists on the patient care units of a hospital might be to measure the incidence of adverse drug reactions. This would be an outcome measure in an inverse way, with reduction in adverse reactions becoming a positive measure of effectiveness. Of course, all other influential factors would have to be carefully controlled during the period of the study.

CONCLUSION

The documentation of effective pharmacy programs (12,13), the introduction of innovative services (14,15), or improvements in the efficiency and effectiveness (16,17) of existing programs require that pharmacists become familiar with the process of program evaluation. The process of program evaluation enables the pharmacy manager to choose from among alternative courses of action and to defend that choice in a rational and logical manner. Program evaluation and evaluative research provide the pharmacy practitioner with the tools needed to address important problems. Properly planned and executed program evaluation can document pharmacist effectiveness and quantify their impact. In a period of vigorous cost containment and critical review of established programs, program evaluation may be the most valuable tool at the disposal of pharmacists.

REFERENCES

1. James G: Administration of community health services. Chicago, International City Managers Association, 1961.
2. Cronbach LJ: *Essentials of Psychological Testing,* ed 3. New York, Harper and Row, 1969.
3. Rossi P, Wright JD, Anderson AB: *Handbook of Survey Research.* New York, Academic Press, 1983.
4. Knapp DE, Knapp DA, Edwards JD: The pharmacist as perceived by physicians, patrons and other pharmacists. *J Am Pharm Assoc* NS9:80-84, 1969.
5. Flay BR, Best JA: Overcoming design problems in evaluating health behavior programs. *Eval Health Prof* 5:43-69, 1982.
6. Knapp DA, Knapp DE, Brandon BM, West S: Development and application of criteria in drug use review programs. *Am J Hosp Pharm* 31:648-656, 1974.
7. Donabedian A: *The Criteria and Standards of Quality.* Ann Arbor, Health Administration Press, 1982.
8. Suchman EA: *Evaluative Research.* New York, Russell Sage Foundation, 1967, p 112-123.
9. Donabedian A: Evaluating the quality of medical care, Part 2. *Milbank Mem Fund Quart* 44:166-203, 1966.
10. Suchman, *op. cit.,* p 51-73.
11. King RC: Evaluating pharmaceutical service in community health centers. *Contemp Pharm Pract* 2:30-38, 1979.
12. Kiresuk TJ, Lund SH, Larsen NE: Measurement of goal attainment in clinical and health care programs. *Drug Intell Clin Pharm* 16:145-153, 1982.
13. Fink A, Kosecoff J, Oppenheimer PR, et al: Assessing whether a clinical pharmacy program is meeting its goals. *Am J Hosp Pharm* 39:806-810, 1982.
14. Almond SN, Caiola SM, Huff PS: Pharmacist-managed allergy desensitization program. *Am J Hosp Pharm* 39:284-288, 1982.
15. Mutchie KD: Pharmacist monitoring of parenteral nutrition: Clinical and cost effectiveness, *Am J Hosp Pharm* 36:785-787, 1979.
16. Brakebill JI, Robb RA, Ivey MF, et al: Pharmacy department costs and patient charges associated with a home parenteral nutrition program. *Am J. Hosp Pharm* 40:260-263, 1983.
17. Chrischilles EA, Helfing DK, Rowland CR: Clinical pharmacy services in family practice: Cost-benefit analysis. I. Physician time and quality of care. *Drug Intell Clin Pharm* 18:333-341, 1984.

ADDITIONAL READING

Abramson JH: The four basic types of evaluation: Clinical reviews, clinical trials, program reviews, and program trials. *Pub Health Rep* 94:210-215, 1979.
Pathak DS: Evaluation of clinical programs: An operational framework. *Drug Intell Clin Pharm* 15:459-463, 1981.
Suchman EA: *Evaluative Research: Principles and Practice in Public Service and Social Action Programs.* New York, Russell Sage Foundation, 1974.
Veney JE, Kaluzny AD: *Evaluation and Decision-Making for Health Services Programs.* Englewood Cliffs, NJ, Prentice-Hall, 1984.
Weiss CH: *Evaluation Research: Methods for Assessing Program Effectiveness.* Englewood Cliffs, NJ, Prentice-Hall, 1972.

CHAPTER 42

Using Statistics

ARTHUR A. NELSON and C. EUGENE REEDER

One cannot read a contemporary pharmacy journal without encountering an author's reference to statistics or statistical significance. Statistics are the tools that researchers use to analyze and evaluate data; they are the essence of a researcher's attempts to develop and test scientific theories. A cynic once commented that he could take statistics and prove anything he wished to prove. Although he was exaggerating, there is an element of truth in the claim. The novice (or even seasoned) researcher may make statements about his or her research which are not totally accurate descriptions. Such cases often result from the inadvertent use of inappropriate statistical procedures.

The purpose of this chapter is to organize commonly used statistical concepts in a logical analysis of the nature and role of statistics in the research process. We assume that you possess a general understanding of introductory statistics. Consequently, the mathematics underlying statistics will not be discussed. If you are interested in the mathematical aspects, refer to any introductory level statistics text listed at the end of the chapter.

Statistics are invaluable to any meaningful attempt to analyze or interpret data. The initial step in our process of understanding is to classify, or categorize, data. In the realm of research, this classification process is characterized by the use of *descriptive statistics*. As shown in Table 42.1, descriptive statistics are used to summarize a large set of data. Indices are computed to describe the data and make it more manageable. Once summarized, the next step in the research process is to use the data from the sample to extrapolate to the population of interest. Extrapolation uses the methods of inferential statistics. While descriptive statistics summarize our data, inferential statistics permit us to generalize our findings to a population larger than our sample. Moreover, inferential statistics permit us to test research hypotheses.

MEASUREMENT

Measurement is a familiar concept to all pharmacists regardless of their practice site. Pharmacists have been using drams, grams, and milliliters for many years. The concept of measurement as it relates to statistics has a much broader interpretation than the traditional assessment of weight or volume. Pharmacists are now concerned with a range of topics from patients' attitudes and behaviors to the serum levels of medications. Serum levels can be accurately measured with appropriate instrumentation and reported in familiar units. Likewise, attitudes and behaviors can be measured and analyzed statistically. Central to an appreciation of how abstractions such as attitudes can be quantified is an understanding of levels of measurements and measurement scales.

Measurement usually refers to the assignment of numbers to observations according to a set of rules. The rules which are applied in the assignment of numbers are known as *scales* or *levels of measurement*. Measurement can be made at four levels: nominal, ordinal, interval, and ratio. The scales or levels vary depending on the degree of mathematical properties that are applied in the measurement process.

Nominal Measurement. The weakest or lowest level of measurement is nominal measurement. Nominal measurement, also referred to as categorical or qualitative measurement, assigns numbers or symbols to an observation (person, object, or property) simply to identify or classify the observation. The numbers do not impart any meaning to the observation other than serving as a label. Examples of nominal measurements include social security numbers, patient identification numbers, and automobile license tags. The measures are nominal because they identify a particular observation and can be assigned arbitrarily. Nominal measures are not required to be numbers; classifying a person by sex, race, or political party is also nominal measurement.

In applying nominal measures, a group of observations is divided into mutually exclusive groups. The only formal mathematical property that exists between groups is that of equivalence or nonequivalence. *Equivalence* means nothing

TABLE 42.1 Frequency Distribution of Specimen Data

Age (yr)	No. in Category	% of Total Patients
0-10	66	27.8
11-21	14	5.9
21-40	45	19.0
41-60	49	20.7
> 60	63	26.6
	237	100.0

more than the members of one group are equal with respect to the property being measured (e.g., sex or political party). Categorical measures cannot be ordered, added, subtracted or divided. This lack of mathematical manipulation limits the types of statistical techniques that can be applied to nominal measurement.

Ordinal Measurement. The second level of measurement, ordinal, assigns numbers or symbols to observations so that the observations cannot only be categorized but can also be ranked, or ordered, in relation to each other. In addition to the equivalence property discussed before, ordinal measurement has the additional property of transitivity (if a > b and b > c, then a > c). Examples of ordinal measures include military rankings and the UPI top ten basketball teams in the United States.

Although ordinal measurement permits statements about the order or ranking of groups, you cannot compare groups relative to quantities of the property measured. For example, we may know that two hospitals are ranked first and second in a city with respect to innovative clinical services (ordinal measurement). However, we do not know how much distance there is between the top two institutions in clinical innovation. They may be very close or very far apart. Hence, ordinal measurement indicates relative position and not the magnitude of differences between groups.

Interval Measurement. In addition to having all the characteristics of nominal and ordinal measures, interval measurements also have equal distances between the scale points or intervals. In an interval scale, however, both the unit of measure and the zero point are determined arbitrarily. The characteristic of equal intervals makes this level of measurement considerably stronger than nominal or ordinal levels.

A familiar example of interval level measurement is temperature. A thermometer measures temperature in degrees, and the interval, or distance between degrees, is the same over the range of the thermometer. The zero point for the thermometer is determined arbitrarily. To illustrate, the freezing point for water is 32 degrees on the Farenheit scale and zero degrees on the centigrade scale.

In interval level measurements, the ratio of any two intervals is independent of the arbitrary zero point and the unit of measurement. The mathematical operations of addition, subtraction, multiplication, and division can be used with interval level data. Consequently, statistics that utilize these mathematical operations may also be used with this level of measurement.

Ratio Measurement. The highest level of measurement is ratio. Ratio level measures have all the characteristics of interval level measures with the additional property of a true zero point. A true zero point provides an actual quantity to be measured. The values or numbers on the measurement scale indicate the actual quantities of the property being measured, and the values themselves, rather than the intervals between them, can be compared. For example, since money is measured on a ratio scale, a value of 100 dollars represents an actual amount of money.

Ratio level measurement contains all the properties of the real number system. Hence, all mathematical operations, and consequently all statistics, may be applied when this level of measurement is achieved. Other examples of ratio

level measures are numbers in the physical sciences: weights, volumes, time, and distance. Ratio level measures, however, are not as common in social sciences research except for some demographic data such as income, age, and years of education.

Measurement and Statistics. An important correspondence exists between the level of measurement and the type of statistics that can be used appropriately with that level. As discussed, the level of measurement of the data should be the major determinant in the selection of types of statistical techniques. However, it is not uncommon to read a paper in which the researcher has employed a statistical procedure that is inappropriate for the level of the data. In the following sections we will review some of the more popular statistical data in detail.

DESCRIPTIVE STATISTICS

As stated in the introduction, descriptive statistics summarize and characterize a large data set. Descriptive statistics may also be used to describe the relationship of two or more variables in a data set. Large amounts of data can be concisely presented by using tables, graphs, figures, and summary statistical measures.

One of the most commonly used methods of summarizing data is a frequency distribution. A frequency distribution displays the data in a set of predetermined intervals with the number, or frequency of observations within each interval. Frequency distributions may be illustrated in tables or graphically in the form of histograms or frequency polygons. Histograms, or ''bar graphs,'' are formed by plotting the intervals along the horizontal (x) axis and the frequencies along the vertical (y) axis. Frequency polygons are constructed by plotting the actual values, or the midpoints of the intervals, along the horizontal axis and the frequencies along the vertical axis and above the horizontal axis. Either method permits you to determine the number of observations in a particular interval or group by reading the frequency directly from the graph.

To illustrate, suppose you wanted to describe the census of a hospital by the ages of the patients. The Admissions Office provides you a list of names and ages of the patients. To summarize this data, you could prepare a table similar to Table 42.1 depicting the number of patients by ages in 10-year intervals. Likewise, you could construct a histogram (bar graph) or frequency polygon (line graph) (Figs. 42.1 and 42.2). From any of these summary measures, it is clear that the larger number of the patients in the hospital are in the age range of 0-10 years and over 60 years. Notice that both the histogram and the frequency polygon use the midpoint of the age range to anchor values along the horizontal axis.

In addition to displaying data in tables or figures, several summary statistics may be computed to describe the data. Measures of central tendency, such as averages, are useful in describing the location of data and in comparing two groups. The three most common measures of central tendency are the mean, median, and mode. The *mean* is the arithmetic average of a group of data. The *median* reports the value that divides the data into two halves. Last, the *mode* represents the most frequently occurring value in a

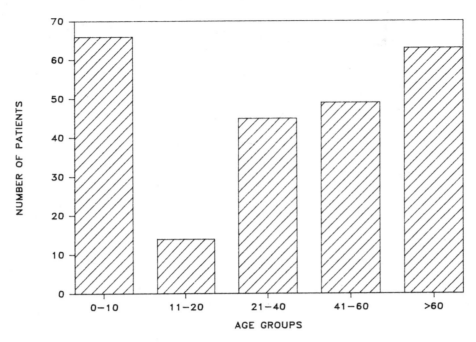

FIGURE 42.1 Example of histogram.

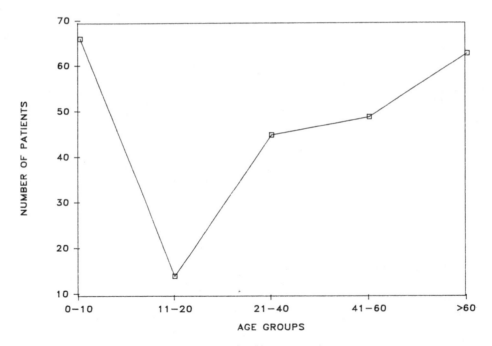

FIGURE 42.2 Example of frequency polygon.

set of data. To illustrate, suppose the blood glucose levels of five patients were as follows: 90, 120, 150, 180, and 180. The mean blood glucose level for the group is 144, whereas the median is 150 and the mode is 180.

It is possible for a distribution of numbers to have the same value for the mean, mode, and median. When this occurs, the distribution is said to be symmetric or *normally distributed*. More often, however, the measures are unequal and the distribution is asymmetric or *skewed*. If the mean is greater than the mode of the data, the distribution has a "positive skew." If the mean is less than the value of the mode, the distribution has a "negative skew." These mea-

sures of skewness or symmetry that help to describe the shape of a frequency polygon are depicted in Figure 42.3.

In addition to measures of central tendency and skewness, data may be further characterized by measures of dispersion or variation. If a group of values are very similar to each other, there is little variation or dispersion in the group. On the other hand, a high degree of dissimilarity would result in a high degree of variation.

The simplest measure of the dispersion of a distribution of data is the range. The *range* is usually reported as the difference between the highest and lowest values in a distribution. Occasionally, the range may be reported simply

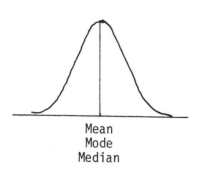
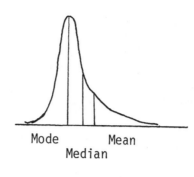
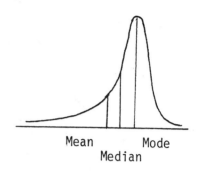

FIGURE 42.3 Examples of symmetric and skewed distributions. *a*, Symmetric; *b*, positive skew; *c*, negative skew.

as the two extreme values. In the example of the blood glucose data, the range would be 90 (180-190).

Because the range does not reveal any details about the variation of scores between the two extremes, it is not a very strong indicator of dispersion. Two superior measures of variability are the variance and the standard deviation. These statistics are better indicators because they are computed from all the data rather than two extreme points. The *variance* (σ^2 or s^2) is computed as the average of the squared deviations of the values about the mean of the *group*. The *standard deviation* (σ or s) is simply the square root of the variance. In addition to describing the spread of a distribution of values, the variance and standard deviation are quite useful in comparing the variability of two separate distributions. For example, in evaluating the bioavailability data for two "equivalent" antibiotics, you should be concerned not only with the mean or average blood levels of the two products, but also with the variance in the blood levels among patients. Both products may produce acceptable mean blood levels, but one patient's blood levels may vary so greatly that the product could produce subtherapeutic levels.

Before leaving the topic of descriptive statistics, one final area deserves discussion: correlation. *Correlation* describes a relationship between two variables. A relationship may be positive, negative, or zero. Two variables are positively correlated when their values systematically move together in the same direction. A negative correlation exists when two variables are inversely related. Finally, a zero correlation exists when no systematic relationship is apparent between two variables.

The strength and the direction of the relationship of two variables is indicated by a statistic known as the correlation coefficient. The range of the correlation coefficient is from -1.00 to $+1.00$, with the sign indicating a negative (inverse relationship) or positive (direct relationship) between variables. The strength of the relationship is suggested by the magnitude of the correlation coefficient. The closer the coefficient is to $+1$ or -1, the stronger the relationship. A coefficient near zero indicates no systematic relationship.

Examples of commonly used correlation techniques include Pearson product-moment correlation (r), Spearman's rho, point-biserial technique, biserial technique, phi correlation, and tetrachoric correlation. Basically, these techniques differ only in the level of measurement required.

A note of caution regarding interpretation of correlations is worthwhile. Correlation indicates that two variables move together in a systematic manner; it does not indicate *causality* between the variables.

Descriptive statistics are invaluable tools in summarizing and characterizing a set of data. Unfortunately, authors frequently fail to include an adequate exploration of their data using descriptive statistics. Effective presentation of descriptive statistics can provide meaningful insight into the nature and structure of a researcher's data.

INFERENTIAL STATISTICS

Whereas descriptive statistics are concerned with describing or characterizing a set of data, inferential statistics are used to infer the characteristics of a larger group, the population, from a smaller group, the sample. Often, inferential statistics are the only feasible techniques available to characterize a large group. The alternative of taking a census of the population may be too costly, too time consuming, or even impossible.

If a researcher makes inferences from a sample, it is essential to have a sample that is *representative* of the population. That is, all the characteristics that are present in the population are evenly distributed among the units in the sample. One technique researchers use to make a sample representative is random selection of the sample units from the population. *Random sampling* means that every member of the population has an equal chance of being selected for the sample. To the extent that random selection is violated, inferences and generalizations to the population are limited.

Although inferential statistics are used to estimate population characteristics from a sample, a more common use for these techniques is in hypothesis testing. Inferential statistics aid the researcher in making decisions between alternative hypotheses. For example, a researcher may wish to compare two or more groups of diabetic patients to determine if they differ in their mean blood glucose levels. The hypothesis is the guide for the researcher wishing to answer these types of questions. Based on theory, prior experience, and the literature, a hypothesis is a statement of the *proposed relationship* between two or more variables. Hypotheses are stated in measurable terms and hence, the relationships states in hypotheses can be evaluated or tested.

The statistical analysis of hypotheses involves a determination of whether two statistics, such as means, are truly different, or if the observed differences are due purely to

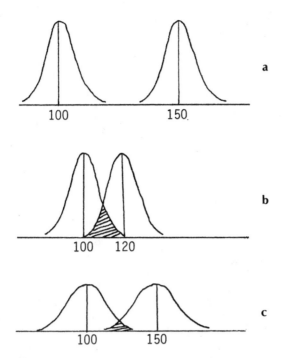

FIGURE 42.4 Comparison of means and variances of two population distributions.

chance. In essence, we are comparing two mean scores and asking the question: "Are these values from the same or different population?" To answer this question and test our hypothesis of different means, we must rely on our earlier discussion of variance or dispersion and the standard deviation. The greater the difference between two mean values, the greater the likelihood they came from two different populations, or distributions, and are, therefore, *significantly different*. Consider, for example, Figure 42.4, which depicts the relationship between populations of blood glucose levels with differing means and variances. Whether two means are significantly different depends on the magnitude of the difference between the two means and the variance of distributions to which the means belong. Figure 42.4*a* illustrates two significantly different means. These two mean blood glucose levels are considered statistically different because the distributions of the two populations do not overlap. When no overlap is present, there is no chance that two means belong to the same population group. In contrast, Figure 42.4*b* shows that two means which have a "chance" of belonging to the same population. Because the two distributions share a common area, depicted by the shaded area, the two observed mean blood glucose levels (100 and 120) may actually fall within the same population distribution. The more overlap, or shared variation between two distributions, the greater the chance or probability that the observed means are not truly different.

Figure 42.4*c* shows the relationship of variance and significant differences between means. Although the means in this figure are identical to those in Figure 42.4*a*, the means in Figure 42.4*c* have a chance of being from the same population. This possibility occurs in the latter but not in the former because the variances of dispersions of the values in Figure 42.4*c* are greater.

TABLE 42.2 Types of Statistics

Type of Statistics	Example Procedures	Function
Descriptive	Mean, median, mode variance, standard deviation, skewness	1. Summarize data 2. Describe distribution
Inferential	Chi square, *t*-test, ANOVA, regression	1. Infer values from samples to populations 2. Test hypotheses

The essence of significant differences relies on a comparison of observed differences to a measure of variation. If the variance of the data is large relative to the magnitude of the difference, the result will not be statistically significant. On the contrary, if the difference between two means is large relative to the dispersion of the data, the observed difference is likely to be "statistically significant." (Computations of these measures are beyond the scope of this chapter, but the reader may refer to any good elementary statistics text for a detailed discussion of the calculations.)

In summary, descriptive statistics are used to characterize and describe large data sets, whereas inferential statistics are used to test hypotheses and make inferences about the population. Various procedures are available to the researcher using either type of statistics. Both descriptive and inferential statistics are of strategic importance in proper data analysis. Table 42.2 summarizes and compares the two types of statistics.

PARAMETRIC VS NONPARAMETRIC STATISTICS

Statistical tests can be divided into two types depending on the assumptions that underlie their application: parametric and nonparametric. Parametric statistical procedures are the most popular and assume that the data are from populations that are normally and independently distributed. Also, the populations must have similar variances (known as homogeneity of variance). Furthermore, parametric statistics require that data be measured in at least interval level. Examples of parametric statistical tests include the mean, standard deviation, *t*-test, and Pearson's correlation coefficient.

Nonparametric statistical procedures, commonly referred to as "distribution-free" statistics, do not require the assumptions of normality and homogeneity of variance. The major underlying assumption of nonparametric statistics is that the observations are independent. Also, nonparametric statistics may be used with lower level measurements, such as nominal or ordinal level data. Some examples of frequently used nonparametric statistics are the mode, median, Spearman's rho, and the chi-square test.

SELECTED STATISTICAL TECHNIQUES

The purpose of this section is to briefly review some of the more frequently used statistical procedures and their appropriate application. This treatment is by no means exhaustive and the researcher is encouraged to pursue a more in-depth exploration of these selected procedures in an appropriate statistics text.

Chi Square. The chi square (χ^2) statistic is a nonparametric technique that is used when the data are expressed in frequencies or proportions. This procedure is typically employed to test whether observed differences are significantly different from what might be observed by chance alone. As a nonparametric technique, the chi-square statistic may be appropriately used with nominal level data. As an illustration, a researcher is interested in knowing if the number of males and females in a sample was significantly different from the distribution of sexes in the population. The chi square would be an appropriate statistic.

t-Test. Although the *t*-test can be used for several purposes, it is most commonly used to test the significance of a difference between two group means. If two sample means are far enough apart on the variances or the two means are very small, the *t*-test will demonstrate a significant difference. Due to the mathematics involved in the *t*-test, at least interval level data are required for analysis.

Analysis of Variance. Whereas the *t*-test is limited to testing differences between two group means, an analysis of variance (ANOVA) may be used to test for significant differences between two or more group means. For example, ANOVA may be utilized to detect significant differences between two or more group means. For example, ANOVA may be utilized to detect significant differences among the peak serum concentrations of five different brands of a drug product. The test statistic in ANOVA is the *F* statistic. If the value of the *F*-test is large, it means that most of the variance in the data is accounted for by differences between the groups; hence true differnces do exist. At least interval level data are needed for an analysis of variance.

Regression. One of the most useful statistical techniques in behavioral science research is regression analysis. This parametric procedure is used to determine how the change in one variable is related to the change in another variable. Regression analysis is a very powerful procedure in that it can be used to test for statistical significance, determine degrees of relationship, evaluate effects of changes in variables, and predict values. A regression model typically contains one dependent variable and one or more independent variables.

Researchers who deploy regression analysis are most often concerned with the signs and magnitudes of the regression coefficients. The sign of the regression coefficients indicates the direction of the relationship between the independent variable and the dependent variable. A positive sign suggests a direct relationship, whereas a negative sign indicates an inverse relationship. Whether or not a particular regression coefficient is significant depends on the size of the coefficient when compared to its variance. Either *t*-test or ANOVA is traditionally used to determine if a coefficient is significantly different from zero. Another statistic that is generated in regression analysis is the coefficient of determination, R^2. This statistic provides an estimate of the amount of variation in the dependent variable that can be explained by the one or more independent variables. Regression analysis should only be used with interval or ratio levels of measurement.

STEPS IN STATISTICAL ANALYSIS OF DATA

Statistical analysis of data is not simply the computation of a *t*-statistic or correlation coefficient. Rather, it is an organized process whereby researchers use statistical procedures to interpret, or explain, the meaning of a collection of numbers. Kerlinger (1) contrasts *statistics* and *statistical analysis* as follows:

Analysis means the categorizing, ordering, manipulating and summarizing of data to obtain answers to research questions. The purpose of analysis is to reduce data to intelligible and interpretable form so that the relations of research problems can be studied and tested. A primary purpose of statistics . . . is to manipulate and summarize numerical data and to compare the obtained results with chance expectations.

Statistical analysis should proceed stepwise:
1. State the null hypothesis
2. Choose the appropriate statistical test for the level of measurement of the data
3. Specify the level of statistical significance
4. Define the region of rejection
5. Compute the statistic to test the null hypothesis
6. Interpret the results of the test

The remaining sections of this chapter will consider each step in detail.

State the Null Hypothesis

We never directly test the statistical proposition (or hypotheses) we believe is true. For example, you would never statistically test the hypothesis that score 1 > score 2, or it may be that the two are equal. A statistical analysis of the relationship between score 1 and score 2 takes the form of a prediction of which alternative is most likely. Because of this, we state the null form of the hypothesis and test it rather than the research hypothesis.

Although not always true, a null hypothesis is usually a statement of *no relationship*. Statistical tests are primarily directed to the purpose of rejecting or disproving the null hypothesis. If it is rejected, the alternative or research hypothesis may be accepted.

This probably seems rather confusing. Perhaps an example will clarify the concept. Suppose you are studying the relationship between pharmacists' productivity in a hospital practice setting and the use of supportive personnel. From your study, you state a theory that proposes that a worker's job satisfaction determines his productivity. Hence, your theory would lead us to believe that if we incorporate technicians into the work force, we could release pharmacists to perform more clinical functions, thereby increasing overall satisfaction for pharmacists. Thus, your theory proposes that use of technicians will increase productivity. This prediction would be our *research hypothesis*. Confirming this hypothesis would support the theory of the relationship between use of supportive personnel and productivity. To carry the illustration further, assume that we test this hypothesis directly by measuring some productivity index in two groups of pharmacists. The group using technicians has a mean productivity index of 80, whereas the mean productivity index for the group without technicians is 70. From this, it would seem that your hypothesis is upheld. Productivity is higher in the group with technicians. However, this may not actually be true. As explained in the first part of the chapter, the differences observed may be due to *chance*. Even though the mean productivity indices of the two groups differ by 10 units, the actual indices may be equal (i.e., they came from the same population of means). This is the reason we have only two possible outcomes in hypothesis testing: (1) reject the null hypothesis or (2) not able to reject the null hypothesis. We never accept a (null) hypothesis when the statistical test results in a value that is not significant.

By testing the null hypotheses, we are, in reality, testing the proposition that the mean of the first group is not different than the mean of the second ($M_1 = M_2$). Thus, we build our theory by rejecting the null hypothesis in favor of the alternative $M_1 \neq M_2$. If the theory suggests that the productivity of one group is greater than the other (e.g., the group with technicians will have greater productivity than the group without technicians), then the alternative is expressed in a like manner ($M_1 > M_2$).

Choose the Appropriate Statistical Test

One of the most frustrating aspects of statistical analysis to the novice researcher or evaluator of research papers is the decision on which statistical test is appropriate for a particular data set. It is easy to learn the computational formula of the various statistical procedures, but somehow the topic of selecting the correct "tool" for the analysis is often overlooked in elementary statistics classes. Then, the day arrives when data are collected and the moment of decision is at hand. Will it be a *t*-test? Is ANOVA more appropriate? What about a correlation coefficient? How do I choose from such a menu?

There are two criteria generally used in selecting a statistical procedure: (1) the level of measurement of the data and (2) the power of the procedure. The concept of level of measurement was presented earlier. Let us now turn our attention to the criteria of power.

The *power of a test* is defined as the probability of rejecting a null hypothesis when in fact it is *false*. This concept is closely related to the third step in statistical analysis, specifying the level of significance. This will be explained in the next section, but generally, the parametric procedures (those used with interval and ordinal data) are also the more powerful procedures. It is beyond the scope of this chapter to elaborate further, other than to say power becomes most critical when selecting *nonparametric* statistical tests. As a general rule, if you select a statistical procedure that is applicable to the level of measurement of the data, then you will probably have the maximum level of power available from statistical procedures given their intended purposes.

The importance of level of measurement on choice of statistical procedure is illustrated in Table 42.3. This diagram relates statistical tests to the level of measurement and the type of sample, either *related* or *independent*. Independent samples are those for which observations in one group are not related in any important way to those in the other group(s). Stated more succinctly, samples are independent when the selection of one subject does not bias (influence) the selection of any other subject in the study. Related samples are those in which the observations are for the same subjects (called repeated measures) or matched subjects. The designation of one sample vs two samples vs k samples in the diagram relates to the number of groups or treatments. The tests under the heading "k samples" are for more than two treatment groups.

Perhaps an example will help explain how this information might be used. Suppose a researcher was testing the effect of a new antihypertensive medication on reducing blood pressure. The research design called for measuring a patient's blood pressure at two time intervals: 1 hour before

TABLE 42.3 Level of Measurement, Nature of Sample, and Appropriate Statistical Procedure[a]

Level of Measurement	Statistical Test					Measure of Correlation
		Two-Sample Case		k-Sample Case		
	One-Sample Case	Related Samples	Independent Samples	Related Samples	Independent Samples	
Nominal	Binomial test χ^2 one-sample test	McNemar test for significance of changes	Fisher exact probability test χ^2 test for two independent samples	Cochran Q test	χ^2 test for k-independent samples	Contingency coefficient: c
Ordinal	Kolmogorov-Smirnov one-sample test One-sample runs test	Sign test Wilcoxon-matched-pairs signed-ranks test	Median test Mann-Whitney U test	Friedman two-way analysis of variance	Extension of the median test Kruskal-Wallis one-way analysis of variance	Spearman rank correlation coefficient: r_s Kendall rank correlation coefficient: τ Kendal partial rank coefficient: $\tau_{xy.z}$ Kendall coefficient of concordance: W
Interval and ratio		Student's t-test Paired samples	Student's t-test	Analysis of variance	Analysis of variance	Pearson's correlation coefficient: r Partial correlation coefficient: $r_{ab.c}$ Analysis of covariance

[a]Modified from Siegel S: *Nonparametric Statistics*. New York, McGraw-Hill, 1956.

taking the medication and 1 hour after taking the medication. The same patients are used throughout. To serve as a control, each patient initially receives a placebo. According to the protocol, samples are taken 1 hour before the placebo is administered and 1 hour after. In the next trial, the test drug is administered according to the protocol. There are two groups of data (placebo and test drug); however, since the measures were taken on the *same* patients, the groups are *related samples*. Moreover, since the level of measurement of blood pressure is a ratio measure, the appropriate statistical test would be the *t*-test for matched pairs. This is the most powerful two-sample statistical test for related samples. If, on the the other hand, there had been two different test drugs administered along with the placebo, then the problem would have required a test that considered k-related samples. From Table 42.3, it is clear that the appropriate test would have been ANOVA. It is the most powerful k-sample test and can be used with interval and ratio level data. It is also the only test that may be applied to related or independent samples.

This discussion of how level of measurement influences the statistical test may be confusing to some students who have observed researchers using *t*-tests, ANOVA tests, and Pearson's correlation coefficients with ordinal level data. For example, a researcher may give a series of statements asking the respondent to strongly agree, agree, disagree, or strongly disagree. When the researcher chooses a statistical test, he often picks the *t*-test to compare the difference between the responses of two groups. Clearly, these data are ordinal. How can a *t*-test be used?

Strictly speaking, most rating scales yield an ordinal level of measurement. Even though the scale points have numbers assigned, it is clear that the distance between "agree" and "strongly agree" is probably not equal to the distance between "agree" and "no opinion." Moreover, there is no numerically true zero value. Hence, the numeric identification signifies nothing more than an order to the responses and statistics, such as mean and standard deviation, have no meaning. The conservative researcher will choose those ordinal level statistical tests for the analysis. Yet there are cases when the more powerful parametric tests can be used with assurance that the results are valid. Kerlinger (2) makes the case as follows:

> The argument is evidential. If we have, say, two or three measures of the same variable, and these measures are all substantially and linearly related, then equal intervals can be assumed. This assumption is valid because the more nearly a relation approaches linearity, the more nearly equal are the intervals of the scales.

This caution is to alert you to distortions and errors that may be evident in using interval measures with ordinal data. Results should be interpreted with care to be sure that major errors do not occur. As Kerlinger (3) concludes, " . . . the consequences are evidently not serious."

Specify the Level of Statistical Significance

The level of statistical significance discussed earlier in the chapter is the alpha level. Many researchers treat this step in the process lightly. Since most reports of research choose an alpha level of 0.05, it has become somewhat the standard by default. However, one cannot make a case for an alpha level of 0.05 any more effectively than one can make a case for an alpha of 0.01 or 0.08. The 0.05 level has simply become traditional.

In choosing an alpha level, a researcher should consider the risk of making type I and type II errors. Alpha is the probability of making a type I error. A type I error is defined as the error of rejecting the null hypothesis when, in fact, it is true. An alpha of 0.05 means the researcher is willing to risk five chances out of 100 that the conclusion of his hypothesis test is to reject the null hypothesis when it is actually true. A type II error is the failure to reject the null hypothesis when it is actually false. The probability of making a type II error is beta. The value of beta is determined by the size of the sample and the value of alpha. The relationship is inverse: a decrease in the value of alpha will increase beta for any given sample size.

Alpha and beta should be set before you do the research. The values chosen would set the example size. In reality, most researchers set the alpha level and sample size first and then determine beta. The decision as to the level of significance selected usually depends on the relative cost of making either a type I or type II error. For example, a clinician may not be willing to risk a new drug therapy with a high potential for serious side effects unless it is definitely more effective than the traditional treatments that have fewer severe side effects. This is a case of not wanting to risk rejecting the null hypothesis that the new therapy is equivalent to the traditional therapy when, in fact, the null hypothesis is true. Hence the alpha level would be set at a high level, perhaps 0.01 or 0.001. However, if two treatments carry about the same level of side effects and the cost of therapy is roughly equivalent, then there is less risk associated with making a wrong judgment. An alpha level of 0.05 or 0.10 may be acceptable.

You can see the potential for researcher bias in this process. By selecting a low level of significance, a researcher can support alternative hypotheses he may favor. Likewise, by setting an unrealistically high level for alpha, research can conclude that the null hypothesis cannot be rejected. Hence, you should carefully consider the alpha level in interpreting the results of any hypothesis test.

There is one final factor to consider in determining how extreme the results must be before rejecting the null hypothesis: the number of subjects. Blalock describes the relationship as follows: "With a very large number of cases, it is practically always possible to reject any false hypothesis we might set up, regardless of how far our hypothesized value may be different from the true one" (4). With a large number of cases, say 5,000-10,000, it is quite easy to reject a null hypothesis at the 0.001 level. To illustrate, suppose we hypothesize that the probability of getting heads in a coin toss is 0.5. If we toss the coin only ten times, very extreme results are required to reject the null hypothesis. This suggests that there are major differences between statistical significance and practical significance. Statistical significance can exist because of the minor differences that occur in the way a problem is analyzed. However, statistical differences must be weighed against whether the difference is importance. In some problems it might very well be important. In others it may be meaningless.

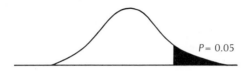

FIGURE 42.5 One-tailed region of rejection (shaded area alpha = 0.05).

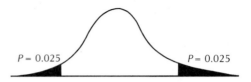

FIGURE 42.6 Two-tailed region of rejection (shaded area alpha = 0.05).

Define the Region of Rejection

As stated before, hypotheses are tested given a controlled probability of error, type I error. That is, we conclude whether a hypothesis is true or false within a specified range of probability called the alpha level. If our particular result falls outside of this range into what is called the *region of rejection*, we reject the null hypothesis with the probability of making a type I error. The probability associated with any value in the region of rejection is equal to or less than alpha.

Figure 42.5 illustrates this concept. The darkened area shows a region of rejection equal to an alpha of 0.05. It is termed a *one-tailed* region since the entire area under the curve relating to the region of rejection is in one tail of the distribution. Figure 42.6 depicts a *two-tailed* region of rejection. There is 2.5% in each end, yeilding a total alpha of 0.05.

The determination of whether the alpha should be in one or two tails is determined by the nature of the hypothesis. If the alternative hypothesis indicates the predicted direction of the difference between the groups, then the one-tail region is chosen. If there is no direction hypothesized, then a two-tail region is used.

Compute the Statistic to Test the Null Hypothesis

The data collected to test the hypothesis is entered into the appropriate formula to compute a value called the *test statistic*. Each test statistic has a corresponding *degree of freedom,* which is a number that represents the number of observations used to compute the statistic. These two values—the test statistic and the degrees of freedom—are then used to determine the results of the hypothesis test.

Interpret the Results of the Test

To draw a conclusion from the statistical analysis, one must analyze the value of the test statistic in relation to the region of rejection. If the test statistic falls within the region of rejection, then the researcher will reject the null hypoth-

esis in favor of the alternative hypothesis. If the test statistic does not fall within the rejection region, then the researcher will conclude that, given the data at hand, he can not reject the null hypothesis.

Statisticians have developed tables of values, called *critical values,* that simplify the process of determining the region of rejection. There is a table for each type of test, i.e., chi square, *t*-test, etc. Critical values are given for each level of significance and degrees of freedom. If the value of the computed test statistics is greater than or equal to the critical value, then the test concludes that the hypothesis is not true. For example, suppose we have analyzed a data set with a *t*-test and the computed test statistic to be 3.54 and 30 degrees of freedom. Further, assume that the research hypothesis indicates the predicted direction of the differences; hence, a one-tail test is appropriate. Looking in a table of critical values for *t*-tests with 30 degrees of freedom and an alpha of 0.01, we find that the critical value is 2.46. Since the test statistic is larger than the critical value, we reject the null hypothesis.

CONCLUSIONS

Statistical procedures are truly tools of the researcher. They help summarize data, detect the nature of the distribution, infer population characteristics from a sample, and test hypotheses. A researcher must exercise care in selecting specific procedures to use, considering the level of measurement, the independence of the samples and the power of the test. When used appropriately, statistics can lead to meaningful, valid conclusions. When used inappropriately, statistics can prove anything.

REFERENCES

1. Kerlinger, FN: *Foundations of Behavioral Research,* ed 2. New York, Holt, Rinehart & Winston, 1973, p. 134.
2. ibid., p 438.
3. ibid., p 441.
4. Blalock HM: *Social Statistics,* ed 2. New York, McGraw-Hill, 1972, p 162.

CHAPTER 43

Utilization Review

DUANE M. KIRKING

The frequent use and significant cost of drugs as health care interventions have been discussed in great detail throughout the pharmacy literature. The morbidity and mortality associated with the less-than-rational prescribing and use of medications is similarly well documented, and estimates of the direct and indirect costs of these problems to society are staggering (1). Although a variety of programs—many of which are pharmacist initiated—have achieved improvements in drug use, major problems remain. The continually growing number of new drugs and the increasing complexity of those drugs and related delivery systems are only two of the reasons for programs that review drug therapy to identify its deficiences and develop strategies for correcting them (2).

Drug utilization review (DUR)* programs are designed to achieve these goals. After defining DUR and identifying more explicitly its objectives, this chapter will outline the formal requirements for conducting DUR. In addition, a perspective of DUR as part of a comprehensive quality assurance program will be provided. A major portion of the chapter is devoted to introducing the steps involved in developing a DUR program. Finally, examples of published DUR activities are briefly reviewed to direct the reader interested in learning more about this important topic.

DEFINITION OF DUR

An important conceptual definition of DUR has been provided by Brodie and Smith: "Drug utilization review is an authorized, structured and continuing program that reviews, analyzes and interprets patterns (rates and costs) of drug usage in a given health care delivery system against predetermined standards" (3). Although elements of this definition will be discussed in detail throughout the chapter, highlighting several phrases here serves to illustrate the nature of DUR.

First, DUR considers "*patterns* . . . of drug usage." In this way, it differs from drug therapy monitoring, which is oriented toward individual patients and their therapy. It is important that this distinction be made clear to all persons involved in a DUR program. This "system" orientation of

DUR, i.e., concern with *aggregate* usage in specified categories of medications, disease states, or prescribers, can be troublesome for health care providers whose training and practice is directed toward helping individuals. Such an orientation does not mean DUR is not concerned with improving patient care, however. Indeed its potential to optimize care is greater than with routine monitoring because DUR seeks to identify and correct inappropriate drug use for an entire institution rather than on a patient-by-patient basis. In addition, if the review is being conducted on a prospective or concurrent basis, results also may be of value to the individual patient.

Second, DUR is more than merely collecting data. A good DUR program "reviews, analyzes and interprets" those data with the goal of improving health care, rather than allowing the results of a review to collect dust on a shelf.

Third, a DUR program should be a well-planned one that uses mutually acceptable, specific measures ("authorized," "structured," "predetermined standards") rather than a haphazardly instituted activity that may yield different results each time it is done, depending upon the biases of the individual reviewer.

Fourth, a particular DUR program must be designed for "a given health care delivery system." Although specific criteria have been developed for widespread use, they should be adapted as necessary to meet the needs of a particular health care setting.

Finally, DUR should be a "continuing program." While individual, one-time DUR *studies* or audits can be valuable in research designed to quantify and describe drug usage, the value of an ongoing *program* is in its ability to monitor drug usage on a continuing basis to determine if there are improvements over time.†

Stolar adds an important element perhaps implied but not explicitly stated in the Brodie and Smith definition of DUR. A DUR program includes "efforts to correct patterns of drug use not consistent with these standards. It includes a mechanism for measuring the effectiveness of these corrective actions" (4). The primary goal of a DUR program is to assure the quality of drug use. This is another distinction

---

*Drug utilization review is generally considered synonymous with "drug use review" and "drug usage review." Fortunately, all three phrases can be represented by the same acronym.

†The distinctions between and purposes of DUR studies vs programs as well as differences between qualitative and quantitative studies are discussed in detail by Stolar (4).

between DUR programs and studies. The latter often do not include efforts to correct deficiencies, such as through educational programs or, if necessary, the institution of sanctions.

In conclusion, it is important to note what is not included in definitions of DUR. The nature of the data collecting and processing system is not specified, nor whether that data should be collected retrospectively, concurrently, or prospectively. The peer review mechanism is not defined. Thus, the uniqueness of every situation is recognized. Decisions of this type are to be made by local health care providers and administrators as individual programs are developed (5).

OBJECTIVES OF DUR

The objectives of DUR with regard to patient care identified by the Health, Education and Welfare Task Force on Prescription Drugs are as appropriate today as when first presented in the late 1960s. "Utilization review is . . . aimed first at rational prescribing and the consequent improvement in the quality of care, and second at minimizing needless expenditures" (6). (Rational prescribing was defined as the right drug, for the right patient, in the right amounts, at the right time [6]). This statement recognizes the central role played by drugs in health care: that if the quality of drug therapy can be optimized, the overall quality of care should improve as well.

Note also that reduction of drug costs is a secondary objective of DUR. It is entirely possible that a well-designed program can lead to cost savings by identifying situations where existing therapy can be replaced by less expensive drugs or even by nondrug therapy with equal or better results. However, this may not always be the case. Indeed, the most appropriate therapy may actually increase medication cost while resulting in a decrease in the total cost of treating a particular disease or illness through, for example, a decreased length of hospital stay (7).

In addition to patient care objectives, there are pharmacy objectives that can also be met by DUR. The implementation of prospective reimbursement systems is forcing hospital administrators to require departments to justify the services they provide (8). For pharmacy this means justification of both distributive and clinical functions. To justify these activities, pharmacy departments must convince administration that (1) the activities of pharmacists can improve the quality of drug use and (2) while cost control of drugs is important, decreased drug use is not necessarily consistent with improved quality of overall care. DUR studies can provide evidence that problems with drug usage may be leading to increased total costs. Subsequent follow-up studies conducted after institution of clinical pharmacy activities may document that intervention by pharmacists can reduce usage problems. Of course, the value of clinical pharmacy services can be shown only if that value does indeed exist. Assuming this situation is true, a DUR program can help provide the necessary documentation for justification of clinical pharmacy services.

Because DUR requires active interaction of pharmacists with other health care providers in the hospital or other institution, there is the potential for increased interdisciplinary cooperation and recognition of the knowledge and skills of pharmacists by other professionals. It should not be assumed that DUR teamwork will necessarily improve existing negative relationships, but it does have the potential to strengthen images and relations that are already positive or perhaps neutral.

One important strategy advocated by hospital administrators in reaction to the constraints of prospective reimbursement is to increase physician awareness of and involvement in cost and quality of care issues (9). This is clearly one of the objectives of DUR and may be used to justify expansion of DUR activities.

Although the orientation of this chapter is toward the use of DUR as a means of improving the quality of care within a given institution, DUR has been widely and legitimately used as a research tool. The pharmacy and health care literature is replete with studies describing what drugs are used, who uses them, and who prescribes them. Other reports document the extent of misprescribing or the incidence of adverse drug effects or other problems of therapy. Such activities, when well conducted, can contribute substantially to our understanding of drug use. Before undertaking a descriptive DUR study as a research project, the pharmacist should determine if the results are likely to add significantly to the existing literature and, if so, if the study is designed with sufficient scientific rigor.

Some DUR activities are likely to meet the needs of both research and patient care. An analysis of drug use in a population or practice environment not yet adequately described in the literature, a compilation of newly created or revised DUR criteria resulting from a recently completed review, or a novel method of conducting review activities such as through computerization of a certain aspect of the review are all examples of results that might appropriately be shared via pharmacy and other health care journals. In most cases, however, DUR activities should be designed primarily to improve the quality of drug use in the institution.

REQUIREMENTS FOR DUR

Although concern for the quality of health care and, in particular, drug usage is not new, the development of formal review requirements and accompanying terminology is largely a product of the past two decades. Commencing with the passage of the Medicaid-Medicare legislation of 1965, which required utilization review and medical audits, a variety of organizations have developed review requirements, each having its own unique terminology.‡

Current requirements for DUR in the institution derive from two major sources: the Medicare-Medicaid regulations and the accreditation standards of the JCAH. Although JCAH standards state that DUR is ultimately a responsibility of the medical staff, the requirement for direct involvement by the pharmacy department is clearly identified in at least two standards (10):

---

‡For example, the Joint Comission on Accreditation of Hospitals (JCAH) has "patient care audits" and "patient care evaluation"; the now defunct professional standards review organizations (PSROs) used "medical-care evaluation studies." The interrelationship of these and other review activities has been discussed by Stolar (5).

1. The development and surveillance of pharmacy and therapeutics policies and practices, particularly drug utilization within the hospital, shall be the responsibility of the medical staff and shall be carried out in cooperation with the pharmacist and with representatives of other disciplines as required. (Interpretation of Medical Staff Standard IV, p 102.)

2. [T]he director of the pharmaceutical department/service should be responsible for at least the following: . . . participating in those aspects of the overall hospital quality assurance program that relate to drug utilization and effectiveness. This may include determining usage patterns for each drug according to clinical department/service or individual prescribers, and assisting in the setting of drug-use criteria. (Interpretation of Pharmaceutical Services Standard III, pp 136, 137.)

While pharmacy involvement in DUR action is mandated by JCAH standards, the nature and extent of the involvement are not prescribed but only suggested. Thus, how involved the pharmacy department becomes in DUR activities is determined within each individual institution. This situation generally requires the pharmacy department to help determine how it will become involved in DUR as well as perhaps defining the very nature and extent of the entire DUR program.

Three particular areas described by JCAH standards are worthy of additional note. First, although specific drugs subject to review are not identified in the standards, antibiotic usage review is mandated and often serves as a starting point for a DUR program (Medical Staff and Infection Control Standards, pp 103 and 70, respectively). In addition, as hospitals expand their activities beyond traditional inpatient situations, review functions expand accordingly. Thus, DUR is to be conducted for ambulatory care patients treated by the staff although, as above, only antibiotics are mentioned specifically (Hospital-Sponsored Ambulatory Care Services Standard VI, p 67). Finally, review of a hospital's home care activities must include drug review: "This review and evaluation shall also include review of all medications a patient is known to be taking. . . . Consultation with a registered pharmacist should be available as needed" (Interpretation of Home Care Services Standard IV, p 57). While the home care requirement appears to be more related to drug therapy monitoring than formal DUR, it is clear that JCAH considers review of drug therapy important for both inpatient and outpatient settings and that pharmacists should be a part of that review process (10).

Until recently, monitoring an institution's adherence to the Medicare-Medicaid utilization review regulations was the responsibility of PSROs. However, PSROs have been replaced by a new structure, utilization and quality control peer review organizations (PROs), which have a similar function (11). The specific activities of PROs and their activities regarding DUR are not known at this time. What is known, however, is that hospitals must contract with a PRO to be eligible to participate in Medicare. Thus, some organization outside of the hospital itself will continue to regularly monitor the hospital's utilization review activities. The interested reader is encouraged to contact the local (usually statewide) PRO to determine its activities regarding DUR.

Finally, although adherence to its standards is not a requirement for hospital accreditation or third-party reimbursement, the American Society of Hospital Pharmacists (ASHP) has included DUR as one of the clinical functions of the pharmacist and has endorsed such review as a function of the Pharmacy and Therapeutics Committee, a Drug Utilization Review Committee, and/or other appropriate bodies within the institution (ASHP Guideline on Hospital Drug Control Systems, Statement on the Pharmacy and Therapeutics Committee, and Statement on Clinical Functions in Institutional Pharmacy Practice) (12).

QUALITY ASSURANCE AND DUR

Pharmacy departments should have a departmental quality assurance (QA) program that is part of the hospital-wide QA program mandated by the JCAH Quality Assurance Standards. As shown in Figure 43.1, DUR can be considered one component of the pharmacy QA program. Most pharmacy QA activities are directed toward functions that are primarily departmental in nature. The quality of drug usage, however, is a function of the actions of several departments in the hospital, and thus, as discussed in the previous section, DUR is a joint obligation of pharmacy, the medical staff, and often other departments. Actual conducting of reviews is frequently done by the pharmacy department, however.

In designing a comprehensive pharmacy QA program, it is important to examine the entire drug use process even though it may be necessary to separate intradepartmental activities from interdepartmental activities such as DUR when operationalizing the program. The six steps of this process, as enumerated by Knapp et al (13), are:

1. Determination of a need for a drug by the prescriber. This involves diagnosis and a choice in general terms between drug and nondrug therapy.

2. Selection of a specific drug product. This involves decisions as to therapeutic category, active ingredient, and specific drug product.

3. Selection of regimen. This involves determination of route of administration, dosage form, strength, dosage quantity, and length of therapy.

4. Obtaining the drug product. The chosen product must be obtained by or procured for the patient.

5. Administration/consumption of the drug product. Ambulatory patients or their family are responsible for self-administration of therapy.

6. Effects of drug therapy and feedback to all concerned. These effects are perceived and interpreted by the patient, the prescriber, and relevant others.

DUR is directed primarily toward the first three steps of this process, which are usually the physician's responsibility in the inpatient setting. Generally, it is assumed that establishing the diagnosis, a part of step one, has been done correctly. Increasingly, the pharmacist is involved in portions of the first three steps (e.g., through generic and therapeutic substitutions, provision of pharmacokinetic consults, and other therapy recommendations as well as actual prescribing to a limited extent).

Review of the pharmacist's actions in these areas is likely to be done as part of pharmacy's intradepartmental QA activities rather than through DUR. In what specific part of a comprehensive QA program this review is accomplished

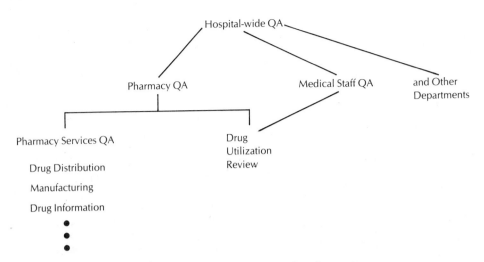

FIGURE 43.1   DUR as a component of quality assurance.

is not critical, only that review does indeed occur. Step four, which includes, for example, IV admixture preparation and extemporaneous compounding as well as inventory control and drug distribution, is almost certain to be reviewed as an internal, pharmacy function.

Step five introduces the role of the nurse, although pharmacy has become involved in drug administration to a limited extent. Inclusion of administration criteria have been included in some DUR programs (14,15).

The last step is concerned with the outcomes of drug therapy (either positive or negative). This area is one that has seen only limited review for a variety of reasons, including difficulty in defining specific therapeutic outcomes and relating these outcomes directly to specific therapy.

Successful therapy requires that the entire drug use process be conducted appropriately. This appropriateness can be assured only if all steps and personnel involved are reviewed in some way. Although some elements of a review of this process are clearly part of DUR, the distinction is not as clear with other parts. The specific assignment of review functions to DUR vs other aspects of a comprehensive QA program is best guided by the particular situation at a given institution as long as it is understood that a review of drug usage is not complete unless all steps of the drug use process are evaluated.

A conceptual definition of quality, as applied to any aspect of health care, including drug use, is extremely difficult to develop. In his latest exposition on what is included in such a definition, Donabedian concludes "that there are several definitions of quality, or several variants of a single definition; and that each definition or variant is legitimate in its appropriate context" (16). Similarly, quality can be *measured* in several ways, and while an unambiguous conceptual definition of quality may not be necessary to develop a DUR program, an understanding of the ways of measuring quality is essential.

Perhaps the best known classification scheme for measuring quality of health care is the structure-process-outcome typology developed by Donabedian (16). This typology is discussed in some detail in Chapter 41, and the reader who is not well aware of it is encouraged to review that material. Most DUR activities evaluate process measures of

drug use (e.g., appropriate use of renal function tests for patients with renal dysfunction receiving aminoglycoside antibiotics), although outcome assessment is being used with increasing frequency, especially when specific therapeutic endpoints are measureable (e.g., blood pressure reduced to less than 90 mm Hg). A major problem with outcome measures, particularly if they are more general than the above example (e.g., death or recovery), is that outcome can also be influenced by exogenous factors, making it difficult to be certain of the effect of the specific drug being reviewed.

In today's health care environment, cost is a major consideration. Although convincing arguments can be presented for not including costs directly in a definition of quality, the two issues are closely interrelated (16). Both the direct cost of providing a product or service, drug therapy in the present case, and indirect costs (e.g., costs associated with an increased hospital stay secondary to less-than-optimal therapy) are important. Unfortunately, the cost dimension of DUR has not been developed as well as the strictly defined quality assurance dimension. Recently, however, applications of principles of drug cost-benefit and cost-effectiveness analysis and of drug therapy effects on length of stay patterns have been published (7,17). The current economic climate in health care provides the incentive for including cost-benefit consideration in DUR along with traditional quality considerations. However, cost containment must not become the only issue, and both direct and indirect costs must be considered in DUR. Care must be taken to assure that DUR does not become primarily a program, disguised as quality assurance, to contol drug costs. If saving a few dollars by reducing medication costs results in complications and lengthening of a hospital stay, then neither the goals of quality assurance nor cost containment are achieved.

DESIGNING AND OPERATING A DUR PROGRAM

The characteristics of DUR are well illustrated by the quality assurance cycle (Figure 43.2), which has been adapted to pharmacy services by Stolar (5) and others from its origins in the American Hospital Association's Quality As-

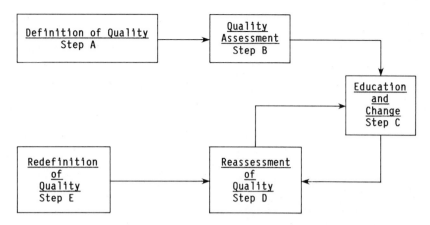

FIGURE 43.2   The quality assurance cycle. (Redrawn by permission from Stolar MH: Conceptual framework for drug usage review, medical audit and other patient care review procedures. *Am J Hosp Pharm* 34:139-145, 1977.)

surance Program. This cycle emphasizes the formal structure of DUR; its need to correct, as well as detect, problems and the iterative nature of a good DUR program. Thus, it provides a general framework that should be the basis for any DUR program.

The process of designing and operating a DUR program is quite complex, however, and is best described by subdividing the categories of the quality assurance cycle. Although the categorization of the steps in a DUR program is somewhat arbitrary, there are certain elements that should be considered. The categorization to be discussed below is shown in Figure 43.3. Space precludes a complete discussion of each of the elements; the remainder of this section serves only to introduce them. Persons interested in developing their own DUR programs should build upon this introduction by reading more in-depth discussions of relevant

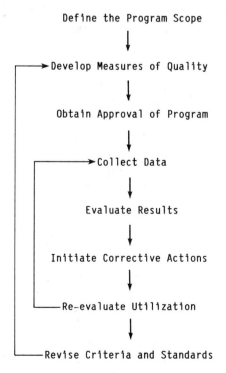

FIGURE 43.3   Steps in developing a DUR review program.

topics and reviewing examples of actual programs referenced below.

Define the Program Scope. No DUR program can review all drug use in an institution, since the resources required would be prohibitive. The program should first consider therapeutic classes of drugs that have the greatest demonstrated potential to cause harm, are most susceptible to the development of problems in achieving optimal usage, and/ or have the most potential for positive impact as a result of improvement in use. Antibiotics and cardiovascular agents are commonly reviewed since they have been shown to be responsible for half of all adverse drug reactions in hospitals (18). While published reports of drug usage problems can be consulted, data from the individual institution provide the best guideline to identifying specific drugs or drug classes for review and for prioritizing the order in which they will be reviewed. In any event, it is best to develop a program around one or two drugs or drug classes and then expand the program after the review system is well established and accepted.

Develop Measures of Quality. Developing appropriate measures of quality is difficult and is one of the most crucial steps of the entire DUR process. Suboptimal measures, including those that are too general, too difficult to operationalize, or are based on incorrect therapeutic principles, can result in incorrect conclusions of may prevent the review from being completed.

A body of terminology has developed that describes measures of quality. *Criteria* are "predetermined elements against which aspects of the quality of a medical service may be compared" (19). There are often several components *(elements)* of the criteria for any given drug that help define quality drug use in a complete way. For example, there may be one or more "indication for use" elements (e.g., patient has documented diagnosis of disease A), "process" elements (e.g., drug was administered within ½ hour of scheduled time), or "outcome" elements (e.g., patient's diastolic blood pressure reduced to less than 90 mm Hg). While criteria may be either *explicit* (objective) or *implicit* (subjective); written, explicit criteria are necessary to assure that they can be applied consistently in different situations and by different reviewers.

Both *screening* criteria and *in-depth* criteria have been

developed. As the name implies, screening criteria are used to identify situations for further, in-depth review. They may be based on, for example, a minimum and maximum daily dose or length of therapy for a specific drug. Screening criteria are not usually part of the institutional DUR, which generally starts directly with in-depth criteria.

Standards are measures of the acceptable deviation from the elements of the criteria. Frequently, no deviations are allowed, and thus the standard is set at 100% or 0%. There may be *exceptions* stated, however, which identify situations in which legitimate clinical variation is recognized. Finally, one may see reference to *norms,* which are measures of the existing situation. Other than providing justification for conducting a specific review (because of evidence of poor-quality drug use in an area), norms have little place in the development of a DUR program. In particular, it is important that criteria be designed toward achieving the optimal situation and not perpetuating the existing one.

Criteria may be developed by the institution or it may draw upon previously developed criteria. The second approach is generally preferable for at least two reasons: First, developing criteria when they already exist is a major waste of valuable time. Second, and perhaps less obvious but no less important, preexisting criteria are presumably literature based, developed by experts in the field, and have been shown to be valid from previous use. (These assumptions should be confirmed before they are used, however.) They are less likely to reflect the biases and suboptimal usage that may exist in any particular health care setting.

If preexisting criteria are used, they should be reviewed, however, and perhaps modified for use in each specific institution. Not only the content, but also the form for collecting information and availability of that information may vary from place to place. In addition, published criteria should be reviewed to assure they are consistent with current therapy recommendations, since there may be a significant time delay between development of criteria, their publication, and subsequent use by another institution. Modification of criteria should be undertaken with care, however, so that their objectivity is not destroyed.

Sources of existing DUR criteria include published studies describing DUR programs and compilations of sets of criteria. In the former case, if the criteria are not part of the article, they may be available from the author. Examples of compiled criteria sets are available for psychotropic drugs (20), for antibiotic prophylaxis in surgery (21), and for DUR in skilled nursing facilities (22). A two-volume set covering a wide variety of drugs has been published by the ASHP (23,24). The criteria for propranolol review from the ASHP collection are given in Figure 43.4. This example illustrates the various components of DUR criteria as described above. Note that the criteria include "data retrieval instructions" directing the reviewer to sources of the desired information. Finally, sets of screening criteria have also been published (25,26). These particular collections were designed primarily for ambulatory care use and include minimum and maximum dose criteria and/or size-of-prescription limits.

Obtain Approval of Program. Proper authorization and approval of DUR activities not only legitimize the program's existence, they should reflect a commitment of resources to conduct the program and to implement its findings (3). While agreement in principle by the hospital administration, the medical staff, and/or other appropriate administrative bodies should be sought before a program is developed, a reiteration of that support in its fully developed form is valuable as well.

Successful DUR programs are rarely developed solely by pharmacy because the ultimate authority for conducting DUR does not rest in this department. It is important that the program be developed along with existing committees with review functions (e.g., pharmacy and therapeutics or antibiotic surveillance committees). The support of these committees should facilitate program approval by the administrator and medical staff. Techniques to create an environment conducive to interdisciplinary cooperation have been described (27).

Collect Data. Collection of data to compare existing patterns of drug usage to the approved measures of quality may be done either retrospectively (after therapy is completed), concurrently (during the course of therapy), or prospectively (prior to initiation of therapy). All three time frames have advantages and disadvantages, which have been discussed in detail elsewhere (24). The majority of DUR programs utilize a retrospective approach. By concentrating on previous events, the review can be conducted at a convenient time and does not interfere with the daily activities of the pharmacy staff. In retrospective reviews, however, the quality of the data collected cannot be better than the quality of the written patient records upon which the review is based.

Prospective review has the distinct advantage of being able to benefit the particular patient for whom suboptimal therapy is ordered. It must, however, be integrated into the daily pharmacy routine, which can be disruptive, particularly if not all relevant patient variables are easily retrievable. In addition, prospective review limits the use of relatively inexpensive nonprofessional personnel. Concurrent review, if initiated early in the course of therapy, may be able to benefit the affected patient while removing some of the disruptive influence of prospective review.

The similarity of both prospective and concurrent review to the concept of drug therapy monitoring should be obvious, and it is at this point that the differences between DUR and drug therapy monitoring become less distinct. This overlap of activities is not inappropriate, since both have the goal of optimizing drug therapy. One distinction that is important, however, is that DUR has the added dimension of being concerned with *patterns* of care within the institutions and not only the therapy of an individual patient. In addition, DUR activities are usually based upon more explicit criteria than is drug therapy monitoring.

The timing of the review is also a function of the type of assessment being conducted. For example, outcome measures cannot be done on a prospective basis nor generally on a concurrent basis. Thus, a DUR program that includes an outcome assessment component must be conducted at least in part on a retrospective basis. Also, a DUR program that measures more than the prescribing aspect of the drug use process (e.g., proper drug administration) cannot be conducted on a prospective basis.

When collecting data, it is important to obtain descriptions of the providers and the services provided, as well as demographic characteristics of the patients that are reviewed

Audit Criteria:

Propranolol for Hypertension

No.	Elements	Standard 100% 0%	No.	Exceptions	No.	Data Retrieval Instructions
	Justification of Use					
1	One of the following: a) essential hypertension not controlled by diuretics[1-4] (blood pressure remains 160/90 mm Hg or greater on diuretic therapy) b) initial therapy for essential hypertension[1,2,5,6] (blood pressure 160/90 mm Hg or greater)	X	1A	None	1	History, progress notes, nursing notes, order sheet, medication administration record (MAR)
	Critical (Process) Indicators					
2	Patient does not have asthma, chronic obstructive pulmonary disease, chronic bronchitis, emphysema, second- or third-degree atrioventricular block, congestive heart failure, or bradycardia (heart rate <45 beats/min)[2,4,6-8]	X	2A	Artificial pacemaker in place in patients with second- or third-degree atrioventricular block	2 2A	History, progress notes History
3	Salt-restricted diet[9]	X	3A	None	3	Order sheet, progress notes
4	No concurrent administration of other beta-blockers (e.g., nadolol, atenolol, timolol, metoprolol)[1,3,10]	X	4A	None	4	Order sheet, MAR

FIGURE 43.4 DUR criteria for propranolol. (Reprinted by permission from Henricks JN: *Audit Criteria for Drug Utilization Review.* Bethesda, American Society of Hospital Pharmacists, 1981.)

Audit Criteria:

Propranolol for Hypertension (continued)

No.	Elements	Standard 100%	Standard 0%	No.	Exceptions	No.	Data Retrieval Instructions
5	Pretreatment hematocrit or hemoglobin; serum creatinine (SCr) or blood urea nitrogen (BUN); serum potassium, glucose, uric acid, cholesterol, SGOT, SGPT, and alkaline phosphatase; urinalysis; and electrocardiogram[11,12]	X		5A	Studies obtained in previous 12 months	5 / 5A	Order sheet, lab reports / History, clinic or office notes
6	Monitor blood pressure three times daily and heart rate once daily (hospitalized patients)	X		6A	None	6	Order sheet, nursing notes, progress notes
7	Usual maintenance dosage range and administration schedule: 80-480 mg/day in two to four divided doses[2-5,13]	X		7A	Dosages up to 960 mg/day required to maintain blood pressure less than 160/90 mm Hg	7 / 7A	Order sheet, MAR / Progress notes, nursing notes, blood pressure records, order sheet
8	Dosage increases at least 1 week apart[3]	X		8A	None	8	Order sheet, progress notes
9	Propranolol discontinued over at least 1-2 weeks[3,7]	X		9A	Discontinued abruptly due to adverse reaction (see Criteria 11-16)	9 / 9A	Order sheet, progress notes / Progress notes, nursing notes, order sheet
10	Patient instructed not to discontinue propranolol abruptly	X		10A	None	10	Progress notes, nursing notes
	Complications				<ins>Critical Preventative/ Responsive Management</ins>		
11	Bronchospasms or wheezing[1-4,7,8]		X	11A / 11B	Discontinue propranolol / Consider beta-agonist inhalations	11 / 11A-D	Progress notes, nursing notes / Order sheet, progress notes

FIGURE 43.4, cont'd

Audit Criteria: Propranolol for Hypertension (continued)

No.	Elements	Standard 100%	Standard 0%	No.	Exceptions	No.	Data Retrieval Instructions
				11C	Consider aminophylline		
				11D	Institute alternative antihypertensive therapy (may try metoprolol or atenolol if bronchospasms are considered minor)		
12	Fatigue[3,7]	X		12A	Decrease dose or try another beta-blocker	12	Progress notes, nursing notes
						12A	Order sheet, progress notes
13	Cold extremities, worsening claudication, or Raynaud's disease[2,3,7]	X		13A	Decrease dose or try a cardioselective beta-blocker (metoprolol, atenolol)	13	Progress notes, nursing notes
						13A	Order sheet, progress notes
14	Vivid dreams, dizziness, hallucinations, or depression[2-4,7,8]	X		14A	Decrease dose or try another beta-blocker	14	Progress notes, nursing notes
						14A	Progress notes, order sheet
15	Congestive heart failure[1-4,7,8]	X		15A	Decrease dose or discontinue propranolol	15	Progress notes
				15B	Institute therapy for congestive heart failure	15A-C	Order sheet, progress notes
				15C	Consider alternative non-beta-blocker antihypertensive therapy		
16	Aggravation or precipitation of angina when propranolol is discontinued[3,7,14]	X		16A	Reinstitute propranolol therapy and taper over 1-2 weeks	16	Progress notes, nursing notes
						16A	Order sheet, progress notes
	Outcome Measures						
17	Blood pressure less than 160/90 mm Hg[1,15]	X		17A	None	17	Progress notes, nursing notes

FIGURE 43.4, cont'd

(3). Examples of this type of data include age, training, and specialty of providers; length of stay data for specific diseases and related patient status variables; and age, sex, and socioeconomic characteristics of patients. Although some of this information may seem irrelevant to the drug use process, it does provide a more complete base from which to interpret results and search for the sources and causes of drug use problems.

The growth of computer use in hospitals will have major implications for DUR programs in the future. Their major use to date has been to sort data and identify cases for review. Thus, a computer can identify in seconds all patients in the last 3 months receiving heparin, for example, a procedure that could take hours when done manually. The time-saving capability of computerized searching and sorting can be optimized only if the computer has a good data base management system that allows the user to generate reports using any desired configuration of drugs, diagnostic related groups (DRGs), diseases, patients, prescribers, or other characteristics. This capability only exists on some systems and is a feature that should be investigated before a computer is purchased.

Although they have not generally been used in this way for DUR activities, computers do have the capability to accept data directly from a terminal—not unlike entering medication orders directly into a terminal from written orders. This capability can eliminate much of the need for data collection forms, punch cards, or other methods of entering data into a computer for statistical analysis. Until such capability is widespread, however, data collection forms will have to be prepared that guide the data collector toward the information needed to determine if the quality criteria have been met. An example of a form for antibiotic review is shown in Figure 43.5 and one for nursing home use in Figure 43.6. Note that completing the form does not require making major therapeutic decisions, and therefore data could be collected by someone other than a pharmacist.

The ultimate value of the computer in data collection is to program criteria directly into its memory in a manner similar to the way potential drug interactions are programmed into many existing computer systems. When a problem arises through order entry or when another event occurs that violates a standard (e.g., a week passing without a particular lab test being conducted), the pharmacist would be notified to determine the need for corrective action, and a permanent record of the event would be made. Thus, there is no real data collection required other than recording the incidence and resolution of problems. This type of program would greatly facilitate the feasibility of prospective and concurrent review.

The use of such sophisticated technology will probably be initiated with the inclusion of relatively simple screening criteria that will alert the pharmacist to the need for more in-depth review. A prerequisite for incorporating in-depth criteria into computerized review is an institution-wide computerized information system that includes as a minimum the medical record and laboratory results in addition to drug therapy. A comparison of two types of computer-assisted DUR and a manual system has shown that, particularly as a screening system, the computer can be of value and can decrease the time required for review. Although this research was done in outpatients, the authors state that the system would appear to be useful in an inpatient setting as well (28).

Although such sophisticated computerized review is not imminent, the astute pharmacy department will be aware of developing technology in this area. The development of more complete hospital management information systems as an offshoot of newly implememted prospective reimbursement systems provides the pharmacy department with an opportunity to update all of its computerized functions, including DUR. While most newly developed DUR programs will most likely continue to involve manual data collection systems, programs should be developed with the goal of adapting to various levels of computerization as that capacity becomes available.

Evaluate Results. The first step in using the collected data is to display it in ways that will reveal patterns of drug use. Presentation of use by prescriber type, by disease or DRG, or by patient characteristics and particularly highlighting situations that deviate drastically from the criteria all provide clues to interpreting the results. Development of these profiles are only the first and the easiest step in the evaluation process, however. Because interpretation of usage patterns is more difficult, it may not always be done. The result is that too many DUR studies never achieve the greater purpose of ulilization review and are perceived, quite appropriately, as ''meaningless busywork'' (24).

Interpretation involves examining the results for evidence of specific problems. If none are found and the criteria are valid, then the analysis is finished. Unfortunately, however, problems usually exist. They can be of many types. They may be in improper prescribing vs improper monitoring once therapy is initiated, improper dosing vs use for the wrong indication, lack of use of less expensive alternatives where appropriate, or in individual prescribers vs certain types of prescribers or a hospital-wide problem.

Problem identification is followed by determining why problems exist. This activity may require close cooperation with other health professionals, particularly those working in the involved area. Some possible causes of deviation from criteria include lack of information, presence of misinformation, errors due to haste or lack of concern, and lack of adequate resources to monitor therapy correctly.

Initiate Corrective Actions. Without a concerted effort to correct the problems that have been identified, the DUR program is also of limited value. Many different actions are possible and the correct one for any situation is that action which most closely addresses the scope and cause of the problem. If the deficiency is limited to one practitioner, consultation by letter or in person—usually by a peer—may be sufficient. A more widespread problem may require a more extensive educational program. Occasionally, merely sharing the findings of the DUR program may result in positive change. Sometimes systemwide actions such as formulary modifications or limitations on prescribing are necessary.

Three general rules can be stated with regard to corrective actions. First, if possible, behavioral change should be attempted through educational means and only with punitive actions if necessary. Not all changes induced by education or reminder programs may be permanent, however, and reinforcement may be necessary to avoid the return to previous habits (29). Second, the plan of action should be as

I. DEMOGRAPHIC DATA

| | | | | | | Patient Unit Number

1   6

| | | Patient age in years: (99 = not given)

7 8

| | Patient sex: Male (1)   Female (2)   Other (9)

9

| | | Service:

10 11

(01) Med   (05) Ophthal   (09) Neurosurg
(02) Gen   (06) Other   (10) Urol
    Surg   (07) Dental   (11) Gyn
(03) Ent   (08) Psych
(04) Ortho

| | | | | Primary diagnosis (9999 = not given)

12   15

| | | | | | Admission date (mo/dy/yr)

16   21

II. INFECTIOUS DISEASE CONTEXT OF USE

Is the choice or use of antibiotic consistent with active infectious disease process?

| | Evidence of active infectious disease process: Yes (1)   No (2)

22

| | | | Temperature: Code actual data or 999 for not given or not applicable

23   25

| | | | | | WBC

26   31

| | WBC differential: Normal (1)   Shift to left (2)

32

| | NBT test: Yes (1)   No (2)

33

| | | Locus of infection:

34 35

(01) Pulmonary   (05) Burns   (11) Ent
(02) Skin and   (06) Blood   (12) Oral
    Soft Tissue   (07) UTI   Lesions
(03) Enteric Dis- (08) Ortho
    ease   (09) Ophthal
(04) Wound In-   (10) CNS
    fection
    (Surg.)

| | Suspected locus (1)   Proven locus (2)   Not given (9)

36

| | | Causative organism (see Coding Sheet)

37 38

| | Suspected organism (1)   Proven organism (2)

39

| | Were culture and sensitivity studies ordered prior to the initiation of therapy? Yes (1)   No (2)

40

| | | | | | Date of culture (mo/dy/yr)

41   46

| | | Source of culture:

47 48

(01) Blood   (05) Tracheal   (09) Urethra
(02) CSF   aspirate   (10) Urine
(03) Ear   (06) Sputurn   (11) Vaginal
(04) Eye   (07) Stool   (12) Wound
              (08) Throat

| | Were disc sensitivities done? Yes (1)   No (2)

49

| | Were quantitative susceptibility studies ordered: Yes (1)   No (2)

50

| | Were antibiotic blood levels ordered: Yes (1)   No (2)

51

| | Were cultures obtained during treatment: Yes (1)   No (2)

52

| | | Could another drug have been used on the basis of the sensitivity results:

53 54

(01) Gentamycin   (08) Dicloxacillin
(02) Kanamycin   (09) Streptomycin
(03) Carbenicillin (10) Colistin
(04) Sulfas   (11) Clindamycin
(05) Tetracycline (12) Erythromycin
(06) Penicillin   (13) Nitrofurantoin
(07) Oxacillin   (99) None

| | Was the antibiotic used prophylactically: Yes (1)   No (2)

55

III. GENERAL CHARACTERISTICS OF HOST STATUS

| | Does the patient present overt evidence of major debilitating and/or active disease in addition to infection? Yes (1)   No (2)

56

| | | | If yes to above question, specify

57   60

| | Does patient have history of penicillin allergy: Yes (1)   No (2)

61

IV. DRUG FACTORS

| | Drug used: Cephaloridine (1)   Cephalexin (2)   Cephalothin (3)

62

| | Dosage: .25 grams (1)   0.50 grams (2)   1.0 grams (3)   2.0 grams (4)

63

| | Dosage intervals: Every 4 hours (1)
                      Every 6 hours (2)
                      Every 8 hours (3)
                      Every 12 hours (4)
                      Single dose (5)

64

| | | Duration of therapy in days:

65 66

| | | | | | Date therapy was initiated (mo/dy/yr)

67   72

| | If the drug used was Cephalexin, was it used within the guidelines set forth by the Pharmacy and Therapeutics Committee: Yes (1)   No (2)

73

| | | Did patient receive any other antibiotics prior to or during Cephalosporin therapy?

74 75

(01) Gentamycin   (08) Dicloxacillin
(02) Kanamycin   (09) Streptomycin
(03) Carbenicillin (10) Colistin
(04) Sulfas   (11) Clindamycin
(05) Tetracycline (12) Erythromycin
(06) Penicillin   (13) Nitrofurantoin
(07) Oxacillin   (99) None

V. OUTCOME

| | Was there evidence of bacteriological and/or clinical cure? Yes (1)   No (2)   Uncertain (3)

76

| | Evidence of follow-up evaluation: None (1)
Continue medication (2)   Follow-up culture (3)
Return to clinic (4)

77

Additional comments:

FIGURE 43.5 Cephalosporin utilization study. (Reprinted with permission from Pierpaoli PG, Coarse JF, Tilton RC: Antibiotic use control—an institutional model. *Drug Intell Clin Pharm* 10:258-267, 1976.)

```
┌─────────────────────────────────────────────────────────────────────┐
│                                                                       │
│        Drug Utilization Review          Patient_____       │
│            Abstract Form                                              │
│                                         Physician_____       │
│           NITROGLYCERIN                                              │
│              (NTG)                       Room_____Date_____     │
│                                                                       │
├─────────────────────────────────────────────────────────────────────┤
│  If in doubt over some item, please note in the margin for further review.
│                                                                       │
│    I.  Indication for Use                                            │
│        Does patient have angina pectoris?  (See hospital discharge   │
│        summary, MD's orders and MD's notes)                          │
│        (If not, check square------------------------------------- □  │
│                                                                       │
│   II.  Administration                                                │
│                                                                       │
│        A.  How is nitroglycerin ordered?  (See original MD's orders) │
│            _____                       │
│            (Dose, schedule)                                          │
│                                                                       │
│        B.  What does patient actually receive?  (See med sheet and   │
│            nurse's notes)                                            │
│            _____                       │
│            (Be specific)                                            │
│                                                                       │
│        C.  Is nitroglycerin administered as ordered?                │
│            (If not, check square----------------------------------- □│
│                                                                       │
│        D.  Is NTG being given sublingually?                          │
│            (If not, check square----------------------------------- □│
│                                                                       │
│  III.  Monitoring                                                    │
│                                                                       │
│        Are the following test results and vital sign determinations  │
│        being taken and recorded at the indicated intervals?  If not, │
│        check appropriate square.                                     │
│                                                                       │
│        A.  See patient's hospital discharge summary, MD's notes,     │
│            vital signs and lab test records:                         │
│            1)  EKG - AT LEAST ONCE----------------------------------- □│
│            2)  Hemoglobin (Hgb) - AT LEAST ONCE--------------------- □│
│                                                                       │
│        B.  See MD's and nurse's notes and vital signs records:       │
│            1)  Blood pressure (BP) - WEEKLY, AND ONCE FOLLOWING EACH  │
│                EPISODE OF NTG USE RECORDED ON THE PATIENT'S MED SHEET------ □│
│            2)  Pulse - WEEKLY, AND ONCE FOLLOWING EACH EPISODE OF NTG │
│                USE RECORDED ON THE PATIENT'S MED SHEET--------------- □│
│            3)  Weight - MONTHLY------------------------------------- □│
│                                                                       │
└─────────────────────────────────────────────────────────────────────┘
```

FIGURE 43.6 Data collection form for nitroglycerin DUR in long-term care facilities. (Reprinted by permission from Kabat HF et al: *Drug Utilization Review in Skilled Nursing Facilities*. Washington, DC, U.S. Government Printing Office, November 1975.)

simple as possible and directed toward the cause of the problem. Finally, implementation of the action should be done by the persons and/or committees who have the proper authority to do so. Corrective action is rarely an exclusive function of the pharmacy department and often may not involve pharmacy directly at all.

Reevaluate Utilization. The success of a program of corrective action cannot be determined unless the review is repeated and comparison made of the two (or more) sets of utilization patterns. While there is probably no common, optimal time interval for reevaluation, a range of 3 to 12 months has been suggested. Allowing sufficient time for the plan of action to have an effect and to generate a sufficient sample for reevaluation must be balanced against natural attrition of providers and the lack of impact that feedback from the results of reevaluations can have if they are far removed in time from the original assessment (24). While reevaluations may be prospective or concurrent, it is generally important that at least the initial review be retrospective. From a retrospective review, it should be easier to obtain all the information needed (including drug use, disease, patient, and provider characteristics) to generate baseline profiles of drug utilization for subsequent comparisons.

Revise Criteria and Standards. Because of the fast-

NITROGLYCERIN

C. Is a description of the episode being entered in the patient's records each time the use of nitroglycerin is noted on the med sheet?
(If <u>not</u>, check square--- ☐

IV. <u>Possible Problem Areas</u>

A. If <u>yes</u> to any of the following, check appropriate square.
(See MD's and nurse's notes)
1) Does the patient's chest pain last 5 minutes or longer after the administration of nitroglycerin?------------------- ☐
2) Have there been times when nitroglycerin was administered and the patient experienced no relief from angina?---- ☐
3) Has there been an increase in the frequency and/or severity of the patient's angina attacks?------------------- ☐

If there is a positive response to any part of A, please continue. Otherwise, stop.

B. Is patient diabetic and showing signs of insulin reactions? (Weakness, stupor, convulsions, etc.) (See MD's and nurse's notes)
(If <u>yes</u>, check square and note symptoms in margin-------------- ☐

C. Does patient have a thyroid condition? (See MD's notes and hospital discharge summary)
(If yes, check square and note type and treatment in margin----- ☐

D. Is patient currently receiving any of the following medications? (See MD's orders, patient Kardex and med sheet)
If <u>yes</u>, check appropriate square and note exact name of drug and amount in margin.
1) Propranolol (Inderal^R)--- ☐
2) Apresoline^R--- ☐
3) D-thyroxine (Choloxin^R)----------------------------------- ☐
4) Sympathomimetic agents (Isoproterenol, epinephrine, amphetamines, cold medications including decongestants, Neosynephrine^R, ephedrine, etc.)-------------------------- ☐

E. If <u>no</u>, check appropriate square
1) Are the nitroglycerin tablets being stored in their original container? (Check medication cabinet and bedside container if there is one)------------------------- ☐
2) Is the unused nitroglycerin being replaced by fresh stock at least every 6 months? (Check dispensing date on bottle)--- ☐

Abstractor's signature_____

FIGURE 43.6, cont'd

changing nature of drug therapy, it is often necessary to revise the criteria and standards before they are used subsequent to the original review. The need for such revision may be identified during a review itself (e.g., a prescriber is found to be using a medication in a way consistent with recently published research but inconsistent with the current DUR criteria). In addition to revising measures of quality to keep them consistent with current definitions of optimal therapy, it may be possible, over time, to develop measures that are more exacting or allow fewer deviations from the criteria (i.e., higher standards if currently less than 100%).

Developing a quality DUR program is a difficult task requiring a commitment to excellence and the interaction of persons representing a variety of positions. While one should be as methodical and complete as practicable in developing a program, it is not always possible to meet every detail of the ideal program. If one examines the reports of the examples of DUR programs discussed in the next section, it will be concluded that none are ideal, but each has been successful in its particular setting and has contributed to the improvement of the DUR process.

EXAMPLES OF DRUG UTILIZATION REVIEW PROGRAMS

Antibiotic review is perhaps the most commonly performed type of DUR. Pierpaoli et al (30) describe a successful antibiotic review program that categorizes therapy as being for treatment of an active infection, for prophylaxis or for "symptomatic" treatment as an initial screen for further review (30). Durbin et al (31) used a similar categorization (therapeutic, prophylactic, and empirical). A prospective program that concentrated on parenteral antibiotics and did not require an unwieldy amount of pharmacist time is outlined by Cohen (32). Selection of specific antibiotics for review and various education options for improvement in drug use are presented by Klapp and Ramphal (33). Several older studies also describe antibiotic DUR activities (34-37).

Examples of DUR programs for specific therapy other than antibiotics include Keys and Narduzzi's report on warfarin, digoxin, and total parenteral nutrition reviews (18). Two lithium reviews have been published: Gill (38) presents a set of criteria with documentation for their selection. The report by Feldman et al (29) on lithium showed that educational programs and reminder notices had to be provided on a continuing basis to maintain their effect. Alexander et al (39,40) demonstrated significant cost savings as well as improvements in the quality of therapy in their DUR program for parenteral albumin use.

Kelly et al (15) developed a program for a community hospital that was not drug specific, but rather provided a monthly, retrospective review of randomly selected charts for patients discharged within the previous 60 days. This review, which was not based on explicit criteria but did utilize up to three levels of review per chart, involved both drug prescribing and drug administration reviews and thus included active involvement by pharmacy, medicine, and nursing.

At the University of Wisconsin Hospitals DUR is comprehensive in its scope. A DUR committee composed of both administrative and staff pharmacists as well as the clinical coordinator and the drug information pharmacist meets monthly to identify and review problem areas. Their actions may include conducting specific drug audits, making recommendations to the Pharmacy and Therapeutics Committee, or providing educational programs. In addition to this retrospective review, all orders are reviewed using specific criteria before any medications are dispensed. These criteria, which are developed for approximately 300 drugs, generally include elements for proper indication, features of the regimen, presentation and correction of adverse effects, interactions (drug, food, and laboratory), patient information, therapy monitoring parameters, administration considerations, and other pharmacy implications. A major key to the success of this program is the decentralized pharmacists who are responsible for transcribing all medication orders after consideration of the above factors. The computer also contributes to the review process both by monitoring for drug interactions and other adverse effects and by its capability to print records of a patient's course of therapy for in-depth review. Finally, the pharmacy department interfaces with the hospital-wide QA program by participating on its quality assurance committee (14).

While most of the previous examples are from inpatient settings, some of the earliest DUR activities were conducted in an ambulatory care setting (41). These activities become more relevant to hospitals as programs are expanded beyond inpatient care. Several reviews using screening criteria composed of maximum and minimum dosage quantities and length of therapy have been reported (25,26), including one study that compared results of applying several sets of criteria to the same data (26). King and Cheung (42) describe their involvement with a multidisciplinary medical care audit team. While they were able to review a patient's entire therapy, implicit criteria had to be used frequently as explicit criteria were not available for the large number of drugs involved.

Although there is less literature available on DUR in long-term care facilities, a guide to DUR in this environment has been published that includes criteria for a limited number of drugs as well as data collection forms (22). Some examples of actual reviews are also available (43,44).

As a final example, Knapp et al (7) have added a dimension that has rarely, if ever, been applied to DUR. In their reviews of drug therapy for pyelonephritis and pneumococcal pneumonia, they demonstrated that appropriate therapy was associated with a shorter length of stay in the hospital. Such a finding can be converted directly into a measure of reduced health care cost. Interestingly, underdosing was reported in a substantial number of the uses of inappropriate therapy. Thus, as suggested earlier, optimal therapy resulting in significant overall cost saving could require an increase in the drug therapy component of the total cost.

CONCLUSION

The integration of drug quality and health care costs as developed by Knapp et al (7) is one example of the improvements needed in DUR methodology. Another is the inclusion of computer capabilities and other methods for increasing the efficiency of the DUR process. The costs of providing comprehensive DUR services can be substantial, particularly if the process is highly labor intensive and uses primarily professional personnel. The cost should not exceed the total benefit received.

The costs of providing them notwithstanding, there will continue to be increased interest in DUR activities. Not only formal requirements, but also concern by health professionals, administrators, and patients for quality health care at a reasonable cost will encourage the growth of DUR. Pharmacists can benefit from this trend by striving to achieve recognition as monitors of drug therapy at the aggregate level and by using DUR findings to identify problem areas where the role of educator and consultant for drug therapy can be justified.

REFERENCES

1. Silverman M, Lee PR, Lydecker M: *Pills and the Public Purse*. Berkeley, University California Press, 1981.
2. Kirking DM: New horizons in pharmaceutical technology. *Ann Am Acad Polit Soc Sci* 468:182-195, 1983.
3. Brodie DC, Smith WE: Constructing a conceptual model of drug utilization review. *Hospitals* 50:143-144, 6, 8, 150, March 1976.

4. Stolar MH: Drug use review: Operational definitions. *Am J Hosp Pharm* 35:76-78, 1978.

5. Stolar MH: Conceptual framework for drug usage review, medical audit and other patient care review procedures. *Am J Hosp Pharm* 34:139-45, 1977.

6. Department of Health, Education and Welfare: *Final Report, Task Force on Prescription Drugs*. Washington, DC, U.S. Government Printing Office, 1969.

7. Knapp DA, Knapp DE, Michocki RJ, et al: Drug prescribing and hospital cost containment. *Top Hosp Pharm Mgt* 3:7-14, 1982.

8. Enright SM: Understanding prospective pricing and DRGs. *Am J Hosp Pharm* 40:1493-1494, 1983.

9. Bonney RS: *Survival Strategies for the Future*. Presented at the Sixteenth Annual Seminar in Hospital Pharmacy, Toledo, November 12, 1983.

10. Joint Commission on Accreditation of Hospitals: *AMH/84-Accreditation Manual for Hospitals*. Chicago, Joint Commission on Accreditation of Hospitals, 1983.

11. Health Care Financing Administration: Medicare program: Utilization and quality control peer review organizations (PRO) area designations and definition of eligible organizations. *Fed Reg* 49:7202-7208, 1984.

12. American Society of Hospital Pharmacists: *Practice Standards of the American Society of Hospital Pharmacists*. Bethesda, American Society of Hospital Pharmacists, 1983.

13. Knapp DA, Knapp DE, Brandon BM, West S: Development and application of criteria in drug use review programs. *Am J Hosp Pharm* 31:648-656, 1974.

14. Grant KL, Ploetz PA, Thielke TS: *Drug Utilization Review: A Second Look*. Presented at the American Society of Hospital Pharmacists Midyear Clinical Meeting, New Orleans, December 7, 1981.

15. Kelly WM, White JA, Miller DE: Drug usage review in a community hospital. *Am J Hosp Pharm* 32:1014-1017, 1975.

16. Donabedian A: *The Definition of Quality and Approaches to its Assessment*. Ann Arbor, Health Administration Press, 1980.

17. McGhan WF, Rowland CR, Bootman JL: Cost-benefit and cost-effectiveness: Methodologies for evaluating innovative pharmaceutical services. *Am J Hosp Pharm* 35:133-140, 1978.

18. Keys PW, Narduzzi JV: Drug audit: A component of quality assurance. *QRB* 5:17-23, January 1979.

19. Department of Health, Education and Welfare: *P.S.R.O. Program Manual*. Washington, DC, Department of Health, Education and Welfare, 1974, p 16.

20. Dorsey R, Ayd FJ, Cole J, et al: Psychopharmacological screening criteria development project. *JAMA* 241:1021-1031, 1979.

21. Veterans Administration Advisory Committee on Antimicrobial Drug Usage: Guidelines for peer review: 1. Prophylaxis in surgery. *JAMA* 237:1001-1008, 1977.

22. Kabat HF, Kidder SW, Marttila JK, et al: *Drug Utilization Review in Skilled Nursing Facilities*. Washington, DC, U.S. Government Printing Office, November 1975.

23. Henricks JN: *Audit Criteria for Drug Utilization Review*. Bethesda, American Society of Hospital Pharmacists, 1981.

24. Henricks JN: *Audit Criteria for Drug Utilization Review*, vol 2. Bethesda, American Society of Hospital Pharmacists, 1983.

25. Brandon BM, Knapp DA, Klein LS, et al: Drug usage screening criteria. *Am J Hosp Pharm* 34:146-151, 1977.

26. Helling DK, Norwood GJ, Donner JD: An assessment of prescribing using drug utilization review criteria. *Drug Intell Clin Pharm* 16:930-934, 1982.

27. Tremblay J: Creating an appropriate climate for drug use review. *Am J Hosp Pharm* 38:212-215, 1981.

28. Helling DK, Hepler CD, Herman RA: Comparison of computer assisted medical record audit with other drug use review methods. *Am J Hosp Pharm* 36:1665-1671, 1979.

29. Feldman J, Wilner S, Winickoff R: A study of lithium carbonate use in a health maintenance organization. *QRB* 8:8-14, 1982.

30. Pierpaoli PG, Coarse JF, Tilton RC: Antibiotic use control—an institutional model. *Drug Intell Clin Pharm* 10:258-267, 1976.

31. Durbin WA, Lapidas B, Goldman DA: Improved antibiotic usage following introduction of a novel prescription system. *JAMA* 246:1796-1800, 1981.

32. Cohen SS: A pharmacy-based antibiotic utilization review program. *QRB* 10:22-25, 1984.

33. Klapp DL, Ramphal R: Antibiotic review performed by a pharmacy and therapeutics subcommittee. *QRB* 8:15-29, 1982.

34. Roberts W, Visconti JA: The rational and irrational use of systemic antimicrobial drugs. *Am J Hosp Pharm* 828-834, 1972.

35. Scheckler NE, Bennett JV: Antibiotic usage in seven community hospitals. *JAMA* 213:264-267, 1970.

36. Moody ML, Burk JP: Infections and antibiotic usage in a large private hospital. *Arch Intern Med* 130:261, 1972.

37. McGowan JE, Finland M: Effects of monitoring the usage of antibiotics: An inter-hospital comparison. *South Med J* 69:193-195, 1976.

38. Gill DH: Critique of an audit of beginning lithium therapy. *QRB* (special edition on integrated quality assurance), 1979, pp 71-80.

39. Alexander MR, Alexander B, Mustion AL, et al: Therapeutic use of albumin. 2. *JAMA* 247:831-833, 1982.

40. Alexander MR, Ambre JJ, Liskow BI, et al: Therapeutic use of albumin. *JAMA* 241:2527-2529, 1979.

41. Maronde RF: *Drug Utilization Review with On-Line Computer Capability*. Washington, DC, Department of Health, Education and Welfare, 1973.

42. King RC, Cheung AMK: Drug therapy review as part of a medical audit process. *Am J Hosp Pharm* 35:578-580, 1978.

43. Cheung A, Kayne R: An application of clinical pharmacy services in extended care facilities. *Calif Pharm* 23:22-28, September 1975.

44. Vlasses PH, Lucarotti RL, Miller DA, et al: Drug therapy review in a skilled nursing facility: An innovative approach. *J Am Pharm Assoc* 1977; NS17:92-94, 1977.

CHAPTER 44

The Research Report and the Published Paper

GEORGE P. PROVOST*

No research project is complete until the report has been written. The most carefully designed and conducted study is of little importance unless the findings are transmitted to others. With these points in mind, this chapter will attempt to relate some of the information in the preceding chapters of Section V to the end point of a research project: communicating results to colleagues in the field. It is impossible to attempt this without discussing four interrelated topics: (1) basic writing skills, (2) research design and methodology, (3) the specialized subject of scientific or technical writing, and (4) the editorial policies and practices of scientific journals. The reader should realize that these topics cannot be treated exhaustively in one brief chapter of a book; references listed at the end of the chapter should be reviewed as necessary. Further, this chapter, as the title indicates, is restricted to a discussion of research reports intended for journal publication. The investigator who must develop a report for several different groups—e.g., for oral presentation at a meeting, for a grant sponsor, for a hospital administrator, or for submission as a thesis—must be prepared to write several entirely different reports, each oriented toward the particular audience or medium.

PRINCIPLES OF CLEAR WRITING

The teaching of basic writing skills has been sadly neglected through all levels of our educational system (1). Therefore, it is no surprise that scientific writing, in general, is weak. Some of the faults which abound are poor organization and flow of idea, a preference for complexity over simplicity, redundancy, the passive voice, sloppy syntax, jargon, unnecessary words, excessive abstraction, clichés, and rhetoric. Too many researchers, it seems, equate pretentious language with profundity. In a critical article on medical writing, Crichton suggested that the literature may have reached the point of "obligatory obfuscation," at which "medical obscurity may now serve an intra-group recognition function . . ." (2).

The first aim of scientific writing is to be understood; it

is not "to produce the greatest number of papers from the minimal amount of data using the maximum number of words" (3). As general rules, authors should write to express (not impress) and they should choose words carefully and correctly, express thoughts clearly and logically, keep style intact and sentences short and clear, and use action verbs. For an elaboration of these and other principles, the reader is referred to several texts on scientific and technical writing (4-8).

Although admittedly a negative approach, our discussion will focus on what to *avoid* in writing a research report. In view of the limitations in the length of this chapter, readers may find emphasis on some selected "don'ts" more helpful than an attempt to relate all the "do's" of basic writing principles.

Fourteen Selected "Don'ts"

1. Don't use the passive voice if you can avoid it, and you usually can. The passive voice, although dull and often unclear, pervades much scientific writing. Be careful of verbs that can be changed into nouns, and put action into verbs.

Example: We made an analysis of . . . (passive); We analyzed . . . (better).

2. Don't use jargon; it is the dry rot of literate writing (9).

Example: Orientation toward improvement of the gratificational-deprivation balance of the actor. (Translation: the pleasure principle) (10).

3. Although some manuals on technical writing advise otherwise, don't write the way you talk. There are differences in standards of grammar used in writing and those that have gained acceptance in speaking.

Example: You might say "It's me" in speaking, but only "It is I" in writing.

4. Don't use rhetoric in scientific writing; don't try to persuade or impress. Realistically, rhetoric cannot be eliminated entirely, but observations and conclusions should be presented with a minimum of emotional or moral bias (11).

*Deceased. This chapter reprinted in memory of this respected leader's contribution to pharmacy.

5. Avoid abstract or vague words and terms when a specific or concrete word or term should be used; choose words carefully and precisely.

6. Don't use modifiers excessively. They can be confusing. Question: What is the size of a small hospital pharmacist?

7. Don't use long sentences; keep sentences short and clear.

8. Don't use clichés: last but not least, beyond the shadow of a doubt, etc.

9. Avoid vogue words: hopefully, finalize, utilization, etc.

10. Avoid vague words: fine, horrible, actually, really, etc.

11. Don't phrase comparative statements in a confusing manner.

Example: Men are more interested in engineering than women. (Could have two meanings.)

12. Don't use a long and pointless phrase when one or two words will do.

Examples: In a situation when; within the realm of possibility; few in number; in regard to; the profession of pharmacy; at this point in time.

13. Don't omit a necessary verb or auxiliary in writing.

Example: Students never have (liked) and never will like Mickey Smith's course.

14. Don't use conjunctions (while, since, as, etc) that have two meanings if they can be avoided. Be careful when *while* is used to mean *whereas* or *although,* and when *since* or *as* is used to mean *because.*

This list is obviously incomplete but it represents some of the most common errors in writing. Writing style is beyond the scope of this discussion.

THE RESEARCH REPORT

The content of a research report can be no better than the design, methodology, and conclusions of the study on which the report is based. If a clear definition of the problem is lacking from the outset of the project, if sampling techniques are inappropriate, if statistical tests are misapplied, or if the investigator draws results that outstrip his data, there is nothing he can do to overcome the problem in his written report. The best writing in the world cannot mask poor research, but the best research can be obscured by a poor report.

Outlining a research report even before the project begins can help to organize the study itself, and the very act of writing the final report can help to clarify thinking (12).

The Outline

The three broad components of a research report are:
1. The problem (introduction)
2. The methodology (experimental section)
3. Results, conclusions, and interpretations (discussion)

In preparing a preliminary outline for a report, it may help to pose the following questions: What was the question (problem statement)? What were the answers obtained? What was the purpose of the study and what is the significance of the conclusions? Answers should not be given without first posing corresponding questions, and the purpose and significance of the study should always be stated.

The "IMRAD" structure (13) is another helpful guide to outlining a research report:

Introduction: Why did you start?
Method: What did you do?
Results: What did you find?
And
Discussion: What does it mean?

This structure ties in well with the following discussion.

A more detailed outline of a research report is shown in Table 44.1; variations may be in order depending on the type of study conducted.†
1. The problem (introduction)
   The introduction should briefly describe the basis for the research project, refer to pertinent work previously reported in the literature, and point out the need for the present investigation.
   a. General problem
      The identification of a broad general problem, often in the form of a question, comes first. At this stage, the author has not yet begun to discuss all the variables that may be involved in the study.
   b. Literature review/significance of study
      The purpose of this section is to explain the significance of the problem and the theoretical rationale for the investigator's approach to the problem. Too many authors appear to have a subconscious desire to write a review article at this point (14). Use good judgment here; if you are reporting the results of a study of particulate contamination in parenteral solutions, there is no need to use five pages to describe the work of Garvan and Gunner 13 years ago. Their work has had time to become well known. Restrict this section to a brief summary of the *pertinent* literature. Justify your study by telling the reader what has *not* been done, as well what has been done, by previous investigators. Primary reference should always be used.
   c. Scope
      This section should tell the reader, in a sentence or two, "who, what, and when."

      Example: The scope of this study was limited to medication errors committed by pharmacists in three voluntary general hospitals during July 1977.

   d. Problem statement
      The specific problem that was investigated and the hypotheses that were tested should be clearly stated.

†This outline and other information in this section of the chapter are adapted from material developed by Kenneth N. Barker, PhD., Professor of Pharmacy Administration, School of Pharmacy, Auburn University, for presentation at Institutes on Research Methods conducted by the American Society of Hospital Pharmacists Research and Education Foundation. The author extends thanks to Dr. Barker for permission to use the material.

Operational definitions should always be used for terms which may be unclear or subject to differences in interpretation. "Pharmacy technician" is an example of a term that always requires an operational definition.

2. Methodology (experimental section)

A section devoted to the experimental aspects of the study usually follows the introduction. This section, which provides the details of procedures, equipment, and materials used in the project, should be addressed to colleagues in the general field.

a. Design

This part of the experimental section advises the reader what variables were manipulated and, if applicable, what controls were used.

b. Population and sample

The author should identify the population to which the results are to be related, and he should specify the sample size and describe how the sample was selected. If the sample studied and reported on differs from the sample originally selected, the difference should be noted and clarified.

c. Data collection techniques

Enough information should be included in this section to permit replication of the study. Complete information on materials and equipment should be given. If an interview technique is used, all questions that were asked, as well as information on the experience and training of the interviewers, should be included. However, if the procedures or techniques that are used have been previously described in the literature, the author may simply cite the literature reference and describe any modifications that were made. In some cases, it may be preferable for the materials description or the copy of the data collection instrument to appear as an appendix.

d. Statistical hypotheses and tests

If a standard statistical analysis is used, the writer should simply identify the test and the level of significance. When a pre-test is used, merely to try out the procedure, it may be mentioned only briefly. More information should be supplied if the results of the pre-test heavily influenced the methodology.

3. Results, conclusions, and interpretations (discussion section)

This section is sometimes divided into two or three parts, depending on its length and the complexity of the data and the data analysis. The most important function of this section is to show how the data do or do not support the hypothesis, and how the results bear on the hypothesis. The section is usually organized in the sequence shown in Table 44.1. The results should include all evidence for and against the hypothesis. The author should note any apparent nonsensical results or obvious inconsistencies, or any failure to obtain results that were sought. In deciding what results are relevant, the investigator should continually return to the problem statement and hypothesis.

When tables are used to depict results, they should include as much of the numerical data as possible. At the same time, they should illuminate the text but not substitute for it. Although tables should be self-explanatory, the text should refer to each table and briefly summarize its meaning.

Limitations of the study, an important element of a research report, too often are omitted or buried in the discussion section. Depending on the nature of the research, these limitations may include sampling inadequacies (e.g., nonrandom sampling), subject assignment inadequacies, methodologic weaknesses, and statistical deficiencies that were impossible for the investigator to overcome.

Four Major Weaknesses

The four most prevalent weaknesses of research reports are:

1. Absence of a clear problem statement
2. Lack of operational definitions adequate to permit replication of the study
3. Inappropriate sampling (e.g., nonrandom assignment)
4. Conclusions that are not justified on the basis of the study

THE PUBLISHED ARTICLE

Since journals are an important and widely used vehicle for research reports, let us now relate the structure of a research report to that of a published article. This discussion will also present some tips for preparing a manuscript for publication, as well as information on the general requirements of scientific journals and the procedures used in reviewing and evaluating manuscripts submitted for publication.

The core of the published research paper corresponds to the major elements of a research report outlined in the previous section: the introduction, the experimental section, and the discussion section. A few words about additional elements surrounding this core are now in order.

Table 44.1   Elements of a Research Report

1. The problem (introduction)
   a. General problem
   b. Literature review/significance of the study
   c. Scope: who, what, when
   d. Problem statement/operational definitions/hypotheses
2. Methodology (experimental section)
   a. Design
   b. Population and sample
   c. Data collection techniques
   d. Statistical hypotheses and tests
3. Results, conclusions, and recommendations (discussion section)
   a. Data obtained
   b. Analysis, including statistical tests
   c. Conclusions
   d. Interpretations
   e. Limitations

Title, Author Listing, Abstract, and References

Title. Keep the title short, don't clutter it with unnecessary words, and make sure it conveys what you mean. An actual example of how not to title a paper was a manuscript originally entitled, "The Development and Implementation of a Rational Pediatric Parenteral Hyperalimentation Solution Capable of Being Individualized to Patient's Needs and Accurately Adjustable Daily by Utilization of the Computer." Clearly (or rather, unclearly) the title tried to say too much. A more appropriate title for this paper might be, "Computer-Assisted Pediatric Total Parenteral Nutrition."

Author Listing. Try to keep the list of authors to a minimum by including only the names of the people who actually developed the manuscript. Editors realize that many individuals may have been involved in a research project and that they all deserve credit for their participation. However, the credit can often be given via a footnote rather than by listing everyone as a co-author. Obviously, this removes a person's name from indexes and secondary references and prevents him from including the article in his *curriculum vitae* (15). However, when a journal receives a manuscript listing more than four or five authors, the editor can't help but wonder how many names really deserve to belong there.

Abstract. Many scholarly journals include a prefatory abstract following the title and the authors' names. The abstract is often either too long, or too brief, to give the proper information. Further, to the dismay of editors, it is often indicative rather than informative. "The treatment of hypertension is described and the results of therapy are discussed" does not mean much to the reader who is looking for a brief but informative synopsis. A truly informative abstract can be prepared by responding to four questions: (1) What was the problem? (2) How was it solved? (3) What was found? (4) What was learned? Stated another way, the elements of an abstract can be put into four words that conform to the structure of the entire article: problem, methods, results, and conclusions (16). If the article itself has been clearly written, a sentence or two answering each of the four questions is often sufficient.

Some journals include "key words" along with prefatory abstracts. These tie in with standardized index terms. As a rule, the key words are assigned by the editorial staff and need not be proposed by the author.

References. The discussion of the literature review under "The Research Report" emphasized that references should be limited to pertinent papers. It is not necessary to reference the sentence, "Clinical services are becoming an important part of the hospital pharmacist's activities," with 37 citations to back up the statement. Only primary references should be used, and they should be completely accurate. More outright errors appear in the references of the average manuscript than in all other parts of the paper combined (14). This reflects a lack of appreciation of the importance of accurate literature citations on the part of many authors. A common error is the failure to give the complete date rather than just the month for a weekly or biweekly journal. Finally, references should be cited in the proper style for the journal to which the manuscript will be submitted, using accepted abbreviations for journal titles and the prescribed order of information for a complete citation. *JAMA* and *JAPhA* are not acceptable abbreviations. When in doubt, *Index Medicus* style should be used.

Journal Policies and Practices

There is considerable variation in editorial policies and practices among scientific journals, but any journal worthy of that adjective evaluates manuscripts through peer review. (This author is now guilty of using a vogue term; see the "don'ts" under "Principles of Clear Writing.") Usually, manuscripts are initially reviewed inhouse to some degree before they are sent to outside referees for in-depth evaluation. For example, the editorial staff may first screen papers to determine if they (1) fall within the scope of the journal, (2) appear to be unique enough to warrant consideration, and (3) are structured and written in an acceptable manner. The heavy demands placed on expert referees call for this initial screening. Otherwise, referees are burdened with manuscripts that the editor could have judged unacceptable for one clear reason or another.

Referees are generally recognized to be expert in the subject matter of the paper under consideration. Depending on the topic of the manuscript and the editor's experience with a particular referee or author, only one referee may be called on. Usually, however, critiques are solicited from two, and sometimes three, referees. Some journals that have an editorial advisory board use members of that board for this purpose, either exclusively or as a core group of reviewers. In other cases, manuscript review is outside the scope of the editorial advisory board.

The referee system serves as a mechanism for reviewing and criticizing the methodology and conclusions of a research report. The referee's critique may also identify points that require clarification, suggest expansion or elimination of parts of the report, identify questions or omissions that may have escaped the author, or propose other means of improving the paper. The referee may see a way to improve a paper when the author (or the editor) cannot (17).

There are two schools of thought on maintaining the anonymity of authors and referees. The identity of the author may or may not be withheld from the referee, but the referee is never identified to the author. The referee's written critique is sent "blind" to the author with a request for a rebuttal. The critique and the author's response are then weighed by the editorial staff. Sometimes the author's response is forwarded to the referee for consideration and a further "blind" exchange is coordinated through the editorial office. On occasion, when a stalemate is reached (as may happen when two referees are used), the manuscript and the author-referee exchange may be sent to an additional referee for arbitration. The editorial advisory boards of some journals function in this capacity when the editor is faced with a difficult decision resulting from conflicting referee evaluations.

In the final analysis, it is almost always the editor who makes the decision to accept or reject a paper based on the referee's commentary and the author's rebuttal. When the referee's critique has identified inherently poor experimental design or methodology and there appears to be no hope of

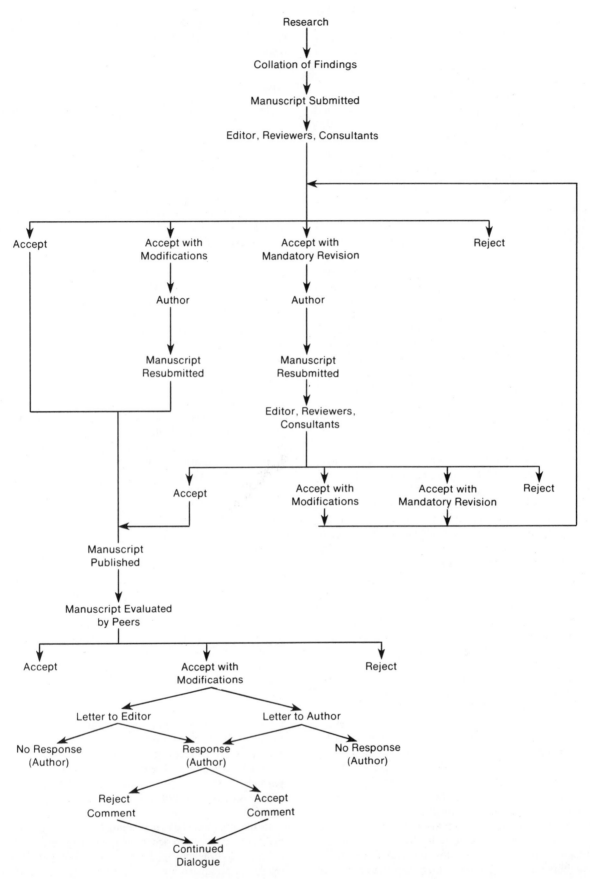

FIGURE 44.1 Typical literature chain of events.

salvaging the report short of repeating the study and preparing a new paper, the manuscript may be rejected outright. If the methodology is basically sound but the paper is revised by the author upon recommendation of the referee, the revised version often can be accepted by the editor without again calling on the referee. Sometimes, however, the editor must submit the version to the original referee in order to make an informed judgment.

Figure 44.1 depicts a possible chain of events beginning with a research project and continuing through publication consideration and postpublication evaluation of the report.

A journal's primary responsibility is to the reader, not to the author. A firm tradition of editors is to consider authors equal; friend and stranger alike receive a critical review of a manuscript. After all, the primary purpose of this review is to assist the author through an impartial analysis of his data (18). A paper revised in accordance with a good critique is invariably an improved paper. The referee process assists the author and the journal in meeting their responsibility to the reader. The most discouraging and frustrating experience for an editor is to have an author interpret an unfavorable critique or a rejection notice as a personal affront without understanding that the process is designed to be constructive and to benefit the author as well as the reader.

CONCLUSION: A DOZEN "DO'S"

The following suggestions are offered as sequential steps for researchers who aspire to be good writers and to have their manuscripts fare well in the hands of editors and reviewers:

1. Plan and outline your report in the manner previously recommended.
2. Write a rough draft.
3. Cool it; wait a few hours or a day so you will be more likely to view the draft as another reader would view it.
4. Prepare the first revision. Go over the draft in detail to ensure accuracy of data, correct terminology, and proper organization.
5. Revise it again. Consider how much material can be removed without jeopardizing reader understanding and needs. Strive for clarity and brevity, eliminate verbose expressions, and check grammar and spelling.
6. Revise it a third time with emphasis on improving the writing style. Proofread the manuscript carefully.
7. Ask at least one colleague to read the paper critically. If it is revised again as a result, proofread the paper one more time.
8. Choose the one most appropriate journal, keeping in mind the scope of journals that may be potential vehicles and the audiences that would be most interested in and benefitted by your report. On occasion, editors still encounter authors who are apparently unaware that playing the game by the established rules precludes submitting an identical paper to more than one journal at a time. The neophyte author, in particular, is advised not to play "bingo" by scattering one paper to two or more journals and then sitting back to wait for the first acceptance notice. This practice does not endear authors to editors, who usually find

out about such things. It may be difficult for an editor to maintain his objectivity when he receives a manuscript from an author who is known to have played bingo on some past occasion.

9. Resist the temptation to write several reports on one study, each with a different slant, for submission to several journals. This practice is rarely justified and tends to clutter the literature unnecessarily. The investigator's natural desire to get as much "mileage" from his work as possible should be offset by his sense of responsibility to the scientific community and its literature. In the long run, it is in the investigator's interest to avoid being labeled a mileage champion by readers and editors.

10. Follow the prescribed style according to the "Directions to Authors" which nearly all journals publish from time to time. This may require still another revision. Several style guides are also available in libraries; these include the *Style Guide for Biological Journals* of the American Institute of Biological Sciences, the American Chemical Society's *Handbook for Authors* and the American Medical Association's *Style Book*, and *Editorial Manual*. A book by DeBakey (19) may also be helpful in this regard.

11. If you are asked to revise your paper according to a referee's suggestion, it is better to follow the advice and resubmit it to the same journal for further consideration. Ignoring advice and submitting the original paper to a second journal may or may not get your name in print a little faster. Even if it does, your article will be recognized as one which could have been improved.

12. If your manuscript is ultimately rejected, don't be discouraged. Most authors have had this happen to them. Learn from the experience and try harder the next time.

Writing a good research report and developing it into a manuscript for a scientific journal require considerable effort. Too many investigators will spend months, or even years, working on a research project and then try to write a report in a week or less. Any research project worth 6 month's effort is worth devoting 1 month's time to writing the report (14). Because scientific writing can strengthen scientific thinking, because it can be personally challenging and satisfying and professionally rewarding, the time and effort are worthwhile. Good scientific writing is as much the result of the author's attitude toward his work as the result of his knowledge and expertise with words. Try it; you'll like it!

REFERENCES

1. Lyons G: The higher illiteracy. *Harper's* 253:33, 1976.
2. Crichton M: Medical obfuscation: Structure and function. *N Engl J Med* 293:1257, 1975.
3. Reece RL: Space-occupying gambits for medical writers. *JAMA* 200:162, 1967.
4. Trelease SF: *How to Write Scientific and Technical Papers.* Baltimore, Williams & Wilkins, 1958.
5. Gilman W: *The Language of Science: A Guide to Effective Writing.* New York, Harcourt, Brace and World, 1961.
6. Ehrlich E, Murphy D: *The Art of Technical Writing: A Manual for Scientists, Engineers and Students.* New York, Thomas Y Crowell, 1964.
7. Tichy HJ: *Effective Writing for Engineers/Managers/Scientists.* New York, John Wiley & Sons, 1966.

8. Mitchell JH: *Writing for Professional and Technical Journals*. New York, John Wiley & Sons, 1968.

9. Kuehn HR: Resuscitating the scientific paper. *JAMA* 226:452, 1973.

10. Degnan JP: Masters of babble—turning language into stone. *Harper's* 253:37, 1976.

11. Roland CG, Cox BG: Loaded language and drug use (editorial), *JAMA* 226:660, 1973.

12. Woodford FP: Sounder thinking through clearer writing. *Science* 156:743, 1967.

13. Paton A: Writing and speaking in medicine—how I write a paper. Br Med J 2:1115, 1976.

14. Feldmann TG: Technical writing. *Am J Hosp Pharm* 22:329, 1965.

15. Provost GP: One free with a dozen (letter)? *Am J Hosp Pharm* 34:231, 1977.

16. Southgate MT: On writing the synopsis-abstract (editorial). *JAMA* 222:1307, 1972.

17. Pyke DA: Writing and speaking in medicine—how I referee. Br Med J 2:1117, 1976.

18. Soffer A: Is the critical reader dead? *JAMA* 200:141, 1967.

19. DeBakey L: *The Scientific Journal: Editorial Policies and Practices—Guidelines for Editors, Reviewers, and Authors*. St Louis, CV Mosby, 1976.

CHAPTER 45

Investigational Drugs in the Hospital

JOSEPH F. GALLELLI, PAUL K. HIRANAKA, and GEORGE J. GRIMES, Jr.

Since hospitals are the primary centers for conducting clinical investigations with new investigational drugs* and pharmacists have the responsibility for all aspects of drug usage in hospitals, pharmacists should be actively involved in the management of these special drugs.

A primary concern of clinical investigators and research sponsors is that clinical research studies in the hospital be carried out properly. Investigational drug studies, however, are not always managed and conducted as effectively and efficiently as they could be, e.g., drug regimens could be interrupted, drug initiation could be delayed because of poor inventory control, drugs could be stored improperly, resulting in their deterioration, and ineligible patients could receive study drugs.

It is necessary for the pharmacist to develop policies, procedures, and programs to deal with investigational drugs and other drugs as they relate to clinical research activities in the hospital.

The extent of the pharmacist's involvement with investigational drugs will depend on the type of hospital facility, the willingness of the pharmacy to accept the responsibility for investigational drug control, the amount of pharmaceutical services required, and the support and resources provided by the hospital administration.

Clinical investigations in the hospital involve many people—physicians, pharmacists, patients, pharmaceutical manufacturing personnel, nurses, and other hospital personnel. Each individual has shared responsibility and obligation to the study system and all must work together. However, the principal investigator of the study is the person who is legally responsible for its conduct. Thus, the primary role of the hospital pharmacist should be to assist and support the principal investigator in meeting his obligations to the patients in the study, the institution, and the sponsor of the research.

This chapter gives an overview of the investigational drug process as regulated by the Food and Drug Administration (FDA), a description of the role of the hospital pharmacist

*An investigational or new drug is defined as any drug that has not yet been released for general use and has not been cleared for sale in interstate commerce by the FDA. The drug is not necessarily a new chemical substance, but may be an old or approved drug proposed for a new use, a new combination of two or more old drugs, a combination of old drugs in new proportions, or a new dosage form or method of administration, or it may be a new drug because it contains a new component such as an excipient, a coating, or a menstruum.

in handling these special drugs in both the small hospital and the large research hospital, and the type of pharmaceutical investigational drug services that need to be established to deal with the particular needs of the hospital facility.

FDA REGULATIONS

At the present time, the clinical investigation and subsequent marketing of new drugs are governed by the 1938 Federal Food, Drug, and Cosmetic Act and the Kefauver-Harris Amendments of 1962 (1). These statutes have been implemented by a series of FDA regulations in Title 21 of the Code of Federal Regulations. In essence, these laws and regulations define the conditions under which clinical investigational drugs and biologic products may be shipped in interstate commerce and delineate the evidence needed for the claimed safety and efficacy of the new drug that needs to be provided prior to its being marketed (2).

PRECLINICAL STUDIES

Before investigational new drugs are given to human subjects, adequate preclinical research studies must be done in animals or in vitro. This includes conducting pharmacokinetic, pharmacologic, and toxicologic studies to obtain data to show that there will not be unreasonable risks in initiating human research. This is done by extrapolating, when possible, the animal data to humans in order to predict possible therapeutic or toxic effects.

Pharmacokinetic studies determine the new drug's absorptive, distributive, metabolic, and excretory pathways. The general purpose of these studies is to estimate the pharmacokinetic parameters, such as plasma drug concentration, biologic half-life, drug distribution, metabolism, and excretion.

Pharmacologic studies determine the action of the new drug in animals to estimate the magnitude of its intended therapeutic effect.

Toxicologic studies in animals predict relative safety in humans and monitor parameters that will be used in clinical trials. Acute and chronic toxicity are determined in several animal species at varying dosage levels. Initial doses of drug in Phase I clinical studies are often based on the preclinical toxicologic data. Preclinical toxicity studies are important because the initial benefit or risk assessment for use of the drug in humans is made from these studies.

FILING A NOTICE OF CLAIMED INVESTIGATIONAL EXEMPTION FOR A NEW DRUG

After preclinical studies have been completed and favorable results obtained, the new drug may be ready to be studied in humans. Although this is usually done under the sponsorship of a pharmaceutical company, an individual physician may file a "Notice of Claimed Investigational Exemption for a New Drug" (Form FDA 1571), commonly called an investigational new drug application, or IND, with the FDA. This form (Appendix 45.1) contains 16 parts. Some of the information includes:

1. Complete composition of the drug, its source, and manufacturing data to show that appropriate standards exist to ensure safety and give significance to studies conducted with the drug.

2. Results of all preclinical investigations, including animal studies. Initially, these studies should be directed toward defining the drug's safety rather than its efficacy. The data should support the scope and duration of the proposed clinical trial and demonstrate that there will not be an unreasonable risk in initiating human studies. As a minimum, the animal data should include a pharmacologic profile, acute toxicity studies in several species of animals using the route of administration to be used in the clinical investigation, and short-term animal studies to evaluate toxicity from 2 weeks to 3 months, depending on the proposed use.

3. Information regarding training and experience of each clinical investigator. Investigators are responsible to the sponsor and are required to submit to the sponsor either a Form FDA 1572 (Appendix 45.2) for clinical pharmacology studies (Phase I and II) or a Form FDA 1573 (Appendix 45.3) for clinical trials (Phase III) (see "Qualifications of Investigators" and "Obligation of Investigators"). Where the sponsor himself is the sole investigator, submission of his curriculum vitae may be adequate.

4. Copies of informational materials must be supplied to each investigator. This includes an accurate description of prior investigations and experience and their results pertinent to the safety and possible usefulness of the drug under the conditions of the investigation. Also described are all relevant hazards, contraindications, side effects, and precautions suggested by prior investigations and experience with the drug.

5. A detailed outline (protocol) of the planned investigation, including the phase or phases of the study (see "The Clinical Investigation" and "Institutional Review Board").

6. A statement that the sponsor will notify the FDA if the investigation is discontinued and the reasons why.

7. A statement that the sponsor will notify each investigator if a new drug application (NDA) is approved or if the investigation is discontinued.

8. Assurance that the clinical studies will not begin until 30 days after the FDA acknowledges receipt of the IND.

THE CLINICAL INVESTIGATION

The clinical investigation of a new drug is divided into three phases and is directed toward producing substantial proof of the safety and efficacy of the drug (3).

Phase I. Clinical pharmacology studies represent the initial introduction of the new drug in man. The purposes of these studies include the determination of human toxicity, absorption, metabolism, elimination, pharmacodynamics, preferred route of administration, and safe dosage range. Phase I studies involve a small number of persons (20-80) and should be conducted under carefully controlled circumstances by qualified clinical pharmacologists (4).

Phase II. Clinical pharmacology studies are conducted on a limited number of patients (100-200) for the treatment or prophylaxis of a specific disease. Phase II studies are conducted by clinicians familiar with the methods of drug evaluation, as well as the disease being treated, and drugs currently in use for this condition. These carefully supervised studies are designed to demonstrate the new drug's efficacy and relative safety.

Phase III. Studies for this phase, involving extensive clinical trials, may be initiated if the information obtained in the first two phases demonstrates reasonable assurance of safety and effectiveness or suggests that the drug may have a potential value outweighing possible hazards. The Phase III studies are intended to assess the drug's safety, effectiveness, and most desirable dosage in treating a specific disease in a large group of subjects. The studies should also be carefully monitored, even though they are extensive.

The FDA should receive constant reports on the progress of each phase. If the continuation of the studies appears to present an unwarranted hazard to the patients, the sponsor may be requested to modify or discontinue clinical testing until further preclinical work has been done.

QUALIFICATIONS OF INVESTIGATORS

The sponsor (usually a pharmaceutical manufacturer) of an investigational new drug will ask the clinical investigator to supply the following information before shipping the investigational drug to the investigator: a statement of his education, training, and experience and information regarding the hospital or other medical institution where the investigation will be conducted and special equipment and other facilities. This information will be supplied on Form FDA 1572 for clinical pharmacologists engaged in Phase I or II trials or Form FDA 1573 for physicians engaged in Phase III clinical trials. The clinical investigators should be experts qualified by scientific training and experience to investigate safety and effectiveness of drugs.

The training and experience requirements will vary, depending on the kind of drug and the nature of the investigation. In Phase I, the investigator must be able to evaluate human toxicology and pharmacology. In Phase II, the investigator should be familiar with the conditions to be treated, the drugs used in these conditions, and the methods of their evaluation. In Phase III, in addition to the experienced clinical investigators, other physicians not regarded as specialists in any particular field of medicine may serve as investigators. At this stage, a large number of patients may be treated by different physicians to obtain a broad background of experience with the drug.

OBLIGATIONS OF INVESTIGATORS

When the clinical investigator signs either the Form FDA 1572 or Form FDA 1573, he or she agrees to:

1. Maintain adequate records of the disposition of all investigational drugs, including dates and quantities received and their use, and to return unused supply of drug when the investigation is completed, terminated, or suspended.

2. Prepare and maintain adequate and accurate individual case histories designed to record all observations and other pertinent data.

3. Furnish progress reports to the sponsor. The sponsor collects and evaluates the results from various investigators and submits progress reports to the FDA at intervals not exceeding 1 year.

4. Report adverse reactions to the sponsor promptly so that the FDA and other investigators can be notified.

5. Submit annual progress reports and comments regarding disposal of the drug when studies are discontinued.

6. Maintain records of disposition of drugs and case histories for a period of 2 years following the date an NDA is approved, or if the NDA is not filed or approved, 2 years after the investigation is discontinued.

7. Certify that the drug will be administered only to subjects under his personal supervision or under the supervision of physicians responsible to him.

8. Certify that informed consent will be obtained in writing from all patients on whom the drug is to be tested before the test is made, including any person used as a control, or from their representatives, except where this is not feasible or, in the investigator's professional judgment, is contrary to the best interests of the subject.

9. Give assurance that for investigations involving institutionalized subjects the studies will not be initiated until the institutional review board has approved the study.

It should be noted that the FDA does not give formal approval to the submissions in the IND, but it does monitor and review them. The sponsor is notified of any deficiencies, and if a safety problem exists, the IND will be terminated.

PREPARATION OF AN IND APPLICATION

A pharmacist with knowledge of the FDA regulations for new drugs can inform and advise the physician (clinical investigator) on how to file with the FDA or pharmaceutical firm to obtain approval for use of a new drug in the hospital. The extent of responsibility and communication with the FDA will depend on who is the IND sponsor, either the pharmaceutical firm or the physician.

1. *Pharmaceutical firm as sponsor:* If the sponsor is the pharmaceutical firm, then the physician is required to provide the *sponsor* (and not the FDA) with the following information. (In doing so, the sponsor holds the IND for the drug and the physician is a co-investigator.)
   a. Clinical research protocol approved by the institutional review board
   b. A curriculum vitae and bibliography of each physician participating in the study
   c. Signed "Statement of Investigator" (Form FDA 1572 if study is Phase I or II; Form FDA 1573 if study is Phase III)
2. *Physician as sponsor:* If the sponsor is the physician, then he is required to provide the following information to the FDA:

a. Clinical research protocol, approved by the institutional review board
b. A curriculum vitae and bibliography of each physician participating in the study
c. Signed "Statement of Investigator" (Form FDA 1572 if study is Phase I or II; Form FDA 1573 if study is Phase III)
d. Signed Form FDA 1571
e. Manufacturing information

The type and extent of manufacturing data provided will depend on where the drug was obtained and whether or not it has been altered. For example:

a. For marketed drugs that are unaltered prior to use provide:
   (1) Source of drug (name and address of manufacturer)
   (2) Dosage form and strength
   (3) Copy of label as found on the marketed package
b. For nonmarketed drugs and chemicals supplied to the investigator by a manufacturer provide:
   (1) Source of drug (name and address of manufacturer)
   (2) Dosage form and strength
   (3) Copy of label as found on package
   (4) Authorization (in a letter) from the manufacturer for the FDA to refer to its master file, NDA or Investigational New Drug Notice, on file with the FDA for the manufacturing information on the drug
c. For drugs altered by or prepared completely by the investigator or the pharmacy, the following information should be provided:
   (1) Best available descriptive name (including the chemical formula, if known) of the new drug substance and a statement of how it is to be administered
   (2) Statement of the source of the new drug substance, including name and address of supplier
   (3) Brief description of the preparation of the new drug substance together with the methods used to determine its identity, purity, and potency adequate for the purpose and period of clinical trial
   (4) List of inactive ingredients, if used, together with a statement concerning their quality, i.e., USP or NF grade
   (5) A statement of the quantitative composition (including inactive ingredients) of the finished dosage form and a brief description of the preparation of the finished dosage form and methods of analysis together with results obtained on each batch.
   (6) A copy of the label to be used on the bottle, box, ampule, etc (5)

The above information could also be provided in the form of an analytical data sheet (Figs. 45.1 and 45.2).

INSTITUTIONAL REVIEW BOARD (IRB)

The FDA regulations published in Title 21, Part 56, of the Code of Federal Regulations requires that all clinical studies involving investigational drugs in humans be re-

Text continued on p. 487.

Pharmaceutical Development Service   Date:
Pharmacy Department, CC, NIH
Analytical Data Sheet for:

_____

_____

_____

GENERAL INFORMATION:

  Chemical Name: _____

                              _____

                              _____

  Other Names: _____

                              _____

                              _____

  Molecular Formula: _____

  Molecular Weight: _____

  Structural Formula:

SPECIFICATIONS: for _____

                            _____

                            _____

compared with values obtained by the Pharmaceutical
Development Service, Analytical Laboratory, Pharmacy
Department, CC, NIH, that reported in the literature
and _____

_____

_____

1
2
3 Pharmaceutical Development Service, Analytical Laboratory, Pharmacy Department,
CC, NIH

FIGURE 45.1   Format of the analytical data sheet for bulk material.

```
                                                                          -2-
Pharmaceutical Development Service              Date:
Pharmacy Department, CC, NIH
Analytical Data Sheet for:

                              _____

                              _____

                              _____




Description:              Reported[1]        Reported[2]        Found[3]

                          _____

                          _____

                          _____

                          _____

Solubility:               _____

                          _____

                          _____

                          _____

                          _____

                          _____

                          _____

pH:                       _____

Melting Point:            _____

Loss on Drying:           _____

                          _____

Residue on Ignition:      _____

Specific Rotation:        _____

                          _____

                          _____

                          _____

                          _____



_____
```

FIGURE 45.1, cont'd

-3-

Pharmaceutical Development Service   Date:
Pharmacy Department, CC, NIH
Analytical Data Sheet for:

_____

_____

_____

ELEMENTAL ANALYSIS: % Theory   % Found[4]

   % Carbon   _____

   % Hydrogen   _____

   % Nitrogen   _____

_____

_____

INFRARED ANALYSIS: Recorded as _____

_____

Positive for_____

as compared to _____

_____

(See enclosed Spectra).

                 Reported   Found

INFRARED BANDS AT   _____

_____

_____

_____

_____

4

FIGURE 45.1, cont'd

```
                                                                    -4-
Pharmaceutical Development Service              Date:
Pharmacy Department, CC, NIH
Analytical Data Sheet for:


                               1%
ULTRAVIOLET SPECTRA:       E₁ cm =        at _____nm  for _____

                           in         (c = _____%

                           (See enclosed spectra)

THIN-LAYER CHROMATOGRAPHY:

   Stationary Phase:       _____

                           _____

   Mobile Phase:           _____

                           _____

   Spot:                   _____

   Detection:              _____

                           _____

                           _____

   Results:                _____

                           _____

                           _____

                           _____

GAS-LIQUID CHROMATOGRAPHY:

   Instrument:             _____

                           _____

   Column:                 _____

                           _____

   Temperature:            Column - _____° C.

                           Injection port - _____° C.

                           Detector - _____° C.
```

FIGURE 45.1, cont'd

-5-

Pharmaceutical Development Service   Date:
Pharmacy Department, CC, NIH
Analytical Data Sheet for:

Detection: _____ (attenuation x _____)

Carrier Gas: _____ at_____ ml/min (P = _____ psi)

Procedure: _____

_____

_____

_____

_____

_____

Results: _____

_____

_____

_____

_____

_____

HIGH PRESSURE LIQUID CHROMATOGRAPHY:

  Instrument: _____

_____

  Column: _____

_____

  Mobile Phase: _____

_____

  Flow Rate: _____ ml/min (P = _____ psi)

  Detection: Absorbance at _____ nm (attenuation x _____)

FIGURE 45.1, cont'd

```
Pharmaceutical Development Service                    Date:            -6-
Pharmacy Department, CC, NIH
Analytical Data Sheet for:




Procedure:       _____

                 _____

                 _____

                 _____

                 _____

                 _____

Results:         _____

                 _____

                 _____

                 _____

                 _____

                 _____
```

FIGURE 45.1, cont'd

-7-

Pharmaceutical Development Service
Pharmacy Department, CC, NIH   Date:
Analytical Data Sheet for:

_____

_____

_____

ASSAY:

   Procedure:

FIGURE 45.1, cont'd

```
                                                                    -8-
Pharmaceutical Development Service              Date:
Pharmacy Department, CC, NIH
Analytical Data Sheet for:
                              _____

                              _____

                              _____



ASSAY:  (Continued)

   Results:              _____

                        _____

                        _____

                        _____

                        _____

                        _____

                        _____

                        _____

                        _____

                        _____

                        _____

                        _____

   Packaging & Storage:  _____

                        _____

                        _____

   Stability:            _____

                        _____

                        _____


         _____
```

FIGURE 45.1, cont'd

```
Pharmaceutical Development Service                    Date:
Pharmacy Department, CC, NIH
Analytical Data Sheet for:
                        _____ *

                        _____

                        _____


Manufacturer:           Bulk material:    _____


                        _____

                        _____ : Pharmaceutical Development Service
                        Pharmacy Department, NIH, PDS lot _____

Description:            _____

                        _____

                        _____

                        _____

                        _____

                        _____

                        _____

                        _____

                        _____


Sterility:              Meets requirements of test.  Tested by Division of
                        Biologics Standards, NIH, in Accordance with U.S.P.
                        _____ (p.    ).

Pyrogen Test:           Meets the requirements of the test. Tested by
                        Division of Biologics Standards, NIH, in accordance
                        with U.S.P. _____ (p.     ).

Weight Variation        Twenty _____ selected at random passed the U.S.P.
                        weight variation test in accordance with U.S.P. ____,
                        (p.   ).  The mean _____ weight was found
                        to be _____.  The range was from _____
                        above the mean to _____ below the mean.




* _____
```

FIGURE 45.2 Format of the analytical data sheet for finished product.

Pharmaceutical Development Service   Date:
Pharmacy Department, CC, NIH   -2-
Analytical Data Sheet for:

_____ *

_____

_____

Tablet Disintegration Tests: Six tablets, selected at random, were tested by the
                             U.S.P. tablet disintegration test in accordance with
                             _____. The disintegration time
                             was found to be _____.

Dissolution: Six _____, selected at random, were tested by
                             the U.S.P. dissolution test in accordance with U.S.P.
                             _____, (p.   ). The dissolution mediam was
                             _____ and the rotation rate was
                             was _____rpm. The results are summarized
                             below.

                                   Time   % Dissolved

                             _____   _____

                             _____   _____

                             _____   _____

                             _____   _____

                             _____   _____

                             _____   _____

Tablet Hardness: _____

                             _____

                             _____

pH: _____

Tablet Thickness: _____

_____

FIGURE 45.2, cont'd

Pharmaceutical Development Service   Date:
Pharmacy Department, CC, NIH   -3-
Analytical Data Sheet for:
                                          *

_____

_____

_____

<u>Assay</u>:

  <u>Procedure</u>:

FIGURE 45.2, cont'd

```
Pharmaceutical Development Service                    Date:
Pharmacy Department, CC, NIH                          -4-
Analytical Data Sheet for:
                                    _____ *

                                    _____

                                    _____



Assay: (Continued)

   Results:          _____

                     _____

                     _____

                     _____

                     _____

                     _____

                     _____

                     _____

                     _____

                     _____

                     _____

                     _____

   Comments:         _____

                     _____

                     _____

                     _____

                     _____
```

FIGURE 45.2, cont'd

```
Pharmaceutical Development Service                    Date:
Pharmacy Department, CC, NIH                          -5-
Analytical Data Sheet for:
                                    _____  *

                                    _____

                                    _____



Route of Administration:    _____

Packaging & Storage:        _____

                            _____

                            _____

                            _____

                            _____

                            _____

                            _____

                            _____

Stability:                  _____

                            _____

                            _____

                            _____

                            _____

                            _____

                            _____

Label:


                            _____
```

FIGURE 45.2, cont'd

viewed and approved by an IRB in the hospital. When a sponsor submits a signed Notice of Claimed Investigational Exemption for a New Drug (IND) to the FDA, he is assuring (under Part 10 of Form FDA 1571) that an IRB in the hospital will be responsible for the initial and continuing review approval of the proposed clinical study and for assuring the patient's informed consent. The sponsor must also provide assurance that the investigators will report to the IRB all changes in the research activity and all unanticipated problems involving risks to human subjects or others. The sponsors obtain this assurance when the investigator signs the Statement of Investigator, either Form FDA 1572 or 1573. An IRB should be composed of no less than five persons with varying backgrounds, possessing the professional competence necessary to review research studies.

The IRB should ensure that the clinical research meets appropriate scientific, legal, and ethical standards. In addition, the IRB should determine whether subjects will be placed at risk and, if so, determine if the risks outweigh the potential benefits to the subject and the knowledge to be gained. If risks overshadow benefits, no protocol should be approved. Furthermore, the IRB must also see that the rights and welfare of all subjects are carefully protected and that proper informed consent is obtained in accordance with the provision of governmental and hospital requirements.

INFORMED CONSENT

An IRB requires that the investigator give to the patient in the clinical research study information regarding the research, known as the "informed consent document." This document is part of the clinical research protocol that must be approved by the IRB and signed by the patient or the patient's legally authorized representative before the study can begin. The consent form is merely a mechanism for verifying in writing that informed consent exists with respect to a particular research patient. The informed consent document assures that the patient understands the risks, expected outcomes, and procedures when participating in the study and voluntarily agrees to participate in the study under those conditions. The patient should be kept informed of any significant changes in the information originally presented so that he can decide if continued participation is desirable. The language in the informed consent document should be understandable to the patient or the representative and information should be specific and include the eight basic elements of informed consent as provided in the regulations (6).

INVESTIGATIONAL USE OF COMMERCIALLY AVAILABLE DRUGS

The FDA has no authority over the practice of medicine and cannot require a physician to prescribe or not to prescribe a drug for a particular illness. However, physicians are encouraged to submit an IND when they use a drug regularly for purposes other than those approved by the FDA. The FDA can then accumulate data on the safety and efficacy of the drug for such treatment and can share the information with other physicians.

The FDA is proposing to exempt from the IND regulations those clinical investigations using marketed drugs that (1) are not intended to be reported to the FDA as a well-controlled study in support of a new indication nor intended to be used to support any other significant change in the advertising or labeling for the drug and (2) involve a route of administration, dosage level, or use in a patient population that does not significantly increase the risks associated with the use of the drug product. The regulations would also prohibit the sponsor from commercializing the investigation or promoting the drug for its investigated use, except on specific approval by the FDA (10).

USE OF DRUGS FOR LABORATORY PROCEDURES

New drugs used only for in vitro studies or in laboratory animals are exempted from the new drug regulations provided they are labeled *"Caution—Contains a new drug for investigational use only in laboratory research animals or for tests in vitro. Not for use in humans."* The exemption does not apply, however, to a new drug used in vitro when this use will influence the diagnosis or treatment of disease in a human patient—e.g., disks to determine the sensitivity to antibiotics of bacteria in culture or a stick or strip of paper incorporating a reagent to test for sugar in the urine. Apparent ineffectiveness of an antibiotic sensitivity disk or a false negative test for glycosuria might well lead to an incorrect diagnosis and deprive the patient of appropriate treatment (3).

Before such a preparation can be marketed, there must be certification (in the case of antibiotics) or approval of an NDA (in the case of other drugs). For that reason, it is necessary to submit adequate proof of the effectiveness of these preparations before they can be marketed.

PHARMACEUTICAL INVESTIGATIONAL DRUG SERVICE

Basic Activities for the Hospital Pharmacist

The extent of the hospital pharmacists' activities in providing pharmaceutical investigational drug service will depend on the type of hospital, its facilities and equipment, specialized services, and the expertise of the pharmacy department. Before discussing the extent of these different activities, we should discuss what is the minimal or basic activity of all hospital pharmacies handling investigational drugs. These basic activities include the registration, control, storage, dispensing, maintenance of disposition records, and drug information for every investigational drug. In order for hospital pharmacies to carry out even the basic activities, it is imperative that the hospital adopt certain policies and procedures for the use, storage, and control of investigational drugs.

Although the FDA does not require that investigational drugs be stored in and dispensed through a hospital pharmacy (7), the standards of the Joint Commission on Accreditation of Hospitals do require that all drugs used in the hospital, including investigational drugs, be stored, dispensed, and controlled by the pharmacy. Thus, many hospitals require that all investigational drugs for use in patients be registered and stored by the hospital pharmacy and dispensed on orders from specifically authorized physicians. The advantages of this policy, which should be stressed to physicians, are drugs can be stored, dispensed, accounted for, and available 24 hours a day; observed for shelf-life and stability; and returned to the manufacturer when needed by the pharmacy. In addition, some hospitals have established a policy that no investigational drug be administered to a patient by a nurse or physician unless it bears a pharmacy department control or registration number. Armed with these two policies, the hospital pharmacists can now exert some effective control over the use of investigational drugs in the hospital.

Registration and Control

After the physician (clinical investigator) submits his written clinical research protocol (which describes the use of the investigational drug) to the hospital's IRB, obtains approval, and arranges with a pharmaceutical firm for receipt of the investigational drug, he meets with the pharmacist to arrange for the registration, storage, dispensing, and control of the drug. It is at this initial meeting that the subject of drug delivery, control, labeling, ordering, storage, disposition, protocol, and authorized investigators are discussed and an Investigational Drug Service Request form (Figs. 45.3 and 45.4) is completed. The specific information requested on the form includes the name of the drug (chemical and other); dosage form and strength; pharmacology; purpose of the investigation, including a copy of protocol or outline for the study approved by the IRB; route of administration; dosage; side effects, toxicity, and any known antidote; storage conditions; stability of product; pharmaceutical manufacturer and name and telephone number of its medical director with knowledge of the drug; names of the principal investigator and co-investigators authorized to prescribe; nursing units; name of sponsor and IND number for the drug; how the drug will be written (what it will be called); the need to relabel product if necessary; and arrangements for obtaining additional drug along with tentative utilization rates.

The use of this form facilitates the registration process and ensures that complete and consistent information will be obtained. The physician should be informed that the pharmacy will be preparing an Investigational Drug Fact Sheet for the nurses and pharmacists handling the drug and that it will be cleared through him prior to distribution. After the pharmacist meets with the physician, the drug product is labeled with a pharmacy department control number, a drug accountability record prepared, and the drug stored in a separate area from the commercially available drugs. The clinical investigator can then initiate the use of the investigational drug by writing the drug order on a duplicate doctor's order form in the patient's chart or enter the order into a computer terminal and have it electronically transmitted. In either case, the order is received in the pharmacy. Prior to filling the order, a pharmacist checks the Drug Accountability Record to confirm if the physician writing the order is an authorized investigator and, if so, the order is filled (8).

Drug Accountability Record

The physician or clinical investigator is allowed by the FDA to delegate authority to the hospital pharmacist to maintain the investigational drug disposition records. Although the records will differ with each hospital, they usually include the name of the drug, quantity and date received, the dosage form and strength, the name of the manufacturer, lot or control number, and expiration date (Fig. 45.5). As each drug order is filled, the date, patient's name, serial number of the prescription, and name of the prescribing investigator and quantity dispensed are recorded on the form. In addition, a list of the authorized co-investigators, the pharmacology of the drug, the maximum dose and route of administration of the drug, and a description of the dosage form should be included on the form. This form can also be used as an inventory record by maintaining a running balance as each drug order is filled.

Drug Information

Before an investigational drug is administered to a patient, the nurse should have basic information concerning the drug, including dosage forms and strengths available, actions and uses, adverse effects, toxicity, and antidote. This information can be provided in the form of an Investigational Drug Fact Sheet (Fig. 45.6). The data on the sheets is approved by the principal investigator prior to its release and is updated by the pharmacy as more information becomes available. In addition to being provided to the nurses, the data sheets may be distributed to other pharmacists and authorized personnel.

Investigational Drug File

The pharmacy may also maintain an information file on each investigational drug that is registered and used in the hospital. Such a file is useful in helping to answer any inquiries about the drug. Included in each file is the registration form, copy or outline of the protocol, drug fact sheet, drug disposition records, correspondence regarding the drug, and any pertinent articles published on the drug.

Expanded Activities for the Hospital Pharmacist

The expansion of activities for the hospital pharmacists handling and managing investigational drugs depends on whether or not the pharmacy can provide the additional services, special equipment, and expertise. It also depends on the commitment of the department and support received from administration.

These expanded activities include additional administrative, clinical, and research and development activities.

Administrative Activities

Additional administrative activities can include the reordering of investigational drugs, disposal of used or unused drugs, and computerization of drug records.

Reordering of Investigational Drugs. Although the principal investigator usually reorders the investigational drug,

Investigational Drug Service Request

**Submit to Pharmaceutical Development
Service, Pharmacy Dept., NIH 496-1031**

Name of Drug

Other Names

Protocol Title

CC Protocol No.

Name of Manufacturer and Lot No.

Description

Dosage Form

Strength

PDS Control No.

Ordering Physician Limited To:

Principal Investigator

Institute

Nursing Unit/Clinic

IND No.

Sponsor:

Location: In Pharmacy; In Satellite

Associate Investigators

Service and Pkg. Requested:

NCI Assigned Protocol No.:

Route of Administration:

Dosing Regimen:

Please Enter Pertinent Information

Patients will be:

☐ IP   ☐ OP   ☐ Both

Where will they be seen?
(Nursing Unit/Clinic)

Are you entering protocol
screen(s) in MIS?

Are you filing your protocol
with the FDA?

Do you have drug source(s) sponsors(s)? If yes, describe:

Company/Sponsor

Address

Contact Person

Phone No.

Drug Supplies to be Registered with PDS (name and quantity)

For Investigational Drug Provided by NCI/IDB:
NCI Assigned Protocol No:
NSC No.

Physician's Signature

Institute

Pharmacy Department Use Only

	Need	Done
Index	☐	☐
IND No.	☐	☐
MIS Screens	☐	☐
Blinding Plan	☐	☐
Authorizations	☐	☐
Study Write Up	☐	☐
Drug Fact Sheet	☐	☐
Analytical Data Sheet	☐	☐
PDS Minutes	☐	☐
White Sheets	☐	☐
Label Design	☐	☐
Low Balance Card	☐	☐
Low Balance Amt.	☐	☐
_____	☐	☐
_____	☐	☐
_____	☐	☐
_____	☐	☐
_____	☐	☐

Telephone Ext/Beeper No.

Bldg./Room No.

Pharmacy Department Use Only

Received By

Date

Completed By

Date

. ● U.S. GPO: 1984-421-141/116

FIGURE 45.3   First page of the Investigational Drug Service Request form.

FORMULATION DATA

Drug	Quan. Per Unit	Total Quan.	Name of Manufacturer and Lot. No.

Completed by	Checked by		Affix Label Here
Sterility Test		Date Sent	
		Date Comp.	
		Result	
Pyrogen Test	Dose mg/kg	Date Sent	
		Date Comp	
	ml/kg	Result	
Other Test:			
Assay	Date	Completed By	
Reassay	Date	Completed By	
Method and Results			

FIGURE 45.4 Second page of the Investigational Drug Service Request form.

Investigational Drug Service Request
Drug Accountability Record

Submit to Pharmaceutical Development
Service, Pharmacy Dept., NIH 496-1031

Name of Drug	Dosage Form	PDS Control No.
Other Names	Strength	
Protocol Title	Ordering Physician Limited To:	
	Principal Investigator	
	Institute	Nursing Unit/Clinic

CD Protocol No.	IND No.	Associate Investigators
Name of Manufacturer and Lot No.	Location: In Pharmacy; In Satellite	
Description		

Special Instructions:
NCI Assigned Protocol No.:

Date	Patient's Name	R$_x$ No.	Physician	Dose	Quantity	Balance	Pharmacist

Issued by PDS

Minimum Stock Level

Received by

FIGURE 45.5   Third page of the Investigational Drug Service Request form (Drug Accountability Record).

NCS No.:   Institute:

IND No.:   Principal Investigator:

Date Abstract Revised: Clinical Project No.:

Generic Name:

Other Names:

Chemical Name:

Description:

How Supplied:

Stability or Storage:

Availability:

Route of Administration:

Suggested Dose:

Use or Purpose of Investigation:

Title of Protocol & No.:

Mechanism of Action:

Known Toxicology:

References:

FIGURE 45.6 The format of the drug fact sheet.

he may wish to delegate this responsibility to the pharmacist because the pharmacy is already involved in the receipt (acquisition), storage, and maintenance of accountability records for the drug. The pharmacy, therefore, knows when additional supplies are needed and can notify the pharmaceutical company directly. The unavailability of the study drug because the principal investigator was on leave or could not order the drug from the pharmaceutical company in a timely manner could result in the pharmacy and thus ultimately the patient not receiving the drug. This problem can be further compounded when several different authorized physicians are writing drug orders for their patients. All of these problems can be prevented by the principal investigator having the pharmacist call the pharmaceutical company to send the drug directly to the pharmacy department with the words "For the Use of Dr. _____." However, it should be noted that, while most pharmaceutical companies readily accept orders from pharmacists, a few prefer to deal directly with the clinical investigator even though there are no legal requirements to do so.

Disposal of Used or Unused Drugs. Any unused drugs at the end of a study must be returned to the sponsor (or pharmaceutical company) unless the sponsor has indicated the remaining drug be destroyed by the pharmacy. In either case, the principal investigator should be contacted to agree on the drug disposition method and be notified in writing

about the disposal or return of the unused drugs (for their records). Recently, more pharmaceutical companies are requiring the return of all used, partially used, and unused drug containers that remain in the patients' hands at the end of their study regimen. The return of these drug containers has created, particularly with large studies, a huge handling and storage problem for pharmacies. Although more and more pharmaceutical companies are requiring the return of empty containers, there is no legal or FDA requirement to do this. Therefore, before the study begins, pharmacists should attempt to convince the sponsor that alternative procedures, such as specific monitoring and review of returns by the pharmacy, should be conducted.

Computerization of Drug Ordering and Control. A computerized drug ordering and control system can provide several advantages to the pharmacy, principal investigator, and sponsor in the handling and managing of investigational drugs in the hospital. This could include a system that can be programmed so that only authorized physicians, designated by the principal investigator, will have access to the investigational drug. By the use of specific screens constructed by the pharmacy, drugs ordered for a given protocol could be entered into the computer by selecting from a uniform formated screen with a precise name, form, strength, and directions. In addition, before the investigational drug could be ordered, the physician would have to note on the computer screen that a written informed consent was obtained, certain tests were conducted and the results noted, and warnings or contraindication were reviewed.

A computerized investigational drug program could be capable of providing a backup system for drug records or be the primary source of the drug accountability record if the dispenser's initials or name, quantity of drug dispensed, and lot number could be entered for each patient. As changes in logistics, dosage form, strength, contraindications, warnings, adverse drug reactions, and authorized investigators are more frequent with research studies, the capability to correct this information on line would be a more efficient and effective method of communicating changes about drugs in the research study. Since all the data is on line, authorized physicians, nurses, and pharmacists would be eligible to see the corrected or updated information immediately. Further sophisticated computer use could be conducted by combining the computerized drug ordering procedure with the use of an optical character reader or a bar code reader that can record the specific drug container along with the drug name, form, strength, lot number, quantity dispensed date, and dispensing pharmacist's initials. With the use of a computerized drug ordering and control system, the computer could maintain running inventories for each study drug and indicate reorder points; provide daily or periodic drug usage reports to quickly summarize the number of patients receiving a drug and also the drug's total usage for the period; list all other pertinent information about the study that will be needed for annual reports and budgets; and be used to develop workload and staffing estimates of the overall activity or complexity of the study. The computerization of investigational drug ordering and control could be done with a hospital's total information computer system or with a freestanding microcomputer. The system that is chosen will depend on the complexity of what is needed to effectively manage an investigational drug program's activity and on the resources of the hospital.

Clinical Activities

Clinical pharmacists can make important contributions to a pharmaceutical investigational drug service or program. The clinical pharmacist is in an ideal position to coordinate the use of investigational drugs in the study. By virtue of his being in the patient care area, he is in a unique position to monitor what is happening, be a data manager, report adverse drug reaction, provide staff and patient education about the investigational drugs, and be an active member of the IRB.

Member of the IRB. As a member of an IRB, a clinical pharmacist would be in a critical position to learn what study protocols involved which investigational drugs during the initial reviews of the studies. He or she would also have the ability to educate other members of the review board about FDA requirements concerning investigational drug studies, filing of the INDs, and providing information on the drug, e.g., how the drug should be given and its compatibility, contraindications, and stability.

Data Manager. The clinical pharmacist can also be a data manager for the research study. This person would be responsible for seeing that the study is carried out as stated in the protocol, that special procedure tests are conducted, that laboratory values and data are collected, and that patients are monitored for incidents and severity of adverse reactions. The monitoring of patients would involve coordinating the data collection required in the study; therefore, a master data collection form is essential. Standardized procedures for its use must be developed and followed by all investigators in the study, particularly with large studies. The pharmacist is the ideal person to oversee data collection and compile the results in a reportable form. Checking the collected data against a master list of protocol data requirements is a good way to ensure that the reports are complete and correct. The data should be regularly reviewed by principal investigators. In addition to data collection, the pharmacist would be concerned about the monitoring of the authorized physician and patients, informed consents, accuracy of records, reordering and disposing of drugs, and quality control of the data and records.

Adverse Drug Reaction Reporting. Patients entering clinical trials with investigational drugs must be monitored for any and all adverse reactions that might be caused by the drug. These adverse reactions must be documented and reported to the sponsor, who in turn must report them to the FDA. Because of his unique training, the clinical pharmacist can determine the incidence of adverse reactions by developing either questionnaires or other tools for documenting subjective side effects that may have occurred. It follows that he or she should also be responsible for preparing the adverse reaction reports. These reports should be sent to the FDA, the involved pharmaceutical company, the hospital's pharmacy and therapeutics committee, and the IRB. To report adverse drug reactions, most hospitals use the FDA's Drug Experience Report or a derivative of it.

Research and Development Activities

Some hospitals have pharmacies that conduct research and have product development services to assist physicians in their clinical research studies. These unique services or activities include sitting up single- or double-blind studies; formulation, development, and preparation of finished dosage forms stability studies; in vitro and in vivo drug analysis; and the preparation of drug identity documents for the FDA.

Single- and Double-Blind Studies. Pharmacists can be extremely helpful in setting up single- and double-blind studies (5). "Blinded studies" are extremely important as part of a clinical trial and are continually emphasized by the FDA to eliminate subjective evaluations of drug efficacy. The hospital pharmacy can play an integral role with the investigator in the initiation of these studies because the pharmacist has been trained to design such studies and can therefore act as a consultant to the investigator.

Blinded studies objectively evaluate an investigational drug by comparing its actions to those of a placebo or another drug. In a single-blind study, the patient's course of drug therapy is unknown to him. In some cases, it is also unknown to the person (either the nurse or nonprescribing physician) evaluating the patient's response to the drug. In a double-blind study, the patient, nurse, and prescribing physician are unaware of which therapy the patients receive.

The pharmacist can develop a simple system for coding

drugs for single-blind studies. This system involves assigning, after consultation with the investigator, a series number and some letters to the drug or drug and placebo. For example, the drug may be assigned letters A, C, and T and the placebo letters B, E, and Y in compound series 492. If the physician wanted to prescribe the drug for the patient, he would have three choices and could write a prescription for compounds 492A, 492C, or 492T. Likewise, the physician has three choices to prescribe for the placebo: compounds 492B, 492E, or 492Y. More letters and numbers can, of course, be assigned if needed to keep the study blinded.

Double-blind studies are generally more objective than single-blind studies, since the patient's courses of drug therapy are randomized. This randomization helps to eliminate bias and to give more validity to data generated from these studies. For simple double-blind studies, a pharmacist can use a table of random numbers or a calculator with a random number generator to set up the study. For example, a double-blind study may involve ten patients, each of whom is to receive a 2-week course of either drug or placebo. To create the random sequence of treatment regimens, one begins by arbitrarily assigning label numbers 1-5 to treatment regimen A (drug) and label numbers 6-10 to treatment regimen B (placebo) (R.S. Raff, National Heart and Lung Institute, personal communication). Ten consecutive random numbers are then obtained, and the first random number is assigned label number 1, the second random number is assigned label number 2, etc. The random numbers are then rearranged in numerical order, and the corresponding label numbers provide the random sequence of the treatment regimens (Table 45.1).

If the study is more involved, the use of a statistician is imperative, e.g., if a study is divided into phases and the patient receives a placebo in one phase and the drug in the other or if the patient population is divided into special groups. This kind of study design ensures the validity of the study. The consultant statistician may meet with the pharmacist or discuss the study with the physician and then prepare the randomization. In the latter case, the physician presents the pharmacy with the randomization in a sealed envelope. In cases in which a pharmaceutical company is sponsoring the study, the randomization, packaging, and matching placebo are all provided. Here the pharmacist is only involved in the drug distribution, data collection, and record maintenance aspects of the study.

At the meeting between the pharmacist and the physician to prepare a double-blind study, certain basic information must be obtained. First, the study is assigned a name—this is to alert pharmacy personnel that this is a special study when they receive a copy of the physician's order sheet. The study is usually named after the drug being used or the disease being treated. The pharmacist then ascertains the number of patients to be studied, the number and frequency and courses of therapy, the randomization (as discussed above), and the directions to the patient. If the directions to the patient will not change throughout the study, a preprinted label may be prepared. The pharmacist then explains to the physician the format in which the order should be written. This format should be standard for all physicians participating in the study, and the importance of adhering

TABLE 45.1 Assigning Random Numbers to Treatment Regimens

Label No.	Random Numbers	Random Numbers in Numerical Order	Label No. and Corresponding Treatment Regimens	
1	36	11	4	A
2	69	19	5	A
3	72	26	8	B
4	11	36	1	A
5	19	43	9	B
6	56	56	6	B
7	82	62	10	B
8	26	69	2	A
9	43	72	3	A
10	62	82	7	B

to this format should be stressed. The more rigid the format, the less likelihood there is for error.

A form for use in the preparation of a "double-blind" study is seen in Figures 45.7 to 45.9. The use of this form greatly simplifies the preparation of a study. It details all of the information necessary for the pharmacist to accurately dispense drug or placebo. The form consists of three pages. Page one (Fig. 45.7) identifies the principal investigator and any other investigators on the study; the institute involved; the nursing unit on which the study will be conducted; the description, i.e., the appearance of the dosage form and its strength (this sometimes includes the manner of packaging); the purpose of the investigation; the dose to be used throughout the study; and the dispensing information. The dispensing instructions include all the information that should appear on the written prescription for the drug to be used in the study. Page two (Fig. 45.8) outlines information concerning the storage of the drug and placebo in the pharmacy, how they will be labeled, and how the dispensing label should appear. Dispensing labels are preprinted with as much information as possible to reduce the time the pharmacist must spend typing the label and dispensing the study drugs. The following information is usually preprinted: name of study, patient number (followed by a blank to be filled in), course number (also followed by a blank), patient instructions, and a blank for the date and physician's name. At the bottom of page two is a statement that is incorporated into all double-blind studies and is self-explanatory. Page three (Fig. 45.9) is the randomization sheet used in the study. This randomization sheet can be designed to provide whatever information is needed.

Formulation, Development, and Preparation of the Dosage Form. When an investigator wishes to conduct a study with a new drug that no manufacturer is interested in preparing or sponsoring, he can often obtain assistance for the development and formulation of the dosage form from the pharmacist (9). The service the pharmacist can provide varies from the reformulation of commercial tablets into matching drug and placebo capsules, to the preparation of a suitable effective dosage form from a bulk powder. If this service is needed, the investigator will meet with the pharmacist, discuss the study, and provide the pharmacist with certain information. The information is recorded on the Investigational Service Drug form, which is the same docu-

FORMAT FOR STUDY WRITE-UP
NAME OF STUDY

Principal Investigator: Institute: Nursing Unit:

Other Investigators:

Description:

Purpose of Investigation:

Dose:

Dispensing Instructions:

1. The following information should appear on prescriptions received for this study:
    a. Name of patient and nursing unit (if inpatient)
    b. Name of study
    c. Patient number or letter
    d. Course number
    e. Directions for the patient
    f. Physician's signature

FIGURE 45.7   Page one of the double-blind protocol form listing descriptive information.

Date _____
Page 2

FORMAT FOR STUDY WRITE-UP

2. Upon receipt of the Rx for the _____ study determine whether drug or placebo is to be given. See Randomization Sheet. Drugs are located in _____.

3. The drug or placebo will be packaged under _____.

4. Record the necessary information on the log sheet and randomization sheet.

5. The drug (Name of Study) will be found labelled as: (Give sample of label on container, as brought to Pharmacy Service).

6. The placebo will be found labelled as follows: (Give sample of label on container as brought to Pharmacy Service).

7. Give information as to how Pharmacy Service is to dispense drug. Label it as follows: (Give sample label as to how you want label to appear when it is dispensed by Pharmacy Service).

FIGURE 45.8 Page two of the double-blind protocol form listing dispensing information for investigational drug and placebo.

FORMAT FOR STUDY WRITE-UP

Additional Background Information:

This is a double-blind study. Under no circumstances should physicians dealing with the patients be able to ascertain the identity of the drugs. If for any reason it is necessary to identify the drug a certain patient is receiving, write the name of the doctor making the request, the date, and the time the code is broken, and the reason for breaking the code on the randomization sheet.

RANDOMIZATION SHEET FOR _____STUDY

Patient Number	Patient Name	Course 1	Date Received	Course 2	Date Received
1		Drug		Placebo	
2		Placebo		Drug	
3		Drug		Placebo	
4		Placebo		Placebo	
5		Placebo		Drug	
6		Drug		Drug	
7		Drug		Drug	
8		Drug		Placebo	
9		Placebo		Placebo	
10		Placebo		Drug	
11		Placebo		Drug	
12		Drug		Drug	
13		Drug		Placebo	
14		Placebo		Drug	
15		Drug		Drug	

FIGURE 45.8, cont'd

ment used for the registration of a drug (in the finished dosage form) obtained from the pharmaceutical manufacturer sponsoring it (Fig. 45.3). The portion of the form marked "service and packaging requested" will include specifics: dosage form, potency per dose, route of administration, quantity, method of packaging and labeling, certification of analysis, and any other information, chemical or otherwise, that may be available about the drug.

Initially, the analytical and quality control section in the pharmacy conducts studies to ensure the identity, strength, quality, and purity of the compound. With this information, and guided by the investigator's stated desires, the pharmacist is ready to proceed with the formulation. To provide an optimal rate of absorption in the body, the pharmacist concerns himself with particle size, solubility, pH, disintegration and dissolution time, and other factors. The pharmacist will reject distasteful, objectionable combinations, because a medication is useless if the patient cannot or will not take it. Therefore, the physical form and dose, possible pain on injection, odor, and appearance of the drug are considered. The pharmacist must also test for a parenteral drug's sterility, pyrogenicity, and safety. When the formulation is complete, it is noted on the back of the Investigational Drug Service Request sheet, which also contains package specification, all lot or control numbers, and a copy of the label (Fig. 45.4).

If the clinical investigator is satisfied with the dosage form, the pharmacist can now prepare the formulation as a pilot plant batch. If no suitable assay method for the active ingredient is available, it should be noted that another pharmacist from the quality control section may monitor the manufacturing to provide a double check, thus ensuring that the proper amount of active drug is used. However, if an assay method does exist or has been developed, then the pharmacists in the analytical and quality control section will determine the active drug content. This group also determines pharmaceutical quality and specifications for the drug. The specifications for the fill weight for hard gelatin capsules and tablets, pH, and specific gravity, when appropriate, should be included. The completed Investigational Drug Service Request sheet and the master formula card are "drug checked" to ensure that the proper control-approved ingredients were employed.

Stability. Along with the preparation of the drug dosage form, some knowledge of its stability is required in order to use it effectively. Also, since most investigational and many marketed drugs have not been adequately evaluated for stability and compatibility, particularly as prescribed by the physician, stability studies should be conducted by the research pharmacist. He may study the rate and mechanism of the drug's decomposition, develop assay methods, and predict long-range stability under various storage conditions. He may have to experiment further with the formulation and packaging to achieve the desired stabilization. He may also conduct studies on drugs stored in the frozen state, thawed, and in various diluents, with other drugs, in different pHs and temperature, and in different containers and packaging materials.

If possible, a stability profile should be obtained at every stage in the formulation in order to support standards of identity, strength, quality, and purity being proposed for the drug. The analytical methods used to obtain this data should be capable of measuring characteristic physical and chemical properties associated with the intact drug. Stability characteristics of the drug under extreme conditions of temperature (e.g., 5°, 50°, and 75° C), humidity (90% RH at 25° C), and light (UV 3500 to 4000 Å) could be carried out to satisfy FDA requirements of stability and shelf-life if the sponsor—in this case, the physician—is filing for the IND. The degradation products encountered during stability studies should be quantitatively and qualitatively identified, if possible, and the source (e.g., reactants) and mechanisms considered. The stability studies of the dosage form subsequently developed should include the behavior of the degradation products as well as other impurities associated with the drug. The test methods should be capable of distinguishing the intact molecule from the degradation products.

Drugs that are susceptible to heat, light, and air should be carefully monitored, and changes in manufacturing procedures may introduce trace quantities of metal that may affect the stability of the drug product.

The most carefully produced dosage form can be no better than the quality of the container in which it is held. The safety, effectiveness, and stability of the product depends to a significant extent on the suitability of the packaging materials and the adequacy of the packaging. Therefore, stability studies that do not include temperatures and conditions beyond room temperature with the drug form in its container are usually not satisfactory.

Drug Analysis and Quality Control. Some comments about the need for a drug analysis and quality control laboratory in the pharmacy when dealing with the preparation of dosage forms and the filing of an IND are necessary.

The analytical and quality control laboratory of the pharmacy can ensure the identity and quality of an investigational drug. Its primary objectives should be to determine methods for testing the bulk investigational materials and the chemical formulation. The physician or clinical investigator, pharmaceutical manufacturer, or screening group supplying the bulk investigational material is requested to submit information on the chemical and physical properties of the drug. The research pharmacist in the analytical and quality control laboratory then conducts a literature search on the assay methodology for the major component, anticipated minor components, and degradation products. When possible, the bulk material may be examined by gas-liquid chromatography, high-pressure liquid chromatography, and thin-layer chromatography to detect unexpected minor components. Other data sought for a given material may include the results of elemental analyses; heavy metal determination; loss on drying; optical rotation, infrared, ultraviolet, and nuclear magnetic resonance spectra; and the results of functional group or minor component determinations. A pharmacist then reviews the data for each lot before it is used. Any bulk supply stored for 6 months or more is reexamined before it is formulated for clinical testing.

If possible, the analytical group defines a standard reference sample of known purity. This can be used in preparing specifications for the drug when it is processed for clinical formulation and for eventual large-scale manufacturing.

In addition to conducting in vitro drug analyses and quality control, a research pharmacist, in a pharmacy-based clinical pharmacokinetic research laboratory, can assist in supporting the physician in his clinical research studies by developing analytical methods to rapidly determine plasma levels of drugs and their metabolites, carry out clinical pharmacokinetic and bioavailability studies for understanding and interpreting the response of a patient to a given regimen, and collaborate with the physician in following and fine-tuning the drug therapy plans.

Drug Identity Documents. The drug analysis and quality control laboratory is also responsible for the preparation of drug identity and purity documents for submission to the FDA to support an IND. These documents, or data sheets, are prepared for both the bulk investigational drug and the finished product. The data for the bulk drug may include its clinical and other names, the empirical and structural formula, molecular weight, solubility, melting point, pH, identification, assay, packaging, and storage. The document for the finished product may include source and batch or control of bulk drug, control or research number of finished dosage form, the manufacturer, and such characteristics as pH, weight variation, and dissolution and disintegration time (if applicable), sterility, pyrogenicity, identification, assay, moisture determination (if applicable), stability testing and shelf-life, packaging, and storage (Figs. 45.1 and 45.2).

All assay and stability studies to determine expiration date and shelf-life of the finished dosage form, including its use in intravenous additive admixtures, are carried out by the analytical and quality control laboratory. The effects of variables such as temperature, air, light, and autoclaving are considered. Accelerated storage conditions are used, such as elevated temperatures, increased humidity, or exposure to ultraviolet light. Although data obtained in this way may not be translated directly into shelf-life data, they serve as guides for immediate working conditions.

SUMMARY

The hospital pharmacist has a definitive role in the handling and monitoring of all investigational drugs by virtue of his or her expertise in the labeling, storage, and dispensing of all drugs in the hospital. Also, the pharmacy is the logical place for the central repository of all investigational drug information, including IND numbers. The basic services that could be provided by the pharmacist in the handling of investigational drugs are the registration, control, storage, dispensing, maintenance of drug accountability records, and drug information for every investigational drug evaluated for use in humans. If the drug dosage form is prepared in the hospital by the pharmacist, he plans an even larger role as a manufacturer of the drug product as well as advisor on filing the necessary drug information for an IND with the FDA. The expanded roles will depend on the pharmacist's expertise in formulation, development, and preparation of finished drug dosage forms; setting up single- and double-blind studies; assaying the drug and confirming its identity; and preparing documents as the manufacturer for submission to the FDA in support of the IND. The pharmacist also has a responsibility to provide information to the physician on how and what to submit to the FDA in compliance with the new drug regulations. This includes information for both roles the physician plays, i.e., as a co-investigator and as the sponsor. As long as investigational drugs are used in clinical investigations in the hospital, some type of pharmacy involvement will be needed in the management of these special drugs.

REFERENCES

1. Kelsey FO: The Kefauver-Harris amendments and investigational drugs. *Am J Hosp Pharm* 20:515-517, 1963.
2. Abrams WB: Introducing a new drug into clinical practice. Anesthesiology 35:176-192, 1974.
3. Food and Drug Administration: *Clinical Testing for Safe and Effective Drugs.* DHHS Publication No. (FDA) 74-3015, Washington, DC, U.S. Government Printing Office.
4. Kumkumian CS: *Manufacturing and Controls: Guidelnes for IND's and NDA's.* Presented at the Fifteenth Annual International Industrial Pharmacy Conference at the University of Texas, Austin, February 24, 1976.
5. Kleinman LM, Tangrea JA: Involvement of the hospital pharmacist in single- and double-blind studies. *Am J Hosp Pharm* 31:979-981, 1974.
6. *Federal Register* 46:8651, 1981.
7. Bureau of Medicine, Food and Drug Administration: Investigational drug circular. *Am J Hosp Pharm* 22:69-70, 1965.
8. Kleinman LM, Tangrea JA, Gallelli JF: Control of investigational drugs in a research hospital. *Am J Hosp Pharm* 31:368-371, 1974.
9. Gallelli JF, Skolaut MW: Pharmaceutical development: New concept in pharmacy service. *Hospitals* 41:95-101, December 1967.
10. *Federal Register* 48:26720,1983.

DEPARTMENT OF HEALTH AND HUMAN SERVICES PUBLIC HEALTH SERVICE FOOD AND DRUG ADMINISTRATION	*Form Approved OMB No. 0910-0014*
NOTICE OF CLAIMED INVESTIGATIONAL EXEMPTION FOR A NEW DRUG	**NOTE:** No drug may be shipped or study initiated unless a complete statement has been received. *(21 CFR 312.1(a)(2)).*

Name of Sponsor _____   Date _____

Address _____   Telephone (   ) _____

Name of Investigational Drug _____

FOR A DRUG:

Food And Drug Administration
Office of New Drug Evaluation *(HFN-106)*
5600 Fishers Lane
Rockville, Maryland 20857

FOR A BIOLOGIC:

Food and Drug Administration
Office of Biologics *(HFN-823)*
8800 Rockville Pike
Bethesda, Maryland 20205

Dear Sir:

The sponsor, _____, submits this notice of claimed investigational exemption for a new drug under the provisions of section 505(i) of the Federal Food, Drug, and Cosmetic Act and § 312.1 of Title 21 of the Code of Federal Regulations.

Attached hereto in triplicate are:

1. The best available descriptive name of the drug, including to the extent known the chemical name and structure of any new-drug substance, and a statement of how it is to be administered. (If the drug has only a code name. enough information should be supplied to identify the drug.)

2. Complete list of components of the drug, including any reasonable alternates for inactive components.

3. Complete statement of quantitative composition of drug, including reasonable variations that may be expected during the investigational stage.

4. Description of source and preparation of, any new-drug substances used as components, including the name and address of each supplier or processor, other than the sponsor, or each new-drug substance.

5. A statement of the methods, facilities, and controls used for the manufacturing, processing, and packing of the new drug to establish and maintain appropriate standards of identity, strength, quality, and purity as needed for safety and to give significance to clinical investigations made with the drug.

6. A statement covering all information available to the sponsor derived from preclinical investigations and any clinical studies and experience with the drug as follows:

a. Adequate information about the preclinical investigations, including studies made on laboratory animals, on the basis of which the sponsor has concluded that it is reasonably safe to initiate clinical investigations with the drug: Such information should include identification of the person who conducted each investigation; identification and qualifications of the individuals who evaluated the results and concluded that it is reasonably safe to initiate clinical investigations with the drug and a statement of where the investigations were conducted and where the records are available for inspection; and enough details about the investigations to permit scientific review. The preclinical investigations shall not be considered adequate to justify clinical testing unless they give proper attention to the conditions of the proposed clinical testing. When this information, the outline of the plan of clinical pharmacology, or any progress report on the clinical pharmacology, indicates a need for full review of the preclinical data before a clinical trial is undertaken, the Department will notify the sponsor to submit the complete preclinical data and to withhold clinical trials until the review is completed and the sponsor notified. The Food and Drug Administration will be prepared to confer with the sponsor concerning this action.

b. If the drug has been marketed commercially or investigated (e.g. outside the United States), complete information about such distribution or investigation shall be submitted, along with a complete bibliography of any publications about the drug.

c. If the drug is a combination of previously investigated or marketed drugs, an adequate summary of preexisting information from preclinical and clinical investigations and experience with its components, including all reports available to the sponsor suggesting side-effects, contraindications, and ineffectiveness in use of such components: Such summary should include an adequate bibliography of publications about the components and may incorporate by reference any information concerning such components previously submitted by the sponsor to the Food and Drug Administration. Include a statement of the expected pharmacological effects of the combination.

d. If the drug is a radioactive drug, sufficient data must be available from animal studies or previous human studies to allow a reasonable calculation of radiation absorbed dose upon administration to a human being.

7. A total (one in each of the three copies of the notice) of all informational material, including label and labeling, which is to be supplied to each investigator: This shall include an accurate description of the prior investigations and experience and their results pertinent to the safety and possible usefulness of the drug under the conditions of the investigation. It shall not represent that the safety or usefulness of the drug has been established for the purposes to be investigated. It shall describe all relevant hazards, contraindications, side-effects, and precautions suggested by prior investigations and experience with the drug under investigation and related drugs for the information of clinical investigators.

8. The scientific training and experience considered appropriate by the sponsor to qualify the investigators as suitable experts to investigate the safety of the drug, bearing in mind what is known about the pharmacological action of the drug and the phase of the investigational program that is to be undertaken.

9. The names and a summary of the training and experience of each investigator and of the individual charged with monitoring the progress of the investigation and evaluating the evidence of safety and effectiveness of the drug as it is received from the investigators, together with a statement that the sponsor has obtained from each investigator a completed and signed form, as provided in subparagraph (12) or (13) of this paragraph, and that the investigator is qualified by scientific training and experience as an appropriate expert to under-

take the phase of the investigation outlined in section 10 of the "Notice of Claimed Investigational Exemption for a New Drug." (In crucial situations, phase 3 investigators may be added and this form supplemented by rapid communication methods, and the signed Form FD-1573 shall be obtained promptly thereafter.)

10. An outline of any phase or phases of the planned investigations and a description of the institutional review committee, as follows:

a. Clinical pharmacology. This is ordinarily divided into two phases: Phase I starts when the new drug is first introduced into man - only animal and in vitro data are available - with the purpose of determining human toxicity, metabolism, absorption, elimination, and other pharmacological action, preferred route of administration, and safe dosage range; phase 2 covers the initial trials on a limited number of patients for specific disease control or prophylaxis purposes. A general outline of these phases shall be submitted, identifying the investigator or investigators, the hospitals or research facilities where the clinical pharmacology will be undertaken, any expert committees or panels to be utilized, the maximum number of subjects to be involved, and the estimated duration of these early phases of investigation. Modification of the experimental design on the basis of experience gained need be reported only in the progress reports on these early phases, or in the development of the plan for the clinical trial, phase 3. The first two phases may overlap and, when indicated, may require additional animal data before these phases can be completed or phase can be undertaken. Such animal tests shall be designed to take into account the expected duration of administration of the drug to human beings, the age groups and physical status, as for example, infants, pregnant women, premenopausal women, of those human beings to whom the drug may be administered, unless this has already been done in the original animal studies. If a drug is a radioactive drug, the clinical pharmacology phase must include studies which will obtain sufficient data for dosimetry calculations. These studies should evaluate the excretion, whole body retention, and organ distribution of the radioactive material.

b. Clinical trial. This phase 3 provides the assessment of the drug's safety and effectiveness and optimum dosage schedules in the diagnosis. treatment, or prophylaxis of groups of subjects involving a given disease or condition. A reasonable protocol is developed on the basis of the facts accumulated in the earlier phases, including completed and submitted animal studies. This phase is conducted by separate groups following the same protocol (with reasonable variations and alternatives permitted by the plan) to produce well-controlled clinical data. For this phase, the following data shall be submitted:

i. The names and addresses of the investigators. (Additional investigators may be added.)

ii. The specific nature of the investigations to be conducted, together with information or case report forms to show the scope and detail of the planned clinical observations and the clinical laboratory tests to be made and reported.

iii. The approximate number of subjects (a reasonable range of subjects is permissible and additions may be made), and criteria proposed for subject selection by age, sex, and condition.

iv. The estimated duration of the clinical trial and the intervals, not exceeding 1 year, at which progress reports showing the results of the investigations will be submitted to the Food and Drug Administration.

c. Institutional review board (IRB). The sponsor must give assurance that an IRB that complies with the requirements set forth in Part 56 of this chapter will be responsible for the initial and continuing review and approval of the proposed clinical study. The sponsor must also provide assurance that the investigators will report to the IRB all changes in the research activity and all unanticipated problems involving risks to human subjects or others, and that the investigators will not make any changes in the research without IRB approval, except where necessary to eliminate apparent immediate hazard to the human subjects. FDA will regard the signing of the Form FDA-1571 as providing the necessary assurances above.

(The notice of claimed investigational exemption may be limited to any one or more phases, provided the outline of the additional phase or phases is submitted before such additional phases begin. A limitation on an exemption does not preclude continuing a subject on the drug from phase 2 to phase 3 without interruption while the plan for phase 3 is being developed.)

Ordinarily, a plan for clinical trial will not be regarded as reasonable unless, among other things, it provides for more than one independent competent investigator to maintain adequate case histories of an adequate number of subjects, designed to record observations and permit evaluation of any and all discernible effects attributable to the drug in each individual treated, and comparable records on any individuals employed as controls. These records shall be individual records for each subject maintained to include adequate information pertaining to each, including age, sex, conditions treated, dosage, frequency of administration of the drug, results of all relevant clinical observations and laboratory examinations made, adequate information concerning any other treatment given and a full statement of any adverse effects and useful results observed, together with an opinion as to whether such effects or results are attributable to the drug under investigation.

11. A statement that the sponsor will notify the Food and Drug Administration if the investigation is discontinued, and the reason therefor.

12. A statement that the sponsor will notify each investigator if a new-drug application is approved, or if the investigation is discontinued.

13. If the drug is to be sold, a full explanation why sale is required and should not be regarded as the commercialization of a new drug for which an application is not approved.

14. A statement that the sponsor assures that clinical studies in humans will not be initiated prior to 30 days after the date of receipt of the notice by the Food and Drug Administration and that he will continue to withhold or to restrict clinical studies if requested to do so by the Food and Drug Administration prior to the expiration of such 30 days. If such request is made, the sponsor will be provided specific information as to the deficiencies and will be afforded a conference on request. The 30-day delay may be waived by the Food and Drug Administration upon a showing of good reason for such waiver; and for investigations subject to institutional review committee approval as described in item 10c above, and additional statement assuring that the investigation will not be initiated prior to approval of the study by such committee.

15. When requested by the agency, an environmental impact analysis report pursuant to § 25.1 of this chapter.

16. A statement that all nonclinical laboratory studies have been, or will be, conducted in compliance with the good laboratory practice regulations set forth in Part 58 of this chapter, or, if such studies have not been conducted in compliance with such regulations, a statement that describes in detail all differences between the practices used in conducting the study and those required in the regulations.

Very truly yours,

SPONSOR	PER
	INDICATE AUTHORITY

(This notice may be amended or supplemented from time to time on the basis of the experience gained with the new drug. Progress reports may be used to update the notice.)

ALL NOTICES AND CORRESPONDENCE SHOULD BE SUBMITTED IN TRIPLICATE.

INSTRUCTIONS FOR FILING A NOTICE

A new drug for investigational use in human subjects may not be in insterstate commerce unless some responsible individual or firm sponsors clinical studies with the drug and submits a Notice of Claimed Investigational Exemption for a New Drug, Form FD-1571.

A Notice should include the facts that satisfy the sponsor that the agent may be justifiably administered to man as proposed. Thus the claim for exemption should contain information on appropriate prior animal studies for safety evaluation, any available clinical data, adequate drug identification and manufacturing information necessary to support safety and give significance to a clinical trial, and a detailed outline of the proposed clinical study to include dosage ranges, routes of administration, approximate number of patients involved, and approximate duration of treatment.

The sponsor should provide a statement of the scientific training and experience he will require investigators to demonstrate. Further, the names and a summary of the training and experience of each investigator should be a part of the filed Notice. Where the sponsor himself is the sole investigator, submission of his curriculum vitae may be adequate.

Additionally, the sponsor is required to obtain statements from clinical investigators (Form FD-1572 for clinical pharmacology and Form FD-1573 for other clinical studies) and retain them in his files. Copies of the completed statements may be included as part of the material filed for an exemption. Specimens of these forms are included.

If a sponsor does not himself perform manufacturing and control operators for new drug substances or final dosage forms, this information (required by parts 1 through 5 of the Notice Form FD-1571) can be furnished on his behalf by suppliers performing those operations. Similarly, a supplier may provide pre-clinical or clinical study data. The sponsor may forward such supporting information or arrange to have it sent directly to us.

A Notice is to be filed in triplicate with the Food and Drug Administration. The information filed may be in narrative form but should be presented as outlined in the enclosed Notice form.

In addition to the name of the drug, please be sure to indicate the dosage form.

Mail Completed Applications to:
Food and Drug Administration
Document Control Section, HFN-106
Office of Drug Research and Review
5600 Fishers Lane
Rockville, Maryland   20857

MAIL IN TRIPLICATE
INCLUDING COVER LETTER

Appendix 45.2

DEPARTMENT OF HEALTH AND HUMAN SERVICES PUBLIC HEALTH SERVICE FOOD AND DRUG ADMINISTRATION **STATEMENT OF INVESTIGATOR** *(Clinical Pharmacology)*	*Form Approved* *OMB No. 0910-0015*

NOTE: No drug may be shipped or study initiated unless a completed statement has been received *(21 CFR 312.1(a)(12)).*

TO: SUPPLIER OF THE DRUG *(Name and address, include ZIP Code)*	NAME OF INVESTIGATOR *(Print or Type)*
	DATE
	NAME OF DRUG

Dear Sir:

   The undersigned, _____
submits this statement as required by section 505(i) of the Federal Food, Drug, and Cosmetic Act and § 312.1 of
Title 21 of the Code of Federal Regulations as a condition for receiving and conducting clinical pharmacology
with a new drug limited by Federal (or United States) law to investigational use.

1. A STATEMENT OF THE EDUCATION AND TRAINING THAT QUALIFIES ME FOR CLINICAL PHARMACOLOGY

2. THE NAME AND ADDRESS OF THE MEDICAL SCHOOL, HOSPITAL, OR OTHER RESEARCH FACILITY WHERE THE CLINICAL
PHARMACOLOGY WILL BE CONDUCTED

3. The investigator assures that an IRB that complies with the requirements set forth in Part 56 of this chapter will be responsible
for the initial and continuing review and approval of the proposed clinical study. The investigator also assures that he/she will
report to the IRB all changes in the research activity and all unanticipated problems involving risks to human subjects or others,
and that he/she will not make any changes in the research that would increase the risks to human subjects without IRB approval.
FDA will regard the signing of the Form FD 1572 as providing the necessary assurances stated above.

4. THE ESTIMATED DURATION OF THE PROJECT AND THE MAXIMUM NUMBER OF SUBJECTS THAT WILL BE INVOLVED

FORM FDA 1572 (10/82)   PREVIOUS EDITIONS ARE OBSOLETE.

5. GENERAL OUTLINE OF THE PROJECT TO BE UNDERTAKEN *(Modification is permitted on the basis of experience gained without advance submission of amendments to the general outline, but with the approval of the review committee and upon notification of the sponsor.)*

6. THE UNDERSIGNED UNDERSTANDS THAT THE FOLLOWING CONDITIONS GENERALLY APPLICABLE TO NEW DRUGS FOR INVESTIGATIONAL USE GOVERN HIS RECEIPT AND USE OF THIS INVESTIGATIONAL DRUG

a. The sponsor is required to supply the investigator with full information concerning the preclinical investigation that justifies clinical pharmacology.

b. The investigator is required to maintain adequate records of the disposition of all receipts of the drug, including dates, quantity, and use by subjects, and if the clinical pharmacology is suspended, terminated, discontinued, or completed, to return to the sponsor any unused supply of the drug. If the investigational drug is subject to the Comprehensive Drug Abuse Prevention and Control Act of 1970, adequate precautions must be taken, including storage of the investigational drug in a securely locked, substantially constructed cabinet, or other securely locked, substantially constructed enclosure access to which is limited, to prevent theft or diversion of the substance into illegal channels of distribution.

c. The investigator is required to prepare and maintain adequate case histories designed to record all observations and other data pertinent to the clinical pharmacology.

d. The investigator is required to furnish his reports to the sponsor who is responsible for collecting and evaluating the results, and presenting progress reports to the Food and Drug Administration at appropriate intervals, not exceeding 1 year. Any adverse effect which may reasonably be regarded as caused by, or is probably caused by, the new-drug shall be reported to the sponsor promptly; and if the adverse effect is alarming it shall be reported immediately. An adequate report of the clinical pharmacology should be furnished to the sponsor shortly after completion.

e. The investigator shall maintain the records of disposition of the drug and the case reports described above for a period of 2 years following the date the new-drug application is approved for the drug; or if no application is to be filed or is approved until 2 years after the investigation is discontinued and the Food and Drug Administration so

notified. Upon the request of a scientifically trained and specifically authorized employee of the Department, at reasonable times, the investigator will made such records available for inspection and copying. The names of the subjects need not be divulged unless the records of the particular subjects require a more detailed study of the cases, or unless there is reason to believe that the records do not represent actual studies or do not represent actual results obtained.

f. The investigator certifies that the drug will be administered only to subjects under his personal supervision or under the supervision of the following investigators responsible to him,

_____

_____

_____

_____

and that the drug will not be supplied to any other investigator or to any clinic for administration to subjects.

g. The investigator certifies that he will inform any patients or any persons used as controls, or their representatives, that drugs are being used for investigational purposes, and will obtain the consent of the subjects, or their representatives, except where this is not feasible or, in the investigator's professional judgment, is contrary to the best interests of the subjects.

h. The investigator is required to assure the sponsor that for investigations subject to an institutional review requirement under Part 56 of this chapter the studies will not be initiated until the institutional review board has reviewed and approved the study. (The organization and procedure requirements for such a board as set forth in Part 56 should be explained to the investigator by the sponsor.)

Very truly yours,

Name of Investigator _____

Address _____ Telephone ( ) _____

Appendix 45.3

DEPARTMENT OF HEALTH AND HUMAN SERVICES PUBLIC HEALTH SERVICE FOOD AND DRUG ADMINISTRATION **STATEMENT OF INVESTIGATOR**	*Form approved OMB No. 0910–0013*
	Note: No drug may be shipped or study initiated unless a completed statement has been received *(21 CFR 312.1(a)(12)).*

TO: SUPPLIER OF DRUG *(Name, address, and Zip Code)*	NAME OF INVESTIGATOR *(Print or Type)*
	DATE
	NAME OF DRUG

Dear Sir:

    The undersigned, _____

submits this statement as required by section 505(i) of the Federal Food, Drug, and Cosmetic Act and §312.1 of Title 21 of the Code of Federal Regulations as a condition for receiving and conducting clinical investigations with a new drug limited by Federal *(or United States)* law to investigational use.

1. THE FOLLOWING IS A STATEMENT OF MY EDUCATION AND EXPERIENCE:

a. COLLEGES, UNIVERSITIES, AND MEDICAL OR OTHER PROFESSIONAL SCHOOLS ATTENDED, WITH DATES OF ATTENDANCE, DEGREES, AND DATES DEGREES WERE AWARDED

b. POSTGRADUATE MEDICAL OR OTHER PROFESSIONAL TRAINING. GIVE DATES, NAMES OF INSTITUTIONS, AND NATURE OF TRAINING.

c. TEACHING OR RESEARCH EXPERIENCE. GIVE DATES, INSTITUTIONS, AND BRIEF DESCRIPTION OF EXPERIENCE.

d. EXPERIENCE IN MEDICAL PRACTICE OR OTHER PROFESSIONAL EXPERIENCE. GIVE DATES, INSTITUTIONAL AFFILIATIONS, NATURE OF PRACTICE, OR OTHER PROFESSIONAL EXPERIENCE.

e. REPRESENTATIVE LIST OF PERTINENT MEDICAL OR OTHER SCIENTIFIC PUBLICATIONS. GIVE TITLES OF ARTICLES, NAME OF PUBLICATIONS AND VOLUME, PAGE NUMBER, AND DATE.

    IF THIS INFORMATION HAS PREVIOUSLY BEEN SUBMITTED TO THE SPONSOR, IT MAY BE REFERRED TO AND ANY ADDITIONS MADE TO BRING IT UP-TO-DATE.

FORM FDA 1573 (10/82)   PREVIOUS EDITIONS ARE OBSOLETE.

2a. The investigator assures that an IRB that complies with the requirements set forth in Part 56 of this chapter will be responsible for the initial and continuing review and approval of the proposed clinical study. The investigator also assures that he/she will report to the IRB all changes in the research activity and all unanticipated problems involving risks to human subjects or others, and that he/she will not make any changes in the research that would increase the risks to human subjects without IRB approval. FDA will regard the signing of the Form FDA 1573 as providing the necessary assurances stated above.

b. A description of any clinical laboratory facilities that will be used. (If this information has been submitted to the sponsor and reported by him on Form FDA 1571, reference to the previous submission will be adequate).

3. *The investigational drug will be used by the undersigned or under his supervision in accordance with the plan of investigation described as follows: (Outline the plan of investigation including approximation of the number of subjects to be treated with the drug and the number to be employed as controls, if any; clinical uses to be investigated; characteristics of subjects by age, sex and condition; the kind of clinical observations and laboratory tests to be undertaken prior to, during, and after administration of the drug; the estimated duration of the investigation; and a description or copies of report forms to be used to maintain an adequate record of the observations and test results obtained. This plan may include reasonable alternates and variations and should be supplemented or amended when any significant change in direction or scope of the investigation is undertaken.)*

4. **THE UNDERSIGNED UNDERSTANDS THAT THE FOLLOWING CONDITIONS, GENERALLY APPLICABLE TO NEW DRUGS FOR INVESTIGATIONAL USE, GOVERN HIS RECEIPTS AND USE OF THIS INVESTIGATIONAL DRUG:**

a. The sponsor is required to supply the investigator with full information concerning the preclinical investigations that justify clinical trials, together with fully informative material describing any prior investigations and experience and any possible hazards, contraindications, side-effects, and precautions to be taken into account in the course of the investigation.

b. The investigator is required to maintain adequate records of the disposition of all receipts of the drug, including dates, quantities, and use by subjects, and if the investigation is terminated, suspended, discontinued, or completed, to return to the sponsor any unused supply of the drug. If the investigational drug is subject to the Comprehensive Drug Abuse Prevention and Control Act of 1970, adequate precautions must be taken including storage of the investigational drug in a securely locked, substantially constructed cabinet, or other securely locked substantially constructed enclosure, access to which is limited, to prevent theft or diversion of the substance into illegal channels of distribution.

c. The investigator is required to prepare and maintain adequate and accurate case histories designed to record all observations and other data pertinent to the investigation on each individual treated with the drug or employed as a control in the investigation.

d. The investigator is required to furnish his reports to the sponsor of the drug who is responsible for collecting and evaluating the results obtained by various investigators. The sponsor is required to present progress reports to the Food and Drug Administration at appropriate intervals not exceeding 1 year. Any adverse effect that may reasonably be regarded as caused by, or probably caused by, the new drug shall be reported to the sponsor promptly, and if the adverse effect is alarming, it shall be reported immediately. An adequate report of the investigation should be furnished to the sponsor shortly after completion of the investigation.

e. The investigator shall maintain the records of disposition of the drug and the case histories described above for a period of 2 years following the date a new-drug application is approved for the drug; or if the application is not approved, until 2 years after the investigation is discontinued. Upon the request of a scientifically trained and properly authorized employee of the Department, at reasonable times, the investigator will make such records available for inspection and copying. The subjects' names need not be divulged unless the records of particular individuals require a more detailed study of the cases, or unless there is reason to believe that the records do not represent actual cases studied, or do not represent actual results obtained.

f. The investigator certifies that the drug will be administered only to subjects under his personal supervision or under the supervision of the following investigators responsible to him,

_____

_____

_____

and that the drug will not be supplied to any other investigator or to any clinic for administration to subjects.

g. The investigator certifies that he will inform any subjects including subjects used as controls, or their representatives, that drugs are being used for investigational purposes, and will obtain the consent of the subjects, or their representatives, except where this is not feasible or, in the investigator's professional judgment, is contrary to the best interests of the subjects.

h. The investigator is required to assure the sponsor that for investigations subject to an institutional review requirement under Part 56 of this chapter the studies will not be initiated until the institutional review board has reviewed and approved the study. (The organization and procedure requirements for such a board as set forth in Part 56 should be explained to the investigator by the sponsor.)

Very truly yours,

Name of Investigator_____

Address_____ Telephone ( )

(This form should be supplemented or amended from time to time if new subjects are added or if significant changes are made in the plan of investigation.)

Patient-Oriented Services

DEVELOPMENT AND CONDUCT OF PATIENT-ORIENTED SERVICES

Pharmacy, as practiced in health care institutions, is developing a wide spectrum of clinical services that have become part of overall pharmaceutical service but may not be directly associated with drug distribution. Fundamental to these clinical services is the pharmacist's knowledge of drugs, diseases, and patient and drug variables, and his ability to interact closely on a personal basis with other health professionals. Academic training in such areas as toxicology, pathophysiology, and therapeutics, as well as extensive clinical experience, provide the background for a pharmacist to function in this clinical role.

These services include (1) drug information, which encompasses the collection, organization, retrieval, interpretation, and evaluation of the applicable literature and the ability to present the excerpted data in an appropriate fashion; (2) collecting the pharmacy patient data base; (3) patient education; (4) monitoring (either subjectively or objectively) and auditing therapeutic regimens; (5) drug use review; (6) monitoring of specific adverse drug reactions to decrease their incidence; and (7) other similar functions designed to improve patient care by optimizing drug use. Further, clinical functions may extend to the pharmacist's role in primary care as well as in the management of chronic care patients.

CHAPTER 46

Clinical Services and Ambulatory Care

THOMAS P. REINDERS

Ambulatory care is emerging as the dominant theme in health care delivery for the 1980s. Prompted by patient demands for available, accessible, and less costly health care, organized health care settings are rapidly increasing the availability of ambulatory patient care services.

Ambulatory care generally refers to providing health care to patients who are not restricted to bed. The level of care may be primary, secondary, or even tertiary. Traditionally, ambulatory care was provided by physicians in their community-based office practices. Patients were referred to a hospital if their condition warranted close monitoring or if special technology was needed for diagnosis or treatment. Although some hospitals maintained an outpatient clinic, most patients were referred to their private physician's office on hospital discharge. This trend began to change following the passage of the Hill-Burton Act in 1946, as hospitals began to direct resources to the development of ambulatory care services.

The provision of pharmacy services paralleled the evolution of hospital-based ambulatory care services. As hospitals began to establish clinics, hospital pharmacists were encouraged to develop outpatient pharmacy services. Because the mission of most hospitals was primarily directed toward inpatient care, the resource allocations for outpatient services were often inadequate. Pharmacists working in the outpatient settings of hospitals seldom left their assigned work stations and patient contact was nonexistent (1).

Little effort was made to upgrade the level of services until the 1970s. The advent of patient-oriented services such as maintaining medication profiles and counseling patients about their drug therapy began to influence the quality of outpatient pharmacy services. Also during the 1970s, the American Society of Hospital Pharmacists (ASHP) devoted significant resources to improve the standard of ambulatory care pharmacy practice. The trend for improvement continues, with an increasing number of institution-based pharmacy practitioners seeking to provide comprehensive pharmacy services to ambulatory patients.

PRACTICE ENVIRONMENT

Ambulatory care pharmacy programs vary in their description, depending on the sponsoring organization and the patient population served. Universally, successful programs offer the pharmacist access to patient data and the ability to interface with other health providers in managing the patient's drug therapy plan.

Hospital-based Clinics. Hospital-based clinics usually reflect the specialty (e.g., medicine, surgery, pediatrics) and subspecialty (e.g., cardiology, orthopedics, allergy) practice interests of the hospital's medical staff. Either centralized or decentralized pharmaceutical services may be available. Most institutions rely on a centralized pharmacy for drug distribution to ambulatory patients. Maintaining medication profiles and providing patient counseling are frequently described in conjunction with centralized services. At the same time, clinical pharmacy services may be decentralized by placing a pharmacist in the clinic setting.

Most reports of clinical pharmacy involvement in ambulatory care have originated from pharmacists' participation in decentralized clinic operations, usually located within a university hospital. In cardiovascular therapy, pharmacists have described their participation in the management of patients receiving antihypertensive (2-5) and anticoagulant therapy (6-7). Other pharmacists have outlined their management approaches to patients with pulmonary disorders including asthma (8), allergic conditions (9-10), and chronic obstructive pulmonary disease (11). Similar management approaches have been applied to other chronic disease management situations for patients with diabetes (2,12) and tuberculosis (13). Protocols have also been identified for pharmacist management of patients with acute disease conditions such as streptococcal throat infections (14). Patients receiving chronic hemodialysis (15-16), methadone (17), and chemotherapeutic agents (18) have also been identified as groups to receive comprehensive ambulatory care pharmacy services. Additionally, patients attending general service clinics such as pediatrics (19) and obstetrics (20) have been shown to benefit from the level of care provided by pharmacists.

Recognizing that only special ambulatory patient groups are the usual recipients of clinical pharmacy services, several investigators have established general service clinics to serve any patient with special drug needs. One example is a pharmacist-managed clinic where patients with medication compliance problems are referred by physicians for management (21). Another example of a pharmacy-operated clinic is the assessment and refill clinics established in several large outpatient facilities (22-24). In this setting, pharmacists provide medication refills between regularly scheduled clinic visits. Such contributions have been shown to improve patient compliance with medication therapy and future clinic appointments. Depending on the institution, drug distribution services may be centralized or decentralized into the clinic area to make them convenient for the patient.

Decentralized Primary Care Clinics. Ambulatory care clinics located outside of the hospital also afford the pharmacist opportunities to provide clinical services. Often located in medically underserved areas, and geographically separated from the sponsoring institution, primary care is provided by a small staff of health professionals. The remoteness of the sites and the limited resources are usually ideal for establishing interdisciplinary approaches to patient care. In these settings, pharmacists have contributed to the drug management of patients with acute and chronic diseases, as well as participating in disease prevention problems (25-26).

Family Practice Settings. Family practice became a medical specialty in 1969 with the establishment of the American Board of Family Practice. The resulting effect has been described as the resurrection of the family doctor (27). Residency training programs for family practice physicians have increased dramatically and several programs have established professional relationships with clinical pharmacists (28-34). Most often, the pharmacist is an interdisciplinary health team member who provides drug therapy consultation. Drug distribution may also be provided, especially at remote clinic sites.

Other pharmacists have established similar professional practices, yet function as independent community practitioners. Eugene V. White's concept of the office-based family practice has been a reality for several decades in Berryville, Virginia. Patients receive comprehensive pharmacy services in a professional pharmacy office setting, rather than the characteristic drugstore (35). Still another model exists in Lexington, South Carolina, where Robert Davis has established a joint office practice with several family practice physicians. Again, comprehensive pharmacy services are provided to ambulatory patients in a professional pharmacy office (36).

Health Maintenance Organizations. Health maintenance organizations (HMOs) have been endorsed as an alternative form of medical care organization that focuses on providing preventive care rather than episodic care. To achieve quality and economy, the HMO requires an enrolled population of patients, a financial plan, and a managing organization that assures legal, fiscal, public, and professional accountability. This organized health care delivery system also includes pharmacy services to ambulatory patients. Pharmacy services may be centralized in the HMO facility or decentralized to community pharmacies (37-38).

Community Mental Health Centers. Pharmacy services have been provided to ambulatory patients through the development of community mental health center programs (39-45). A variety of arrangements exist for providing drug distribution and clinical services. Often, drug distribution services may be contracted to hospital or community pharmacy practitioners, whereas consultation services are provided by a pharmacist with specialized training in mental health.

Home Health Care Programs. Home care as an alternative to institutional care is an established part of our health care system. Traditionally, pharmacist involvement has been limited in the provision of services to home health care programs. More recently, hospital pharmacists have initiated a spectrum of services for home care agencies, especially those that are hospital based (46-51). Pharmacists are generally used as consultants for drug information and staff education, and infrequently visit a patient's home to evaluate the drug therapy.

SCOPE OF SERVICES

The scope of clinical pharmacy services varies with the practice site, but generally includes those services outlined in the ASHP Statement on the Provision of Pharmaceutical Services in Ambulatory Care Settings (52). These services are outlined below.

Obtain and Document Medication Histories. The pharmacist's responsibility in obtaining and documenting medication histories is an accepted clinical pharmacy service for ambulatory patients. The history includes the past and present use of prescription and nonprescription medications, drug allergies, previous adverse effects associated with medication use, and an estimate of the patient's compliance with medication regimens.

Maintain Medication Profiles. A complete listing of acute and chronic medications, their dosage, and dispensing information assists the pharmacist in monitoring the safety and efficacy of a patient's drug therapy. Additionally, the availability of personal computers has facilitated the maintenance of medication profiles for ambulatory care patients.

Provide Drug Information. The pharmacist's ability to provide accurate drug information to prescribers and other health professionals in the ambulatory care setting is essential. Because of physical space limitations in the clinic, limited information sources (e.g., the *American Hospital Formulary Service,* a pharmacology textbook and drug interaction reference) may be useful in answering many questions (53).

Assist in Drug Prescribing. Assisting prescribers in the proper selection and adjustment of drug therapy is a clinical pharmacy service provided by an increasing number of pharmacists practicing in ambulatory care settings. By using drug level determinations and applying pharmacokinetic principles, ambulatory care pharmacists may readily assist in optimizing drug therapy regimens (54).

The role of pharmacists as prescribers has also recently emerged. In 1977, the approval of California Assembly Bill 717 allowed pharmacists to prescribe drugs when engaged in an experimental health manpower project. The general competencies of pharmacists in the University of Southern California School of Pharmacy project included (1) the ability to select an appropriate drug based on the diagnosis established by the physician; (2) knowledge of drugs in the basic formulary, including classification, therapeutic use, dose, dosage schedules, modes of administration, adverse effects and toxicity, drug interactions, and contraindications; (3) the ability to educate the patient about the drugs being prescribed; (4) knowledge of reliable sources of current drug information; (5) knowledge of appropriate state and federal laws and regulations and limitations under AB 717 regarding legal prescribing; (6) knowledge of evaluation processes developed by the sponsoring project and the State Department of Health; and (7) physical assessment skills necessary to assess disease state changes and drug-induced adverse effects of drugs represented in the project's basic formulary (55). Evaluation of the project has demonstrated the advantages that prescribing authority offers the profession of pharmacy and the health care system, as well as the limitations that should exist (56).

Monitor Patient Response. The pharmacist's ability to use assessment skills in the management of acute and chronic diseases has been the basis for developing a wide array of these previously mentioned clinics. Generally the pharmacist works as an interdisciplinary team member with other health professionals to monitor the patient's total treatment plan. Various pharmacy practitioners have relied on protocols or algorithms to monitor patient response and adjust drug therapy (57). Protocols have been found to be useful as a foundation for problem solving, defining the data to be collected, and specifying therapeutic approaches to be considered. A knowledge of physical assessment skills has also been beneficial in allowing the pharmacist to competently monitor drug response. Once considered a limitation of the pharmacist, pharmacy curricula and continuing education efforts have adequately provided a knowledge of physical assessment (58-59).

The pharmacist's detection of adverse drug reactions, drug interactions, and noncompliant behavior is also an important component of patient response monitoring. Ambulatory care pharmacists are responsible for documenting positive occurrences and developing effective management approaches.

Provide Patient Information. Providing information to patients about their drug therapy is a major clinical function of the ambulatory care pharmacist. Specific drug information to be communicated to patients has been outlined in the ASHP Statement on Pharmacist-Conducted Patient Counseling (60). It is also important for ambulatory care pharmacists to be a resource for information about health promotion and disease prevention for members of the public.

Conduct Drug Utilization Review. Although drug utilization review has been conducted in hospital settings, only limited investigations have been conducted in ambulatory environments (61-62). Such reviews and audits are essential to assure the quality of drug use in ambulatory patients and to contain drug costs.

Participate in Clinical Drug Investigations. The ambulatory care setting is a frequently used area for conducting clinical drug investigations. Pharmacists practicing in this setting are ideally suited for collaborating with physician investigators in conducting clinical drug trials.

Assure Proper Drug Dispensing Controls. Pharmacists involved in ambulatory care practice should be responsible for assuring the adequacy of the drug dispensing environment. Supervision should be provided for the storage, preparation, and dispensing of medications for use by ambulatory patients.

Participate in the Education of Health Care Providers. Formal and informal education pertaining to the safe and effective use of drug therapy may be readily provided to other health care providers by pharmacists in the ambulatory care setting. In particular, drug education programs directed toward nurses and physicians have been described (28,47).

MINIMUM PRACTICE STANDARD

Recognizing that the preceding services may not be routine for all ambulatory settings, the ASHP has established a minimum standard for ambulatory care pharmaceutical services (63). The five pharmacy services that should be expected in all ambulatory care facilities include the following: (1) the ambulatory care pharmacy must be directed by a qualified pharmacist; (2) the appropriateness of the choice of drug and its dosage, route of administration, and amount must be verified by the pharmacist; (3) all medications dispensed to patients will be completely and correctly labeled and packaged in accordance with all applicable regulations and accepted standards of practice; (4) on dispensing a new medication to the patient, the pharmacist will ensure that the patient or his or her representative receives and understands all information required for proper use of the drug; and (5) all drugs in ambulatory care service areas will be properly controlled.

RESIDENCY TRAINING

To assist in preparing pharmacy practitioners to provide comprehensive pharmaceutical services in an ambulatory care setting, the ASHP approved a Supplemental Standard of Learning Objectives for Residency Training in Ambulatory-Care Pharmacy Practice in 1982 (64).

The following specific requirements have been identified for the ambulatory care service program.

Medical Records. All patient-related records must be accessible before, during, and after the provision of pharmaceutical services.

Drug Information Resources. Each facility shall maintain a centralized body of pharmaceutical and medical literature, containing current primary, secondary, and tertiary literature sources.

Scope of Service. The ASHP Statement on the Provision of Pharmaceutical Services in Ambulatory Care Settings sets forth the fundamental scope of services that should be provided by such a program. Although provision of nonprescription drugs and health-related devices and appliances is included within the intent of this requirement, the sale of sundries and general merchandise is specifically excluded.

Preceptors as Independent Proprietors. In those instances in which the preceptor may also be the sole proprietor of an independent (noninstitutional) ambulatory health care setting, particular attention should be focused on the Accreditation Standard for Specialized Pharmacy Residency Training. Administrative and business concerns of the preceptor in such a setting should not be allowed to detract from the objectives of the residency program.

Review of Quality. There shall be an ongoing quality assurance program to evaluate the pharmacy services being provided.

Residency Objectives. To complete successfully the specialized residency training program, the resident shall be able to:

1. Develop an appreciation for the organization and operation of an ambulatory care pharmacy service, including physical accommodations, reference sources, computer applications, professional and supportive personnel, budgeting, relationships with other health care departments, patient flow, assumed or designated responsibilities, and documentation of services

2. Obtain and document, in the patient's medical record, medication histories, medication profiles, and other pertinent information that may directly affect the intended therapeutic plan

3. Manage a patient's drug therapy by advising prescribers about the design of a drug therapy treatment plan, using established therapeutic protocols, or independently prescribing or adjusting drug therapy in instances where supportive legislation allows

4. Monitor the safety and efficacy of drug therapy through the use of physical assessment skills, interpretation of laboratory data, patient interview, and medical record review

5. Provide drug information to prescribers and other health care practitioners

6. Refer the patient, when necessary, to other appropriate health care providers

7. Supervise the storage, preparation, and dispensing of medications and the provision of surgical and ostomy supplies

8. Participate in, or recommend alternative methods of, administering medications to ambulatory care patients in either the medically supervised or home health care setting

9. Identify and initiate strategies to correct noncompliant patient behavior

10. Establish functional systems for detecting, reporting, and managing adverse drug reactions, interactions, allergies, and other untoward drug-related effects

11. Educate and counsel patients, the general public, and health care providers in the proper use of medications and drug delivery systems

12. Establish criteria for safe and effective drug use and coordinate drug use reviews and patient care audits

13. Organize an ongoing educational program directed toward the professional advancement of all health care staff members

14. Develop and defend a proposal for obtaining reimbursement for patient care activities

15. Establish a quality assurance program directed toward continuous assessment of the patient care pharmaceutical services being provided

16. Participate in the management of medical emergencies

Additionally, certain areas of emphasis have been identified to provide an optimal experience for the resident. To meet the criteria of the training program, the resident should acquire clinical problem-solving experiences in many of the areas listed below.

A. Acute illness
   1. Upper respiratory infections
   2. Headaches
   3. Diarrhea
   4. Otitis media
   5. Skin allergies
   6. Acne
   7. Local fungal infections
   8. Hay fever
   9. Viral gastroenteritis
  10. Streptococcal pharyngitis
  11. Parasitic infections
  12. Venereal disease
  13. Urinary tract infections

B. Chronic illnesses
   1. Diabetes mellitus
   2. Hypertension
   3. Seizure disorders
   4. Parkinsonism
   5. Rheumatoid arthritis
   6. Tuberculosis
   7. Chronic obstructive pulmonary disease
   8. Asthma
   9. Angina pectoris
  10. Congestive heart failure
  11. Thrombosis
  12. Neoplastic disease
  13. Renal failure and transplantation
  14. Peptic ulcer disease
  15. Ulcerative colitis
  16. Thyroid disorders
  17. Gout
  18. Anemias
  19. Glaucoma
  20. Intractable pain

C. Preventive care
   1. Nutrition
   2. Hygiene
   3. Exercise programs
   4. Alcohol abuse rehabilitation program
   5. Smoking cessation program
   6. Weight reduction program
   7. Stress reduction program

D. Self-care (nonprescription medication use)

E. Emergency care
   1. Cardiopulmonary resuscitation
   2. Acute burn therapy
   3. Shock
   4. Trauma

F. Family planning
   1. Contraception
   2. Pregnancy testing
   3. Teratogenicity
   4. Maternogenicity

G. Devices
   1. Nutrition delivery systems
   2. Drug delivery systems
   3. Prosthetic devices
   4. Home health care supplies
   5. Ostomy supplies
   6. Oxygen systems
   7. Surgical appliances
   8. Durable medical equipment

H. Communication skills
The resident shall have numerous assignments throughout the year aimed at developing written and verbal communication skills. The residency preceptor shall be specifically responsible for setting goals for the resident's growth and development in these areas,

monitoring the resident's progress, and counseling the resident on a regular basis concerning communication abilities.

CONCLUSION

The delivery of hospital-based ambulatory care pharmaceutical services will continue to expand during the 1980s. Hospital pharmacists will be encouraged to provide the previously outlined clinical services to ambulatory patients, in the same manner they are currently provided to hospitalized patients. Pharmacists in the ambulatory setting will also continue to be interdisciplinary health team members and will likely assume new program responsibilities, including health promotion, disease prevention, and advising the patient about safe and effective self-care measures. Efforts will also continue to resolve current practice limitations, including professional turf issues, the limited number of specialty trained practitioners, and inadequate reimbursement. These changes will ultimately afford hospital pharmacists unique opportunities to provide quality clinical services to ambulatory patients.

REFERENCES

1. Baumgartner RP: Ambulatory care pharmacy services: The long range view. Paper presented at the American Society of Hospital Pharmacists' Institute on Ambulatory Care Pharmacy Services, New Orleans, March 10, 1982.
2. Hawkins DW, Fiedler, FP, Douglas HL, Eschbach RC: Evaluation of a clinical pharmacist in caring for hypertensive and diabetic patients, *Am J Hosp Pharm* 36:1321-1325, 1979.
3. Mattei TJ, Balmer JA, Corbin LA, Gonzales Duffy Sr M: Hypertension: A model for pharmacy involvement. *Am J Hosp Pharm* 30:683-686, 1973.
4. McKenney JM, Slining JM, Henderson HR, Devins D, Barr M: The effect of clinical pharmacy services on patients with essential hypertension. *Circulation* 48:1104-1111, 1973.
5. Reinders TP, Rush DR, Baumgartner RP, Graham AW: Pharmacist's role in management of hypertensive patients in an ambulatory care clinic. *Am J Hosp Pharm* 32:590-594, 1975.
6. Bernstein D, Harrison EC, McCarron MM: A patient profile system for monitoring long-term anticoagulant therapy. *Am J Hosp Pharm* 31:258-261, 1974.
7. Reinders TP, Steinke WE: Pharmacist management of anticoagulant therapy in ambulant patients. *Am J Hosp Pharm* 36:645-648, 1979.
8. Ekwo E, Hendeles L, Weinberger M: Those who make decisions about management of children with asthma: Pharmacist-physician interaction. *Am J Hosp Pharm* 35:295-299, 1978.
9. Hunter RB, Osterberger DJ: Role of the pharmacist in an allergy clinic. *Am J Hosp Pharm* 32:392-395, 1975.
10. Almond SN, Caiola SM, Huff PS: Pharmacist-managed allergy desensitization program. *Am J Hosp Pharm* 39:284-288, 1982.
11. Miller MB, Conrad WF: Pharmacist involvement in an education program for patients with chronic obstructive pulmonary disease. *Am J Hosp Pharm* 32:909-911, 1975.
12. Sczupak CA, Conrad WF: Relationship between patient-oriented pharmaceutical services and therapeutic outcomes of ambulatory patients with diabetes mellitus. *Am J Hosp Pharm* 34:1238-1242, 1977.
13. Dayton CS. Pharmacist involvement in a tuberculosis outpatient clinic. *Am J Hosp Pharm* 35:295-299, 1978.
14. Davis S: Evaluation of pharmacist management of streptococcal throat infections in a health maintenance organization. *Am J Hosp Pharm* 35:561-566, 1978.
15. Conrad W, Sczupak C, Forman H, Gal P: Consultant approach to improving drug-related services to chronic hemodialysis patients. *Am J Hosp Pharm* 35:558-561, 1978.
16. Skoutakis V, Sergio A, Martinez D, Lorisch D, Wood GC: Role-effectiveness of the pharmacist in the treatment of hemodialysis patients. *Am J Hosp Pharm* 35:62-65, 1978.
17. Harrison WL, Flinkow SP: Clinical pharmacy in a methadone program. *Am J Hosp Pharm* 35:62-65, 1973.
18. See E, Bergquist S: Pharmacist as a provider of oncology ambulatory care services. *Am J Hosp Pharm* 34:1238-1242, 1977.
19. Levin RH: Clinical pharmacy practice in pediatric clinic. *Drug Intell Clin Pharm* 6:171-176, 1972.
20. Ericson AJ, Shainfeld FJ: The pharmacist in an obstetrical service. *Am J Hosp Pharm* 35:295-299, 1978.
21. Scheider P, Cable G: Compliance clinic: An opportunity for an expanded practice role for pharmacist. *Am J Hosp Pharm* 35:288-295, 1978.
22. D'Achille KM, Swanson LN, Hill WT: Pharmacist-managed patient assessment and medication refill clinic. *Am J Hosp Pharm* 35:66-70, 1978.
23. Gardner ME, Trinca CE: The pharmacy clinic: A new approach to ambulatory care. *Am J Hosp Pharm* 35:429-431, 1978.
24. McKenney JM, Witherspoon JM, Pierpaoli PG: Initial experiences with a pharmacy clinic in a hospital-based group medical practice. *Am J Hosp Pharm* 38:1154-1158, 1981.
25. Erickson SH: Primary care by a pharmacist in an outpatient clinic. *Am J Hosp Pharm* 34:1086-1090, 1977.
26. Johnson RE, Tuchler RJ: Role of the pharmacist in primary health care. *Am J Hosp Pharm* 32:162-164, 1975.
27. Canfield PR: Family medicine: An historical perspective. *J Med Educ* 51:904-911, 1976.
28. Love DW, Hodge NA, Foley WA: The clinical pharmacist in a family practice residency program. *J Fam Pract* 10:67-72, 1980.
29. Juhl RP, Perry PJ, Norwood GJ, Martin LR: The family practitioner–clinical pharmacist group practice: A model clinic. *Drug Intell Clin Pharm* 8:572-575, 1974.
30. Maudlin RK: The clinical pharmacist and the family physician. *J Fam Pract* 3:667-668, 1976.
31. Moore TD: Pharmacist faculty member in a family medicine residency program. *Am J Hosp Pharm* 34:973-975, 1977.
32. Perry PJ, Hurley SC: Activities of the clinical pharmacist practicing in the office of a family practitioner. *Drug Intell Clin Pharm* 9:129-133, 1975.
33. Helling DK: Family practice pharmacy service: Part I. *Drug Intell Clin Pharm* 15:971-977, 1981.
34. Helling DK: Family practice pharmacy service: Part II. *Drug Intell Clin Pharm* 10:35-48, 1982.
35. White EV: *The Office-Based Family Pharmacist: E. V. White, Pharmacist.* Berryville, VA, Eugene White, 1978.
36. Dolan M: Family practice: A new approach in the new south. *Am Pharm* NS18:489-493, 1978.
37. Kidder W, Isack G: Health maintenance organizations and pharmaceutical services. *J Am Pharm Assoc* NS12:8-12, 14-15, 1972.
38. Johnson RE, Campbell NH: Drug services and costs in HMO prototypes. *Am J Hosp Pharm* 30:405-421, 1973.
39. Ivey MF: The pharmacist in the care of ambulatory mental health patients. *Am J Hosp Pharm* 30:599-602, 1973.
40. Coleman JH, Evans RL, Rosenbluth SA: Extended clinical roles for the pharmacist in psychiatric care. *Am J Hosp Pharm* 30:1143-1146, 1973.
41. Miller WA, Corcella J: Professional pharmacy functions in community mental health centers. *J Am Pharm Assoc* NS12:68-73, 1972.
42. Evans RL, Kirk RF, Walker PW, Rosenbluth SA, McDonald J: Medication maintenance of mentally ill patients by a pharmacist in a community setting. *Am J Hosp Pharm* 33:635-638, 1976.
43. Gray DR, Namikas EA, et al: Clinical pharmacists as allied health care providers to psychiatric patients. *Contemp Pharm Pract* 2:108-116, 1979.
44. Stimmel GL: Clinical pharmacy practice in a community mental health center. *J Am Pharm Assoc* NS15:400-401, 418, 1973.
45. Rosen EC, Holmes S: Pharmacist's impact on chronic psychiatric outpatients in community mental health. *Am J Hosp Pharm* 35:704-708, 1978.
46. Baumgartner RP, Glascock J, Smith R, Weissman AM: Home health agencies and the pharmacist. *J Am Pharm Assoc* NS14:355-357, 377, 1974.
47. Cardoni AA, Pierpaoli PG, Abbott RD: Drug information consultation service for visiting nurses. *Am J Hosp Pharm* 31:1063-1065, 1974.
48. Eastman PF: Pharmaceutical services for home health agencies. *J Am Pharm Assoc* NS11:391-394, 1971.
49. Gerson CK: The team approach to home health care. *Am Pharm* NS18:621-624, 1978.

50. Solomon DK, Baumgartner RP, Weissman AM, Briscoe ME, Smith RM, McCormick WC: Pharmaceutical services to improve drug therapy for home health care patients. *Am J Hosp Pharm* 35:553-557, 1978.

51. White SJ, Godwin HN: Pharmacist-community nurse liaison services. *Am J Hosp Pharm* 31:1063-1065, 1974.

52. Anon: ASHP statement on the provision of pharmaceutical services in ambulatory care settings. *Am J Hosp Pharm* 37:1096, 1980.

53. Babington MA, Robinson LA, Monson RA: Requests for drug information in a university hospital medicine clinic. *Am J Hosp Pharm* 39:127-128, 1982.

54. Robinson JD: Pharmacokinetic service for ambulatory patients. *Am J Hosp Pharm* 38:1713-1716, 1981.

55. Stimmel GL, McGhan WF: The pharmacist as prescriber of drug therapy: The USC pilot project. *Drug Intell Clin Pharm* 15:665-672, 1981.

56. Stimmel GL, et al: Comparison of pharmacist and physician prescribing for psychiatric inpatients. *Am J Hosp Pharm* 39:1483-6, 1982.

57. Brands AJ: Treating ambulatory patients. *US Pharm* 2:70-74, 1977.

58. Downs GD, Vlasses PH, Cali TJ, Gans JA: Physical parameters for monitoring patient care—a new direction in clinical pharmacy education. *Am J Pharm Educ* 40:407-410, 1976.

59. Longe RL, Calvert JC: Physical assessment and the clinical pharmacist. *Drug Intell Clin Pharm* 11:200-203, 1977.

60. Anon: ASHP statement on pharmacist-conducted patient counseling. *Am J Hosp Pharm* 33:644, 1976.

61. D'Achille KM, Flickinger DB, Riethmiller MK, Facey WK: Antimicrobial use review in a family practice setting. *Am J Hosp Pharm* 38:696-699, 1981.

62. Reed DM, Hepler CD, Helling DK: Antibiotic use review in ambulatory care using computer-assisted medical record audit. *Am J Hosp Pharm* 39:280-284, 1982.

63. Anon: ASHP guidelines: Minimum standard for ambulatory-care pharmaceutical services. *Am J Hosp Pharm* 39:316, 1982.

64. Anon: ASHP supplemental standard and learning objectives for residency training in ambulatory-care pharmacy practice. *Am J Hosp Pharm* 39:1967-1969, 1982.

ADDITIONAL READING

Allen RJ, Eckel FM: The pharmacist's role in a hospital-based outpatient clinic. *Drug Intell Clin Pharm* 6:278-284, 1972.

Anderson JM, Ostry S, Uhl HS, Smith RE: Evaluation of a limited drug formulary in an adult internal medicine clinic. *Am J Hosp Pharm* 39:1184-1186, 1982.

Anderson PO, Taryle DA: Pharmacist management of ambulatory patients using formalized standards of care. *Am J Hosp Pharm* 31:254-257, 1974.

Anon: *Report of the Task Force on Health Planning and Pharmacy Practice in North Carolina*. Chapel Hill, School of Pharmacy, University of North Carolina, 1978.

Bass M: The pharmacist as a provider of primary care. *Can Med Assoc J* 112:60-64, 1975.

Baumgartner RP, Land MJ, Hauser LD: Rural health care—opportunity for innovative pharmacy service. *Am J Hosp Pharm* 29:394-400, 1972.

Beasley JW, Moskol FE: The clinical community pharmacist. *Drug Intell Clin Pharm* 13:351-353, 1979.

Bell CJ, Wiser TH, Kerr RA: Oral anticoagulant management by pharmacy clinicians. *Contemp Pharm Pract* 2:101-107, 1979.

Bernstein LR, Klett EA, Jocoby KE: Physicians' attitudes toward the use of clinical pharmaceutical services in private medical practice. *Am J Hosp Pharm* 35:715-717, 1978.

Black HJ, Kastendieck SD, Hedges AC: Duplicate prescription system to facilitate communication between a hospital pharmacy and community pharmacies. *Am J Hosp Pharm* 35:1528-1530, 1978.

Boucher BA, Metzler DM, Baxter H, et al: Improving revenue collection for ambulatory pharmaceutical services. *Am J Hosp Pharm* 39:610-612, 1982.

Bosso JA: Serving on the health team at summer camp for diabetic children. *J Am Pharm Assoc* NS16:463-464, 1976.

Boykin SP, Burkart V, Lamy PP: Drug use in a day treatment center. *Am J Hosp Pharm* 35:155-159, 1978.

Brands AJ: Innovative pharmacy services in the Indian Health Service. *Hosp Formul* 10:402-406, 1975.

Brodie DC, Knoben JE, Wertheimer AI: Expanded roles for pharmacists. *Am J Pharm Ed* 37:591-600, 1973.

Brown DJ, Helling DK, Jones ME: Evaluation of clinical pharmacist consultations in a family practice office. *Am J Hosp Pharm* 36:912-915, 1979.

Burns LA: Trends and initiatives in hospital ambulatory care. *Am J Hosp Pharm* 39:799-805, 1982.

Canada AT, Iazzetta SM: Pharmacy care for ambulatory patients. *J Am Pharm Assoc* NS14:18-20, 1974.

Carmichael JM, Hak SH, Edgman SM, Caiola SM: Emergency-room services for a community health center. *Am J Hosp Pharm* 38:79-83, 1981.

Chubb JM, Winship III HW: The pharmacist's role in preventing medication errors made by cardiac and hyperlipoproteinemia outpatients. *Drug Intell Clin Pharm* 8:430-436, 1974.

Cooper JW, Campbell NA: Community-hospital practitioner consultation. *J Am Pharm Assoc* NS15:484-487, 533, 1975.

Covington TR: Toward a rational approach to the issue of prescribing authority for pharmacists. *Drug Intell Clin Pharm* 17:660-666, 1983.

Crootof LM, Veal JH, Brunjes SD: Pharmacy information system for a health maintenance organization. *Am J Hosp Pharm* 32:1058-1062, 1975.

Davis RE, Crigler WH, Martin H: Pharmacy and family practice—concept, roles and fees. *Drug Intell Clin Pharm* 11:616-621, 1977.

Dolan M: Clinical pharmacy in the coal fields—holistic health care at cabin creek. *Am Pharm* NS18:22-25, 1978.

Dugas JE, Brown S: Community mental health centers. A milieu for expansion of pharmacist services. *Hosp Pharm* 13:78-87, 1978.

Eckel FM: Community-oriented pharmacy services. *Am J Hosp Pharm* 30:425-427, 1973.

Ellinoy BJ, Mays JF, McSherry PV, Rosenthal LC: A pharmacy out-patient monitoring program providing primary medical care to selected patients. *Am J Hosp Pharm* 30:593-598, 1973.

Erickson SH, Romano JA, Barrett JE: Telephone management of drug-related problems in a family practice clinic. *Am J Hosp Pharm* 39:101-104, 1982.

Eshelman FN, Campagna KD: Pharmaceutical services for the primary care health team. *Hosp Pharm* 11:295-300, 1976.

Fink JL, Myers MJ: Compensating pharmacists for new roles. *J Am Pharm Assoc* NS17:168-172, 1977.

Francke D: The pharmacist's outpatient role. *Drug Intell Clin Pharm* 6:277, 1972.

Gebhart MC, Caiola SM, Eckel FM: An ostomy patient care program. *Drug Intell Clin Pharm* 6:374-379, 1972.

Geyman JP: Clinical pharmacy in family practice. *J Fam Pract* 10:21-22, 1980.

Greenberg D, Winship HW: Pharmaceutical services provided to outpatients by U.S. military, public health service and veterans administration hospitals. *Mil Med* 41:307-315, 1976.

Greifenhagen R, Pearlman JJ: Pharmacy system for screening ambulatory patients. *Am J Hosp Pharm* 36:916-920, 1979.

Greiner GE: The pharmacist's role in patient discharge planning. *Am J Hosp Pharm* 29:72-76, 1972.

Griffin GD: The pharmacist as primary provider of maintenance health care. *Hosp Pharm* 9:84-101, 1974.

Guernsey BG, Ingrim NB, Grant JA, et al: Use of a medication cart to integrate pharmaceutical services in an outpatient clinic. *Am J Hosp Pharm* 40:1539-1540, 1983.

Gurwich EL, Swanson LN: Clinical pharmacy practice in an outpatient clinic. *J Am Pharm Assoc* NS15:392-399, 1975.

Hart L, Evans DC, Welker RG, Fritz JN: The clinical pharmacist on an interdisciplinary primary health care team. *Drug Intell Clin Pharm* 13:414-419, 1979.

Hawkins D: Clinical pharmacy functions in ambulatory patient care. *J Clin Pharmacol* 21:251-252, 1981.

Helling DK, Hepler CD, Jones ME: Effect of direct clinical pharmaceutical service on patients' perceptions of health care quality. *Am J Hosp Pharm* 36:325-329, 1979.

Hood JC, Murphy JE, Gee JC: Characteristics of outpatient medications and implications with hospitalizations. *Drug Intell Clin Pharm* 2:362-365, 1977.

Holt RJ, Gaskins JD: Neuroleptic drug use in a family-practice center. *Am J Hosp Pharm* 38:1716-1719, 1981.

Huff PS, Hak SH, Caiola SM: Immunizations for international travel as a pharmaceutical service. *Am J Hosp Pharm* 39:90-93, 1982.

Hull JH, Murray WJ, Brown HS, et al: Potential anticoagulant drug interactions in ambulatory patients. *Clin Pharmacol Ther* 24:644-649, 1978.

Irgens TR, Henderson WM, Shelves WH: A mini-computer approach to outpatient pharmacy information system. *Hosp Formul* 12:413-415, 1977.

Jinks MJ, Hansten PD, Hirschman JL: Drug interaction exposures in an ambulatory medical population. *Am J Hosp Pharm* 36:923-927, 1979.

Jinks MJ: Reaching the rural elderly through the council on aging network. *Am J Hosp Pharm* 38:1778-1779, 1981.

Kushner D: Hospital expansion of ambulatory-care services: Implications for pharmacy. *Am J Hosp Pharm* 39:863-864, 1982.

Latiolais CJ, Berry CC: Misuse of prescription medications by outpatients. *Drug Intell Clin Pharm* 3:270-277, 1969.

Leedy JB, Schlager CE: A unique alliance of medical and pharmaceutical skills. *J Am Pharm Assoc* NS16:460-462, 1976.

Lesshafft CF: An exploration of the pharmacist's role in outpatient clinics. *J Am Pharm Assoc* NS10:205-209, 1970.

Ludy JA, Gagnon JP, Caiola SM: The patient-pharmacist interaction in two ambulatory settings—its relationship to patient satisfaction and drug misuse. *Drug Intell Clin Pharm* 11:81-89, 1977.

Madden EE: Evaluation of outpatient pharmacy patient counseling. *J Am Pharm Assoc* NS13:437-443, 1973.

Matte DA, McLean WM: Self-medication—abuse or misuse? *Drug Intell Clin Pharm* 603-611, 1978.

Mattei TJ: Clinical involvement for the pharmacist in chronic care. *Am J Hosp Pharm* 31:1053-1056, 1974.

Matiella A, Nease KO, Caplan MF: Portrait of a pharmacy primary care program. *J Am Pharm Assoc* NS16:455-459, 1976.

McConnell WE: A twenty-twenty vision: Alternative futures for hospital pharmacy. *Am J Hosp Pharm* 40:1315-1322, 1983.

McKay AB, Jackson RA: Attitudes of primary care physicians toward utilization of the pharmacist versus the physician's assistant in patient care. *Am J Pharm* 148:157-167, 1976.

McKelvey CP, Lamy PP: Patient care information in an ambulatory health care environment. *Am J Hosp Pharm* 29:401-406, 1972.

McKenney JM, Wyant SL, Atkins D, et al: Drug therapy assessment by pharmacists. *Am J Hosp Pharm* 37:824-828, 1980.

McLeod DC: Clinical pharmacy practice in a community health center. *J Am Pharm Assoc* NS11:56-59, 1971.

Mehl B, Kissner EA: Ambulatory pharmaceutical services in a changing urban community. *Am J Hosp Pharm* 29:407-410, 1972.

Miller RF, Herrick JD: Modernizing an ambulatory care pharmacy in a large multi-clinic institution. *Am J Hosp Pharm* 36:371-375, 1979.

Mitchell GW, Stanaszek WF, Nichols NB: Documenting drug-drug interactions in ambulatory patients. *Am J Hosp Pharm* 36:653-657, 1979.

Parks PM: A patient medication counseling group in an adult psychiatric facility. *Hosp Pharm* 12:63-64, 1977.

Parrish RH, Mirtallo JM, Fabri PJ: Behavioral management concepts with application for home parenteral nutrition patients. *Drug Intell Clin Pharm* 16:581-586, 1982.

Podell LB: U.S. supreme court decision in *Jefferson County Pharmaceutical Association versus Abbott Laboratories et al. Am J Hosp Pharm* 40:1537-1538, 1983.

Provost GP: The pharmacist as a primary practitioner: A guarded view. *Am J Hosp Pharm* 28:238-239, 1971.

Roberts RW, Steward RB, Doering PL, Yost RL: Contributions of a clinical pharmacist in a private group practice of physicians. *Drug Intell Clin Pharm* 12:210-214, 1978.

Rany PB, Johnson CA, Rapp RP: Economic justification of pharmacist involvement in patient medication consultation. *Am J Hosp Pharm* 32:389-392, 1975.

Scott DM, Nordin JD: Pharmacist's role in projects for children and youth. *Am J Hosp Pharm* 37:1339-1342, 1980.

Shasky HG: A guide to taking medication for outpatients and discharge patients. *Hosp Pharm* 7:221-222, 1972.

Smith DL, Hill DS, Page EA, Pylatuk KL: A patient information system in an outpatient clinic. *Can J Hosp Pharm* 27:165-169, 1974.

Solomon DK, et al: Use of medication profiles to detect potential therapeutic problems in ambulatory patients. *Am J Hosp Pharm* 31:348-354, 1974.

Spencer E: The attitudes of ambulatory patients toward a hospital-based pharmacy service: The patient as consultant. *Drug Intell Clin Pharm* 8:710-716, 1974.

Spruill WJ, Cooper JW, Taylor WJR: Pharmacist coordinated pneumonia and influenza vaccination program. *Am J Hosp Pharm* 39:1904-1906, 1982.

Steil CF, Lesshafft CT, Martin DA, Crass RE: Pharmacy in family practice: A description and evaluation. *Contemp Pharm Pract* 2:166-169, 1979.

Stewart RB, Cluff LE: Studies on the epidemiology of adverse drug reactions: Part VI, utilization and interactions of prescription and nonprescription drugs in outpatients. *Johns Hopkins Med J* 129:319-331, 1971.

Stewart RB: A study of outpatients' use of medication. *Hosp Pharm* 7:108-117, 1972.

Stewart RB, Cluff LE: A review of medication errors and compliance in ambulant patients. *Clin Pharmacol Ther* 13:463-468, 1972.

Streit RJ: A program expanding the pharmacist's role. *J Am Pharm Assoc* NS13:434-443, 1973.

Temkin LA, Jeffrey LP, Gallina JN, Ingalls KK: Communicating information to the ambulant patient. *J Am Pharm Assoc* NS15:488-493, 1975.

Wallner JN, Stitt RP: Survey of outpatient pharmaceutical services in university hospitals. *Am J Hosp Pharm* 36:1193-1196, 1979.

Weissman AM, et al: Computer support of pharmaceutical services for ambulatory patients. *Am J Hosp Pharm* 33:1171-1175, 1976.

Zellmer WA: Hospital-based care for ambulatory patients. *Am J Hosp Pharm* 37:801, 1980.

CHAPTER 47

Pediatrics

WELTON O'NEAL, Jr., and JOHN J. PIECORO, Jr.

The pharmacologic management of pediatric patients is a unique and challenging specialty in clinical pharmacy. Many considerations within this population may influence drug recommendations. These factors include a rapidly changing body weight, height, and composition, the maturity of organ systems to eliminate various drug products, and the nutritional status and requirements of the patient.

Because drugs are dosed on the basis of size (e.g., mg/kg, mg/m²), a rapidly changing body weight and height play an extremely important role in proper dosing. Of additional importance is the change of body water as an infant matures. For example, water represents 80% and 60% of total body weight (TW) in the premature infant and 1-year-old, respectively. In general, drugs that are hydrophilic (like water) will distribute to a larger volume in the younger infant. Thus, the percentage of body water may influence the pharmacokinetic properties of a drug. It should also be noted that small changes in body weight are much more significant in neonates than in older infants and children. For example, a weight change of 100 g in an 800-g preterm infant is more significant than the same weight change in an 8-kg infant. Day-to-day increases in TW result from fluid intake, fluid retention, or growth. Losses in TW may result from dehydration or inadequate caloric intake. However, many other factors may influence weight gain or loss (e.g., infections, burns, surgery).

The responsibilities of the clinical pharmacist require him or her to be knowledgeable of these previously mentioned factors, as well as other clinical and distributive skills. Included is a clear perception of the IV administration of drugs, the emergency use of drugs, the preparation of dosage forms, and the use of medical surgical supplies. Therefore, a rational approach to attain competence in pediatric service is necessary. Psychologic adjustment, technical competence, and academic preparation must be combined and must flow together to make the "complete" pediatric practitioner. The purpose of this chapter is to discuss the facets of clinical service and to examine areas of proper drug therapy in pediatrics.

CLINICAL PEDIATRIC PHARMACIST SERVICE RESPONSIBILITIES

The service responsibilities of the pediatric clinical pharmacist are challenging because they demand a wide range of skills. In general, the primary responsibilities should include (1) selecting medical surgical supplies, (2) rounding with physicians and students, (3) attending daily medical conferences, (4) monitoring drug therapy, (5) providing drug information and in-service training, (6) providing drug counseling for patients and their parents, (7) participating in teaching conferences, and (8) participating on cardiopulmonary resuscitation teams.

SELECTING MEDICAL SURGICAL SUPPLIES

At our institution, the pharmacy and central supplies departments are combined and decentralized. Each clinical pharmacist is designated an assistant director of pharmacy central supply (PCS). The clinical pharmacist is responsible for assisting with the selection of various medical and surgical supplies that are routinely used in their area. In their evaluation, several questions are answered. What are the alternative products? Which manufacturer's brand is the most cost effective? Should a newly marketed product(s) be chosen or evaluated? The choice of products involves a multidisciplinary agreement. Because physicians, nurses, and respiratory therapists are the primary users of the supplies, their input in the selection of these products is very valuable. For example, a nurse employed in the neonatal intensive care unit (NICU) may request special high-pressure tubing. The nurse or supervisor will communicate the desired tubing qualities to the clinical pharmacist. The clinical pharmacist will report this information to the supervisor(s) of medical surgical supplies in the central PCS area. Different brands of tubing will then be evaluated for the desired qualities by the clinical pharmacist and the supervisors. With the advent of diagnosis related groups (DRGs), the cost of the items has gained even more importance. Once an item is selected, the product will be given a clinical trial involving actual patient use. Any problems with the item will be communicated to the clinical pharmacist for resolution. The addition of newly marketed medical surgical supplies requires a final approval by the hospital's Product Selection Committee.

Some supply items, such as IV infusion control devices, present a number of problems associated with their use that warrant input by the clinical pharmacist. Whether an infusion control device possesses the qualities of various alarms (e.g., occlusion, low-flow volume), ease of use, and accuracy has become increasingly important in the 1980s. An ideal infusion control device would possess these qualities as well as versatility. Versatility in pediatric patients means being capable of administering IV fluids and total parenteral nutrition (TPN), enteral feedings, and drugs (e.g., aminoglycoside antibiotics, dopamine drips, aminophylline drips) without waste. Blood or blood products present a special problem in NICU patients. On many occasions the blood products will be dispensed in a syringe, thereby requiring a syringe pump for administration. Thus, syringe pumps are needed, as well as other infusion devices for the administration of other drugs and fluids. The choice of infusion devices must be based on clinical evaluations and cost effectiveness. In our institution, a hospital infusion device committee has been established and includes representatives from nursing, medical staff members, and the hospital administration. A clinical pharmacist serves as the chairman. The committee receives input from all involved areas before a decision on which infusion device(s) should be purchased and used. Communications between the pediatric clinical pharmacist and the infusion device committee are obviously necessary to ensure the proper recognition of special situations (e.g., blood administration in the NICU) occurring in pediatrics.

ROUNDING

The purpose of rounds is to discuss the general condition or diagnosis of each patient and then review the treatment plans. More specifically, the patient's diagnosis, assessment, laboratory parameters, nutritional status, and pharmacologic management are reviewed. The rounding team is composed of health care professionals, including physicians (medical interns and residents), clinical pharmacists, students (medical and pharmacy), and occasionally nurses or clinical nutritionists. Input from the clinical pharmacist involves discussion on drug selection, proper dosages, adverse effects, drug interactions, drug administration (e.g., rate of infusion, IV compatibility) and TPN. The pharmacist also provides a computer printout that includes each patient's complete medication profile during hospitalization.

Three types of pediatric rounds occur in our institution. First, *work rounds* are done every morning between 7:30 and 8:30 AM. Each patient and his or her management are discussed. Any pertinent changes in present therapy are made. Thus, the health care team approach is employed. Second, *attending rounds* are held at least 3 days per week between 10:00 AM and 12:00 noon. The team's attending physician presents and leads the patient care discussions. Often only two to three patients are thoroughly discussed with emphasis on teaching. The pathophysiology of their diseases is presented along with a more in-depth discussion of pharmacologic management, desirable laboratory tests, and other modes of therapy (e.g., respiratory therapy, physical therapy). The third kind of rounds is *daily checkout rounds,* which generally occur in the late afternoon or early evening. Here the medical interns and residents give brief summaries of their patients' conditions and therapy plans to the house staff physicians on call for the night. The clinical pharmacist is again present to advise and comment on drug therapy and pharmacokinetics where appropriate.

Rounding is strongly encouraged by the director of PCS because rounds foster positive interaction and rapport among the clinical pharmacist, physicians, and other allied health professionals. The clinical pharmacist is present to participate in firsthand decisions within the multidisciplinary approach to patient care.

MONITORING DRUG THERAPY

Medication dosage monitoring is a function performed throughout the day. In the morning (preferably before 9:00 AM), the clinical pharmacist reviews the computer printout of each patient's medication profile against the actual physician's order. Orders are examined for appropriate dosages, length of therapy, potential drug-drug interactions, and correct computer entry. When an error is found, it is corrected by one of three means. First, the physician may be contacted to completely rewrite the order or to obtain a verbal order. Second, a medication discrepancy form may be completed by the pharmacist that would be treated as a physician's order. The discrepancy form is used to correct computer entry errors, to add omitted orders to the patient profile, or to change the specific time schedules (hours) for drug administration. Third, a drug order clarification form may be initiated, which primarily serves to change a nonformulary drug to a formulary product where appropriate. To obtain nonformulary drugs, the attending physician must write the medication order or a nonformulary request form must be completed. The nonformulary request form must be signed by the attending physician.

During the day, the physician's orders are closely reviewed for drugs that are pharmacokinetically monitored (e.g., digoxin, theophylline, aminoglycosides). When identified, appropriate dosage accessments and adjustments are recommended to the physician. The suggestions are communicated verbally, by written comments in the patient's chart, or typically both. It is the opinion of the authors that pharmacokinetics is one of the most unique areas of clinical practice.

ATTENDING CONFERENCES

In general, at least two pediatric conferences are held daily. The conferences include morning report, pediatric grand rounds, and noon conferences. Morning report is usually held four times each week. The attending physicians, the house staff physicians (e.g., interns, residents), the clinical pharmacists, and both medical and pharmacy students attend this conference. The most interesting two or three patients admitted during the past 24 hours are presented to the group by one of the house staff members. A discussion of the diagnosis and planned therapy will generally be initiated by one of the attending physicians. Any drug-related questions are referred to the clinical pharmacist.

Pediatric grand rounds are held once each week in lieu of morning report. The topics are formally presented and vary in content from disease states to current ethics. The presenter is typically a physician who has special training or subspecialization in the area of discussion. The audience generally consists of attending physicians, house staff, pharmacists, nurses, medical and pharmacy students, and any other interested health professionals. Grand rounds is a conference common to many teaching hospital institutions.

Noon conference is held daily and is directed toward house staff physicians. The presentations may be formal or informal and cover a variety of topics. The presenter is usually a physician. The clinical pharmacist, however, makes frequent presentations at this conference. Topics presented by the pharmacist have included cough and cold products, antihypertensive therapy in pediatrics, prostaglandins E_1 and E_2, plasma volume expanders, and the uses of steroids.

Pharmacy residents and students assigned to a pediatrics rotation are strongly encouraged to attend the various conferences. All of the conferences may be called teaching conferences and are therefore good tools of the learning process. Additionally, conference presentations or comments by the clinical pharmacist aid in building and establishing physician rapport.

MEDICATION COUNSELING

Patient medication counseling is performed where appropriate or when requested by either nurses or physicians. Most patients or parents (or guardians) will receive medication counseling from their local pharmacist or the outpatient pharmacist with dispensing of the medication. Because our hospital is a tertiary care institution, many of the patients have chronic diseases requiring multiple hospital admissions and continuous medication therapy. The clinical pharmacist will encourage compliance and answer questions concerning drug side effects (e.g., cystic fibrosis patients prescribed prophylactic antibiotics). Pharmacy students and residents are encouraged to participate in patient counseling.

A unique patient or parent medication counseling situation involves the Parent Care Unit (PCU). Patients admitted to the PCU have chronic diseases (e.g., malignancies, hypertension, convulsive disorders) and parents are trained to care for their children. Medications prescribed for these patients are handled as outpatient prescriptions and delivered by the pharmacist. The parents are given routine counseling concerning (1) medication identification, (2) dosing schedules, (3) typical adverse effects, and (4) special administration techniques (e.g., the use of oral syringes). Generally a 5-day supply of medicine is dispensed and the parents are encouraged to contact the clinical pharmacist if questions arise. The nurse assigned to the PCU acts as the liaison between the pharmacist and the parents.

PEDIATRIC TASK FORCE

The Pediatric Task Force is a special administration committee that meets once each month. The members of the committee include the departmental chairman of pediatrics, the pediatric chief resident, the clinical pharmacist, the pediatric director of nursing, a representative of the hospital administration, invited chiefs of various pediatric specialities, and other department heads. Duties of the committee include (1) recommend new policies and procedures to the hospital clinical board, (2) routinely discuss and resolve problems related to hospital admissions and isolation policies, (3) make suggestions to the Product Evaluation Committee for new medical surgical supplies, and (4) review requests for new drug items or changes in drug therapy for the pediatric population. Because medical and surgical supplies and drugs are the responsibility of the PCS, the clinical pharmacist plays a key role in the task force. A copy of the committee meeting minutes are given to each member. Also, the director of the PCS will receive a copy of the minutes to inform him of any actions taken that will affect the PCS. One of the key decisions involving drug therapy was initially proposed and subsequently refined by this task force. This decision involved the pediatric drug dose standardization program to be described later.

THE UNIT DOSE SYSTEM

The necessity of accurate dosing, especially when administering small volumes of solutions, warrants an efficient and organized pharmacy operation. Hospitals serving pediatric patients should employ a unit dose drug distribution system for several reasons. Unit dose systems are more accurate and are associated with fewer medication errors. In our hospital, as in many other institutions, the unit dose system is complemented by computerized patient medication profiles and nursing administration sheets. This computerization allows for the rapid retrieval of hospital formulary drugs and medications requiring special preparation as well as for billing purposes.

Unit dose systems should be designed to handle around-the-clock services. Services include the preparation of oral medications, IV or IM medications, IV fluids, and TPN. For example, in the preparation of oral medications, palatability is extremely important. Therefore, many oral medications must be made into solutions or suspensions and flavored with sweetening agents such as cherry syrup. Parenteral products usually require small dispensing units (e.g., 1- and 3-ml syringes, 250-ml IV bags or bottles). Because the preparation of medications may be tedious, conscientious technical support is essential. Physicians and nurses are usually very cooperative. They depend on the pharmacy to provide drug products that are accurate and easy to use.

Unit dose systems are often considered one of the clinical services that promote physician and nursing rapport with the pediatric pharmacist. Numerous questions arise concerning dosages and dosage formulations. Most clinical pharmacists seize the opportunity to answer formulation questions or problems. In addition, they provide drug information regarding adverse effects, contraindications, and drug interactions or compatibilities.

There are several guidelines for administering medications to children. Generally, children under 5 years of age cannot take solid oral dosage forms. There are some children, however, who are able to swallow small tablets. In situations where liquid forms are not commercially available, solutions can be prepared from tablets or capsules. Some commonly used diluents include cherry syrup, simple syrup, aromatic elixir, and methylcellulose, 1-2%. Sorbitol, 70%, is sometimes used; however, frequent use may cause osmotic diarrhea. Another alternative is to crush the tablet or open the capsule and sprinkle it onto pleasant tasting food (e.g., applesauce, ice cream).

When accurately measuring liquid dosage forms, oral

syringes are preferred. In our institution, Pediatric Drug Dose Standardizations have been developed and approved by the Pediatric Task Force Committee. In the standardizations, unusual dosages are rounded off to a volume that can be accurately prepared (1). In general, the minimum increments are set at 0.05 ml for an injection or 0.5 ml for an oral liquid. Most injectable drugs are prepared in 1-, 3-, and 5-ml plastic syringes or 1- and 2.5-ml glass tubexes.

Extemporaneous oral dosages formulas should be compiled in a bound notebook for consistency of preparation. A list of dosage formulations can be obtained by contacting the ASHP Pediatric Special Interest Group (SIG) or a pediatric hospital. Careful attention must be paid to expiration dates and formulations requiring refrigeration.

PEDIATRIC DOSING

It has long been recognized that the pediatric patient is not simply a "little adult" and should not be dosed or treated in that manner. The relative immaturity of various organ systems make drug effects and drug disposition vastly different. Also, the continuous state of rapid growth and metabolic change makes the dosing of many therapeutic agents interesting and challenging.

To become a competent and respected clinical pediatric pharmacist one must master various pharmacokinetic principles that alter drug disposition. These principles include drug absorption, distribution, metabolism, and excretion. The maturity of the gastrointestinal, renal, and hepatic systems are very important for drug disposition. The influence of hepatic system changes is demonstrated in the pharmacokinetic elimination of theophylline (2). Additionally, the changes in body water percentages as the infant grows into an adolescent or adult must be recognized as a very important factor in drug distribution and dosing (3).

The drugs that are commonly dosed based on known and calculated pharmacokinetic parameters include digoxin, theophylline, phenytoin, phenobarbital, carbamazepine, valproic acid, ethosuximide, primidone, aminoglycoside antibiotics, and aspirin. In general these drugs possess narrow therapeutic indexes, thus requiring pharmacokinetic dosing and monitoring (Table 47.1) (4). However, for the majority of drugs used in pediatrics, doses are determined on the basis of mg/kg of body weight or mg/m^2 of body surface area. Body surface area (BSA) can most easily be determined using a nomogram when the body height and weight are known (5). Noting that numerous rules or formulas have been developed to calculate a pediatric dose as a proportion of the adult dose shows there is no universal equation (i.e., Clark's rule, Young's rule, Fried's rule, Starkenstein's rule). The various rules should no longer be used. Thus, a good reliable set of reference books with dosing tables or recommendations is required to aid in making a sound clinical dosing recommendation (Table 47.2). To keep abreast of new dosing recommendations, therapeutic effects, and side effects, a review of the current pediatric literature is strongly advised (Table 47.3).

Pharmacokinetic principles will be briefly discussed here but deserve extensive study for specific application. Absorption can be defined as the passage of a substance through some surface of the body into body fluids and tissues. The rate at which a drug enters the bloodstream depends on the route of administration (i.e., oral, IM), and physiochemical properties of the drug (pKa, lipid solubility, molecular weight) (2,7). More important, factors such as membrane properties, rate and magnitude of organ perfusion, and pH of biologic fluids at the site of contact determine a drug's absorption (6). Newborn infants have relative gastrointestinal dysfunction with respect to gastric pH, gastric emptying time, intestinal motility, and the maturation of intestinal enzyme systems necessary for proper absorption. Lipophilic substances (i.e., diazepam, phenobarbital, carbamazepine, imipramine), as well as the vitamins A and D, are generally faster absorbed during infancy than at any other time in life (7). However, beyond infancy and early childhood there are no functional differences between

TABLE 47.1 Normal Pharmacokinetic Serum Ranges of Drugs Commonly Used in Pediatrics[a]

Drug	Units	Therapeutic Range
Amikacin	μg/ml	5–10 (trough)
		25–35 (peak)
Gentamicin	μg/ml	<1–2 (trough)
		5–10 (peak)
Tobramycin	μg/ml	<1–2 (trough)
		5–10 (peak)
Phenytoin	μg/ml	10–20
Phenobarbital	μg/ml	15–40
Carbamazepine	μg/ml	8–12
Primidone	μg/ml	5–12
Ethosuximide	μg/ml	40–100
Valproic acid	μg/ml	50–100
Lidocaine	μg/ml	1.5–6.5
Digoxin	ng/ml	0.8–2.0
Theophylline	μg/ml	10–20
Caffeine	μg/ml	3–15
Aspirin	mg/dl	15–30
		(antiinflammatory)
Methotrexate	μmol/liter	48 hr <0.5

[a]Reprinted by permission from *Policy and Procedure Manual.* Department of Pathology, Albert B. Chandler Medical Center, Lexington, University of Kentucky, 1984.

TABLE 47.2 Reference Books Suggested for Clinical Pediatric Pharmacy Practice

Benitz WE, Tatro DS: *The Pediatric Drug Handbook.* Chicago, Year Book Medical Publishers, 1981.

Ford DC, Leist ER, et al: *Guidelines for the Administration of Intravenous Medications to Pediatric Patients.* Bethesda, American Society of Hospital Pharmacists, 1982.

Klein JO, Brunell PA, et al: *Report of the Committee on Infectious Disease,* ed 19. Evanston, IL, American Academy of Pediatrics, 1982.

Nelson JD: *Pocketbook of Pediatric Antimicrobial Therapy,* ed 5. Dallas, Jodone Publishers, 1983.

Nelson WE, et al: *Textbook of Pediatrics,* ed 12. Philadelphia, WB Saunders, 1983.

Pagliaro LA, Levin RH: *Problems in Pediatric Drug Therapy.* Hamilton, IL, Drug Intelligence Publications, 1982.

Shirkey HC: *Pediatric Therapy,* ed 6. St Louis, CV Mosby, 1980.

Winters RW (ed): *The Body Fluids in Pediatrics.* Boston, Little, Brown, 1973.

TABLE 47.3 Suggested Pediatric Journals Used to Keep Abreast of Current Practice

Pediatrics, American Academy of Pediatrics, Evanston, IL 60204.
The Journal of Pediatrics, CV Mosby, St Louis, MO 63146.
The American Journal of Diseases of Children, American Medical Association, Chicago, IL 60610.
Pediatric Clinics of North America, WB Saunders, Philadelphia, PA 19105.
Clinical Pediatrics, JB Lippincott, Philadelphia, PA 19105
Clinics in Perinatology, WB Saunders, Philadelphia, PA 19105.

the healthy child and adults that would alter gastrointestinal absorption (2,8).

In general, absorption of drugs from IM or SC sites depends on tissue perfusion. Because of decreased amounts of subcutaneous and muscular tissues in the premature and newborn infant, absorption is substantially diminished. After 2-3 weeks of life, the newborn infant has better IM absorption (2,7), In contrast, the thin and vulnerable skin of premature infants, newborns, and infants permits better absorption of topical lipophilic drugs (i.e., corticosteroid-containing creams or ointments) (7).

Drugs circulate in the body either free or bound. The distribution of drugs in the body depends on physiochemical properties of the drugs (i.e., partition coefficient, pka), protein binding, and the percentage of the total body weight made up by water. The physiochemical properties of drugs remain at constant values. However, both the amount of protein binding and the amount of body water changes in growing pediatric patients (6).

Albumin is the serum protein that constitutes the majority of drug protein binding. The normal adult albumin serum concentration ranges from 2.5-5.0/dl. Neonatal serum contains approximately 80% of adult serum albumin levels (6). Thus, the amount of unbound drug or free drug available for interaction with receptor sites is greater in neonates. It should also be noted that bilirubin, an endogenous substance, also binds to serum albumin. Drugs that are highly protein bound may compete with bilirubin for albumin binding sites. For example, sulfisoxazole significantly displaces bilirubin. Kernicterus caused by hyperbilirubinemia may lead to central nervous system damage.

The size of the extracellular water (ECW) space influences serum drug concentrations because most drugs distribute throughout the ECW to reach their sites of action and effect. Total body water (TBW) comprises up to 85% of body weight in premature infants, 75% in full-term infants, 60% in 1-year olds, and 55% in adults. TBW is composed of intracellular water (ICW) and ECW. The ECW as a percentage of TBW decreases from up to 57% in neonates to 32% in adults. The shift of water into the ICW and decrease in the TBW as the child grows into an adult account for a smaller volume of ECW where drugs may distribute (2,6-7). The term "apparent volume of distribution" (AV_d) then describes the volume that must be filled with drug before the desired plasma concentration can be achieved. For several drugs that have been studies (i.e., digoxin, aminoglycoside antibiotics), the AV_d is relatively larger in newborns and children than in adults. It is worth pointing

out that the AV_d may be greater than the TBW if a drug is highly tissue bound (i.e., diazepam is highly lipid bound) because the tissue sites become saturated first, then the ECW space filled.

Thus, in the neonate, the AV_d for a drug can be increased because of larger amounts of TBW and ECW, smaller amounts of serum proteins, and less binding by available serum proteins. The AV_d will decrease as the neonate matures into a child and then an adult.

Elimination of drugs from the body is determined by metabolism (hepatic) and excretion (primarily renal). Drug metabolism is primarily affected by hepatic microsomal enzyme systems. The reactions involve mainly oxidation but also include some reduction and conjugation reactions. Most enzymatic microsomal systems responsible for various biotransformations are present at birth, but are not fully developed. The maturation of the various enzymatic systems occurs at different rates. When a drug undergoes more than one metabolic step, the overall characterization of hepatic metabolism is difficult. A point worth noting is that the microsomal enzyme systems present at birth can be enhanced by intrauterine or postnatal exposure to enzyme inducers such as phenobarbital. Phenobarbital induces the cytochrome oxidase system (P-450), as well as the glucuronyl transferase systems that allow newborns to metabolize bilirubin at a higher rate. Additionally, conjugation with glucuronic acid and amino acids (e.g., glycine, cysteine, glutathione) probably mature about the second and third months of life, respectively (6). In general, most drugs will be metabolized at slower rates in premature and newborn infants than in older children and adults. In late infancy and childhood, however, many drugs are eliminated via hepatic metabolism at greater rates than in adults (e.g., theophylline).

Excretion is the ultimate route for elimination of drugs or metabolites from the body. Most drugs or metabolites are excreted in the urine by renal mechanisms. However, excretion can occur through the bile, feces, or lungs. The renal mechanisms primarily involved are glomerular filtration (GFR) and tubular secretion (TS). These functions are relatively poorly developed in the newborn infant and even less developed in premature infants. Much of the initial reduction in renal excretion may be accounted for by the significantly lower neonatal GFR (2,6-7). At 2-3 days of life the GFR may be 8-20 ml/min/1.73 m^2 in a term infant. Full adult values for GFR and TS are not reached until 5-7 months of age (6,8). Decreased renal function can lead to drug accumulation. Therefore, dosage adjustments must be made to avoid excessive accumulation. This is certainly true for the aminoglycoside antibiotics and digoxin, which are commonly dosed pharmacokinetically.

The proper dosing of drugs in pediatrics is thus a complex and challenging facet of clinical pediatric pharmacy practice. It involves the use of multiple reference books, a good understanding of pharmacokinetics, and a sound background in pediatric pathophysiology. The use of rules to calculate pediatric dosages from adult dosages is outdated, dangerous, and should be avoided. Further clinical trials are still needed to determine the pharmacokinetic parameters and dosages of many drugs for pediatric patients. The future of pediatric pharmacy is filled with numerous challenges.

INTRAVENOUS ADMINISTRATION OF DRUGS

When drugs are administered intravenously they are introduced directly into the bloodstream to quickly achieve high serum levels. However, despite the achievement of a rapid clinically desirable effect the possibility of adverse reactions is more likely and the severity is greater with the IV route of administration. With this route of administration one must know if a drug can be safely given by IV push or if it requires infusion over an extended time period. It is also necessary to know if a drug can be safely given by a nurse or if it should be administered by a physician. One of the most difficult questions involving pediatric patients concerns the amount of fluid used to dilute a drug before IV use. Because many patients have limited fluid maintenance requirements, the amount of diluent used becomes very important. If the dilution guidelines for adult patients are employed in pediatrics, then the possibility of eventual fluid overload is inevitable. Therefore, balancing the amount of diluent needed to minimize phlebitis and toxicity with amounts that will not significantly alter serum electrolyte and fluid status is essential.

To answer most questions concerning the IV administration of drugs in pediatric patients, the practitioner should refer to the ASHP Guidelines for the Administration of Intravenous Medications to Pediatric Patients (9). This guide will usually apply to pediatric patients up to 17 years of age. Additional information may be obtained from a publication by Rapp et al, ''Guidelines for the Administration of Commonly Used Intravenous Drugs—1984 Update'' (10). Although this reference applies mainly to adults, it does contain useful data applicable to general pediatric patients and adolescents.

At many institutions, the use of metered chambers (e.g., Buretrols, Solusets) to dilute IV drugs is a common practice. They are also used to determine the total amount of fluids given to patients and to control fluid administration. The introduction of highly technical and extremely accurate infusion devices will eventually replace metered chambers. Minibags, minibottles, and manufacturers' partial-fill bottles are frequently not employed because of fluid limitations among pediatric patients.

EMERGENCY USE OF DRUGS IN PEDIATRIC PATIENTS

The use of pharmacologic agents in pediatric emergency situations is often confusing and frightening to pharmacists and other health care practitioners. An emergency situation, for our purposes, can be defined as a respiratory arrest or a cardiac arrest. In progressive hospitals, the pharmacist attends emergency situations (codes). He or she is often responsible for preparing the drugs and calculating dosages and administration rates. The drugs are usually stored in a cart or box (e.g., a tackle box), which is taken to the site of the code. It is useful to have a pocket-sized reference card or book readily available that describes the proper use of emergency drugs.

Most pediatric emergencies are respiratory arrests. Cardiac arrest in infants and children is rarely the primary event. It is usually the result of hypoxia secondary to respiratory arrest. Therefore, establishment of the airway and correction of the metabolic acidosis produced by hypoxia are of primary concern (11). The pediatric pharmacist should be certified in cardiopulmonary resuscitation (CPR). Additional knowledge about intubation equipment (e.g., various sized endotracheal tubes, laryngoscopes with varying blade sizes, lubricating gels, suctioning equipment) is beneficial.

Because respiratory arrest is the most common pediatric emergency, endotracheal intubation is often performed. Generally, the size of the trachea is approximately the size of the patient's fifth or little finger; thus, the proper endotracheal tube (ET) can be chosen. The 3.5-mm ET tube is most commonly employed. The tube should be made of nonirritating material. Tubes with a uniform diameter are preferred to those that are tapered. In children younger than 7 or 8 years of age, uncuffed tubes are used. Cuffed tubes are employed in older children (11). When selecting an ET tube, one size larger and one size smaller should be also obtained to allow for individual patient variation. Because of the flexibility of the ET tube and the smallness of the trachea, a stylet or plastic-coated metal guidewire is often needed for proper placement of the ET tube.

The selection of a laryngoscope and size of the laryngoscopic blade is made in large part by the physician's own preference. Once intubation is successful, oxygenation should follow using 100% oxygen by facemask and Ambu bag attached to the ET tube (11).

Proper emergency drug dosing is very important. The clinical pharmacist is expected to be proficient in the use of emergency medications. Useful dosing guidelines established at the University of Kentucky are presented in Table 47.4 (12). On first arriving at a pediatric emergency, it is important to assess the patient's weight and underlying disease. In general, the primary goals of drug therapy are to correct hypoxemia, acidosis, heart rate, and hypotension.

Hypoxemia should be corrected initially with 100% oxygen until proper blood gas determinations are available. Both the degree of hypoxemia and degree of metabolic acidosis will be determined by blood gas analysis. A heparinized syringe is typically used to obtain a blood sample (11). The heparinized syringe is often prepared by the clinical pharmacist; a 3-ml syringe containing 0.1 ml of 1:1000 heparin is recommended.

During a cardiopulmonary arrest, metabolic acidosis results from the accumulation of lactic acid. Correction of the acidosis can be achieved with one of two pharmacologic agents. First, sodium bicarbonate ($NaHCO_3$), 1-3 mEq/kg body weight, is given as a solution diluted 1:1 or 1:2 with sterile water for injection. Drug dilution decreases the amount of severe vein irritation produced by sodium bicarbonate and aids in the calculation of the proper dose (premixed solution diluted 1:1 is commercially available). After administration of the initial $NaHCO_3$ dose, a blood gas determination should be made to guide further $NaHCO_3$ doses. (NOTE: If blood gas determinations are not possible, additional dosages may be given every 5-10 minutes) (11). It is important to note that catecholamines are inactivated by $NaHCO_3$ and therefore should not be mixed for administration. Additionally, $NaHCO_3$ forms a white precipitate with calcium salts (e.g., calcium gluconate, calcium chloride (13). Sodium bicarbonate may be contraindicated in patients with preexisting cardiac disease or sodium imbalance. When

TABLE 47.4   Pediatric Emergency Medications During Cardiopulmonary Resuscitation (12)

Drug	CPR Indications	Pediatric Emergency Drug Information	
Sodium bicarbonate	Acidosis	1-2 mEq/kg IV, ½ initial dose q 5-10 min; may dilute in premature and newborn	1 mEq/cc; use sterile H_2O for dilution (1:1 or 1:2)
Epinephrine	Asystole, bradycardia, hypotension—acute	0.1 ml/kg of 1:10,000 IV, IT, IC Adolescent: 5-10 cc of 1:10,000	Stock epinephrine 1:1,000; dilute 1:10 to get 1:10,000
Atropine	Bradycardia	0.01 mg/kg/dose, repeat q 5 min, up to 4× Adolescent: 0.5 mg/dose, up to 4 doses	0.2 mg/0.5 cc = 0.4 mg/cc; if needed, dilute 1-10 for 0.04 mg/cc
Calcium	EMD, hypotension, asystole, hyperkalemia	CA gluconate, 100 mg/kg, slow, max 10 cc CA CL_2, 0.2 cc/kg, slow, max 10 cc (CA CL_2: 1 cc/5 kg)	100 mg/cc, CA gluconate, max Push: 1 to 2 ml/min; caution in digitalized patients
Dextrose	Hypoglycemia	250-500 mg/kg/dose, adolescent, 50 cc D_{50}	D_{25} = 250 mg/cc D_{50} = 500 mg/cc Dilute at least 1:2
Regular insulin	Hyperkalemia	Give with dextrose; dose is 0.2 u/kg/ dose IV	
Lidocaine	VT, VF	1 mg/kg, drip 20-50 µg/kg/min Adolescent: 50-100 mg bolus, 1-4 mg/ min	1 gm in 500 = 2 mg/ml
Electroshock	VT, VF, SVT, atrial FIB *or* flutter	1-4 watt-sec/kg, ↑50-100% each time; Newborn: start at 25 W-S Adolescent: 400 W-S	SYN off for VF SYN on for all other arrhythmias
Furosemide	↑ICP, fluid overload, pul edema	1 mg/kg IV	
Sodium nitroprusside	Acute hypertensive crisis	0.5-8.0 µg/kg/min (but much lower dosage in the range of 10.0 µg/min; total dose may be adequate in pump failure) (t½ = 30 sec-1 min)	1 vial = 50 mg 50 mg in 250 ml = 200 µg/ml 50 mg in 500 ml = 100 µg/ml Dilute in D_5 only Thiocyanate toxic level is 3-15 mg% but want it less than 10 mg%—primary toxicity seen in RF after use for 2-3 days
Digoxin	SVT, atrial FIB, atrial flutter, CHF	40 µg/kg IV, PO, divide ½, ¼, ¼ over 8 to 48 hr; maintenance 10 µg/kg/ day ÷ q 12	Do not load premature
Propranolol	SVT, atrial FIB, atrial flutter	0.1 mg/kg IV, slow	
Verapamil	SVT	0.1-0.2 mg/kg/dose; may repeat in 30 min (max dose = 10 mg)	1 amp = 5 mg/2ml
Mannitol	↑ICP, early ATN	0.25-0.50 g/kg/dose	0.25 g/cc
Tromethamine	Acidosis	0.3 M, 1-2 ml/kg, drip 10-50% v/v	Watch for ↓ glucose, respiratory depression
Phenytoin	Anticonvulsant	Up to 20 mg/kg IV as load; 10 mg/kg/ day ÷ q 12 hr for maintenance	IV rate: 10 mg/min, ppts easily, flush with NS
Isoproterenol drip	Bradycardia, hypotension	1-5 µg/min or 0.1-1.5 µg/kg/min; do not use concurrently with epinephrine	5 ml = 1 mg (vial) 1 mg/500 D_5W = 2 µg/ml
Epinephrine drip	Bradycardia, hypotension, agonal heart	1-4 µg/min or 0.1-1.5 µg/kg/min	5 ml of 1:1000 in 500 = 10 µg/ml
Levoterenol drip	Bradycardia, hypotension	0.1-1.5 µg/kg/min	4 ml = 4 mg (vial) 4 mg/500 ml D_5W = 8 µg/ml
Dopamine drip	Hypotension, agonal heart	Start 2-5 µg/kg/min, ↑q 15 min up to max 50 µg/kg/min (t½ = 2-4 min)	1 amp = 200 mg 200 mg in 250 = 800 µg/ml 200 mg in 500 = 400 µg/ml Do not mix with alkaline solutions; dilute in D_5W, NS, D_5NS, D_5LR, LR
Dobutamine drip	Cardiogenic shock, hypotension due to refractory CHF	Low dose: 0.5 µg/kg/min Usual dose: 2.5-15 µg/kg/min; ↑q 10 min up to max of 40 µg/kg/min (t½ = 2 min)	1 vial = 250 mg 250 mg in 500 ml = 500 µg/ml 250 mg in 1000 ml = 250 µg/ml Do not mix with alkaline solutions; dilute in D_5W, NS, lactated Ringer's
Naloxone	Narcotic OD	0.01 mg/kg IV, IM, can ↑ dose also; Adolescent: 0.4 mg IV, IM	q 2 to 3 min prn, then q 1 hr, available as 0.02 mg/ml (neonatal) and adult, 0.04 mg/ml
Morphine	Pain, pul edema	0.2 mg/kg IV, IM, SC	Watch for ↓ BP, respiratory depression
Paraldehyde	Anticonvulsant	0.2 cc/kg, IM, pr or 1 ml/yr	

ATN = acute tubular necrosis; BP = blood pressure; CPR = Cardiopulmonary resuscitation; EMD = electromechanical dissociation; FIB = fibrillation; HTN = hypertension; ICP = intracranial pressure; IDM = infant of diabetic mother; RF = respiratory failure; SVT = supraventricular tachycardia; VF = ventricular fibrillation; VT = ventricular tachycardia; W-S = watt seconds.

TABLE 47.4, cont'd

Drug	CPR Indications	Pediatric Emergency Drug Information	
Diazepam	Anticonvulsant	0.1-0.3 mg/kg/dose, IV, or 1 mg/yr Adolescent: 5-10 mg IV (max)	Watch for respiratory depression
Phenobarbital	Anticonvulsant	10-20 mg/kg IV load Maintenance: 5 mg/kg/day ÷ q 12	Watch for respiratory depression (esp if diazepam given first)
Glucagon	IDM with hypoglycemia	0.025 mg/kg IV, IM, SC; IDM, 300 μg	
Diazoxide	HTN	5 mg/kg IV, can repeat × 1 in 30 min	IV push, monitor BP
Hydrocortisone	Bacteremic shock?	50-150 mg/kg q 6 hr	
Methylprednis-olone	Bacteremic shock?	30 mg/kg q 6 hr or one dose only	

$NaHCO_3$ is contraindicated or the physician prefers a second drug, tris-hydroxymethyl amino methane (THAM) can be used. The dosage of THAM is shown in Tabel 47.4. The main advantage of THAM is that it is sodium free. However, its disadvantages must be recognized. THAM can produce side effects such as hypoglycemia, respiratory depression, hyperkalemia, vasospasm, and intracranial hemorrhage. Vessel irritation and tissue necrosis may result from extravasation because of the drug's alkalinity (14). One must recognize that it is easy to overshoot the correction of acidosis; therefore, THAM dosing should be closely monitored using blood gas analysis.

The scope of the present chapter does not allow for a discussion of all of the drugs employed in pediatric CPR. Therefore, a brief description of a limited number of agents used will be presented.

The use of IV catecholamines or sympathomimetic agents is often a part of emergency situations involving the cardiovascular system. (A primary cardiac arrest with its concomitant dysrhythmias is rare in infants and children.) The sympathomimetic agents typically used include epinephrine, isoproterenol, dopamine, dobutamine, and, occasionally, tolazoline. In general, epinephrine (adrenalin) is used when there is no heart action or when the action is very slow and ineffective. Its actions will result in an increased heart rate, an increased inotropic effect, and an increased blood pressure. Isoproterenol is often used following the initial use of adrenalin. Isoproterenol causes an increase in heart rate and a positive inotropic effect, but a decrease in arterial vascular resistance because of its pure beta-adrenergic effects. Both epinephrine and isoproterenol cause tachycardia and dysrhythmias at toxic doses and therefore should not be used concomitantly (or use with extreme caution). Cardiac monitoring is strongly recommended when administering either drug. Dobutamine should be used in the event of cardiac shock; it is an inotropic agent resulting in an increased myocardial contractile force and an increased blood pressure. Dopamine is used in a low dose of 2-5 μg/kg/min to induce increased renal output or in doses of 15-20 μg/kg/min to induce primarily alpha-adrenergic effects resulting in an increased heart rate and an increased blood pressure. Dosages in the range of 5-15 μg/kg/min give primarily beta-adrenergic effects. The alpha effects can also be seen at doses as low as 5 μg/kg/min in very young infants and children (11,15).

Calcium is often given as either the gluconate or chloride salt. Calcium ion is necessary for proper myocardial contraction and may be given in electromechanical dissociation of the heart, hyperkalemia, hypotension, and asystole. Calcium chloride is the preferred salt to employ; however, it is very irritating to vessels. Calcium gluconate may be a better alternative in premature and newborn infants. Both salts are recommended to be administered via slow IV infusion. (NOTE: 1 g of calcium chloride gives 13.6 mEq calcium ion; 1 g of calcium gluconate gives 4.8 mEq calcium ion.) Also, calcium salts should be administered cautiously to digitalized patients because of potential synergistic inotropic effects (10,11,15).

Atropine is administered to accelerate the cardiac rate of contraction in clinically significant bradycardia. The dose is 0.01 mg/kg/dose, which may be repeated every 5 minutes for a maximum of four doses. Atropine is an anticholinergic drug that decreases vagal tone and thereby increases the heart rate (11,14,15).

Table 41.4, a course in CPR, and references such as the *Textbook of Advanced Cardiac Life Support* (11) or *Problems in Pediatric Drug Therapy* (16) provide a data base for developing skills in the use of pediatric emergency drugs.

FLUIDS AND ELECTROLYTES

The administration of fluids and electrolytes to pediatric patients is significantly different from that in the adult. They differ by infusion rates, amounts infused, and the types of fluids infused. In general, (1) the amount infused should equal the amount lost (input equals output), (2) changes in the concentration of electrolytes can lead to profound changes in organ function (i.e., hyponatremia may cause convulsions), and (3) the rate of change (losses) is more important than the total loss.

Fluid loss leading to dehydration is an important concept in pediatric patients. Dehydration may occur because of decreased accessibility to water, excessive vomiting or diarrhea, or a defect in the thirst mechanism. Normal losses are composed of sensible losses (urinary and feces) and insensible losses (water lost through breathing and sweating). The sensible losses account for approximately 1000 ml/m²/day of fluid loss, whereas the insensible losses account for an additional 500 ml/m²/day. Therefore, the total amount of fluids normally lost per day is 1500 ml/m². There are several situations resulting in additional losses; however, for a discussion of these situations refer to the text, *The Body Fluids in Pediatrics* (17).

Fluid excess can also be an important problem. Many

physiologic conditions or diseases may lead to fluid overload. Physiologic states that may contribute to fluid overload include acute renal failure (ARF), chronic renal failure (CRF), congestive heart failure, advanced liver disease, and ascites. To obtain a proper perspective on fluid excess see *The Body Fluids in Pediatrics* (17).

Electrolyte requirements in fluid administration must be carefully observed (18). Appropriate monitoring of serum electrolyte concentrations should guide increases or decreases in further administration. In our institution, the standard pediatric fluid and electrolyte solution is D_5 1/4 NS with 20 mEq KCl added per liter.

PEDIATRIC TOTAL PARENTERAL NUTRITION

Total parenteral nutrition also presents the pediatric clinician with a challenge. Parenteral nutrition solutions in premature infant, neonate, and general pediatric patients differ significantly from the adult. Special considerations in the pediatric population relate to a smaller body size, rapid growth rates, and highly variable fluid requirements. Additionally, premature and newborn infants have immature organ systems. TPN is frequently used in hospitalized pediatric patients who cannot tolerate enteral nutrition because of the stress of trauma, major surgery, or severe infection. A lack of nutrition in these patients could possibly lead to complications such as depressed central nervous system function, increased susceptibility to infection, and increased difficulty weaning patients from mechanical ventilators because of weakening respiratory muscles.

Because of the potentially severe problems that may result from malnutrition, TPN should be initiated as early as possible when it is determined that an infant or small child is malnourished. Most normal newborns establish positive nitrogen balance with weight stabilization or weight gain by the second to fourth postpartum day (18). Therefore in newborn infants and older children unable to tolerate adequate enteral nutrition, sufficient nutrients can usually be provided by IV infusions of dextrose and amino acid solutions and fat emulsion.

The choice of a commercially available amino acid solution must receive proper attention. For example, it is known that premature infants and neonates are unable to synthesize cysteine from methionine because of a deficiency of cystathionine synthetase (18,19). Cysteine then becomes an essential amino acid in these patients whereas in older children and adults it is nonessential. At present the only marketed amino acid solution containing cysteine is Neopham.* However, there is a commercially available solution of cysteine that can be added to amino acid solutions (e.g., Aminosyn). Therefore, the selection of a crystalline amino acid solution for use in TPN must include consideration of the amino acid content and concentration.

Sufficient thought must be given to physiologic conditions in pediatric patients. The percentages of protein, fat, and water that make up total body weight differ among the premature infant, term infant, child, and adult. In addition,

*Neopham was voluntarily withdrawn from the market because of instability problems.

TABLE 47.5 Indications for TPN[a]

Neonates
  Surgical
  Low birth weight (<1500 g)
  Necrotizing enterocolitis (NEC)
General pediatrics
  Surgical
  Inflammatory bowel disease
  Intractable diarrhea
  Anorexia nervosa
  Failure to thrive (FTT)
  Burn patients

[a] Modified from Kerner JA (ed): *Manual of Pediatric Parenteral Nutrition*. New York, John Wiley & Sons, 1983.

the number of days of survival without nutrition by a premature infant is 4-12 days whereas a 1-year-old child may survive up to 42 days. Also without good nutrition the development of various organ systems may be slowed or impeded (e.g., central nervous system, hepatic and renal systems, gastrointestinal tract) (18,19).

The complete nutritional assessment of the pediatric patient should include a medical history, diet history, anthropometric measurements, skin testing, and laboratory values such as nitrogen balance and serum transferrin. In addition to nutritional assessments, the medical indications for TPN should be emphasized (Table 47.5). Surgery requiring hospitalization is a common indication for TPN. Examples of surgically treated conditions that make TPN essential include gastroschisis, omphalocele, tracheoesophageal fistula, diaphragmatic hernia, and meconium ileus.

The requirements of the various nutrients (i.e., fluids, proteins, carbohydrates) change with increasing age and weight. A good reference book such as the *Manual of Pediatric Parenteral Nutrition* (18) edited by Kerner, or the *Textbook of Pediatric Nutrition* (19) edited by Suskind, should be used for a more complete understanding of these requirements and pediatric TPN. Generally, 1 g of carbohydrate yields 3.4 Kcal, 1 g of fat yields 9 Kcal, and 1 g of protein yields 4 Kcal. Several authors (17-19) provide guidelines for nutrient requirements in pediatrics (e.g., fluids, electrolytes, carbohydrates, proteins, fats, trace elements).

TPN infusion is not without complications. The complications are both technical and metabolic. The technical problems are related to catheter insertion or placement and maintenance. Catheters are inserted into either a peripheral vein or the subclavian vein (central vein). Central vein placement carries the most complications (e.g., pneumothorax, air embolism, bacteremia, septicemia). The major problem associated with peripheral vein TPN infusion relates to maintenance of the catheter site (e.g., thrombophlebitis, infiltration) (18-19).

Metabolic complications include electrolyte disturbances caused by infusion of too much or not enough of a specific electrolyte (e.g., hypernatremia). Metabolic acidosis is sometimes seen as a complication of TPN in premature and newborn infants. Fluid overload can occur resulting in pulmonary edema. Many other complications are possible and a full discussion can be found in the *Textbook of Pediatric*

Nutrition and the *Manual of Pediatric Parenteral Nutrition* (18,19).

PEDIATRIC INFECTIOUS DISEASE AND IMMUNIZATIONS

Children typically may harbor many infectious diseases (e.g., colds, flu, diarrhea). In the hospital, good hand-washing techniques are the cornerstone for preventing the spread of infections from patient to patient. Also employed are various isolation procedures when more serious infections (e.g., meningitis, hepatitis, TB) are involved. Specific information on most pediatric infectious diseases and special preventative measures may be found in the American Academy of Pediatrics 1982 Red Book, *Report of the Committee on Infectious Diseases* (22).

Proper immunizations for the common childhood diseases such as diphtheria, measles, mumps, rubella, polio, and pertussis are essential for good health. The 1982 Red Book provides guidelines for immunizations. Comments on the safety and possible adverse effects of immunizing agents are also included. In our institution, as in many other institutions, an immunization history is obtained regarding each patient on admission. If it is discovered that no immunizations have been given or if the child is behind in the immunization schedule then the physician will initiate an appropriate regimen. The *Report of the Committee on Infectious Diseases* gives a correction schedule for the immunization of children who are behind or off schedule (22).

Hospital isolation and handwashing techniques in conjunction with proper immunizations help to control pediatric infectious disease. The observance of these practices should be strongly encouraged.

COMMONLY EMPLOYED PHARMACOLOGIC AGENTS USED IN LABOR AND DELIVERY AND THEIR EFFECTS ON THE NEWBORN

Several pharmacologic agents are used to inhibit labor or induce labor. These agents are not without side effects maternally, fetally, or in the neonate. Agents that inhibit contractions of the uterine smooth muscle, thus inhibiting labor, are termed "tocolytics." The categories of drugs routinely used as tocolytic agents include the betamimetics primarily (e.g., ritodrine, terbutaline), the calcium channel antagonist, and ethanol, which is of historical interest. Drugs that stimulate uterine contraction, thus accelerating childbirth, are termed "oxytocics." The most commonly used oxytocic agents include oxytocin and prostaglandin E₂ (PGE₂).

Not all of the tocolytics or oxytoics have been thoroughly studied; therefore, specific adverse effects in the fetus and neonate need further investigation. Further information regarding the tocolytic agents (23), as well as the oxytocic agents (22-25) is available.

The clinical pharmacist can therefore provide useful information to the physician concerning oxytocics and tocolytics. Insight can be gained involving the adverse effects or abnormal behavior of these agents in the neonate. The ideal tocolytic or oxytocic agent would obviously have no effect on the fetus or neonate. It is worth noting that many

new tocolytics (e.g., fenoterol, hexoprenaline) are being presently investigated. The use of newer oxytocics, such as PGE₂, has not been very popular but could possibly be useful in the future. Presently, PGE₂ is primarily employed in the management of missed abortions and intrauterine fetal death (26).

DRUG AGENTS TRANSMITTED BY BREAST MILK

During lactation several drugs may be transmitted to the infant via the mother's milk. It is important to recognize that untoward pharmacologic effects may occur in infants unless we are aware of the large number of drugs transferable via breast milk. Some drugs are contraindicated during breast feeding because of potential severe adverse effects in the infant (e.g., gold salts, thiouracil) (27). In this context, there are also some drugs that require temporary cessation of use by the mother while breast feeding (e.g., radiopharmaceuticals, metronidazole) (27). A large number of agents can be used safely during breast feeding (e.g., secobarbitol, captopril) (27). However, one should be aware that in general most categories of drugs are transmitted by breast milk. Numerous foods and environmental agents may also have an effect on breast-fed infants (e.g., aspartane) (27).

In conclusion, it should be noted that all antibiotics are transferred into breast milk in limited concentrations. Generally, the penicillins are safe both during pregnancy and breast feeding. If possible, drugs and environmental agents should be avoided during breast feeding. If a pharmacologic agent is administered, the benefits must heavily outweigh the risks.

CONCLUSION

The practice of pediatric clinical pharmacy in the 1980s involves the combined use of pharmacokinetics, communication skills, clinical experience, and a great deal of altruism. An individual who is pursuing a career in this area is strongly encouraged to obtain a pharmacy degree and complete a clinical residency or fellowship. Clinical research and the use of computers are two areas where expertise is of growing importance.

Pediatric clinical pharmacists have varied service responsibilities. They must become proficient in TPN, fluids and electrolytes, proper immunization schedules, and the emergency use of drugs. Knowledge of IV administered drugs, extemporaneous formulations, and unit dose systems facilitate proper dosing and monitoring of drug therapy.

One area of pediatric subspecialization encompasses the intriguing world of neonatology. Clinical pharmacists must be knowledgeable of drugs used in labor and delivery because these agents may produce untoward effects in the fetus and newborn. Additional knowledge about drugs that are transmitted in breast milk is important. Much clinical drug

Special acknowledgment is due to Nan M. Hendrickson, Pharm. D., for her valuable assistance in editing this chapter, and our wives Joyce and Sue for their patience and understanding while writing and composing this chapter.

research is needed in this area. Our opinion is that neonatology is the frontier of pediatric clinical pharmacy for the 1980s.

REFERENCES

1. Albert B: Chandler Medical Center: *University Hospital Formulary.* Lexington, KY, May 1984.
2. Udkow G: Pediatric clinical pharmacology. *Am J Dis Child* 132:1025-1032, 1978.
3. Finberg L, Kravath RE, Fleischman AR: *Water and Electrolytes in Pediatrics.* Philadelphia, WB Saunders, 1982.
4. *Policy and Procedure Manual.* Department of Pathology, Albert B. Chandler Medical Center, Lexington, University of Kentucky, 1984.
5. Shirkey HC: *Pediatric Therapy,* ed 6. St Louis, CV Mosby, 1980, p 1229.
6. Hilligoss DM: Neonatal pharmacokinetics. In Evans WE, Schentag JJ, Jusko WJ (eds): *Applied Pharmacokinetics.* San Francisco, Applied Therapeutics, 1980, pp 76-94.
7. Martin E, Guignard JP: Pediatric clinical pharmacology. *Helv Paediat Acta* 37:509-517, 1982.
8. Zenk KE: An overview of perinatal clinical pharmacology. *Clin Lab Med* 1/2:361-375, 1981.
9. American Society of Hospital Pharmacists: *Guidelines for the Administration of Intravenous Medications to Pediatric Patients.* Bethesda, American Society of Hospital Pharmacists, 1982.
10. Rapp RP, Wermeling DP, Piecoro JJ: Guidelines for the administration of commonly used intravenous drugs—1984 update. *Drug Intell Clin Pharm* 18:218-232, 1984.
11. Chameides L, Melker R, Raye JR, Todres D, Viles PH: Resuscitation of infants and children. In McIntyre KM, Lewis AJ, (eds): *Textbook of Advanced Cardiac Life Support.* Dallas, American Heart Association, 1981, pp 1-18.
12. *Policy and Procedure Manual.* Pediatrics and Pharmacy Departments, Albert B. Chandler Medical Center, Lexington, KY, May 1984.
13. Trissel L: *Handbook on Injectable Drugs,* ed 3. Washington, DC, American Society of Hospital Pharmacists, 1983.
14. Benitz WE, Tatro DS: *The Pediatric Drug Handbook,* Chicago, Year Book Medical Publishers, 1981.
15. Goodman LS, Gilman A: *The Pharmacological Basis of Therapeutics,* ed 6, New York, Macmillan, 1982.
16. Pagliaro LA, Levin RH: *Problems in Pediatric Drug Therapy.* Hamilton, IL, Drug Intelligence Publications, 1979.
17. Winters RW (ed): *The Body Fluids in Pediatrics.* Boston, Little, Brown, 1973.
18. Kerner JA (ed): *Manual of Pediatric Parenteral Nutrition.* New York, John Wiley & Sons, 1983.
19. Suskind RM (ed): *Textbook of Pediatric Nutrition.* New York, Raven Press, 1981.
20. Stegink LD: Amino Acids in pediatric parenteral nutrition. *Am J Dis Child* 137:1008-1016, 1983.
21. The University of Michigan Hospitals: Parenteral and enteral nutrition manual, ed 2, Ann Arbor, The University of Michigan Hospitals, 1982.
22. American Academy of Pediatrics: *Report of the Committee on Infectious Diseases* (The Red Book), ed 7, Evanston, IL, American Academy of Pediatrics, 1982.
23. Niebyl JR: *Drug Use in Pregnancy.* Philadelphia, Lea & Febiger, 1982.
24. Souney PF, Kaul AF, Osathanondh R: Pharmacotherapy of preterm labor. *Clin Pharm* 2:29-44, 1983.
25. Ulmstem U, Wingerup L, Ekman G: Local application of prostaglandin F_2 for cervical ripening or induction of term labor. *Clin Obstet Gynecol* 26/1:95-105, 1983.
26. Andersson KE, Forman A, Ulmstem U: Pharmacology of labor. *Clin Obstet Gynecol* 26/1:56-77, 1983.
27. Boyd JR (ed): *Facts and Comparisons.* St Louis, Facts and Comparison, Inc, January 1983, pp 118-118c.
28. Boyd JR (ed): *Facts and Comparisons.* St Louis, Facts and Comparisons, Inc, November 1981, pp 732c-732d.
29. American Academy of Pediatrics Committee on Drugs: The transfer of drugs and other chemicals into human breast milk. *Pediatrics* 72:375-383, 1988.

CHAPTER 48

Geriatric Therapy

W. GARY ERWIN

The graying of America has begun. The over 65 years of age group, which in 1900 represented only 4.1% of the population, today accounts for 11.2% or approximately 25 million people. Current projections for the year 2040 place these figures at 18% or approximately 55 million persons (1-3). Of all individuals who have ever been over 65 years of age, more than 50% are alive today (4). Significant shifts are also occurring within the over 65 years of age population. In 1900, only 1.2% or 0.9 million persons were over 75 years of age; today an estimated 4.2% or 9.4 million persons are in this group. Projections for 2040 place the figures at 9% or approximately 28 million persons. Currently, of the over 65 years of age population, 38% are over 75 years of age and 9% are over 85 years of age. Projections for the year 2010 are that these figures will be 45% over 75 years of age and 12% over 85 years of age (1,2,5). These individuals are now classified as young-old (65-75 years of age) or old-old (over 75 years of age).

The elderly population is predominantly female, with 68 males per 100 females over 65 years of age, 58 males per 100 females over 75 years of age, and 48 males per 100 females over 85 years of age (1,2).

Life expectancy is currently 73.3 years as compared to 49 years in 1900 (6). This prolongation is attributable to several factors, including control of childhood infectious diseases, improved living standards, and higher quality prenatal and postnatal care.

The stereotype of the elderly person as frail, alone, and institutionalized is incorrect. The majority of the elderly live at home with spouses, family, or friends. Approximately 38% live alone (7). Studies have demonstrated that most older persons manage quite well, with little limited mobility and a high degree of functional capacity. A major contributing factor to this success is the level of maturity and degree of adaptability of this population. Only with greatly advancing age (over 85 years of age) does their functional capacity and well-being decline significantly.

NORMAL AGING: A REVIEW OF SYSTEMS

Although from a legal perspective the elderly population is composed of those persons over 65 years of age, this arbitrary demarcation has little basis in physiology. It is difficult to make generalizations about the elderly population because it is a much more heterogeneous group than the young. This heterogenicity is the result of wide interpatient variation in the deterioration of organ system function. Aging or senescence must therefore be viewed as a spectrum of biologic degradation beginning in the twenties but with little significance until a person reaches the mid-seventies. A detailed review of aging is beyond the scope of this chapter and the reader is referred elsewhere (8,9). A basic review of aging, by organ system, is presented to differentiate normal from pathologic aging.

Eyes, Ears, and Mouth. Astigmatism, caused by a flattening of the lens, and presbyopia, or farsightedness, caused by a reduced elasticity of the lens and a reduced ability to focus on near objects, are common in elderly persons. Wrinkles, enophthalmos, and ptosis occur commonly as a result of skin and muscle changes around the eye. The quantity of tear secretions decreases with increasing age. Arcus senilis, a deposition of fat at the corneoscleral junction, occurs commonly but has no known pathologic significance.

Partial hearing loss is common, both as result of a decrease in conductive hearing and a loss of ability to hear the highest frequencies because of degenerative processes.

Changes in salivary glands lead to dry mouth, and a decrease in the number of taste buds leads to a diminished perception of taste. Loss of teeth usually is secondary to poor peridontal hygiene rather than aging.

Skin. The skin loses moisture, strength, and elasticity. There is a decrease in vascularity and an increase in capillary fragility. Subcutaneous fat, hair, and seborrheic glands are lost. Seborrheic keratosis, or hyperpigmentation spots, are common. Actinic keratosis, which are rough, scaly, pink to reddish premalignant lesions, may occur and are related to sun exposure.

Cardiovascular System. Loss of elasticity as a result of collagen aging in the arterial system, especially the aorta, leads to an increase in peripheral vascular resistance. The issue of whether the rise in blood pressure, which may accompany the increase in peripheral vascular resistance, is normal is unclear and controversial. The Framingham study demonstrated that elevated blood pressure in the elderly was a contributing factor to morbidity and mortality from cardiovascular and cerebrovascular disease. Cardiovascular function at rest is usually adequate in the elderly; however, there is a lack of reserve to develop an appropriate response in stroke volume to increased stress on the system. A decrease in baroreceptor response makes postural hypotension a problem in the elderly.

Pulmonary System. The lungs also work well in normal

conditions. However, changes such as decreased elasticity, diminished alveolar capillary surface area, and decreased numbers of alveoli may decrease the functional capacity of the lungs. Musculoskeletal changes within the chest wall can decrease expansion of the lungs. These changes are characterized by a decrease in mean inspiratory pressure and mean expiratory pressure. There is a decrease in residual volume as a result of airway collapse at higher lung volumes.

Gastrointestinal System. Changes within the gastrointestinal tract are usually insignificant. There may be a decrease in the active transport mechanisms of some substances such as iron, calcium, and vitamin B_{12}. A decrease in gastric hydrochloric acid production occurs and there is some degree of gastric mucosa atrophy.

Hepatic System. Liver function is thought to decrease with increasing age; however, the significance of this is unclear. Liver blood flow diminishes, most likely as a result of a decreased cardiac output. Liver weight and size decreases. There is much controversy concerning a possible decrease in metabolic enzymatic activity. Phase one enzymatic reactions, such as oxidation, reduction, and hydroxylation, are thought to be affected to a greater degree by aging than are phase two reactions such as conjugation.

Renal System. Kidney function steadily declines with advancing age. There is both a decrease in renal blood flow and a loss of cortical renal mass as a result of intrarenal vascular changes. Despite this decrease in function the kidneys are still capable of maintaining appropriate electrolyte and acid-base status under normal conditions.

Genitourinary System. Prostatic enlargement occurs frequently in elderly males. This process typically is benign, but there is a great propensity toward malignancy. This enlargement may interfere with bladder emptying. Reduced muscle tone in the bladder wall and urethra can also impair bladder emptying and thus increase residual urine. Nocturia may be common as a result of a decreased bladder capacity and loss of stretch impulse.

There is atrophy of testicular tissue in elderly males. Erection may be slower and weaker, ejaculation slower, ejaculatory volume decreased, and ejaculatory refractory period increased. Despite these changes, elderly males are still quite capable of maintaining a normal sex life.

The female genital system is characterized by atrophic vaginitis resulting from lack of estrogen after menopause. This in conjunction with reduced vaginal secretions may create difficulties with sexual function. Orgasms are of shorter duration and are less intense. Prolapse of the uterus may occur as a result of childbirth and the laxity of supporting ligaments.

Musculoskeletal System. There is a decrease in lean body mass per kilogram of body weight and an increase in body fat. Calcium is lost from bones, leading to osteopenia.

Endocrine System. There is a decrease in glucose tolerance because of a change in insulin response to blood glucose concentrations. This change is not considered significant and is accepted as normal. Atrophy of the thyroid gland is common, and secondary hypothyroidism may occur.

Hematopoietic System. There is a great amount of controversy whether the decreased hemoglobin concentrations found in elderly persons reflects a diminished bone marrow function. Total leukocyte count is decreased, but absolute granulocyte counts do not change significantly.

Immune System. Changes in the immune system are likely related to involution of the thymus gland, which occurs with aging. The total number of T and B lymphocytes in peripheral blood does not change; however, there is an increase in immature T lymphocytes and inducer T lymphocytes and a decrease in suppressor T lymphocytes. These findings suggest a disturbance in regulation rather than a change in cell numbers. There are increased autoantibodies and decreased cell-mediated and humoral immune responses to foreign antigens with increasing age.

Central Nervous System. Changes within the central nervous system that are directly attributable to aging are unclear. The changes that occur resulting in decreased intellectual function are thought to be quantitative rather than qualitative. These changes include loss of brain weight, neurons, horizontal dendrites and spines, and synaptic contact. Neuritic plaques and neurofibrillary tangles may be present, as well as possible neurotransmitter deficiencies.

Current Health Status

Individuals over 65 years of age are the greatest consumers of health care services today. The elderly visit physicians on an ambulatory basis more frequently than do young patients. It is projected that in the year 2020 the greatest percentage of an internist's time will be spent with persons over 65 years of age (10). One of the health care services under-used by elderly persons is dental care. This is most likely because of the lack of third-party coverage for these services.

Persons over 65 years of age spend more days in the hospital than those in younger age groups and have longer lengths of stay (11). Individuals over 65 years of age spend an average of 4.2 days per year in an acute care hospital compared to 0.8 days per year for persons 15-44 years of age and 1.6 days for persons 45-64 years of age. These figures can be further broken down to 3.2 days per year for persons 65-74 years of age and 5.9 days per year for persons 75 years of age and older. Persons over 65 years of age will spend 11 days in the hospital per admission vs 5.3 days per admission for persons 15-44 years of age. It is estimated that 44% of acute care beds are occupied by persons over 65 years of age.

The figures for nursing home care are even more staggering. There are currently more nursing home beds in the United States than acute care beds and approximately 86% of all nursing home residents are over 65 years of age (12). It is estimated that 20-25% of persons over 65 years of age will die in a nursing home (13). As mentioned previously, only a small percentage of persons over 65 years of age will reside in a nursing home on any given day, approximately 5%. This figure is misleading, however, for several reasons. First, statistics demonstrate a great heterogenicity within this group (13), 1% over 65 years of age, 6% over 75 years of age, and 20% over 85 years of age. Second, it is estimated that as many as 40% of persons over 65 years of age will reside at some time in a nursing home (14).

The reasons for this consumption of health care services are many and complex but two are worth mentioning in detail. First, although elderly persons have fewer acute illnesses than young persons, they have many more chronic diseases. Approximately 8% of persons over 65 years of age have one or more chronic diseases (15). These chronic conditions require extensive follow-up by health care personnel and are often so severe and debilitating that adequate care of these persons cannot be accomplished at home. The second reason is access to third-party reimbursement, specifically Medicare and Medicaid. In 1979, approximately 90% of Medicare enrollees were 65 years of age or older (16). The majority of Medicare and Medicaid expenses, currently representing approximately 10% of the federal budget, are paid to hospitals and nursing homes. Estimates vary, but approximately 40-50% of Medicaid expenditures and 2% of Medicare expenditures go to nursing home care (17,18). In 1976, almost 60% of all days in nursing homes were financed totally or in part by Medicaid (19). This reliance on Medicaid, which is a welfare program, must be viewed in conjunction with the fact that only 14% of the over 65 years of age population is below poverty level, as compared to 11.6% of the general population (7,20). Many more persons end up on Medicaid in nursing homes than when they enter. Current reimbursement policy requires the exhaustion of personal funds before being eligible for Medicaid, which has a great impact on the financial security of many families.

APPROPRIATE CARE FOR THE ELDERLY

Partially as a result of this massive consumption of health care dollars to care for the aged, and partially because society has taken a more compassionate view toward the plight of the aged, the emphasis of health care services for the elderly is evolving into one of health maintenance. Current programs are aimed at keeping the elderly independent and out of long-term care facilities for as long as possible. A rapidly expanding knowledge base in geriatric medicine and an awareness of the potential contributions of other members of the health care team are helping to reshape the medical care of this population.

Because one of the major causes of disability in the elderly

population is the increased incidence of chronic disease, much effort is being spent on preventive medicine in the hopes of alleviating or at least delaying the onset of some of these diseases. Elderly patients are being requested to exercise more, adjust dietary habits, and participate more frequently in social and group activities. Included in the preventive care plan are routine medical and sociologic health checks. These interactions with the health care system may help uncover previously undiagnosed illnesses and risk factors. The frequency of these evaluations must be determined by the patient's general health and ability to pay because most third-party reimbursement plans will not cover these expenses. It is also recommended that elderly patients be vaccinated against the influenza virus and pneumococcal pneumonia on a regularly scheduled basis.

As medicine's knowledge of physiologic changes that occur with aging and how these affect drug disposition increases (Table 48.1), so does the ability to better manage many of the chronic diseases of aging. Drug therapy in the aged, which in the past was mainly by trial and error, is becoming more precise as studies of drug pharmacokinetics become available (Table 48.2). However, when one considers that the elderly account for 25% of all drug expenditures and consume larger numbers of drugs per person than any other age group, there is still much that needs to be learned. The data that are available must also be viewed with caution for several reasons. Differences in study design and data evaluation often lead to conflicting results. Study designs may not take into account such differences as gender, smoking, or environment, which may have significant affects on drug disposition. Findings of increased serum concentrations of drugs do not explain what pharmacokinetic variables may be affected and thus offer little useful information. Most important, changes in pharmacokinetic parameters do not always fully account for altered responses in the elderly. This is evident with such drugs as narcotic analgesics, benzodiazepine anxiolytics and hypnotics, and beta-adrenergic blocking agents, where there is an increased pharmacologic effect as a result of increased sensitivity to the drugs.

Based on the uncertainty of drug disposition, drug effect,

TABLE 48.1   Physiologic Changes as Determinants of Drug Disposition in the Elderly

Effect	*Altered Physiology*	*Clinical Significance*
Absorption	Increased gastric pH	Rate of absorption: no change in time to peak
	Decreased gastrointestinal blood flow	Extent of absorption: no change in steady state
	Decreased active transport mechanisms	concentrations
Distribution	Body composition	Decreased volume of distribution of polar drugs
	Decreased total body water	Increased volume of distribution of nonpolar drugs
	Decreased lean body mass per kilogram body weight	
	Increased body fat	
	Decreased serum albumin	Increased free fraction of highly bound drugs
	Decreased red blood cell binding	
Metabolism	Decreased liver blood flow	Unclear: environmental factors may be more important
	Decreased liver size	portant
	Possible decreased enzymatic activity	
Excretion	Decreased glomerular filtration rate	Prolonged half-life and decreased clearance of renally eliminated drugs
	Decreased renal blood flow	nally eliminated drugs
	Decreased tubular function	

TABLE 48.2 Summary of Selected Studies of Altered Pharmacokinetics in the Elderly

Reference	Drug	Pharmacokinetic Change
21	Acetaminophen	Volume of distribution decreased Elimination half-life and clearance not significantly different
22	Acetaminophen	Elimination half-life prolonged Volume of distribution and clearance not significantly different
23	Amitriptyline	Plasma concentration increased
24	Aspirin	Elimination half-life prolonged Volume of distribution increased Clearance not significantly different
25	Aspirin	Metabolite concentrations increased Mean serum concentrations not significantly different
26	Atenolol	Total body clearance decreased Positive correlation with creatinine clearance Peak concentration and time to peak not significantly different
27	Atenolol	Clearance, volume of distribution, and elimination half-life not significantly different
28	Chlordiazepoxide	Elimination half-life prolonged Clearance decreased Volume of distribution increased
29	Cimetidine	Clearance decreased
30	Cimetidine	Clearance decreased
31	Desipramine	Plasma concentrations not significantly different
32	Desmethyldiazepam	Elimination half-life prolonged Clearance decreased Volume of distribution not significantly different
33	Diazepam	Elimination half-life prolonged Volume of distribution increased Clearance not significantly different
34	Digitoxin	Elimination half-life, clearance, and volume of distribution not significantly different
35	Digoxin	Plasma half-life prolonged Plasma clearance decreased Volume of distribution not significantly different
36	Diphenhydramine	Volume of distribution, elimination half-life, and clearance not significantly different
37	Flurazepam	Elimination half-life prolonged in elderly males only Steady state concentration increased in elderly males only
38	Furosemide	Volume of distribution increased Clearance decreased Elimination half-life rpolonged
39	Gentamicin	Mean clearance, volume of distribution, and elimination half-life not significantly different
40	Imipramine	Elimination half-life prolonged Clearance decreased
23	Imipramine	Plasma concentration increased
41	Lidocaine	Volume of distribution increased Elimination half-life increased Clearance not significantly different
42	Lithium	Clearance decreased
43	Lorazepam	Volume of distribution decreased Clearance decreased Elimination half-life not significantly different
44	Lorazepam	Volume of distribution, clearance, and elimination half-life not significantly different
45	Lorazepam	Free fraction increased Unbound volume of distribution increased Unbound clearance decreased
46	Meperidine	Unbound plasma concentration increased
47	Meperidine	Plasma concentration increased Red blood cell binding decreased

TABLE 48.2, cont'd

Reference	Drug	Pharmacokinetic Change
48	Meperidine	Clearance decreased
		Elimination half-life prolonged
		Volume of distribution not significantly different
49	Metoprolol	Volume of distribution, elimination half-life, and clearance not significantly different
50	Morphine	Volume of distribution decreased
		Elimination half-life prolonged
		Clearance decreased
51	Nortriptyline	Plasma concentration not significantly different
52	Oxazepam	Elimination half-life and clearance not significantly different
53	Penicillin	Elimination half-life increased
		Positive correlation to creatinine clearance
54	Penicillin	Serum concentration increased
55	Phenylbutazone	Elimination half-life not significantly different
22	Phenylbutazone	Elimination half-life and volume of distribution not significantly different
56	Phenytoin	Percentage unbound drug increased
57	Phenytoin	Maximum rate of metabolism decreased
		Plasma concentration at which rate of metabolism is one half of the maximum not significantly different
58	Phenytoin	Protein binding decreased
		Clearance increased
59	Prazepam (desmethyldiazepam)	Volume of distribution increased
		Elimination half-life prolonged in elderly males
		Clearance decreased in elderly males
60	Procainamide	Clearance decreased
		Positive correlation to creatinine clearance
61	Propoxyphene	Elimination half-life not significantly different
26	Propranolol	Peak concentration, time to peak, and clearance not significantly different
62	Propranolol	Plasma concentration increased
63	Propranolol	Clearance decreased
		Elimination half-life prolonged
		Plasma concentration increased
64	Propranolol	Steady state plasma concentration increased
		Elimination half-life prolonged
		Clearance and volume of distribution not significantly different
65	Quinidine	Elimination half-life prolonged
		Clearance decreased
66	Sulfisoxazole	Plasma half-life prolonged
		Clearance decreased
		Positive association with creatinine clearance
		Volume of distribution not significantly different
67	Temazepam	Elimination half-life, volume of distribution, and clearance not significantly different
68	Tetracycline	Serum concentration increased
69	Theophylline	Elimination half-life, volume of distribution, and clearance not significantly different
70	Theophylline	Clearance not significantly different
71	Theophylline	Clearance, elimination half-life, and volume of distribution not significantly different
72	Tolbutamide	Unbound fraction increased in vitro
73	Warfarin	Elimination half-life, clearance, and volume of distribution not significantly different
74	Warfarin	Binding capacity decreased in vitro

and potential for adverse effects with increasing numbers of drugs consumed, guidelines need to be established to assure proper drug utilization. These guidelines should include the following:

1. Whenever possible, drug therapy should be based on a conclusive diagnosis. Often little documentation or history is available to determine why medications may be prescribed.

2. Drugs should be prescribed only when necessary. Society's view that medicine has a pill for every problem can have devastating effects on an elderly patient. Appropriate counseling by health care providers is exceedingly important.

3. Before the prescription of a drug, a thorough drug history should be obtained.

4. The individual responsible for monitoring drug therapy should have a thorough knowledge of drug pharmacology and how the previously mentioned physiologic changes that occur with aging may affect that drug's disposition.

5. Drug therapy should be initiated at low doses and increased gradually. The most significant change affecting drug therapy is the decrease in glomerular filtration rate with age, and thus renally excreted drugs may accumulate without proper dosage adjustments. Decreases in liver enzymatic activity and the affect this has on drug metabolism are not as certain.

6. Drug therapy can produce adverse effects. Symptoms such as confusion, lethargy, or depression may be caused by drugs and, if they appear, should not be considered as the inevitable consequences of aging.

7. Drug regimens should be simplified as much as possible. Noncompliance is well known to be a significant component of drug taking behavior in the elderly.

8. Pharmacokinetic services should be used to monitor serum drug concentrations. The uncertainties of how much renal or hepatic function is lost in an elderly patient can be overcome by appropriate therapeutic drug monitoring.

9. Adequate explanation should be given to elderly patients concerning why and how to take medications. These instructions should be continually reinforced by health care providers.

10. Compliance should be evaluated. Communication between health care providers concerning drug consumption is imperative for appropriate therapy.

11. Drug regimens should be continually evaluated to remove any unnecessary medications.

As in all other patients, a logical and organized treatment plan for drug therapy can prevent many problems from occurring in the elderly population and can produce a much more effective outcome.

EXTRAORDINARY CARE: ETHICAL CONSIDERATIONS IN LONG-TERM CARE

Society is just beginning to exert influence over medical care in patient responsibilities and rights. Many legislative bodies are being requested to pass into law the right of the patient to deny heroic measures to maintain life. Individuals in the health care system are also beginning to look at the ethics involved in the high technology of medicine. In no group of people is this dilemma more relevant than in the elderly. The focus of this controversy has centered on the acutely ill, hospitalized elderly patient, where the severity and rapid progression of the disease may dominate all decisions. The focus is shifting to the nursing home where the chronic nature of the diseases may not be as rapidly progressive but is no less devastating. Also, some degree of dementia is so common among nursing home residents that it may render the patient unable to participate in decisions concerning quality of life.

The ethical consideration usually centers on whether a disease or illness should be treated in a patient where successful treatment will not improve quality of life and may actually prolong suffering. The same holds true in the case of costly or invasive diagnostic tests where the results of the tests will not affect the therapy or outcome in any way.

The decision to withold commonly accepted treatments in incurable or critically ill nursing home residents requires ongoing communication among the physician, family, and patient, if possible. Decisions to withhold treatment should be made in advance and continually assessed as the patient's condition changes. All members of the health care team caring for the patient should be made aware of what decisions have been made and how they may possibly influence or be influenced by the decision. Finally, the decision must be made with the best interest of the patient in mind and should not be absolute, especially if the treatment, although not life prolonging, may increase the patient's comfort.

OPPORTUNITIES FOR PHARMACISTS IN GERIATRICS

The opportunities for pharmacists to influence the care of elderly patients are unlimited. The only federally mandated use of clinical pharmacy services involves drug regimen reviews in long-term care facilities, the majority of which are nursing homes. For pharmacists to be able to meet the challenges inherent in these opportunities, they must receive adequate training, both academically and experientially. Colleges of pharmacy must incorporate geriatrics into their curriculums and should require all students at least to be exposed to nursing homes on a clerkship basis. Geriatrics must also become a viable research area for pharmacists, especially basic pharmacokinetic and pharmacology studies and clinical drug use. Postgraduate experiences must be developed in geriatrics. The American Society of Consultant Pharmacists and the American Society of Hospital Pharmacists have been instrumental in helping to initiate programs of this type. Finally, the attitudes of pharmacists, as those of society in general, must change to understand that institutionalization and the loss of intelligence are not inevitable consequences of aging. This can only be accomplished by adequate education and the opportunity for interaction.

REFERENCES

1. US Bureau of the Census: *Prospective Trends in the Size and Structure of the Elderly Population, Impact of Mortality Trends, and Some Implications.* Washington, DC, Current Population Reports, 1979, Series P-23, No. 78.
2. US Bureau of the Census: *Demographic Aspects of Aging and the Older Population in the United States.* Washington, DC, Current Population Reports, 1976, Series P-23, No. 59.

3. Lowenstein SR, Schrier RW: Social and political aspects of aging. In Schrier RW, (ed): *Clinical Internal Medicine in the Aged*. Philadelphia, WB Saunders, 1982, p 2.

4. Dames PE, Kerr MR: Gerontology and geriatrics in medical education. *N Engl J Med* 300:228-232, 1979.

5. Federal Council on Aging: *Public Policy and the Frail Elderly. A Staff Report*. Washington, DC, Department of Health and Human Services, 1978, DHHS Publication No. (OHDS) 79-20959.

6. National Center for Health Statistics: *Health, United States*. Washington, DC, US Department of Health and Human Services, 1980, DHHS Publication No. (PHS) 81-1232.

7. US Bureau of the Census: *Social and Economic Characteristics of the Older Population*. Washington, DC, Current Population Reports, 1979, Series P-23, No. 85.

8. Finch CE, Hayflick L: *Handbook of the Biology of Aging*. New York, Van Nostrand Reinhold, 1977.

9. Cape RTD, Coe RM, Rossman I: *Fundamentals of Geriatric Medicine*. New York, Raven Press, 1983.

10. Butler RN: The doctor and the aged patient. *Hosp Pract* 13(3):99-106, 1979.

11. National Center for Health Statistics. *Utilization of Short-Stay Hospitals, Annual Survey of the United States 1978*. Washington, DC, Department of Health and Human Services, 1980, DHHS Publication No. (PHS) 80-1797.

12. Campion EW, Bang A, May MI: Why acute care hospitals must undertake long term care. *N Engl J Med* 308:71-75, 1983.

13. Kane RL, Kane RA: Care of the aged. Old problems in need of new solutions. *Science* 200:913-919, 1978.

14. Vicente L, Wiley JA, Carrington RA: The risk of institutionalization before death. *Gerontologist* 19:361-366, 1979.

15. Federal Council on Aging: *The Need for Long Term Care: Information and Issues*. Washington, DC, Department of Health and Human Services, 1981, DHHS Publication No. (OHDS) 81-20704.

16. Mose DN, Sawyer D: *Medicare and Medicaid Data Book, 1981*. Washington, DC, Department of Health and Human Services, 1982, DDHS Publication No. (HCFA) 82-03128.

17. Kane RL, Kane RA: A guide through the maze of long term care. *West J Med* 135:503-510, 1981.

18. Gibson RM, Waldo DR: National Health Expenditure, 1980. *Health Care Financ Rev* 3(1):1-54, 1981.

19. Vital & Health Statistics: *The National Nursing Home Survey: 1977 Summary for the United States*. Hyattsville, MD, Department of Health and Human Services, 1979, DHHS Publication No. (PHS) 79-1794.

20. Administration on Aging: *Facts about Older Americans, 1979*. Washington, DC, Department of Health and Human Services, 1980, DDHS Publication No. 80-20006.

21. Divoll M, Abernethy DR, Ameer B, Greenblatt DJ: Acetaminophen kinetics in the elderly. *Clin Pharmacol Ther* 31:751-756, 1982.

22. Triggs EJ, Nation RL, Long A, Ashley JJ: Pharmacokinetics in the elderly. *Eur J Clin Pharmocol* 8:55-62, 1975.

23. Nies A: Relationship between age and tricyclic antidepressant plasma levels. *Am J Psychiatry* 134:790-793, 1977.

24. Cuny G, Royer RJ, Mur JM, Serot JM, Faure G, Netter P, Maillard A, Penin F: Pharmacokinetics of salicylates in the elderly. *Gerontology* 25:49-55, 1981.

25. Montgomery PR, Sitar DS: Increased serum salicylate metabolites with age in patients receiving chronic acetylsalicylic acid therapy. *Gerontology* 27:329-333, 1981.

26. Barber HE, Hawksworth GM, Petrie JC, Rigby JW, Robb OJ, Scott AK: Pharmacokinetics of atenolol and propranolol in young and elderly subjects. *Brit J Clin Pharmacol* 11:118P-119P, 1981.

27. Robin PC, Scott PJW, Micheau K, Pearson A, Ross D, Reid JL: Atenolol disposition in young and elderly subjects (letter). *Brit J Clin Pharmacol* 13:235-237, 1982.

28. Roberts RK, Wilkinson GR, Branch RA, Schenker S: Effect of age and cirrhosis on the disposition of elimination of chlordiazepoxide. *Gastroenterology* 75:479-485, 1978.

29. Drayer DE, Romankiewicz J, Lorenzo B, Reidenberg MM: Age and renal clearance of cimetidine. *Clin Pharmacol Ther* 31:45-50, 1982.

30. Gugler R, Somogyi A: Reduced cimetidine clearance with age (letter). *N Engl J Med* 301:435, 1979.

31. Cutler NR, Zavadil AP, Eisdorfer C, Ross RJ, Potter WZ: Concentrations of despiramine in elderly women. *Am J Psychiatry* 138:1235-1237, 1981.

32. Klotz U, Miller-Seyolitz P: Altered elimination of desmethyldiazepam in the elderly (letter). *Br J Clin Pharmacol* 7:119-120, 1979.

33. Klotz U, Avant GR, Hoyumpa A, Schenker S, Wilkinson GR: The effects of age and liver disease on the disposition and elimination of diazepam in adult man. *J Clin Invest* 55:347-359, 1975.

34. Donovan MA, Castleden CM, Pohl JEF, Kraft CA: The effect of age on digitoxin pharmacokinetics. *Br J Clin Pharmacol* 11:401-402, 1981.

35. Cusack B, Kelly J, O'Malley K, Noel J, Lavan J, Horgam J: Digoxin in the elderly: Pharmacokinetic consequences of old age. *Clin Pharmacol Ther* 25:772-776, 1979.

36. Berlinger WG, Goldberg MJ, Spector R, Chiang CK, Ghoneim MM: Diphenhydramine: Kinetics and psychomotor effects in elderly women. *Clin Pharmacol Ther* 32:387-391, 1982.

37. Greenblatt DJ, Divoll M, Harmatz JS, MacLaughlin DS, Shader RI: Kinetics and clinical effects of flurazepam in young and elderly non-insomniacs. *Clin Pharmacol Ther* 30:475-486, 1981.

38. Kerremans ALM, Tan Y, VanBaars H, Van Ginneken CAM, Gribnau FWJ: Furosemide kinetics and dynamics in aged patients. *Clin Pharmacol Ther* 34:181-189, 1983.

39. Bauer LA, Blouin RA: Gentamicin pharmacokinetics: Effect of aging in patients with normal renal function. *J Am Ger Soc* 30:309-311, 1982.

40. Hrdina PD, Rovei V, Henry JF, Hervy MP, Gomeni R, Forette F, Morselli PL: Comparison of single dose pharmacokinetics of imipramine and maprotiline in the elderly. *Psychopharmacology* 70:29-34, 1980.

41. Nation RL, Triggs EJ: Lignocaine kinetics in cardiac patients and aged subjects. *Br J Clin Pharmacol* 4:439-448, 1977.

42. Hewick DDS, Newbury PA, Hopwood S: Age as a factor in lithium therapy. *Br J Clin Pharmacol* 4:201-205, 1977.

43. Greenblatt DJ, Allen MD, Locniskar A, Harmatz JS, Shader RI: Lorazepam kinetics in the elderly. *Clin Pharmacol Ther* 26:103-113, 1979.

44. Kraus JW, Desmond PV, Marshal JP, Johnson BS, Schenker S, Wilkinson GR: Effects of aging and liver disease on disposition of lorazepam. *Clin Pharmacol Ther* 24:411-419, 1978.

45. Divoll M, Greenblatt DJ: Effect of age and sex on lorazepam protein binding. *J Pharm Pharmacol* 34:122-123, 1982.

46. Mather LE, Tucker GT, Pflug AE, Lindop MJ, Wilkerson C: Meperidine kinetics in man. Intravenous injection in surgical patients and volunteers. *Clin Pharmacol Ther* 17:21-30, 1975.

47. Chan K, Kendall MJ, Mitchard M, Wells WDE, Vickers MD: The effect of aging on plasma pethidine concentrations. *Br J Clin Pharmacol* 2:297-302, 1975.

48. Holmberg L, Odar-Cederlof I, Boreus LO, Heyner L, Ehrnebo M: Comparative disposition of pethidine and norpethidine in old and young patients. *Eur J Clin Pharmacol* 22:175-179, 1982.

49. Lundborg P, Regardh CG, Landahl S: The pharmacokinetics of metaprolol in healthy elderly individuals (abstract). *Clin Pharmacol Ther* 31:246, 1982.

50. Owen JA, Sitar DS, Berger L, Brownell LB, Duke PC, Mitenko PA: Age related morphine kinetics. *Clin Pharmacol Ther* 34:364-368, 1983.

51. Montgomery S, Braithwaite R, Dawling S, McAuley R: High plasma nortriptyline levels in the treatment of depression. *Clin Pharmacol Ther* 23:309-314, 1978.

52. Shull HJ, Wilkinson GR, Johnson R, Schenker S: Normal disposition of oxazepam in acute viral hepatitis and cirrhosis. *Ann Intern Med* 84:420-425, 1976.

53. Kampmann J, Molholm-Hansen J, Siesbaek-Nielsen L, Laursen H: Effect of some drugs on penicillin half-life in blood. *Clin Pharmacol Ther* 13:516-519, 1972.

54. Leikola E, Vartia KO: On penicillin levels in young and geriatric subjects. *J Gerontol* 12:48-52, 1957.

55. O'Malley K, Crooks J, Duke E, Stevenson IH: Effect of age and sex on human drug metabolism. *Br Med J* 3:607-609, 1971.

56. Patterson M, Heazelwood R, Smithurst B, Eadie MJ: Plasma protein binding of phenytoin in the aged: In vivo studies. *Br J Clin Pharmacol* 13:423-425, 1982.

57. Bauer LA, Blovin RA: Age and phenytoin kinetics in adult epileptics. *Clin Pharmacol Ther* 31:301-304, 1982.

58. Hayes MJ, Langmann MJS, Short AH: Changes in drug metabolism with increasing age. 2. Phenytoin clearance and protein binding. *Br J Clin Pharmacol* 2:73-79, 1975.

59. Allen MD, Greenblatt DJ, Harmatz JS, Shader RI: Desmethyldiazepam kinetics in the elderly after oral prazepam. *Clin Pharmacol Ther* 20:196-202, 1980.

60. Reidenberg MM, Camacho M, Kloger J, Drayer DE: Aging and renal clearance of procainamide and acetylprocainamide. *Clin Pharmacol Ther* 28:732-735, 1980.
61. Melander A, Bodin NO, Danielson K, Gustalsson B, Haglund G, Westerlund D: Absorption and elimination of d-propoxyphene, acetyl salicylic acid and phenazone in a combination tablet (Doleron): Comparison between young and elderly subjects. *Acta Med Scand* 203:121-124, 1978.
62. Castleden CM, Kaye CM, Parsons RL: The effect of age on plasma levels of propranolol and practolol in man. *Br J Clin Pharmacol* 2:303-306, 1975.
63. Castleden CM, George CF: The effect of aging on the hepatic clearance of propranolol. *Br J Clin Pharmacol* 7:49-54, 1979.
64. Vestal RE, Wood AJJ, Branch RA, Shand DG, Wilkinson GR: Effects of age and cigarette smoking on propranolol disposition. *Clin Pharmacol Ther* 26:8-15, 1979.
65. Ochs HR, Greenblatt DJ, Woo E, Smith TW: Reduced quinidine clearance in elderly persons. *Am J Cardiol* 42:481-485, 1978.
66. Boisvert A, Barbeau G, Belanger PM: Pharmacokinetics of sulfisoxazole in young and elderly subjects. *Gerontology* 30:125-131, 1984.
67. Divoll M, Greenblatt DJ, Harmatz JS, Shader RI: Effect of age and gender on disposition of temazepam. *J Pharm Sci* 70:1104-1107, 1981.
68. Vartia KO, Leikola E: Serum levels of antibiotics in young and old subjects following administration of dihydrostreptomycin and tetracycline. *J Gerontol* 15:392-394, 1960.
69. Antal EJ, Kramer PA, Mercik SA, Chapron DJ, Lawson IR: Theophylline pharmacokinetics in advanced age. *Br J Clin Pharmacol* 12:637-645, 1981.
70. Bauer LA, Blouin RA: Influence of age on theophylline clearance in patients with chronic obstructive pulmonary disease. *Clin Pharmacokinetics* 6:469-474, 1981.
71. Blouin RA, Erwin WG, Foster TS, Scott S: Pharmacokinetics of theophylline in young and elderly subjects. *Gerontology* 28:323-327, 1982.
72. Adir J, Miller AK, Vestal RE: Effects of total plasma concentration and age on tolbutamide plasma protein binding. *Clin Pharmacol Ther* 31:488-493, 1982.
73. Shepard AMM, Hewick DS, Moreland TA, Steveson IH: Age as a determinant of sensitivity to warfarin. *Br J Clin Pharmacol* 4:315-320, 1977.
74. Hayes MJ, Langman MJS, Short AH: Changes in drug metabolism with increasing age: 1. Warfarin binding and plasma proteins. *Br J Clin Pharmacol* 2:69-72, 1975.

CHAPTER 49

Mental Health Pharmacy

GLEN L. STIMMEL and MICHAEL Z. WINCOR

During the first half of the 1970s, psychopharmacy practice developed into a well-defined clinical role model of direct patient care services. The term "psychopharmacy" is now the preferred term to refer to this area of practice, replacing the earlier terms "mental health pharmacy" and "psychiatric pharmacy practice." Practitioners in this area are most commonly called psychiatric pharmacists, and the American Society of Hospital Pharmacists Special Interest Group (ASHP SIG) on Psychopharmacy Practice recently proposed the term "clinical pharmacy specialist in psychiatry." The earlier terms "mental health pharmacist" and "psychopharmacist" have been abandoned. In this chapter we will describe why psychopharmacy services are needed, describe the development of such a service, describe organizational activities of psychiatric pharmacists, and detail the psychopharmacy training programs available.

THERE IS A NEED

The primary goal of clinical pharmacy services is to improve the quality and safety of patients' drug therapy. The independent emergence of virtually identical psychopharmacy practices in geographically distinct areas supports the view that in the early 1970s practitioners responded to such a need in mental health facilities. Several factors can be identified that have facilitated the development and implementation of clinical pharmacy services in mental health facilities. First, whereas most other medical specialties are practiced in large, urban, institutional facilities or private medical practices, much of mental health care is provided in smaller and more numerous facilities. Virtually every county of each state in the country has some type of mental health care system for ambulatory and hospital treatment. Second, because the public sector has adopted the concept of providing necessary mental health care, the burden of delivering appropriate care is great. The budgets of most mental health facilities are very limited. Mental health care must compete with public education, transportation, housing, welfare, and other health programs for public funds. One result of this reality is that much of mental health care is provided by a variety of disciplines, with the psychiatrist usually providing consultation and administrative support. Medication evaluation and maintenance may not be done by the psychiatrist, but by the patients' assigned therapist. The psychologist, social worker, nurse, or aide may often

be responsible for assessing the response to a medication or its adverse effects. This information is reported to the psychiatrist, who then writes or approves the order. Both the psychiatrist and therapists are usually not pleased with this system, but budgetary limitations prevent using psychiatrists for all medication assessment. Thus, this system points to a need for an available individual with drug therapy skills.

Third, the need for an available drug information source and consultant is greatest in mental health facilities. The majority of staff members are of nonmedically oriented disciplines, yet most patients are treated with medication. Psychiatrists and nurses constitute a minority of staff members in mental health facilities, being outnumbered by psychologists, psychiatric social workers, medical case workers, occupational therapists, recreational therapists, community workers, and aides. Because the latter group provides a significant amount of direct patient care, yet knows little about the drugs their patients are taking, the need is created for an available drug consultant.

For the three reasons just cited, psychiatric pharmacists are used for their direct patient care capabilities and contributions relative to psychotropic drug therapy. For the same reasons, the potential for full implementation of clinical psychopharmacy practice in mental health facilities also exists.

Recognition of the need for a clinical pharmacy specialist in psychiatry is not limited to our profession alone. Physician acceptance has been excellent in the many facilities where pharmacists have initiated clinical services. Pharmacists experience resistance only when they attempt to implement services independent of the team approach to patient care that is the standard of practice in psychiatric institutions. Acceptance by other staff is characteristically positive because the pharmacist represents an available source of information and consultation for drug therapy concerns. Patient acceptance is also uniformly good. Most patients appreciate the availability of the pharmacist to answer questions and counsel them regarding their medication.

A final aspect of the recognition of need is the legislative and regulatory activities concerning the use of psychotropic drugs. In the 1970s there was the peak of public concern about psychotropic drug misuse, and evidence of these concerns still exists now. News reports and newspaper headlines regularly continue to be seen that report on patient deaths

---

VOLUNTARY PATIENT'S CONSENT TO SPECIFIED MEDICATIONS

Please read this form carefully. If you have problems reading it, ask to have it read to you. There is also a Spanish version.

Dr. _____ met with me and we talked about the following items:
(Please Print)

We discussed my mental problems. The doctor told me of medications which are known to be of help in treating mental problems such as mine. The doctor also discussed with me the likelihood of my improving or not improving without such medication(s). I understand that in agreeing to take medication(s) that I may participate in other forms of treatment.

The doctor told me that there are three major groups of medications used for serious mental problems and that the medication(s) I take will be from the group(s) checked below:

_____ Major Tranquilizers (neuroleptics)

_____ Lithium

_____ Anti-depressants

We also discussed the range of amount(s) and frequency of medication(s) including possible additional doses as needed (PRN), the method, and the probable duration of taking the medication(s).

He or she discussed with me the more common side effects that my particular medication(s) may cause, as well as side effects which may occur because of any physical conditions that I may have. If the doctor prescribed a major tranquilizer, he or she discussed with me a condition called "tardive dyskinesia", a possible side effect caused by major tranquilizers.

I understand that if I have any further questions or want to know more about my medication(s), I can ask the pharmacist, nursing staff, social workers, psychologists or doctors for further information.

I understand that I have the right to accept or to refuse medication(s) ordered for me by telling the doctor, the nursing staff, social workers, psychologists, etc., at any time.

I HAVE READ THIS FORM, I UNDERSTAND IT, AND I CONSENT TO TAKE THE MEDICATION(S) PRESCRIBED BY THE DOCTOR.

_____
Date and Time

_____
Patient's Signature

_____
Physician's Signature

_____
Date and Time

_____
Witness

NS-2027 (3/83)   ORIGINAL—CHART   CANARY—PATIENT

FIGURE 49.1 Informed consent to receive psychotherapeutic medications.

and the misuse of psychotropic medications in mental health facilities, or report on the irreversible consequences of long-term drug use such as tardive dyskinesia and renal damage. The history of misuse and abuse of other psychiatric treatments (psychosurgery, electroshock therapy) in the public mind now includes psychotropic drugs. Some states have enacted legislation to limit psychosurgery and electroconvulsive therapy, and several states have enacted legislation restricting psychotropic drug use. Legislation and regulations in California can serve as examples of how this public concern can be channeled into constructive efforts to improve patients' drug therapy and that includes pharmacists.

In 1978, Assembly Bill 3644 (Chapter 1393, 1978 statutes) was passed, which mandates an ongoing medication monitoring system as part of the quality assurance program of California's public mental health facilities. This legislation resulted from 2 years of investigation by the Department of Health and legislative hearings on the alleged misuse and abuse of psychotropic drugs in mental health facilities. The more radical patient advocacy groups argued that psychotropic drugs should be severely restricted in use because they only control behavior and damage the brain, whereas physicians' groups argued they are not misusing drugs. Testimony by clinical pharmacists acknowledged that misuse does occur, but the solution can be found in assuring adequate monitoring of drug therapy on a continuing basis. The latter argument was accepted and incorporated into AB3644. A continuous medication monitoring system is mandated, "including procedures to review the appropriateness of the medications prescribed, the effectiveness of the medications for the client, the occurrence of any adverse effects, the extent of patient compliance, and the level of patient information and ability to manage his own medication regimen." Such monitoring "is to be carried out by, be in conjunction with, or be under the supervision of, a person licensed to prescribe or dispense prescription drugs." This legislation, which contains an excellent description of clinical pharmacy services (drug therapy monitoring, patient education), was directly responsible for the creation of full-time positions for psychiatric pharmacists within several county mental health centers, and part-time consultative positions for pharmacists in their local mental health facilities (1).

In 1980, the California Department of Mental Health established regulations mandating that voluntary patients in inpatient psychiatric settings give informed consent before receiving psychotherapeutic agents. The drugs included are neuroleptics, antidepressants, and lithium. The areas that the physician is required to discuss with the patient include the nature of the particular mental disorder; the nature of the medications to be prescribed; the likelihood of improving with or without the medications; alternative treatments; the dosage range, frequency of dosing (including prn orders), route of administration, and probable duration of treatment; the common short-term side effects, as well as any particular side effects expected because of concurrent physical conditions; possible longer term side effects (in particular, tardive dyskinesia with the neuroleptics); and that alternative treatments will not be withheld if the patient refuses medications. The patient must also be informed that medication can be refused at any point in the course of treatment by

simply telling any member of the treatment team. A sample form that the patient signs following such a discussion is shown in Figure 49.1. Again, this regulation, although initially identifying the physician as the provider of information, has provided an opportunity for pharmacists to initiate or expand their existing patient education activities. Indeed, one wonders if the pharmacist who dispenses psychotherapeutic agents would not be legally liable to be certain first that the patient has given informed consent. One of the authors (M.Z.W.) designed a form for an inpatient psychiatric unit that included an extra copy of the informed consent form; this was to be sent directly to the pharmacy department and kept with the patient's drug profile and monitoring paperwork. States other than California have established similar regulations; other states have considered and are considering extending the regulations to include both voluntary and involuntary patients. And it would not be at all surprising if, at some point, such regulations include all patients—both inpatients and outpatients—who receive psychotherapeutic agents.

DEVELOPMENT OF A PSYCHOPHARMACY SERVICE

The purpose of this section is to describe the step-by-step development of a psychopharmacy service. Much of this discussion is based on the personal experience of one of the authors (M.Z.W.) in developing such a service in a 55-bed mental health unit (with an average census of 35) within a 566-bed private medical center. In addition to specific activities and ideas related to this one setting, general comments are offered for extrapolation to other settings and other conditions. For other descriptions of such services, the reader is referred to Coleman et al (2), Kohan et al (3), Ellenor and Frisk (4), Parks (5), Stimmel (6), and Kubica and Gousse (7).

Before describing the three-phase development of a service, three basic ingredients for success should be mentioned. These are (1) the availability of a knowledgeable and skilled psychiatric pharmacist; (2) administrative support; and (3) optimal use of educational and marketing techniques.

Availability implies physical presence; without it, the impact is significantly reduced. Knowledge and skill, combined with some degree of diplomacy, can result in the rapid development of respect for the psychiatric pharmacist by all members of the multidisciplinary team. Administrative support must come from the pharmacy and/or the hospital administration. Without it the service cannot even begin to develop. Initially, the administration, as with any new program, must be willing to take a risk, directing more staff time into the service than can be justified on the basis of current distributive and/or clinical needs. The pharmacist may also have to invest more time than his or her basic 40-hour week. Finally, education and marketing may be more important than either of the other two basic ingredients. The current state of affairs is not one in which every psychiatric unit is searching for a psychiatric pharmacist; therefore, the administration as well as each member of the multidisciplinary team must be educated regarding and "sold" the notion of pharmacist involvement.

Phase I—Setting the Foundation

Initially, one must assess baseline strengths and weaknesses within the existing system. Needs must be identified. At the same time, the practitioner must have some clear idea of what the service should ideally look like for the specific site. This practitioner-specific and site-specific endpoint may change over time, but at least there is an initial endpoint toward which to strive. This initial assessment of needs may involve a number of activities in the first few weeks. Formal and informal meetings with members of other disciplines must take place to identify their perceived needs, as well as to educate them regarding the training, capabilities, and interests of a psychiatric pharmacist. Such meetings would include the medical director and other attending psychiatrists, clinical psychologists, social workers, the nursing supervisor and other members of the nursing staff, and members of the adjunctive therapies department. At this point, power sources and decision-making groups must be identified; the development of a service is not only a professional but is also a highly political affair.

One should pay attention to the existing distribution system. Will the pharmacist be involved to some degree with distributive services? If so, does the existing distribution system add to the development of a clinical service or detract from it? What type of distribution system would be of greatest potential benefit to a developing clinical service?

It may be of major benefit to assess prescribing patterns in this initial phase. This requires that the pharmacist collect data while having as little impact on prescribing as possible. Questions must be asked that can be answered quantitatively. For instance, one can look at what drug categories are being used in treating each of the major psychiatric disorders. Dosage ranges can be assessed. Are anticholinergics being used prophylactically with neuroleptics? How frequently are anticonvulsant levels being drawn, and, if subtherapeutic, are there corresponding changes in dosage? A number of questions can be asked regarding lithium: (1) How frequently are baseline laboratory parameters being ordered before initiating treatment? (2) How frequently are levels drawn following initiation of treatment or any dosage change? (3) How frequently do patients reach toxic levels? (4) How frequently do patients remain at subtherapeutic levels for more than ten days? (5) How often is a neuroleptic tapered once a patient has a therapeutic level and is showing a clinical response?

It is advantageous to collect data on prescribing patterns and needs as quantitatively as possible. This not only provides a clear idea of one's starting point, but also allows for easier measurement later of the impact of psychopharmacy intervention.

Once the assessment of needs has been completed and marketing is under way, the pharmacist can set priorities. These priorities should be based on degree of need, estimated time required and time available, and, of course, the individual practitioner's own interests.

Phase II—Intervention and Evaluation

The bulk of the active developmental work occurs in this phase. This is a multifaceted phase in which a number of activities occur in parallel. With needs assessed and priorities set, it is ideal if interventions can be designed in a way that their impact can later be evaluated quantitatively. Although development of a service may involve marketing and politics, quantitative measures can accomplish considerably more than anecdotes.

If prescribing patterns have been assessed, as described above, the findings may be presented formally to the Department of Psychiatry. They can be presented as general trends and compared with current standards of practice with reference to the psychiatric literature. This may accomplish several goals. First, it provides the attending psychiatrists an opportunity to see how drugs are being used in general. Second, it provides an educational experience with respect to current standards of practice. Third, it provides an excellent forum in which the pharmacist can demonstrate his or her knowledge of psychopharmacology, scientific approach, and tact. Finally, it can be a major step toward developing genuine professional respect for the psychiatric pharmacist as a member of the treatment team.

Presentation of this type of data may generate such concern over specific prescribing patterns that the pharmacist may become involved in the formal establishment of appropriate interventions. Such was the case with lithium use in one institution. Hospital-wide guidelines were written, approved by the Department of Psychiatry and the Pharmacy and Therapeutics Committee, and established as official hospital policy. A copy of these guidelines is shown in Figure 49.2. In addition to such guidelines, written and/or verbal reminders to physicians constitute the intervention. Evaluation of impact then involves simply collecting data similar to the initial data and statistically analyzing for changes between before- and after-intervention data.

A variety of clinical services can be provided during this second phase of the developmental process. One might expect that a clinically oriented pharmacist would complete a basic workup for every patient admitted to the hospital. Such a workup would include age, sex, height, and weight; psychiatric diagnoses; medical diagnoses; a brief history of present illness; information on past psychiatric hospitalization, treatments, and responses to treatment; names of attending psychiatrist and consultants; and a brief drug history including information on medication taken before admission, past psychotherapeutic agents used, use of street drugs, tobacco, alcohol, and caffeine, allergies, adverse and therapeutic effects, and degree of compliance. All of this information, along with a drug profile, can aid the pharmacist in assuring appropriate drug therapy and optimizing recommendations.

The drug profile is a continually running record of all drugs ordered in the hospital. Ideally, this drug profile is an integral part of a unit dose distribution system. If such a system does not already exist, the pharmacist, again, can design and implement the system in such a way that the impact can later be measured in terms of medication errors, cost savings, etc. With such a distribution system, including a satellite within the patient care area, the pharmacist is physically present and available to provide clinical services formally and informally. Assignment of an experienced technician to the satellite also helps because it can free up considerable time for pharmacist involvement in clinical activities. If no such technician exists, it may be very worth-

---

LITHIUM PROTOCOL

Approved by Psychiatric Subcommittee
Approved by P&T Committee

I. MANDATORY PROCEDURES

A. Baseline Data

The following baseline data must be ordered or assessed prior to initiation of lithium:

1. BUN
2. Serum creatinine
3. Urinalysis with specific gravity
4. Electrolytes
5. Thyroid function studies (T3, T4, TSH)
6. CBC with differential
7. Cardiovascular status

In the case of the first six parameters, the samples (blood or urine) must be collected before the first dose of lithium; results need not be available, however, before starting the drug.

Cardiovascular work-up consists of (1) a physical examination for patients under age 40 or (2) an electrocardiogram for patients 40 years of age or older or any patient with a history or evidence by physical exam of cardiovascular disease.

B. Lithium Levels

Lithium levels must be obtained within the following guidelines:

1. Upon admission, if the patient had previously been receiving lithium.
2. Within 5 days of initiating lithium treatment.
3. Within 5 days of any change in dosage.
4. At least once weekly until steady state plasma level, at the desired end point, is achieved.

II. RECOMMENDED DOCUMENTATION

The physician is strongly encouraged to provide adequate documentation in the progress notes regarding:

1. Clinical response (i.e., observed changes in symptomatology).
2. Adverse effects, including significance and any actions taken.
3. Point at which desired steady state level is achieved in the patient.

III. OPTIONAL SERVICE—"Lithium Flow Sheet"

The physician may request, by chart order, that the psychopharmacist place a "lithium flow sheet" (includes dose ordered, dose ingested, lithium levels) in the chart and update it on a daily basis.

FIGURE 49.2 Lithium guidelines.

---

while in the long run to invest the time and energy required to train someone. The drug profile in such a system can be used for monitoring, unit dosing, and billing.

Each patient's drug therapy can be monitored by the pharmacist and priorities can be set in regard to which patients require the greatest attention. Review of the drug profile enables the pharmacist to identify drug-drug interactions, questionable doses of drugs, instances of polypharmacy, and inconsistencies between the amount of drug ordered and the amount administered (as reflected by the amount remaining in the patient's medication bin at the time of unit dosing, as well as entries in the nursing medication administration record). With a satellite in the patient care area, the pharmacist can immediately discuss possible problems with the medication nurse. Therapeutic and adverse effects are monitored primarily through direct interaction with the patient. A list of target symptoms—the patient's specific symptoms expected to respond to drug therapy—is generated by the pharmacist and followed through the course of treatment.

As part of drug therapy monitoring, the pharmacist may attend and participate in rounds, community meetings, and nursing reports. Individual discussions regarding patients may become common with other members of the treatment team. These activities not only provide the pharmacist with patient information but also educate members of the other disciplines.

Other clinical activities in which the pharmacist may become involved include (1) providing drug information to members of the various disciplines; (2) new drug reviews for the Pharmacy and Therapeutics Committee with recommendations regarding formulary considerations; (3) in-service presentations to the psychiatric staff as well as the nonmedical staff; (4) teaching and role modeling for pharmacy students who can be integrated into the clinical service; and (5) research along the lines of drug utilization review, pharmacy impact, or clinical drug studies.

A number of formal clinical services may be offered. These could include initial drug histories, medication counseling, discharge counseling, specialty groups such as a substance abuse group, lithium monitoring, pharmacokinetic consultations, and other miscellaneous consultations. In fact, with the agreement and under the supervision of a psychiatrist, the pharmacist may, in some settings, provide the primary pharmacologic treatment of a specified caseload. There are some good reasons to offer these types of services on the basis of chart-ordered requests by physicians. In some settings, particularly the private setting, the treating physician decides which services and consultants he or she wants for the patients. Patients without such orders are not neglected; in fact, for some, the pharmacist or some other member of the treatment team may want to recommend that an order be written. Another reason for chart-ordered requests is that the pharmacist is then seen as a consultant and has a means of documenting the work and input in the patient's medical record. Saving copies of these orders is a simple way of collecting data regarding demand for services and provides a quantitative measure of what the psychiatric pharmacist is doing with his or her time. A final reason for formal requests is that services provided may then have a greater potential for reimbursement.

An initial drug history, if offered, should be completed within 24-48 hours after admission. Based on data obtained from interviewing the patient, review of past medical records, and, at times, telephone contact with relatives or others, it should be as complete an account as possible of the patient's current and past use of medications—both prescription and nonprescription agents. In psychiatry, the history of past response to psychotherapeutic agents is a major factor in drug selection. Sometimes in the initial drug history current nonpsychotherapeutic agents are first identified (e.g., antihypertensives, thyroid products). For each drug identified, the dose, regimen, duration of use, and perceived therapeutic and adverse effects are noted. An assessment is made of tobacco, caffeine, alcohol, and street drug use. At times, a drug-induced psychiatric disorder may be identified or a possible drug-withdrawal syndrome may be foreseen. Allergy information is elicited and an assessment is made as to whether the patient is describing a true allergy; if not, the patient is educated. An assessment should be made of

PROGRESS RECORD

PATIENT DRUG HISTORY

Date	Note Progress of Case, Complications, Consultations, Change in Diagnosis, Condition on Discharge, Instructions to Patients
	ALLERGIES AND ADVERSE EFFECTS
	PRESCRIPTION MEDICATIONS — Start — Stop
	NONPRESCRIPTION DRUGS (Used Regularly)
	No — Yes
	Analgesics ____ ____
	Antacids ____ ____
	Laxatives ____ ____
	Cold Preps ____ ____
	Sleep Aids ____ ____
	Skin Products ____ ____
	Hemorrhoidal Preps ____ ____
	Diet Preps ____ ____
	Tobacco ____ ____
	Caffeine ____ ____
	Alcohol ____ ____
	Street Drugs ____ ____
	Other ____ ____
	COMMENTS

FIGURE 49.3 Standard form for reporting findings of initial drug history.

the patient's compliance with prescribed regimens; this will be important with regard to follow-up with medication counseling, discharge counseling, and perhaps even posthospital placement. Finally, as with any data obtained primarily from the patient, a note should be included regarding his or her reliability as a historian. Because a great deal of information is collected and one would ideally want it presented in a concise and easily readable way, a standard form may be adopted for placement into the chart. One example of such a standard format may be seen in Figure 49.3.

Medication counseling is provided relatively early in treatment. It may be provided on an individual basis or within a group setting (depending on the ward schedule, the number of patients requiring counseling, and the number of patients receiving similar medications). After assessing the patient's existing knowledge base, the pharmacist provides information regarding the nature of the medication, expected therapeutic effects, common adverse effects and how to deal with them, the probable course of treatment, special precautions and instructions, and the importance of compliance. In addition, an assessment is made of the patient's understanding of the information and the opportunity is provided for the patient to ask any questions then or in the future. Medication counseling is of particular importance in psychiatry for several reasons. First, the patient is given the opportunity to take some responsibility in his or her own treatment by understanding the medications. Second, society in general has moved toward increased patient education. And third, noncompliance is probably greatest in the psychiatric population; hence, the psychiatric pharmacist may have some impact on compliance.

Discharge counseling covers many of the same areas as initial medication counseling but at this point specific directions for taking the medications may be discussed. When possible, relatives should be involved in the session. Extra emphasis is placed on compliance. More information is provided regarding drug-drug, drug-alcohol, and drug-food interactions. Also, any special instructions may be given (e.g., importance and timing of lithium levels, initial signs of lithium toxicity, what to do once they are recognized).

Specialty groups may be developed as needs are identified. One such group could be a substance abuse group for patients with problems of substance abuse. The psychiatric pharmacist may have a recreational therapist, psychologist, social worker, or nurse as a co-leader to provide complementary skills and knowledge. The group can cover such topics as the pharmacology of the abused agents, medical and psychosocial sequelae, as well as reasons for becoming involved in and alternatives to substance abuse.

Lithium monitoring involves maintenance on a daily basis of a record of dose ordered, dose ingested, lithium levels, and comments regarding inconsistencies between the dose ordered and ingested, as well as observed therapeutic and adverse effects. In addition, notes are made regarding baseline parameters and lithium levels may be plotted in a graphic display of the treatment course. One example of a lithium flow sheet is given in Figure 49.4.

Miscellaneous consultations may include a variety of requests by both attending psychiatrists and internists. These may involve an assessment of possible adverse effects or treatment recommendations in particularly complicated cases. This type of consultation may require a great deal of time and energy in that an extensive patient interview may be required, past records need to be reviewed, a literature search may be necessary, and then the findings, assessment, and recommendations must be entered into the chart.

The final aspect of intervention within this second phase of development of the psychopharmacy service is that of availability and dialogue. This cannot be overemphasized. Ongoing dialogue between the pharmacist and others improves patient care. A final aspect of availability and involvement concerns the pharmacist's involvement in various policy making committees. Such committees may include the Pharmacy and Therapeutics Committee, Unit Management Committee, and others.

A number of interventions have now been described. Within this second phase of development there should be ongoing evaluation of the impact of psychopharmacy involvement. One can look at changes in prescribing patterns and changes in demand for service. In general, one simply needs to ask questions that can be answered relatively quantitatively.

Phase III—Continuation and Further Development

Assuming that the first two phases of the developmental process are successful, the next phase consists of the continuation and expansion of all existing services coupled with the further evaluation and development of new programs, as well as new ways of looking at old programs.

Justifying additional staff positions can be fairly straightforward when data on demand for service are being collected. By estimating times needed to provide various services, one can approximate the amount of time needed for a psychiatric pharmacist to meet the existing needs, as well as any projected needs. For example, the average time involved in completing a drug history (from the time of locating the patient to the point of entering the completed product into the chart) may be 30 minutes. Medication counseling and discharge counseling may require 20 minutes each if done on an individual basis. Each lithium flow sheet may require 15 minutes initially and then 5 minutes daily. The range of time required for more complicated clinical pharmacology consultations may be 90-120 minutes. Along these lines, time estimates can be attached to every activity (including distributive activities) in which the pharmacist is involved. The result is then a fairly clear indication of time and staff needs.

In expanding the service, one may decide to make rounds on a regular basis with the medical director, nursing supervisor, or others. There may be multidisciplinary treatment planning sessions to attend; especially in a private setting, where the private attending psychiatrist might not be able to attend every treatment planning session, the pharmacist is an ideal member of the team to provide the needed medical and pharmacologic input.

Evaluation is an ongoing process through this third phase of development. The impact of psychopharmacy services can be measured along various lines. The growth of demand for service can continue to be monitored. Other areas of interest, but somewhat difficult to measure, would be ques-

LITHIUM FLOW SHEET

Baseline Data

Parameter	Date	Result
BUN	____	____
Ser. Creat.	____	____
Spec. Grav.	____	____
'Lytes	____	____
Thyr. Fcn.	____	____
CBC	____	____
Cardiovasc.	____	____

Date	Lithium Ordered (mg/day)	Lithium Received (mg/day)	Plasma Lithium (mEq/L)	RBC Lithium (mEq/L)	RBC/Plasma Ratio (%)	Comments

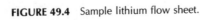

FIGURE 49.4 Sample lithium flow sheet.

tions of psychopharmacy impact on length of hospital stay, cost of drug treatment, medication compliance after discharge, and rehospitalization rate.

Finally, issues of reimbursement and cost justification must be addressed. Many services have the potential for generating revenue for the institution and/or the individual practitioner. However, with the current push toward cost containment, it may actually become more profitable for the psychiatric pharmacist and the institution to demonstrate how psychopharmacy involvement can decrease the length of a hospital stay, rehospitalization rates, and total drug costs (through simplification of drug treatments and regimens).

ORGANIZATIONAL ACTIVITIES

Psychiatric pharmacists were among the first pharmacy practice area groups to organize national meetings. In 1973, the First National Conference for Mental Health Pharmacists was held in Athens, Georgia. These national conferences were also held in 1974 and 1975. In these early years, practice models were compared, common problem areas identified, and a strong sense of identity developed among these psychiatric pharmacists. In 1974, the ASHP established an Advisory Panel on Pharmacy Services in Mental Health Facilities. When the ASHP SIG was established in 1975, the group chose to discontinue the National Conferences and channel all efforts through the SIG on Psychopharmacy Practice. Although initially limited to planning educational programing, the Psychopharmacy SIG began work on accreditation standards for psychopharmacy residency programs. With the completion of these activities in 1980, the SIG has more recently focused on developing standards of practice for psychiatric pharmacists, addressing the controversial issue of specialty recognition, and updating the residency accreditation standards.

TRAINING PROGRAMS

The early psychiatric pharmacists acquired their training through their own ingenuity and experience. Once a general, widely applicable role model was established, however, attention turned toward developing a specific psychopharmacy clerkship for pharmacy students and, eventually, a post-pharmacy degree residency in psychopharmacy practice.

Many schools of pharmacy offer a psychopharmacy clerkship, and in some schools it is required rather than elective. These clerkships are unique in that psychotropic drug therapy monitoring is less dependent on charted laboratory and physical findings; rather, extensive and frequent patient interviewing is necessary to assess changing mental status and to detect many of the adverse effects. The skills of extracting and assessing pertinent information from direct patient interaction are highly applicable to all health care settings and are needed for students in any type of future pharmacy practice. Students also develop skills in communicating with patients in such uncomfortable areas as suicide assessment, sexual problems, and substance abuse. Whereas such a clerkship is insufficient to train a psychiatric pharmacist, it provides a solid foundation for the pharmacist who wishes to pursue further training in the area. Until psychopharmacy residency programs become more numerous, these clerkships will serve as the training for many pharmacists who wish to pursue employment in mental health facilities.

The need for a specialized clinical pharmacy residency program in psychiatry became evident once jobs for psychiatric pharmacists became available. Many generalist clinical pharmacists found great difficulty in switching from a medical or surgical area to psychiatry. When a pharmacy satellite would open on the psychiatric ward, many directors of pharmacy found that the expected level of clinical services could not be provided by pharmacists transferred from medical areas. The result was that the transferred pharmacist would provide only distributive and drug information services; or after rotating three or four pharmacists through the area, one would be found who was motivated to develop some direct patient care services.

A clinical pharmacist can usually easily transfer from a medical ward to a surgical ward or to a cardiac care unit; the knowledge base required may be somewhat different, but the skills needed for monitoring drug therapy are essentially the same. The primary obstacle in psychiatry is that the vast majority of clinical skills needed are not developed in other areas of practice. These factors contributed to the search for pharmacists with specific clinical training in psychiatry.

Specialized clinical pharmacy residency programs in psychiatry evolved during the early 1970s and became standardized in the late 1970s. The first psychopharmacy residency was developed by one of the authors (G.L.S.) in 1972, at the University of California–San Francisco. The general clinical pharmacy residency program was converted into a 1-year residency in psychiatry at the Langley Porter Neuropsychiatric Institute and University of California Psychiatric Clinic. In 1974 and 1975, several psychopharmacy educators began to discuss how to implement training programs and determine the content of such a training program. One of the workshops of the 1975 National Conference for Mental Health Pharmacists addressed the issue of training programs. During 1975, the ASHP Task Force on Advanced Residency Training and Accreditation asked a panel of psychopharmacy practitioners and educators to prepare specialty practice and training analyses. In 1975, two formalized psychopharmacy residency programs were available— one at the University of Southern California School of Pharmacy (Glen Stimmel) and one at the University of Tennessee College of Pharmacy (James Coleman). Other residencies were later developed at the University of Missouri–Kansas City (R. Lee Evans), the University of Nebraska (James Wilson), and the University of Texas–San Antonio (Larry Ereshefsky). Preceptors of these five programs developed standards and learning objectives for the residencies. These standards were finalized by the ASHP SIG on Psychopharmacy Practice in 1979 and were approved by the ASHP Board of Directors in 1980 as the first standards for Specialized Residency Training (8,9). (A copy can be obtained from the ASHP.) These five programs were subsequently accredited by the ASHP in the early 1980s. As of June 1984, approximately 50 pharmacists have completed formal psychopharmacy residency training programs.

REFERENCES

1. Stimmel GL: Pharmacy services in California community health centers. *Calif Pharm* 27:23-30, 1979.
2. Coleman JH, Evans RL, Rosenbluth SA: Extended clinical roles for the pharmacist in psychiatric care. *Am J Hosp Pharm* 30:1143-1146, 1975.
3. Kohan S, Chung SY, Stone J: Expanding the pharmacist's role in a psychiatric hospital. *Hosp Community Psychiatry* 24:164-166, 1973.
4. Ellenor GL, Frisk PA: Pharmacist impact on drug use in an institution for the mentally retarded. *Am J Hosp Pharm* 34:604, 1977.
5. Park PM: A patient medication counseling group in an adult psychiatric facility. *Hosp Pharm* 12:63-64, 1977.
6. Stimmel GL: Clinical pharmacy services in mental health facilities. *Hospitals* 51:71-74, 1977.
7. Kubica AJ, Gousse GC: Expansion of pharmacy services in a mental health center. *Hosp Pharm* 14:125-133, 1979.
8. ASHP Board of Directors: ASHP accreditation standard for specialized pharmacy residency training (with guide to interpretation). *Am J Hosp Pharm* 37:1229-1232, 1980.
9. ASHP Special Interest Group on Psychopharmacy Practice: ASHP supplementary standard and learning objectives for residency training in psychiatric pharmacy practice. *Am J Hosp Pharm* 37:1232-1234, 1980.

ADDITIONAL READING

General References

Bassuk EL, Schoonover SC, Gelenberg-AJ, (ed): *The Practitioner's Guide to Psychoactive Drugs,* ed 2. New York, Plenum, 1983.
Kaplan HI, Freedman AM, Sadock BJ: *Comprehensive Textbook of Psychiatry/III*. Baltimore, Williams & Wilkins, 1980.

Diagnostics

American Psychiatric Association: *Diagnostic and Statistical Manual of Mental Disorders,* ed 3. Washington, American Psychiatric Association, 1980.
Goodwin DW, Guze SB: *Psychiatric Diagnosis,* ed 2. New York, Oxford University Press, 1979.

Selected Articles

Coyle JT: The clinical use of antipsychotic medications. *Med Clin North Am* 66:993-1009, 1982.
Erehefsky L, Gilderman AM, Jewett CM: Lithium therapy of manic depressive illness. *Drug Intell Clin Pharm* 13:403-408, 492-497, 1979.
Feighner JP: The new generation of antidepressants. *J Clin Psychiatry* 44:49-55, 1983.
Gelenberg AJ: Prescribing antidepressants. *Drug Therapy* 4:95-115, 1979.
Greenblatt J, et al: Benzodiazepines: A summary of pharmacokinetic properties. *J Clin Pharm* 11:11S-16S, 1981.
Schuckit MA: Current therapeutic options in the management of typical anxiety. *J Clin Psychiatry* 42:15-24, 1981.
Wincor MZ: Insomnia and the new benzodiazepines. *Clin Pharm* 1:425-432, 1982.

CHAPTER 50

Nuclear Pharmacy

WILLIAM B. HLADIK III, JAMES A. PONTO, and RODNEY D. ICE

Regardless of the practice setting, nuclear pharmacy is considered to be "a patient-oriented service that embodies the scientific knowledge and professional judgment required to improve and promote health through assurance of the safe and efficacious use of radioactive drugs for diagnosis and therapy" (1). The purpose of this chapter is to elaborate on this definition to familiarize hospital pharmacists with the basic principles of nuclear pharmacy practice. Whenever possible, the chapter will emphasize components of this specialty area that are unique to the institutional setting.

An obvious place to begin is with an understanding of the term "radioactive drug," which is generally used interchangeably with the term "radiopharmaceutical." The Food, Drug, and Cosmetic Act has defined "radioactive drug" as a drug "which exhibits spontaneous disintegration of unstable nuclei with the emission of nulcear particles or photons and includes any non-radioactive reagent kit or nuclide generator which is intended to be used in the preparation of any such substance" (2).

Most nuclear pharmacies restrict their services to those related to radiopharmaceuticals used in vivo for diagnosis. Although some nuclear pharmacies are involved in providing radiotherapy and in vitro diagnostic services, the use of radionuclides for these purposes is usually the responsibility of the radiation therapy department and the pathology or clinical laboratory departments, respectively.

Because of the current widespread use of radiopharmaceuticals, nuclear pharmacists practice in both institutional and community settings. Institutional nuclear pharmacists are primarily meeting the needs of large hospitals, especially in those university hospitals where research on radiopharmaceuticals is conducted. Community nuclear pharmacists, on the other hand, are providing radiopharmaceutical services for numerous hospitals located within their distribution area. Regional (centralized) nuclear pharmacies of this type often service hospitals that use radiopharmaceuticals, but do not require the services of a full-time nuclear pharmacist on staff. However, even hospitals that employ their own nuclear pharmacist may obtain certain radiopharmaceuticals from centralized nuclear pharmacies to allow the in-house nuclear pharmacist more time to perform research and consultative activities. Moreover, in some cities, hospital-based nuclear pharmacies also function as regional nuclear pharmacies, distributing radiopharmaceuticals and providing consultation to other hospitals and clinics in the area.

HISTORY

Natural radioactivity was first observed in 1867 by Niepce de Saint Victor who noticed "fogging" in a silver chloride emulsion while working with uranium salts. However, it was not until 1898, after Marie Curie had studied the radiation emitted by uranium, that the phenomenon of radioactivity was truly recognized. By 1899, Rutherford had determined the existence of two distinct types of radiation, which he called alpha and beta. One year later, Curie and Villard identified a third type of radiation, which they called gamma. The theory of radioactive disintegration was advanced in 1903 by Rutherford and Soddy (3,4). The discovery of artificially produced radioactive nuclides occurred on New Year's Eve 1933 in a positron experiment conducted by Joliot and Curie (5). By the end of July 1934, Fermi had produced radioisotopes of 40 elements by neutron bombardment (6). Also in 1934, Lawrence invented the cyclotron and produced numerous radionuclides by bombarding stable atoms with artificially accelerated particles (7).

The development of the cyclotron resulted in an increased availability of radionuclides and a corresponding increase in the medical use of radioactive compounds. The development of the nuclear reactor permitted the production of still larger quantities of radioactive materials at reduced costs. In 1946, radionuclides produced in the Oak Ridge reactor were made available for biologic and medical purposes. Abbott Laboratories began marketing a line of radioactive pharmaceuticals in 1948. Two years later, the vice-chairman of the Joint Committee on Atomic Energy suggested that atomic energy should be a matter of concern to practicing pharmacists (8). In that same year, Christian, a professor of pharmacy, stated unequivocally that hospital pharmacists should be prepared to provide information and assistance in the establishment of radioisotope facilities and programs (9). In 1954, Hutchinson indicated that preparations containing radioactivity that are intended for human use are indeed pharmaceuticals and should fall under the purview of pharmacists (10). A report of the first Committee on Isotopes of the American Society of Hospital Pharmacists (ASHP), appointed in 1954, presented pictorially the first functional radiopharmacy in this country, established at the University of Chicago Clinics (11).

With the advent of the technetium-99m generator in the late 1960s (12), a source of a versatile radionuclide became readily available to thousands of hospitals. As technetium was found to be complexed and chelated by a number of organ-specific compounds, pharmaceutical manufacturers began supplying kits designed for the simplified compounding of ^{99m}Tc-labeled radiopharmaceuticals. ^{99m}Tc radiopharmaceutical use spread rapidly and pharmacists became increasingly involved in the preparation and dispensing of short-lived radiopharmaceuticals for human use. Institutional and regional nuclear pharmacies were established, and the practice of nuclear pharmacy began to emerge as a specialty (13-21). On August 6, 1974, nuclear pharmacists first met as a group in Chicago at the ''Nuclear Pharmacy '74'' Symposium conducted under the auspices of the American Pharmaceutical Association's (APhA) Academy of General Practice of Pharmacy (now the Academy of Pharmacy Practice). The Section on Nuclear Pharmacy in the APhA's Academy of Pharmacy Practice was established in 1975. In that same year, a Special Interest Group (SIG) on Nuclear Pharmacy Practice was formed within the ASHP. Nuclear pharmacy was officially recognized as a specialty in pharmacy practice by the Board of Pharmaceutical Specialties in 1978.

The growth of nuclear pharmacy has lagged somewhat behind the growth of nuclear medicine. A survey by Jones in 1970 showed that in only 3% (6/205) of hospitals surveyed were radiopharmaceuticals dispensed by pharmacists; radiopharmaceuticals were dispensed in the majority of hospitals by technologists (22). In 1972, only about 300 pharmacists were practicing nuclear pharmacy in the United States compared with 4500 physicians practicing nuclear medicine (23). According to the Lilly Hospital Pharmacy Survey conducted in 1982, 0.9% of the 2169 reporting hospitals indicated that their Department of Pharmacy was involved with dispensing radiopharmaceuticals (24). This low figure may in part be the result of the high percentage of small and medium-sized hospitals in the United States (approximately 85%), which likely have no nuclear pharmacy services whatsoever. However, even if the assumption is made that nuclear pharmacy services are provided exclusively in large hospitals (over 400 beds), the figures still do not change drastically; through extrapolation it is calculated that only 7% of these large hospitals provide such services. It is evident, then, that nuclear pharmacy is one area of hospital pharmacy practice that still has much potential for growth.

ORGANIZATIONAL STRUCTURE

Like most other hospital departments, a typical hospital-based nuclear pharmacy is, by necessity, interdisciplinary in function. Therefore, to assure the optimal provision and use of radiopharmaceuticals within the hospital, the nuclear pharmacy must interact regularly with other organizational sections within the hospital including the nuclear medicine unit (which if not autonomous, is usually organized within the internal medicine, radiology, or diagnostic imaging departments); the imaging modality divisions of radiology other than nuclear medicine (particularly if the nuclear pharmacy handles various types of contrast material or paramagnetic agents); the clinical laboratory and/or pathology department (especially if the nuclear pharmacy is involved with in vitro procedures); the health physics division (which may be another section of the radiology department); the

pharmacy department; central services; and hospital administration, among others. Within this interactive framework, three basic types of organizational structure may exist for hospital-based nuclear pharmacies:

- The nuclear pharmacy as part of the nuclear medicine department
- The nuclear pharmacy as part of the pharmacy department
- The nuclear pharmacy as an independent, separately licensed entity

In reality, most hospital-based nuclear pharmacies are presently under the administrative jurisdiction of the nuclear medicine department alone, primarily because of the close physical proximity and degree of daily interaction between these two disciplines. Equally important is that nuclear medicine personnel have frequently been more willing than pharmacy administrators to foster the development of a nuclear pharmacy service, probably because of the direct benefits that are realized by the nuclear medicine department as a result of the existence of such a satellite pharmacy. In addition, nuclear medicine personnel have traditionally been more extensively trained in the use of radiopharmaceuticals than hospital pharmacists, which would naturally make these individuals more comfortable and confident about justifying the establishment of a nuclear pharmacy to hospital administrators. Another practical advantage in favor of nuclear medicine is that authorization by the Nuclear Regulatory Commission (NRC) or agreement state agency licensing to possess, handle, and use radioactive materials is most easily obtained with this organizational structure. Because of these factors and others, a low percentage of institutional nuclear pharmacies report solely to the director of pharmacy, although in some hospitals the nuclear medicine and pharmacy department heads share administrative responsibilities for the nuclear pharmacy. Rarely is the nuclear pharmacy an administratively independent department reporting directly to the hospital administration.

In contrast to what has just been discussed, the accreditation standards for pharmaceutical services promulgated by the Joint Commission on Accreditation of Hospitals (JCAH) (25) lend support to the opinion that the pharmacy department should have administrative authority over the nuclear pharmacy. According to the JCAH standards, it is the responsibility of the pharmacy department to control all drugs within the institution, which would include radiopharmaceuticals. Two interpretive statements seem to be particularly relevant to nuclear pharmacy:

- ''When the hospital pharmaceutical department/service is decentralized, a licensed pharmacist, *responsible to the director of the pharmaceutical department/service* [emphasis added], shall supervise each satellite pharmacy or separate organizational element involved with the preparation and dispensing of drugs and with the provision of drug information and other pharmaceutical services'' (25). (Most hospital-based nuclear pharmacies could be considered as a satellite of the central pharmacy department.)
- ''Hospitals with an organized pharmaceutical department/service shall have the necessary space, equipment and supplies for the storage, preparation (compounding, packaging, labeling), and dispensing of drugs. As appropriate, this shall include the preparation and dispensing of paren-

teral products and *radiopharmaceuticals''* (25) [emphasis added].

In the absence of an already established nuclear pharmacy, the JCAH standards should *not* be interpreted to mean that the pharmacy department must be directly involved with the provision and use of radiopharmaceuticals, particularly if there is no pharmacist on the staff with appropriate training in nuclear pharmacy. The accreditation standard for nuclear medicine services states that "appropriate credentials shall be required for any pharmacist involved in the preparation of radiopharmaceuticals" (26). However, the pharmacy department probably should have input into the development of the policies and procedures that control radiopharmaceutical use in the hospital, even if the nuclear medicine department is more directly involved with handling the radiopharmaceuticals on a daily basis.

Within the nuclear pharmacy itself, the scope of services provided will determine the number of employees required by the department. Nuclear pharmacies provide a variety of services, depending on the needs expressed by the physicians at the institution and by the capabilities of the available nuclear pharmacist(s). If multiple individuals are needed to operate the nuclear pharmacy, virtually any combination of nuclear pharmacists, basic medical scientists, and/or technologists may comprise the unit. This situation would obviously necessitate some sort of intradepartmental organizational structure, which should be individualized according to the needs, priorities, and regulations of the specific hospital.

THE PRACTICE OF NUCLEAR PHARMACY

The Nuclear Pharmacy Practice Standards suggest that the practice of nuclear pharmacy is composed of the following eight general areas (1):
1. Procuring radiopharmaceuticals
2. Compounding radiopharmaceuticals
3. Performing routine quality control procedures
4. Dispensing radiopharmaceuticals
5. Distributing radiopharmaceuticals
6. Implementing basic radiation protection procedures and practices
7. Consulting and educating the nuclear medicine community, patients, pharmacists, other health professionals, and the general public
8. Researching and developing new formulations

Each of these areas will be briefly discussed in terms of hospital-based nuclear pharmacy practice.

Procuring radiopharmaceuticals involves determining specifications for purchase orders, initiating purchase orders, logging in radiopharmaceutical shipments, maintaining good inventory control, and assuring proper storage conditions for the radiopharmaceuticals.

Determining specifications for purchase orders and ordering radioactive drugs and supplies is similar to a regular hospital pharmacy with the exception that the decay of the radiopharmaceuticals must be taken into account. In addition, many radiopharmaceuticals must be specially ordered for specific patients. Both of these factors make it essential to designate exact delivery instructions. Receiving radioactive drugs differs from a regular hospital pharmacy pri-

marily because all incoming shipments must be monitored for conformance to labeled radioactivity levels and for signs of radiocontamination caused by improper filling techniques, faulty closures, or container damage (27).

Because of the short physical half-lives of most common radiopharmaceuticals, the nuclear pharmacy must establish and use inventory and cost control procedures. Inventory and cost control are best effected after a thorough study of differences among similar products supplied by various manufacturers, the ability of a manufacturer to guarantee delivery at requested times (even if an airline strike and adverse weather conditions should occur), shipping costs, bidding procedures, calibration date of the radionuclide, special promotions or "deals," etc. The nuclear pharmacist should be constantly in communication with nuclear medicine staff to determine the preferred radiopharmaceutical for a given procedure and the level of use anticipated for each radiopharmaceutical. In addition to the radioactive materials in the pharmacy's inventory, adjunct pharmaceuticals and nonradioactive kits and/or kit components must also be inventory controlled.

Once the quantities and types of commercial radiopharmaceuticals, adjunct pharmaceuticals, and kits or kit components have been determined, a systematic purchasing arrangement can be worked out with the various suppliers. From this point, routine inventory control procedures should assure a smooth operation of the nuclear pharmacy.

The effective inventory control of radiopharmaceuticals permits a nuclear pharmacy to be self-supporting and economically practical. Reports by Quinn (16), Porter et al (23), and Gnau et al (28) verify this important aspect of nuclear pharmacy operations. Only a minimal inventory should be stocked because product half-lives are short. Furthermore, inventory turnover is more profitable than inventory on the shelf. A nuclear pharmacy should have an inventory turnover of greater than 30 times per year.

Storage of radiopharmaceuticals must take into consideration the chemical state of the radioactive drug, the quantity and type of radiation involved, and any special storage and stability requirements (27). For example, gaseous or volatile radiopharmaceuticals should be kept in specially vented areas, whereas certain other radioactive drugs require refrigeration. Storage conditions are normally specified in product package inserts and USP monographs (29). In addition, appropriate shielding must be used for storage areas to minimize personnel exposure.

Compounding radiopharmaceuticals incorporates a wide range of activities, from the relatively simple task of reconstituting reagent kits with ^{99m}Tc sodium pertechnetate solution to the complex job of radiolabeling blood cellular components (3) or monoclonal antibodies (31). Compounding protocols should be established by the nuclear pharmacy and consolidated into a procedures book. These protocols may be modified as necessary to reflect any changes in radiopharmaceutical kit components, different radionuclide generators, etc that which may influence the compounding methods. Strict aseptic technique must be observed in compounding procedures, because most radiopharmaceuticals are administered parenterally.

A majority of the radiopharmaceuticals prepared on a daily basis are compounded with the radionuclide ^{99m}Tc.

When preparing ^{99m}Tc radiopharmaceuticals using the eluate from a ^{99}Mo/^{99m}Tc generator and reagents kits, several factors should be considered including (1) the number of patients who will receive doses from the kit, (2) the amount of active ingredient and radioactivity required per patient study, (3) the optimal administration volume, (4) the minimum volume required to dissolve the ingredients, (5) the maximum amount of radioactivity permissible to add to the kit, (6) time required for maximum radiolabeling efficiency to occur, (7) the radiolabeling efficiency as a function of time, (8) the shelf life of the radiolabeled radiopharmaceutical, and (9) the number and volume of samples required for quality assurance testing (27). Many of these same factors must also be considered when dispensing the drug once it is compounded.

A complete record of each radiopharmaceutical compounded by the nuclear pharmacy must be maintained. Most nuclear pharmacies record complete compounding, quality assurance, and product disposition data on a common document.

In some instances, nuclear pharmacies that prepare and dispense radiopharmaceuticals may also be subject to FDA registration as a drug establishment (manufacturer). Much confusion exists concerning interpretation of some nuclear pharmacy activities as pharmacy practice (compounding) or as manufacturing. To aid in clarification, the FDA has published a guideline describing criteria for determining when to register as a drug establishment (32). In general, nuclear pharmacies that dispense radiopharmaceuticals on the receipt of a valid prescription or hospital order are not considered to be manufacturers.

Quality control of radiopharmaceuticals entails performing the appropriate chemical, biologic, and physical tests on potential radiopharmaceuticals and the interpretation of the resulting data to determine the suitability of the products for use in humans and animals, including internal test assessment and authentication of product history. This definition includes not only completion of the test, but clinical professional interpretation of results, evaluation of analytical test methods, and maintenance of records to identify the product from its initial production to its ultimate use.

Quality control procedures are required at every stage of radiopharmaceutical preparation, from the production of the radionuclide to final dispensing. The extensive tests and measurements performed on radiopharmaceuticals to assure chemical, radiochemical, and radionuclidic purity, sterility, freedom from pyrogens, and conformance to stated efficacy have been described in detail by Tubis (33).

The nuclear pharmacist must be fully assured of the physical quality of the materials received and dispensed by the nuclear pharmacy. Radionuclidic purity may be assured by establishing the identity of the radionuclide and any impurities by determining the type and energy of radiation emitted and the half-life. Routine health physics procedures will determine whether leakage has occurred during shipment and if the radiation exposure level of the package conforms to that indicated on the package label. Foreign particles, abnormal color, etc may be detected by a quick visual examination of parenteral solutions after placing them behind leaded glass.

Chemical and radiochemical purity must meet USP monograph standards in the case of the official radiopharmaceuticals, or comparable well-established standards in the case of nonofficial radiopharmaceuticals. Often used techniques for chemical and radiochemical purity determination include spectrophotometry, thin-layer chromatography (34), and refractive index.

The considerations and procedures for generator eluate quality assurance used in compounding most radiopharmaceuticals are indicated in the manufacturer's drug insert, NRC regulations, and the USP (29).

Particulate-containing radiopharmaceuticals (e.g., technetium sulfur colloid, human albumin microspheres) are used in suspension form. Such preparations require assurance of correct particle size distribution.

Sterility and freedom from pyrogens of parenteral radiopharmaceuticals must be assured by the use of appropriate aseptic techniques. USP tests for sterility and the absence of pyrogens (29) are required for all materials used to compound radiopharmaceuticals. Because most radiopharmaceuticals are compounded and used within a period of a few hours, it is often impossible to perform USP tests on the final products before dispensing. Thus, aseptic techniques must be adhered to rigorously and the technique, rather than the product, tested for integrity. As a check on the nuclear pharmacist's technique in assuring sterility and freedom from pyrogens, unused portions of all radiopharmaceuticals should be saved for testing ipso facto. Both the radiometric test for sterility, using the BACTEC (Johnston Laboratories, Cockeysville, MD) system and the limulus amebocyte lysate test for endotoxin pyrogens are more rapid than official tests. Thus, these tests are often used in the nuclear pharmacy.

All quality control procedures that apply to nonradioactive pharmaceuticals are also applicable to radiopharmaceuticals (e.g., pH, isotonicity).

The quantity of radioactivity in a radiopharmaceutical dose must be measured and compared to calculated or labeled values before dispensing, and any discrepancies must be identified and corrected.

Two other forms of quality control not directly associated with the radiopharmaceutical product are environmental and instrumentation quality control (27). Monitoring for radiocontamination of work stations should be performed routinely. As in the IV admixture area, the laminar flow clean benches must be certified according to manufacturer's specifications. Accuracy, precision, and linearity of the dose calibrator should be performed as specified in the pharmacy's radioactive materials license. Likewise, other radioactivity measuring devices must be calibrated periodically to assure proper function.

All quality assurance tests and measurements should be systematically recorded and filed. Access to quality assurance information is valuable in the case of questions that may arise if any unusual results should occur following the administration of a radiopharmaceutical to a patient. Figure 50.1 illustrates a case where radiochemical purity test results were helpful in determining the cause of altered radiopharmaceutical biodistribution.

Dispensing radiopharmaceuticals occurs on the request of a physician, usually via a prescription order. In a hospital with a full-time nuclear pharmacist, radiopharmaceuticals

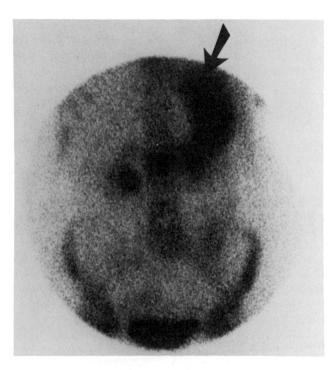

FIGURE 50.1 Anterior "spot view" of a bone scan. Arrow points to the accumulation of a radiochemical impurity, ^{99m}Tc pertechnetate, in the stomach of the patient. This pattern of biodistribution indicates degradation of the bone imaging agent ^{99m}Tc medronate.

are usually dispensed in unit doses, ready for administration to the patient.

The nuclear pharmacist is responsible for assuring that the radiopharmaceutical dose is consistent with preestablished dosage schedules based on patient history, age, weight, sex, and surface area, as well as gamma camera sensitivity. To determine the correct volume of a radiopharmaceutical that will contain the desired number of millicuries prescribed for the patient, the pharmacist must calculate the extent of the radioactive decay that has occurred from the time that the radiopharmaceutical was first assayed to the time that the dose is needed. This calculation is easily facilitated by using decay correction charts, programmable calculators, and/or radionuclide calibrator instruments equipped with an automatic volume calculation function. The pharmacist must also take into account the amount of radiopharmaceutical that is likely to be retained in the administration vehicle to allow for the prescribed dose to be delivered to the patient. With some radiopharmaceuticals, it is necessary for the pharmacist to consider not only the amount of radioactivity in the radiopharmaceutical dose, but also the amount of chemical.

Doses must be drawn aseptically from properly shielded containers, using remote dispensing where appropriate. The volume and dose of each radiopharmaceutical dispensed and the time for which the dose was calibrated must be recorded on the radiopharmaceutical disposition sheet and the prescription label.

The ultimate goal of radiopharmaceutical dispensing is to ensure that the right drug, in the right dose, in the right dosage form is received by the right patient at the right time by the right route of administration (1).

Distributing radiopharmaceuticals within an institution is subject to institutional policies and regulations. In general, each radiopharmaceutical dose is labeled with the patient's name, radiopharmaceutical identification information, and a radioactivity warning. Lead-lined boxes or other shielded containers are used when transporting these doses to other areas within the institution.

Distribution of radiopharmaceuticals to other institutions is subject to local, state, and federal regulations, including those promulgated by state Boards of Pharmacy, the Department of Transportation (DOT), and the Food and Drug Administration (FDA).

Many state boards of pharmacy have adopted the National Association of Boards of Pharmacy (NABP) Model Regulations for Nuclear Pharmacy (35). Although specific regulations may vary between states, NABP recommendations include the following labeling requirements: the immediate outer container shall be labeled with (1) the standard radiation symbol; (2) the words "Caution—Radioactive Material"; (3) the radionuclide; (4) the chemical form, (5) the amount (activity) of radioactive material contained; (6) if a liquid, the volume; and (7) the calibration time for the amount of radioactivity contained. The immediate inner container shall be labeled with (1) the standard radiation symbol; (2) the words "Caution—Radioactive Material"; (3) the name, address, and telephone number of the nuclear pharmacy; and (4) the prescription number.

Transport of radiopharmaceuticals must comply with DOT regulations (36,37). Key items of compliance include (1) type A packaging, (2) presence of absorbent material if the contents are liquid; (3) presence of security seal; (4) appropriate labeling based on radiation exposure rates at the surface and at 1 meter; (5) control of removable radioactive contamination; (6) placarding of the delivery vehicle if necessary; (7) completion of shipping papers classifying, describing, and certifying packages containing radioactive materials. Additionally, packaging of radioactive materials must comply with specific NRC requirements (38). Licensing requirements for carriers who transport radioactive materials are also specified by the NRC (38).

Transfer of radiopharmaceuticals to another institution must comply with NRC regulations (39,40). Before transporting radioactive materials, the shipper must verify that the transferee is authorized to receive the type, form, and quantity of radioactive material to be shipped. This requirement is most easily satisfied by keeping on file a current copy of the transferee's radioactive materials license. Additionally, records of the transfer must be maintained for at least 5 years.

Basic radiation protection procedures and practices are crucial elements of nuclear pharmacy practice. Nuclear pharmacists should practice with the philosophy of keeping radiation exposures as low as reasonably achievable (41,42).

Specific procedures and practices regarding radiation protection and the safe handling of radioactive materials have been recommended by the National Council on Radiation Protection and Measurements (43-45). The NRC has established standards for protection against radiation (46) that include permissible radiation doses, levels of radiation, concentrations of radioactivity, waste disposal, and precautionary procedures.

Nuclear pharmacists have an integral role in implementing a sound radiation safety program. Specific areas of responsibility may include (1) establishing a floor plan that separates radioactive areas from nonradioactive areas (47,48); (2) storing and handling radioactive materials in accordance with the principles of time, distance, and shielding; (3) radioactive waste disposal; (4) posting radioactive areas; (5) monitoring radiation exposure to personnel; (6) monitoring environmental radioactive contamination; (7) decontamination; and (8) general laboratory safety and security (49-52).

Consulting and educating constitute the framework of clinical nuclear pharmacy, an important aspect of nuclear pharmacy practice. Pioneering activities in this area involved selecting radiopharmaceutical products and doses, identifying radiopharmaceutical-radiopharmaceutical and radiopharmaceutical-drug interactions, and advising patients on radiologic safety (53-56). Additional patient-oriented services now commonplace in hospitals include review of the patient's medical and drug history, application of pharmacokinetic and pharmacodynamic principles for radiopharmaceutical dosage assessment and adjustment, monitoring the safety and effectiveness of radiopharmaceuticals through patient follow-up and nuclear medicine scan review, providing technical drug information to physicians and allied health personnel, and maintaining patient records of accumulated radiation absorbed doses (27).

The ASHP Accreditation Standard for Residency Training in Nuclear Pharmacy (57) lists several other areas in which nuclear pharmacists can provide clinical consultation and input:

- Troubleshooting unanticipated or unusual radiophar-

maceutical biodistribution patterns which result from various iatrogenic causes, radiopharmaceutical formulation problems, variations in human pathology, physiology, or anatomy, etc

- Assistance with interpreting radiometrically determined drug serum levels
- Advice on timely and appropriate radioactive drug use and administration
- Investigating and reporting adverse reactions to radiopharmaceuticals
- Advice on using radiotracer techniques for evaluating the pharmacokinetics of therapeutic drugs
- Monitoring the safety and efficacy of a patient's therapeutic drug regimen using radiometric methods
- Assuring the proper preparation of patients for nuclear medicine studies
- Administering therapeutic radiopharmaceuticals to patients (with appropriate follow-up of these patients)

In addition, Hladik et al have recently compiled information relevant to the clinical aspects of nuclear pharmacy practice (58).

The hospital-based nuclear pharmacist is in a unique position to be involved in a variety of both educational and consultant activities. On a daily basis, there is direct interaction with physicians and nuclear medicine technologists. For example, most hospital nuclear pharmacists attend daily scan conferences to obtain feedback on the in vivo performance of radiopharmaceuticals. Also, there is usually the opportunity for interaction with patients and their families. Most hospital nuclear pharmacists are involved in presenting seminars or in-service programs directed to nuclear medicine technologists, nurses, pharmacists, and other health professionals. Many hospital nuclear pharmacists are also involved in teaching nuclear medicine technology students, radiology and nuclear medicine residents, pharmacy students, and others.

Research and development is vital for the viability and future growth of the nuclear pharmacy profession. Areas of nuclear pharmacist involvement may include radiopharmaceutical product development and clinical testing, clinical evaluation of new uses for existing radiopharmaceuticals, investigation of methods for improving the diagnostic accuracy and therapeutic effectiveness of routine nuclear medicine procedures, utilization review of nuclear medicine procedures, development of new or improved methods for testing the quality of radiopharmaceuticals, and investigation of potential causes for the altered biodistribution of radiopharmaceuticals. In addition, nuclear pharmacists often serve as members on institutional radioactive drug research committees and radiation protection and human uses subcommittees.

FINANCIAL CONSIDERATIONS

Before implementing a nuclear pharmacy service, thorough consideration must be given to initial costs, operating costs, and prescription pricing as they affect profitability. These costs will vary depending on the scope of operations and the prescription volume.

Initial costs include equipment, inventory, remodeling costs, and initial operating costs until such time as cash flow

TABLE 50.1   Basic Nuclear Pharmacy Equipment List[a]

1. Gamma well scintillation counter
2. Dose calibrator
3. Laminar airflow clean bench
4. Fume hood
5. G-M survey meter, Cutie Pie meter, air monitor
6. Refrigerator (lead-lined)
7. Typewriter
8. Programmable calculator
9. Ultrasound water bath
10. Variable temperature hot water bath (up to 100°C)
11. Lead bricks and sheet lead (for shielding)
12. Lead syringe transfer pigs, vial containers
13. Lead radioactive waste containers
14. Lead-glass syringe holders
15. Lead-glass drawing station and shield
16. Analytical balance
17. Quality control testing supplies
    a. Sterility testing
    b. Pyrogen testing
    c. Molybdenum-99 breakthrough testing
    d. Aluminum ion breakthrough testing
    e. Stannous ion concentration testing
    f. Radiochemical purity testing
    g. Particle sizing
    h. pH testing
    i. Instrumentation calibration (sealed reference sources)
18. Sterile, disposable syringes and evacuated glass vials
19. Laboratory glassware

[a]Modified by permission from Laven DL: Nuclear pharmacy (Part III): Quality assurance of radiopharmaceuticals. *Fla J Hosp Pharm* 3:217-234, 1983.

TABLE 50.2   Equipment Requirements for Expanded[a] Nuclear Pharmacy Practice

1. Pyrogen oven
2. Autoclave
3. Centrifuge
4. Shaker/water bath unit
5. Multichannel analyzer
6. Radiochromatogram scanner
7. Germanium-lithium detector or cadmium telluride detector
8. HPLC
9. Spectrophotometers
10. Lyophilizer
11. Computer system
12. Automated gamma counter (if the nuclear pharmacy is involved with in vitro diagnostic testing)

[a]Includes nuclear pharmacy research, manufacturing, preparation of investigational drugs, and automated record keeping

allows a stabilization of operating costs. The major initial cost is equipment. Basic equipment items to meet certain state regulatory requirements (59,60) are minimal standards and cost approximately $20,000-$25,000. The basic regulatory equipment requirements assume that the only products dispensed are FDA approved. Although these requirements vary somewhat from state to state, a fairly complete list is given in Table 50.1. The need to prepare investigational new drug (IND) products and custom-made radiopharmaceuticals can increase equipment costs to over $50,000. Involvement in basic research and the manufacture of reagent kits, as well as the use of automated record-keeping systems, will also boost equipment costs over the $50,000 level. Table 50.2 lists some of the equipment required for expanded nuclear pharmacy services.

Inventory costs, unlike those of a regular pharmacy, are minimal, usually not more than $5000. Short physical half-lives preclude large inventories and thus most radiopharmaceuticals are ordered for not more than 1 week at a time. Inherent in this inventory level is the need for well-established purchasing procedures, rapid product delivery, rapid product check-in, and high product turnover.

Operating costs, either associated with initiation or maintenance of services, parallel typical hospital pharmacy costs with the following exceptions:

• Salaries for nuclear pharmacists, because of their specialty training, are often 10-15% higher than other pharmacists' salaries. Specialty certification may also eventually have some impact on salary demands.

• Radiation safety costs must be considered. Included under safety costs are film badges, waste disposal, safety surveys, record keeping, and decontamination supplies.

• Instrumentation maintenance and regular calibration are essential. Nuclear pharmacies must periodically purchase gamma reference sources for quality assurance testing of certain equipment. In addition, some equipment must be routinely serviced and/or calibrated by outside commercial firms who provide standards and unknowns for testing.

• The use of radioactive material increases supply costs because many items used are disposable (e.g., gloves, absorbent paper, pipettes, beakers). Although the purchase of disposable supplies is often more expensive than the decontamination of nondisposable items, the radiation hazard is significantly reduced.

• Shielding materials, lead pigs, leaded glass, and syringe holders must be obtained regularly. Some of these costs can be recovered by selling to salvage operators the lead containers from incoming shipments or by returning decayed generators to the manufacturer.

• If a regional nuclear pharmacy is established in the hospital, the cost for the delivery of radiopharmaceuticals to other hospitals must be taken into account.

Pricing of radioactive prescriptions, like regular pharmacy operations, depends on the prescription volume, the professional services provided, the cost of the components, and the desired profit. Prices vary with all manufacturers; thus, bids can often assist in establishing the best price. Each pharmacist should carefully consider available services and the quality of the product before selecting a particular brand. Furthermore, using a formulary system can help to minimize inventory and enhance bid volume.

Radiopharmaceuticals are usually priced using a professional fee added on to the cost of the product and the overhead of the pharmacy. Because most products are compounded, the professional fee is usually a sliding scale based on the actual amount of pharmacist's time involved in compounding and delivering clinical services. Thus, the prescriptive product price is made up of: Cost of product (including incoming freight) + Operation costs (business overhead on a per prescription basis) + Professional fee (sliding scale).

The volume of ^{99m}Tc products has brought about a significant decline in technetium prices. Often, nuclear pharmacies will simplify pricing structures by pricing all technetium products similarly (e.g., $15-$20 a dose).

In most hospitals with nuclear pharmacies, there is not

presently a mechanism established that allows the nuclear pharmacist to charge a separate fee for consulting services performed, even if these services significantly contribute to a patient's diagnostic workup or therapeutic management. If reimbursement for clinical pharmacy services already exists or is being considered in a hospital, the nuclear pharmacy should be included as part of the overall clinical program.

EDUCATIONAL PROGRAMS

The American Association of Colleges of Pharmacy (AACP) has indicated that all pharmacists should be instructed in radiopharmaceutical information and communication skills (61). To meet that need, a number of textbooks provide a comprehensive introduction to nuclear pharmacy (62-66). Voices 12/60, available from ASHP, has a series of tapes regarding nuclear pharmacy operations. A series of articles in the *U.S. Pharmacist* (67-72) and *Florida Journal of Hospital Pharmacy* (73-77)* describe the basic radiopharmaceutical knowledge needed by all pharmacists.

To meet the need for future nuclear pharmacists, educators currently direct academic programs to meet five different levels of competency (78,79).

General education in nuclear pharmacy includes the basic information skills in nuclear pharmacy required by all pharmacists. This information is usually attained in a few hours of lectures and covers general nuclear pharmacy, radiologic health, radiation safety, and the clinical uses of radiopharmaceuticals (80,81). At the completion of the general education nuclear pharmacy program, a pharmacist should be able to (1) communicate effectively with both patient and physician about the use of radiopharmaceuticals, (2) understand the interaction of radiopharmaceuticals with other medical procedures or other pharmaceuticals, and (3) understand the properties of well-established radiopharmaceuticals.

Undergraduate specialization in nuclear pharmacy involves 8-20 semester hours of nuclear pharmacy course work, including a radiopharmaceutical dispensing laboratory. In this type of program, each student takes upper division courses in radiation biology, radiologic physics, health physics and instrumentation, radiopharmaceutical chemistry and kinetics, clinical uses of radiopharmaceuticals, management, and nuclear pharmacy practice (80). At the completion of the undergraduate specialization program, the pharmacist should be able to function in a hospital or community nuclear pharmacy and, as the need arises, be able to compound, dispense, and advise on the use of radiopharmaceuticals in patients. In its report to the AACP, however, the 1982-1983 Argus Commission rejected the concept of an elective-track approach within the undergraduate curricula in favor of specialized postgraduate programs (82).

Postgraduate traineeships in nuclear pharmacy offer short-term, intensive training. In this type of a program, the pharmacist obtains 1-2 months of didactic instruction and practicum experience (83). At the completion of the traineeship, the pharmacist should be able to assist in the preparation and distribution of radiopharmaceuticals.

Advanced training in nuclear pharmacy is available in postgraduate residency programs or in graduate programs specializing in nuclear pharmacy. In a residency program, the pharmacist obtains 9-12 months of didactic, laboratory, and clinical course work and training (84). Residency programs in nuclear pharmacy are subject to accreditation by the ASHP (57). In PharmD or MS programs, the pharmacist obtains 9-18 months of didactic and laboratory work followed by 3-12 months of clerkship or clinical training in nuclear pharmacy (85,86). At the completion of these programs, the pharmacist is capable of preparing, dispensing, and advising about radiopharmaceuticals, be they approved, investigational, or research. These graduates are fully capable of operating any commerical or institutional nuclear pharmacy.

Research and education training in nuclear pharmacy involves 3-4 years of specialized education leading to the PhD degree. The emphasis in such programs spans the entire scope of nuclear pharmacy knowledge, including radiopharmaceutical design and development (87). Graduates of such programs usually go into academic settings to teach and do research or into industry to be involved with the design and development of new radiopharmaceuticals.

CERTIFICATION

The Board of Pharmaceutical Specialties (BPS) was created on January 5, 1976, when the APhA membership approved the BPS Bylaws. The BPS was first appointed by the APhA Board of Trustees in January 1976. It is composed of pharmacists, other health professionals, and a member of the public. The BPS has developed procedures for considering and recognizing specialties in pharmacy practice (88). In 1978, the BPS approved a petition submitted by the APhA Academy of Pharmacy Practice Section on Nuclear Pharmacy and recognized nuclear pharmacy as a specialty. Nuclear pharmacy thus became the first officially recognized specialty in pharmacy practice. A Specialty Council on Nuclear Pharmacy was appointed and charged to develop a certification program for the new specialty.

A committee of pharmacists practicing contemporary nuclear pharmacy first identified areas of responsibility that were considered unique to nuclear pharmacy, a specialty practice within the profession of pharmacy. After this task analysis was completed, a cross section of nuclear pharmacists was sampled to determine the extent to which they were involved in such activities. The analysis of these data resulted in a draft of the Nuclear Pharmacy Practice Standards, which were subsequently reviewed and adopted by the APhA Academy of Pharmacy Practice Section on Nuclear Pharmacy (1). The BPS Specialty Council on Nuclear Pharmacy has adopted these standards as the standards for the specialty. The standards, because they represent agreed on functions that are the responsibilities of nuclear pharmacists, were used as the basis for determining areas of knowledge and skills to be addressed in developing the certification examination. The processes involved in the development and implementation of the nuclear pharmacy certification examination, including item writing, test assembly, test administration, and score interpretation, have been described in detail by Grussing et al (89).

---

*Additional articles in this series are in press.

Eligibility for nuclear pharmacy certification includes both educational and experiential requirements. An applicant must be a graduate of a school of pharmacy accredited by the American Council on Pharmaceutical Education and must possess a valid license to practice pharmacy. Moreover, an applicant must have acquired at least 4000 hours of experience in nuclear pharmacy practice. Experience credit may be obtained in the following ways:

1. Up to 2000 hours may be obtained from nuclear pharmacy coursework completed in academic settings.
2. Up to 2000 hours may be obtained from nuclear pharmacy residency programs.
3. Up to 2000 hours may be obtained from internships in licensed nuclear pharmacies or health care facilities.
4. Up to 4000 hours may be obtained from nuclear pharmacy practice in a licensed nuclear pharmacy or health care facility.

The fee to sit for the certification examination was set at $400 (90).

The Nuclear Pharmacy Certification Examination was offered for the first time on April 24, 1982, in conjunction with the APhA annual meeting. Of the 72 practitioners who sat for the 1-day examination, 63 were subsequently awarded Certification in Nuclear Pharmacy (91). The Nuclear Pharmacy Certification Examination is offered annually in conjunction with the APhA Annual Meeting.

PROFESSIONAL ORGANIZATIONS

Three major national professional organizations are structured to provide for the special needs of nuclear pharmacists. The ASHP has organized a SIG for nuclear pharmacy, the APhA's Academy of Pharmacy Practice (APP) has a Section on Nuclear Pharmacy (SNP), and the Society of Nuclear Medicine (SNM) has a Radiopharmaceutical Scientists Council (RSC). Each of these organizations speaks to specific needs within nuclear pharmacy.

The SIG on Nuclear Pharmacy is one of 11 such groups within the ASHP that allows specialty practitioners to have a voice in hospital pharmacy at a national level. Advisory working groups of the SIG are established as needed to address various issues facing nuclear pharmacy. Major projects that members of the SIG have undertaken include the development of the ASHP Accreditation Standard for Residency Training in Nuclear Pharmacy (57) and a revision of section 78:00 (radioactive agents) of the American Hospital Formulary Service (92). SIG members also review papers relevant to the practice of nuclear pharmacy that are submitted for presentation at the ASHP Midyear Clinical Meeting. Additionally, a 3-contact-hour continuing education program is sponsored by the SIG each year at the ASHP Midyear Clinical Meeting and at the ASHP Annual Meeting. A separate fee is assessed by the ASHP for membership in the SIG, which is open to nuclear pharmacists from all practice settings. Members receive a newsletter entitled the *Signal* on a bimonthly basis.

The SNP is one of five divisions of the APP. Because the SNP has a larger membership of nuclear pharmacists than either the SIG or the RSC, it is probably the most representative group for nuclear pharmacists in the United States. Six standing committees comprise the primary work-

force of SNP along with its officers, including committees for educational affairs, regulatory affairs, communications, nontraditional radiopharmaceuticals, programs, and nominations. Each year at the Annual APhA Meeting, the SNP hosts a 2-day conference consisting of several continuing education sessions, a business meeting, and a contributed papers session. Important contributions of the SNP to nuclear pharmacy include the Nuclear Pharmacy Practice Standards (1) and the development of the nuclear pharmacy certification examination, both of which have already been discussed in detail. Members must pay additional dues to the APP in addition to the regular APhA dues. Like the ASHP SIG, membership is open to nuclear pharmacists working in hospital, industry, education, and community practice. The newsletter *Pharmacy Practice* is received by members monthly.

The RSC is the branch of SNM that serves members involved primarily with radiopharmaceutical research and development and is one of seven councils of the SNM. Seminars on various topics of interest to members are sponsored by the RSC in conjunction with the parent society; these seminars are normally held at the Annual Meeting of the SNM, and proceedings of these conferences are frequently published in either written or cassette tape format by the SNM. Business meetings of the RSC are usually held at the Annual and/or Midwinter Meetings of the SNM. Membership is limited to members of the SNM and a nominal fee is required.

POTENTIAL INVOLVEMENT OF HOSPITAL PHARMACISTS IN NUCLEAR MEDICINE

The need for employing a nuclear pharmacist in a hospital depends on a combination of factors, including (1) the number and type of nuclear medicine procedures performed each day; (2) the number and type of physicians, technologists, and other nuclear medicine scientists already employed by the nuclear medicine department; (3) the degree to which the nuclear medicine department is involved with, or concerned about, basic and clinical research, manufacturing reagent kits and investigational drugs, quality assurance, radiation safety, cost containment, patient education, and clinical nuclear pharmacy activities; (4) the quality of the relationship between the nuclear medicine department and the pharmacy department; and (5) the availability of radiopharmaceuticals from a nearby centralized nuclear pharmacy.

Pursuant to NRC licensing regulations (93), most community hospitals rely on existing nuclear medicine personnel to provide nuclear pharmacy services, because pharmacists in these hospitals have not received adequate training in nuclear pharmacy. Nonetheless, the hospital pharmacist can make a positive contribution to health care delivery by helping to ensure optimum radiopharmaceutical use. Most of these contributions may be in the form of assistance (i.e., working together with nuclear medicine personnel) and education (i.e., in-service presentations, etc). Ponto and Hladik (94) have previously described a number of potential areas of hospital pharmacist involvement in nuclear medicine.

Policy and Procedure Manual. The hospital pharmacist

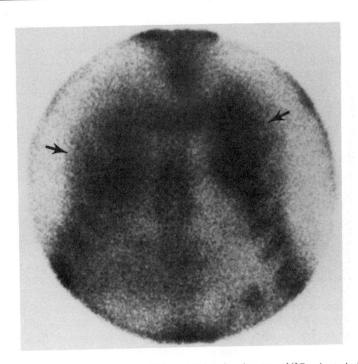

FIGURE 50.2 Anterior chest image shows abnormal diffuse localization of ⁶⁷Ga citrate in both lungs (arrows) in a patient with cyclophosphamide-induced pulmonary toxicity.

can be a valuable source in the development of a nuclear pharmacy policy and procedure manual. The hospital pharmacist can work together with nuclear medicine personnel to assure that the manual meets all of the requirements of the JCAH, etc.

Record Keeping. Similarly, the hospital pharmacist can work together with nuclear medicine personnel to develop appropriate log books, forms, or computer programs to record radiopharmaceutical receipt, inventory, disposition, disposal, etc (54,65,95-97).

Aseptic Technique. The pharmacist is often the authority on aseptic technique in the hospital. The hospital pharmacist can use his or her knowledge and expertise in this area to review and reinforce the objectives, procedures, and limitations of alcohol disinfection, laminar flow hoods, and other aspects of aseptic technique as should be practiced in the nuclear medicine area (98-100). A further step would be to assist in developing quality control procedures for verifying the maintenance of sterility and apyrogenicity in the laminar flow hood, pooled product samples, etc. (101,102).

Investigational New Drugs. The hospital pharmacist is frequently the individual most familiar with the regulatory aspects of investigational new drugs (INDs). The hospital pharmacist can use this knowledge to assist nuclear medicine personnel in the preparation of clinical protocols, obtaining institutional review board approval, developing patient consent forms, recording case report results, etc (103-105).

Drug Information. The hospital pharmacist can be a valuable source of drug information for nuclear medicine personnel. The hospital pharmacist is in a unique position to help in the identification of potential drug-radiopharmaceutical interactions (106,107). For example, abnormal pulmonary accumulation of gallium-67 citrate has been re-

ported in patients with bleomycin-induced pulmonary interstitial fibrosis. The pharmacist can alert nuclear medicine personnel that pulmonary accumulation of ⁶⁷Ga citrate may also be anticipated in patients treated with other drugs known to cause pulmonary fibrosis, viz, busulfan, cyclophosphamide, melphalan, methotrexate, mitomycin, nitrofurantoin, and procarbazine (107,108) (Fig. 50.2). The hospital pharmacist can also disseminate information on newly marketed drugs. For example, propranolol is known to affect exercise radionuclide ventriculograms by virtue of its pharmacologic effects on the heart. The hospital pharmacist can alert nuclear medicine personnel that similar effects may be anticipated with other beta-blockers that have recently been marketed, viz, atenolol, metoprolol, nadolol, and timolol (109). Finally, the hospital pharmacist can provide information about nonradioactive drugs used in nuclear medicine studies (110) such as dose selection, pharmacologic effects, contraindications, warnings and precautions, and adverse reactions. For example, the hospital pharmacist can advise on the use of synthetic analogs of cholecystokinin for stimulating gallbladder contraction and emptying in the evaluation of gallbladder function during hepatobiliary imaging studies (Fig. 50.3).

FUTURE TRENDS

Radiopharmaceutical imaging of the brain decreased significantly in the past decade because of the introduction of CT scanners. This trend is now reversing with the introduction of radiopharmaceuticals that penetrate the blood-brain barrier and assess physiologic function and pathology. The introduction of radiopharmaceuticals that demonstrate regional cerebral metabolism (e.g. ¹⁸F deoxyglucose) (111), regional cerebral blood flow (e.g., ¹²³I iodoamphetamine,

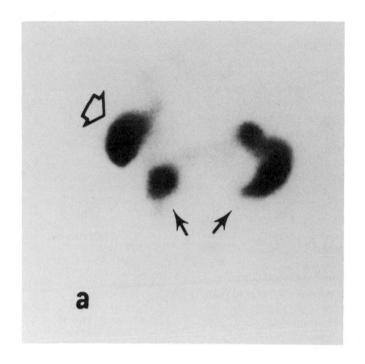

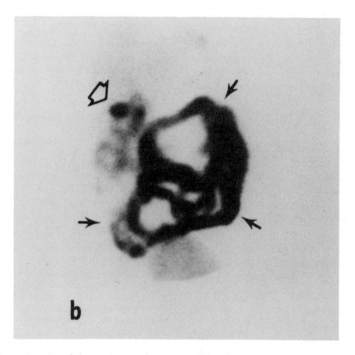

FIGURE 50.3   *a,* Anterior abdomen image shows normal localization of ⁹⁹ᵐTc disofenin in gallbladder (open arrow) and small intestine (arrows). *b,* A second image shows emptying of gallbladder activity (open arrow) into small intestine (arrows) 10 minutes after the injection of 0.3 μg/kg sincalide.

[123]I HIPDM, ^{99m}Tc diamines) (112-114), and distribution of specific receptors (e.g., ^{123}I iodoquinuclidines for muscarinic receptors) (115) indicate a future increase in brain function studies. These drugs not only measure pathologic function, but are capable of measuring cognitive responses to verbal, visual, and auditory inputs. Clinical areas under evaluation include learning disabilities (e.g., dyslexia), senility (e.g., dementia, Alzheimer's disease), and psychiatric disorders (e.g., depression, psychosis). It is currently estimated that in 5 years, 40% of all nuclear medicine procedures will be involved with brain function studies.

Other potential pharmaceuticals currently being labeled for specific organ diagnostic imaging and function evaluation include monoclonal antibodies (116,117), specific enzyme inhibitors (118), and fatty acid (119).

Positron emitting radiopharmaceuticals will be available in 1985 in 30 U.S. installations (60 worldwide). Potential radionuclide generators for [82]Ru and ^{68}Ga could make this technique available nationwide. These short half-life products are detected using positron emission tomography (PET) cameras. The reconstructed tomographic images, obtained from a variety of angles from the patient, provide significantly increased diagnostic information when compared to planar imaging. The use of positron emitting radiopharmaceuticals enhances the diagnosis of physiologic function. Using ^{18}F deoxyglucose, current clinical studies are assessing diffuse and focal epilepsy, Huntington's disease, Alzheimer's disease, and muscular dystrophy (111).

Single photon emission computerized tomography (SPECT) procedures use currently available radionuclides (e.g., ^{123}I or ^{99m}Tc) and are capable of describing radiopharmaceutical localization based on the movement of the camera in relation to the location of the radionuclide. Computer reconstruction of the data permits imaging of different slices of the organ imaged, thus improving significantly the clinician's information from which to make decisions. These SPECT systems are currently replacing many standard gamma cameras in hospitals.

Nuclear magnetic resonance imaging (NMR or MRI) has recently been approved by the FDA. An estimated 100-140 units were installed in the United States during 1984. These instruments pertubate the normal magnetic field that controls proton spin, thus causing the protons to release energy that can be measured. Different images result from altered proton spins associated with pathologic conditions.

Additional information about the pathologic tissue can be obtained using either paramagnetic or spectroscopic agents as drugs (120,121). Paramagnetic contrast agents alter the magnetic properties of the nuclei (usually water protons) being imaged. Thus, paramagnetic agents (unlike X-ray contrast agents) are not imaged, but their presence affects the image from the observed protons. Potential metal ions with paramagnetic moments include Gd, Mn, Fe, Co, V, Cr, Cu, and Ti. Mn-antimyosin has been observed in myocardial infarcts in dogs. These agents may also attach to monoclonal antibodies. Gd-DTPA is currently being used in clinical trials. In addition to protons ^{31}P, ^{13}C, ^{2}H, [23]Na, ^{19}F, and [17]O have the requisite spectroscopic property of spin moment. The presence of abnormal metabolites or chemical peaks, shifted from their normal resonance position, may indicate pathologic states.

Pharmacists will have the opportunity to be heavily involved with the research, development, supply, and clinical use of the pharmaceuticals used in conjunction with these newer imaging modalities. Some pharmacists are also becoming more active in the provision of contrast agents used for traditional X-ray procedures. Because of this expansion of responsibilities into areas other than strictly nuclear medicine, it is likely that over the next few years the term "nuclear pharmacy" will take on a new meaning, or rather, may even be changed to "radiologic pharmacy" or "diagnostic imaging pharmacy."

REFERENCES

1. Academy of Pharmacy Practice, Section on Nuclear Pharmacy: *Nuclear Pharmacy Practice Standards.* Washington, DC, American Pharmaceutical Association, 1976 (currently under revision).
2. Title 21 Code of Federal Regulations, Part 310.3(n).
3. Chase GD, Rabinowitz JL: *Principles of Radioisotope Methodology,* ed 3. Minneapolis, Burgess, 1967.
4. Hevesy GC: Marie Curie and her contemporaries. *J Nucl Med* 25:118-131, 1984.
5. Joliot F, Curie I: Artificial production of a new kind of radio-element. *Nature* 133:201, 1934.
6. Brucer M: *Trilinear Chart of the Nuclides.* St Louis, Mallinckrodt, 1979.
7. Lawrence EO: Evolution of the cyclotron. Nobel Prize lecture, December 11, 1951. In *Nobel Lectures: Physics, 1922-1941.* New York, Elsevier, 1965, pp 430-443.
8. Durham CT: Pharmaceutical aspects of atomic energy. *J Am Pharm Assoc* 11:346-350, 1950.
9. Christian JE: Radioactive isotopes in hospital pharmacy. *Bull Am Soc Hosp Pharm* 7:178-183, 1950.
10. Hutchinson GB: Some aspects of radioisotope therapy of interest to pharmacists. *J Am Pharm Assoc* 15:361-377, 1954.
11. Latiolais CJ, Parker PF, Hutchinson GB, et al: Radioisotopes in hospital pharmacy. *Bull Am Soc Hosp Pharm* 12:372-379, 1955.
12. Richards P: The technetium-99m generator. In Andrews GA, Kniseley RM, Wagner HN, Jr (eds): *Radioactive Pharmaceuticals.* Oak Ridge, U.S. Atomic Energy Commission, 1966, pp 323-334 (USAEC Symposium Series No. 6, Report CONF-651111).
13. Briner WH: Nuclear medicine has come of age. *Am J Hosp Pharm* 17:333-338, 1960.
14. Rubin I: Who will dispense radioactive drugs? *Am Prof Pharm* 30:28-29, 1964.
15. Briner WH: Radiopharmacy, the emerging young specialty. *Drug Intell* 2:8-13, 1968.
16. Quinn JL III: The role of the hospital radiopharmacy. In *Yearbook of Nuclear Medicine.* Chicago, Yearbook Medical Publishers, 1970, pp 5-13.
17. Wolf W, Tubis M, Marcus CS: The radiopharmacist, a new professional specialty. *Proc Am Nucl Soc* 15:132, 1972.
18. Dirksen JW: Nuclear pharmacy, a new pharmaceutical specialty. *NE Mortal Pestle* June 1973.
19. Wolf W: Radiopharmacy, a new profession. *Hospitals* 47:64-68, 1973.
20. Hamilton DR, Barnett M: Radiopharmacy: The challenge of an emerging specialty. *Hosp Formul* 11:364-365, 1976.
21. Rhodes BA, Friedman B: Why nuclear medicine spurs the need for more radiopharmacists. *Pharm Times* 44:94-96, April 1978.
22. Jones FE: Current handling procedures of radiopharmaceuticals in U.S. hospitals. *Am J Hosp Pharm* 27:38-49, 1970.
23. Porter WC, Ice RD, Hetzel KR: Establishment of a nuclear pharmacy. *Am J Hosp Pharm* 32:1023-1027, 1975.
24. Deiner CH (ed): *Lilly Hospital Pharmacy Survey.* Indianapolis, Eli Lilly, 1983.
25. Joint Commission on Accreditation of Hospitals: Pharmaceutical services. In *Accreditation Manual for Hospitals,* 1984 ed. Chicago, JCAH, 1983, pp 133-142.
26. *ibid.*: Nuclear medicine services. In *Accreditation Manual for Hospitals,* 1984 ed. Chicago, JCAH, 1983, pp 105-109.

27. Kawada TK, Tubis M, Ebenkamp T, et al: Review of nuclear pharmacy practice in hospitals. *Am J Hosp Pharm* 39:266-274, 1982.

28. Gnau TR, Maynard CD: Reducing the cost of nuclear medicine: Sharing radiopharmaceuticals. *Radiology* 108:641-645, 1972.

29. United States Pharmacopeial Convention: *The United States Pharmacopeia,* rev 20, and *The National Formulary,* ed 15. Easton, PA, Mack Publishing, 1979.

30. Freeman LM, Blaufox MD (eds): Cell labeling (part 1). *Semin Nucl Med* 14:68-140, 1984.

31. Burchiel SW, Rhodes BA (eds): *Radioimmunoimaging and Radioimmunotherapy.* New York, Elsevier, 1983.

32. Food and Drug Administration: *Nuclear Pharmacy Guideline Criteria for Determining When to Register as a Drug Establishment.* Washington, DC, Department of Health, Education and Welfare, April 1980.

33. Tubis M: Quality control of radiopharmaceuticals. In Tubis M, Wolf W (eds): *Radiopharmacy.* New York, John Wiley & Sons, 1976, pp 555-577.

34. Shen V, Hetzel KR, Ice RD: *Radiochemical Purity of Radiopharmaceuticals.* Ann Arbor, Gelman Instrument Co, 1974 (Gelman Technical Bulletin No. 32).

35. National Association of Boards of Pharmacy: *Model Regulations for Nuclear Pharmacy,* rev ed. Chicago, National Association of Boards of Pharmacy, March, 1983.

36. Title 49 Code of Federal Regulations, Parts 170-189.

37. Department of Transportation: *A Review of the Department of Transportation (DOT) Regulations for Transportation of Radioactive Materials.* Washington, DC, Department of Transportation, October, 1977.

38. Title 10 Code of Federal Regulations, Part 71.

39. Title 10 Code of Federal Regulations, Part 30.

40. Title 10 Code of Federal Regulations, Part 35.

41. National Council on Radiation Protection and Measurements: *Review of the Current State of Radiation Protection Philosophy.* Bethesda, National Council on Radiation Protection and Measurements, 1975 (NCRP Report No. 43).

42. Nuclear Regulatory Commission: *Guide for the Preparation of Applications for Medical Programs.* Washington, DC, Nuclear Regulatory Commission, 1980 (Regulatory Guide 10.8).

43. National Council on Radiation Protection and Measurements: *Safe Handling of Radioactive Materials.* Bethesda, National Council on Radiation Protection and Measurements, 1964 (NCRP Report No. 30).

44. National Council on Radiation Protection and Measurements: *Radiation Protection for Medical and Allied Health Personnel.* Bethesda, National Council on Radiation Protection and Measurements, 1977 (NCRP Report No. 48).

45. National Council on Radiation Protection and Measurements: *Nuclear Medicine—Factors Influencing the Choice and Use of Radionuclides in Diagnosis and Therapy.* Bethesda, National Council on Radiation Protection and Measurements, 1982 (NCRP Report No. 70).

46. Title 10 Code of Federal Regulations, Part 20.

47. Kawada T, Wolf W, Seibert S: Planning a radiopharmacy. *Am J Hosp Pharm* 31:153-157, 1974.

48. Spicer JA, Phelps MR, Leary M, et al: Optimization of radiopharmacy by redesign. *J Nucl Med Technol* 5:90-93, 1977.

49. Ice RD, Hetzel KR: Nuclear pharmacy health physics. In *Selected Papers on Nuclear Pharmacy.* Washington, DC, American Pharmaceutical Association, 1976, pp 39-44.

50. Gandsman E, North D, Spraragen SC: Radiation safety in a nuclear medicine department. *Health Physics* 38:399-407, 1980.

51. Baker WJ, Beightol RW, Christian PE, et al: Common sense radiation protection in the radiopharmacy: Utilization of existing resources. *J Nucl Med Technol* 9:143-145, 1981.

52. Bureau of Radiological Health: *Workshop Manual for Radionuclide Handling and Radiopharmaceutical Quality Assurance.* Rockville, MD, Department of Health and Human Services, 1982 (HHS Publication FDA 82-8191).

53. Distefano RM, Herandez L: Clinical radiopharmacy. *Drug Intell Clin Pharm* 4:209-212, 1970.

54. Bowen BM: Radiopharmaceutical patient profile: A clinical approach. In *Selected papers on Nuclear Pharmacy.* Washington, DC, American Pharmaceutical Association, 1976, pp 28-30.

55. Ice RD, Hetzel K: Clinical nuclear pharmacy. In *Selected Papers on Nuclear Pharmacy.* Washington, DC, American Pharmaceutical Association, 1976, pp 31-37.

56. Wolf W: A system for the delivery of radiopharmaceutical services. *Hosp Formul* 11:376-378, 1976.

57. American Society of Hospital Pharmacists: ASHP Accreditation Standard for Residency Training in Nuclear Pharmacy. *Am J Hosp Pharm* 38:1964-1971, 1981.

58. Hladik WB III, Saha GB, Study KT (eds): *Essentials of Nuclear Medicine Science.* Baltimore, Williams & Wilkins, 1986 (in press).

59. *Florida Board of Pharmacy Regulations, Rules.* Chapter 21S (21S-3.03 to 3.04), January 1981.

60. *Regulations on Radiopharmaceuticals.* Arizona State Board of Pharmacy, Regulation No. R1-23 501-K, adopted November 30, 1974.

61. *House of Delegates Resolutions.* American Association of Colleges of Pharmacy Annual Meeting, Lake Kiamesha, NY, July 1975.

62. Tubis M, Wolf W (eds): *Radiopharmacy.* New York, John Wiley & Sons, 1976.

63. Rhodes BA, Croft BY: *Basics of Radiopharmacy.* St Louis, CV Mosby, 1978.

64. Phan T, Wasnich R: *Practical Nuclear Pharmacy,* rev 2. Honolulu, Banyan Enterprises, 1981.

65. Vandergouw HF: *Guidelines to Radiopharmacy.* Floral Park, MD, Scientific Publishing, 1982.

66. Saha GB: *Fundamentals of Nuclear Pharmacy,* ed 2. New York, Springer-Verlag, 1984.

67. Behm HL, Ice RD: An introduction to nuclear pharmacy. *US Pharm* 1:29-33, 1976.

68. Behm HL, Ice RD: Radiological physics of nuclear pharmacy. *US Pharm* 2:50-57, 1977.

69. Behm HL, Ice RD: Nuclear pharmacy radiological health. *US Pharm* 2:42-47, 1977.

70. Behm HL, Ice RD: Nuclear pharmacy: Organ imaging radiopharmaceuticals. *US Pharm* 2:64-74, 1977.

71. Behm HL, Ice RD: In vitro radiopharmaceuticals. *US Pharm* 2:64-74, 1977.

72. Behm HL, Ice RD: Nuclear pharmacy: Radiological function studies. *US Pharm* 2:70-80, 1977.

73. Laven DL: Nuclear pharmacy: An introduction to a new specialty. *Fla J Hosp Pharm* 3:33-63, 1983.

74. Laven DL: Nuclear pharmacy (Part II): Radiopharmaceuticals—facts and uses. *Fla J Hosp Pharm* 3:97-166, 1983.

75. Laven DL: Nuclear pharmacy (Part III): Quality assurance of radiopharmaceuticals. *Fla J Hosp Pharm* 3:217-234, 1983.

76. Laven DL: Nuclear pharmacy (Part III continued): Quality assurance of radiopharmaceuticals. *Fla J Hosp Pharm* 4:9-58, 1984.

77. Laven DL: Nuclear pharmacy (Part IV): Radiopharmaceutical—drug interactions and altered biodistribution. *Fla J Hosp Pharm* 4:17-64, 1984.

78. Ice RD, Shaw SM, Born GS, et al: Nuclear pharmacy education. *Am J Pharm Ed* 38:420-425, 1974.

79. Schlegel JF, Shaw SM: Nuclear pharmacy education. *Am Pharm* NS21:38-39, 1981.

80. Coupal JJ: The basic undergraduate nuclear pharmacy program. *Am Pharm* NS21:40, 1981.

81. Shaw SM, Bartlett JM, Bennett RW: Medical applications of radiation: An introductory course for pharmacists. *Am J Pharm Ed* 47:53-55, 1983.

82. Anon: Argus commission calls for marketing of colleges of pharmacy. *Am J Hosp Pharm* 40:1596-1598, 1983.

83. Kawada T, Wolf W, Mochizuki D: Hospital radiopharmacy training program. *Am J Hosp Pharm* 32:587-589, 1975.

84. Breslow K: The residency in radiopharmacy. *Am Pharm* NS21:46-47, 1981.

85. Pollock ML, Strane TR, Brown GJ, et al: Nuclear pharmacy: A student's perspective. *Contem Pharm Prac* 2:190-194, 1979.

86. Wolf W, Tubis M, Kawada TK: The master of science in radiopharmacy. *Am Pharm* NS21:41-43, 1981.

87. Ice RD, Basmadjian G: Nuclear pharmacy Ph.D. programs. *Am Pharm* NS21:44-45, 1981.

88. Board of Pharmaceutical Specialties: *Petitioner's Guide for Specialty Recognition.* Washington, DC, American Pharmaceutical Association, 1974.

89. Grussing PG, Allen DR, Callahan RJ, et al: Development of pharmacy's first specialty certification examination: Nuclear pharmacy. *Am J Pharm Ed* 47:11-18, 1983.

90. Board of Pharmaceutical Specialties: *Nuclear Pharmacy Certification Examination Candidate's Guide*. Washington, DC, American Pharmaceutical Association, 1982.

91. Penna RP: Pharmacy's first specialty. *American Pharmacy* NS22: 612-615, 1982.

92. McEvoy GK (ed): *American Hospital Formulary Service*. Bethesda, American Society of Hospital Pharmacists, published annually.

93. Del Medico J: NRC's approach to nuclear pharmacy education. *Am Pharm* NS21:48-49, 1981.

94. Ponto JA, Hladik WB III: Providing pharmacy services in the small hospital: Nuclear pharmacy services. Paper presented to 129th annual APhA meeting, Las Vegas, April 26, 1982.

95. Warbick A: A product standards form for new radiopharmaceuticals. *Am J Hosp Pharm* 31:165-166, 1974.

96. Cole CN: An efficient radiopharmaceutical record keeping system. *Hosp Formul* 11:385-389, 1976.

97. Baker WJ, DeBlanc HJ: A multipurpose record-keeping system for the centralized radiopharmacy. In *Selected Papers on Nuclear Pharmacy*. Washington, DC, American Pharmaceutical Association, 1976, pp 21-27.

98. Trapnell LK, Robinson LA: Developing a comprehensive training program in aseptic technique. *Hosp Pharm* 13:431-436, 1978.

99. Kirschner AS: Radiopharmaceuticals. In Turco S, King RE (eds): *Sterile Dosage Forms*. Philadelphia, Lea & Febiger, 1979, pp 321-332.

100. Avis KE, Levchuk JW: Special considerations in the use of vertical laminar-flow workbenches. *Am J Hosp Pharm* 41:81-87, 1984.

101. Frieben WR: Control of the aseptic processing environment. *Am J Hosp Pharm* 40:1928-1935, 1983.

102. Boylan JC: Essential elements of quality control. *Am J Hosp Pharm* 40:1936-1939, 1983.

103. Arbit HM: Regulatory aspects of investigational new drugs. *Am J Hosp Pharm* 35:81-85, 1978.

104. Food and Drug Administration: *Guidelines for the Clinical Evaluation of Radiopharmaceutical Drugs*. Rockville, MD, Health and Human Services, 1981 (HHS(FDA) 81-3120).

105. American Society of Hospital Pharmacists: ASHP guidelines for the use of investigational drugs in institutions. *Am J Hosp Pharm* 40:449-451, 1983.

106. Hladik WB III, Ponto JA, Stathis VJ: Drug-radiopharmaceutical interactions. In Thrall JH, Swanson DP (eds): *Diagnostic Interventions in Nuclear Medicine*. Chicago, Yearbook Medical Publishers, 1985, pp 226-246.

107. Hladik WB III, Nigg KK, Rhodes BA: Drug-induced changes in the biologic distribution of radiopharmaceuticals. *Semin Nucl Med* 12:184-218, 1982.

108. Lentle BC, Scott JR, Noujaim AA, et al: Iatrogenic alterations in radionuclide biodistributions. *Semin Nucl Med* 9:131-143, 1979.

109. Ponto JA, Holmes KA: Discontinuation of beta blockers before radionuclide ventriculograms. *J Nucl Med* 23:456-457, 1982.

110. Ponto JA, Hladik WB III: Common uses of nonradioactive drugs in nuclear medicine. *Am J Hosp Pharm* 41:1189-1193, 1984.

111. Fox JL: PET scan controversy aired. *Science* 224:144-145, 1984.

112. Kung HF, Tramposch KM, Balu M: A new brain perfusion imaging agent: I-123 HIPDM: N,N,N'-trimethyl-N'-hydroxy-3-methyl-5-iodobenzyl-1,3-propanediamine. *J Nucl Med* 24:66-72, 1983.

113. Holman BL, Hill TC, Magistretti PL. Brain imaging with emission computed tomography and radiolabeled amines. *Invest Radiol* 17:206-215, 1982.

114. Troutner DE, Volkert WA, Hoffman TJ, et al: A tetradentate amine oxime complex of Tc-99m. *J Nucl Med* 24:P10, 1983.

115. Eckelman WC, Reba RC, Rzeszotarski WJ, et al: External imaging of cerebral muscarinic receptors. *Science* 223:291-293, 1984.

116. Edwards DC. Targeting potential of antibody conjugates. *Pharmacol Ther* 23:147-177, 1983.

117. Goldenberg DM: Tumor imaging with monoclonal antibodies. *J Nucl Med* 24:360-362, 1983.

118. Stark GR, Bartlett PA: Design and use of potent, specific enzyme inhibitors. *Pharmacol Ther* 23:45-78, 1983.

119. Ercan M, Senekowitsch R, Bauer R, et al: In vivo and in vitro studies with W-[p-^{123}I-phenyl]-Pentadecanoic acid in rats. *Int J Appl Radiat Isot* 34:1519-1524, 1983.

120. Koutcher JA, Burt CT, Lauffer RB, et al: Contrast agents and spectroscopic probes in NMR. *J Nucl Med* 25:606-613, 1984.

121. Chilton HM, Ekstrand KE: Principles and applications of nuclear magnetic resonance imaging. *Am J Hosp Pharm* 41:763-768, 1984.

CHAPTER 51

Oncology Services

WILLIAM J. DANA

The increasing use of cytotoxic agents in the treatment of cancer has given the pharmacist new challenges and opportunities to provide care to the oncology patient. An estimated 200,000-400,000 patients yearly are receiving chemotherapy, producing either a complete or partial response in a significant number of cases (1). At least a dozen tumor types have been identified in which chemotherapy has produced a high percentage of cures (2). An equal number of cancers also show partial response and improved survival rates with the addition of cytotoxic agents to the treatment regimen. These numbers are having a significant impact on institutional pharmacy practice in both the inpatient and outpatient oncology environment. The purpose of this chapter is to review and discuss the various aspects of pharmacy services to the cancer patient.

IV ADDITIVE SERVICES

A majority of the 40 commercially available and approximately 65 investigational cancer chemotherapeutic agents are administered parenterally. Traditionally these products have been administered by the IV bolus method or by intermittent infusion. Tables 51.1 to 51.3 list guidelines for the preparation and administration of both chemotherapeutic agents, as well as antibiotics that are also commonly prescribed for the cancer patient.

The recent literature has indicated that certain cytotoxic agents are more effective when administered by continuous infusion, whereas others are best given by short-term infusion or bolus (3-9). The use of various flow control devices to ensure the accuracy of the delivery of these agents is commonly employed in many institutions. Recently the addition of portable small-volume devices for both hospitalized and outpatient administration is having an impact on pharmacy services (3,4,6). Besides allowing for continuous chemotherapy administration, major advantages for the patient include decreased hospitalization time and cost and greater mobility. The latest addition to this technology is the development of implantable pumps secured subcutaneously, thereby eliminating patient maintenance of the device (10,11).

This recent technology has also produced a tremendous need for chemotherapy stability and compatibility data in numerous types of containers and when mixed with other drugs. As of this writing only a limited amount of chemotherapy stability and compatibility data can be found in the literature (12-15). The reader should refer to Chapter 34 for a detailed discussion on IV admixture systems.

EXPOSURE RISK TO HANDLING CYTOTOXIC AGENTS

The increased awareness to the potential risks of preparing, administering, and disposing of cancer chemotherapeutic agents has produced numerous studies, reviews, and recommendations on this topic. Table 51.4 lists the September 1984 recommendations of the National Study Commission on Cytotoxic Exposure. These are reasonable and prudent guidelines to protect the worker and the environment from needless exposure to cytotoxic agents. Many issues remain unanswered and are currently being addressed by various commissions, agencies, and individual institutions. These include the issues of pregnant personnel handling cytotoxic substances, appropriate disposal of waste products from cancer patients, optimal glove material for employee protection, and the legal ramifications for both employer and employee. Pharmacists must keep current on this issue through communication with other institutions and with the

TABLE 51.1 Guidelines for Chemotherapy IV Push Administration (Administration within 2-3 Minutes)

Agents	Caution Label
L-Asparaginase	Observe for allergic reactions
Cyclophosphamide	
Cytarabine	
Dacarbazine	
Dactinomycin	*Avoid extravasation*
Daunorubicin	*Avoid extravasation; too rapid infusion may cause flushing and other allergy like symptoms*
Doxorubicin	*Avoid extravasation; too rapid infusion may cause flushing and other allergy like symptoms*
Fluorouracil	
Mechlorethamine	*Avoid extravasation*
Methotrexate	
Mitomycin	*Avoid extravasation*
Streptozocin	
Thiotepa	
Vinblastine	*Avoid extravasation*
Vincristine	*Avoid extravasation*

TABLE 51.2 Chemotherapy Fluid Standardizations

Drug	Dose	Fluid	Volume	Rate
Asparaginase	All	D5W	50 ml	Over 15 min
Bleomycin	All	D5W	50 ml	Over 15 min
Carmustine	All	D5W	250 ml	Over 1 hr
Cisplatin	All	NS	1000 ml	Over 2 hr
Cyclophosphamide	All	D5W	100 ml	Over 15 min
Cytarabine	Conventional doses only	D5W	50 ml	Over 15 min
Dacarbazine	All	D5W	100 ml	Over 30 min
Dactinomycin	All	D5W	50 ml	Over 15 min
Daunorubicin	All	D5W	50 ml	Over 15 min
Doxorubicin	All	D5W	50 ml	Over 15 min
Etoposide	All	D5W	500 ml	Over 2 hr
Fluorouracil	All	D5W	50 ml	Over 15 min
Methotrexate	Conventional doses only	D5W	50 ml	Over 15 min
Mitomycin	All	NS	50 ml	Over 15 min
Plicamycin	All	D5W	250 ml	Over 2 hr
Streptozocin	All	D5W	50 ml	Over 15 min
Thiotepa	All	D5W	50 ml	Over 15 min
Vinblastine	All	D5W	50 ml	Over 15 min
Vincristine	All	D5W	50 ml	Over 15 min

TABLE 51.3 Antibiotic Fluid Standardizations

Drug	Dose	Fluid	Volume	Rate
Acyclovir	All	D5W	100 ml	Over 1 hr
Amikacin	All	D5W	100 ml	Over 30 min
Amphotericin-B	All	D5W	500 ml	Over 6 hr
Ampicillin	0-1 g	NS	50 ml	Over 30 min
	1.01 g & over	NS	100 ml	Over 30 min
Carbenicillin	All	D5W	100 ml	Over 1 hr
Cefamandole	0-1 g	D5W	50 ml	Over 30 min
	1.01 g & over	D5W	100 ml	Over 30 min
Cefazolin	0-1 g	D5W	50 ml	Over 30 min
	1.01 g & over	D5W	100 ml	Over 30 min
Cefotaxime	0-1 g	D5W	50 ml	Over 30 min
	1.01 g & over	D5W	100 ml	Over 30 min
Cefoxitin	0-1 g	D5W	50 ml	Over 30 min
	1.01 g & over	D5W	100 ml	Over 30 min
Cephalothin	0-1 g	D5W	50 ml	Over 30 min
	1.01 g & over	D5W	100 ml	Over 30 min
Chloramphenicol	All	D5W	50 ml	Over 30 min
Clindamycin	0-300 mg	D5W	50 ml	Over 30 min
	301 mg & over	D5W	100 ml	Over 30 min
Colistin	All	D5W	50 ml	Over 30 min
Doxycycline	All	D5W	250 ml	Over 1 hr
Erythromycin	All	D5W	100 ml	Over 30 min
Gentamicin	All	D5W	50 ml	Over 30 min
Kanamycin	All	D5W	100 ml	Over 30 min
Methicillin	All	D5W	50 ml	Over 30 min
Metronidazole	All	D5W	250 ml	Over 1 hr
Mezlocillin	All	D5W	100 ml	Over 1 hr
Miconazole	All	D5W	250 ml	Over 2 hr
Moxalactam	0-1 g	D5W	50 ml	Over 30 min
	1.01 g & over	D5W	100 ml	Over 30 min
Nafcillin	All	D5W	50 ml	Over 30 min
Netilmicin	All	D5W	50 ml	Over 30 min
Oxacillin	All	D5W	50 ml	Over 30 min
Penicillin-G	All	D5W	100 ml	Over 1 hr
Piperacillin	All	D5W	100 ml	Over 1 hr
Tetracycline	All	D5W	100 ml	Over 1 hr
Ticarcillin	All	D5W	100 ml	Over 1 hr
Tobramycin	All	D5W	50 ml	Over 30 min
Trimethoprim/sulfamethoxazole	All	D5W	125 ml/Amp	Over 30 min
Vancomycin	All	D5W	100 ml	Over 30 min

TABLE 51.4 Recommendations for Handling Cytotoxic Agents[a] (September 1984)

Preamble

The increasing use of cytotoxic agents and the growing awareness of potential hazards requires special attention to the procedures utilized in the handling, preparation, and administration of these drugs. Equally important is the proper disposal of chemical residues and wastes. These recommendations are intended to provide information for the protection of personnel participating in the clinical process of chemotherapy. The mutagenic and carcinogenic potential of many cytotoxic agents is well established and is a possible hazard to the health of exposed individuals. It is the responsibility of institutional and private health care providers to adopt and use appropriate procedures for protection and safety.

I. Environmental protection

1. All mixing of cytotoxic agents should be performed in a Class II, biological safety cabinet. Type A cabinets are the minimal requirement. Type A cabinets which are vented (some now classified as Type B3) are preferred.
2. Special techniques and precautions must be utilized because of the vertical (downward) laminar airflow (see Supplement I).
3. The biological safety cabinet must be certified by qualified personnel annually or any time the cabinet is physically moved.
4. The biological safety cabinet should be operated with the blower on, 24 hours per day—seven days per week.
5. Drug preparations must be performed only with the view screen at the recommended access opening. Professionally accepted practices concerning the aseptic preparation of injectable products should be followed.

II. Operator protection

1. Disposable surgical latex gloves are recommended for all procedures involving cytotoxic drugs. Polyvinyl chloride (PVC) gloves should not be worn while handling cytotoxic agents. Several types of PVC gloves are permeable to a variety of drugs.
2. Gloves should routinely be changed approximately every 30 minutes when working steadily with cytotoxic agents. Gloves should be removed immediately after overt contamination.
3. Double gloving is recommended for cleaning up of spills.
4. Protective barrier garments should be worn for all procedures involving the preparation and disposal of cytotoxic agents. These garments should have a closed front, long sleeves and closed cuff (either elastic or knit).
5. All potentially contaminated garments must not be worn outside the work area.

III. Compounding procedures and techniques

1. Hands must be washed thoroughly before gloving and after gloves are removed.
2. Care must be taken to avoid puncturing of gloves and possible self-inoculation.
3. Syringes and IV sets with Luer-lock fittings should be used whenever possible.
4. Vials should be vented with a hydrophobic filter to eliminate internal pressure or vacuum.
5. Before opening ampules, care should be taken to insure that no liquid remains in the tip of the ampule. A sterile, disposable alcohol dampened gauze sponge should be wrapped around the neck of the ampule to reduce aerosolization.
6. For sealed vials, final drug measurement should be performed prior to removing the needle from the stopper of the vial and after the pressure has been equalized.
7. A closed collection vessel should be available in the biological safety cabinet or the original vial may be used to hold discarded excess drug solutions.
8. Special procedures should be followed for acute exposure or spills (Supplement II).
9. Cytotoxic agents which are handled within the treatment area should be properly labeled (e.g., "Chemotherapy: Dispose of Properly").

IV. Precautions for medication administration

1. Disposable surgical latex gloves should be worn during all cytotoxic drug administration activities.
2. Syringes and IV sets with Luer-lock fittings should be used whenever possible.
3. Special care must be taken in priming IV sets. The distal tip cover must be removed before priming. Priming should be performed into a sterile, alcohol-dampened gauze sponge, which then is disposed of appropriately.

V. Disposal procedures

1. Place contaminated materials in a leakproof, puncture-proof container appropriately marked as hazardous waste.
2. Cytotoxic drug waste should be transported according to the institutional procedures for contaminated material.
3. There is insufficient information to recommend any single preferred method for disposal of cytotoxic drug waste.
   - 3.1 One method for disposal of hazardous waste is by incineration at a temperature considered sufficient by the Environmental Protection Agency (EPA) to destroy organic compounds. Incineration should be done in an EPA permitted hazardous waste incinerator.
   - 3.2 Another method of disposal is by burial at an EPA permitted hazardous waste site.
   - 3.3 A licensed hazardous waste disposal company may be consulted for information concerning available methods of disposal in the local area.

VI. Personnel policy recommendations

1. All personnel working with cytotoxic agents must receive special training.
2. Access to the compounding area must be limited to only necessary authorized personnel.
3. The personnel working with these agents should be observed regularly by supervisory personnel to insure compliance with procedures.
4. Acute exposure episodes must be documented. The employee must be referred for professional medical examination.

VII. Monitoring procedures

1. Procedures to monitor the equipment and operating techniques of the personnel should be performed on a regular basis and documented. Specific methods of monitoring should be developed to meet the complexities of the function.
2. It is recommended that personnel involved in the preparation of cytotoxic agents on a full time basis be given periodic health examinations in accordance with institutional policy.

[a]Reprinted by permission of the National Study Commission on Cytotoxic Exposure, Department of Pharmacy, Providence, RI.

TABLE 51.4, cont'd

SUPPLEMENT I
Special Techniques and Precautions for Use in the Class II Biological Safety Cabinet

1. All equipment needed to complete the procedure in the Class II Biological Safety Cabinet should be placed into the cabinet before beginning and the view screen should be placed at the recommended operating position. A wait of at least two to three minutes before beginning work to allow the unit time to purge itself of airborne contaminants is recommended.
2. The proper procedures for use in the Biological Safety Cabinet are not the same as those used in the horizontal laminar hood. In many cases they seem contradictory, although in theory they are not. This is because of the nature of the airflow pattern in the Biological Safety Cabinet. Clean air descends through the work zone from the top of the cabinet toward the work surface. As it descends, the air is split, with some leaving through the rear perforation and some leaving through the front perforation. The region where the airflow splits is known as the "smoke split" because smoke introduced into this area appears to split into two directions.
3. It is recommended that the smoke split be determined and marked on each cabinet after it is purchased even if the manufacturer states its location. This can be easily done by using an incense stick to generate smoke and moving it gently from front to rear laterally along the work surface of the cabinet near the center.
4. Routinely used large equipment should be placed in the cabinet in its normal position when the determination of the smoke split is made. The equipment should then be placed in the same position every time the cabinet is used.
5. Personnel should refrain from applying any face powder, eye make-up, rouge, fingernail polish, hairspray or other cosmetics in the work area. These cosmetics may provide a source of prolonged exposure if contaminated.
6. Eating, drinking, chewing of gum, storage of food or smoking in, around or near the Biological Safety Cabinet should be prohibited. Each of these are sources of ingestion if they are accidentally contaminated by the cytotoxic agent or other hazardous products.
7. Sterile products should be arranged in the cabinet so as to minimize the possibility of contamination. This may mean locating them in the immediate vicinity of the smoke split. If appropriate, due to quantity or configuration, the sterile items should be kept only in the center and nonsterile items on either side.
8. For additional operator protection, it is recommended that the area behind the smoke split be used whenever possible since the airflow direction in that area is away from the operator, lessening the chance of accidental exposure.
9. The least efficient area of the cabinet in terms of product and personnel protection is within three inches of the sides near the front opening. Therefore, you should not work within three inches of the sides of the cabinet.
10. Periodic evaluation of the smoke split should be performed on a routine basis. A constantly changing smoke split location may be indicative of problems with the operation of the cabinet.
11. Entry into and exit from the cabinet should be in a direct manner perpendicular to the face of the cabinet. Rapid movements of the hands in the cabinet and laterally through the protective air barrier should be avoided.

SUPPLEMENT II
Special Procedures for Acute Exposure or Spills

1.0 ACUTE EXPOSURE
    1.1 Overtly contaminated gloves or outer garments should be removed and replaced immediately after an exposure.
    1.2 Hands should be washed after removing gloves. Gloves are not a substitute for handwashing.
    1.3 In case of skin contact with a cytotoxic drug product, the affected area should be washed thoroughly with soap and water as soon as possible. Refer to professional medical attention as soon as possible.
    1.4 For eye exposure, flush affected eye with copious amounts of water. Refer to professional medical attention immediately.
2.0 SPILLS
    2.1 All personnel involved in the clean-up of a spill should wear protective clothing (e.g. gloves, gowns, etc.). All clothes and other material used in the process should be treated or disposed of properly.
    2.2 Double gloving should be used in the cleaning up of spills.

medical and nursing staff and other departments affected in their own institution. A selected bibliography on the topic prepared by the Pharmacy Department at M.D. Anderson Hospital and Tumor Institute is listed at the end of this chapter.

INVESTIGATIONAL CANCER CHEMOTHERAPEUTIC AGENTS

Many of the agents used in the treatment of malignancies are in a particular phase of investigation and thus may offer the pharmacist the opportunity to participate in protocol development and design, data management, and inventory control. The Investigational Drug Branch of the National Cancer Institute now requires strict accountability of these agents for each protocol. (See Chapter 45 for a detailed discussion of these topics.)

ANCILLARY SUPPORT OF THE CANCER PATIENT

The aggressive nature of cancer and its equally aggressive treatment often produce complications and toxicities requiring ancillary care involving the pharmacy department. Nutritional support of the cancer patient is often required to offset the catabolic nature of the disease and to hasten recovery from treatment toxicities (16). Chapter 36 deals with this subject in detail.

A considerable number of cancer patients suffer pain and require vigorous analgesic therapy (17-19). The pharmacy department must be prepared to handle what may seem an unduly large narcotic inventory and also must assist in the preparation of special dosage forms for continuous infusion narcotic therapy, as well as for intrathecal, epidural, and intraventricular use. Table 51.5 lists a formula for preparing preservative-free morphine solutions for special uses.

TABLE 51.5 Preparation of Preservative-free Morphine Sulfate, 1 mg/ml

1. Place one 10-mg morphine sulfate tablet in a 20-ml syringe.
2. Draw 10-ml preservative-free normal saline solution into syringe.
3. Place a 0.22-μm filter on syringe.
4. Filter solution into a pyrogen-free 10-ml vial.
5. Autoclave vials at 250° F in 15 psi for 25 minutes.
6. Cap and label vials. Refrigerate until used.

TABLE 51.6 Stomatitis Formulas

Nystatin ice popsicles
   60 million units nystatin powder
   300 ml black cherry concentrate
   1,800 ml sterile water

   1. Mix nystatin powder with 300 ml of sterile water to make solution.
   2. Add black cherry concentrate and stir well.
   3. Add sterile water, qs to 1,800 ml.
   4. Stir or shake well and pour into 30-ml unit dose cups (makes 60 cups, 1 million units nystatin each).
   5. Freeze.
   6. Eat with a spoon qid.

Cook's stomatitis ointment
   120 g boric acid ointment, 10%
   120 g tetracaine (Pontocaine) ointment
   30 drops peppermint oil

   1. Mix thoroughly and place in ½-oz (14-g) ointment jars for prn use.

Dr. Powell's mouthwash
   1.2 million units nystatin
   500 mg tetracycline
   100 mg hydrocortisone
   qs 250 ml diphenhydramine (elixir)

   1. Mix thoroughly; swish and swallow qid.

Dr. Sullivan's mouthwash
   16 ml neomycin, 1% solution
   3.2 ml polymyxin B, 2% solution
   32 oz (960 ml) sterile water

   1. Mix medications with water qs to 32 oz (960 ml); swish and swallow tid or qid.

Other special formulas the pharmacy department may be called on to assist with include products for prevention or management of chemotherapy-induced stomatitis (20,21). Table 51.6 lists formulas that may be useful in treating this painful condition. It is important to note that primary mouth care therapy for chemotherapy-induced stomatitis is a mild saline solution (1 tablespoon per quart of water) or peroxide solution (½%) and that the formulas listed that contain antibiotic or antifungal agents be reserved for conditions warranting their use.

ONCOLOGY PHARMACY AS A SPECIALTY PRACTICE

The American Society of Hospital Pharmacists (ASHP) has recognized the oncology pharmacist as a specialist with the formation of the Special Interest Group (SIG) on Oncology Pharmacy Practice. This SIG currently has 319 members and is the third largest of the 11 groups in the society. Discussions with numerous oncology SIG members have revealed a wide diversity of practice and needs. Many members have only recently become involved in oncology pharmacy practice. Major information needs of these groups include exposure risk to handling cytotoxic agents, development of investigational drug inventory control systems, and guidance in pharmacists' involvement in protocol development and maintenance. In addition, a practice standards document is currently being developed to assist the membership in providing optimal patient care.

Specialized training programs in the form of oncology pharmacy fellowships are available to provide both administrative and clinical education in oncology pharmacy services (22).

Numerous opportunities exist for the oncology pharmacist to participate in cancer awareness programs in the community. Cooperative efforts between hospitals, schools, and professional societies, including the American Cancer Society, can provide a useful public service. The Priority Activities in Cancer Education (PACE) program focuses on the early detection and prevention of the most commonly occurring cancers (23). Pharmacists interested in participating in this or similar cancer awareness programs should contact their local or regional American Cancer Society office.

Patient education is yet another area where the oncology pharmacist can provide a much-needed service. Patient aids such as audiovisual material and chemotherapy booklets or cards have been developed to assist the patient and family with their therapy. Figure 51.1 is an example of a chemotherapy information card designed for this purpose and is the result of a multidisciplinary approach to patient education involving the pharmacist.

THE FUTURE OF ONCOLOGY PHARMACY PRACTICE

New technology and the economics of health care will continue to influence pharmacy services to the cancer patient. Studies are currently underway to administer chemotherapeutic agents in delivery systems such as liposomes, starch microspheres, and monoclonal antibodies for specific cell targeting. Outpatient chemotherapy administration has expanded to include therapy for the patient at home. New challenges for the pharmacist include the need to expand patient education to home care, long-term chemotherapy stability and compatibility, and the issues of handling and disposing of cytotoxic materials at home. The oncology pharmacist must be prepared to meet these new challenges and grow with the expanding technology in treating the cancer patient.

MERCAPTOPURINE
(Purinethol® , 6-MP)

1. Early Side Effects

a. Nausea, vomiting, or appetite loss are common.

b. Local blistering may occur at the injection site. Contact your doctor or nurse immediately if pain, redness, or swelling occurs near the injection site.

2. Late Side Effects

a. A drop in blood cell counts i.e., red cells, white cells, and platelets occurs 7-14 days after treatment.

b. Mouth ulcers may occur within several days after treatment. Mouth care is very important. A dilute mouthwash of hydrogen peroxide and water (1 tablespoonful peroxide to 5 tablespoonfuls water) and the use of a soft toothbrush are helpful. Contact your doctor or nurse if ulcers or pain are severe. Avoid use of commercial mouthwashes.

3. Special Instructions

a. This drug **should not** be taken with the drug allopurinol (Zyloprim®) unless under the direction of your doctor at M. D. Anderson Hospital.

b. This drug may be stored at room temperature.

These are the most common side effects; others may occur. Please report any problems to your doctor.

©The University of Texas M. D. Anderson Hospital and Tumor Institute at Houston

FIGURE 51.1 Chemotherapy patient information card on mercaptopurine. (Permission to reprint granted by Department of Patient Education, Box 21, M.D. Anderson Hospital, 6723 Bertner Ave., Houston, TX 77030.)

REFERENCES

1. DeVita VT Jr: Principles of chemotherapy. In DeVita VT Jr, Hellman S, Rosenberg SA (eds): *Cancer, Principles and Practice of Oncology.* Philadelphia, JB Lippincott, 1982, pp 132-155.
2. DeVita VT, Henney JE, Hubbard SM: Estimation of the numerical and economic impact of chemotherapy in the treatment of cancer. In Burchenal JH, Oettgen (eds): *Cancer Achievements, Challenges, and Prospects for the 1980's.* New York, Grune & Stratton, 1981, pp 857-880.
3. Dorr RT et al: Limitations of a portable infusion pump in ambulatory patients receiving continuous infusions of anticancer drugs. *Cancer Treat Rep* 63:211-213, 1979.
4. Bottino J et al: Continuous intravenous arabinosyl cytosine infusions delivered by a new portable infusion system. *Cancer* 43:2197-2201, 1979.
5. Buckles RG: New horizons in drug delivery. *CA* 28:343-355, 1978.
6. Ballentine R et al: Alternatives in outpatient chemotherapy administration. *Cancer Bull* 32:173-176, 1980.
7. Legha SS et al: Reduction of doxorubicin cardiotoxicity by prolonged continuous intravenous infusion. *Ann Intern Med* 96:133-139, 1982.
8. Yap HY, et al: Vinblastine given as a continuous 5-day infusion in the treatment of refractory advanced breast cancer. *Cancer Treat Rep* 64:279-283, 1980.
9. Lawson M et al: Long term I.V. therapy: A new approach. *Am J Nurs* 79:1100-1103, 1979.
10. Weiss GR et al: Long-term hepatic arterial infusion of 5-fluorode-oxyuridine for liver metastases using an implantable infusion pump. *Am J Clin Oncol* 1:337-344, 1983.
11. Ensminger W et al: Effective control of liver metastases from colon cancer with an implanted system for hepatic arterial chemotherapy (abstract). *Proc Am Soc Clin Oncol* 1:94, 1982.
12. Benvenuto JA, et al: Stability and compatibility of antitumor agents in glass and plastic containers. *Am J Hosp Pharm* 38:1914-1918, 1981.
13. Hoffman DM, et al: Stability of refrigerated and frozen solutions of doxorubicin hydrochloride. *Am J Hosp Pharm* 36:1536-1538, 1979.
14. Greene RF, et al: Stability of cisplatin in aqueous solution. *Am J Hosp Pharm* 36:38-43, 1979.
15. Hardin TC, Clibon U: The stability of 5-fluorouracil in a crystalline amino acid solution. *Am J IV Ther Clin Nutr* 9:39-43, 1982.
16. Donaldson SS, Lennon RA: Alterations of nutritional status—impact of chemotherapy and radiation therapy. *Cancer* 43:2036-2052, 1979.
17. Lewis BJ: The use of opiate analgesics in cancer patients. *Cancer Treat Rep* 63:341-342, 1979.
18. Oster MW et al: Pain of terminal cancer patients. *Arch Intern Med* 138:1801-1803, 1978.
19. Coombs DW et al: Relief of continuous chronic pain by intraspinal narcotics infusion via an implanted reservoir. *JAMA* 250:2336-2339, 1983.
20. Peterson DE, Sonis S: Oral complications of cancer chemotherapy: Present status and future studies. *Cancer Treat Rep* 66:1251-1256, 1982.
21. Carl T: Oral complications in cancer patients. *Am Fam Physician* 27:161-170, 1983.
22. Kaul AF et al: Postgraduate pharmacy fellowships (1983-1984). *Drug Intell Clin Pharm* 17:835-839, 1983.
23. *Cancer Facts and Figures.* New York, American Cancer Society, 1983.

ADDITIONAL READING

General

Carter SK, Bakowski MT, Hellman K: *Chemotherapy of Cancer,* ed 2. New York, Wiley Medical Publications, 1981.
Dorr RT, Fritz WL: *Cancer Chemotherapy Handbook.* New York, Elsevier, 1980.
Procedures for Handling Cytotoxic Drugs. Bethesda, American Society of Hospital Pharmacists, 1983.
NCI Investigational Drugs: Pharmaceutical Data 1983. Silver Springs, MD, Pharmaceutical Resources Branch, National Cancer Institute, 1983.
Rubin P: *Clinical Oncology for Medical Students and Physicians: A Multidisciplinary Approach,* ed 5. New York, National Cancer Society, 1981.

Historic milestones. *Semin Oncol* 7:1979.
Toxicity of chemotherapy. *Semin Oncol* 9:1982.

Handling Potentially Biohazardous Drugs*

Anon: *A Guide for the Safe Preparation and Disposal of Antineoplastic Agents.* Ontario, Ontario Hospital Association, 1982.
Anon: *Cytotoxic Drug Safety Cabinets.* Sydney, Australia, Standards Association of Australia, 1982.
Anon: *Draft Australian Standard for Comment.* Sydney, Australia, Standards Association of Australia, 1982.
Anon: Education protects hospital workers who handle toxic cancer drugs. *Hosp Employ Health* 154-156, November 1982.
Adamson RH, Sieber SM: Carcinogenic potential of cancer chemotherapeutic agents in man. *Cancer Bull* 29(6):179, 1977.
Ames BN et al: Methods of detecting carcinogens and mutagens with the salmonella mammalian–microsome mutagenicity test. *Mutation Res* 31:347-364, 1975.
Anderson RW et al: Risk of handling injectable antineoplastic agents. *Am J Hosp Pharm* 11:1881-1887, 1982.
Ballentine R: Cancerphobia—or whatever happened to red M&M's? (editorial) *Drug Intell Clin Pharm* 16:60-61, 1982.
Bacovsky R: Disposal of hazardous pharmaceuticals. *Canad J Hosp Pharm* 34:12-13, 1981.
Bergemann A: Handling antineoplastic agents. *Am J Intrav Ther Clin Nutr* 10(1):13-17, January 1981.
Boice JD Jr: Leukemia and preleukemia after adjuvant treatment of gastrointestinal cancer with semustine (Methyl-CCNU). *N Engl J Med* 309:1079-1084, 1983.
Brier KL et al: Effect of laminar air flow and clean-room dress on contamination rates of intravenous admixtures. *Am J Hosp Pharm* 38:1144-1147, 1981.
Calabresi P: Leukemia after cytotoxic chemotherapy—a pyrrhic victory? (editorial). *N Engl J Med* 309:1118-1119, 1983.
Carrano AV et al: Sister chromatid exchange as an indicator of mutagenesis. *Nature* 271:551-553, 1978.
Clayson DB: Principles underlying testing for carcinogenicity. *Cancer Bull* 29:161-166, 1977.
Crudi CB: A compounding dilemma: I've kept the drug sterile but have I contaminated myself? *NITA* 3:77-78, 1980.
Crudi CB, Stephens BL: Antineoplastic agents: An occupational hazard? *NITA* 4:223-234, 1981.
D'Arcy PF: Reactions and interactions in handling anticancer drugs. *Drug Intell Clin Pharm* 17:532-538, 1983.
Davignon JP, Trissel LA: Disposal of unused anticancer drugs. *The Signal* May 1979.
Davis MR: Guidelines for safe handling of cytotoxic drugs in pharmacy departments and hospital wards (The Society of Hospital Pharmacists of Australia). *Hosp Pharm* 16:17-20, January 1981.
Delaney RA: Guideline needed for handling of carcinogenic antineoplastics (letter). *Am J Hosp Pharm* 38:166, 1981.
Denton DR: Are we killing the healers? *Occup Health Safety* 52:11-16, 50, December 1982.
Donner AL: Possible risk of working with antineoplastic drugs in horizontal laminar flow hoods (letter). *Am J Hosp Pharm* 35:900, 1978.
Dozier N, Ballentine R: Practical considerations in the preparation and administration of cancer chemotherapy. *Am J Intrav Ther Clin Nutri* 10:6-15, September 1983.
Eriksen IL: Handling of cytotoxic drugs: Governmental regulations and practical solutions. *Pharm Intern* 3(8):264-267, 1982.
Falck K et al: Mutagenicity in urine of nurses handling cytostatic drugs (letter). *Lancet* 1:1250-1251, 1979.
Farber E: Chemical carcinogenesis. *N Engl J Med* 305:1379-1389, 1981.
Fricker MP: IV issues and answers. *Infusion* 4(5):138-139, 1980.
Goldberg LA: The preparation of cytotoxic drugs. *Pharm J* 228:224-225, 1983.
Gousse GC et al: Biological safety cabinets for chemotherapy preparation (letter). *Am J Hosp Pharm* 38:967, 1981.
Gross J et al: Possible hazards of working with cytotoxic agents. *Oncol Nurs For* 8(4):10-12, 1981.

---

*Prepared by the Department of Pharmacy, University of Texas M.D. Anderson Hospital and Tumor Institute at Houston.

Hamilton CW: Risk to personnel admixing cancer chemotherapy. *US Pharm* 7:H1-H8, July 1982.

Hamilton CW, Avis KE: Selection criteria for biological safety cabinets for chemotherapy preparation (letter). *Am J Hosp Pharm* 39:968, 1982.

Harris CC: A delayed complication of cancer therapy cancer. *JNCI* 63:275-277, 1979.

Harris CC: The carcinogenicity of anticancer drugs: A hazard in man. *Cancer* 37:1014-1023, 1976.

Harrison BR: Developing guidelines for working with antineoplastic drugs. *Am J Hosp Pharm* 38:1686-1693, 1981.

Hirst M et al: Caution on handling antineoplastic drugs (letter). *N Engl J Med* 309:188-189, 1983.

Hoffman DM: The handling of antineoplastic drugs in a major cancer center. *Hosp Pharm* 15:302-304, 1980.

Hoffman DM: Handling cytotoxic drugs (letter). *Am J Hosp Pharm* 38:1284-1286, 1981.

Hoffman DM: Lack of urine mutagenicity of nurses administering pharmacy prepared doses of antineoplastic agents. *Am J Intrav Ther Clin Nutr* 10:28-32, September 1983.

Honda D, Ignoffo RJ, Power LA: Safety consideration in the preparation of parenteral antineo-plastics. *CSHP Voice* 8:94-96, Winter 1981.

Hoover R, Fraumeni JD: Drug-induced cancer. *Cancer* 47(suppl):1071-1080, 1981.

International Agency for Research on Cancer: *IARC Monographs on the Evaluation of the Carcinogenic Risk of Chemicals to Humans*. Geneva, Switzerland, World Health Organization, May 1981.

Jagun A et al: Urinary thioether excretion in nurses handling cytotoxic drugs (letter). *Lancet* 2:443-444, 1982.

Johnson BL: Handling methotrexate—a safety problem? *Am J Nurs* 10:1531, 1982.

Jones RB: Safe handling of chemotherapeutic agents: A report from the Mount Sinai Medical Center. *CA* 33:258-263, September/October 1983.

Kleinberg ML, Quinn MJ: Airborne drug levels in a laminar-flow hood. *Am J Hosp Pharm* 38:1301-1313, 1981.

Kleinberg ML, Quinn MJ, Lee P: Effects of pharmaceutical packaging on antibiotic levels in the environment. *Partic Microb Contr* 2(3):56-60, May/June 1983.

Knowles RS, Virden JE: Handling of injectable antineoplastic agents. *Br Med J* 281:589-591, 1980.

Krikorian G et al: Occurrence of non-Hodgkin's lymphoma after therapy for Hodgkin's disease. *N Engl J Med* 401:452-458, 1979.

Kruse RH: Microbiological safety cabinetry. *Pathologist* :641-647, 1983.

Ladik CF et al: Precautionary measures in the preparation of antineoplastics (letter). *Am J Hosp Pharm* 37:1184-1186, 1980.

Lambert B, Ringborg U, Harper E, Lindblad A: Sister chromatid exchanges in lymphocyte cultures of patients receiving chemotherapy for malignant disorders. *Cancer Treat Rep* 62:1413-1419, 1978.

LeRoy ML et al: Procedures for handling antineoplastic injections in comprehensive cancer centers. *Am J Hosp Pharm* 40:661-663, 1983.

Macek C: Hospital personnel who handle anticancer drugs may face risks. *JAMA* 247(1):11-12, 1982.

Marquardt H: Introduction of malignant transformation and mutagenesis in cell cultures by cancer chemotherapy agents. *Cancer* 40(suppl):1930-1934, 1977.

Matney TS et al: Genotoxic classification of anticancer drugs, *Teratogenicity, Carcinogenicity, and Mutagenicity*. (In press.)

McLendon BE, Bron AJ: Corneal toxicity from vinblastine solution. *Br J Ophthalmol* 62:97-99, 1978.

National Institutes of Health: *Recommendations for the Safe Handling of Parenteral Antineoplastic Drugs*. Washington, DC, Superintendent of Documents, Government Printing Office, 1982 (NIH Publication No. 83-2621).

National Sanitation Foundation: *Standard No. 49 for Class II (Laminar Flow) Biohazard Cabinetry*, rev ed. Ann Arbor, National Sanitation Foundation, May 1983.

National Study Commission on Cytotoxic Exposure: *Recommendations for Handling Cytotoxic Agents*. Providence, RI, Rhode Island Hospital, Department of Pharmacy, September 1984.

Neal A et al: Exposure of hospital workers to airborne antineoplastic agents. *Am J Hosp Pharm* 40:597-601, 1983.

Nevstad NP: Sister chromatid exchanges and chromosomal aberrations induced in human lymphocytes by the cytostatic drug Adriamycin in vivo and in vitro. *Mutation Res* 57:253-258, 1977.

Ng LM: Possible hazards of handling antineoplastic drugs (letter). *Pediatrics* 46:648-649, 1970.

Nguyen TV, Theiss JC, Matney TS: Exposure of pharmacy personnel to mutagenic antineoplastic drugs. *Cancer Research* 42:4792-4796, 1982.

Norppa H et al: Increased sister chromatid exchange frequencies in lymphocytes of nurses handling cytostatic drugs. *Scand J Work Environ Health* 6(4):299-301, 1980.

Perlman M, Walker R: Acute leukemia following cytotoxic chemotherapy (letter). *JAMA* 224:250, 1973.

Pharmaceutical Society (Great Britain), Working Party Report: Guidelines for the handling of cytotoxic drugs. *Pharm J* 228:230-231, 1983.

Power LA, Pech JG: Particulate matter possible in type B vertical flow hoods (letter). *Am J Hosp Pharm* 39:574, 1982.

Power LA: Regulated handling of parenteral antineoplastic agents. *Partic Micro Contr* 2:79-82, July 1983.

Puckett WH Jr: Guidelines for handling antineoplastic agents. *Ohio Pharmacist* 30:324-326, 1982.

Raposa T: Sister chromatid exchange studies for monitoring DNA damage and repair capacity after cytostatics in vitro and in lymphocytes of leukaemic patients under cytostatic therapy. *Mutat Res* 57:241-251, 1978.

Redfearn J: 'Safety' cabinets are not safe, says UK study. *Nature* 278:384, 1979.

Reich SD: Antineoplastic agents as potential carcinogens: Are nurses and pharmacists at risk? *Cancer Nurs* 4:500-502, 1981.

Reimer RR et al: Acute leukemia after alkylating agent therapy of ovarian cancer. *N Engl J Med* 297:177-181, 1977.

Reynolds RD et al: Adverse reactions to AMSA in medical personnel. *Cancer Treat Rep* 66:1885, 1982.

Rosner F: Acute leukemia as a delayed consequence of cancer chemotherapy. *Cancer* 37:1033-1036, 1976.

Sieber SM: Cancer chemotherapeutic agents and carcino-genesis. *Cancer Chemo Rep* 59:915-918, 1975.

Solimando DA: Preparation of antineoplastic drugs: A review. *Am J Intrav Ther Clin Nutr* 10:16-27, September 1983.

Sotaniemi EA et al: Liver injury in subjects occupationally exposed to chemicals in low doses. *Acta Med Scand* 212:207-215, 1982.

Staiano N et al: Lack of mutagenic activity in urine from hospital pharmacists admixing antitumor drugs (letter). *Lancet* 1:615-616, 1981.

Stiller A et al: No elevation of the frequencies of chromosomal alterations as a consequence of handling cytostatic drugs: Analyses with peripheral blood and urine of hospital personnel. *Mutation Res* 121:253-259, 1983.

Stolar MH, Power LA, Viele CS: Recommendations for handling cytotoxic drugs in hospitals. *Am J Hosp Pharm* 40:1163-1171, 1983.

Stuart DG et al: Survey, use, and performance of biological safety cabinets. *Am Ind Hygiene Assoc J* 43:265-270, 1982.

Theiss JC: Detection of carcinogens. In Bucchenal JH, Oettgen HF (eds): *Cancer—Achievements, Challenges, and Prospects for the 1980's*, vol 1. New York, Grune & Stratton, 1981, pp 281-290.

Thompsen DF: PVC gloves for handling anti-neoplastics (letter). *Am J Hosp Pharm* 39:227, 1982.

Thomsen K, Mikkelsen HI: Protective capacity of gloves used for handling of nitrogen mustard. *Contact Dermatitis* 1:268-269, 1975.

Tortorici MP: Precautions followed by personnel involved with the preparation of parenteral antineoplastic medications. *Hosp Pharm* 15:293-301, 1980.

Waksvik H et al: Chromosome analyses of nurses handling cytostatic agents. *Cancer Treat Rep* 65:607-610, 1981.

Weisburger JH et al: The carcinogenic properties of some of the principle drugs used in clinical cancer chemotherapy. *Rec Res Cancer Res* 52:1-17, 1975.

Weiss RB, Brunning RD, Kennedy BJ: Lymphosarcoma terminating in acute myelogenous leukemia. *Cancer* 30:1275-1277, 1972.

Wells JM: A policy for intravenous drugs. *Nurs Mirror* 142:45-46, March 25, 1976.

Wiernik PH, Duncan JH: Cyclophosphamide in human milk (letter). *Lancet* :912, 1971.

Willcox GS et al: A comparison of laminar airflow cabinetry. *Cancer Chemother Update* 1:1-3, September/October 1983.

Wilson JP, Solimando DA: Antineoplastics: A safety hazard? (letter). *Am J Hosp Pharm* 38:624, 1981.

Wilson JP et al: Aseptic technique as a safety precaution in the preparation of antineoplastic agents. *Hosp Pharm* 16:575-581, 1981.

Zellmer WA: Reducing occupational exposure to potential carcinogens in hospitals (editorial). *Am J Hosp Pharm* 38:1679, 1981.

Zimmerman PF et al: Recommendations for the safe handling of injectable antineoplastic drug products. *Am J Hosp Pharm* 38:1693-1695, 1981.

CHAPTER 52

Pharmacokinetic Services

RAY R. MADDOX

Pharmacokinetics is the study of the time course of drug and metabolite disposition in the body. It is an outgrowth of the scientific discipline of biopharmaceutics and involves the development of mathematic relationships that quantitatively describe the processes of drug absorption, distribution, metabolism, and excretion. On the other hand, clinical pharmacokinetics is a health sciences discipline that deals with applying pharmacokinetics to the safe and effective therapeutic management of the individual patient (1). It involves the evaluation and interpretation of several kinds of information, which include physical and metabolic characteristics of the patient; the presence and significance of diseases for which the drug therapy is being provided, as well as those conditions for which no treatment is being used; the route(s) by which drugs are being given and their dosage formulations; the contribution of drug interactions to patient response; and the pharmacodynamics of drug action in the patient.

Clinicians who practice clinical pharmacokinetics generally have scientific and clinical training in biopharmaceutics, pharmacokinetics, and clinical pharmacokinetics in addition to an educational background in the pathophysiology of disease, clinical pharmacology, and patient care assessment. These individuals are often clinically trained pharmacists who have attained the PharmD or MS degree; however, clinical pharmacokinetics is practiced by clinical pharmacologists (MD/PhD), as well as other appropriately trained bioscientists.

The number of pharmacy departments in the United States that provide a clinical pharmacokinetic service (CPS) increased by 135% (27-63) in the years 1979-1983 (2). This dramatic growth is probably related to the increased emphasis given to pharmacokinetic training in pharmacy colleges and to the professional identity fostered by the support of organizational pharmacy for the inclusion of CPSs in contemporary institutional pharmacy practice (3). However, at the same time a significant number of educational programs within other medically related disciplines, specifically clinical chemistry and clinical pharmacology, have resulted in a growth in the application of therapeutic drug monitoring (TDM), the use of measurements of drug concentrations to guide dosage adjustments, in settings where pharmacists may not be directly involved.

The purpose of this chapter is to describe the evolution, organization, and composition of CPSs in institutional phar-

macy practice. Resources necessary for the provision of a CPS will be described and reference sources will be documented. Finally, an assessment of the contribution to patient care of this activity and the potential for the continued development of clinical pharmacokinetics as a specialty practice will be made.

EVOLUTION OF PHARMACOKINETIC SERVICES

Clinical pharmacokinetic services have developed primarily as outgrowths of research programs in pharmacy colleges or departments of clinical pharmacology within medical colleges. Early service programs such as those at the State University of New York at Buffalo were limited in scope and were supported by National Institutes of Health research monies (1). Later programs similar to that of the University of Kentucky were begun as demonstration projects of the College of Pharmacy with the intent of transferring the drug analysis responsibility to a hospital departments of pathology or clinical chemistry when feasible. This evolutionary path was necessary because of the relative lack of ability in most divisions of clinical chemistry within hospitals to provide quantitative drug analysis. Many analytical procedures were expensive and were not automated.

Within the recent past, there have been significant developments in analytical methodologies and equipment that have improved the ability to measure drug concentrations in biologic specimens. These measurements can now be made on very small sample volumes (≤ 50 μl) rapidly, efficiently, and accurately, and have directly contributed to an increase in TDM services offered by clinical laboratories. In most hospitals in which there is a high use of a drug with a narrow therapeutic index and an established concentration–effect relationship, an in-house method for measuring its concentration will be available.

Paralleling the developments in analytical technology, the number of clinically trained pharmacists graduating from pharmacy colleges has increased. These individuals, who generally have attained the PharmD degree, may pursue clinical residency or fellowship training that significantly strengthens their patient care skills and their ability to manage drug therapy using pharmacokinetic principles.

Whereas CPSs were originally located primarily in teaching hospitals, they are now becoming more common in the community hospital setting. Most often the CPS is a collaborative effort of two departments: the clinical chemistry laboratory in the department of pathology provides drug analysis and the pharmacy department provides clinical pharmacists who perform pharmacokinetic evaluations of patients. This arrangement is not always a formalized service where a coordination of effort is apparent between the two groups. There are examples of programs in which clinical pharmacists have been hired by pathology departments to provide a clinical interpretation of drug concentration measurements. In some cases, clinical laboratories have attempted to increase the use of drug analysis by providing the physician with additional information relating to drug dosage and blood sampling times; these efforts have usually failed to significantly improve the pharmacokinetic management of patients by the physician.

ADMINISTRATIVE ORGANIZATION OF A CPS

The administrative structure through which a CPS may be offered in most institutions is relatively straightforward: a collaborative relationship between the departments of pharmacy and pathology (laboratory medicine). A formal administrative agreement between these two departments ensures that the use of resources in each is maximized. Pathology departments have generally invested large sums of money in analytical equipment, supplies, and technologists, which support the drug analysis needs of a CPS. The pharmacy department, on the other hand, has clinically trained professional staff members who can provide the clinical interpretive component of a CPS.

In selected institutions, it may be advantageous for a pharmacy department to provide drug analysis in addition to the pharmacokinetic interpretation. In small community hospitals or specialty clinic facilities where there is no ability in the laboratory to measure drug concentrations, the pharmacy department may offer a CPS that incorporates a drug analysis system such as the EMIT. The pharmacy in this setting would then be responsible for establishing a mechanism for phlebotomy, quality assurance of drug analysis, reporting of analytical results (and pharmacokinetic interpretations), and a patient charge for the analysis procedure. This approach to offering a CPS may be limited because many states require that an individual with an MD or PhD direct laboratories that produce results used to manage patients clinically. Pharmacists should avoid competing with a preexisting drug analysis laboratory in the hospital if at all possible.

There are several examples of institutions in which TDM activities continue to be provided within the framework of research. These programs are generally located in research hospitals or in clinical settings where specialty patient groups (e.g., neurology) are served by a small research laboratory. Occasionally, clinical pharmacologists will offer this kind of TDM program to selected patient populations.

COMPONENTS OF A CPS

There are basically three primary elements of a clinical pharmacokinetic service: personnel, a drug analysis laboratory, and patient information. Each of these elements is essential to providing high-quality pharmacokinetic assessments of patients and meaningful input into their pharmacologic management.

Personnel

Personnel who significantly contribute to the routine functions of a CPS consist of clinical pharmacists, laboratory employees (chemists, technologists, phlebotomists), nurses, and ward clerks.

Pharmacists who participate in a CPS must have an educational and experiential background in several areas. This background will include training in biopharmaceutics, pharmacokinetics, and clinical pharmacokinetics. These individuals will need a thorough understanding of pharmacotherapeutics, an ability to evaluate and/or perform limited physical assessments of patients, an ability to interpret the results of laboratory tests, and an ability to communicate effectively verbally and in writing. Although specialized clinical residency or fellowship training is not necessary for all pharmacists who participate in a CPS, there is a need for a resource person who may have such training. Most PharmD curricula provide the components outlined above; additionally, well-designed staff development programs for the baccalaureate-level practitioner may satisfy these requirements.

The clinical chemist is a professional who is instrumental in evaluating periodic problems with assay methodology that may require modifications in an analysis procedure because of an assay interference or the need for drug measurements in body fluids other than serum or plasma. Technologists are responsible for the routine analysis of drugs; there should be sufficient numbers of these individuals to ensure that drug concentration measurements are provided efficiently and in a timely manner. It is desirable that the laboratory be staffed at a level that allows the assignment of one technologist to each analytical procedure or instrument. Phlebotomists who can be assigned to obtain blood specimens at nonroutine times of the day are necessary for a CPS to function effectively.

There are two important resource people to the CPS who work in the patient care area: nurses and ward clerks. Whereas they do not perform drug analyses or pharmacokinetic evaluations of patients, they have a significant role in scheduling and administering drugs for which the TDM is of benefit. The informed cooperation of these individuals is of paramount importance to a successful CPS.

Laboratory

Drug analysis, as noted earlier, may be provided by the pharmacy or more commonly by the clinical laboratory. Small analytical systems such as those that support EMIT are useful in a pharmacy-based drug analysis service. On the other hand, the clinical chemistry section within the laboratory may employ a variety of methodologies, including high-performance liquid chromatography (HPLC), gas chromatography (GC), radioimmunoassay (RIA), enzyme immunoassay (EIA), fluoroimmunoassay (FIA), flame photometry, and microbiologic assay. A well-equipped lab may have several hundred thousand dollars invested in analytical equipment and supplies in addition to the space necessary to accommodate the equipment and personnel. Rapid ana-

TABLE 52.1 Analytical Procedures for TDM Drugs

Anticonvulsants	
Phenytoin, primidone, phenobarbital, ethosuximide, carbamazepine, valproic acid	GC, EIA, FPIA, FIA, HPLC
Antibiotics	
Chloramphenicol	HPLC
Aminoglycosides	RIA, EIA, FPIA, FIA
Vancomycin	HPLC, FPIA, EIA
Antiarrhythmics	
Lidocaine, procainamide, n-acetyl procainamide, quinidine, propranolol, disopyramide	GC, HPLC, EIA, FPIA
Digitalis glycosides	
Digoxin, digitoxin	RIA, EIA, FPIA
Tricyclic antidepressants	HPLC
Miscellaneous	
Lithium	Flame photometry
Theophylline	HPLC, EIA, FPIA, FIA
Methotrexate	FPIA, EIA
Salicylic acid	TLC, HPLC
Acetaminophen	EIA

GC = gas chromatography; EIA = enzyme immunoassay (EMIT, Syva); FPIA = fluorescent polarization immunoassay (TDX, Abbott); FIA = fluorescent immunoassay (Optimate, Ames); HPLC = high-performance liquid chromatography; RIA = radioimmunoassay; TLC = thin-layer chromatography.

lytical procedures that require minimal sample preparation and are automated, such as the TDX, provide excellent turnaround times. Methodologies such as EIA, FIAS, and RIA, however, require reagents with relatively short shelf lives. If low numbers of specimens are available for analysis, these kits may expire before they are completely used and necessitate a relatively high cost for drug analysis. Table 52.1 is a list of most of the drugs for which TDM is important and the commonly used analytical procedures for these agents.

Regardless of where the drug analysis is performed, a method of quality assurance is essential. Errors in measurements of drug concentrations will be amplified in pharmacokinetic calculations and subsequent dosage adjustments. These errors will quickly compromise the credibility of a CPS. Commonly, large laboratories will participate in quality assurance programs such as those of the American Association for Clinical Chemistry and the American Academy of Clinical Pathologists. These laboratories are generally certified by a state and/or federal certification agency. Additionally, there are usually internal procedures within the laboratory that are designed to ensure the reliability of standard curves and technologist performance.

Patient Information

Pharmacists who provide pharmacokinetic input into a patient's therapy require access to relevant patient information that is generally located on the nursing unit. It is clinically inappropriate for dosage manipulations to be made routinely from a central pharmacy area over the telephone even when these regimens have been designed with computer assistance. In formulating a pharmacokinetic evaluation the pharmacist must have access to the following types

of information: (1) the medical record (chart) that provides data concerning the patient's medical history, the physician's treatment plan, and is the record on which observations and recommendations are recorded; (2) the medication administration record (MAR) and other documents that record the times of drug administration; (3) the results of laboratory analysis for drug concentration and other biochemical markers; and (4) the patient interviews from which one can assess compliance, over-the-counter drug use, and otherwise undiscovered side effects and toxicities of therapy.

It might also be necessary for the pharmacist to evaluate the drug administration system when there are discrepancies between actual and expected analytical results. These differences may be caused by variations or interruptions in IV infusion rates or inadvertent mixing of incompatible drugs by the nurse. A physical presence by the pharmacist in the patient care setting has an incalculable positive influence on all clinical services, including a CPS.

DRUGS FOR WHICH PHARMACOKINETIC MONITORING IS IMPORTANT

Currently TDM and the subsequent pharmacokinetic manipulation of therapy is useful for only a limited number of drugs. Measurements of drug levels are clinically appropriate when there is an established relationship between the serum (or plasma) concentration and the intended therapeutic effect; i.e., a therapeutic range is defined. The therapeutic concentration range of a drug is that set of values between which most patients exhibit a pharmacologic response. It can be used as a guide to dosage manipulation with the expectation that (1) dose increases made when the concentration is low will likely produce an increase in efficacy without side effects and (2) dose increases made when the concentration is high will likely produce an increase in side effects with a minimal change in efficacy. Table 52.2 lists the generally accepted therapeutic range of drugs for which TDM is clinically useful.

The therapeutic range of a drug in a patient may be influenced by a number of patient-specific variables such as the state of hydration, the concentrations of serum or plasma proteins, the presence of other drugs or endogenous biochemicals, and the ability of receptors to bind drug molecules. These characteristics, as well as others, contribute to the pharmacodynamics of drug effect—an area of study closely related to pharmacokinetics but less understood.

The selection of which drugs to monitor in an institution is influenced by drug use patterns in the hospital. These patterns are directly determined by the medical specialties represented and the patient populations that they serve. Drugs commonly included in a CPS are antibiotics (aminoglycosides, chloramphenicol, vancomycin), anticonvulsants, theophylline, and antiarrythmics. Aminoglycoside antibiotics are the most frequently monitored drugs.

COMPUTER SUPPORT OF A CPS

The use of electronic data processing (EDP) equipment to support clinical pharmacokinetic evaluations of patients has allowed clinical pharmacists to translate relatively abstract concepts into meaningful input into patient care. Sig-

TABLE 52.2 Therapeutic Concentration Range for Selected Drugs

Acetaminophen	10-20 μg/ml	Lithium	0.6-1.2 mEq/L
Amikacin	Peak 20-30 μg/ml; trough < 10 μg/ml	Methotrexate	$>0.01 \times 10^{-6}$ M
Amitriptyline	80-200 ng/ml	Netilmicin	Peak 6-12 μg/ml; trough <2 μg/ml
Carbamazepine	5-10 μg/ml	Nortriptyline	50-150 ng/ml
Chloramphenicol	10-20 μg/ml	Phenobarbital	10-35 μg/ml
Desipramine	75-160 ng/ml	Phenytoin	10-20 μg/ml
Digoxin	0.9-2.0 ng/ml	Primidone	5-12 μg/ml
Digitoxin	15-25 ng/ml	Procainamide[b]	4-10 μg/ml
Disopyramide	2-4 μg/ml	Propranolol	50-100 ng/ml
Doxepin	>110 ng/ml	Protriptyline	70-240 ng/ml
Ethosuximide	40-80 μg/ml	Quinidine	2-5 μg/ml
Flucytosine	50-100 μg/ml	Salicylic acid	150-300 μg/ml
Gentamicin	Peak 5-10 μg/ml; trough < 2 μg/ml	Theophylline	10-20 μg/ml
Heparin[a]		Tobramycin	Peak 5-10 μg/ml; trough < 2 μg/ml
Imipramine	>180 ng/ml	Valproic acid	50-100 μg/ml
Lidocaine	1.5-5.0 μg/ml	Vancomycin	2.5-40 μg/ml

[a]Heparin is best monitored by maintaining the activated partial thromboplastin time (APTT) at 1.5-2.0 times that of the control value.
[b]Procainamide (PA) is metabolized to n-acetylprocainamide (NAPA). The sum of concentrations of PA and NAPA should be in the range of 10-30 μg/ml.

nificant advances in hardware and software have provided powerful, yet compact, equipment that can be easily used in the clinical setting.

Systems that support a CPS require several characteristics to maximize their utility to the clinical pharmacist. Many of the mathematic equations used to "model" patients are employed repetitively; the solution of these equations is made easier if they are programmed into the EDP equipment. Systems should be capable of storing predetermined pharmacokinetic variables from population data so that dosage regimens can be designed before any measurements of drug concentration in the patient. Clinical pharmacokinetic assessments are generally made in patient care areas; therefore, the clinical pharmacist needs a system that is small, portable, and durable, yet versatile. Preferably the system will accommodate the storage of patient-specific pharmacokinetic information and will allow the selective retrieval of both patient and population data. Computer-printed consults and graphs of drug serum concentration vs time relationships improve the clinical pharmacist's ability to communicate the pharmacokinetic assessment of the patient to the physician.

A variety of hardware and software is available that supports pharmacokinetic practice and research. These systems range from hand-held programmable calculators to advanced data analysis software on mainframe computers. Hand-held programmable calculators such as the Hewlett-Packard (HP) 65, HP41CV, and the Texas Instruments (TI) 59 series are the most commonly used EDP systems by pharmacists. There are a number of programs that have been written and published (4) or offered for sale for these instruments. The personal-sized microcomputer will likely become the EDP system of choice for pharmacokinetic monitoring, because it provides essentially all of the elements required to support a CPS. Pharmacokinetic software for microcomputers such as the Apple II and the IBM PC has been developed, tested, validated, and marketed.

Several vendors (5) of minicomputer systems that support the drug distribution functions of an institutional pharmacy offer pharmacokinetic enhancements to their users. These enhancements usually have a limited capacity to model pa-

tient data and provide little more than an electronic screening of the appropriateness of a drug dose based on the patient's weight or age. Other software such as NONLIN (6) and ESTRIP (7) are designed to analyze research data and of necessity operate on larger computers generally located on a university campus or in a pharmaceutical firm.

Most pharmacokinetic data for patient monitoring can be evaluated using relatively nonsophisticated compartmental modeling, i.e., the one-compartment open model. However, there are patient populations, such as renal failure patients, that may require two-compartmental modeling for selected drugs. The majority of software for hand-held calculators uses single compartmental mathematic relationships, whereas microcomputer technology allows multicompartment analysis. Drugs such as phenytoin, which obey nonlinear (Michaelis-Menton) pharmacokinetics, require the use of software designed for this type of analysis. More sophisticated projection techniques, such as Bayesian pharmacokinetic modeling, are still in the development stages, but software has been written for the microcomputer and larger systems.

IMPACT OF PHARMACOKINETIC MONITORING ON PATIENT CARE

There is insufficient evidence to document clearly that most clinical pharmacy activities improve patient outcomes; clinical pharmacokinetic monitoring is no exception. On the other hand, there is direct evidence that suggests that TDM activities coordinated with clinical pharmacists involved with pharmacokinetic monitoring improves the use of drug concentration measurements from the laboratory and reduces the cost associated with unusable results.

Pharmacokinetic monitoring of aminoglycoside antibiotics in critically ill patients results in a reduction in morbidity and mortality (8,9). It may also reduce the number of days that patients require therapy in an intensive care unit (8). The involvement of clinical pharmacists in this activity has been shown to be cost effective through the use of a statistical model appropriate to the nature of the data (8). Pharmacokinetic monitoring of theophylline therapy, however, improves patient outcomes (10) but can be cost prohibitive in some clinical settings (11). It should be expected that pharmacokinetic monitoring can result in a more rapid optimization of a patient's drug therapy; this effect can lead to a reduction in the potential for adverse drug reactions and in the length of therapy and hospitalization. These changes should produce an overall improvement in health care with the potential for a reduction in its cost.

ORGANIZATIONAL IDENTITY AND SPECIALTY TRAINING

The development of clinical pharmacokinetics and therapeutic drug monitoring cannot be credited to one single group of health scientists nor to one organization that represents them. As mentioned previously, clinical pharmacokinetics evolved primarily from biopharmaceutics and pharmacokinetics, but its use in clinical medicine has been influenced greatly by advances in analytical chemistry and clinical pharmacology.

The initial identity of clinical pharmacokinetics as a health sciences discipline can be traced to the Academy of Pharmaceutical Sciences of the American Pharmaceutical Association (1). It was this group that set the direction for the routine use of clinical pharmacokinetic principles in patient care. The American Society for Clinical Pharmacology and Therapeutics is a focus for the dissemination and publication of research concerning clinical pharmacokinetics. The American Association for Clinical Chemistry provides educational programming for its members to increase their competency in TDM and provides a quality assurance monitoring program for drug analysis services.

Within institutional pharmacy practice, the American Society of Hospital Pharmacists (ASHP) has given direction to the routine involvement of pharmacists in clinical pharmacokinetic monitoring as part of comprehensive clinical services (3). Various special interest groups (SIGs) of ASHP provide educational programs for their members on the use of pharmacokinetic principles in selected patient populations. Additionally, the SIG on Clinical Pharmacokinetics Practice provides identity to individuals who concentrate their practice and research interests on the broader discipline and directs educational programs that appeal to the society and its members in general.

The need for specialists in clinical pharmacokinetics is probably quite limited. As mentioned earlier, clinical pharmacokinetics is an important tool in the management of all patients; thus, specialized training in other practice entities such as pediatrics, geriatrics, and others will include this resource. However, specialized residency and fellowship training in clinical pharmacokinetics is available. The ASHP administers an industry-supported fellowship and a number of institutions provide support for their own fellowship and residency programs. These postgraduate experiences generally give strong emphasis to the use of pharmacokinetics in all patient populations, laboratory technology, pharmacokinetic modeling of data, the use of computers, and the administrative management of an interdisciplinary service. The recognition of clinical pharmacokinetics as a specialty in pharmacy practice probably will not occur, although the need for the availability of residency and fellowship training

is important to the provision of a small number of expertly qualified individuals with a broad base of knowledge in this area.

REFERENCES

1. Levy G: An orientation to clinical pharmacokinetics. In Levy G (ed): *Clinical Pharmacokinetics: A Symposium*. Washington, DC, American Pharmaceutical Association, 1974, pp 1-9.
2. Rich DS, Jeffrey LP: Pharmacokinetic consultation services: 1979 versus 1983 (letter). *Am J Hosp Pharm* 41:56, 1984.
3. American Society of Hospital Pharmacists: ASHP statement on the role of the pharmacist in clinical pharmacokinetic services. *Am J Hosp Pharm* 39:1369, 1982.
4. Robb, RA, Bauer LA, Koup JR: *Manual of Integrated HP41C Calculator Programs for Pharmacokinetic Calculations*. Bethesda, American Society of Hospital Pharmacists, 1982.
5. Swanson DS, Broekemeier RL, Anderson MW: Hospital pharmacy computer systems—1982. *Am J Hosp Pharm* 39:2109-2117, 1982.
6. Metzler CM, Elfring GL, McEwen AJ: *A User's Manual for NONLIN and Associated Programs*. Kalamazoo, MI, Upjohn, 1974.
7. Brown RD, Manno JE: ESTRIP, a BASIC computer program for obtaining initial polyexponential parameter estimates. *J Pharm Sci* 67:1687, 1978.
8. Bootman JL, et al: Individualizing gentamicin dosage regimens in burn patients with gram negative septicemia: A cost-benefit analysis. *J Pharm Sci* 68:267-272, 1979.
9. Moore RD, Smith CR, Lietman PS: Association of aminoglycoside plasma levels with mortality in gram-negative bacteremia. *Clin Pharmacol Ther* 35:260, 1984.
10. Mungall D, et al: Individualizing theophylline therapy: The impact of clinical pharmacokinetics on patient outcomes. *Ther Drug Monit* 5:95-101, 1983.
11. Lehmann CR, Leonard RG: Effect of theophylline pharmacokinetic monitoring service on cost and quality of care. *Am J Hosp Pharm* 39:1656-1662, 1982.

ADDITIONAL READING

Books

Evans WE, Schentag JJ, Jusko WJ: *Applied Pharmacokinetics*. San Francisco, Applied Therapeutics, 1980.
Gibaldi M, Perrier D: *Pharmacokinetics*, ed 2. New York, Marcel Dekker, 1982.
Gibaldi M, Prescott L: *Handbook of Clinical Pharmacokinetics*. New York, ADIS Health Science Press, 1983.
Sadee W, Beelen GCM: *Drug Level Monitoring—Analytical Techniques, Metabolism, and Pharmacokinetics*. New York, John Wiley & Sons, 1980.
Winter ME. *Basic Clinical Pharmacokinetics*. San Francisco, Applied Therapeutics, 1980.

Journals

Clinical Chemistry. Winston-Salem, American Association for Clinical Chemistry.
Clinical Pharmacokinetics. Newtown, PA, ADIS Press International.
Clinical Pharmacology and Therapeutics. St Louis, CV Mosby.
Clinical Pharmacy. Bethesda, American Society of Hospital Pharmacists.
Drug Intelligence & Clinical Pharmacy. Cincinnati, Drug Intelligence & Clinical Pharmacy.
Therapeutic Drug Monitoring. New York, Raven Press.

Journal Articles

General References

Bollish SJ, Kelly WN, Miller DE, Timmons RG: Establishing an aminoglycoside pharmacokinetic monitoring service in a community hospital. *Am J Hosp Pharm* 38:73-76, 1981.
Koup JR: Clinical pharmacokinetic service and research—present status and future goals at SUNY–Buffalo. *Am J Pharm Educ* 40:400-406, 1976.
Lawson LA, Blouin RA, Parker PF: Quality assurance program for a clinical pharmacokinetic service. *Am J Hosp Pharm* 39:607-609, 1982.

Maddox RR, Lampasona V: Administrative aspects of clinical pharmacokinetic services. *Top Hosp Pharm Manag* 2:61-73, 1982.

Maddox RR, Vanderveen TW, Jones EM, et al: Collaborative clinical pharmacokinetic services. *Am J Hosp Pharm* 38:524-529, 1981.

Rietscha WJ, Heissler JF, Paulson MF, et al: Collaborative clinical pharmacokinetics service in a community hospital. *Am J Hosp Pharm* 41:473-477, 1984.

Taylor JW, McLean AJ, Leonard RG, et al: Initial experience of clinical pharmacology and clinical pharmacy interactions in a clinical pharmacokinetics consultation service. *J Clin Pharmacol* 19:1-7, 1979.

Evaluation of Patient Outcomes

Bootman JL, Wertheimer AI, Zaske D, et al: Individualizing gentamicin dosage regimens in burn patients with gram-negative septicemia: A cost-benefit analysis. *J Pharm Sci* 68:267-272, 1979.

Moore RD, Smith CR, Lietman PS: Association of aminoglycoside plasma levels with mortality in gram-negative bacteremia (abstract). *Clin Pharmacol Ther* 35:260, 1984.

Mungall D, Marshall J, Penn D, et al: Individualizing theophylline therapy: The impact of clinical pharmacokinetics on patient outcomes. *Ther Drug Monit* 5:95-101, 1983.

Cost Benefit

Bootman JL, Zaske DE, Wertheimer AI, Rowland C: Cost of individualizing aminoglycoside dosage regimens. *Am J Hosp Pharm* 36:368-370, 1979.

Elenbass RM, Payne VW, Bauman JL: Influence of clinical pharmacist consultations on the use of drug blood level tests. *Am J Hosp Pharm* 37:61-64, 1980.

Flynn TW, Pevonka MP, Yost RL, et al: Use of serum gentamicin levels in hospitalized patients. *Am J Hosp Pharm* 35:806-808, 1978.

Greenlaw CW, Blough SS, Hauger RK: Aminoglycoside serum assays restricted through a pharmacy program. *Am J Hosp Pharm* 36:1080-1083, 1979.

Levin B, Cohen SS, Birmingham PH: Effect of pharmacist intervention on the use of serum drug assays. *Am J Hosp Pharm* 38:845-851, 1981.

Slaughter RL, Schneider PJ, Visconti JA: Appropriateness of the use of serum digoxin and digitoxin assays. *Am J Hosp Pharm* 35:1376-1379, 1978.

Vlasses PH, DePiro CR, Chalupa D, et al: Appropriateness of sampling time for selected serum drug assays. *Hosp Pharm* 17:371-373, 1982.

Reimbursement

Kelly WN, Gibson GA, Miller WE: Obtaining reimbursement for clinical pharmacokinetic monitoring. *Am J Hosp Pharm* 39:1662-1665, 1982.

Maddox RR: Update on clinical pharmacokinetic service (letter). *Am J Hosp Pharm* 39:40-41, 1982.

Moore TD, Schneider PJ, Nold EG: Developing reimbursable clinical pharmacy programs: pharmacokinetic dosing service. *Am J Hosp Pharm* 36:1523-1527, 1979.

Nold EG: Third-party payer reimbursement for patient education and pharmacokinetic dosing services (letter). *Am J Hosp Pharm* 35:1337, 1978.

Patterson LE, Huether RJ: Reimbursement for clinical pharmaceutical services. *Am J Hosp Pharm* 35:1373-1375, 1978.

Smith WE, Weiblen JW: Charging for hospital pharmaceutical services: Product cost, per diem fees and fees for special clinical services. *Am J Hosp Pharm* 36:355-359, 1979.

CHAPTER 53

The Patient Profile System

MICHAEL F. POWELL

The patient medication profile (PMP) has been an integral part of the evolution of pharmacy practice from a product-oriented to a patient-oriented discipline. The PMP consolidates all relevant information about a patient's drug therapy into a single source from which the pharmacist can make professional judgments about the drug use process (1) and control drug-related tasks. With the PMP, the pharmacist maintains data for many purposes (1-12):

1. To monitor the drug distribution process
2. To document the dispensing and accuracy of dispensing medications
3. To document work performed
4. To bill medication charges
5. To monitor and prevent potential drug interactions, adverse reactions, and side effects
6. To help ensure the appropriateness of drug selection by monitoring for drug or therapeutic duplications or for drug indications
7. To detect and prevent potential drug toxicities caused by overdoses or allergic reactions
8. To help detect and prevent physical and chemical incompatibilities between drugs and solutions or between drug additives in IV solutions
9. To monitor drug administration to help ensure compliance with prescribed regimens
10. To provide information supporting the instruction of patients regarding medication use
11. To evaluate the effects of drug therapy (i.e., effectiveness)

In summary, the PMP serves as a tool with which the pharmacist assures appropriateness, safety, and effectiveness of drug therapy.

The PMP has evolved physically, as well as in its uses. Originally, PMPs were record-keeping documents for such diverse functions as tax records, prescription dispensing, and drug monitoring in community pharmacies. Generally, the PMP was a card-weight document on which the pharmacist made handwritten entries. As use became more widespread, efforts to improve the efficiency in using PMPs led to the development of pressure-sensitive duplicate labels that could be affixed to the PMP card in lieu of written entries. Contemporary PMPs are frequently computerized records. Whatever the form, PMPs still consist of elements common to the original PMPs and the applications have changed relatively little.

ELEMENTS OF THE PMP

There are three broad categories of information common to PMPs: (1) patient demographic data, (2) patient medical history data, and (3) drug-related data. Patient demographic data should minimally include the patient's name, age (date of birth), sex, telephone number, and address. The patient's height and weight are potentially critical information, especially in children for verifying dosing. Hospital inpatient records should include the medical record or billing number and bed location as part of the demographic information. Insurance carrier information and patient's social security number should be included for ambulatory patients to aid billing and patient identification. The patient's race or ethnic background may be useful information when certain classes of drug are prescribed because certain genetic traits affect the metabolism or the elimination of drugs.

Patient medical history data is used in evaluating the appropriateness of drug use, detecting drug-related incidents, and monitoring drug effects. A patient medication history is the starting point for the PMP. In addition to recording demographic data, the pharmacist taking a medication history should note all medical problems for which the patient is being treated, drug allergies or sensitivities, and social drug use (alcohol, tobacco, etc). Information regarding the familial history of disease may also be useful in evaluating drug therapy. Another element of data that should be included where possible is diagnostic data, particularly in hospitals. Although not obtained as part of the medication history, pharmacists should routinely document laboratory data that may indicate the effect of the drug on the patient or the potential effectiveness of drugs ordered. Serum electrolytes, enzymes, or metabolic by-product levels, for instance, are important in monitoring the effects of drugs, whereas culture and sensitivity data may be important in the selection of antibiotics (13).

Drug-related data obtained during the patient medication history and for the duration of the patient–pharmacist relationship should include both current and past medication use. Moreover, over-the-counter and legend medication use should be recorded. Elements of drug-related data to be documented are drug name, dose strength, dosage form (or route of administration), directions for administration, refill information, and the prescriber's name and address. For hospital inpatients, administration times should be documented in lieu of directions, and duration of therapy or stop dates should be recorded where specified or dictated by policy. In teaching institutions, the patient's attending physician should be identified on the PMP. Quantities, brand names, and costs of medications should be maintained in ambulatory care settings.

The pharmacist should obtain the patient medication history directly from the patient whenever possible. By asking the appropriate questions, the pharmacist can determine whether reported drug allergies were truly allergies or dose-related toxicity or hypersensitivity reactions. In other words, the pharmacist can verify the accuracy of historic data rather than relying on the patient's interpretation of a drug-related event. Moreover, direct questioning relating to specific nonprescription drugs or foods can elicit more complete documentation of drug use because patients frequently fail to identify certain types of medications or consumer products as drugs or drug-containing (2,14,15). In the hospital, interns and residents generally include drug use in their history

---

To Our Patients:

Please take a moment to assist your pharmacist by supplying information about you and the medications you take. The pharmacy service will maintain a record of all prescriptions received by you from this pharmacy. This record, which we call the Patient Medication Profile, will help the pharmacist to assist the physician with your drug therapy. Information will be considered confidential. Thank you.

1. Name _____
    (if child - specify also parent or guardian name)

2. Address _____

3. Social Security Number _____

4. Date of Birth _____

5. Are you allergic to any medication? Yes _____   No _____

    a. If yes, please list name of medication(s) _____

        _____

6. Please list any prescription or non-prescription medication you
    take (such as vitamins, aspirin, laxatives, antacids, etc.)

    _____   _____   _____

    _____   _____   _____

    _____   _____   _____

    _____   _____   _____

FIGURE 53.1 Patient medication profile.

Patient Name

Phone Number

MRN

Address

Birthdate

Insurance Information

Allergies/Sensitivities (Food and Drug)

Problem List

Current Legend/Non Legend Medications

Family History
_____ Ca -
_____ Cardiac-   DOH   by
_____ DM-
_____ HNT-
Tobacco Usage   _____ Stroke-
ETOH Intake   _____ TB-

Date Issued	Prescription Number	Trade Name, Strength, Quantity or Generic Name, Company Strength, Quantity	Physician	Refill Record	R. Ph.	Fee	Cost

HEALTH CARE INSTITUTE
DEPARTMENT OF PHARMACY

MEDICATION PROFILE

FIGURE 53.2   Outpatient PMP.

taking. Still, the pharmacist should supplement this information because research has shown that pharmacists obtain more complete drug use histories (14,15). However, if a verbal history cannot be obtained, a written form completed by the patient or a family member can serve as a secondary source of medication history, especially for demographic and patient medical history data components (Fig. 53.1).

PMP SYSTEMS

In general, PMP systems improve the pharmacist's accessibility to patient medication history data by centralizing the accumulated history of a patient's medication use at a common source. Three basic types of systems are employed in the storage, filing, retrieval, use, and purging of PMP data: (1) manual systems, (2) manual systems with mechanical filing devices, and (3) electronic data processing. Manual systems generally are based on an index card with defined spaces for recording the data elements. The cards are then filed in alphabetic sequence by the patient's last name and by the first name secondarily where common surnames are encountered. Manual PMP systems are the most common, especially in the ambulatory care setting, and generally the least costly when patient and prescription volumes are relatively small. PMP cards may be stored in file cabinets or tub files, with the types of storage units depending on card size and patient volume. As patient and prescription volume increases, storage, filing, and retrieval of PMP cards becomes more time consuming and demands increasingly greater storage capability. A sequela of the space and filing demands is that records must be purged and replaced with updated PMP cards more frequently. In hospital settings, the need to place PMP cards in secondary storage limits accessibility, thus eliminating a potentially valuable information source on readmissions. Color coding of PMP cards can facilitate both retrieval and purging. By rotating card color or tab colors, PMP card status is readily apparent to permit retrieval of active records and purging inactive records without screening multiple records. Tickler file systems have been described to permit retrieval of manual PMPs according to certain data criteria for purposes of drug use review, refill reminder systems, or compliance review (16-18). Mechanical retrieval systems are available to facilitate record retrieval when the patient volume is sufficient. The use of pressure-sensitive labels affixed to the PMP card can diminish the pharmacist's time commitment to maintaining manual systems by minimizing the need for handwritten entries (19). Several commercially available PMP systems have been described (20). Figures 53.2 and 53.3 provide illustrations of outpatient and inpatient systems (manual), respectively.

Electronic data processing or computerized PMP systems provide several important advantages. First, accessibility of information is more rapid. Retrieval, data entry, and filing of PMP data can be accomplished in essentially one step. Another advantage is reduced storage space requirements. Computerized PMP systems generally must be purged less frequently and when data must be placed in storage off-line (i.e., tape storage), it can still be accessed more easily than in manual or combined manual and mechanical systems. Moreover, the computerized PMP system consolidates other tasks associated with the medication use process. Label generation, patient and third-party billing, inventory adjustment, medication pricing, adverse drug reaction screening, drug interaction screening, and dose delivery scheduling are tasks that can be automated as part of computerized PMP systems (13,21-25). Automation of the PMP reduces personnel time associated with medication handling and patient record handling, improves charge capture and inventory records, and expands the pharmacist's ability to monitor drug therapy in terms of numbers of patients. As a result, the computerized PMP system enhances the effectiveness

Inpatient PMP

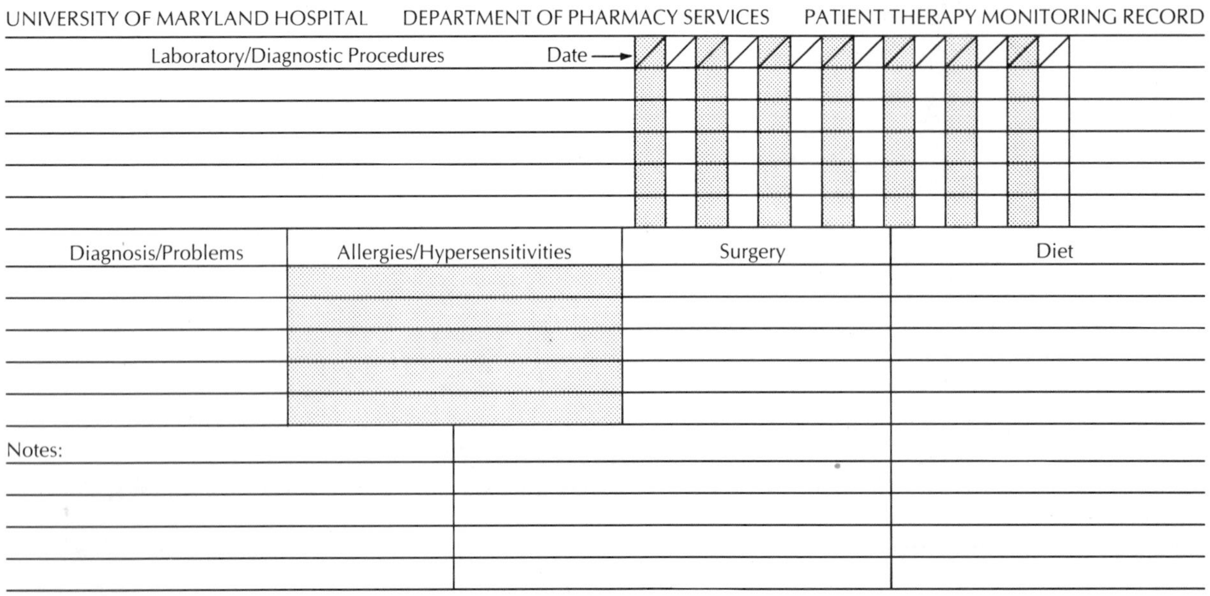

FIGURE 53.3A. Inpatient PMP.

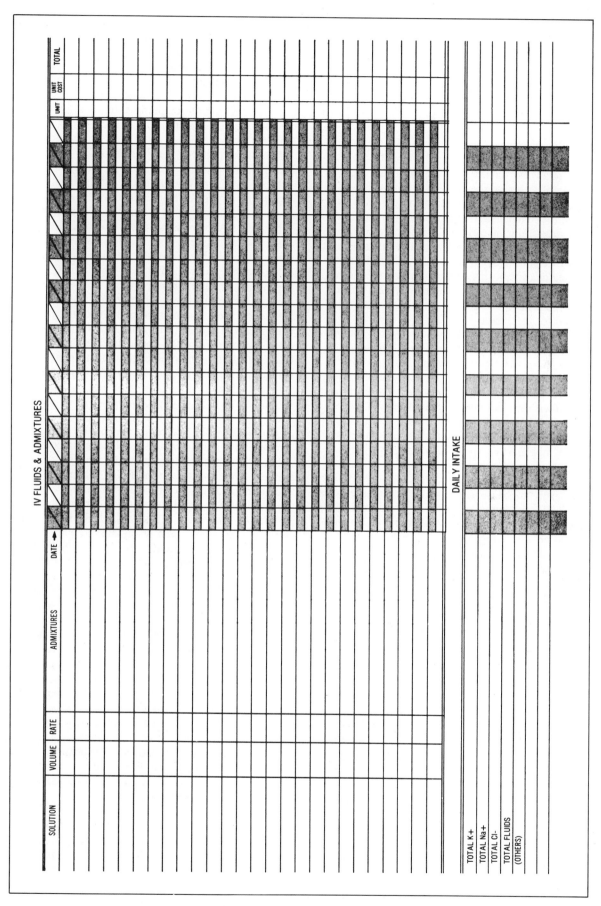

FIGURE 53.3B. Inpatient PMP—cont'd.

and efficiency of the pharmacist, both for medication handling and for clinical tasks. Finally, the computerized PMP increases the accessibility of specific drug use data for clinical evaluation of a drug use review.

PMP UTILIZATION

As a tool, the pharmacist uses the PMP with the overall objective of of monitoring patient drug therapy to avert and/or solve potential drug therapy–related problems such as (1) duplication of an active prescription for the same drug, (2) duplication of an active prescription for a similar therapeutic entity, (3) patient under- or overutilization of a drug, (4) potential drug-drug interactions, (5) potential disease-drug contraindications, (6) drug allergies or hypersensitivity, or (7) prescription discrepancies (26). In the hospital setting, the pharmacist may also use the PMP in monitoring for drug-food and drug–laboratory test interactions because the patient's medical record provides the additional information needed for these tasks.

The PMP should be monitored prospectively, i.e., before dispensing the medication. In reviewing the PMP, the pharmacist should ask a series of routine questions: (1) Is the medication indicated based on the diagnosis? (2) Is the medication selected the most effective with the least potential for adverse effects? (3) Is the dosage and route of administration correct based on the patient's physical size and condition? (4) Is the duration of therapy appropriate (i.e., too short, too long)? More specific questions may be included with specific categories of drugs, such as antibiotics. For instance, the pharmacist should determine whether the organism is likely to be sensitive to the drug based on diagnosis, whether culture and sensitivity results indicated the organism was susceptible to the antibiotic, or whether the culture was obtained properly (i.e., from the correct site based on diagnosis). Retrospective review of the PMP will diminish the benefits to the patient because intervention will take place after any problems have occurred. Retrospective review of the PMP is an element after the prescription is renewed. The PMP can then be used to review for (1) compliance with medication regimens, (2) therapeutic success or failures of the drug regimen, and (3) adverse drug reactions and drug interactions.

If a problem is detected in prospective review, the pharmacist is responsible for effectively communicating the nature and the mechanism of the problem to other health professionals. Moreover, simply recognizing a problem is not enough. The pharmacist must be able to make recommendations regarding the resolution of the therapeutic problem. The clinical significance of a therapeutic problem is always of importance, especially relating to drug interactions. The pharmacist should be prepared to discuss the likelihood that a potential therapeutic problem will occur when presenting it to other health professionals or advising a patient.

APPLICATIONS OF THE PMP

Although the PMP is a single source for consolidation of a patient's drug-related information, the effectiveness of

PMPs is limited by the completeness of drug histories and continuity. Patients receive health care in multiple locations and thus receive prescriptions from many sources. Moreover, patients obtain medications from many different pharmacies and from nonpharmacies. Presently, there is no practical method of transmitting a patient's medication records as he or she moves through the different levels of the health care setting (i.e., hospitals, extended care facilities, ambulatory care).

Some continuity of the PMP information can be maintained when patients use one facility for all health care. For instance, a patient who uses a health maintenance organization's facility for both ambulatory and hospital care would receive medications from essentially the same pharmacy in either case. Another instance is the patient who receives medications routinely from the hospital's outpatient pharmacy after discharge from the hospital. In such cases, the patient's PMP information can routinely be transferred between inpatient and outpatient areas for drug therapy monitoring. Pocket medication profiles for the patient to carry have been used as a method of transferring patient medication records between a hospital and community pharmacy after discharge from the hospital (27). Other methods include transferring the profile from the hospital to a primary care physician or to a pharmacy selected by the patient (28).

INPATIENT SERVICES

The PMP is the central document for both drug distribution and clinical services in the contemporary hospital setting. The pharmacist maintains a record of drugs prescribed and dispensed on the PMP. When new medication orders are received, the pharmacist reviews the order against medications already documented for potential therapeutic problems. Once the order is verified, the order is recorded and the pharmacist signs or initials the entry to verify its accuracy. Medication refills are initiated from the PMP in both individual patient prescription and unit dose drug distribution system (29,30). The pharmacist indicates approval of doses dispensed on the PMP, making the record a quality control document, and records doses dispensed for use in billing and tracking drug use. The status of drug orders is noted by procedures for canceling orders so that the pharmacist can evaluate both active and inactive medication treatment. IV admixture services use PMPs to detect physical chemical incompatibilities between fluids and additives and to schedule workload (2). The PMP helps to reduce medication errors, missed doses, and incorrect doses (31). Clinically, the benefit of the PMP in reducing medication-related incidents has been demonstrated (5,13,24). The pharmacist screens the patient's medication use records along with laboratory and diagnostic findings for drug interactions, toxicities, allergies, duplications, etc to help avoid therapeutic problems.

PMP use has also been reported as a key element in decentralization of pharmacists in patient care areas (25,32). A combination PMP and medication administration record (MAR) eliminates the duplication of recording orders between pharmacy and nursing and the need to reconcile records. The pharmacist is placed directly in the patient care area at the disposal of other disciplines. The pharmacist uses the same document for monitoring drug therapy as the nurse uses for documenting administration.

OUTPATIENT SERVICES

The use of the PMP for outpatients has been widely discussed (33,34). Solomon et al (26) studied the effectiveness of the PMP in aiding the pharmacist to detect potential therapeutic problems. In phase I of the study, patient information was recorded on PMP cards. Data were collected on 23,657 prescriptions from 14,069 patients. During this phase, the pharmacist's ability to detect therapeutic problems without the PMP was measured. During phase II, the PMP cards were used for detection and documentation of potential therapeutic problems. In phase II, 1497 potential therapeutic problems were identified from 25,197 prescriptions presented by 14,975 patients. This compared to only 13 potential therapeutic problems identified in phase I.

A particularly important element of PMP use in outpatient services is compliance with therapeutic drug regimens. Reports have indicated that from 20-82% of patients fail to take their medications as prescribed (35). The PMP enables the pharmacist to detect over- or underutilization of medications based on refill frequency. Moreover, reminder systems based on both manual and computerized PMPs have been described that improve a patient's compliance with obtaining refill medications (15,16).

PRIMARY CARE AND SPECIALTY CLINICS

The PMP has been used in support of nontraditional roles performed by pharmacists in primary care and specialty clinics (36-41). Bernstein et al (41) described the use of a PMP system in monitoring the anticoagulant therapy of patients with prosthetic heart valves. PMPs have also been used by pharmacists in the management of hypertensive patients (43) and endocrinology clinic patients (44). In these roles, the pharmacist obtains medication histories, evaluates the patient for drug-related problems, instructs patients in the use of medications, orders laboratory tests, and recommends or develops treatment plans for their patients. Other tasks have included screening patients for respiratory and dermatologic conditions. In these cases, the PMP is a key resource in fulfilling these roles.

COMPUTERIZED PMPs

In recent years, PMPs have been computerized with greater frequency. In the inpatient drug distribution systems, entry of a medication order into the computerized PMP accomplishes the tasks of drug charges and inventory adjustment simultaneously (21,22,25). Wareham et al (25) described a decentralized pharmacy distribution system combining a mobile cart with a computerized order entry system. The pharmacist enters orders into the patient's medication record on a cathode ray tube mounted on a mobile pharmacy cart. The pharmacist screens the profile, checks for drug allergies or other problems, and bills the patient in a single function. Derewicz and Zellers (22) reported on a computerized system in which the pharmacist enters medications and schedules doses in the patient's computerized profile. The computer then automatically generates a list of all doses due at hourly intervals and charges the patient for doses. Because the system permits dispensing of doses only immediately before being due, costs associated with pilferage and obsolesence are minimized and the need for a redundant controlled substance system are eliminated. Automation of drug therapy monitoring via the computerized PMP expands the number of beds or patients a single pharmacist can monitor (13,24,45). The computerized PMP automatically screens new orders against existing orders for problems such as adverse drug reactions, drug interactions, therapeutic duplications, etc and warns the pharmacist. Systems integrated with hospital-wide information systems also provide the pharmacist with the opportunity to screen the PMP against clinical laboratory and other diagnostic data.

The computerized PMP also provides the pharmacist with the ability to collate and analyze drug use review information prospectively (46-48). Computerized PMP systems similarly support medication dispensing, medication monitoring, and drug use review in ambulatory care (23,47-49).

PHARMACOLEGAL ASPECTS OF THE PMP

The maintenance of a PMP is legally required in only eight states (Table 53.1). However, 25 states have regulations regarding the computerized storage of prescription records (50). In these states, computerized prescription records must include the same data elements and be retrievable in the same fashion as PMP records.

As PMPs become more widely accepted as a standard of practice, the question arises whether the pharmacist will incur more or less liability through their use. One legal authority in Food, Drug, and Cosmetic Law has commented that pharmacists will be expected by consumers and the courts to perform to new standards as they evolve. Moreover, he contends that pharmacists will be expected to perform to the highest applicable standard regardless of locality (51). Today, more potent and toxic drugs are increasing the potential for adverse drug effects, consumers are more knowledgeable, pharmacists lack the time to establish personal relationships with patients, malpractice insurance is more accessible, and pharmacists are taking on new responsibilities such as consultation and patient therapy monitoring. All of these factors are expanding the pharmacist's liability according to Joseph Fink III, assistant dean of the University of Kentucky School of Pharmacy (52). On the other hand, Frank Gartland, vice president and general counsel of Druggists Mutual Insurance Company, cited a patient receiving excessive medications as one of six major areas leading to pharmacy litigation. The implication is that a patient who suffers harm because of irrational drug therapy, refilling medications too often, or drug interactions will seek

TABLE 53.1 States Requiring Patient Medication Profiles

Delaware	New Jersey
Idaho	North Dakota
Iowa[a]	Washington
Maine	Wisconsin[b]

[a]If interns on premises.
[b]For schedule II controlled substances only.

damage against someone in a position to prevent these events, i.e., the pharmacist (52). In the case of computerized profiles, a special liability factor is a concern. In computerized PMP systems with automatic drug monitoring features, overriding the system increases the potential liability (52).

In general, it is clear there is some legal impetus for the use of PMPs in general pharmacy practice. First, some states require their use. Second, the legal environment of pharmacy practice is such that the PMP both increases and decreases the pharmacist's liability exposure. Still, with the greater potential for adverse drug effects and overexposure to drug therapy, drug therapy monitoring via the PMP generally improves the liability exposure of pharmacists. Koepsell et al (53) found that the probability of a patient receiving seriously interacting drugs was generally less when profiles were maintained on patients. Moreover, the study findings further indicated that PMPs enabled the earlier detection and elimination of drug combinations that were therapeutically redundant or potentially interacting. Clearly, such findings imply that the liability risk is greater in not using PMPs. Further, as the prevalence of PMPs continue to increase— and it is estamated that nearly two thirds of US pharmacies have either paper or computerized PMPs (54)—both consumers and the courts will expect pharmacists to use PMPs as a standard of practice.

IMPLICATIONS

The need for PMPs is based on the health status of the public. Outpatient prescription drug sales for 1983 totaled $1.5 billion, and total drug sales account for approximately 9% of total health care expenditures when hospital-prescribed drugs and over-the-counter drugs are considered (55). Moreover, drug allergies and adverse reactions are relatively common. In one study (56), 22% of patient profiles screened in one PMP system indicated patients were allergic to one or more medications. Further, it has been estimated (57) that adverse drug reactions account for from 4-7% of hospital admissions annually. The pharmacist, by virtue of the frequency of contact with the public, is obviously in a key position to influence these events through the use of PMPs.

The cost of PMPs and who will pay for the services should be considered, however. A recent survey showed that 66% of consumers would not pay for the pharmacist to maintain PMPs, although 71% considered the maintenance of PMPs a desirable service (58). Despite the public's unwillingness to pay for the service, PMPs have been shown to be cost effective (59). The desirability of PMPs to the consumer was shown to produce an increase in prescription volume offsetting the costs of implementing the PMP with new revenues by more than two to one.

In the hospital setting, the PMP also takes on several clinical management applications that are particularly relevant in this cost containment era. PMPs are essential sources of prospective drug use review programs (46). Drug use review that does not take place before a drug order is implemented will simply be ineffective. Effective drug use review will be critical to successful formulary management and drug cost containment.

SUMMARY

The PMP is a central component of comprehensive pharmacy services. The PMP supports the pharmacist both in drug distribution and in clinically related tasks. It is the central source for applying the pharmacist's knowledge to the drug use process.

REFERENCES

1. O'Hara GL: Patient medication profile monitoring. *J Pharm Assoc* NS16(5):248-249, 270, 1976.
2. Goldman L: The pharmacist's role in monitoring drug therapy. *Hosp Pharm* 6(6):5-13, 1971.
3. Berquist SC: Patient profile card used in clinical pharmacy services. *Am J Hosp Pharm* 32:597-598, 1975.
4. Cooper JW, Campbell NA: Community-hospital practitioner consultation. *J Am Pharm Assoc* NS15:484-533, 1975.
5. Smith WE: Using the patient profile. *Drug Intell Clin Pharm* 4:73-76, 1970.
6. Painter JA, Archambault GF, Dodds AW: Pharmacist monitoring of prescribed medications. *Hosp Formul Mgt* 123-132, 1975.
7. Cain R: New prescription practices . . . patient record systems. NS4:*J Am Pharm Assoc* 164-168, 1964.
8. Stevens R, Wolfert R: Three years experience with a patient medication record and charge ticket. *Am J Hosp PHarm* 25:569, 1968.
9. Stevens R, Wolfert R: A random filing system for inpatient medication records. *Am J Hosp Pharm* 26:290-293, 1969.
10. Slining J, Cole P, Sister Emmanuel: Development of a drug incompatibility file and its use in patient medication profile reviews. *Am J Hosp Pharm* 27:459-467, 1970.
11. Cain RM, Kahn JS: The pharmacist as a member of the health care team. *Am J Pub Health* 61:2223-2228, 1971.
12. Gibson PA, Gloutier G: Epilepsy: Patient education and services. *Am Pharm* NS24(4):39-43, 1984.
13. Hulse RK, Clark SJ, Jackson C, Warner HR, Gardner RM: Computerized medication monitoring system. *Am J Hosp Pharm* 33:1061-1064, 1976.
14. Wilson RS, Kabat HF: Pharmacist initiated drug histories. *Am J Hosp Pharm* 28:49-53, 1971.
15. Covington RT, Pfeiffer FG: The pharmacist-acquired medication history. *Am J Hosp Pharm* 29:692-695, 1972.
16. Kruger M: A follow-up system for hypertensive patients. *Mich Pharm* 13:48-49, 1975.
17. Simpkins CV, Wenzloff NJ: The evaluation of a computerized "tickler system" in the enhancement of patient medication refill compliance. Paper presented at the American Society of Hospital Pharmacists' Midyear Clinical Meeting, Atlanta, December 1984.
18. Becker M, Maiman L: Strategies for enhancing patient compliance. *J Commun Health* 6:113-135, 1980.
19. Srnka QM, Rosenbluth SA, Niedelman W: Evaluation of a patient medication profile based on the use of duplicate labels. *Am J Hosp Pharm* 31:79-83, 1974.
20. Anon: Patient record systems. *J Am Pharm Assoc* NS13:360-374, 1973.
21. Freund RG: Evolution of a computerized drug profile. *Am J Hosp Pharm* 30:160-164, 1973.
22. Derewicz HJ, Zellers DD: The computer-based unit dose system in the Johns Hopkins Hospital. *Am J Hosp Pharm* 30:206-212, 1973.
23. Weissman AM, et al: Computer support of pharmaceutical services for ambulatory patients. *Am J Hosp Pharm* 33:1171-1175, 1976.
24. Greenlaw CW, Zellers DD: Computerized drug-drug interaction screening system. *Am J Hosp Pharm* 35:567-570, 1978.
25. Wareham DV, Johnson SR, Typrell T: Combination medication cart and computer terminal in decentralized drug distribution. *Am J Hosp Pharm* 40:976-978, 1983.
26. Solomon DK, et al: Use of medication profiles to detect potential therapeutic problems in ambulatory patients. *Am J Hosp Pharm* 34:348-354, 1974.
27. Zilz DA, Silbert R: Drug profile follows patient into the community. *Hospitals* 46:63-72, 1972.
28. Toal DR: Development of an efficient pharmacy drug record system. *J Am Pharm Assoc* NS13:375, 1978.

29. Almquist DD: Manual patient drug profiles as part of a drug distribution system. *Am J Hosp Pharm* 27:988-993, 1970.

30. Davis NM: Patient profiles draw the whole picture. *Hosp JAHA* 45:110-115, 1971.

31. Minor MF: Patient drug profile. *Hosp Pharm* 5:10-13, 1970.

32. Lipman AG, et al: Decentralization of pharmaceutical services without satellite pharmacies. *Am J Hosp Pharm* 36:1513-1519, 1979.

33. Hernandez Land Boutet JC: Outpatients get better service. *Hospitals* 46:81-85, 1972.

34. Tice LF: Outpatient pharmacy services. *J Am Pharm Assoc* NS7:622-623, 1967.

35. Steward RB, Cluff LE: A review of medication errors and compliance in the ambulant patient. *Clin Pharmacol Ther* 13:463-468, 1972.

36. Ivey MF: The pharmacist in the care of ambulatory mental health patients. *Am J Hosp Pharm* 30:599-602, 1973.

37. Evans RL, et al: Medication maintenance of mentally ill patients by a pharmacist in a community setting. *Am J Hosp Pharm* 33:635-638, 1976.

38. Anderson PO, Taryle DA: Pharmacist management of ambulatory patients using formalized standards of care. *Am J Hosp Pharm* 31:254-257, 1974.

39. Ellinoy BJ, et al: A pharmacy outpatient monitoring program providing primary medical care to selected outpatients. *Am J Hosp Pharm* 30:593-598, 1973.

40. Ellinoy BJ, et al: Pharmacy audit of patient health records—feasibility and usefulness of a drug surveillance system. *Am J Hosp Pharm* 29:749-754, 1972.

41. Greifenhagen R, Pearlman TT: Pharmacy system for screening ambulatory patients. *Am J Hosp Pharm* 36:916-920, 1979.

42. Bernstein D, Harrison EC, McCarron MM: A patient profile system for monitoring long-term anticoagulent therapy. *Am J Hosp Pharm* 31:258-261, 1974.

43. Reinders T, et al: Pharmacist's role in the management of hypertensive patients in an ambulatory care clinic. *Am J Hosp Pharm* 32:590-594, 1975.

44. Miller KO: Pharmacist involvement in an endocrinology clinic. *Am J Hosp Pharm* 38:1720-1721, 1981.

45. Ford DR, Rivers NP, Wood GC: A computerized detection system for potentially significant adverse drug-drug interactions. *J Am Pharm Assoc* NS17:354-357, 1977.

46. Stolar MH: Model for a formal, prospective antibiotic use review program. *Am J Hosp Pharm* 35:809-811, 1978.

47. Maronde RF, et al: Physician prescribing practices—a computer based study. *Am J Hosp Pharm* 26:566-573, 1969.

48. Maronde RF: Drug utilization review with on-line computer capability, selected methodology and findings from a demonstration. Department of Health, Education and Welfare Publication No. (SSA)73-11853, May 1972.

49. McEvilla JD: A computerized prescription recording system. *J Am Pharm Assoc* NS7:636-638, 1967.

50. *Survey of Pharmacy Law—1983-84.* Chicago, National Association of Boards of Pharmacy, 1983, p 24.

51. Willig SH: Legal considerations for the pharmacist undertaking new drug consultation responsibilities. *Food Drug Cosmet Law J* 25:444-452, 1970.

52. Messnick R: Seminar tackles pharmacists' new legal liability exposure. *Drug Top* 128(11):42,44, 1983.

53. Koepsell TD, et al: The Seattle evaluation of computerized drug profiles: Effects on prescribing practices and resource use. *Am J Public Health* 73:850-855, 1983.

54. Wertheimer AI: A prescription is not a simple matter anymore. *Am J Public Health* 73:844-845, 1983.

55. Anon: 1983 National prescription audit. *Pharm Times* 50(4):27-35, 1984.

56. Huffman DC: The feasibility of modern managerial systems and innovative professional services in a community pharmacy: A case study. PhD dissertation, Oxford, University of Mississippi, 1970.

57. Kennedy EM: Vital roles for the pharmacist. *J Am Pharm Assoc* NS13:563, 1973.

58. Laverty RF: Payment for services? Don't hold your breath. *Drug Top* 128(11):18-19, 1984.

59. Smith HA: Application of cost-effectiveness analysis to patient record systems. *J Am Pharm Assoc* NS13:15-16, 1973.

CHAPTER 54

Decentralized Pharmacy Services

WILLIAM E. SMITH and DENNIS W. MACKEWICZ

The development and implementation of decentralized pharmacy services are responses by hospital pharmacists to the drug-related needs of patients, physicians, and nurses in the hospital setting. The two components of decentralized services are drug distribution and the pharmacist's clinical practice. Each is directed at different needs. The drug distribution component is directed at minimizing medication system errors and emphasizing drug availability and accountability. The pharmacist's clinical practice is directed at individual patient drug therapy problems and the informational needs of the physician and nurse for safer drug prescribing and administration and the aggregate review of drug use and patient outcome.

Inherent in implementation of a decentralized pharmacy service is the answer to an important question: What are the necessary roles and responsibilities of the pharmacist in the hospital? The pharmacist's roles and responsibilities include ensuring that patients' drug therapy is the safest and most effective possible. To accomplish this requires competent pharmacists, systems, and services for practice in patient care areas and cooperation among physicians, pharmacists, and nurses. A decentralized service maximizes the pharmacist's contributions to the patient and to the professional staff members of the hospital.

The need for the decentralization of pharmacy services will usually increase with the size of the hospital. Some large hospitals with central pharmacies may, in fact, provide many of the services discussed, whereas a smaller hospital may not. The position of the authors is that the decentralization of pharmacy staff facilitates providing necessary inpatient pharmaceutical services. Although to some this may appear self-evident, the issues revolve around what the definition of basic pharmacy inpatient services should be. From a more pragmatic point of view, the question is whether the cost of a decentralized pharmacy service is justified. The rationale for providing clinical pharmaceutical services and the alternative central and decentral approaches to providing these services will be discussed in this chapter.

PATIENT NEEDS

Several aspects of drug use in the hospital setting have been studied and reported in the literature since the 1950s. These reports illustrate patients' drug-related needs in the hospital setting.

Medication Errors. Hospital medication systems have been reported to have 8-20% of doses in error, errors being defined as wrong patient, wrong drug, wrong dose, and wrong time (1,2).

Drug Effects. Complications in patients resulting from drug use that have been reported include hospital admissions caused by drugs—2-5% of patients (3), adverse drug reactions—5-30% of patients (4), prolonged hospitalization from adverse drug reactions (5), drug-modifying laboratory tests (6), drugs inducing blood dyscrasias (7), drugs affecting liver function tests (8), and drugs and teratology (9). Drugs by definition "alter the structure and function of parts of the body." It is not surprising, then, that if someone seeks complications arising from the drug effects, he finds they frequently occur. The key question is how to minimize these effects through the clinical application of drug knowledge and better hospital medication systems.

Medication System Costs. Of the total daily patient cost in the hospital, 8-12% may be for the hospital medication system. The real medication system cost to the patient includes the nursing time involved in medication-related activities plus pharmacy department patient charges (10).

From the patient's point of view, hospital medication systems, in which the physician prescribes, the pharmacist dispenses from a central location, and the nurse administers the medications, results in a high rate of errors, significant drug complications, and considerable expense. In the future, more drugs will be available that will be more complicated to prescribe and administer and will be of greater potency and toxicity. If the hospital medication system and the pharmacist's practice are not modified, even greater drug-related complications may be anticipated in the hospital setting.

NURSING NEEDS

The nurse has a major role in the hospital medication system. Depending on the scope of services provided by the pharmacy department the nurse may have to requisition drugs from a central pharmacy, prepare and reconstitute doses for administration, administer medications, record each drug administered, keep additional records for narcotics and other controlled drugs received and administered, and be knowledgeable about storage, dosage forms and strengths, and the effects of each drug prepared and administered. As a result, a great deal of nursing time, frequently more than 20%, has been reported spent in medication-related activities (11). The nurse may also have to procure IV solutions and add drugs as needed using aseptic technique. Medication errors that occur in a nurse-controlled parenteral admixture program have been reported (12).

The question is which drug-related activities in the hospital should be performed by the nurse in a given hospital from an efficiency and quality of care point of view? Is it realistic to expect nurses to be knowledgeable about all the drugs administered even with nurse specialization and at the same time devote adequate time to maintain their nursing knowledge and skills? Generic drug names, therapeutic substitutions, variable dosages depending on the salt form, drugs that are administered through direct IV push, and more dangerous drugs such as oncology agents are examples of continuing areas of confusion and potential errors without adequate pharmacy support for the nurse. A centralized hospital pharmacy service cannot provide adequate doublechecks in the system, which leads to many unanswered questions by a busy nurse. Decentralized pharmacy services more readily allow the transfer of many drug-related activities and clinical drug information. Decentralized drug distribution using a satellite pharmacy has been associated with more efficient use of nursing time compared with centralized drug distribution (13).

PHYSICIAN NEEDS

The physician diagnoses the patient's medical problem and then prescribes a plan of therapy. Today the length of patient stay and overall cost is a major concern. Patients in the hospital today are likely to require more intensive care with the goal to discharge each patient as soon as possible. Drug prescribing is frequently a critical aspect of the therapy plan for both medical and surgical patients. Drug complications identified previously illustrate the physician's need for general and specific clinical drug information. Management of the patient's drug therapy by the pharmacist, such as the anticoagulant, antibiotic, and other drug regimens requiring close monitoring, reduces the chances of costly drug reactions and quickens the discharge of the patient. The high degree of medical staff specialization has increased the pharmacist's role in assessing newly admitted patient's medications that the patients had been taking at home.

Although much effort has been expended on behalf of patient drug education, the sources of drug information for the physician has changed little over the years. Usual sources of drug information to the physician include the medical service representative, *Physician's Desk Reference,* journal articles, textbooks, and professional conferences. These usual sources are inadequate to meet the physician's needs for clinical drug information, particularly as it relates to unique hospital drug therapies. Pharmacists must practice in patient care areas to apply clinical drug knowledge skills and to provide their knowledge to help physicians meet their drug therapy related needs.

PHARMACIST NEEDS

Pharmacists' time in a centralized pharmacy system is likely to be used inefficiently (14). Participation in the drug information needs of the hospital staff is minimal. Personal professional relationships with physicians, nurses, and patients are limited. The lesson to be learned from the past is that the traditional pharmacist's practice in the central pharmacy does not serve or meet patient, physician, and nurse drug-related needs. Decentralized pharmacy services have evolved to meet these needs by providing clinical pharmacy services and a more efficient and less error-prone medication distribution system.

In a decentralized environment, the pharmacist is no longer underutilized and is able to relate directly to patient's drug therapy needs, provide drug use control, and meet legal requirements and standards for the accreditation of the hospital. Initial doses for a new order can be provided quickly. Pharmacist-regulated drug therapy can be instituted effectively. Pharmacists develop experience and knowledge for particular patient care areas such as pediatrics, obstetrics and gynecology, medicine, and surgery, which represents a concentration of hospital drug therapeutics compared to any one physician. The pharmacist is able to effectively inform and communicate with the nurse and physician as needed. A rapport can be developed with the medical staff such that the pharmacist's input into drug therapy orders can be made before orders are written instead of just responding to problems after the fact.

The pharmacist cannot meet professional responsibilities and maintain personal growth and development practicing while in a central pharmacy that is remote from the patient care areas where prescribing therapy decisions are made, where drugs are used and controlled, and where legal requirements must be met.

SERVICES AND EXPECTED PATIENT BENEFITS— PHARMACISTS' CLINICAL PRACTICE

During the 1960s and 1970s, pharmacists practicing in hospitals took an active role in developing new pharmaceutical services directed toward reducing the problems associated with drug use. Such services included unit dose drug distribution, patient medication profiles, drug information services, pharmacists practicing in patient care areas, and clinical pharmacokinetics. Advocates of these new services identified as "clinical pharmacy" services contended that significant benefits, including improved patient care at a reasonable cost, would result. However, because of the absence of documentation on the total costs of the traditional medication system and the benefits of providing clinical pharmacy services, implementation of the concept in hospitals has been slow.

The characteristics of a pharmacist's practice in a decentralized clinical pharmacy are described below. Expected patient benefits for each characteristic are also described.

Patient Care Rounds. Pharmacists accompany physicians making patient rounds, primarily teaching rounds. Participation occurs in providing drug information on the request of physicians or by the initiation of the pharmacist. The drug information provided to the physician frequently deals with improvements in the patient's treatment plan.

Patient Interviews. Patient drug history information is obtained verbally by the pharmacist to complete pharmacy records. Information may include drugs being taken, both prescription and over-the-counter, drug allergies, and attitudes about drugs as to which drugs worked or did not work. Previous patient drug therapy problems, attitudes, and misconceptions as to what drugs worked or did not work are identified and can be avoided during hospitalization.

Patient Medication Therapy Monitoring. Patient charts are reviewed to determine if the patient is receiving safe and effective drug therapy. Drugs administered, pertinent laboratory tests, and patient's diagnosis and medical condition are essential parts of the monitoring process. If changes in the drug therapy are desirable, the pharmacist discusses these with the physician. Potential and actual drug therapy problems are identified and communicated to the physician by the pharmacist. Safer and more effective drug therapy should result.

Physicians' Inquiry. Physician-initiated patient drug therapy and general drug information questions are answered by the pharmacist. Safer and more effective drug therapy can result if questions are answered satisfactorily and implemented in patient therapy.

Nurses' Inquiry. Nurse-initiated patient drug therapy, general drug information, and drug order clarification questions are answered by the pharmacist. More accurate drug administration and nursing medication records and greater drug knowledge of the nurse results in safer drug administration for the patient.

Drug Information. The physician and pharmacist will initiate drug information questions involving a particular patient's drug therapy problem requiring a search of the available literature for information to provide a response. The answers should result in safer and more effective drug therapy.

Cardiac Arrest Emergency Participation. The pharmacist is a member of the hospital's cardioresuscitation team and participates by providing drug therapy assistance and needed drugs. Pharmacist assistance with drug availability and drug therapy questions can greatly facilitate resuscitation procedures.

Special Drug Therapy Services. The pharmacist will develop and perform special drug therapy services as requested by the physician, such as anticoagulation, dosing of drugs in patients with compromised renal status, drugs affecting blood and liver, aminoglycoside dosing, pain control, hyperalimentation, and aminophylline therapy. Safer, more patient-specific and effective drug therapy can result.

Clinical Pharmacokinetics. The pharmacist schedules the appropriate time for drug levels to help ensure the test results are usable. Consultation services using the drug level and kinetic knowledge can be provided for modification of the dose and dosing interval to meet specific patient drug needs.

Drug Utilization Review. Special drug case studies are conducted and educational programs provided to the medical, nursing, and pharmacy staffs by the pharmacist. Incorrect and inappropriate drug prescribing of physicians can be corrected via educational programs. Costs of drug therapy can be defined and documented.

PHARMACIST PERFORMANCE CHARACTERISTICS

A goal of a pharmacist in clinical practice is to develop knowledge and skills for patient service, teaching, and re-

search. Patient services were described previously as the pharmacist's clinical practice. Teaching should be provided to physicians, nurses, pharmacists, and students of each profession about drugs and drug use. Clinical drug research activities can range from patient drug therapy quality assessment to the evaluation of new drug therapy regimens (e.g., drug utilization review, phase II, III, and IV drug trials, the application of pharmacokinetics). The pharmacist's clinical drug knowledge and skills, services to patients, and teaching programs are all enhanced and improved with some ongoing involvement in clinical drug research.

To accomplish this goal requires pharmacists with a commitment to high standards of patient services who are interested in teaching and research. It requires knowledge and skill, a commitment to life-long learning, but also the important characteristics of initiative and motivation, self-accountability, and productivity. It requires planning and the organization of time, patience, and persistence toward a goal. It requires specialization or concentration of time and energy into selected areas of clinical drug use.

Pharmacy education should direct programs toward a goal in which students will develop the knowledge and skills to become competent scientific clinical practitioners. The student should learn methodologies and available resources to develop the style of an independent, competent pharmacist who can continue to learn and expand knowledge and skills during a professional career. The alternative to accomplishing these goals is to continue the pharmacist in the role of a dispenser and perpetuate a system incapable of meeting the drug-related needs of patients, physicians, and nurses.

PHARMACIST CLINICAL PRACTICE RELATIONSHIP

What departmental organizational plan or structure is the most effective in providing these services? The first necessary element is a drug distribution system that maximizes the use of nonpharmacists in the inpatient drug distribution of the hospital. Many unit dose systems have been described in the literature. The benefits of unit dose distribution are more than just providing more doublechecks within the drug distribution system making it less error prone. It also allows the pharmacist to delegate many of the manual drug distribution tasks to technicians and still maintain the necessary responsibility and supervision. Unit dosing and the use of technicians have been readily accepted in hospitals that have tried them because of the difficulties experienced with traditional systems. Also, because the hospital drug distribution system interfaces with the licensed nurse (i.e., drugs are being issued to a licensed health professional and not to a patient for self-administration), the use of technicians has been more readily accepted. The primary point is that the use of technicians in conjunction with a unit dose system allows pharmacists time for clinical services that otherwise would not have been available.

The unit dose system also can provide a drug therapy record that can become the basis for the pharmacist's patient drug therapy monitoring system. Patient names, current drug therapy, and other appropriate information can be organized to easily review ongoing and new drug orders.

ADVANTAGES AND DISADVANTAGES OF A DECENTRALIZED PHARMACY SERVICE

Given a unit dose drug distribution system using technicians and patient drug therapy profiles, what are the advantages and disadvantages of centralized and decentralized pharmacy services? The following discussion will deal first with this question and then examine alternative departmental organizational structures.

Although the topic being considered centers on clinical pharmacy services with regard to decentralization, how the rest of the nonclinical pharmacy services are organized may bear directly on the options available as to the scope of the clinical services provided. Pharmacy departments are usually referred to as either centralized or decentralized. This is an oversimplification, however, of the actual situation in most cases. In fact, most decentralized pharmacy departments are organized into a mix of some centralized and some decentralized functions. Decentralized pharmacies are frequently quite different from one another as to exactly how and what is decentralized. The way services are provided may also vary from shift to shift and from weekday to weekend. The following functions are all possibilities for either a centralized or a decentralized approach:

1. New order review by the pharmacist
2. First dose preparation
3. Unit dose preparation of ongoing orders
4. Unit dose checking by a pharmacist or technician
5. IV order review by the pharmacist
6. IV order preparation including admixtures and TPNs
7. IVPB order reconstitution
8. IVPB order review by a pharmacist
9. IVPB order distribution to the patient
10. Discharge and inpatient prescription filling by the pharmacist
11. Unit dose packaging
12. Pharmacokinetic consults by pharmacist
13. Drug level ordering and/or scheduling by pharmacist
14. Drug information questions directed to the pharmacist
15. Answering drug information questions
16. Nonformulary drug request follow-up by the pharmacist
17. Pharmacist-patient interviewing as needed
18. Drug therapy regulation by the pharmacist
19. Drug therapy monitoring by the pharmacist
20. Drug reaction monitoring by the pharmacist
21. Pharmacy charge processing

Several observations can be made of the activities listed above. First, some of these activities must be performed by the pharmacist whereas others can be performed by a technician or clerk. Second, some of these activities that are to be done require the pharmacist to be outside the physical confines of the "pharmacy," whether located centrally or decentrally. Third, some of the nonpharmacist activities require immediate supervision whereas others require minimal pharmacist supervision. An ideal configuration of a given pharmacy department must start first with a statement of the scope of pharmacy services. This should include not only what services are to be provided but also when they will be available (24 hours a day, day shift only, etc). Then one can start addressing where these services should be provided to be as efficient as possible.

Another issue to be considered is the relationship of any clinical services provided to that of the drug distribution system provided. In particular, the review of new drug orders usually is a part of the clinical pharmacist's responsibility prospectively or it becomes a part of the clinical pharmacist's responsibilities to review retrospectively new drug orders from a clinical perspective beyond the "drug distribution pharmacist." The size of the institution may be a factor concerning the use of pharmacy technicians as a whole and this may vary from day to day and shift to shift. The availability of space in decentralized areas or the lack of it for centralized pharmacies may dictate how the drug distribution system is organized. The clinical services provided must then be woven into the basic configuration of the drug distribution system.

There are many advantages to decentralization of the pharmacy personnel responsible for providing drugs and drug information services to inpatients.

1. Immediate availability of drugs for administration to the patient. Satellite pharmacists provide drugs to patients more quickly following a new drug order.
2. Greater drug control and accountability.
3. Direct pharmacist communication with physicians and nurses, resulting in better rapport.
4. More space for the pharmacy as a whole and providing flexibility in reallocating or designing existing space in the central pharmacy.
5. Implementation of unique drug distribution systems designed to issue drugs to the nurse are more readily acceptable.
6. The pharmacist can review the chart or talk with the patient in an efficient manner.
7. Drug information through the pharmacist is readily available to physicians and nurses.
8. Nursing time involved with drug distribution is reduced (13). Having the initial dose of a new order available for the nurse when needed provides the nurse more flexibility in organizing time. Transferring the drug administration task to pharmacy personnel would further influence nursing time.
9. Pharmacist drug therapy specialization by patient care area is more easily accomplished.
10. Specialized clinical services can be developed and efficiently provided by the pharmcist, such as regulating a specific patient's drug therapy as ordered by the physician (e.g., heparin and oral anticoagulants, digoxin, aminophylline, aminoglycosides, TPN).
11. Pharmacists can more readily perform clinical drug research and patient drug therapy quality assessment studies.

The disadvantages of decentralized inpatient pharmacy services are as follows:

1. All pharmacists must become proficient as supervisors to deal effectively with technicians.
2. Pharmacists are responsible for both drug distribution and clinical services. Their time in nondrug distribution activities is dependent on the availability and quality of pharmacy technicians and their ability ef-

fectively to organize their time between both responsibilities.

3. Staffing flexibility is reduced when only one pharmacist with or without a technician is providing all
inpatient pharmacy services for a specific patient care
area when census levels are above or below normal.
Vacation, sick leave, etc coverage must be carefully
planned and provided for, including contingencies for
personnel replacement when required.

4. Unrealistic expectations from nurses and physicians
and excessive interruptions of the pharmacist and/or
technician.

5. Drug inventory control within the department is more
complex because of multiple pharmacy locations for
the same drug, particularly those prescribed infrequently.

6. Communications within the pharmacy department are
somewhat more difficult.

7. More space and equipment is required (e.g., drug
information references, refrigerators, etc).

8. Patient acuity and resulting drug distribution workload
may exceed the capacity of space and personnel in
decentralized pharmacy units.

9. Utilization of technology to automate and mechanize
the drug distribution system component of pharmacy
services will require more hardware.

The advantages of a centralized pharmacy are few if it
is to provide equivalent clinical pharmaceutic services.

1. Drug inventory control within the department is easier.
2. Less pharmacy space and equipment is needed.
3. Pharmacy staff flexibility is greater.
4. More efficiency for tasks requiring a minimum of interruptions.

The disadvantages of a centralized pharmacy service that
attempts to provide equivalent clinical services center on
the problem of providing drugs and services from a centralized location in an efficient and timely manner to patients, physicians, and nurses who are decentralized. The
disadvantages and/or problems listed below deal with trying
to provide pharmacy services equivalent to those of a decentralized operation from a centralized pharmacy location:

1. There is less effective communication between pharmacists and the nurses and patients who are physically
separated from them.

2. Because the pharmacist is not directly accessible to
the physician, the demand for clinical drug information is low.

3. Pharmacist's clinical services are minimal and less
efficient because patient information is not readily
available and physician-pharmacist contact is minimal.

4. Current patient information is not readily available to
the pharmacist even when the pharmacist distributes
drugs and processes drug orders.

5. Ongoing patient drug-related problems are likely to
continue and increase in complexity and severity as
more complex drugs and drug administration evolve
in the future.

In the central location, pharmacists will not fully use their
drug knowledge because the patient's clinical information,

nurse, and physician are not readily available. Pharmacists'
drug knowledge will not grow and develop to any reasonable
degree because their practice in the central area does not
demand growth and development. A centralized pharmacy
is likely to concentrate on drug distribution requests where
requests for drugs are received and not evaluated relative to
other drug orders for the same patient. Typically, the most
significant demands placed on the pharmacist in the central
pharmacy system is to process the greatest number of items
in the least amount of time, a situation that does not provide
the time or opportunity for drug knowledge judgments or
growth in clinical drug knowledge.

The alternatives to the organizational structure of a pharmacy department must relate to the functional requirements
and goals of the department. The various components of
the pharmacy in the organizational chart will probably be
similar whether it is centralized or decentralized so long as
the pharmacy services are to provide both drug information
and drug distribution tasks. However, the location of each
component of the pharmacy department may be different.
The basic components of a pharmacy department organization providing drugs and drug information to the hospital
will generally be organized in the following manner:

1. Organizational management: Budgeting, department
goals, and objectives

2. Business management: Purchasing/bidding, receiv-
ing/issuing, charging system

3. Inpatient services: New order processing, ongoing
medication orders, IV additives, IVPBs, patient drug
therapy monitoring

4. Outpatient services: Clinics, discharge, bedside/pass
prescriptions, surgery, emergency room, drug counseling

5. Drug information services: Referral questions, Pharmacy and Therapeutics Committee, newsletters, drug
formulary

6. Narcotics control: Intradepartmental and interdepartmental transactions

7. Manufacturing and packaging: Manufacturing, unit
dose packaging, prepackaging

8. Clinical pharmacokinetic services: Schedule drug
levels, provide consultations for drug dose and dosing

Employing a hypothetical example in which the inpatient
pharmaceutical services of a 200-bed hospital will be provided with six pharmacists and six technicians, there are
two alternative plans one might compare. Assume that services are to be provided for two shifts, each day, 7 days a
week. A centrally located pharmacy would provide staffing
of two pharmacists and two technicians on both the day and
evening shifts 7 days per week. If clinical activities did arise
requiring the pharmacist to see the chart or talk with the
patient, one pharmacist would be available to go to the floor.
Alternately, one pharmacist could float and make rounds
covering all of the patient care areas for the 200 beds. This
plan tends to split the pharmacists' responsibilities functionally (i.e., one providing drug distribution, the other
providing clinical services). Some of the difficulties encountered with such an approach are listed as follows:

1. The pharmacist in the patient care area will maintain
monitoring records that are physically located away

from the central pharmacy, thus not available centrally for the dispensing pharmacist to review new drug orders. The pharmacist on the floor will not be able to review the majority of new drug orders.

2. The pharmacist on the floor will have to triage drug distribution problems encountered. For 200 patients a great deal of time would be involved with drug distribution.

3. A pharmacist's area of drug therapy expertise and interest will probably influence the amount of time spent with different categories of patients instead of being based on patient needs.

4. The drug information demands on the pharmacist would be diverse, covering all categories of patients and drug therapy regimens in which the 200 patients encompass (e.g., pediatrics, internal medicine).

5. The pharmacist's availability for physicians' and nurses' questions on the floors will amount to one full-time equivalent pharmacist per shift.

A decentrally located pharmacy would provide the same two pharmacists and two technicians per day and evening shift 7 days a week. They would, however, be able to provide services from two satellite pharmacies. In this example, each pharmacist is responsible for supervising technicians and providing both drugs and drug information. The pharmacist's areas of clinical expertise need only address the unique needs of 100 patients, instead of 200. The pharmacist would have closer communications with both the physician and nurses by providing twice as many pharmacist manhours on the patient floors to handle questions as they arise.

The above advantages relate primarily to providing clinical pharmacy services. Providing drug distribution from a satellite pharmacy also eliminates the need for special delivery systems to send initial doses for new orders and IV admixtures from a central location to the floor. The above example, dealing with 200 patients, could be extrapolated to a 300-, 500-, or 700-bed hospital. The key assumption being made is that those pharmacists who supervise centrally located technicians are the same pharmacists who would otherwise be providing additional pharmacist manhours on the floor in a decentralized pharmacy.

RELATIVE COSTS OF A CENTRALIZED AND DECENTRALIZED PHARMACY SERVICE

The question of costs is a very important part of the hospital's decision as to what form of pharmacy services to support. Costs can be divided into patient benefits, such as reduction in mortality, morbidity, and patient hospital days. There has not been an ideal study to relate these types of patient benefits from clinical pharmacy services to the cost of these services. This type of study would have to be hospital-wide or for all patient types because drug use needs and problems are different by patient types. This study would require a long period of time to obtain data for both before and after implementing clinical pharmacy services. The problem created is how to hold variables constant that affect patient stay, such as new drugs, changes in nursing care and surgical procedures, to allow for the determination of the benefits directly from the pharmacy services and the

pharmacists' clinical practice. Such a study has not been designed, nor have any funds been made available to support one. Costs can also be divided into equipment and facilities, and personnel, with personnel costs being the more significant.

Equipment and Facilities

Equipment needs will depend primarily on the drug distribution systems employed. The equipment required for unit dose drug packaging and medication carts would be common whether centralized or decentralized. If there are differences, they would be minor in scope and cost. IV admixtures and other sterile reconstitution and packaging done in decentralized areas of the hospital would involve purchasing more clean air hoods.

Space availability in patient care areas is usually difficult to obtain, which has resulted in the development of several approaches to providing a decentralized presence. Satellite pharmacies in hospitals was first described in 1960 (15). Hospitals that were originally built or remodeled with satellite pharmacies in mind generally have little trouble providing enough space to do all of the drug distribution and clinical activities planned.

The size of a typical decentralized or satellite pharmacy would be in the 200-300 square foot range for approximately 100 beds. Other variables that enter into discussions of space are: the size of the hospital, the physical layout of the hospital, the number of patients per hospital floor, and the number of nursing stations per hospital floor and per hospital. These are important because all are determining factors for the number of dose preparation or dispensing areas. In the final analysis, the space for a decentralized pharmacy system may or may not be greater than the space for a centralized pharmacy. The cost difference is also affected if adequate space already exists in the nursing station area that can easily be converted into a satellite pharmacy. When space is not available for a satellite pharmacy, pharmacists have used a mobile cart system. Such a system still focuses on the decentralized clinical pharmacist to provide the immediate drug distribution needs of the patient (e.g., in providing the initial doses). Ongoing drug needs may also be provided from the mobile cart or from a centralized drug distribution system (16).

Computer systems can provide better communications within the hospital such as patient tracking from the admitting department and pathology results. Computer systems also allow transmittal of pharmacy orders from the patient care area to virtually any location in or even outside the hospital building. The key issue concerning an order entry computer system is whether the pharmacist ever sees the original physician's order. Unless the physician enters orders into a terminal directly, having a nurse enter this information is error-prone and loses the control provided by a pharmacist's interpretation of the order. Pharmacy computer systems can be used in both decentralized and centralized pharmacy operations to better communicate within the department. For decentralized pharmacy operations, computer systems offer more flexibility in splitting those functions that can be more effectively done centrally.

Personnel

The determination of personnel costs may rest within the pharmacy department or may also include the impact of the pharmacy services on nursing time in the hospital mediation system. It is suggested that comparative personnel costs for alternative systems and services be factored to a cost per patient day. In this way, personnel costs are reduced to a common factor for comparisons.

Several cost comparisons could be made as follows:
1. Centralized pharmacy service personnel costs per patient day
2. Decentralized pharmacy service personnel costs per patient day
3. Nursing personnel costs in medication-related activities before clinical pharmacy services (central and decentral)
4. Nursing personnel costs in medication-related activities after clinical pharmacy services (central and decentral)
5. Pharmacist and nonpharmacist personnel costs (central and decentral)
6. Pharmacy personnel costs based on program elements (e.g., unit dose, IV admixtures, clinical services)

All of these cost breakdowns will enable comparisons as to what the overall financial results for personnel would be, depending on the pharmacy service system configuration.

Where these costs have been determined, there has been overall actual personnel costs savings (17). For example, at Memorial Medical Center, Long Beach, California, in a study done in 1971-1972, nursing time in medication activities was reduced 19.2 minutes per patient day at $1.63 per patient day. Pharmacy personnel costs increased $1.11 per patient day. The nursing time was actually reduced so an overall savings of $0.52 per patient day or $98,900 per year was achieved, based on 521 patients per day. Other hospitals in the United States have implemented decentralized clinical pharmacy services on a reasonable cost basis.

If the overall personnel costs are increased from previous levels, key factors to consider include the starting level of pharmacy services, and pharmacy staff and nursing time not reduced or adjusted for the time saved.

Ultimately, it is up to each hospital to determine from its own operational characteristics whether personnel costs will be greater or if savings can be achieved from implementing a decentralized pharmacy service. The assumption that it will cost more because of increases in the size of the pharmacy staff cannot be made until studies on costs are completed.

Why not separate drug distribution from clinical services and have the drug distribution centralized and the pharmacist decentralized? This is an alternative to be considered. The key question is allocation of the available pharmacists' time. For example, if 100 hours of pharmacists' time are available, how much time would be needed to supervise and staff the central areas? The central area cannot be staffed without pharmacists' supervision. It is believed that a majority of the 100 pharmacist hours would be required to staff the central area, which would leave a minority of the hours for clinical practice. This also means the pharmacists' time in the patient care area is not fulltime but will be limited to the hours left available. This is in contrast to decentralized

staffing, where it is realistic to have a majority of the pharmacists' time (perhaps as much as 75%) available for clinical services and 25% for drug distribution. The determination of this time allocation of the pharmacists' hours should be done when a hospital management is trying to decide between central vs decentral services.

Another important factor is the job satisfaction of the pharmacists when they are in the central area and really desire to be in the patient care area. Rotation of the staff is not a satisfactory solution, because of the difficulty in developing relationships between pharmacists, nurses, and physicians. Also, the growth and development of the pharmacists' clinical expertise is slowed while they are in the central area. Another factor is what kind of pharmacists do we educate? All for clinical practice? Some for clinical practice and a majority for the central pharmacy operation? These are not easy questions to answer.

FORCES THAT PREVENT OR INTERFERE WITH DECENTRALIZED PHARMACY SERVICES

Several forces prevent and interfere with providing clinical pharmacy services. They are described briefly as follows.

Attitudes and Behavior. Negative attitudes and behavior by the physician and nurse to the pharmacist will not allow for the implementation of the pharmacist's information and knowledge. A negative attitude by hospital management as reflected in inadequate pharmacist staff, pharmacy facilities, and equipment will not allow the pharmacist to even attempt to provide drug knowledge and information. A negative attitude and behavior by pharmacists will prevent their providing drug knowledge and information.

Pharmacy Department Facilities. If pharmacy department facilities are lacking in terms of space and equipment, adequate clinical services cannot be easily provided. An ample amount of space in the patient care area is needed for the pharmacist to function effectively.

Drug Information Resources. Without well-educated and interested pharmacists in clinical practice, these services cannot be provided.

Pharmacists' Time for Information Functions. The hospital administration must approve a pharmacist staffing pattern to provide time for information functions.

Legal Requirements. Present pharmacy state laws may limit the use of nonpharmacists in providing services that minimize the amount of pharmacists' time available for information functions. Federal laws continue to increase pharmacy time required for drug stock accountability, which reduces the time available for information and knowledge functions.

FUTURE CONSIDERATIONS—1980s

The new financial era for hospitals in the 1980s, led by cost containment, diagnosis related groups (DRGs), state rate setting commissions, and price competition, may adversely affect the growth of clinical and decentralized pharmacy services. Pressures to reduce operational costs for providing care to inpatients is intense in US hospitals. Idealistic thinking with realistic planning is needed by all hospital managers to provide the most cost-efficient care with a high level of quality. Decentralized pharmacy services, like all other hospital services, will need to redefine and defend operational objectives and results.

It is the opinion of the authors that decentralized pharmacy services will still be a cost-effective method for providing clinical pharmacy services. Hospitalized patients will require a significant amount of drug therapy. Modern drug therapy will increase in complexity. Medication systems will need to be responsive in a manner to help keep patient stay to a minimum. Automation, mechanization, and continued use of pharmacy technicians will be necessary to cope with the volume of drug use in a hospital. New drugs and drug delivery systems will require pharmacists in clinical practice with greater drug knowledge and skills than currently is practiced (18).

SUMMARY

The usual assumption is that centralized pharmacy services are less costly. This assumption is not true in all cases and probably is wrong for many situations. Each hospital must determine its own profiles regarding costs, the provision of clincal pharmacy services, and the level of safety desired for patients and their drug therapy.

The pharmacists' responsibilities in a modern hospital are to distribute drugs safely and accurately and to provide drug information to meet the needs of patients, physicians, and nurses. To most effectively meet these responsibilities requires that pharmacists practice in the patient care areas of the modern hospital.

REFERENCES

1. Hynniman CE, et al: A comparison of medication errors under the University of Kentucky unit-dose system and traditional drug distribution systems in four hospitals. *Am J Hosp Pharm* 27:803, 1970.
2. Davis NM, Cohen MR: *Medication Errors: Causes and Prevention.* Philadelphia, Stickley, 1981.
3. Brodie DC: *Drug Utilization and Drug Utilization Review and Control.* Washington, DC, Department of Health, Education and Welfare, Public Health Service, Health Services and Mental Health Administration, National Center for Health Services Research and Development, 1970.
4. Oglivie RI, et al: Adverse drug reactions during hospitalization. *Can Med Assoc J* 97:1450, 1967.
5. Barr DP: Hazards of modern diagnosis and therapy, the price we pay. *J Am Med Assoc* 159:1452, 1955.
6. Young DS, Pestaner LC, Gibberman V: Effects of drugs on clinical laboratory tests. *Clin Chem* 21(5):1D-432 D, 1975.
7. Swanson M, et al: *Drugs, Chemicals and Blood Dyscrasias.* Cincinnati, Drug Intelligence Publications, 1977.
8. Cluff LE: 5 Liver manifestations. *Major Prob Intern Med* 5:131-227, 1975.
9. Briggs G, et al: *Drugs in Pregnancy and Lactation,* Baltimore, Williams & Wilkins, 1983.
10. Smith WE: The drug component for inpatient care in the hospital setting. (Unpublished.)
11. Helmlund BA: *Drug Distribution Study—VI, a Computer Assisted Satellite Pharmacy System for Hospital Drug Distribution.* Saskatoon, Saskatechewan, University of Saskatoon.
12. Thur MP, et al: Medication errors in a nurse-controlled parenteral admixture program. *Am J Hosp Pharm* 29:298, 1972.
13. Wadd WB, Blissenbach TJ: Medication-related nursing time in centralized and decentralized drug distribution. *Am J Hosp Pharm* 41:477, 1984.
14. Barker K: The work of the pharmacist and the potential use of auxilliaries. *Am J Hosp Pharm* 29:25-53, 1973.
15. Carner DC: *New Concept in Hospital Pharmacies.* Indianapolis, Tile and Till, 1960.
16. Lipman AG, et al: Decentralization of pharmaceutical services without satellite pharmacies. *Am J Hsop Pharm* 36:1513, 1979.
17. Smith WE: *The Economic Feasibility of Clinical Pharmacy in the Hospital Setting.* HSM 110-711208. Springfield, VA, National Technical Information Service, U.S. Department of Commerce, 1973.
18. Smith E: Clinical pharmacy in the 1980's. *Am J Hosp Pharm* 40:223-229, 1983.

Educational Activities

CONDUCT OF AND PARTICIPATION IN EDUCATIONAL ACTIVITIES

A wide range of educational activities is performed routinely in the institution and involves all health practitioners and students of the various health professions. The director of pharmacy services, or his designee, is responsible for coordinating the department's contribution to these educational activities. Further, he is responsible for training new personnel and for carrying on a continuous educational program for pharmacists and pharmacy supportive personnel. In institutions having a pharmacy residency program, the pharmacist must develop a well-planned and coordinated program so that the residency is a meaningful educational experience in the development of future practitioners. In institutions offering a pharmacy residency program in conjunction with an academic program, the phamacist must have a thorough understanding of his own program and the course material and objectives of the academic phase to assist in coordinating one with the other.

CHAPTER 55

Pharmacy Technicians

LOUIS P. JEFFREY and CHARLES D. MAHONEY

Supportive personnel have been used in pharmacy practice for nearly four decades. They are extensively used in both community and hospital pharmacy practice. A review of the literature over the past decade reveals a wealth of information and data that documents the need and justification of a secondary level pharmacy practitioner (1-4). This secondary health care practitioner, commonly referred to as a "pharmacy technician," is differentiated from other types of supportive personnel ("aide," "clerk," "helper," etc) by the degree of education and training and the level of responsibility at which he or she performs.

With the advent of more sophisticated and direct approaches to providing pharmaceutical services to the patient, pharmacists are recognizing there is an increasing need for supportive personnel specifically trained to assist the pharmacist. Pharmacists are placing less emphasis on traditional distributive services because modern pharmacy is becoming more directly involved and integrated into the health care delivery system. Pharmacists must, therefore, be relieved of many traditional tasks to make room for newer ones.

Currently, little uniformity exists in individual state statutes or regulations concerning pharmacy supportive personnel. Pharmacy technicians are not registered or licensed at either the state or national level, nor is there any certification process for pharmacy technicians nationally. Interestingly, the Michigan Pharmaceutical Association has taken the initiative to certify pharmacy technicians by examination statewide (5): the title "pharmacy certified technician" is granted.

Basically, the two methods of training pharmacy technicians are informal on-the-job training and formal education and training programs that integrate didactic instruction with on-the-job experience. The majority of technicians in pharmacy practice today are not graduates of formal pharmacy technician training programs, but received their training on the job. The structured, hospital-based technician training programs have demonstrated that competent pharmacy technicians can be trained in a concentrated course of instruction.

It has become evident that the current health manpower dilemma will not immediately be solved by increasing the number of practicing physicians, nurses, or pharmacists, but that to attain this goal, while maintaining the highest quality in medical care, optimal use of allied health personnel will be needed (6).

Because the job description of a technician varies with the location and size of the hospital and is compounded by the scope and span of professional and other services provided by the pharmacy department, there are varying opinions from directors of pharmacy services as to the function and responsibility of this category of personnel. Thus, if there are divergent attitudes on the use of the technician, of necessity there will also be varying opinions on a host of other factors related to their qualifications, education, and evaluation.

TYPICAL TRAINING

Historically, the lack of national standards for the education and training of supportive personnel for pharmacy has resulted in a proliferation of concepts. The American Society of Hospital Pharmacists (ASHP) established in 1982, and subsequently revised in 1983, a standard for pharmacy technician training programs (7). It is anticipated that the ASHP standard will assist practitioners and educators in restructuring and standardizing the numerous types of pharmacy technician training programs throughout the country.

Within the past several years, numerous junior colleges, technical colleges, and other types of educational institutions have offered specialized courses of instruction to prepare students for a career in pharmacy as a pharmacy technician. Colleges of Pharmacy are also becoming involved (8). The Massachusetts College of Pharmacy and Allied Health Sciences was the first and is currently the only college of pharmacy that offers a hospital pharmacy technician program. A certificate is awarded by the college on the successful completion of the program.

After almost four decades of experience with the use of supportive personnel in hospital pharmacy practice, the general consensus of pharmaceutical organizations and institutional practitioners is that technicians should be educated and trained in a hospital.

The type of program may vary from an informal concept based on a brief orientation and work experience to a formalized and organized regimen of didactic instruction and work experience, combined with quizzes, examinations, and laboratory exercises. The length of a training program also varies from a few days to 600 hours to 1 year. A typical hospital-based program is outlined below (9). The length of the program is 15 consecutive 40-hour weeks.

Curriculum	Hours
Orientation	24
Classroom instruction	45
Conference (1 hour per week)	15
Seminars (2 hours per month)	8
Study and examination periods (3 hours per week)	42
On-the-job instruction	115
Work experience assignments	351
	600

QUALIFICATIONS

As an illustration, the Rhode Island Hospital Personnel Department established the following guidelines for pharmacy technician applicants:

1. Applicant may be male or female.
2. Applicant must be a high school graduate or possess a high school equivalency certificate. He or she should have passed a course in algebra and chemistry. Algebra exposes a student to abstract concepts in mathematics (i.e., how to solve for an unknown). This background helps a student solve ratio and proportion problems. A brief exposure to chemistry is necessary for the student to understand the fundamental principles of the pharmaceutical sciences (i.e., chemical formulas and names, molecular changes, temperature, weight, and density, particulate matter in the environment).
3. It is desirable, but not required, that applicants have completed 2 years of college or be a high school graduate with employment experience comparable to college training.
4. An official transcript of high school grades and those of other educational institutions are required.
5. Applicant must be of good moral character.
6. Applicant's proficiency to read, write, and speak English must be acceptable.
7. Applicant must satisfactorily pass a written admission test.
8. Applicant must meet all of the requirements for employment set forth by the hospital.

ENTRY LEVEL

The entry level pharmacy technician should be viewed as an individual in the training or learning process. At this level, the technician receives the basic instruction and the on-the-job training in the skills the technician is expected to possess. Depending on the type of professional setting (community or institutional practice) and the degree of sophistication of the services provided, the entry level will require various times for completion. For example, the entry level in some departments of pharmacy is a formal training program. This type of program is often conducted over a 15- to 30-week period. Other primary level technicians receive nearly all of their instruction and experience on the job and therefore spend longer periods of time at this level, perhaps as long as 12 or 18 months.

A sample job description for entry level pharmacy technicians in an institution appears below. There are many such job descriptions, which will vary slightly from one institution to another. Entry level technicians in community practice may have no written job description, but the scope of their responsibilities will be similar in most instances.

Sample job description
Entry level pharmacy technician
General
Receives instruction and training in all areas or sections of the department of pharmacy. Assists the pharmacist and learns methods and procedures for dispensing, packaging, and labeling drugs, bulk pharmaceutical formulation, distribution of floor stock, and clerical record-keeping duties.
Supervision received
Under direct supervision of the pharmacy supervisor. Receives functional guidance from the pharmacist assigned to the work area.
Supervision exercised
None.
Typical duties
1. Assists the pharmacist in various sections of the department according to assignment. The following duties are illustrative of the level of work performed during the training period:
   a. Learns procedure for stocking and maintaining inventory in stockroom and supply cabinets.
   b. Assists with stocking mobile drug cart for distribution of medication to patient care units.
   c. Assists with dispensing, packaging, and labeling drug orders and prescriptions under direct supervision of a pharmacist.
   d. Assists with record keeping in the area assigned.
2. Attends lectures and classes as directed.
   a. Fulfills reading assignments.
   b. Submits weekly reports on training received.

INTERMEDIATE LEVEL

After a period at the entry level, either in a formal training program or an informal, on-the-job program, the technician often assumes responsibility for more complicated tasks and performs more job functions with a goal of productivity rather than of learning. This phase of the technician's career may be called the "intermediate level," and usually involves a wide range of functions. Quite often, especially in larger institutions, an individual technician is assigned to perform only a specific number of functions because of the specialization of the tasks to be performed. The important thing to keep in mind is that technicians at the intermediate level are generally expected by their supervisors to be able to perform *all* functions if they are requested to do so. A sample job description follows.

Sample job description
Intermediate level pharmacy technician
General
Performs various rotating functions in inpatient and outpatient dispensing, product formulation, unit dose distribution, or distribution of controlled substances, to become familiar with all aspects of pharmacy operations; follows well-defined instructions to assist the pharmacist in the area assigned. Compounds and dispenses medications and pharmaceutical supplies under direct supervision of a pharmacist. Maintains pertinent operational records in accordance with legal requirements or hospital policy. Orders supplies from bulk storage and restocks dispensing bins and service areas as needed. Stocks medication carts and delivers contents to patient care areas according to

schedule. Compiles and computes prescription charges. Processes credits.

Education

High school graduation or equivalent.

Experience

No prior experience necessary. Requires completion of 500-hour training course, plus 3 to 6 months of on-the-job training.

Supervision received

Under direct supervision of the pharmacist assigned (all work is checked by a pharmacist).

Supervision exercised

Responsible for own work only. May give functional guidance to new employees in the position.

Principal duties

1. Reviews written prescriptions to determine ingredients needed. Compounds ingredients through such processes as filtering, emulsifying, or triturating, to prepare medications.
2. Fills prescriptions from bulk stock.
3. Uses clean air center and sterile technique in filling and labeling syringes for delivery to patient dispensing units. May sterilize injectable preparation if prepared in the pharmacy or purchased in nonsterile prepared forms.
4. Fills bottles or other package forms with measured amounts of medications according to prescription specifications. Types and affixes labels to containers showing identification data and directions for use.
5. Assists pharmacist in maintaining records on all prescriptions of inpatient or ambulatory patient use. Transcribes medication orders to patient profiles. Computes and records prescription charges; may collect charges from outpatients.
6. Maintains all control records on narcotics, poisons, and controlled substances as required. Responsible for exercising maximum security precautions.
7. Maintains perpetual inventory of pharmaceuticals and supplies in the dispensing area assigned, storing under proper conditions in refrigeration and security. Orders supplies and restocks shelves and bins as necessary.
8. Fills, packages, and labels prescriptions, and stocks the master medication cart. Brings the cart to patient dispensing stations according to a predetermined schedule. Responsible for preparation and delivery of extemporaneous medications on an as needed basis.
9. Serves as intermediary between patient care units and pharmacy.
10. Maintains work area in clean and neat condition.
11. Performs other duties as required.

ADVANCED LEVEL

After a period of obtaining primary skills through a formal training program or through extensive on-the-job training, and after experience at the intermediate level, some pharmacy technicians acquire considerable skill and expertise. To function at an advanced level, it is assumed the pharmacy technician is proficient in all of the duties normally assigned to technicians at the entry and intermediate levels (10). This advanced level may be achieved when the technician acquires a specialized skill through training, such as computer programming or scientific writing, or through a combination of advanced training and experience, such as skills in personnel management, sterile techniques, quality control, or drug distribution. An advanced position provides for career extension, recognition of performance, and increased salary potential to meet the personal and social needs of a tech-

nician performing in a professional environment. A sample job description follows.

Sample job description

Advanced level pharmacy technician

General

Must be a high school graduate. Two years of college training or its equivalent preferred. Must have graduated from a formal pharmacy technician training program. Required to successfully complete an advanced level technician training program conducted by the department of pharmacy. Must be able to function proficiently in all duties normally assigned to pharmacy technicians. Over and above these proficiencies, however, may possess a single specialized skill, or a combination of skills in various areas that permits functioning at an advanced level of responsibility with a pharmacist.

Supervision received

Functions under the direct supervision of a pharmacist or pharmacy supervisor.

Supervision exercised

Provides routine supervision of technical functions of other supportive personnel assigned to the same area. Acts as a coordinator between the activities of supportive personnel and the pharmacist or pharmacy supervisor of the assigned area.

Assists the pharmacy supervisor in performance appraisal reviews of other supportive personnel. The personnel so supervised may include pharmacy technicians, pharmacy technician trainees, machine operators, clerks, keypunch operators, and work experience students (volunteers).

Principal duties

1. Functions as a pharmacy technician in all the areas that technical personnel are usually assigned.
2. Gathers and compiles workload and other statistics for departmental reports.
3. Conducts surveys under the guidelines established by a member of the supervisory or administrative staff.
4. Orders and controls all necessary supplies from hospital stores.
5. Monitors preventive maintenance of all equipment in the assigned area.
6. Assists the supervisor in the appraisal of supportive personnel.
7. Assigns and regulates the routine work production performed by supportive personnel in the assigned areas. Determines priorities for established production procedures.
8. Maintains adequate working levels of inventory in the assigned areas. Monitors the expiration dates of the working inventory.
9. Serves as communications liaison between the pharmacy supervisor and supportive personnel.
10. When functioning at a decentralized pharmacy location, must be able to take suitable action(s) or provide answers to questions of routine pharmacy procedure. Interacts with physicians, nurses, and other hospital personnel and must be able to refer questions to the proper authorities.
11. Monitors the compliance of subordinates to pharmacy policies and procedures on behalf of the director of pharmacy services.
12. Coordinates the technical functions of an assigned area with those of other pharmacy service areas. (e.g., coordination of sterile formulations with distribution, distribution with packaging and labeling, decentralized pharmacy with sterile formulations, or decentralized pharmacy with distribution.
13. Coordinates the orientation of trainees and new employees to the technical functions of the assigned areas.
14. Keeps all records and log sheets used in the assigned areas accurate and up to date.
15. Performs other duties as assigned.

Areas of assignment

1. Distribution services
2. Sterile and nonsterile product formulations

3. Packaging, printing, and labeling
4. Pharmacy service unit
5. Purchasing and inventory control
6. Quality control systems

SUMMARY

None of the currently identified clinical roles being assumed by pharmacists throughout the country could have been implemented and maintained as viable, economically feasible services without the support of secondary level pharmacy practitioners. We believe it is essential for pharmacy to continue developing programs to properly identify and train technicians. Technicians are currently performing vital roles in both institutional and community practice. Differentiating technicians from other supportive personnel and establishing advancement opportunities for technicians will alleviate the frustration that thousands of trained technicians experience.

REFERENCES

1. ASHP Workshop on subprofessional personnel in hospital pharmacy. *Am J Hosp Pharm* 26:224-232, 1969.
2. Jeffrey LP, Mahoney CD: Training, utilization and motivation of pharmacy technicians—a five-year analysis. *Am J Hosp Pharm* 32:491-494, 1975.
3. Letcher KI: Supportive personnel in the health professions—hospital pharmacy. *Am J Hosp Pharm* 30:507-510, 1973.
4. Shoup LK: Recruitment, selection and training of pharmacy technicians. *Am J Hosp Pharm* 27:907-910, 1970.
5. Mysiewicz TM: Technicians update: Michigan grabs the ball. *Drug Top* 125:68-70, 1981.
6. Hanan ZI: Technicians in health care. In Durgin JM, Hanan ZI, Ward CD (eds): *Pharmacy Technicians' Manual,* ed 2. St Louis, CV Mosby, 1978, pp 215-216.
7. ASHP accreditation standard for pharmacy technician training programs. *Am J Hosp Pharm* 41:333-334, 1984.
8. Smith TP: Supportive personnel training program based at a technical college. *Am J Hosp Pharm* 39:443-446, 1982.
9. Jeffrey LP, Mahoney CD: *Pharmacy Technician Manual,* ed 4. Providence, Rhode Island Hospital Department of Pharmacy, 1982, pp 182-187.
10. Jeffrey LP, Mahoney CD: Pharmacy technician specialist: A career opportunity. *Am J Hosp Pharm* 32:491-494, 1975.

ADDITIONAL READING

Barker KN, Smith MC, Winter ER: The work of the pharmacist and the potential use of auxiliaries. *Am J Hosp Pharm* 29:35-50, 1972.
Durgin JM, Hanan ZI, Ward CD (eds): *Pharmacy Technicians' Manual,* ed 2. St Louis, CV Mosby, 1978.
Friedman E: Ebb tide for allied health. *Hospitals* 57:66-71, 1983.
Jeffrey LP: Impact of the pharmacy technician upon pharmacy service in the year 2000. *Drug Intell Clin Pharm* 9:430-432, 1975.
Pevonka MP, Lemberger MA: Legal status and organizational attitudes toward use of supportive personnel in pharmacy. *Am J Hosp Pharm* 38:1702-1705, 1981.

CHAPTER 56

Continuing Education

LOUIS P. JEFFREY and CHARLES D. MAHONEY

Next to integrity, competence is the first and most fundamental moral responsibility of all the health professions . . . .
Each of our professions must insist that competence
will be reinforced through the years of practice. After the
degree is conferred, continuing education is society's only
real guarantee of the optimal quality of health care (1).
EDMUND D. PELLEGRINO

The pharmacist, as a health care professional, has an inherent moral responsibility to maintain a high level of knowledge and professional competence through a process of lifelong learning.

It has become increasingly obvious to faculties of colleges of pharmacy, graduates who are participating in an internship or residency, and pharmacists who practice in a community pharmacy or in a hospital environment that the traditional role of the practitioner is continually undergoing change. During the past decade, a host of new services have been identified as functions of the pharmacist. A review of these activities makes it abundantly clear that the acceptance of these duties demands, in addition to the legal responsibilities of the pharmacist, a personal commitment to continuing education (2). Because of the changing role of the pharmacist and of a professional requirement for continuing education, an absolute need exists to develop a level of competence that will improve patient care.

PROFESSIONAL REQUIREMENTS

The need for the continuing education of pharmacists has been increasingly emphasized during the past two decades. As the concept developed, a great deal was written concerning the subject. Thus, it seems appropriate to include the following philosophy of continuing education expressed by a prominent pharmacy leader of that period (3).

The concept of continuing education has existed among scholars for hundreds of years but only in recent times has it evolved conspicuously as an intregral part of the education process of those who enter the professions. Lifelong learning is becoming part of the philosophy of professional education and through it a sustaining influence for the nurture of the professions is being supplied. We accept the thesis, albeit with difficulty in a materialistic world, that the primary motivation for a career in the professions is to serve. The drive to serve is a spiritual one—it reflects an attitude of the mind and of the heart. The concept of continuing education,

therefore, becomes one of re-enforcement of the primary objective in the life of a professional person.

As a personal credo, the authors have always felt that continuing education should be a self-imposed responsibility and, therefore, have supported the concept of voluntary continuing education. There are those who feel that continuing education should be a fringe benefit of employment. There are still others who feel that mandatory continuing education should be essential and indispensable, whereas opponents are equally adamant. Obviously, the various opinions concerning these subjects do not necessarily chart a clear path for the future. The voices of individual practitioners, educators, professional associations, regulatory agencies, and, most recently, legislators often clash in a dissonant chorus of opinion and conjecture about the need for mandatory continuing education and how it should be implemented. State boards of pharmacy have been invested with the authority to ensure public health and safety via laws, regulations, and a licensing procedure for pharmacists. Several states reinforce these basic safeguards through a concept of compulsory continuing education (Appendix 56.1).

The responsibility to maintain professional excellence is inherent in the pharmacist's role. Continuing education programs offer valuable and essential means of fulfilling this obligation. The prevailing attitude is that pharmacy practitioners should pursue their own continuing education. But although this is true, they may not be solely responsible. Management also has a commitment to provide continuing education programs (4).

The preamble to the ASHP Statement on Continuing Education reads in part (5):

While every practitioner should assume personal responsibility for maintaining and improving professional competence . . . he may often require assistance in identifying gaps between actual and desired performance, in setting priorities, and in selecting learning activities which will contribute most toward achieving these objectives.

The Joint Commission on the Accreditation of Hospitals (JCAH) shares the philosophy that a commitment to education and training can assist in the quest for improved pharmacy and patient care services. In the interpretation of Standard III of the JCAH Standard on Pharmaceutical Services, it is stated that the director of pharmacy should be responsible for (6):

Requiring and documenting the participation of pharmacy personnel in relevant education programs, including orientation of new employees, as well as in-service and outside continuing educational programs. Frequency of programs and participation shall be related to the scope of the pharmaceutical services offered and shall be established with the approval of the chief executive officer.

There is a great deal of justification for supporting the position that continuing education be provided as a fringe benefit of employment. In the mid-1950s, Dr. Jeffrey inaugurated education programs at the Albany Medical Center Hospital (Albany, New York) during the workday as part of a complete pharmaceutical service. This successful 10-year program served as the foundation for the similar, but expanded, program at Rhode Island Hospital, which has been in effect for 15 years. We believe that the individual pharmacist practitioner should make the determination as to what the needs are and what steps are essential to maintain professional competence. A "Pharmacist Standard for Maintaining Professional Competence" was developed as a guideline for pharmacists in meeting established objectives (Fig. 56.1). This activity of the department of pharmacy is conducted by its division of education and training. For example, each week a minimum of four 1-hour continuing education programs are prepared and presented by both intra- and extradepartmental personnel for the professional staff. In addition to these departmental in-service programs, the continuing education commitment is supplemented by the multiple staff conferences, medical grand rounds, or pediatric grand rounds. Almost all of these activities are scheduled during the workday, as physicians, pharmacists, educators, and others offer their expertise to their colleagues.

Some examples of the type of continuing educational activities that may be desirable for a group of pharmacists are described below.

Drug Information Conference. A list of selected questions that have been processed by the Drug Information Service during the previous month is the agenda for this 1-hour conference conducted monthly. The purpose of this conference is to share with professional staff the information disseminated by the Drug Information Service. These conferences also contribute to the objective of building a drug information capability in all our professional staff.

Pharmacy Clinical Conference. The pharmacy clinical conference is conducted twice weekly. The conference is conducted by a member of the staff or a pharmacy resident and uses case studies or information on clinical subjects of interest with which the staff is involved.

Professional Health Conference. The professional health conference is a 1-hour program conducted each week that features guest presentations by physicians, nurses, pharmacists, visiting dignitaries, and other speakers. All members of the professional staff are required to attend. Indeed, even those pharmacists who may not be on duty on that particular day or that particular time invariably attend this important continuing education program.

Pharmacists' Committee. The pharmacists' committee meeting is conducted each month. It provides a forum for peer dialogue as all professional members of the department gather in a social atmosphere to discuss professional matters. This meeting provides a medium for open discussions concerning a broad range of issues and answers.

Other Aids to Continuing Education. Other aids include a self-study area equipped with current journals, reprints, and cassette tape presentations; participation in the extensive hospital medical, surgical, and pediatric conferences; and numerous other conferences conducted by other divisions of the pharmacy.

Pharmacist Standard for Maintaining
Professional Competence

Preamble

Pharmaceutical Services are an essential health care service. Pharmacists, therefore, have a moral obligation to continuously maintain and improve their professional competence. The Department of Pharmacy offers a number of in-service educational programs to assist the pharmacist in increasing his/her knowledge.

Each pharmacist is required to attend and actively participate in education and training programs. The dynamic nature of the pharmacy services at the Rhode Island Hospital, however, makes it difficult to schedule these activities and events so that they will be equally convenient to all pharmacists. Some aspects of the program are conducted while the pharmacist is on duty, while others are expected to be an individual effort on personal time.

Therefore, it is necessary for each pharmacist to exercise professional self-discipline in complying with the "Pharmacist Standard for Maintaining Professional Competence."

FIGURE 56.1

SUPPORTIVE PERSONNEL

For almost four decades, leaders within the profession have advocated delegating some of the technical functions of the pharmacist to supportive personnel. The most commonly designated title for this classification of personnel is pharmacy technician. Regardless of the work setting, this formally educated and trained group of secondary practitioners serves a vital role and performs some of the pharmacist's technical functions. Because technicians have assisted with some of the pharmacist's tasks, there is an inherent obligation to assist in maintaining the skills of these trained people. Thus, continuing education is desirable and necessary for the secondary practitioner, as well as for the pharmacist (7). Improvements and modifications are constantly being assimilated as new techniques are developed. Therefore, two opportunities are offered at Rhode Island Hospital to the technicians to maintain their technical skills and knowledge.

Technician Educational Seminar. The technician educational seminar is a continuing education program held weekly. The meeting is conducted by a technician or a technician specialist and provides a forum for pharmacists, technicians, and other health care practitioners to discuss topics of interest to technicians.

Technician's Committee. In addition to the formal educational atmosphere of the technician educational seminar, the technicians meet as a group once each month as the Technician's Committee. The educational process here is less formal as the technicians participate in a "give and take" atmosphere. The committee is chaired by a member of the administrative staff and all aspects of departmental operations are open for discussion.

OTHER PERSONNEL

Within the personnel classifications of a pharmacy, in addition to pharmacists and technicians, are other categories of employees. These include such positions as secretary, clerk, aide, stock clerk, machine operator, and other similar titles. If the employer provides continuing education as a benefit of employment for pharmacists and technicians, then this benefit also should be considered for all employees. Therefore, an educational program of general but related interest is prepared and presented monthly. These general staff meetings are open to all personnel classifications in the pharmacy.

General Staff Meeting. Once a month, a topic of broad educational value to the entire staff, both professional and supportive, is presented. These meetings may include presentations by representatives of the State Health Department, Alcoholics Anonymous, another hospital department, etc. The general staff meetings are valuable for their educational content and the feeling of "family" they foster in the department.

CONCLUSION

Continuing education is a responsibility of all personnel who are responsible for some component of the health care delivery system. The late Dr. George Urdang said, "It is through education that the professions originated, and it is through programs in education that what we call 'professional progress' comes about." The pharmacist has an obligation to the public to maintain a high level of competence, and the employer has a parallel obligation to provide support.

REFERENCES

1. Pellegrino ED: Continuing education in the health professions. *Am J Pharm Educ* 33:712, 1969.
2. Jeffrey LP, Gallina JN: Pharmacist standard for maintaining professional competence. *Am J Hosp Pharm* 31:943-946, 1974.
3. Griffenhagen GB (ed): Whoso neglects learning. *J Am Pharm Assoc* 5:415, 1965.
4. Mahoney CD: Management's commitment to continuing education. *Curr Concepts Hosp Pharm Mgt* 1:4-12, 1978.
5. American Society of Hospital Pharmacists: Statement on continuing education. *Am J Hosp Pharm* 35:815-816, 1978.
6. *Accreditation Manual for Hospitals 1983.* Chicago, Joint Commission on Accreditation of Hospitals, 1983.
7. Mahoney CD, Gallina JN, Jeffrey LP: A comprehensive program to increase job satisfaction among pharmacy technicians. *Am J Hosp Pharm* 17:547-550, 1982.

ADDITIONAL READING

Anderson EL, Garrett EB, Lemaistre CA, et al: Continuing competence of pharmacists. *J Am Pharm Assoc* 15:432, 1975.
Grussing PG: Mandatory public relicensure examinations: Alternatives and recommendations. *Am J Pharm Educ* 43:244-249, 1979.
Jeffrey LP, Gallina JN, Mahoney CD, et al: The pharmacy troika: A participative approach to the development of professional competency standards. *Curr Concepts Hosp Pharm Mgt* 5:9-15, 1983.
Jeffrey LP, Mahoney CD: Continuing education for pharmacy staff in a large hospital. *Hosp Pharm* 10:56-58, 1975.
Lilly GN, Kirk KW: Adult education theory and its application to pharmacy continuing education. *Can Pharm J* 108:345, 1975.
Mergener MA, Weinsing MM: Motivations of pharmacists for participating in continuing education. *Am J Pharm Educ* 43:195-199, 1979.
Moore RL: Continuing education for the improvement of professional intervention in patient care. *Drug Intell Clin Pharm* 14:415-419, 1980.
Smith MA, Guerrant JM, Vogt DD: Assessment of continuing education needs for pharmacists. *Am J Pharm Educ* 45:139-148, 1981.
White AI: Report of the special tripartite committee on education. *Am J Pharm Educ* 35:467, 1971.

Appendix 56.1

STATES THAT REQUIRE PROFESSIONALS TO CONTINUE THEIR EDUCATION

	Nurses[a]	Physicians[b]	Pharmacists[c]		Nurses	Physicians	Pharmacists
Alabama			X	Nebraska	X		X
Alaska			X	Nevada	X		X
Arkansas			X	New Hampshire		X	X
Arizona		X	X	New Jersey			X
California	X	X	X	New Mexico	X	X	X
Colorado	X			New York			
Connecticut				North Carolina			
Delaware				North Dakota			
Florida	X		X	Ohio		X	X
Georgia				Oklahoma			X
Hawaii		X		Oregon			X
Idaho			X	Pennsylvania		X	
Illinois				Rhode Island		X	
Indiana			X	South Carolina			
Iowa	X	X	X	South Dakota	0		X
Kansas	X	X	X	Tennessee			X
Kentucky	X		X	Texas			
Louisiana	0		X	Utah		X	
Maine		X	X	Vermont			
Maryland		X		Virginia			
Massachusetts	X	X	X	Washington		X	X
Michigan		X	X	West Virginia			
Minnesota	X	X	X	Wisconsin		X	
Mississippi			X	Wyoming			X
Missouri							
Montana			X	TOTAL	11	18	30

X = states that require continuing education for relicensure; O = states in which required continuing education may be instituted at the discretion of the state professional association ("enabling legislation").
[a]Information on continuing education for nurses was obtained from the *American Journal of Nursing*, November 1982, pp 1668-1675.
[b]Information on continuing education for physicians was obtained from the American Medical Association.
[c]Information on continuing education for pharmacists was obtained from the National Association of Boards of Pharmacy.

CHAPTER 57

Patient Education and Compliance

TIM R. COVINGTON

The fundamental and ubiquitous problem of patient noncompliance continues to be significant in the management of disease processes in the ambulatory patient. Much time, effort, and money are expended in diagnosing and subsequently selecting the appropriate drug therapy (1,2). What occurs beyond this point is often left to chance with the consequence, in many instances, being either drug toxicity or therapeutic failure.

Some authors consider noncompliance to be the single most significant problem facing medical practice today (3,4). One reviewer states with discouragement that in an era where efficacious therapies exist or are being developed at a rapid rate, only approximately one half of the patients for whom an appropriate therapy is prescribed will receive full benefit through strict adherence to treatment.

The term "noncompliance" implies that the patient is solely responsible for the appropriate use of a prescribed regimen and is at fault when the medication is not properly consumed. In fact, the largest responsibility for ensuring that the patient complies rests with the physician and the pharmacist. To improve therapeutic compliance, health professionals must more fully appreciate the incidence, the clinical implications, and the variable causes of noncompliance. The purpose of this chapter is to explore these aspects of noncompliance and to suggest methods for improving patient compliance. Once these factors are put in the proper perspective, more vigorous and meaningful efforts can be used to combat this public health menace.

INCIDENCE OF NONCOMPLIANCE

Wide variations in the reported incidence of noncompliance appear in the literature. Estimates of noncompliance for short-term medication regimens have varied from 11-92% (1-27). This wide range may be the result of different criteria used to define noncompliance, use of different measuring instruments (e.g., dosage unit counts, interview, urine testing, serum analysis), and different demographic and pathologic factors in the various study populations.

Dramatic manifestations of noncompliance also have been demonstrated in chronically ill patients. Approximately 50% of patients with hypertension fail to follow referral advice, and over 50% drop out of care within 1 year. Only about two thirds of those who remain under care consume enough medication adequately to control their blood pressure (28).

A typical range of noncompliance in the ambulatory population at large is 25-50%. In an analysis of 12 studies that employed the dosage unit count method of determining compliance, the weighted mean revealed noncompliance of approximately 47% (6). A review of more than 50 compliance studies concluded that between one fourth and one half of all outpatients often failed to take prescribed medication (20). In addition to failing to take medication, patients might take medication for the wrong purpose, make errors in dosage or timing of dosage intervals, employ an improper technique of administration, and/or consume outdated medication. The therapeutic dilemma is complicated further because patients may take medications (legend and over-the-counter) not prescribed or recommended by the physician that are capable of interacting with other drugs, often with clinical consequences.

CLINICAL IMPLICATIONS OF NONCOMPLIANCE

Noncompliance with a prescribed regimen frequently produces adverse sequelae, the nature of the consequence depending on the type of error. In a study of 134 patients who received 380 prescriptions, it was determined that 118 (31%) of the prescriptions were being misused in a manner that posed a serious threat to the patient's health (13).

One of the more common errors of compliance is *underutilization* of a medication. The implications of underutilization of medications are obvious and account for a large number of therapeutic failures. Numerous studies document the incidence of underutilization of prescribed medication regimens (21-26). Many documenting underutilization of medications used for acute infectious diseases. Patients with chronic infections, such as tuberculosis, have on many occasions been classified as refractory to treatment with traditional drug therapy when relapses occurred. In a number of such cases the relapse caused by a failure to consume medications as prescribed (29,30).

The ultimate in underutilization occurs when patients fail to have prescriptions filled. Hammel and Williams (33) found that of 2000 prescriptions issued, 3% were not filled within 10 days. Boyd et al (14) found, in the analysis of compliance patterns of 134 socioeconomically deprived patients who received 380 prescriptions, that 24 (6.3%) were never filled.

Noncompliance that results in the *overutilization* of a medication presents an infinite number of obvious health hazards. In an analysis of the value of medication profiles to detect potential therapeutic problems, the overutilization of medications accounted for 65% of the potential problems identified (34). Overutilization of medications predisposes patients to dose-related adverse drug reactions. These situations often occur out of ignorance or misinformation. For example, many overzealous patients believe if one dose is good, two or more doses will be better, and will hasten a cure. Because most patients are unaware of the biopharmaceutics and pharmacokinetics of medications, they may double the dose at the next dosing interval if the prior dose was omitted.

Although the most common errors of compliance are overutilization, underutilization, and administering medications at inappropriate time intervals, other compliance errors have clinical implications. These include an improper technique of administration, using a medication for the wrong purpose, and consuming outdated medication. To maximize absorption, it is essential that appropriate techniques of administration be employed. This is not as critical with most oral dosage forms as with ophthalmics, otics, and suppositories (vaginal, rectal). Additionally, many patients may self-diagnose and use prescription medication to treat symptoms perceived to be similar to those for which the prescription was originally issued. If a drug is to be used to treat similar symptoms, at a later date, it should have been properly stored and not aged to the point of degradation to inactive or toxic constituents.

REASONS FOR NONCOMPLIANCE TO PRESCRIBED REGIMEN

The correlation between noncompliance and a number of variables has been tested; significant relationships appear to exist between noncompliance and advancing age, duration of therapy, number of drugs in the regimen, frequency of administration, drug-induced adverse effects, relief of symptoms, fear of drug dependancy, unpalatable dosage form, absence of a viable patient-physician relationship, excessive waiting to see the physician or pharmacist, nature of the illness (e.g., psychiatric disorders), and cost of the medication (2,3,6,12-14,19,31-38). A thorough discussion of the details of these relationships is beyond the scope of this chapter.

The most important aspects of therapeutic compliance appear to be the complexity of the regimen, and the understanding by patients of the nature of their illness, the importance of therapy, and the instructions for use (2,20). Time spent explaining these issues pays multiple dividends.

Compliance is generally reduced when the drug regimen is complex. In an evaluation of patients with diabetes or congestive heart failure, errors of compliance were less than 15% when only one drug was prescribed. When two or three drugs were prescribed, the noncompliance rate increased to 25% and exceeded 35% when five or more drugs were taken (39). Some pharmaceutical manufacturers have moved toward simplifying regimens by producing drug combinations, longer acting drugs, and a regimen requiring less frequent dosing. Such activity is to be encouraged if therapeutic outcomes are not compromised in the name of convenience and simplicity.

Evidence of patient failure to comprehend the importance of medications, directions for use, and potential consequences if the medication is not used according to instructions, is found often in the literature (40). Hermann (41) suggested that ambulatory patients lacked expertise in establishing an appropriate schedule for medications to be administered bid, tid, or qid. Approximately 15% of the patients were unable to interpret the implied schedule, and the interpretation of 33.3% of the directions varied greatly among patients. For example, the misinterpretation of a prescription for furosemide with the instruction, "Take one tablet as needed for fluid retention," may lead to the belief that the drug would cause one to retain fluid. The warning "force fluids" on prescriptions for sulfonamides may be interpreted as an order to "strain during urination" by some patients.

In a study by Mazzullo et al (42), 67 patients were asked to interpret instructions on each of ten prescription labels, and in no case was a label uniformly interpreted by all patients. The frequency of interpretive error ranged from 9-64%. In a study by Schwartz et al (43), it was revealed that 43 of 105 patients who made errors with regard to medications did not comprehend the general purpose of the medication, and 22 of the 43 patients had inaccurate knowledge about their drugs that could have dangerous consequences.

Obviously, it is not always enough to provide written and/or verbal instructions. Validation of patient understanding is essential. Pratt et al (44) found that physicians overestimate the level of medical knowledge of patients, and patients generally make no aggressive demand for more information. If misunderstanding occurs when explicit written and/or verbal instructions are provided, one must wonder how patients cope with "as directed" or "when needed" as a component of the written instructions.

To determine the frequency with which "as directed" was used as the only instruction on prescription labels and "when needed" was employed as all or part of the label instructions, 400 consecutive prescriptions from 50 community pharmacies in Oklahoma City were monitored. "As directed" was recorded most frequently as the sole instruction to the patient on prescription for topicals (14.3%) and vaginal preparations (14.24%).

Topicals are complex formulations; proper administration can do much to enhance the bioavailability of the active ingredients, whether steroids, nitroglycerin, or anti-infectives. The assumption that the patient knows how to apply vaginal preparations properly is certainly not without risk, as reflected by the female who consumed phenylmercuric acetate douche liquid orally on receiving "as directed" instructions on the prescription label. Certainly ophthalmics and otics require special instructions for application to maximize the absorption of the therapeutic agent(s).

There is considerable room for misinterpreting the proper technique for administering oral dosage forms. In one particular case, a teaspoonful of ampicillin oral suspension was instilled into a child's aching ear by a well-intentioned mother who received inadequate instructions for administering the drug.

Powell et al (45) found that of 115 "as directed" prescriptions without auxiliary instructions, there were 44 instances where the patient gave a different interpretation of the direction from that intended by the physician. Even the interpretation of detailed written instructions presents a significant problem (41). It appears inappropriate to presume that patients will be able to recall what was intended by "as directed." Proper use of potent legend drugs should not be left to chance.

"When needed" was frequently encountered as a component on the prescription label in the Oklahoma City Study. This is alarming because the instruction to use a drug "when needed" encourages self-assessment, self-diagnosis, and the abuse of potent legend drugs. Few patients are capable of assessing their clinical situation and subsequent therapeutic needs accurately and objectively. This situation is further complicated because in many instances all of the dosage units prescribed for a given illness may not be taken. If patients experience similar symptoms after a period of weeks, months, or even years, they may go to the medicine cabinet and conclude that "when needed" gives them license to use the medication for a condition that may be totally unrelated to the condition for which the medication was initially prescribed.

ROLE OF THE PHARMACIST IN PATIENT EDUCATION

Stewart and Cluff (1) have suggested that in our society better instructions are provided for the proper use and maintenance of a new camera or automobile than when patients receive medications with the potential to cause illness and even death if not properly consumed. The successful management of ambulatory, self-medicating patients requires greater effort by the health care team, particularly the pharmacist, in ensuring therapeutic compliance.

That pharmacists may more effectively educate patients with regard to the importance of their drug therapy, we must communicate, both verbally and in writing. Counseling patients regarding the safe and appropriate use of legend and nonprescription drugs is one of our greatest professional responsibilities. We have a professional and moral obligation to share our knowledge with the patient. Failure to voluntarily communicate therapeutic information deprives the public of a vital health service and results in a narrow view of the pharmacist by the public. Additionally, with pharmacies across the country implementing patient education and counseling services, the service is evolving as a "standard of practice." Failure to provide information to patients concerning the safe and appropriate use of their medication regimen leaves the pharmacist open to lawsuits, alleging negligence or breach of contract, if damage and/or direct cause can be proved.

A good start towards enhancing compliance can be made by basing instructions on these points: patients remember best the first instructions presented; instructions that are emphasized are better recalled; and the fewer the instructions given the greater will be the proportion remembered (3).

Essential elements of information that might be provided to patients (or their representative or guardian) for each medication in the therapeutic regimen are enumerated in the American Society of Hospital Pharmacist's Statement on Pharmacist-Conducted Patient Counseling. These elements include:

1. Name (trademark, generic, common synonym or other descriptive name[s])
2. Intended use and expected action
3. Route, dosage form, dosage, and administration schedule
4. Special directions for preparation
5. Special directions for administration
6. Precautions to be observed during administration
7. Common side effects that may be encountered, including their avoidance and action required if they occur
8. Techniques for self-monitoring the drug therapy
9. Proper storage
10. Potential drug-drug or drug-food interactions or other therapeutic contraindications
11. Prescription refill information
12. Action to take in the event of a missed dose
13. Any other information peculiar to the specific patient or drug

The pharmacist, in cooperation with other members of the health care team, can determine what specific information listed above is appropriate, to maximize compliance and therapeutic success. The prescription label should be comprehensive and should be reinforced by verbal instructions.

When health professionals verbally instruct patients, they should recognize the distinction between "providing information" and "educating." Instructions must be communicated on a level the patient can comprehend, and questions and comments from the patient should be encouraged so that an assessment of comprehension can be made.

Considering therapeutic failures, the economic consequences of hospitalization, missed workdays because of illness, and increased numbers of prescriptions needed to treat the complications of noncompliance, one must conclude that it is better to avoid the problem of poor compliance than to treat its consequences. Compliance appears to be primarily dependent on comprehension and recall in instructions. Fundamental to an understanding of proper medication use are appropriately written and labeled prescriptions with verbal and written auxiliary instructions supplemented by counseling.

CONCLUSION

Because inadequate comprehension and incomplete recollection of prescription instructions by patients is often a common denominator in drug defaulting, health practitioners should be aware of the means to maximize compliance. Verbal counseling, auxiliary written instructions, and the prescription label are most likely to have the greatest influence on comprehension and recall. Instructions for proper use should not be restricted to fit the dimensions of a prescription label. Rather, supplemental labeling should be affixed to the container. A detailed prescription label may have a strong influence on comprehension and memory. In studies conducted to compare the effects of various educational media, subjects were found to retain only 10% of the information provided solely by verbal communication, compared to 20% by visual means. When information was presented by both visual and verbal means, the 3-day recall level was 65% (6). A complete prescription label, in addition to appropriate verbal counseling by the physician or pharmacist, is an important factor in improving recall and compliance.

REFERENCES

1. Stewart RB, Cluff LE: Commentary: A review of medication errors and compliance in ambulant patients. *Clin Pharmacol Ther* 13:463-468, 1972.
2. Blackwell B: Patient compliance. *N Engl J Med* 289:249-252, 1973.
3. Haynes RB: Introduction. In Haynes RB, Taylor DW, Sackett DL (eds): *Compliance in Health Care.* Baltimore, Johns Hopkins University Press, 1979, pp 1-7.
4. Dunbar JM, Stunkard AJ: Adherence to diet and drug regimen. In Levy R et al: *Nutrition Lipids and Coronary Heart Disease.* New York, Raven Press, 1979, pp 391-423.
5. Haynes RB: A critical review of the "determinants" of patient compliance with therapeutic regimens. In Sackett DL, Haynes RB, (eds): *Compliance with Therapeutic Regimens.* Baltimore, Johns Hopkins University Press, 1976, pp 26-39.
6. Boyd JR et al: Drug defaulting—Part I: Determinants of compliance. *Am J Hosp Pharm* 31:362-367, 1974.
7. Clinite JC, Kabat HF: Errors during self-administration. *J Am Pharm Assoc* NS9:450-452, 1969.
8. Leistyna JA, Macaulay HJC: Therapy of streptococcal infections. Do pediatric patients receive prescribed oral medications? *Am J Dis Child* 111:22-26, 1966.
9. Maddock RK: Patient cooperation in taking medicines. *JAMA* 199:137-140, 1967.
10. Marrow R, Rabin DL: Reliability in self-medication with isoniazid. *Clin Res* 14:362, 1966.
11. Latiolais CJ, Berry CC: Misuse of prescription medications by outpatients. *Drug Intell Clin Pharm* 3:270-277, 1969.
12. Rickels K, Briscoe E: Assessment of dosage deviation in outpatient drug research. *J Clin Pharmacol* 11:153-160, 1970.
13. Malahy B: The effects of instruction and labeling on the number of medication errors made by patients at home. *Am J Hosp Pharm* 23:283-292, 1966.
14. Boyd JR et al: Drug defaulting—part II: Analysis of noncompliance patterns. *Am J Hosp Pharm* 31:485-491, 1974.
15. Geersten HR et al: Patient non-compliance within the context of medical care for arthritis. *J Chronic Dis* 26:689-698, 1973.
16. Weintraub M et al: Compliance as a determinant of serum digoxin concentration. *JAMA* 224:481-485, 1973.
17. Sheiner LB et al: Differences in serum digoxin concentrations between outpatients and inpatients: An effect of compliance? *Clin Pharmacol Ther* 15:239-246, 1974.
18. Brook RH et al: Effectiveness of inpatient follow-up care. *N Engl J Med* 285:1509-1514, 1971.
19. Hare EH, Wilcox DC: Do psychiatric inpatients take their pills? *Br J Psychiatry* 113:1435-1439, 1967.
20. Hussar DA: Patient noncompliance. *J Am Pharm Assoc* NS15:183-190, 201, 1975.
21. Blackwell B: The drug defaulter. *Clin Pharmacol Ther* 13:841-848, 1972.
22. Willcox DR et al: Do psychiatric outpatients take their drugs? *Br Med J* 2:790, 1965.
23. Joyce CRB: Patient cooperation and the sensitivity of clinical trials. *J Chronic Dis* 15:1025, 1962.
24. Colcher ES: Penicillin treatment of streptococcal pharyngitis. *JAMA* 222:657, 1972.
25. Charney E et al: How well do patients take oral penicillin?: A collaborative study. *Pediatrics* 40:188, 1967.
26. Green JL et al: Recurrence rate of streptococcal pharyngitis related to oral penicillin. *J Pediatr* 75:292, 1969.
27. Bergman AB, Werner RJ: Failure of children to receive penicillin by mouth. *N Engl J Med* 268:1334-1338, 1963.
28. Rudd T et al: Hypertension continuation adherence—natural history and role as an indicator condition. *Arch Intern Med* 39:545-549, 1979.
29. Moulding T et al: Supervision of outpatient drug therapy with the medication monitor. *Ann Intern Med* 73:559, 1970.
30. Preston DF, Miller FL: The tuberculosis outpatients' defection from therapy. *Am J Med Sci* 247:21-25, 1964.
31. Fox W: The problem of self-administration of drugs with particular reference to pulmonary tuberculosis. *Tubercle* 39:269, 1958.
32. Pfeiffer FG et al: Analysis of the pharmacist's role in improving therapeutic compliance in ambulatory hypertensive outpatients. Thesis, University of Oklahoma, May 1975.
33. Hammel RW Williams PO: Do patients receive prescribed medication? *J Am Pharm Assoc* NS4:331-334, 1964.
34. Solomon DK et al: Use of medication profiles to detect potential therapeutic problems in ambulatory patients. *Am J Hosp Pharm* 31:348, 1974.
35. Mazzullo JM, Lasagna L: Take thou. . . . *Drug Ther* 2:11, 1972.
36. Ayd FJ Jr: Once-a-day neuroleptic and tricyclic antidepressant therapy. *Int Drug Ther Newsletter* 7:33, 1972.
37. Marshal EJ: Why patients do not take their medications. *Am J Psychiatry* 128:656, 1971.
38. Francis V et al: Gaps in doctor-patient communication. *N Engl J Med* 80:534-540, 1969.
39. Hulka BS et al: Medication use and misuse: Physician-patient discrepancies. *J Chronic Dis* 28:7-21, 1975.
40. Davis MS, Eichhorn RL: Compliance with medical regimens: Panel study. *J Health Hum Behav* 4:240-249, 1963.
41. Hermann F: The outpatient prescription label as a source of medication errors. *Am J Hosp Pharm* 30:155-159, 1973.
42. Mazzullo JM et al: Variations in interpretation of prescription instructions. *JAMA* 227:929, 1974.
43. Schwartz D, et al: Medication errors made by elderly, chronically ill patients. *Am J Public Health* 52:2018-2029, 1962.
44. Pratt L et al: Physicians views on the level of medical information among patients. *Am J Public Health* 47:1277-1283, 1957.
45. Powell RJ, Cali TJ, Linkewich A: Inadequately written prescriptions, "as directed" prescriptions analyzed. *JAMA* 226:999, 1973.

CHAPTER 58

Hospital Pharmacy
Residency Programs

HERMAN LAZARUS

A pharmacy residency is an organized, directed, post-graduate program of training in some area of pharmacy practice.* Each of these adjectives bears some comment.

Organized. A residency program is planned in advance with specific outcome objectives in mind, and structured in such a way that those objectives may be attained. Pharmacy residencies commonly consist of several discrete blocks of training, or rotations, each devoted to one particular aspect of practice. Further, a residency is structured in such a way that all the outcome objectives can be accomplished within the allotted time for the program. (The minimum length of a pharmacy residency is 12 months, fulltime.)

Directed. Director of Pharmacy Services in the institution in which the residency is conducted is the director of the residency program. He or she is responsible for establishing overall program goals, specific learning objectives, training schedules, adequate preceptorship, and resident evaluation.

Postgraduate. A pharmacy residency occurs subsequent to graduation from pharmacy school (i.e., following completion of an entry level for pharmacy practice).

It is important to distinguish between a residency and other types of professional practice education and training. A residency may be distinguished from externships and clerkships in that these two experiences are associated with degree requirements and typically represent the student's initial exposure to various professional practice settings. Although these experiences are designed to demonstrate the principles of pharmacy practice, they do not provide opportunities for independent judgment by the student. A residency, by contrast, is a program in which one learns to practice; it provides opportunities for a graduate pharmacist to build on his or her undergraduate clerkships and internships.

A residency differs from an internship in that an internship is a training program meeting the requirements established by boards of pharmacy for licensure. The amount of internship training required subsequent to graduation varies considerably from state to state. A residency program, on the other hand, seeks to develop skills and knowledge far

beyond that required for licensure. As noted earlier, a residency is a minimum 12-month program.

Finally, a residency may be distinguished from a fellowship in that residencies exist primarily to teach one how to practice, whereas fellowships concentrate on clinical research.

ORIGIN AND EVOLUTION OF PHARMACY RESIDENCIES

Hospital pharmacy as a distinct form of practice began to take shape in the 1930s, paralleling the growth of the hospital industry in general. The history of this development lies outside the scope of this chapter; however, by the end of the 1930s there was considerable interest in forming a national association of hospital pharmacists. The American Society of Hospital Pharmacists (ASHP) was finally established in 1942.

Pharmacy schools in that era concentrated almost exclusively on training community practitioners, and hospital pharmacy pioneers found that they had to establish their own postgraduate apprenticeship programs to prepare pharmacists for institutional practice. Several hospital pharmacy "internships" (this is the term that was used at that time) were established in various parts of the country before the formation of the ASHP. There were no standards for such training programs at that time, however, and the quality of these early internships must have varied greatly.

The need for standardized guidelines for training hospital pharmacists was identified early in the ASHP's existence, and the first set of standards was published in 1948 (1).

As the demand for qualified hospital pharmacy manpower grew, it became increasingly more apparent that a program of accreditation of hospital pharmacy internships was needed. The ASHP established such a program in 1962, predicated on the first accreditation standard for hospital pharmacy residency training. (This marked the first time the term "residency" was used in an official ASHP document, and this term was adopted to distinguish between an internship, which had come to be used in referring to the practical experience required for licensure, and the formal 12-month training program required in the new accreditation standard.) The hospital pharmacy residency accreditation

---

*Definition adopted by the Department of Accreditation Services of the American Society of Hospital Pharmacists.

program represented the first effort in American pharmacy practice to ensure, through external review, adherence to a minimum standard in postgraduate professional practice training programs.

Many believe that the development of residency programs has been one of the most important factors contributing to the dramatic growth in institutional pharmacy during the past 30 years. Residency preceptors, by and large, have aspired to train not merely technically competent practitioners, but also people with leadership potential. The ideal for residency training expressed by Latiolais (2) some years ago has influenced an entire generation of preceptors and residents:

There are essentially four phases through which a new resident graduate must progress before he becomes a knowledgeable hospital pharmacist . . .:

(1) The first phase revolves around gaining experience in basic practice situations. The pharmacist learns how to perform the basic functions of everyday practice in each division of the hospital pharmacy.
(2) The second phase revolves around gaining experience in learning how to coordinate the various functions and divisions within the hospital pharmacy so that a meaningful service can be provided.
(3) The third phase revolves around gaining experience in learning how to coordinate this total pharmacy service with the needs of the total institution.
(4) The fourth phase revolves around gaining experience in learning how to conceptualize his accumulated experiences and knowledge of practice and to transform these concepts into new and improved types of pharmaceutical services.

ACCREDITATION OF RESIDENCY PROGRAMS

Accreditation is the process by which an agency or organization evaluates and recognizes a program of study or an institution as meeting certain predetermined qualifications or standards. The accrediting body for residencies in institutional pharmacy practice is the ASHP. The ASHP's accreditation program has as its objectives the following: (1) to improve the professional competence of pharmacists practicing in institutional and related health care settings, or to prepare pharmacists for entry into these practice settings, through organized educational training programs; (2) to guide, assist, and recognize health care institutions and related organizations that wish to support the profession by operating such programs; (3) to provide criteria for the prospective resident in selecting a program by identifying those institutions or organizations conducting accredited residency programs; and (4) to provide prospective employers a basis for determining the level of competence of pharmacists in institutional practice by identifying those pharmacists who have successfully completed accredited residency programs.†

In 1980, the ASHP adopted a position paper "ASHP Position on Long-Range Pharmacy Manpower Needs and Residency Training" (3), which related the residency accreditation program to specific manpower needs in institu-

tional practice. Specific categories of manpower needs identified in this document are institutional pharmacy generalists, clinical practitioners, specialized practitioners, managers, and administrators. Accordingly, the ASHP has developed residency accreditation standards in clinical practice and several specialized areas of practice (e.g., ambulatory care, drug information, geriatrics, nuclear pharmacy, nutrition support, oncology, pediatrics, psychopharmacy), in addition to general hospital pharmacy practice (4-14).‡ It is expected that an accreditation standard for an advanced level residency in institutional pharmacy administration will soon be approved.

The Commission on Credentialing

The body within the ASHP structure responsible for administering its accreditation program is the Commission on Credentialing. The Commission comprises eight practitioners who are directors of accredited residency programs, two public members, and a staff secretary (the ASHP's Director of Accreditation Services). Its charges are to develop accreditation standards for institutional pharmacy training programs and to carry out a program of accreditation based on those standards. The Commission meets twice a year; its agenda typically includes considering new accreditation application, reviewing programs for reaccreditation, and reviewing interim progress reports from residency directors, among other items.

Members of the Commission typically serve, along with a member of the staff of the ASHP Department of Accreditation Services, on accreditation site visit teams. Each commissioner presents reports on programs he or she has surveyed at the next Commission meeting following the survey. That surveyor's recommendation is then considered by the full Commission. Commission members are appointed by the ASHP president; the normal term of appointment is 3 years.

Applying for Accreditation. The procedures for making an application for the accreditation of a pharmacy residency training program are given in the ASHP document, "ASHP Regulations on Accreditation of Pharmacy Residencies" (15). The application may be submitted any time after the first resident has started the training program. After all application materials have been received by the ASHP, arrangements are made with the institution for a site evaluation by the accreditation survey team. Because survey visits are scheduled in the order of receipt of completed applications, there may be a delay of as long as 6 months or more before the site visit can be scheduled.

The Accreditation Survey. A typical accreditation site visit is completed in 2 days and includes interviews with designated individuals (e.g., hospital director, chairman of the Pharmacy and Therapeutics Committee and other members of the medical staff, the director of nursing service, the director of pharmacy services, and members of the pharmacy staff, including the residents). There is also an intensive review of the documentation of the pharmacy service

---

†These objectives paraphrase those set forth in the former ASHP Statement on Accreditation of Pharmacy Residencies, but they have been broadened here to reflect more recent interpretations by the ASHP.

‡The reader who is interested in other related positions of the ASHP should refer to the position paper already cited (3).

and the residency program and of the institution's facilities, with primary emphasis on the pharmacy department and the areas it serves. The survey is conducted by a two-member team, as described above.

The purpose of the site evaluation is to determine the degree of compliance with the requirements of the appropriate accreditation standard. The evaluation is conducted in the spirit of offering recommendations and advice for meeting the requirements of the accreditation standard and not primarily to criticize existing shortcomings or deficiencies.

The Accreditation Survey Report. Following the site evaluation the survey team prepares a report summarizing its findings, listing significant deficiencies, and offering specific recommendations for correcting deficiencies and for improving pharmacy services and the residency training program. The report is sent to the chief executive officer of the institution and to the director of pharmacy services for their review. They are invited to submit their written comments responding to any deficiencies listed in the report and to correct any factual errors. The report, along with comments submitted by the institution, are considered by the Commission on Credentialing when it acts on the accreditation application submitted by the hospital.

Reaccreditation and Interim Self-Audit. Accreditation is granted for a maximum period of 6 years; however, the Commission on Credentialing may request a site evaluation at any time if it becomes evident that there has been a major change in the residency training program. Each accredited residency is required to submit every 2 years a self-audit and status report on progress made in correcting deficiencies cited in the previous survey report. Each self-audit and status report is reviewed by the Commission on Credentialing, which then makes a determination on any required followup action, such as requesting additional documentation or an early site reevaluation.

SELECTING A RESIDENCY PROGRAM

Any pharmacist or pharmacy student interested in a career in institutional pharmacy practice should give serious consideration to residency training. Because of the formal structure and concentrated nature of the training in a pharmacy residency program, the resident should develop competence in a broader scope of pharmacy practice in a 1- or 2-year residency program than might be possible in several years as a staff pharmacist with a fixed assignment. Generally speaking, completing an accredited residency training program will greatly increase the employment opportunities for the individual; furthermore, residency preceptors will usually assist the resident in locating suitable employment on completing the training program.

Types of Residencies. Pharmacy residency programs may be categorized in two ways: by practice area and by academic affiliation status. With respect to practice area, there are three broad categories of accredited residencies: hospital pharmacy, clinical practice, and specialty practice; a fourth category, institutional pharmacy administration, will soon be added.

Hospital pharmacy residencies are designed to prepare a generalist in institutional pharmacy who can practice com-

fortably in a variety of settings or assignments, and who is sufficiently diversified that he or she can continually grow professionally. Clinical practice residencies are designed to prepare a pharmacist for an advanced level of clinical practice. These programs are predicated on completing pharmacy degree level clerkships and emphasize the development of independent decision-making abilities. Experiences are gained in providing clinical services to a wide range of patients. Specialty residencies concentrate on developing skills in some very specific area of practice, such as nuclear pharmacy, drug information, oncology, psychopharmacy, etc. These, too, for the most part require completing doctoral level clerkships as a foundation. Pharmacists completing such residencies should qualify to direct such service areas in most pharmacy departments.

The need for well-trained administrative pharmacists has led to the efforts now under way to develop an accreditation standard for an advanced level residency in institutional pharmacy administration. Such a program, it is envisioned, will prepare individuals who can move immediately into key administrative positions (assistant director level or higher) in institutional pharmacy departments.

Residency programs that are offered only in conjunction with an advanced degree (MS or PharmD) are referred to as academically affiliated residencies. These programs are taken concurrently with course work required for the degree, and the combined program typically requires 2 years to complete. The residency requires a minimum of 2000 hours. Approximately 15% of the currently accredited residency programs are academically affiliated.

Nonaffiliated residencies (i.e., those not associated with a degree program) require a full-time commitment for 1 year (a minimum of 2000 hours).

Entry Level Requirements. Residencies are postgraduate experiences, and therefore one fundamental requirement for admission to any residency is that the resident be a graduate pharmacist. Most hospital pharmacy residencies are open to baccalaureate graduates; however, some programs have additional entry requirements that must be met. Completing a PharmD degree is generally required for admission to clinical and specialty residencies. Information on specific entry requirements may be found in the annual *Residency Directory* published by the ASHP.

Residency Stipends. All accredited residency programs provide the resident with a stipend, although the amount varies from program to program, depending on such factors as number of actual training hours per year, the value of any fringe benefits provided, geographic location (cost of living), and related factors. Cash stipends generally are inadequate to cover living costs for a resident with significant family support responsibilities. Furthermore, a residency, whether affiliated or nonaffiliated, requires a full-time commitment on the part of the resident and usually does not permit supplementing income through part-time employment. For these reasons, applicants with family support obligations generally must have financial resources in addition to the residency stipend on which they can rely during the residency training period. The ASHP Residency Directory lists in the description of each program the annual stipend paid to the resident, as well as applicable fringe benefits and prerequisites.

Enrolling in the Resident Matching Program. In 1977 the ASHP initiated the Resident Matching Program. The purpose of the matching plan is to bring about a free and competitive but orderly choice between residency applicants and pharmacy residencies in hospitals and to avoid unwarranted competition between hospitals and undue pressures or coercion being exercised on residency applicants. The Resident Matching Program does not alter significantly, for either the applicant or the hospital, existing application, interview, and selection procedures, except for observing certain time deadlines for completing applications and submitting the required matching plan documents.

The ASHP Resident Matching Program is open to all qualified applicants and to all pharmacy residency training programs in hospitals accredited by the ASHP. To participate, applicants must sign a form contracting to accept any residency position listed by them to which they are matched. They are free to apply or accept positions at any other hospital if they are not matched by the announced deadline. Similarly, hospitals must agree to accept any candidate whose name they have submitted and ranked and who is matched with them by the deadline. A hospital must also agree not to appoint any applicants outside of the matching plan before the announced deadline. Both the applicant and the hospital are assessed a nominal fee for participation in the Resident Matching Program. On receipt by ASHP of the Applicant Agreement (contract) form and the required fee, a copy of the annual Residency Directory will be mailed to the applicant, along with an acknowledgment letter showing the applicant's assigned code number. This number identifies the applicant in all subsequent communications with residency programs and with the ASHP matching plan office.

Application for admission to an accredited residency is made directly to the hospital, not to the ASHP. The ASHP Residency Directory contains information on the procedures to be followed in applying for admission to accredited residencies.

Residency Showcase. Each year at the ASHP Midyear Clinical Meeting (conducted during the first full week of December), directors of accredited residency programs participate in an organized exhibit program that allows each to showcase his or her program and to meet potential applicants. The annual Residency Showcase is a unique opportunity for those interested in applying to residencies, in that they have access to most program directors all in one location.

The assistance of the staff of the American Society of Hospital Pharmacists in preparing this chapter is acknowledged.

REFERENCES

1. Standards for internships in hospital pharmacies. *Bull ASHP* 5:233-234, 1948.
2. Latiolais CJ: *Objectives for Hospital Pharmacy Residency Training.* Paper presented at the Second Special Conference on Hospital Pharmacy Residency Training, Columbus, OH, October 12-14, 1966.
3. ASHP position on long-range pharmacy manpower needs and residency training. *Am J Hosp Pharm* 37:1220, 1980.
4. ASHP accreditation standard for pharmacy residency in a hospital (with guide to interpretation). *Am J Hosp Pharm* 36:74-80, January 1979.
5. ASHP accreditation standard for residency training in clinical pharmacy (with guide to interpretation). *Am J Hosp Pharm* 37:1223-1228, 1980.
6. ASHP accreditation standard for specialized pharmacy residency training (with guide to interpretation). *Am J Hosp Pharm* 37:1229-1232, 1980.
7. ASHP supplemental standard and learning objectives for residency training in ambulatory-care pharmacy practice. *Am J Hosp Pharm* 39:1967-1969, 1982.
8. ASHP supplemental standard and learning objectives for residency training in drug information practice. *Am J Hosp Pharm* 39:1970-1972, 1982.
9. ASHP supplemental standard and learning objectives for residency training in geriatric pharmacy practice. *Am J Hosp Pharm* 39:1972-1974, 1982.
10. ASHP accreditation standard for residency training in nuclear pharmacy (with guide to interpretation). *Am J Hosp Pharm* 38:1964-1971, 1981.
11. ASHP supplemental standard and learning objectives for residency training in nutritional support pharmacy practice. *Am J Hosp Pharm* 38:1971-1973, 1981.
12. ASHP supplemental standard and learning objectives for residency training in oncology pharmacy practice. *Am J Hosp Pharm* 39:1214-1215, 1982.
13. ASHP supplemental standard for residency training in pediatric pharmacy practice. *Am J Hosp Pharm* 41:334-337, 1984.
14. ASHP supplemental standard and learning objectives for oncology residency training in psychiatric pharmacy practice. *Am J Hosp Pharm* 37:1232-1234, 1980.
15. ASHP regulations on accreditation of pharmacy residencies. *Am J Hosp Pharm* 37:1221-1223, 1980.

Appendix 58.1
POINTS TO CONSIDER IN SEEKING A RESIDENCY

The following self-assessment questions, interview tips, and other pointers were developed in cooperation with a Resident Advisory Committee of the ASHP Special Interest Group on Administrative Pharmacy Practice. We believe you will find them helpful in organizing your thoughts about residency programs.

1. *Why take a residency?*

   Can you make a clear statement about why you want to take a residency?

   Do you have specific career goals in mind that a residency will help you attain?

   Can you list several specific outcomes you would expect to achieve by taking a residency?

2. *What type of residency should you consider?*

   Hospital pharmacy residencies (the white pages in the Directory) provide training in the general practice of hospital pharmacy. Areas of training included are set forth in Standard V of the Accreditation Standard for Pharmacy Residency in a Hospital (a copy is included in the Directory). Hospital pharmacy residencies may emphasize some specific area of practice (e.g., administration, clinical practice); however, some training in each prescribed area must be included. Information about areas of emphasis is provided in each program listing.

   Some hospital pharmacy residencies are offered only in conjunction with an advanced degree (MS or PharmD), and these generally require 2 years for completion. Others are offered as 1-year programs, with no academic degree affiliation.

   Clinical pharmacy residencies (blue pages) and specialty residencies (yellow pages) concentrate heavily on the clinical elements of pharmacy practice, and are generally offered only as post-PharmD programs (exceptions can be made to this rule, however, depending on the applicant's background).

   The nature of a residency will be greatly influenced by various characteristics of the institution in which it is conducted: size (number of beds), responsibiluty for teaching (university hospital or nonuniversity hospital), ownership (state, federal, community, for-profit corporation, other), and types of medical services provided (general hospital vs specialty hospital).

   We encourage you to study all information in the Directory carefully before you begin scheduling interviews.

3. *Points to consider during the interview.*

   Most residency program directors look at interviews with prospective residents as a two-way process. You will be expected to ask questions, and should go prepared to do so. Please note that we have no predetermined "right" or "wrong" answers in mind for any of the following questions. We believe it is important, however, that the residency applicant understand clearly what the program director's expectations are and how demanding the program is. It will be up to you, once you have all the information, to decide if you are willing, or will be able, to meet the requirements of a given program.

The following questions may help you in planning for your interview visits:

   a. What level of service commitment is required of residents (i.e., hours of coverage in a staff pharmacist capacity)? Are there any other special duties residents are expected to perform?

   b. How much time does the residency require (average number of hours per week)?

   c. How accessible is the program director? Is there a scheduled meeting time between him/her and the resident?

   d. To what extent are other members of the staff involved in the resident's training?

   e. What opportunities for research does the program afford? (NOTE: All residency programs have a "research" or "special project" requirement. Some require the completion of one major project; others require several short-term projects. These experiences are aimed at developing the resident's problem-solving skills.)

   f. What opportunities does the resident have to visit other hospitals, attend professional meetings, etc? Is financial assistance provided for such activities?

   g. Is an advanced degree required? Are there other special requirements for admission? (This information is provided in the Directory, but you might wish to discuss such requirements with the program director during the interview, especially if you feel you have a level of experience that might qualify for a waiver of some specific requirement you do not meet.)

   h. Are residents expected to become licensed in the state in which the residency is conducted? If so, by what date?

   Most residency directors make provision for residency interviewees to meet with the current residents. If you find no such arrangements have been made, you might want to ask to be allowed to do so.

4. *Financial considerations.*

   Will you be able to live on the stipend provided by the residencies in which you are interested? In the case of residencies offered in conjunction with advanced degrees, does the resident receive a tuition waiver? (Note that the amount of stipend shown in the Directory may have been increased for next year. Information concerning other benefits and prerequisites is provided in the Directory.)

5. *Relocation.*

   Are you willing, and financially able, to move to the areas where the residencies you are interested in are located?

6. *Resident-preceptor relationship.*

   Nothing is more crucial to the success of a residency program than a good resident-preceptor relationship. You should be satisfied in your own mind that you can form a good, productive liaison with the preceptor of any program you may be considering. (The director of pharmacy is considered the major preceptor in most residency programs. In some cases, however, someone other than the director of pharmacy may be the individual to whom residents relate most closely on a day-to-day basis.) It

goes without saying that you will also be "sized up" during the interview in terms of how the preceptor feels about the prospect of a healthy resident-preceptor relationship with you.

Quality Assurance

DEVELOPMENT AND CONDUCT OF A QUALITY ASSURANCE PROGRAM FOR PHARMACEUTICAL SERVICES

A major responsibility of the department must be the assurance of the quality of its services and of products dispensed, coupled with a control program for the distribution of drugs throughout the institution.

The pharmacist must conduct service audits, either by process or outcome, or both, to assure the quality of patient care services rendered and to assure the appropriate patient benefit of all pharmaceutical services offered.

CHAPTER 59

The Pharmacy and Therapeutics Committee/Formulary System

CHARLES E. DANIELS

The Joint Commission on Accreditation of Hospitals (JCAH) accreditation manual notes (1):

> The development and surveillance of pharmacy and therapeutics policies and practices, particularly drug utilization within the hospital, shall be the responsibility of the medical staff and shall be carried out in cooperation with the pharmacist and with representatives of other disciplines as required.

One method to accomplish this function is through the use of an appropriate medical staff committee. This committee is the Pharmacy and Therapeutics (P&T) Committee.

The P&T Committee is a key organizational component for institutional pharmacists. It is important for the pharmacist to have a full understanding of the P&T Committee role and function within institutions in general and specifically within the organization where he or she practices. The intent of this chapter is to discuss the committee organization and operation as well as a number of special topics and issues. The formulary system will receive special consideration as a major charge of the committee.

The P&T Committee serves as an advisory group to the medical staff. It represents a formalized organizational line of communication between the pharmacy department and the medical staff. Its charge is to recommend policy to the medical staff and hospital administration regarding the therapeutic use of drugs and related matters (2). These recommendations must then be acted on by the larger medical staff governing body to become policy. The use of a P&T Committee is one option provided for by JCAH to meet their standards and is endorsed by the American Society of Hospital Pharmacists (ASHP).

COMMITTEE STRUCTURE

The P&T Committee is appointed by the medical staff. This is usually done in conjunction with other medical staff committee appointments on an annual basis. It is wise for the pharmacy department head to determine when the medical staff appointment cycle begins so it is possible to plan for changes.

Membership

There are differing opinions regarding optimal size and composition of the committee (3,4). Group dynamics studies suggest that smaller committees may be more productive; conversely, larger committees have potential for greater staff representation. This may be valuable in hospitals with large medical staffs or several specialties with differing needs, perspectives, and expertise. Furthermore, the workload demand on a given committee member will be less if the committee is large. The significance of this workload distribution will be discussed later. The important consideration is that the medical staff members must be representative and interested in the committee activity. The committee obtains its power from the medical staff ranks and will function best if perceived to be a tool of that body. It is necessary to incorporate representatives from major medical services at the minimum.

JCAH standards incorporate participation by nursing, hospital administration, and pharmacy services (1). The question of voting status of nonmedical staff members is not generally agreed on; however, the key is for each of these groups to have an adequate influence in the committee decision-making process.

Committee Chair

As the "formal" group leader, the chairperson is in a position to exert significant influence on group activities and direction. It is generally recognized that the committee chair should be a full medical staff member. This is consistent with the medical staff power base of the committee. The chairperson should have respect as a strong clinician and should also understand the administrative and political workings of the institution. Selection of a P&T Committee chairperson may occur in a number of ways. In some cases, the chair may be automatically associated with some other function (e.g., chief of internal medicine); alternatively, a medical staff election may be used to select the chair. In most cases, however, the chair is appointed by the president or chief of the medical staff (5).

Committee Secretary

The secretary of the committee is usually a pharmacist. Based on the key nature of this role, the director of pharmacy commonly takes this responsibility. Tasks of the secretary include administrative activities as well as providing advice to the committee regarding issues and background where necessary. This usually requires scheduling meetings, taking minutes, preparing agenda packets, and assisting the chairperson in implementation of committee decisions. In most cases, the pharmacist who serves as secretary to the P&T Committee should plan to function as the coordinator of day-to-day committee activities.

Committee Meetings

The P&T Committee should meet frequently enough to conduct regular business. This may mean quarterly, as recommended by JCAH, but more frequent meetings will be required in most cases. The ASHP recommends at least six meetings per year. Frequent meetings allow enough time to handle housekeeping tasks as well as address policy-related issues. The "issue" related activities are more likely to encourage the committee members to become interested. They also tend to make the committee more valuable to the hospital.

Agenda

The chairperson and secretary are responsible for assessment of the committee work to be accomplished. They must also determine the time frame for completion of the work. The decisions are translated into work orders through development of the meeting agenda. Agenda setting can be a routine and technical function. Conversely, meetings of an effective P&T Committee should be well planned and organized to avoid wasted time. This requires work on the part of both the chairperson and secretary. The secretary should file all old and new business items in a specific committee agenda file. In advance of the committee meeting, the chairperson and secretary should confer to plan the meeting and set the agenda. At this agenda meeting, all of the items that are pending should be reviewed. If the item will be addressed at the upcoming meeting, its place on the agenda should be determined. The chairperson and secretary must also understand the reason that each item is added to the agenda. For example, is the item for information, for action, or for some other reason? At the end of the agenda planning meeting, the secretary should be prepared to create the agenda packet for the committee members. In many cases, the sequence of full committee activities will remain similar from meeting to meeting. This makes planning the agenda easier and may be of value to participants of the full committee meeting.

The agenda packet should include the schedule of business (Appendix 59.1) and any supporting documents for business to be conducted, including a copy of minutes from the previous meeting when appropriate. The packet should be sent to members of the committee early enough to allow them to review the supporting documents. One week in advance of the meeting represents a reasonable goal for packet distribution.

Meeting Minutes

It is important to maintain accurate records of committee activities for practical and technical reasons. Responsibility for these records is usually that of the committee secretary. The records should be built around the minutes of committee meetings. The style and content of minutes may vary by location. It is important that the minutes are an accurate reflection of the content and tone of the meeting and that key elements of any discussion are included in summary form. Appendix 59.2 is one format for meeting minutes but is not necessarily the only one.

Meeting minutes should always be included in the agenda packet and approved by the committee at the next meeting. Approved meeting minutes should be forwarded to the appropriate medical staff governing body and kept on file by the secretary. The method for record storage should allow easy access for future needs. The records should be accessible by month and year. The use of a loose-leaf binder is one recommended method for record maintenance. A separate binder for each year, with monthly dividers, makes it easy to gain access to all necessary records.

Attendance

Well-attended meetings are essential to effectively complete business. A committee with consistently poor attendance cannot adequately deal with important issues on behalf of the entire medical staff. In order to ensure regular good attendance at committee meetings, several points should be considered:

1. Meetings should be regularly scheduled far in advance. This allows members to work around these meetings in their scheduling procedures.
2. Meetings should be scheduled for a time that is convenient for most committee members (i.e., early morning or during lunch).
3. Meetings should be interesting enough to encourage attendance. This includes providing a meeting environment where participation is encouraged.
4. Committee work must be viewed as important by members, and committee recommendations must be implemented by the medical staff government and department of pharmaceutical services.

Poor meeting attendance is usually due to failure to address one of the above points. Chronic nonattendance should be investigated and corrected in an appropriate manner.

FORMULARY SYSTEM

One of the major responsibilities of the P&T Committee is the development and maintenance of the institutional formulary. The formulary is "a continually revised compilation of pharmaceuticals . . . that reflects the current clinical judgement of the medical staff" (6). The formulary is intended to aid the medical staff in improving quality and controlling prescribing costs. This is done through the creation of a formulary system. The formulary system is a method for evaluation, appraisal, and selection of drug products that are of most value in routine patient care at a particular institution. In short, the formulary is the document.

The formulary system is the way in which the document is developed.

The printed formulary is a document that must effectively convey the wishes and judgment of the P&T Committee. It is also the visible result of a major P&T Committee work component. It is a document that will be used by multiple work groups, for multiple purposes and must therefore be organized for clarity. It is recommended that the formulary include a list of approved products with basic therapeutic information on each. It also should contain information on P&T Committee and hospital drug use policies along with other types of special information regarding drugs or dosing (7).

The format for listing drug names in a formulary is a reflection of P&T Committee–endorsed hospital policy. Generic names should be used when possible; this endorses the interchangeable nature of generic equivalent products. Cross references from brand names to generic equivalents are likely to make the formulary more useful. Use of a listing of approved products by therapeutic class endorses the concept of rational product selection and may be a reasonable place to include relative price considerations. More detailed suggestions on document format can be found in the ASHP Technical Assistance Bulletin on Hospital Formularies (7). A number of authors have discussed the relationships between formulary style, usability, and effectiveness (8,9). It is often assumed that a pocket-sized formulary will be more convenient to carry and use, thus increasing its effectiveness. It is essential that the formulary be updated often enough to accurately reflect current formulary contents. The formulary should be available on all nursing stations and in other places where drug orders are likely to be written (1). It is customary to place a more comprehensive drug information source, such as the *American Hospital Formulary Service,* in the permanent formulary locations. This serves the basic drug information needs that may come up during the use of the hospital formulary.

In order to perform necessary formulary maintenance, several procedures must be standardized and codified. These include procedures for addition and deletion of drugs and periodic review of the entire formulary and nonformulary drug use.

Formulary Additions

As new products are introduced and new uses are found for currently marketed products, it is necessary to consider the needs for these products to be added to the institution's formulary. Clearly defined policies and procedures for the addition of products will make the process simple and standard. Requests for addition of new products should come from the medical or pharmacy staff who are likely to use it. Requests from other hospital personnel (i.e., nursing, respiratory therapy) should be referred to a physician or pharmacist practicing in that area for consideration and request.

The request should be formalized. This may be accomplished through the use of a letter, official formulary request form (Appendix 59.3), or some other variation of that concept. Regardless, there should be a permanent record of who made the request and when it was made. This should become a permanent part of the P&T Committee records. If there are questions regarding the request, it is the responsibility of the committee secretary to ensure that they are resolved before the committee can take action. All legitimate requests should be scheduled for the agenda of the earliest practical committee meeting. Supporting documentation should be required for each request for addition to the formulary. This documentation may be required of the requester or prepared by the pharmacy department and should serve as the basis of discussion. P&T Committee members with expertise in the specific therapeutic category or the requester should provide information to supplement the available documentation.

It may be desirable to review new product requests in light of products already on the formulary and products that are expected to be available in the near future. New products should be added for a probationary period (e.g., 6 months). At the end of the probation, the committee should review relative aspects of the drug and its use during the probationary period. Products that are deemed by the Committee to be valuable should become permanent additions; all other items should be removed from the formulary at that time.

There may be instances where unique product characteristics such as cost, side effects, or potency make it necessary to look at formulary addition as a special item. These special items may be placed on the formulary but restricted to prescribers with a special expertise to ensure that they are used correctly. Typical examples of this approach are found in restriction of certain antibiotics (10-12).

Deletions

Requests for formulary addition are usually received on a regular basis. Deletions are usually a less automatic process and must be programmed. In order to maintain a trim and useful formulary, it is necessary to delete products that are no longer seen as necessary. There are three basic reasons why a drug should be removed from the formulary: (1) it is no longer available from the manufacturer, (2) it is no longer being used, and (3) it should no longer be used. The first two reasons are fairly obvious and noncontroversial. If an item is no longer available or no longer being used, simple housekeeping activities should be done to remove it and help prevent confusion; i.e., the name of the product(s) should be removed from the formulary listing. This may allow the hospital to return unused deleted products to the manufacturer for credit and have a reduced on-hand inventory.

The third reason for deletion is the most difficult and controversial. It is not always clear when a product that is still being used on a regular basis should be deleted from the formulary. Suggestions for possible deletions may be solicited from requesters of formulary additions. They should be considered at the end of the probationary period for a new addition. If a new drug is added to the formulary, strong consideration should be given to the drug or drugs it may replace. If it is beneficial or cost effective to delete some products, this should be done. Drug deletion should also be a prime objective when formularies are reviewed.

Formulary Review

In addition to month-to-month additions and deletions, it is necessary to perform periodic reviews of all products in each therapeutic category. This may be accomplished in several ways but always relies on the comparison of products currently on the formulary to those that should be on it. The review should evaluate drugs based on their relative therapeutic merit, safety, and cost. Total formulary review is a major time-consuming effort. The work should be divided among all committee members and should be certain to utilize other medical and pharmacy staff members with expertise or interest in a specific area of therapeutics (13). The use of subcommittees or task forces for given groups may be valuable. Each task force may be chaired by a committee member with other interested people involved as members of the group. Specific timetables should be developed to place clear expectations on the task force and avoid having several reports completed at one time. Task force reports and recommendations should be formalized in writing. The task force should also consider the educational needs of prescribers for the drug class being reviewed and incorporate any conclusions in their report.

Nonformulary Drugs

There will always be a need for limited use of drugs that are not on the formulary. These nonformulary items are usually one-time or special items. Requests for nonformulary items may be processed in several ways (14). Before they are processed for use, an attempt should be made by the pharmacist to investigate possible use of a formulary alternative. When the need arises to use a drug product that is not on the formulary and therefore not held in inventory, a supply that is sufficient to complete a course of therapy for that particular patient should be obtained. The product should be charged to the patient and labeled for specific use by him or her. Periodic review of nonformulary drug use patterns should be part of P&T Committee meetings.

Adverse Drug Reaction Monitoring

The P&T Committee is expected to develop policies and to monitor the incidence and severity of adverse drug reactions (ADR) in the institution (1). Policy and procedures should define an ADR and clearly specify how it will be reported and who shall be involved in its reporting. ADR summaries should become a regular component of the committee meeting agenda. When repeated and correctable ADRs are identified, the committee should take action to correct them.

Newsletter

A newsletter issued by the P&T Committee or pharmacy may be an effective way to inform medical, nursing, and other professional staff members of committee activities. The newsletter should include formulary changes and an educational component. The educational component may be based on the work of active P&T Committee task forces, current literature, or commercially available services. The newsletter is typically edited by the pharmacy department and distributed on a regular basis to all medical and professional staff.

Drug Use Review

The P&T Committee is specifically responsible for drug use review (DUR). A plan for completion of this charge should be developed. This will probably involve a combination of regular review activities and specially selected focus efforts. Each year the DUR plan should be reviewed and revised to suit the needs of the institution. The findings of DUR activities should be used to help direct committee educational activities and to focus therapeutic problems that are related to the formulary system or the formulary.

Investigational Drugs

The P&T Committee must take an active role in policies regarding the use of drugs in research within the institution. In this regard, they must work with an appropriate institutional review board. The committee must approve policies regarding the control of drugs used for research, including procurement, storage, and dispensing of these products. Record-keeping formats and sources of information, both emergency and routine, will be of particular importance to the committee. The committee agenda should include a regular summary of investigational drug activities.

Drug Procurement

The P&T Committee must be concerned with drug procurement and its related activities. This includes policies on bid awards, product selection, and vendor sales activities within the institution. The committee must be involved with bid awards from the product quality and suitability perspective. This is most closely related to questions on generic and therapeutic equivalents. It is important that the P&T Committee endorse pharmacy product selection policies in order to create the environment for quality care and price competition. Where possible, committee approval to bid certain categories (i.e., antacids, antibiotics, vitamins) as therapeutically equivalent products greatly facilitates price-based selection options. Questions regarding awards and possible controversial awards should be returned to the committee for resolution and endorsement.

The activities of pharmaceutical vendors should be addressed by the P&T Committee via policy recommendations. Policy and procedures regarding sales representative activities and standards should be reviewed annually by the committee. Disciplinary recommendations against representatives should be based on P&T Committee actions. The committee should be certain to review issues regarding vendor promotional activities, including sales displays, sampling programs, and educational activities.

Pharmacy and Therapeutics Committee Management

The "committee" nature of the P&T Committee makes it easy to overlook the need to apply basic management concepts. However, a well-managed committee is an important tool for the institution and a valuable asset to the pharmacy department. Management of the P&T Committee is a shared responsibility of the chairperson and the secretary. The director of pharmacy must be certain that planning of committee activities occurs at least annually. The committee should develop and agree upon objectives for each year. The chairperson and secretary should organize and direct resources to accomplish these activities.

Objectives that are set should be used as a benchmark for progress throughout the year. Annual progress should be cataloged via a year-end summary report to the medical staff governing body. This may be an appropriate medium to convey objectives for the upcoming year.

Little reference has been made toward the political character of the P&T Committee. All institutions, large or small, have a unique organizational behavior pattern. It is essential that this character be part of all aspects of management of the committee. Failure to adapt the methods to suit the institution will be certain to result in frustration, failure, or both.

REFERENCES

1. *Accreditation Manual for Hospitals—1984*. Chicago, Joint Commission on Accreditation of Hospitals, 1983.
2. *ASHP Statement on the Pharmacy and Therapeutics Committee*. Bethesda, American Society of Hospital Pharmacists, 1984.
3. Roberts KB, Hair JF, Garner DD: Selecting a drug formulary committee using multivariate analysis. *Drugs in Health Care* 2:167-177, 1975.
4. O'Donnell C: Ground rules for using committees. *Mgt Rev* 47:63-67, October 1961.
5. Daniels CE, Wertheimer AI: Analysis of hospital formulary effects on cost control. *Top Hosp Pharm Mgt* 2:32-47, 1982.
6. *ASHP Statement on the Formulary System*. Bethesda, American Society of Hospital Pharmacists, 1983.
7. *ASHP Technical Assistance Bulletin on Hospital Formularies*. Bethesda, American Society of Hospital Pharmacists, 1978.
8. Rucker TD, Visconti JA: *How Effective are Drug Formularies? A Descriptive and Normative Study*. Washington, DC, American Society of Hospital Pharmacists Research and Education Foundation, 1979.
9. Scheiding JL, Sitz MJ: Key inventory to formulary to cut costs. *Hospitals* 54:78-81, September 1980.
10. Torchinsky A: Antibiotic order form decreases use and cost. *Can J Hosp Pharm* 30:30-100, 1977.
11. Ma MY, Goldstein EJC, Meyer RD: Effect of control programs on cephazolin prescribing in a teaching hospital. *Am J Hosp Pharm* 36:1055-1058, 1979.
12. Klapp DL, Ramphal R: Antibiotic restrictions in hospitals associated with medical schools. *Am J Hosp Pharm* 40:1957-1960, 1983.
13. Zilz D: Total medical staff participation in formulary revision. *Drug Intell Clin Pharm* 9:596-600, 1975.
14. May FE, Stewart RB, Cluff LE: Drug use in the hospital: Evaluation of determinants. *Clin Pharmacol Ther* 16:834-845, 1974.

Appendix 59.1

DATE:

TO: Members of the Pharmacy and Therapeutics Committee
FROM: _____ , Secretary
SUBJECT: Pharmacy and Therapeutics Committee Meeting for _____

The next Pharmacy and Therapeutics Committee Meeting will be held on Thursday, _____ from 7:30 to 9 AM in Dining Room III.

If you are unable to attend, please inform the Committee of your alternate.

AGENDA

1. Approval of _____ meeting minutes
2. Drugs for temporary addition to the formulary
    A. DDAVP injection
    B. Golytely
    C. Ortho Novum 7/7/7
3. New dosage form of existing formulary drug
    A. Metaprolol, IV
    B. Loxipine succinate injection
4. Drugs for permanent addition to the formulary
    A. Atropine, pentobarbital, meperidine oral solution
    B. Cefoperazone injection
    C. Clotrimazole oral lozenge
    D. Cyclosporine oral solution and injection
    E. Diflunisal, 500 mg
    F. Erthromycin ethylsuccinate
    G. Insulin, Human U-100
    H. MVI pediatric infusion
    I. Propranolol, sustained release
    J. Urolinase injection
5. Announcements
6. Nonformulary drug request report
7. Policy on medication system
8. Report on changes in approach to cardiopulmonary resuscitation

Appendix 59.2

Pharmacy and Therapeutics Committee
MINUTES

PRESENT:

ABSENT:

GUESTS:

1. The meeting was called to order at 7:30 AM. The minutes of the _____ meeting were approved as written.
2. Report of the Antimicrobial Task Force
   _____ outlined for the committee the process used by this task force. The task force divided its efforts in two major categories: education and communications and formulary recommendations.
   Education and communications
   The committee endorsed the following concepts:
   1. Information on the cost of drugs should be made available on the nursing units and in the medical resident rooms.
   2. The *Pharmacy Bulletin* should be used to present information on the therapeutic actions of drugs with similar biologic activity and to include cost as a component of these comparisons.
   3. Develop informational brochures that can be sent to the medical staff to educate them on less costly but equally effective modes of drug therapy.
   On behalf of the committee, _____ requested that the task force review these recommendations and bring them back to the Committee with more specific ideas on how the various educational programs could be implemented at _____ .
   Formulary recommendations
   The committee voted to create a third category of drugs that require "prior approval" from the pharmacists before the drugs will be dispensed. This group of drugs will be distinguished from nonformulary items in that they will be stored in the pharmacy, but will differ from regular formulary items in that the prescribing physician will need to contact the pharmacist directly to request the drug. The pharmacist will provide the physician with information on nonrestricted alternatives, including cost information. When consistent with criteria approved by the Pharmacy and Therapeutics Committee, the pharmacist will approve the drug order. The pharmacist will document the actions taken regarding all "prior approval" drugs. This information will be presented to the committee 6 months after the program is implemented.
   Attached to the minutes are the recommendations of the task force. They have been revised to reflect the discussion at the committee meeting. These recommendations were accepted pending review and acceptance by the entire task force. The review of the ophthalmic ointments and solutions will be referred to the Department of Ophthalmology.
   At the end of the discussion, the committee thanked _____ and the task force for their efforts to date. The discussion on the task force recommendations will be continued at an upcoming meeting.
3. The meeting was adjourned at 9:10 AM. The next meeting is scheduled for _____ .

Appendix 59.3

Pharmacy and Therapeutics Committee
PHYSICIAN'S REQUEST FOR ADDITION OF A NEW DRUG
TO THE FORMULARY

NOTE: The following information is requested by the Pharmacy and Therapeutics Committee. The form may be completed by any physician, but it must be signed by a physician who is either the head of a division or a department in the health science complex. A new drug will not be stocked by the pharmacy until the request has been approved by the Pharmacy and Therapeutics Committee. Upon acceptance of this drug request by the committee, the drug will be accepted on a trial basis for a period of at least 6 months. At the end of the trial period, the requesting physician will be sent a second form asking him/her to indicate whether he/she wishes to continue or discontinue the use of the new drug. If the physician requests the continued use of this drug, it will be presented to the Pharmacy and Therapeutics Committee for permanent addition to the formulary. Send the completed form to the Secretary of the Committee, _____ . In order for this drug to be on the agenda of _____ , this form must be returned by _____ . To be on the _____ agenda, it must be returned by _____ . Pharmacy fills out items 1 through 6, physician fills out items 7 through 17.

1) Nonproprietary name: _____

2) American Hospital Formulary classification: _____
3) Proprietary name(s) and manufacturer(s): _____
4) Pharmacologic classification: _____
5) To what other drugs is this drug closely related structurally: _____

6) What similar acting drugs are presently stocked in pharmacy: _____

7) Dosage forms and potencies desired stocked: _____

8) Estimated 6-month usage for each dosage form and potency requested: _____

9) What are the indications for the use of this drug: _____

10) What is the proposed mode of action of this drug: _____

11) What are the therapeutic advantages of this drug over similar acting drugs stocked in pharmacy: _____

12) Which of the similar acting drugs stocked in pharmacy should be deleted in favor of this new agent: _____

_____

_____

13) What major side-effects have been reported for this drug: _____

_____

_____

_____

14) What contradictions and precautions have been designated for this new drug: _____

_____

_____

15) List the usual methods of administration, including any special techniques which may be required: _____

_____

_____

16) Are the above answers based on your personal experience of using this drug: _____

No _____   Yes _____   How many patients? _____

17) Indicate the source of your information giving pertinent journal references: _____

_____

_____

_____

_____

Physician requesting	Department	Date

Division or department head	Date

PHARMACIST'S REPORT ON THE DRUG

1. Date request received:

ACTION OF THE PHARMACY AND THERAPEUTICS COMMITTEE

1. Accepted for six-month trial period (   )
2. Approved for admission to the formulary (   )
3. Rejected (   )
4. Other (   )

5. Remarks _____

_____

_____

_____

_____

Secretary	Date

Chairman	Date

CHAPTER 60

Controlled Substance Surveillance

SARA J. WHITE and BRUCE E. SCOTT

The purpose of controlled substance surveillance is three-fold: (1) to ensure compliance with state and federal laws and hospital pharmacy practice standards such as American Society of Hospital Pharmacists' (ASHP) *Technical Assistance Bulletin on Institutional Use of Controlled Substances;* (2) to prevent diversion of these drugs from the hospital into illicit markets and therefore contribute to diversion; and (3) to provide a practical system for controlled substances dispensing and accountability within the hospital. Strict compliance with the applicable laws and regulations is necessary for the hospital to maintain its controlled substances registration. Without the use of controlled substances, many hospital procedures such as surgery would be impossible.

In November and December of 1983, the Drug Enforcement Administration (DEA) (1,2) reported that diversion is now at the retail level rather than at the manufacturer or wholesaler level, with approximately 2% of licensed physicians and pharmacists involved in some type of illicit practice that results in diversion of controlled substances. The DEA recommends that access to controlled substances be prohibited to all employees except those absolutely necessary because employee-related crimes make up 80-90% of the total number of hospital thefts of controlled substances. Hoover et al (3) in 1981 reported a survey of 162 hospitals regarding pilferage of controlled substances. Of the 162 hospitals, 103 (64%) reported at least one documented or suspected case of pilferage in the past year. These 103 hospitals reported 352 separate incidents of controlled substance theft involving 11,285 dosage units. Drug diversion occurred in 76% of hospitals with more than 100 beds and in only 28% of hospitals with fewer than 100 beds. Nurses were implicated in 69% of the incidents; pharmacists and pharmacy technicians in 12%; housekeeping personnel in 4.7%; unit-ward clerks in 3.5%; and physicians in 2.4%. These incidents most frequently involved meperidine, morphine, cocaine, oxycodone, hydromorphone, propoxyphene, pentazocine, diazepam, and codeine products.

Historically, in 1968 the Bureau of Narcotics and Dangerous Drugs (BNDD) was created (4). This was the first formal recognition of the need to establish higher level accountability for selected drugs other than narcotics. When BNDD became the DEA in 1973, the requirements imposed on health care professionals remained intact, namely, to work within a system that would account for the receipt and disbursement of affected drugs. In 1971, these drugs became known as controlled substances (a name that describes the intent of the legislation very well). By legal definition, controlled substances are those drugs that have shown abuse potential and are categorized by their abuse potential, from Schedule II (highest abuse potential) through Schedules III, IV, and V (some of which can be sold over the counter). Schedule I items were of no medical use except for marijuana (THC), which is now being tested as a possible antiemetic agent for cancer patients. Other special programs include methadone maintenance treatment centers for heroin addicts.

The DEA does not provide a detailed protocol on how to maintain a controlled substance system. Instead, it offers a framework that each institution can use as a basis for designing its control system in concert with individual state laws and regulations. The specific federal regulations governing controlled substances can be found in Title 21, *Code of Federal Regulations* (CFR), section 1300 to end, which can be ordered from the Superintendent of Documents, U.S. Government Printing Office, Washington, D.C. Clarification of these regulations can be obtained from the regional DEA office. An excellent discussion of these regulations can be found in *Pharmacy and the Law* by Carl DeMarco and published by Aspen Publications, Germantown, Maryland. The laws are more specific for Schedule II drugs but allow more leeway on handling Schedule III-V drugs; thus, hospital pharmacists must make professional judgements on how systems in their hospitals are set up. A balance must be obtained between a very labor- or paper-intensive system and a pragmatic approach that ensures that no diversion can occur in the pharmacy or on the nursing units.

Norvell et al (5) in 1983 performed a cost analysis on a controlled substance distribution system in a 1000-bed teaching hospital and found that the system cost $0.845 per patient day. The time required by the system included 72.3% from nursing, 26% from pharmacy, and 1.7% from security personnel. These control systems must have ample checks and balances that involve several people, each performing only the functions. If one person performs all the functions in a control system, it would be theoretically possible for that individual to alter the records and divert controlled substances. Once controlled substance systems are set up, they must be constantly monitored by pharmacy management to ensure that all procedures are being followed. This monitoring should also include verification that all reports are accurate and are being maintained for the 2-year requirement (6,7). If the DEA visits the hospital, the pharmacist must be able to produce ordering and disposition records for all controlled substances that have been received and are not currently in stock. The pharmacist should also be responsible for seeing that nursing procedures are appropriate for recording, storing, administering, and charting controlled substances.

Manufacturers are required to indicate the schedule number on their package label, which provides a good reference for the pharmacist. The pharmacist must also be cognizant of applicable state laws. Some drugs may be transferred to more stringent schedules or added to schedules by individual states. The most stringent control always applies. Many hospitals may control some Schedule III and IV drugs as if they were Schedule II drugs, because the pharmacist believes it is the only way to prevent or minimize the potential for pilferage (8-15). Feldman et al (16) in 1983 published the results on an analysis of Massachusetts hospitals that were similar to a nationwide survey. Eighty-one percent of the hospitals control either all or some Schedule III drugs in a manner similar to that used for the distribution and accountability of Schedule II drugs. Seventy-two percent maintained the same systems for Schedule IV agents, in contrast to 42% that controlled Schedule V drugs in a manner similar to Schedule II drugs.

Since hospital pharmacists have to deal with two groups of controlled substances, Schedule II items and Schedule III-V items, this chapter has been divided into two sections. Within each section, the steps involved from the time the drug is ordered through its administration to patients will be discussed.

SCHEDULE II CONTROLLED SUBSTANCES

Registration

Each person, or other legal entity such as the hospital, who handles controlled substances must register annually with the DEA. There are 11 different types of activities, each of which requires a separate registration. Any person registered to engage in one activity may also engage in coincidental activities; for example, a person authorized to dispense controlled substances in Schedules II-V may also conduct research and instructional activities with these drugs. To register, it is necessary to request the original registration form from the regional office of the DEA or by writing Registration Branch, DEA, Box 28083, Washington, D.C. 20005. Hospitals will register as dispensers via DEA form 224. Dispensing is defined (21 CFR 1301) as prescribing, dispensing, and administering controlled substances. When the hospital registers as a dispenser, an exception is made for employees; thus, they need not register provided they are acting in the usual course of their business or employment. The 11 activities are (1) manufacturing, (2) distributing, (3) dispensing (Schedules II-V), (4) conducting research (Schedules II-V), (5) conducting instructional activities (Schedules II-V), (6) conducting narcotic treatment programs (7), research and instruction (Schedule I), (8) chemical analysis, (9) importing, (10) exporting, and (11) compounding for a narcotic treatment center. Authorization

is also given to the hospital that is registered as a dispenser to compound small quantities of controlled substances for internal use without registering as a manufacturer. This authorization would cover preparing IV admixtures but not methadone maintenance program drugs.

Ordering and Receiving

Schedule I and II items require the use of the triplicate DEA order form 222. These order forms are obtained from the DEA Office, Box 28083 Central St., Washington, D.C. 20005, via form 222a. These order forms must be carefully filled out because any strikeovers, erasures, or other mistakes void the form. The hospital pharmacist should store the unused blank forms in a locked place. The ability to sign the forms should be restricted to one or two pharmacists to prevent possible diversion of the forms. The order forms may only be signed by the person whose signature is on the original registration form. Power of attorney may be given to another pharmacist to sign the order forms. The procedures for completing the forms are outlined on the back of the forms. The hospital purchase order will also have to be completed. The top two copies (brown and green) are sent to the manufacturer, and the last copy (blue) is maintained by the pharmacy as record of ordering the items. These blue copies are official records and should be maintained in a secure place by the pharmacist. The pharmacy's copy of the hospital purchase order, which has been stamped "Controlled Substance," should be placed in a date-tickler file by anticipated arrival date. By checking the tickler the pharmacist will be alerted if the order is late so the manufacturer can be contacted, since these drugs may be diverted during shipping. At the end of each month the manufacturer sends the green copy of the DEA order form to the DEA so they have a record of the hospital's Schedule II purchases.

Most hospitals have a receiving dock area where all orders are delivered. Once the receiving dock personnel sign for the package, it is the hospital's property. Appropriate procedures must ensure that controlled substances cannot disappear from the dock or while in transit to the pharmacy. One approach would be to black out on the receiving dock's paperwork the drugs ordered (all pharmacy orders). The dock personnel should only verify the receipt of the package via the purchase order number on the package shipping label and should not open any pharmacy packages. It is critical that no pharmacy packages stay on the dock area overnight, since other personnel may have access to the area.

When the pharmacy packages are received in the pharmacy the controlled substance ones, which are identified by the purchase order number, must be opened immediately and the packing slip verified against the contents, purchase order, and DEA 222 order form. Any discrepancies between what was ordered and received must be documented on the paperwork and signed by the person checking the order in. The pharmacist must complete the receipt area on the blue DEA 222 form, dating and signing it. Once this verification has been completed the drugs should be immediately taken to the pharmacy's locked storage area. To provide a paper trail, it is a good idea to copy the packing skip and have the pharmacist who puts the items in the locked storage area, as well as the receiving technician, sign for the contents. One copy of the signed packing slip can be attached to the purchase order and matched with the invoice for payment. The invoices and completed DEA 222 forms are official records and must be stored separately so they can be readily retrieved if the DEA arrives. The other packing slip copy can be used to enter the items received into the perpetual inventory. Again, the purpose is to ensure that controlled substances do not disappear inside the pharmacy. Although pharmacy hires only trusted employees, they should not be provided with an opportunity to divert controlled substances. From time to time other employees such as housekeeping, maintenance, etc will be in the pharmacy and can, unnoticed, take out controlled substances in trash bags if accessible. Controlled substances can be sold on the street for sizable amounts of money or can be abused.

Storing and Dispensing in Pharmacy

Usually a locked room (vault) is used inside pharmacy for storing Schedule II drugs (17). Security (21 CFR §1301) requires Schedule I drugs to be stored in a securely locked, substantially constructed cabinet, whereas Schedule II-V drugs may be stored in a securely locked, substantially constructed cabinet or may be dispersed throughout the stock of noncontrolled substances. Since Schedule II substances have a very high potential for abuse and diversion, most institutional pharmacies store these as if they were Schedule I drugs. The pharmacist must ensure that the vault cannot be entered by breaking through Sheetrock walls or coming over a drop ceiling; in other words, this storage area must be secure. It is a good idea to keep controlled substances inside locked cabinets inside the locked vault. This double locking would require more time for someone to break in and steal the drugs. Silent alarm systems to security or police and monitoring cameras on the halls outside pharmacy should also be used. Who has access to the key to the vault and inside cabinets and where the key is kept are very important control mechanisms. There should only be one set of keys accessible to the staff pharmacist, and that set should always be carried by a pharmacist. Neither hospital security nor anyone else in the hospital should have a key to the vault. It is possible to get high-security locks and keys that cannot be duplicated. Neither pharmacy students nor supportive personnel should be given the key to the vault. The vault key should never be left in an unlocked box. Since the keys may accidentally get locked inside the vault, a backup key can be kept inside a combination locked box mounted on the wall. A pharmacy manager can then be contacted via telephone or pagemaster and the combination changed the next day. The combination locked box could also be used as a place to leave the keys overnight when no pharmacist is on duty during the midnight shift or weekend hours.

It may be desirable to have only one vault cabinet that the staff pharmacists have access to for dispensing drugs to nursing units. The rest of the locked vault cabinets could be accessible only to one or two pharmacists who are responsible for the controlled substance system. This one dispensing cabinet approach allows for frequent inventories of the cabinet against dispensing records; therapy, diversion would be quickly and easily detected. The DEA requires a biennial inventory that can be taken during the normal business inventory as long as it is within 6 months of May 1. This inventory for Schedule II items must be an exact count, whereas Schedules III-V drugs can be an estimate of broken packages of 1000 units or less. The Schedule II inventory must be a separate document, but Schedule III-V drugs can be interspersed with normal inventory records provided they are readily retrievable. The person taking the inventory must sign it and indicate the exact time it was taken. The DEA does not require that any reconciliation of the physical and perpetual inventory be done or documented, but it is good practice to do so. The higher the number of controlled substance doses that are dispensed each month, the more prudent frequent total vault inventories would be. Obviously frequent visual checks need to be made for ordering purposes because the manufacturers or wholesalers cannot ship Schedule II items until they receive the DEA order form. In many hospitals, the purchase order and order form must be processed in purchasing and accounting before it leaves the hospital, which can take several days to a week.

The pharmacist must request permission from the regional DEA office to dispose of outdated, contaminated, broken packages, etc of controlled substances. This request is made in triplicate, using form 41 and listing each item held for destruction. The DEA regional office will instruct the pharmacist in the manner to be used for destruction of the items. One of the following means will be authorized: (1) transfer to a person registered by the DEA and authorized to possess the substance, (2) delivery to a DEA agent, (3) destruction in the presence of a DEA agent or other authorized person (board of pharmacy inspector), and (4) other means as directed by the DEA. A copy of each form 41 must be maintained for 2 years as proof of the disposition of the items.

The pharmacy may transfer controlled substances to another registered practitioner provided that no more than 5% of the dosage units dispensed per registration year are transferred. To transfer controlled substances other than on a prescription written for a specific patient, a DEA Schedule II order form (DEA 222) must be used. This situation arises when physicians want to stock their offices. The same situation occurs when the local ambulances that bring patients to the hospital's emergency room want to replace their stock. The physician or ambulance must present the brown and green copies of a correctly filled out and signed DEA order form to the pharmacy. At the end of the month pharmacy must send the DEA the green copy and retain the brown copy as proof of the disposition of the drugs.

Nursing Units

For inpatients the physician writes his medication orders in the patient's medical record (chart). The physician does not need to record his registration number on inpatient orders for controlled substances; however, a list of registration numbers and signatures of all physicians who practice in the hospital should be maintained in the pharmacy. Controlled substances may lawfully be dispensed pursuant to an order from individual practitioners (MD, DO, DDS, DVM, etc) acting in the usual course of their professional practice.

The physician's original order or a direct copy should be reviewed by the pharmacist prior to the administration of the controlled substance. There are not specific federal labeling requirements for inpatient use. Pharmacies serving hospitals with a separate registration need not label the medication with all the information necessary for an outpatient prescription provided that (1) the medication is not in the possession of the patient, (2) appropriate records are maintained, and (3) no more than a 7-day supply of a Schedule II drug and a 34-day supply (or 100 dosage units) of a Schedule II-V substance is dispensed.

Because of the need for dose-by-dose accountability, it is prudent to purchase single-use syringes or vials (18). These packages should be tamper proof; e.g., they should have a hard plastic outer container that allows the removal of only one syringe at a time. If the syringes are not so protected, the drug may be pulled out by inserting a needle through the back of the syringe and refilling it with another clear liquid such as hydroxyzine, water, normal saline solution, etc. Obviously vials need similar protection, since the rubber top can be entered with a needle/syringe and an exchange made. With tablets and capsules, individually

packaged ones in reverse numbered roll or card packages are ideal. With these roll packages, a method of visually inspecting the remaining doses (clear window in side of package) is important. It is possible to take out doses at the beginning of a roll, such as numbers 1, 2, 3, and put the roll back in the box with number 25 being the exposed one, indicating that there are 25 in the box. Dial packs can be purchased and refilled by pharmacy for oral dosage forms that are not commercially so packaged. Liquid doses should also be individually packaged. It is difficult to accurately count on the units if there are bulk tablets/capsules in bottles or liquids in multiple-dose containers. Each time a count is made, open packages should be inspected to be sure they have not been tampered with. Drugs that are not commonly used on the unit should be returned to pharmacy as soon as the order is discontinued.

For practical reasons and emergency situations, most hospitals have a small (24-hour) supply of needed Schedule II drugs in locked boxes/cabinets on each nursing unit. A paper record system for pharmacy dispensing/signing out each

FIGURE 60.1 Proof-of-use disposition forms.

item is needed that includes the drug, dosage form, strength, number dispensed, and signatures of those who dispensed it from the vault, delivered it, and received it on the nursing unit. This information can often be incorporated into the disposition form that nurses use on the unit to indicate (in addition to charting) who received each dose. Pharmacy needs to maintain disposition records of which drugs a patient has received. Figure 60.1 is an example of a "proof-of-use" or "certificate of disposition" system. The nurse completes one requisition each time a dose is administered. The completed requisitions are used by pharmacy to verify the nursing unit count, bill the patient, and serve as disposition records (the back hard copy is maintained for 2 years). Another approach is to have the medication administration record (MAR) contain an NCR copy that pharmacy can use for proof of disposition. If the MAR is used, the controlled substances must be readily identified with Schedule II substances separate from the other scheduled substances. This identification can be accomplished by having the nurse check labeled columns representing Schedule II or Schedule III-V drugs as the orders are transcribed. Any wasting, for example a 5-mg dose of morphine being given with an 8-mg syringe, must also be documented. Another nurse must cosign the wastage to prevent a nurse from stealing the wasted drug. It is common practice for nursing to count their controlled substance stock each shift, e.g., at 7 AM, 3 PM, and 11 PM. By counting during each shift, if there is a discrepancy, the nurses can be sure they made out the appropriate paperwork and a short time period is identified if a loss has occurred. It is crucial that the nurses always carry the controlled substance box/cabinet key and that the lock be changed if the key is accidentally taken home by a nurse. It is a good idea if only pharmacy personnel change the locks to prevent other personnel having access to the box.

A system for replacing the nursing units used stock and a record-keeping procedure for an unaccounted dose needs to be developed. Two examples of how unit stock is replaced are (1) the nurse brings down the completed proof-of-use sheet and is issued another supply or (2) pharmacy personnel can inventory each unit daily and restock the items used during the previous 24 hours. To handle the documentation of unaccounted-for doses on the units, a discrepancy form (Fig. 60.2) is generally used. This form documents what the substance is, the facts that the nursing unit has attempted to account for the dose, and what administrative action has been taken. The DEA requires that substantial losses be reported using DEA theft on loss form 106.

There may be other areas of the hospital that need a small stock of Schedule II drugs, such as clinic areas, emergency rooms, and operating rooms (19). The emergency and operating rooms can often be handled just like a nursing unit. Clinic areas that are not staffed around the clock pose special security concerns. All other options such as coming to pharmacy when a dose is needed or picking up a small box each morning and returning it each evening for storage in pharmacy should be explored prior to setting up a stock in unattended areas. If it becomes necessary to set up such a stock, the minimum number of drugs and doses needed for no more than half a week should be stored in a locked cabinet/box inside another cabinet and the keys carried when

the nurses are present and left in a secure hidden spot overnight. It is good procedure for the nurses to check the integrity of the storage area daily, especially if the controlled substances are not administered on a daily basis.

Outpatient

For outpatients the prescription serves as the disposition record. Each outpatient prescription must contain the following information: (1) name of the patient, (2) address of the patient, (3) name of the prescriber, (4) address of the prescriber, (5) registration number of the prescriber, (6) name, strength, and quantity of the medication; and (7) directions for use. All prescriptions must be dated with the day issued, signed manually by the physician, and prepared in ink, indelible pencil, or on a typewriter. Schedule III-V drugs may be dispensed via a verbal order provided that the pharmacist promptly reduces to writing all necessary information except the prescriber's signature. Schedule II drugs may be issued on a verbal prescription only in a bona fide emergency situation. If such a situation exists, the pharmacist may dispense a limited quantity provided he (1) reduced the prescription to writing immediately, (2) knows the prescriber or takes a reasonable effort to ensure the validity of the order, (3) writes across the face of the prescription "Authorized for Emergency Dispensing" and the date, and (4) receives a written prescription from the prescriber within 72 hours. If the pharmacist does not receive this written prescription, he must notify the nearest regional DEA office.

Prescriptions for drugs listed in Schedules III and IV, and in some states Schedule V, may be refilled up to five times provided that no more than 6 months have expired from the date of the original issuance of the prescription and such refills are authorized by the prescriber. When refilling a prescription, the pharmacist should note on the back of the prescription the date of refill, the amount dispensed, and his initials. Schedule II prescriptions may not be refilled. All filled Schedule II prescriptions must be voided by the dispensing pharmacists by signing their names across the face of the prescription.

Prescriptions must be filed with noncontrolled ones but must contain the letter "C" (no less than 1 inch high) stamped, in red ink, in the lower right-hand corner of the prescription. Generally Schedule II prescriptions are filed separately, and Schedule III-V prescriptions are interspersed with the other prescriptions.

The label of a prescription for a controlled substances (21 CFR §1306) must include the date filled, the pharmacy's name and address, the prescription serial number, the name of the patient and prescriber, and the directions for use. A prescription container for a controlled substance must also contain the statement "Caution: Federal law prohibits transfer of this drug to any person other than the patient for whom it is prescribed," generally in the form of an auxiliary label.

A pharmacist (where state law allows) may dispense Schedule V drugs and those nonlegend drugs in Schedule II, III, and IV without a prescription provided the following are done: (1) the pharmacist personally dispenses the drug, (2) a limited quantity is given (opium products, 3 oz or 48

UNIVERSITY OF KANSAS MEDICAL CENTER
DEPARTMENT OF PHARMACY

CONTROLLED SUBSTANCE DISCREPANCY FORM

_51_
UNIT/CLINIC

_8 /24_ _/84_
DATE(mo/day/year)

CONTROLLED SUBSTANCE	STRENGTH	DOSAGE FORM	PREVIOUS # & TIME	CURRENT # & TIME	DISCRP.	REQS.
Diazepam	10 mg	tab	13	10	–2	1

Bill Smith
PHARMACY TECHNICIAN

Nancy Jones
NURSE COUNTING TODAY

NURSING ACTION REQUIRED   (Last copy to pharmacy, rest on unit 24hrs)

☒ SOLVED   Explain (give patient name(s) and hospital #

2 reqs not filled out for patient
John Jones # 8216937-2

Donna Long Head/Charge Nurse

☐ UNSOLVED   I have reviewed all the charts of patients
currently on this drug and can not locate the discrepancy. (Must be signed
by Nursing Assistant Director prior to pharmacy count tomorrow)

_____Head/Charge Nurse
_____Nursing A.D.

PHARMACY ACTION REQUIRED

☐ Billed incorrectly   ☐ Transfered incorrectly

☐ Case filling problem   ☐ Vault adjustment

_____Pharmacy Technician _C. Taylor_ Administrative Res.

PHARMACY MANAGEMENT REVIEW: (Original kept in pharmacy, copy to nursing)

☐ Not entered as a discrepancy

FIGURE 60.2 Discrepancy form for unaccounted-for doses.

dosage units), (3) the purchaser is at least 18 years of age, (4) the purchaser is either known to the pharmacist or proper identification and proof of age is shown, and (5) a bound record book is maintained containing the name and address of the purchaser, date of purchase, name and quantity of controlled substance purchased, and the name or initials of the pharmacist. Many hospitals require, by policy, a prescription for all drugs even if they are over-the-counter or nonlegend drugs.

In hospitals, prescription blank security (forgery), verification of physician signatures, and DEA numbers must be handled with procedures. In hospitals with associated clinics, prescription blanks tend to be left in the treatment/ conference rooms rather than being carried by the physicians, thus making them accessible to patients (20). With blank prescription pads and a valid written prescription for any controlled substance, the patient has the physician's signature and DEA number, facilitating forgeries. In met-

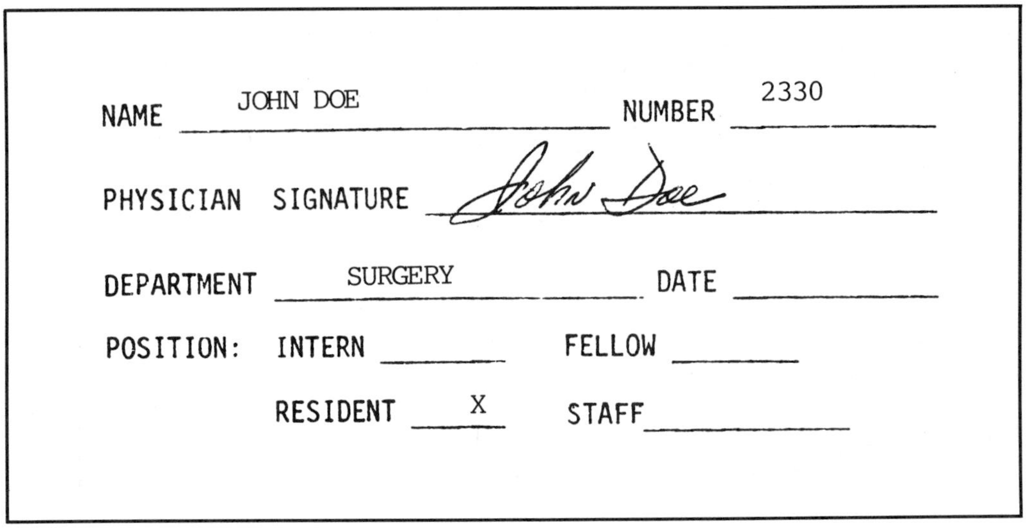

NAME ____JOHN DOE_____   NUMBER ___2330____

PHYSICIAN   SIGNATURE ____*John Doe*_____

DEPARTMENT _____SURGERY_____   DATE _____

POSITION: INTERN _____   FELLOW _____

              RESIDENT ___X___   STAFF_____

FIGURE 60.3   Signature card.

ropolitan areas, it is common for community pharmacists to fill hospital clinic or discharge prescriptions, and these pharmacists are less likely to pick up a forgery. This forgery situation is compounded by hospitals that have medical residents, since they are only present for a few years and rotate through various areas. Medical residents are often not licensed in the state and hence are not eligible for a permanent DEA number. These residents may use the hospital's DEA registration number and be assigned a unique subcode (21,22) provided they are acting in the usual course of their profession and authorized to do so by the hospital. Signature cards (Fig. 60.3) are a must in large hospitals or teaching institutions. Some successful methods used to reduce the chance for forgeries are to have two different prescription blanks (23) that are color coded and indicate ''Valid Only For Schedule II Drugs'' (Fig. 60.4*A*) and ''Not Valid for Schedule II Drugs'' (Fig. 60.4*B*). It is much easier to get the Schedule II blanks locked up on nursing units and sign out only a small quantity, which can be serially numbered, to each physician. Thus, if a forgery does occur, the physician or nursing unit responsible for the blank can be identified. This system does not, however, help prevent Schedule III-V forgeries. Other approaches involve the use of a triple-copy prescription blank (24) or the use of a physician identification card (25).

The outpatient pharmacy area will need a small supply of controlled substances for their dispensing purposes. Secure locked storage, key control, and frequent inventories are necessary to prevent or identify losses. Again, taking two different pharmacists to obtain these drugs from the vault area and transfer them to outpatient areas prevents any altering of the records and possible diversion of the drugs. Once prescriptions are filled, care must be taken to prevent any exchanging of similar looking tablets/capsules or disappearance of them in the delivery process or on the nursing unit. Tamper-evident seals or shrink wrapping, which are not available to nonpharmacists, are one method. Obviously if it is possible for the patient or his agent to pick up the filled prescription and a record of the person's signature is maintained, then the filled prescriptions only have to be

secured in the outpatient pharmacy. Locking them up is the best approach, since personnel such as housekeeping, maintenance, etc may be in the outpatient pharmacy as well as other pharmacy employees. Perhaps the outpatient area is not totally staffed 24 hours a day; if discharge filled prescriptions must be delivered to the nursing units, then a paper trail of who delivered them, who received them on the nursing unit, an available locked place for storage, and the patients signature on receipt are essential to prevent diversion.

Research

The majority of clinical research on new drugs is conducted in hsopitals. No special registration is required to conduct investigations using Schedule II-V drugs provided that the registrant is currently registered to dispense controlled substances. The investigator must also comply with Investigational New Drug (IND) requirements. Schedule I drugs (such as THC) require rigid protocols as outlined in 21 CFR §1301.33.

Records

For Schedule II drugs, all records must be maintained for at least 2 years (21 CFR § 1304-1305); some states may require a longer storage period. The information needed is (1) the name of the substance; (2) a description of each product in finished dosage form and the number of units or volume of finished form in each commercial container; (3) the number of commercial containers of each such finished form received from other persons including the date of receipt, number of containers in each shipment, and the name, address, and registration number of the person from whom the containers were received; (4) the number of units or volume of products in finished form dispensed, including the name of the person to whom it was dispensed, the date of dispensing, the number of units or volume dispensed, and the written or typewritten name or initials of the individual who dispensed or administered the substance on be-

THE UNIVERSITY OF KANSAS MEDICAL CENTER
COLLEGE OF HEALTH SCIENCES AND HOSPITAL

DISMISSAL R$_x$ ☐

RAINBOW BOULEVARD AT 39TH • KANSAS CITY, KANSAS 66103

NAME _James Smith_ AGE _26_ DATE _____

ADDRESS _4312 Madison St K.C. Ks_

DISPENSING BY NON-PROPRIETARY NAME IS AUTHORIZED UNLESS CHECKED HERE ☐

R$_x$

LOT NUMBER

VALID ONLY FOR SCHEDULE II PRESCRIPTIONS

Meperidine 50mg
_# 20_

ī Q6 Hr Prn Pain

FILLED BY

CHECKED BY

LABEL AS SUCH

Dr Olson M.D.
Attending Physician

THIS PRESCRIPTION CANNOT BE REFILLED

DEA NO. _U 134_

73-623

FIGURE 60.4*A*   Prescription blank for Schedule 2 drugs.

THE UNIVERSITY OF KANSAS MEDICAL CENTER
COLLEGE OF HEALTH SCIENCES AND HOSPITAL

DISMISSAL R$_x$ ☐

RAINBOW BOULEVARD AT 39TH • KANSAS CITY, KANSAS 66103

NAME _James Smith_ AGE _26_ DATE _____

ADDRESS _4312 Madison St. K.C., Ks_

DISPENSING BY NON-PROPRIETARY NAME IS AUTHORIZED UNLESS CHECKED HERE ☐

R$_x$

LOT NUMBER

NOT VALID FOR SCHEDULE II PRESCRIPTIONS

Tylenol #3
_#12_

ī - īī Q6 Hr Prn Pain

FILLED BY

CHECKED BY

LABEL AS SUCH

Dr Olson M.D.
Attending Physician

REFILL _Ø_ TIMES

DEA NO. _U 134_

73-623

FIGURE 60.4*B*   Prescription blank for drugs not classified as Schedule 2.

half of the dispenser; and (5) the number of units or volume of product in finished form and/or commercial containers disposed of in any other manner by the registrant, including the date of disposal and the quantity of the substance in finished form disposed. Many hospitals utilize computerization to maintain these records (26-32) provided that the specific information on scheduled drugs may be readily retrieved from the data banks, and the information is stored, either by tape, disc, or any other means for 2 years.

The records that must be maintained are:

1. Used DEA order forms
2. Receiving records and invoices
3. Biennial inventories
4. Proof-of-use disposition records (including any DEA order forms used to purchase/transfer drugs from pharmacy)
5. Destruction, waste, theft, discrepancy records
6. Physician's original orders (inpatient's medical records for inpatients and prescriptions for outpatients)
7. Policy and procedure manuals (both pharmacy and nursing)

SCHEDULES III-V DRUGS

Ordering and Receiving

These drugs can be ordered the same way as any other pharmaceutical provided the controlled substances orders are readily identifiable. Similar procedures as for Schedule II drugs should be used with regard to date tickler files, receiving dock, processing once inside pharmacy, and documenting any discrepancies between what was ordered and received. The invoices for these drugs must be kept separate (invoiced), since they form the basis of receipt for DEA purposes. Agents in these schedules (Tylenol No. 3, Valium, Dalmane, etc) are better known by name because of their wide use than the Schedule II agents; hence, they are just as subject to diversion as Schedule II drugs. Even though the law does not specify locked storage in the pharmacy, the intent is that diversion be prevented.

Storing and Dispensing

Many hospitals have chosen to control some or all of these agents as they do Schedule II (16), whereas other hospitals only control the more common ones. It is prudent to at least keep the back stock of these agents locked up, if not in the vault, then in locked storage areas. Quantities of these drugs on unlocked, open shelves are providing personnel the opportunity to divert them. The dispensing supply may either be interspersed with the other stock or kept in a separate area under the vision of pharmacists, e.g., in a unit dose cart. Obviously the dispensing stock should be kept to a minimum so any significant diversion would be evident.

Unit dose systems are ideal for these agents, since there is only a maximum 24-hour supply available in locked carts on the nursing units, and these are identified for each patient (32). When the doses do not come back in the unit dose carts, they are charged to the patient. A good procedure for pharmacy would be to periodically audit the charging rec-

ords against the patient charting and notify nursing of any discrepancies. Another approach would be to charge off the charting records and verify these against what comes back in the unit dose carts.

These items (generally Valium and/or phenobarbital) are needed in emergency drug boxes, cardiac arrest carts, toxemia trays, or clinics. It is common practice to identify the contents of emergency drugs on the outside of the container and use tamper-evident material on the latches. The emergency drugs need to be in all patient care areas. Pharmacy needs to keep track of where these supplies are, minimize the quantity in each supply, and check them monthly for outdating and the integrity of the container. These areas need to be kept in mind when the official biennial inventory is done.

Records

For Schedule III-V drugs, the following records must be maintained for at least 2 years (refer to "Records" section for Schedule II drugs):

1. Invoices
2. Biennial inventory
3. Proof-of-use disposition records
4. Physician's original order (patient's chart or prescription)
5. Policy and procedure manuals (pharmacy and nursing)

CONCLUSION

Controlled substance surveillance involves having a control system that has built-in checks to prevent any diversion and maintains all the records required by the DEA. Any system must be constantly monitored to ensure that all the procedures are being followed, and the records are complete. Pharmacists must assume the responsibility for the total system, including the nursing drug administration to patients. Pharmacists, in conjunction with nursing, must develop nursing unit procedures and ensure their compliance for controlled substances. Controlled substances are very useful medications and must be appropriately handled to prevent diversion or abuse.

REFERENCES

1. Anon: DEA recommends security measures for pharmacies. *Parenterals* 5:7, 1983.
2. Anon: Most controlled substance diversion is at the retail level. *Kansas State Board of Pharmacy Newsletter* 1983, p 2.
3. Hoover RC, McCormick WC, Harrison WF: Pilferage of controlled substances in hospitals. *Am J Hosp Pharm* 38:1007-1010, 1981.
4. Black HJ: How much control for controlled substances. *Am J Hosp Pharm* 40:788, 1983.
5. Norvell MJ, McAllister JC, Bailey E: Cost analysis of drug distribution for controlled substances. *Am J Hosp Pharm* 40:801-807, 1983.
6. Bergemann DE: Checklist for evaluating management of controlled substances. *Am J Hosp Pharm* 37:1299-1300, 1980.
7. Prosnick JJ: Evaluation of hospital controlled substances distribution systems. *Am J Hosp Pharm* 32:606-608, 1975.
8. Petruconis SK: How to fit Schedule II into the system. *Hospitals* 48:99-125, 1974.
9. Lynsky EL, Richie ND, Taylor RL: A hospital narcotic control system for Schedule II drugs. *Hosp Formul* 12:599-604, 1977.
10. Gerlach AJ: A simple, effective narcotic distribution and control system. *Am J Hosp Pharm* 29:63-67, 1972.

11. Somani SM, Glese RM, Roberts AW: Design of a revised controlled substances distribution system, *Am J Hosp Pharm* 39:612-618, 1982.
12. Smythe HA: Development of a new narcotic and controlled drug system. *Can J Hosp Pharm* 26:109-111, 1973.
13. Pang RJ: Developing an effective institutional compliance program for inventories and records of controlled substances. *Hosp Pharm* 12:220-232, 1977.
14. Proksch RA, Riley AN: Controlled substances system change provides increased accountability. *Hosp Pharm* 17:6-16, 1982.
15. LaMassa PA, Cohen KR, Ruditsky S: How our hospital pharmacy maintains control of controlled substances. *Pharm Times* 48:102-107, 1982.
16. Feldman MJ, Mantel S, Kaill AR: A comparison of the practices used for distribution of controlled substances in Massachusetts hospitals with those reported nationally. *Hosp Pharm* 18:597-599, 1983.
17. Laden SK, White SJ: Satisfaction with controlled substances security systems in university hospitals. *Am J Hosp Pharm* 40:1150, 1983.
18. Preferred packaging for controlled substances. *Am J Hosp Pharm* 40:1150-1152, 1983.
19. McClure-Zola E, Cipolle J, Zaske DE: Distribution system for controlled substances in the operating room. *Am J Hosp Pharm* 38:687-689, 1981.
20. Rapp RP, Sachatello CR: Institutional control of prescription blanks. *Am J Hosp Pharm* 32:52-54, 1975.
21. Alexander V, Lazarus H, McGovern H: Controlled substance registration for nonlicensed physicians. *Hospitals* 53:165-170, 1978.
22. Korn B: Prescribing of controlled substances. *Hospitals* 45:16, 1971.
23. Vanderbush RE, Johnston PE, Whalen FJ: A two-blank system to minimize prescription forgeries. *Hosp Formul* 15:389-395, 1980.
24. Sigler KA, et al: Effect of a triplicate prescription law on prescribing of Schedule II drugs. *Am Hosp Pharm* 41:108-111, 1984.
25. Lee HE: Institutional prescription blank control through use of a physician identification card. *Hosp Pharm* 12:227-228, 1977.
26. Stein RL, Motta LJ, Yee AD: Microcomputer for controlled substance record keeping. *Am J Hosp Pharm* 41:128-132, 1984.
27. Nazzaro JT: A system for automatic data processing of controlled substance disposition. *Hosp Pharm* 13:16-29, 1978.
28. Markin RE, Schwartz JI, Sell AE: Use of a tabletop computer in controlled substances distribution. *Am J Hosp Pharm* 39:1195-1197, 1982.
29. Shaver RG, et al: Computerized controlled drug inventory system. *Am J Hosp Pharm* 35:173-176, 1978.
30. Burleson KW: Review of computer applications in institutional pharmacy 1975-1981. *Am J Hosp Pharm* 39:53-69, 1982.
31. McDaniel HA: Development of a computer-based controlled substances reporting system. *Am J Hosp Pharm* 32:1175-1177, 1975.
32. Larson RL, Muller BA: 24-Hour unit dose distribution of Class III-V controlled substances. *Hosp Pharm* 17:254-259, 1982.

CHAPTER 61

Quality Assurance
and Performance Standards

CLIFFORD E. HYNNIMAN

All of us probably feel comfortable that we understand the word "quality." We know a quality automobile when we see one. Certainly we have participated in discussions regarding the quality of life. While we use such phrases everyday, their meaning varies considerably from one person to another. Quality is a judgment. Common understanding comes about only after more precise definition and the establishment of criteria and standards. Yet, after concentrated study and analysis, the staff of the Joint Commission on the Accreditation of Hospitals (JCAH) concluded that there was no universally accepted definition of quality care (1). Very simply, quality can be defined as conformance to requirements (2). With respect to health care, quality care can be considered the most favorable balance of benefit and risk (3). Qualtiy assurance describes all efforts to measure, assess, ensure, and evaluate health care (4). The word "assurance" suggests action to eliminate substandard performance and improve efficiency of the system of care (5). In a programmatic fashion, Stolar (6) describes quality assurance as deciding what is to be done, measuring how well the job was done after completion, and then, if the results were not acceptable, undertaking corrective action to ensure that in the future they will be acceptable.

Quality assurance efforts have long been associated with health care. Medicine's Flexner report in 1910, credited with revolutionizing medical education, was in part due to the unacceptable care being rendered by graduates of small proprietary schools. In the 1950s, foundations for medical care were established to review the quality of care given by practicing physicians as a prerequisite for reimbursement. The foundations were made up of physicians and were nonprofit. In the early 1970s, the federal government operated experimental medical care review organizations to determine if foundations could improve the quality of care and control services under Medicare and Medicaid. They had little effect on the control of services but may have offered some benefit toward improved quality (7).

The traditional approach thought to ensure quality in health care has been certification, accreditation, or licensure of the practitioner and his or her place of practice. Although having a degree of impact on quality assurance, the effect is only ensured at the time of licensure or accreditation.

Other self-regulatory approaches include codes of ethics and the development of standards of practice. After the formation of the American Society of Hospital Pharmacists (ASHP) in 1942, one of its early and most significant achievements was the development of the Minimum Standard for Pharmacies in Hospitals (8). In describing the philosophy of the standard, Dr. Fischelis stated that committees "labored long and arduously to bring together a consensus of what constitutes good hospital pharmacy practice and the essential elements which must be united to supply the organization which will meet the needs of patients (9)." Over the years the ASHP's statements and guidelines have had a dramatic impact on the quality of institutional pharmacy practice. The current ASHP position is that competency in quality assurance is required for institutional pharmacy practice (10). It is worth noting that self-regulatory approaches such as these are sometimes open to criticism because they depend exclusively on the perceptions of the providers to define appropriate practices.

One of the earliest descriptions of an organized program to monitor pharmacy practice with the goal of eliminating human error was described in 1967. Two reports described the application of the *zero-defects* concept in hospital pharmacy practice (11,12). Zero-defects originated in engineering and production of weapon systems for the U.S. Army. Implementation was directed toward improving the quality of goods and services and reducing the cost by motivating each department to reduce to zero those defects attributed to human error. The pharmacy programs encouraged the staff to report errors, determine the cause and effect, and identify a means to prevent recurrences. One report included a checklist covering environmental, equipment, and procedural factors that could have caused the breakdown (11).

PROFESSIONAL STANDARDS
REVIEW ORGANIZATIONS

Professional standards review organizations (PSRO) were established by the Social Security Amendments of 1972 (P.L. 92-603) (13). These reviews by area-wide physician groups were to ensure that services reimbursed by federal programs met appropriate standards and were effective, efficient, and economical. Responsibilities of the program included reviewing admissions to a health care facility, certifying the necessity for continued inpatient treatment, reviewing extended or costly treatments, conducting medical evaluation studies, and reviewing facility, practitioner, and health care service profiles and other records. PSROs have been challenged in the courts and by many physicians who fear that data collected for the PSRO might be used in malpractice suits. Such factors have contributed to the delayed acceptance by the health care system of this quality assurance approach (4). Although PSROs have placed a heavy emphasis on monitoring efforts to ensure quality of care, their direction over recent years has been more cost oriented (14,15). Private contracts between large corporations and PSROs are growing due to the concern these companies have over escalating medical care premiums (16). Employers want high quality, but also want to be sure they are only paying for medically necessary services.

JOINT COMMISSION ON ACCREDITATION

The American College of Surgeons, a leader in the eventual formation of the JCAH, had standards for tissue review and medical record review at early as 1918. After its founding in 1951, the JCAH's approach to quality review was informal and subjective (17). In the early 1970s, JCAH began to emphasize the use of medical auditing through the implementation of a system called performance evaluation procedure (PEP) (18,19). The system included three phases: criteria development, data extraction, and corrective action. This effort to audit medical practice based on criteria established by the medical staff was complemented by standards requiring reviews by medical and support service departments. By the late 1970s, it became obvious that too much effort was focused on doing audits and too little on resolving identified problems.

In 1979, the JCAH published a standard requiring hospitals to coordinate all of the quality reviews within a facility and to emphasize the identification and resolution of problems (20). Currently the JCAH defines quality assurance as a planned and systematic process for monitoring and evaluating patient care. This focus required ongoing data collection and periodic evaluation to ensure the identification and solution of problems resulting in improved care (17). The *Accreditation Manual for Hospitals* contains a chapter on quality assurance. Standard I in that chapter states (21):

There shall be eivdence of a well-defined, organized program designed to enhance patient care through the ongoing objective assessment of important aspects of patient care and the correction of identified problems.

The chapter on pharmaceutical services also has a standard on quality assurance. Standard VI states (22):

As part of the hospital's quality assurance program the quality and appropriateness of patient care services provided by the pharmaceutical department/service are monitored and evaluated, and identified problems are resolved.

The essential components of the JCAH-defined program shall include identification of problems, objective assess-

ment, and the determination of priorities, implementation of decisions or actions, monitoring to ensure desired results, and documentation to substantiate the effectiveness of the program. Potential data sources for identifying problems are the medical record, morbidity/mortality reviews, monitoring activities of the staffs, hospital committee activities (tissue review, infection control, antibiotic usage review, utilization review, blood utilization review), prescriptions, peer review, process- or outcome-oriented studies, incident reports, clinical reports, insurance claims data, patient billing data, discharge abstracts, patient complaints, and patient surveys. Once problems are identified, actions to eliminate them could include education or training programs, policy or procedure revision, staffing changes, facility or equipment changes, or adjustment of clinical privileges.

QUALITY ASSESSMENT

The classic approach to quality assessment is based on the widely acknowledged classification system devised by Donabedian (3). He categorizes all assessment efforts as either structure, process, or outcome.

Structure is the human, physical, and financial resources needed to provide care. Examples include the number, distribution, and qualifications of personnel; the number, size, and geographic distribution of hospitals or other facilities, medical staff organization; licensure and accreditation; and even the presence or absence of a quality review effort. Examples of structural characteristics in a pharmacy program would include the presence or absence of a unit dose program, IV admixture program, or formulary system. These and other program areas, based on the standards and guidelines of the ASHP, permit the assumption that if the profession's standards exist in a program, quality pharmaceutical care will follow. Structure of proper design and adequate resources may be the most important factor in protecting and promoting quality.

Process activities are those that take place between the patient and the provider. Process measures include the procedures or steps followed in providing care and are the most direct measures of quality. Many pharmacy quality assurance programs utilize process measures. Drug utilization studies, or the auditing of operational criteria for drug distribution are examples of process assessment.

Outcome is a change in the patient's current or future health status that can be attributed to antecedent health care. Outcomes can be classified as clinical, social, psychologic, economic, etc. Outcome assessment is probably the most difficult and costly because of the difficulty in establishing whether the outcome was indeed the result of the care provided. Although most of the literature discusses outcomes in terms of patient outcomes, the concept can also be applied to pharmacy services. Outcome in this case is simply the end result of a set of processes operating within a structure.

There is a fundamental relationship among the elements of structure, process, and outcome (Fig. 61.1). The structural characteristics of the setting influence the process of care, increasing or decreasing its quality. Changes in the process and its quality influence outcome or health status. Elements of the process of care do not signify quality until their relationship to desirable changes in health status has

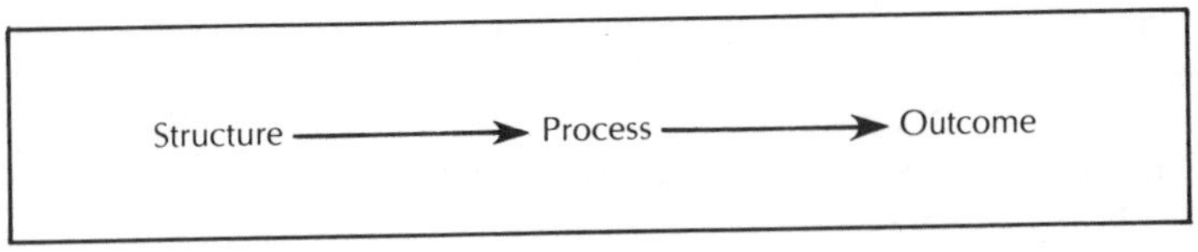

Structure ⟶ Process ⟶ Outcome

FIGURE 61.1 Quality assessment relationships.

been established. If a valid linkage exists, one can assume that the process elements will produce desired outcomes. But one cannot assume that observed outcomes in any situation are the direct result of processes. Patients have been known to improve spontaneously in spite of the care rendered. When measuring outcomes to assess quality be sure that the outcomes can, in fact, be attributed to the care provided. Requiring allergies to be included on patient profiles in the pharmacy will not by itself ensure that drugs to which the patient is sensitive will not be administered. There are numerous other process steps that are important to the achievement of this objective, among which are, of course, the nurse's awareness of the patient's allergies at the time of drug administration and the pharmacist's awareness at the time he releases the drug to the nurse for subsequent administration.

PATIENT SATISFACTION

Patient satisfaction is an outcome measure. According to Donabedian (3), it is a fundamental measure of quality because it provides information on the degree to which the patient's values and expectations are met. It may be difficult for the patient to evaluate the technical or scientific aspects of care, but the amenities of care (cleanliness, privacy, promptness, courtesy, interest) are easily evaluated. Pharmacists and other health care professionals are quick to delineate what is best for the patient, and, therefore, what represents quality care. The patient's perception of the quality provided may be quite different. Some organizations may target their quality assessment only on those measures perceived as important to the patient rather than waste time and money on those "realities" defined by practitioners. According to Donabedian (3), the pharmacist's responsibility is to the patient who, in truth, is the best judge of his own interests if he is properly informed and not mentally impaired. The literature contains numerous examples of efforts to include patient concerns in quality assurance programs (23,24).

DEVELOPING CRITERIA

Because quality is a judgment, it would be impossible to obtain a reproducible level of acceptable quality without criteria and standards. Criteria can be defined as predetermined elements against which aspects of the quality of a medical care may be compared. A variety of classification approaches has been applied. Criteria have been classified as absolute, relative, or pragmatic; subjective or objective; or as structural, process, or outcome (25).

Absolute criteria function as thresholds and are established before data collection. For example, a criterion stating that there will be no positive cultures in a particular sterile product is an absolute criterion. Relative criteria are those that can be related to the distribution of measurements. They describe where to set the regions of acceptance and rejection. For example, the average number of cabinet filling errors per day will not exceed 0.1% of the number of doses administered per day. Pragmatic criteria are developed because they are practically or clinically relevant. Such criteria require a judgment, in the course of practice, regarding when to consider a result significant; e.g., the dose shall be sufficient to maintain a therapeutic blood level.

Subjective (or implicit) criteria are not specifically defined in measurable terms. They do not lend themselves to consistent judgment from person to person or from time period to time period. Objective (or explicit) criteria are specifically defined so that each person applying the criteria will obtain consistent results. Explicit criteria rather than subjective criteria are commonly used in all attempts to measure quality (1,26).

Finally, criteria can also be classified by the already discussed structure, process, or outcome categories. Structural criteria include demographic and ecologic characteristics of the unit of observation. The presence or absence of a program, certification, licensure, and the like are structural criteria elements. Because of the ease in determining whether these criteria are satisfied, such measures may represent the most economical approach to quality assessment. Process criteria measure the what, when, where, and how of care, in other words, the steps followed in performing a service. Outcome criteria are designed to evaluate the end result. If outcome is evaluated based on the patient's status, these criteria are the most difficult to apply because it may not be clear whether the observed result is due to the care rendered (25).

Although measuring quality based on patient outcomes may be difficult, applying outcome criteria in relation to pharmacy services is much more straightforward. For example, consider the following criterion: All stat doses of medication will be delivered ready for administration to the patient within 15 minutes of receipt. The objective is to deliver the dose ready for administration within 15 minutes. The criterion requires a judgment that it either happened or did not happen. The process or steps necessary to achieve this result are not being judged. The process in this example could include transportation, order receipt, interpretation, verification, clarification, transcription, product selection, dose preparation, dose packaging, labeling, packaging control record keeping, and delivery. Outcome criteria used in this fashion are recommended because they are thought to be easier and, therefore, less costly to evaluate (6).

In measuring quality, the criteria applied are usually modified by norms and standards. A norm describes a practice or the frequency of an event as it really exists locally, regionally, or nationally. A standard defines the range of ac-

QUALITY ASSURANCE CRITERIA FOR INPATIENT DRUG DISTRIBUTION (UNIT DOSE)
AT METROPOLITAN MEDICAL CENTER PHARMACY

Elements	Standard	Exceptions	Instructions
1. A pharmacist will review and verify, from the physician's original order, all medication orders prior to the administration of the drug to the patient:	100%	Stat telephone orders: Use special form and record patient name, room No.; medication route, strength, schedule, time needed, No. doses sent; order given by; and pharmacist initials	Pharmacist's initials on order indicates order has been reviewed and verified.
a. Check for patient name and room No. on order.	100%	None	
b. Check for completeness of order (i.e., name of drug, strength, route of administration and schedule).	100%	None	
c. Check for accuracy and appropriateness of order (i.e., appropriate strength, proper dose and route of administration, and possible drug interactions).	100%	None	Refer to list of interactions and procedure for dealing with interactions.
d. Clarification of orders when appropriate.	100%	None	All clarified orders will contain a note of person consulted, action taken, and time of clarification. Unclarified orders should be clipped to shelf in dispensing area and next shift notified.
e. All medication orders on doctor's order are processed.	100%	None	Medication orders starred, circled, underlined, etc. Processed orders have update stickers or profile prepared or medication written on bottom of profile.
2. All drugs dispensed will be checked against the verified order for accuracy.	100%	None	Pharmacist initials profile or medication update stickers, or both, indicating all of elements in Criterion 2 were met.
a. Verify that patient's name and room number on order correspond to that on profile.	100%	None	
b. Medication order on update stickers or profile is transcribed correctly and corresponds with doctor's order.	100%	None	
c. Medication order is checked against profile for allergies and drug interactions.	100%	None	
d. Medication update sticker is properly placed in profile.	100%	None	Scheduled medications at top; PRNs, soporifices and one-time-only at bottom.
e. Verify that name and room No. on medication bag corresponds to that on medication order.	100%	None	
f. Correct drug, strength and route of administration is placed in bag.	100%	None	
g. Medication bag is placed in correct pick-up box.	100%	None	
h. All discontinued drugs and one-time-only orders are "yellowed" out.	100%	None	
i. External drugs are recorded properly in profile.	100%	None	"Other medications" section of profile.
j. Extemporaneous doses are properly labeled with name of drug, strength (if half-tab, written strength per half-tab), company, NDC#, exp. date.	100%	None	
k. Suppositories labeled as in 2j whenever possible.	100%	None	
3. Pharmacy technician properly prepares 24-hour medication exchange box using the pharmacy medication profile.	100%	None	Initials on proper area of profile indicate that Criterion 3 was accomplished by the technician.
a. Correct drug, strength and route of administration is placed in the medication box.	100%	None	
b. Correct number of doses is placed in box (scheduled drugs only).	100%	None	
c. No expired drugs are placed in box.	100%	None	
d. Extemporaneous doses are properly labeled (see 2j).	100%	None	

FIGURE 61.2 Quality assurance criteria for inpatient drug distribution (unit dose) at metropolitan medical center pharmacy. (Reprinted by permission from Brockemier RL, Briner JE, Johnson MK: Audit mechanism for hospital drug distribution. *Am J Hosp Pharm* 37:85-88, 1980.)

MINIMUM STANDARDS OF PRACTICE FOR INPATIENT CARE; ADMISSION DRUG HISTORIES
COMPLIANCE AUDIT: Preliminary ☐   Final ☐

Area _____   Date _____
                                        month/year

Criteria	Standard, %	Exceptions	Procedure	Compliance Yes No	Comments	Recommended action
A. A drug history shall be obtained by a pharmacist on all patients within 48 hours of admission	100	1. Non-English speaking patient 2. Noncommunicative patient 3. Obstetric patient 4. Transferred	1. Patient monitoring form (PMF) review 2. Patient medical record review			
B. The information obtained shall include: 1. Present medications and their use 2. Past relevant drug use 3. Present or past drug-induced problems 4. Present or past drug-related problems 5. Present or past drug side effects 6. Patient allergy 7. Patient's personal physician and pharmacist 8. Street drug use	100		1. Satellite activity observation 2. Patient medical record review			
C. A summary of the medication history shall be placed in the patient's medical record and shall include, in addition to *B* above: 1. Patient's reliability as a historian 2. Patient's compliance to medication instructions 3. Patient's drug knowledge	100		Patient medical record review			

FIGURE 61.3 Audit form used to monitor quality of patient medication histories. (Reprinted by permission from Vogel MS, Gurwich E, Hutchinson RA: The quality assurance of professional staff. *Curr Concepts Hosp Pharm Mgt* 3(2):8-11, 14-17, 1981.)

ceptable variation from a norm or criteria. Both Figure 61.2 and Figure 61.3 list standards. In both illustrations the standard is 100%, meaning there is no acceptable deviation. Criteria and standards should be relevant to the function's actual result; they should be measurable so that the results can be obtained consistently by any auditor; and they should be clear, concise, and achievable.

DESIGNING A PROGRAM

The opportunities for developing quality assurance efforts in institutional practice seem endless. The drug use control process has been described as "that system of knowledge, understanding, judgement, procedures, skills, controls, and ethics that assures optimal safety in the distribution and use of medication (27). Among the professions, the pharmacist is the only individual who devotes his complete attention to these matters. The pharmacist is expected to exert leadership in all aspects of drug use. In developing a quality assurance program, some authors (28,29) have suggested that the pharmacist should give highest priority to those programs for which he is most accountable, e.g., drug distribution. Lowest priority for program development would include areas where the least control is exercised, e.g., determination of drug need and drug selection. When presented with the universe of potential involvements, the advice of these au-

TABLE 61.1 Quality Assurance (QA) Programs for Hospital Pharmacy Reported during 1974-1982[a]

Reference No[b]	States Purpose	Functional Area(s) of Pharmacy	Focus of QA Program			Method of Data Collection	Major Conclusions
			Structure	Process	Outcome		
1	Establish a QA program for all pharmaceutical services in an organized, step-by-step fashion	Inpatient and outpatient dispensing, IV admixtures	x	x		Bimonthly and monthly random selection of audit units	None stated
2	Permit an ongoing evaluation of the quality of pharmaceutical services	Inpatient and outpatient services and IV admixtures	x	x	x	Not specified	Results indicated the need for an ongoing QA program
3	Improve the quality of pharmaceutical services	Unit dose, IV admixtures, outpatient services, drug information, management, purchasing, clinical services, manufacturing, and staff development		x	x[c]	Daily, weekly, monthly, or quarterly retrospective audits or concurrent audits (depending on the service to be audited)	None stated
4	Develop a continuous program of quality assurance	Unit dose			x	Daily completion of cart exception forms	Has allowed continuous monitoring and improvement of the unit dose system
5	Demonstrate how one pharmacy department has used the audit criteria to develop an intradepartmental audit mechanism	Unit dose		x[d]		Random review of 150 physicians' orders, 50 medication profiles, or 50 patient medication drawers	System has not functioned long enough to make judgments concerning effectiveness
6	Describe the department's efforts to comply with aseptic technique in preparing IV admixtures	IV admixtures		x		Random observation over a 2-month period	Program is one component of QA program; expansion to a final product check for sterility is planned
7	Design and implement a QA program for pharmaceutical services provided by a pharmacy management corporation	Multidisciplinary activities, drug distribution, sterile preparations, purchasing and inventory control, management, and clinical functions	x		x[e]	Assessment of pharmacy by director; corrective action planned; no time frame specified	Standards and assessment reporting forms developed are applicable to any hospital pharmacy
8	Develop a hospital pharmacy QA program for use by seven community hospitals	Same as Reference 3		x	x	Periodic or random review (frequency not specified)	Criteria will also serve as guidelines in planning future services; effectiveness will be determined by follow-up
9	Improve the quality of decentralized pharmacy services	Drug distribution, drug information, and limited clinical services	x	x		Not specified	Consistent service and minimum expectations are documented
10	Establish a complete QA program for a pharmacokinetic dosing service	Pharmacokinetic dosing service	x			Competency examination and periodic monitoring of recommendations	Methods will be refined and redefined as program experience increases

[a]Reprinted by permission from Oakley RS, Bradham DD: Review of quality assurance in hospital pharmacy. *Am J Hosp Pharm* 40:53-63, 1983.
[b]See reference list at end of chapter.
[c]The primary focus was on outcome.
[d]Since the medication dispensed is not a patient outcome (although it is a system outcome), the authors did not think criteria were outcome oriented.
[e]While the authors stated that the program was outcome oriented, no specific examples were given.

TABLE 61.1, cont'd

Reference No[b]	States Purpose	Functional Area(s) of Pharmacy	Focus of QA Program			Method of Data Collection	Major Conclusions
			Structure	Process	Outcome		
11	Assist in the development of a QA program for clinical pharmacy services	Clinical services		x		Formal examination, direct observation, and evaluation of written records; no time frames specified	Establishment of QA for clinical pharmacy services is necessary and is an effective management tool
12	Assure the quality and consistency of pharmacokinetic monitoring	Pharmacokinetic dosing service		x		Monthly retrospective chart review of 25% of patients receiving drugs	This program is ongoing, simple, and educational in nature
13	Evaluate the use of particular medications	Drug-specific reviews		x	x	Retrospective chart review; frequency or quantity not specified	Identified deficiencies are presented to the medical and pharmacy staffs
14	Propose and develop a framework and priorities for developing a QA program	Drug-use review and other pharmacy services		x		Not specified	Should adopt this approach because the drug-use process is the primary concern of hospital pharmacist in medical care
15	Influence the quality of care when medications are received	Drug-use review		x		Monthly retrospective chart review	DUR should improve patient health and minimize the resources involved
16	Present a framework within which a QA program for admixture services can be developed	IV admixtures	x	x	x	General guidelines were discussed	Key to quality is adherence to procedure
17	Present guidelines and methods for QA in centralized IV admixture services	IV admixtures	x	x	x	Evaluation of education and training of employees; emphasis on adherence to procedure; end-product testing with sampling using a cumulative-sum procedure	Quality must be built into product during preparation
15.	Discuss methods for establishing an appropriate climate for DUR	Drug-use review		x		Retrospective DUR	An objective, neutral, and confidential climate for DUR will enhance a continuing program
19	Present a method of chart review that focuses on the role of drugs as therapeutic and iatrogenic agents	Drug-use review		x		Retrospective, external medical audit reviewing total care received by the patient	Fully explicit criteria and standards should be developed against which criteria are to be measured
20	Describe a system for reviewing the initial choice of antimicrobial therapy	Drug-use review		x		Development of treatment standards for 12 syndromes, compliance monitored by random audit and exception cases presented and discussed by the medical staff	Effective programs should write standards only for conditions in which there is a consensus of medical opinion

thors may be helpful in the beginning, but the pharmacist's broad responsibility for the total drug use process should be kept in mind. The pharmacist should ensure that program efforts encompass the total drug use process in a way that achieves the highest quality in patient care.

It is desirable to involve as much of the total staff as possible in constructing and maintaining the quality assurance program. If all pharmacists and technicians understand what constitutes quality, and if they regularly receive feedback on performance, quality care will be optimized.

Helpful guidance can be obtained by reviewing the standards and guidelines of the ASHP (30). For example, if one were developing a program in drug distribution, a review of the *ASHP Technical Assistance Bulletin on Hospital Drug Distribution and Control* (31) would be helpful in evaluating the component parts of the distribution system as well as in developing objectives and criteria for evaluating the system. The department's procedure manual could also serve as a basis for program development. In fact, some believe that a quality assurance program should correlate what actually occurs with the established policies and procedures (32). In other words, objectives and criteria might be developed from the department's approved policies and procedures. The quality assurance program would then measure whether performance conforms to the approved requirements.

Table 61.1 provides a list of the pharmacy quality assurance programs reported in the literature between 1974 and 1982. This excellent summary by Oakley and Bradham (33) describes the pharmacy program component and whether the reported quality assurance program focused on structure, process, or outcome measures. The majority of the referenced programs are process oriented. However, the list contains a large number of articles dealing with drug utilization review or clinical services. In areas such as these, which are closely tied to patient status, valid outcome measures are difficult to identify. Notwithstanding this concern, the table outlines the status of quality assurance programs in pharmacy and should prove to be a useful index to the literature for those who are designing programs.

The steps to follow in developing and implementing a program are shown in Table 61.2. The first step is to break the departmental services into their functional components. Such components would include drug distribution, IV admixtures, drug information services, clinical services, etc. Each of these major service areas could be further subdivided. The next step is to define objectives for each of the functional areas. Obviously, each function should have a reason for its existence, and this can be stated in the form of an objective. It may be necessary to assign priorities simply because time and economics may not permit the continuous monitoring of each major function and all of its associated tasks. As discussed earlier, the JCAH encourages emphasis on previously identified problems or suspected or potential problem areas that have a significant impact on patient care. The objectives are next reworded as criteria (outcome criteria if possible), and standards are assigned to each. After defining methods and procedures for measuring compliance, the program should be thoroughly documented and coordinated with the total hospital quality assurance program (6,34).

Often it will not be feasible to measure an outcome be-

cause the result does not occur on a timely basis or is not amenable to valid measure. For example, it is not practical to assay extemporaneously compounded prescriptions; but one can evaluate the process steps, which if conducted properly, could reasonably be expected to produce an efficacious end product. Thus, it may be necessary to revise the program by developing process or structure criteria if the outcome result is not measurable.

QUALITY CIRCLES

The discussion so far has been directed toward identifying problems and measuring the level of quality. After the audits

TABLE 61.2 Sequence of Steps in Carrying Out the Planning Strategy[a]

Sequence of Events	Product
1. Break down the pharmacy service into its primary functions.	1. List of primary service functions.
2. Break down each primary function into its subcomponents.	2. List of tasks comprising each primary function.
3. Prepare objectives for each function and its subcomponents.	3. List of functional objectives.
4. Establish priority of the objectives.	4. List of functional objectives arrayed by assigned priority.
5a. Convert the highest priority objectives into outcome criteria.	5. List of high priority outcome criteria and standards.
b. Set the standard for each criterion.	
6. Develop compliance measurement method for each criterion.	6. List of high priority outcome criteria and standards and their respective compliance measurement methods.
7a. Field-test or otherwise ascertain the workability of the criteria.	7. List of workable priority outcome criteria and standards and their compliance measurement methods.
b. Revise measurement methods as required; delete outcome criteria found not measurable.	
8a. Prepare process or structure criteria to replace those outcome criteria found to be unusable.	8. List of high priority process/structure criteria and standards.
b. Set the standard for each criterion.	
9. Develop compliance measurement method for each criterion of 8a.	9. List of high priority process/structure criteria and standards and their compliance measurement methods.
10a. Field-test or otherwise ascertain the workability of the criteria of 8a.	10. List of workable, priority process/structure criteria and standards and their compliance measurement methods.
b. Revise measurement methods as required.	
11. Design, plan and organize the quality assurance program procedures, incorporating the finished criteria/standards.	11. Quality assurance program policy and procedure manual.
12. Implement the program.	12. A healthier America

[a]Reprinted by permission from Stolar MH: Quality assurance of pharmaceutical services: Objective based planning strategy. *Am J Hosp Pharm* 38:209-212, 1981.

are completed and the problems identified, action must be initiated to reduce or eliminate the identified problems to improve performance. Although many strategies could be effective to achieve this goal, one that has been used to a limited extent in pharmacy is the quality care circle.

A quality care circle consists of up to ten individuals from the same work group who meet voluntarily on a regular basis to solve work-related problems. The group may include supervisors, but the leader is selected by the group. Activities of the circle include training in problem solving, problem solving, identifying and dealing with barriers, setting objectives and goals, monitoring progress, and making recommendations to management. A steering committee or coordinating council is usually established by management to review and evaluate proposals, recommend topics for study, monitor progress, and to communicate management values, opinions, and constraints to the circle (35).

Reports in the pharmacy literature have described quality circles as effective management tools to address employee concerns about work-related problems such as staffing, communications, and training (36,37). There are no reports of their use in association with ongoing audits in pharmacy quality assurance programs, though it would seem a logical application.

DRUG DISTRIBUTION

Most of the quality assurance programs described in the literature employ retrospective audits on a monthly or bimonthly basis (29,32). Specific components of the program may include the IV admixture service, satellite services, the unit dose system, sterile processing, manufacturing and packaging, and outpatient dispensing (29,32,38,39). Some programs are quite specific in their purpose such as the 20-criteria program described by Somani and Giese (40) to audit a newly implemented controlled substances system. A few programs have been reportedly designed for use in multi-hospital systems (41,42). Figure 61.2 shows criteria representative of many programs concerned with quality assurance in drug distribution. The criteria shown evaluate the accuracy of pharmacist order review, drug dispensing, and unit dose cart preparation. The authors of these criteria indicate that audits are conducted by pharmacists and technicians using a sample of physician orders, a sample of profiles, and a sample of patient medication bins. Results are reported to the entire staff and to a staff committee responsible for identifying the appropriate corrective action when deficiencies occur (29).

White and Godwin (43) reported the use of a continuous daily quality assurance audit of the unit dose system. Ten outcome criteria were identified. The criteria were listed on the reverse side of a form provided to nursing personnel. When deviations from the criteria occurred, the form was completed and sent to the responsible pharmacy manager. A pharmacy exception form was used in an identical fashion by the pharmacy staff. Of the ten criteria, those applicable to nursing were primarily concerned with the accuracy and timeliness of distribution, e.g., first doses, stat doses, and medication cassettes. Pharmacy criteria covered accuracy of transcription, scheduling, billing, and audits of whether the nurse administered all scheduled medications or appro-

priately explained any exceptions. In addition to the exception forms, special audits were accomplished through unscheduled visits to the nursing units and the pharmacy dispensing area. Among the areas covered by these audits were medication procedures used by the nurse, security of medication carts, errors made by technicians in filling the unit dose carts, and other pharmacy procedures. All of the data were analyzed monthly and reported to the director of pharmacy and the director of nursing for their information and follow-up.

In addition to ongoing audits based on carefully defined criteria, quality assurance activities can include special studies when problems are identified. One report by utilization review nurses described a study that was motivated because of a concern that physicians were not following the hospital's automatic stop-order policy and becuase it was believed that an effective ASO policy could reduce antibiotic use (44). After an initial audit and an extensive educational program, a second audit showed improved compliance and a 6% decrease in the number of patients receiving antibiotics. It was thought that this result was caused by an increase in patient assessment by physicians before reordering the drug.

IV ADMIXTURE PROGRAMS

The benefits of centralized pharmacist control and preparation of parenteral products are well established. The majority of hospitals now have implemented such programs. Quality assurance in these activities continues to receive more attention than most other pharmacy program areas. Improper storage conditions, contamination of prepared products, improper use of equipment, and compounding errors associated with pharmacy prepared IV admixture products have been documented (45-48). The significance of this route of administration and the fact that it is very difficult to identify problems with these products until they are administered underscores the need for a comprehensive quality assurance program.

Problems associated with the use of parenteral products in hospitals and with their manufacture led to the formation of the National Coordinating Committee on Large Volume Parenterals in the early 1970s (49). Now disbanded, this multidisciplinary group provided considerable direction in assuring quality IV therapy. Among the Committee's publications were *Recommended Methods for Compounding Intravenous Admixtures in Hospitals* (50), *Recommended Guidelines for Quality Assurance in Hospital Centralized Intravenous Admixture Services* (51), and *Recommended Standards of Practice, Policies, and Procedures of Intravenous Therapy* (52). These documents should be consulted in planning a quality assurance program for IV admixtures. The quality assurance guidelines document deals extensively with (1) selection, education, and training of personnel; (2) in-process controls, (3) end-product testing, and (4) sampling guidelines. The standards of practice document considers (1) education of personnel, (2) policies for those who administer IV therapy, (3) practices and procedures, (4) special problem areas, and (5) equipment and supplies.

The JCAH also recognizes that the compounding and admixture of large-volume parenterals should be the responsibility of a pharmacist, and personnel preparing and administering these agents should have special training. If parenteral medications are manufactured, there must be a quality control program to monitor personnel qualifications, training, performance, equipment, and facilities (53).

The objectives of an admixture program around which criteria for evaluation should be constructed are (51,54):

1. To provide products (parenteral admixtures, reconstituted injections, similar preparations) that are therapeutically and pharmaceutically appropriate for the patient
2. To provide products that are free from undesirable levels of particulate or other toxic contaminants
3. To provide products that are free from microbial and pyrogenic contaminants
4. To provide products that contain the correct drug(s) in the correct amount(s)
5. To provide products that are labeled, stored, and distributed in accordance with accepted principles of good drug control.

Criteria can be structurally, procedurally, or end-product oriented. Structural criteria would cover such things as hoods, refrigeration, and other equipment, as well as facilities and the education and training of personnel. Common process criteria might include inspection of supplies, reconstitution of drug additives, or pharmacist review of the physician order. Outcome criteria could include labeling concerns, freedom from contamination, or correct formulation.

One of the most important priorities is to ensure the competency of pharmacists and technicians in aseptic technique and pharmaceutical calculations. After training personnel, evaluation could include written tests or structured performance appraisals (51). However, ongoing audits of personnel performance are desirable, as it has been shown that performance improves when employees know they are being monitored (48). End-product testing also has been reported to be effective in validating operator aseptic technique (55). Another approach described audits of technician performance by trained observers every 2 months (56). Corrective action took the form of one-to-one educational programs by

TABLE 61.3 Elements of Technician Performance[a]

Handwashing
Jewelry removal
Tying hair back
Hood cleaning
Location of work in the hood
Examining supplies for defects
Hood airflow disturbances
Arrangement of items in the hood
Absence of nonessential items in the hood
Technique in assembling syringes and needles
Wiping of ampules and vial tops
Technique in opening ampules
Technique to filter ampule fluids
Syringe technique
Disposal of needles and syringes
Admixture labeling

[a]Adapted from Gurwich EL, Hanold L, Schaeffer PA: First-phase quality assurance program for intravenous admixture aseptic technique. *Hosp Pharm* 17:119-121, 1982.

the pharmacy supervisor. The criteria used covered the topics shown in Table 61.3.

In-process controls and end-product testing should be included in any comprehensive quality assurance program. End-product testing alone is insufficient. In hospital IV admixture programs, the products prepared vary considerably in formulation, composition, packaging, method of preparation, and in the personnel who perform the compounding function. This lack of product-to-product specificity makes it difficult at best to extrapolate the results of end-product testing to all products produced (54). Even the pharmaceutical industry acknowledges that end-product testing does not ensure sterility of aseptically prepared products (57). To ensure quality, more emphasis is placed on the clean room environment, microbiologic environmental monitoring, personnel training, and other special process controls. Given proper operator training and in-process controls, end-product testing has been recommended to validate the compounding process (51,58).

CLINICAL SERVICES

The application of clinical services in hospitals varies in relation to the training and background of the pharmacists, the administrative direction, the individual's interests, and the time available. Knowing whether a service is performed is not enough. The individualized nature of clinical practice makes it difficult to monitor how well the service is being performed. This kind of inconsistency suggests that quality assurance programs in this area may even be more important than those dealing with more traditional pharmacy services (59-61).

Some institutions have developed a comprehensive quality assurance program covering all clinical services. Others have developed a specific program for an individual clinical service or performed a periodic audit of selected activities when problems are identified. Each program developed should follow the principles previously discussed. The University of Illinois (60) started their program by developing minimum standards of practice for the department. Clinical program components included in the standard were providing therapeutic information, drug monitoring, drug histories, discharge counseling, and code participation. The standard for drug histories indicates that, except for those exempted, a drug history will be obtained by a pharmacist for all new admissions. Compliance with all standards is determined through audits of each satellite's activities. Figure 61.3 provides an example of the criteria that are subsequently used to measure the quality of each activity; in this case, drug histories (60).

Pharmacokinetics. A complete program might start with structurally oriented activities, including the development of education and training programs for the staff, the development of guidelines to assist the staff in preparing dosage recommendations, and repeatedly administering written examinations based on case studies until the required performance level is achieved (62).

A second level of program activity could evaluate whether all the appropriate patients are receiving pharmacokinetic dosing services. Criteria and standards can be established for each drug included in the service. One report described monthly reviews of a single drug by evaluating 25% of all patients who received that drug (61). The standard used stated that at least 90% of the patients that should be monitored were monitored.

Additionally, validation of the laboratory's serum analysis procedures should be routinely performed, perhaps as a part of the laboratory's quality program. The pharmacy department should evaluate the quality of the dosing service and recommendations. Also, criteria could be developed to evaluate the pharmacist's charting notations, the assessment of patient data, and the resultant recommendations (63).

Cardiorespiratory Arrest Team. Rather than an ongoing audit program, multidisciplinary efforts such as code blue team performance are frequently evaluated by a special audit. Four areas were included in one such audit (64): adequacy of equipment and medication, written policies and procedures, documentation of activities, and preparedness of team members. One of the results of this audit was the creation of measurable performance standards for team members: (1) policies and procedures must be understood by each team member; (2) each team member must know know to operate code blue equipment; (3) team members must know how to perform and assist in procedures often used during codes; (4) each must know how to identify and interpret various patient monitoring tools; (5) each must understand the use of various therapeutic modalities; and (6) each must know how to work with others as a team.

Nutritional Support Service. Retrospective audits to evaluate the quality of total parenteral nutrition (TPN) have been described (65). One special audit was used to determine the need for a nutritional support service (66). A multidisciplinary committee reviewed the following elements of care: (1) the percentage of patients losing >10% of total body weight since admission; (2) the percentage of patients having an albumin reading of <3.0 mg/dl; (3) whether the head of the bed was elevated during tube feeding; (4) whether daily calorie and protein intake were recorded; (5) whether central line dressings were changed according to protocol; (6) whether TPN was administered in accordance with orders and on schedule; and (7) whether patient nutritional requirements were met by the TPN. Objectives, criteria, and standards could be established for each of these elements permitting their incorporation in a quality assurance program.

Drug Information Service. An excellent review by Amerson and Wallingford (67) indicates the absence of a uniformly accepted and implemented approach to quality assurance for drug information programs. Measurement of physician attitudes, questionnaires, and physician or peer review committees have been used in evaluative studies. One report did attempt to use process and outcome measures to evaluate a sample of written communications that had been implemented by the physician (68). Another approach used a multidisciplinary committee to retrospectively review responses from a drug information center (69). Among other things, the responses were graded as to accuracy and preparation difficulty. Additionally, a one-page questionnaire was sent to the user to determine his satisfaction with the service. The quality assurance program for the Rocky Mountain Drug Consultation Center consists of a nine-physician medical advisory board to retrospectively evaluate responses

by the center (70). Follow-up calls to consumers requesting information was also considered useful to determine if the information was helpful.

The Special Interest Group on Drug and Poison Information Practice of the ASHP is developing a document concerning guidelines for evaluating drug information centers. It is hoped that this effort will provide some needed direction in assuring quality (67,71).

Drug Utilization Review. Drug utilization review has been defined as "an authorized, structured, and continuing program that reviews, analyzes, and interprets patterns (rates and costs) of drug usage in a given health care delivery system against predetermined standards (72). Drug utilization review is an important part of pharmacy's total quality assurance effort. Over the years, it has often been the only quality assurance activity conducted by many pharmacy departments. Even though many of the concepts discussed in this chapter apply to developing drug utilization review programs, this topic deserves more detailed treatment; accordingly, a separate chapter is provided.

PERFORMANCE STANDARDS

This chapter has concerned itself primarily with the services provided by pharmacy departments. Quality assurance assesses the value of the services provided not the performance of individuals. The word "standard" has so far been used to mean the amount of permissible deviation from a norm or criteria. However, throughout the discussion in this chapter references have also been made to standards of practice. Developed by the profession, such standards describe what the pharmacist does in fulfilling his responsibility. Standards also describe what can be expected by regulatory and accrediting agencies and the public. Developing such documents is one of the major responsibilities of the professional organizations. In addition to the already discussed *Practice Standards of the American Society of Hospital Pharmacists* (30), the American Pharmaceutical Association has also published *Standards of Practice for the Profession of Pharmacy* (73).

Some pharmacy departments have developed their own set of practice standards applicable specifically to their department. The previous section on clinical services described such an effort by the University of Illinois (60). Here standards of practice served as a foundation for a quality assurance effort directed toward bringing about consistency and improved quality. In developing the standards, the staff reviewed all activities to determine those with a positive impact on patient safety or drug therapy. Criteria and standards for the quality assurance program were then based on the minimum standards developed as a result of this review. Other who have developed practice standards indicate they have served as a management tools in recruitment, orientation and training, performance planning, and review and in describing staff responsibilities (74). However, standards of practice only address the "what" question; they describe which specific functions or tasks should be performed. A job description also normally deals with what duties and responsibilities are assigned to a position. Neither addresses the question of "how well" the individual is performing the assigned responsibilities. Vogel et al (75) at the University of Illinois acknowledge that audits to determine if the department is in compliance with the minimum standards may describe whether a service is performed but does not determine if it was performed competently. Establishing this fact is possible with the development of individual standards of performance for each person's job.

A performance standard is a statement of conditions that will exist when a job is satisfactorily performed. Performance standards allow the individual to know whether his performance is good or whether further development is needed. The employee does not have to wait until his annual performance appraisal to learn that he was not doing the job expected. It has been estimated that the majority of formal appraisal systems are trait rating systems [76]. Emphasis is on personality characteristics and behavioral patterns. Performance standards, on the other hand, are known and accepted by the employee in advance and focus attention on the desired results.

The standards must be measurable. They should be challenging, but they must also be realistic and achievable. The employee's participation in this process should aid this objective. Each responsibility in the job description may have one or more standards associated with it. However, in the beginning it is best to focus first on the key responsibilities. Standards can be designed to measure quality, quantity, time, or cost associated with the job responsibilities. They should be specific so that one knows when the results are satisfactory; words such as "adequate," "approximate," "few," "reasonable," and "desirable" should be avoided. There are several approaches to results measurement. A standard that is based on the results the organization needs is termed an "engineered standard." One that is based on the results that have been produced previously is a "historical standard." Finally, a standard that is based on the results that others are achieving is a "comparative standard" [76-78].

An example of a standard for a technician in the unit dose cabinet filling process could be that the job is performed satisfactorily if the number of cabinet filling errors identified as a result of the pharmacist's final check does not exceed 0.2% of the total number of doses dispensed during the audit period. This could be considered an engineered standard. Although this standard may indeed satisfy the criteria for a good performance standard, all of the work put into thinking through the job with the technician and establishing agreed upon standards is futile if the data to measure performance is not collected. Sometimes it is too difficult or costly to collect data, or perhaps the way in which to measure good performance is uncertain. Even though one does not know what he wants, he may know what he does not want. In cases such as this it is possible to set a negative standard. An example of another engineered standard is that performance is satisfactory is there is no evidence of aminoglycoside toxicity in patients for which a physician has requested a pharmacokinetic consult and accepted the pharmacist's dosing recommendation.

Establishing standards of performance can be a very time-consuming process. It requires careful review of each job and the participation of the staff. For these reasons the task is often not undertaken. A good set of standards can complement the quality assurance program and serve as a target for the employee and his supervisor to gauge current performance and the need for future improvement.

REFERENCES

1. Vanagunas A, Egelston EM, Hoskins J, et al: Principles of quality assurance. *Qual Rev Bull* 5(2):3-6, 1979.
2. Crosby PB: *Quality is Free.* New York. McGraw-Hill, 1979.
3. Donabedian A: *Explorations in Quality Assessment and Monitoring.* vol I: *The Definition of Quality and Approaches to its Assessment.* Ann Arbor, Health Administration Press, 1980.
4. Stewart JE: Effect of quality assurance efforts on patient care. *Top Hosp Pharm Mgt* 1(3):21, 1981.
5. Jessee WF: Quality assurance systems. Why aren't there any? *Qual Rev Bull* 3(11):16-18, 1977.
6. *Model Quality Assurance Programs for Hospital Pharmacies,* rev ed. Bethesda, American Society of Hospital Pharmacists, 1980, pp 3-9.
7. Lohr KN, Brook RH: Quality assurance and clinical pharmacy: Lessons from medicine. *Drug Intell Clin Pharm* 15:758-765, 1981.
8. Minimum standard for pharmacies in hospitals. *The Bull Am Soc Hosp Pharm* 7:31, January/February 1950.
9. Fischelis RP: The philosophy of the minimum standard. *The Bull Am Soc Hosp Pharm* 7:30, January/February 1950.
10. ASHP guidelines on the competencies required in institutional pharmacy practice. *Am J Hosp Pharm* 32:917-919, 1975.
11. Zero defects in hospital pharmacy service. *Hosp Pharm* 2(3):11-16, 1967.
12. Schwermin FJ: Development of a program concept of zero defects in the hospital. *Hosp Pharm* 2(3):17, 20-21, 1967.
13. *Title XI,* f 249 F.(b), 42 U.S.C. g, 1320c et seq (1974).
14. Schumacher DN: Hospitals and PSROs: Can quality compete with cost? *Qual Rev Bull* 7(11):2-3, 1981.
15. Sandrick KM: PSROs' stormy past and questionable future. *Qual Rev Bull* 7(11):4-8, 1981.
16. Richards G: Business spurs UR growth: Hospitals are coming under increased scrutiny from outside utilization review. *Hospitals* 58(5):96-100, 1984.
17. Roberts JS, Walczak RM: Toward effective quality assurance: The evolution and current status of the JCAH QA standard. *Qual Rev Bull* 10(1):11-15, 1984.
18. Christoffel T, Jacobs ND, Jacobs CM: Audit results. *Qual Rev Bull* 2(4):32-35, 1976.
19. *The PEP Primer.* Chicago: Joint Commission on Accreditation of Hospitals, 1974.
20. *Accreditation Manual for Hospitals.* Chicago: Joint Commission on the Accreditation of Hospitals, 1979.
21. AMH/84: *Accreditation Manual for Hospitals.* Chicago: Joint Commission on the Accreditation of Hospitals, 1983, pp 147-149.
22. AMH/84: *Accreditation Manual for Hospitals.* Chicago: Joint Commission on the Accreditation of Hospitals, 1983, pp 133-142.
23. Thompson RE: Integrating patient concerns into quality assurance activities. *Qual Rev Bull* 8(2):16-18, 1982.
24. Morrison BJ, Rehr H, Rosenberg G, et al: Consumer opinion surveys. *Qual Rev Bull* 8(2):19-24, 1982.
25. Knapp DA, Knapp DE, Brandon BM, et al: Development and application of criteria in drug use review programs. *Am J Hosp Pharm* 31:648-656, 1974.
26. Vanagunas A: Quality assessment: Alternate approaches. *Qual Rev Bull* 5(2):7-10, 1979.
27. Brodie DC: Drug-use control—keystone to pharmacy service. *Drug Intell Clin Pharm* 1:63-65, 1967.
28. Johnson RE, Campbell WH, Christensen DB: Quality assurance of pharmaceutical services in hospitals. *Am J Hosp Pharm* 31:640-647, 1974.
29. Broekemeier RL, Brewer PE, Johnson MK: Audit mechanism for hospital drug distribution. *Am J Hosp Pharm* 37:85-88, 1980.
30. *Practice Standards of the American Society of Hospital Pharmacists 1983-84.* Bethesda, American Society of Hospital Pharmacists, 1983.
31. *Practice Standards of the American Society of Hospital Pharmacists 1983-84.* Bethesda, American Society of Hospital Pharmacists, 1983, pp 88-94.
32. Land MJ, Gaska J, Shull JC, Jones DR: A comprehensive quality assurance program for hospital pharmacy departments. *Top Hosp Pharm Mgt* 1(3):81-89, 1981.

33. Oakley RS, Bradham DD: Review of quality assurance in hospital pharmacy. *Am J Hosp Pharm* 40:53-63, 1983.

34. Stolar MH: Qulaity assurance of pharmaceutical services: Objective based planning strategy. *Am J Hosp Pharm* 38:209-212, 1981.

35. Beddie DJ: Viewpoint. Care circles—an approach to improving quality and controlling costs. *Top Hosp Pharm Mgt* 2(4):78-81, 1983.

36. Parness MI: Quality circles as a management tool for hospital pharmacy. *Am J Hosp Pharm* 39:1189-1192, 1982.

37. Louie C: Experiences in utilizing the quality circle concept. *Hosp Pharm* 18:63-64, 67, 1983.

38. Zelonis A, Fleischer N, Walling RA: Pharmacy quality assurance program. *Hosp Formul* 14:205, 208-209, 211, 1979.

39. Vogel DP, Gurwich E, Campagna K, et al: Pharmacy unit devises quality assurance plan. *Hospitals* 54:83-85, June 1980.

40. Somani SM, Giese RM: Design of a revised controlled substances distribution system. *Am J Hosp Pharm* 39:612-618, 1982.

41. Horowitz K, Lamnin M: Design and implementation of a quality-assurance program for pharmaceutical services. *Am J Hosp Pharm* 37:82-84, 1980.

42. Hoffmann RP, Ravin R, Colaluca DM, et al: Development of a multihospital pharmacy quality assurance program. *Hosp Pharm* 15:365-380, 1980.

43. White SJ, Godwin HN: A unit dose quality assurance program. *Hosp Pharm* 12:90-96, 1977.

44. Zoebelein E, Levy M, Greenwald RA: The effect of quality assurance review on implementation of an automatic stop-order policy. *Qual Rev Bull* 8(8):12-17, 1982.

45. Primary bacteremia—Illinois. *Morbid Mortal Wkly Rep* 25:110, 115, April 16, 1976.

46. Sarubbi FA, Wilson MB, Lee M, et al: Nosocomial meningitis and bacteremia due to contaminated amphotericin B. *JAMA* 239:416-418, 1978.

47. Plouffe JF, Brown DG, Silva J, et al: Nosocomial outbreak of candida parapsilosis fungemia related to intravenous infusion. *Arch Intern Med* 137:1686-1692, 1977.

48. Sanders LH, Mabadeje SA, Avis KE, et al: Evaluation of compounding accuracy and aseptic techniques for intravenous admixtures. *Am J Hosp Pharm* 35:531-536, 1978.

49. Zellmer WA: Solving problems associated with large-volume parenterals I: Pharmacist responsibility for compounding intravenous admixtures. *Am J Hosp Pharm* 32:255, 1975.

50. Recommended methods for compounding intravenous admixtures in hospitals. National Coordinating Committee on Large Volume Parenterals. *Am J Hosp Pharm* 32:261-270, 1975.

51. Recommended guidelines for quality assurance in hospital centralized intravenous admixture services. National Coordinating Committee on Large Volume Parenterals. *Am J Hosp Pharm* 37:645-655, 1980.

52. Recommended standards of practice, policies, and procedures for intravenous therapy. National Coordinating Committee on Large Volume Parenterals. *Am J Hosp Pharm* 37:660-663, 1980.

53. *AMH/84 Accreditation Manual for Hospitals*. Chicago: Joint Commission on Accreditation of Hospitals. 1983, p 136.

54. Stolar MH: Assuring the quality of intravenous admixture programs. *Am J Hosp Pharm* 36:605-608, 1979.

55. Morris BG, Avis KE, Bowles GC: Quality-control plan for intravenous admixture programs. II: Validation of operator technique. *Am J Hosp Pharm* 37:668-672, 1980.

56. Gurwich EL, Hanold L, Schaeffer PA: First-phase qualtiy assurance program for intravenous admixture aseptic technique. *Hosp Pharm* 17:119-121, 1982.

57. Frieben WR: Control of the aseptic processing environment. *Am J Hosp Pharm* 40:1928-1935, 1983.

58. Posey LM: Establishing quality assurance systems for admixture services. *Am J Hosp Pharm* 40:1902, 1983.

59. Ray MD: Administrative direction for clinical practice. *Am J Hosp Pharm* 36:308, 1979.

60. Vogel DP, Gurwich E, Hutchinson RA: The quality assurance of professional staff. *Curr Concepts Hosp Pharm Mgt* 3(2):8-17, 1981.

61. Lawson LA: Quality assurance program for a clinical pharmacokinetics service. *Am J Hosp Pharm* 39:607-609, 1982.

62. Burkle WS, Matzke GR, Lucarotti RL: Development of competency standards of quality assurance in clinical pharmacokinetics. *Hosp Pharm* 15:494-496, 1980.

63. Maddox RR: Administrative aspects of clinical pharmacokinetic services. *Top Hosp Pharm Mgt* 2:61-73, 1982.

64. Duafala ME, Holder LM: Multidisciplinary audit of cardiorespiratory arrest response patterns. *Hosp Pharm* 17:329-330, 335-337, 1982.

65. Schutz DD, Egging P: Quality assurance in TPN. *Nutr Supp Serv* 2:13, 15-16, 1982.

66. Griffin RE: Organization and management of a nutrition support service. *Top Hosp Pharm Mgt* 2:51-60, 1982.

67. Amerson AB, Wallingford DM: Twenty years' experience with drug information centers. *Am J Hosp Pharm* 40:1172-1178, 1983.

68. Keys PW, South JC, Duffy MG: Quality of care evaluation applied to assessment of clinical pharmacy services. *Am J Hosp Pharm* 32:897-902, 1975.

69. Pearson RE, Lauper RD, Davis LJ: Experience with a drug information services review committee. *Am J Hosp Pharm* 32:31-34, 1975.

70. Conner CS, Murphrey KJ, Sawyer D, et al: Drug information services for consumers and health professionals. *Am J Hosp Pharm* 37:1215-1219, 1980.

71. Rosenberg JM: Drug information centers: future trends. *Am J Hosp Pharm* 40:1213-1214, 1983.

72. Brodie DC, Smith WE: Constructing a conceptual model of drug utilization review. *Hospitals* 50:143-144, 146, 148, March 1976.

73. Kalman SH, Schlegel JF: Standards of practice for the profession of pharmacy. *Am Pharm* NS19:133-147, 1979.

74. Neal T: Minimum standards aid performance. *Hospitals* 54:70-73, February 1980.

75. Vogel DP, Gurwich E, Campagna K, et al: Pharmacy unit devises quality assurance plan. *Hospitals* 54:83-85, June 1980.

76. Pickering PH: Using performance standards for employee development. *Health Services Mgt* 13(1):6-9, 1980.

77. Alewine TC: Performance appraisals and performance standards. *Personnel J* 61:210-213, 1982.

78. Wells RG: Guidelines for effective and defensible performance appraisal systems. *Personnel J* 61:776-782, 1982.

Quality Assurance (QA) Programs for Hospital Pharmacy Reported During 1974-1982 (Table 61.1)

1. Land MJ, Gaska J, Shull JC, et al: A comprehensive quality assurance program for hospital pharmacy departments. *Top Hosp Pharm Mgt* 1:81-89, November 1981.

2. Zelonis A, Fleischer MN, Walling R: A pharmacy quality assurance program. *Hosp Formul* 14:205-211, 1979.

3. American Society of Hospital Pharmacists: *Model Quality Assurance Program for Hospital Pharmacies*, rev ed. Washington, DC, American Society of Hospital Pharmacists, 1980.

4. White SJ, Godwin HN: A unit dose quality assurance program. *Hosp Pharm* 12:90-96, 1977.

5. Broekemeier RL, Brewer PE, Johnson MK: Audit mechanism for hsopital drug distribution. *Am J Hosp Pharm* 37:85-88, 1980.

6. Gurwich EL, Hanold L, Schaeffer P: A first-phase quality assurance program for intravenous admixture aseptic technique. *Hosp Pharm* 17:119-121, 1982.

7. Horowitz KN, Lamnin M: Design and implementation of a quality-assurance program for pharmaceutical services. *Am J Hosp Pharm* 37:82-84, 1980.

8. Hoffmann RP, Ravin R, Colaluca DM, et al: Development of a multihospital pharmacy quality assurance program. *Hosp Pharm* 15:365-380, 1980.

9. Vogen DP, Gurwich E: Campagna K, et al: Pharmacy unit devises quality assurance plan. *Hospitals* 1:83-85, June 1980.

10. Burkle WS, Matzke GR, Lucarotti RL: Development of competency standards for quality assurance in clinical pharmacokinetics. *Hosp Pharm* 15:494-496, 1980.

11. Burkle WS: Developing a quality assurance program for clinical services. *Hosp Pharm* 17:125-147, 1982.

12. Lawson LA, Blouin RA, Parker PF: Quality assurance program for a clinical pharmacokinetic service. *Am J Hosp Pharm* 39:607-609, 1982.

13. Keys PW, Giudici RA, Hirsch DR, et al: Pharmacy audit: An aid to continuing education. *Am J Hosp Pharm* 33:52-55, 1976.

14. Johnson RE, Campbell WH, Christensen DB: Quality assurance of pharmaceutical services in hospitals. *Am J Hosp Pharm* 31:640-647, 1974.

15. Visconti JA: Drug use review. In Smith MC, Brown TR (eds): *Handbook of Institutional Pharmacy Practice,* ed 1. Baltimore, Williams & Wilkins, 363-374, 1979.
16. Stolar MH: Assuring the quality of intravenous admixture programs. *Am J Hosp Pharm* 36:605-608, 1979.
17. National Coordinating Committee on Large Volume Parenterals: Recommended guidelines for quality assurance in hospital centralized intravenous admixture services. *Am J Hosp Pharm* 37:645-655, 1980.
18. Tremblay J: Creating an appropriate climate for drug use review. *Am J Hosp Pharm* 38:212-215, 1981.
19. King RC, Cheung AK: Drug therapy review as part of a medical audit process. *Am J Hosp Pharm* 35:578-580, 1978.
20. McGowan JE Jr, Cross ML, Walker HK, et al: Reviewing initial choice of antimicrobial therapy—problems for the individual hospital. *Am J Hosp Pharm* 36:376-378, 1979.

ADDITIONAL READING

Johnson RE, Campbell WH, Christensen DB: Quality assurance of pharmaceutical services in hospitals. *Am J Hosp Pharm* 31:640-647, 1974.
Knapp DA, Knapp DE, Brandon BM, et al: Development and application of criteria in drug use review programs. *Am J Hosp Pharm* 31:648-656, 1974.
National Coordinating Committee on Large Volume Parenterals: Recommended guidelines for quality assurance in hospital centralized intravenous admixture services. *Am J Hosp Pharm* 37:645-655, 1980.
Oakley RS, Bradham DD: Review of quality assurance in hospital pharmacy. *Am J Hosp Pharm* 40:53-63, 1983.
Stolar MH: Quality assurance of pharmaceutical services: Objective based planning strategy. *Am J Hosp Pharm* 38:209-212, 1981.
Vogel MS, Gurwich E, Hutchinson RA: The quality assurance of professional staff. *Curr Concepts Hosp Pharm Mgt* 3(2):8-11, 14-17, 1981.

Special Topics

The designation ''Special Topics'' was chosen carefully. The topics covered are indeed special. Although each might have been ''forced'' into one of the other sections, all deserve special consideration.

CHAPTER 62

Consulting to Long-Term Care Patients

JAMES W. COOPER, Jr.

The need for consultant pharmacist services in long-term care has become much more evident in the past decade. Problems of illicit nursing home practices, poor health care professional performance, and failure to detect and recognize problems in long-term care have been answered, with proposed solutions of expanded pharmacy involvement in the care of the chronically ill patient.

The purpose of this chapter is to summarize the scope and results of consultant activities, their legal and professional bases, and to detail as yet unresolved problems in the pharmacy care of the long-term care patient.

Need for Consultant Services

A recent 2-year study has found that a comprehensive drug regimen review of long-term care facility patients detects a significant drug-related problem (i.e., unwanted effect of drug therapy) every other month throughout their length of stay (1). The rank order of problems and examples found is detailed in Table 62.1. The consultant pharmacist has been shown to decrease overall medication costs, adverse drug reactions and interactions, medication errors, hospitalization, and mortality rates of long-term care patients. In fact, when the consultant is no longer used, overall drug costs have been shown to increase markedly and subsequently decrease when consultant services are reinitiated (2). The results of selected studies are listed in Table 62.2.

Principle. The reduction of drug-related problems and medication-associated costs in long-term care patients is associated with increased consultant pharmacist involvement in comprehensive pharmaceutical services.

Guidelines for Consultant Practice

Consultant pharmacy is a blend of community and institutional practice. The three overlapping areas of professional functions are administrative, distributive, and clinical, as outlined in the guidelines in Table 62.3. The development of guidelines and standards for consultant pharmacy practice concerns three primary forces: regulatory, accreditation, and professional.

Federal regulations require consultant pharmacist activity in long-term care facilities (LTCFs) as a condition of participation (7,8). In addition, there are federal "indicators" for surveyor assessment of the performance of drug regimen review and overall pharmaceutical services (9). On a state level, at least one or more divisions of licensure, regulation, and/or reimbursement inspect each facility at least annually using federal standards and regulations (8-10) as a basis for the facility's annual certification and reimbursement.

Some LTCFs, especially those considered to be an extension of an acute care facility, seek other facility recognition by the Joint Commission on Accreditation of Hospitals (JCAH) (10).

Federal Medicaid regulations also allow the states to work out a mechanism for paying the consultant pharmacist *separate* from the fee paid to the vendor pharmacist. Few states have elected to formalize this payment and most have instructed facilities to pay for this service out of a per diem rate. In addition, federal regulations also allow states to work out a payment mechanism for compensation for unit dose systems, which to date again only a few states have elected.

A common problem occurs when the vendor is also a consultant and the nursing home operator expects the consultant services free or at an unreasonable rate in exchange for the vendor's prescription business. This has been considered illegal and both the pharmacist and the facility operator are subject to federal penalties of fine and/or imprisonment (11). Federal and state surveyor expectations for consultant services, however, are being implemented on a gradual basis as the "state of the art" advances.

Most pharmacists serving LTCFs in any capacity are community pharmacists with little institutional practice training. Two professional organizations serve the consultant pharmacist—the American Society of Consultant Pharmacists (ASCP) and the Long-term Care Section of the American Pharmaceutical Association (APhA) Academy of Pharmacy Practice. Only the ASCP thus far has chosen to advance Guidelines for Consultant Pharmacy Services (Tables 62.3 and 62.4) (12). The APhA has published a text on responsibilities for pharmaceutical services in the LTCF (13). The ASHP has published a supplemental standards and learning objectives guideline for residency training in geriatric pharmacy practice (14). The APhA and the American Association of Colleges of Pharmacy have published comprehensive standards for all areas of pharmacy practice (15). Tables 62.5 and 62.6 detail the ASCP guidelines respectively as to the administrative, distributive, and clinical range of services in the LTCF.

TABLE 62.1 Drug-Related Problems Detected Over a 24-Month Period in 102 Geriatric Long-Term Care Patients[a]

Categories	No (%) of Problems	Example
1. Medication administration and documentation errors	324 (26.5)	Omission of regularly scheduled antihypertensive—blood pressure increased 20-30/10-20 mm Hg
2. Relative contraindication to drug use	202 (10.5)	Use of KCl in patients with moderate renal impairment (CrCl <50 ml/min) and serum K greater than 5 mEq/liter
3. Nutritional/hematinic assessment consideration	128 (10.5)	Patient with consistent weight loss not on restricted caloric intake or who had serum albumin <3.5 g/dl or total lymphocyte count <1500, especially if decubitus or chronic UTI/catheter present
4. Socioeconomic consideration	124 (10.1)	Patient/family unable to pay for medication—recommend less expensive alternative therapy
5. Adverse drug reaction	118 (9.6)	Suspected digoxin toxicity with anorexia, digoxin held because pulse <60 and digoxin level <2 ng/ml
6. Drug duplication	78 (6.4)	Multiple antipsychotic use in patient with dementia
7. Questionable drug efficacy	47 (3.8)	Papaverine use in dementia
8. Therapeutic need by history but treatment modality not ordered	46 (3.8)	History of glaucoma
9. Drug-drug interaction	43 (3.5)	Antacids given with iron salt or tetracycline; anemia still present or bronchitis not improved
10. Lab test or blood level needed to assess drug therapeutic/toxic end point	42 (3.4)	Request serum potassium in patient with Hx hypokalemia on furosemide and digoxin; digoxin level request in suspected toxicity
11. Dosing interval/schedule simplification	24 (2.0)	Drug with >24-hour half-life dosed qid
12. No established diagnosis but drug used or used inappropriately	21 (1.7)	Antidepressant prn for sleep or depression
13. Patient refusal or inability to take chronic care medication	18 (1.5)	Refusal to take antihypertensive with blood pressure increase
14. Dosing modification/length of therapy or change to drug with shorter half-life	9 (0.7)	Request use of shorter rather than longer half-life benzodiazepine in patient with abuse history and carryover sedation
TOTAL	1224 (100)	

[a]Reprinted by permission from Cooper JW: Drug-related problems in geriatric long-term care facility patients. *N Engl J Med* (submitted for publication).

TABLE 62.2 Selected Studies of Consultant Pharmacist Effect on Drug-Related Problems and Drug Use in Geriatric LTCF Patients

Authors	Population Studies	Period of Time	Effects	Projected Cost Savings
Cheung and Kayne (3)	517 SNF patients, 3 facilities	11 mo	Prevented 69 drug-induced hospitalizations or 33 preventable ADRs/1000 patient months	$49,000/yr (1972)
			Reduced medication errors from 20-8% of doses	
			Reduced inappropriate or unnecessary drugs	$20/patient/mo
			Overall savings effect	$0.73/patient/day
Floyd and Thompson (4)	147 SNF patients, 1 facility	31 mo	Prevented 18 ADR-related hospitalizations or 6 ADR/100 patients/month	$9000/yr (1977)
			Overall savings	$0.20/patient/day
Strandberg, et al (5)	10% of 4004 patient records, 3 facilities	8 yr	42.8% decrease in number of pharmacy doses	—
			28.9% decrease in average monthly medication bill	—
Kidder (6)	Review of 7 studies, including ref. 3		Decrease in drugs per patient ranged from 0.9-2.44	Overall (1978) Medicare/Medicaid $3.2-37.2 million/yr

TABLE 62.3   Guidelines for Consultant Pharmacists Practicing in Long-Term Care Facilities[a]

These guidelines for practice pertain to the pharmacist providing consultant services to a long-term care facility.

1. The consultant pharmacist seeks the qualifications, outlined in these guidelines, to practice as a consultant pharmacist.
2. The consultant pharmacist maintains at least 20 contact hours of post-graduate continuing education annually in subjects relative to the practice of consultant pharmacy to assure continued competence.
3. The consultant pharmacist practices within the bounds of all state and federal laws and regulations and the Code of Ethics of the American Society of Consultant Pharmacists.
4. The consultant pharmacist enters into a written contractual agreement with the long-term care facility to which he/she provides service.
5. The consultant pharmacist supervises the entire spectrum of the pharmaceutical services in the long-term care facility, seeking as a goal the attainment and maintenance of the highest quality pharmaceutical services.
6. The consultant pharmacist assesses the drug therapy of each patient at least monthly.

[a]Reprinted by permission from *Guidelines for Consultant Pharmacists Practicing in Long-Term Care Facilities.* Arlington, VA, American Society of Consultant Pharmacists, 1981.

Long-Term Care Patients and Levels of Care

The typical long-term care patient is over 65 years of age and as such is termed "geriatric." Over three fourths of patients in long-term care are in this geriatric group. The most common diseases and conditions found in this group are arthritides, cardiovascular problems, and mental problems.

In a paper that projects the use of medical care forward and backward from 1950 to 2050, institutional care is projected to consume a rapidly expanding share of the medical care budget in the next century, especially in the care of the aged nursing home patient, projected to increase 12.8 per 1000 of the population in 2050, greater than twice the 5.4 per 1000 of 1975 (16). For the immediate future, nursing home expenditures are clearly one of the fastest accelerating categories of medical care expenditures, doubling between 1978 and 1985 ($15.8 to over $32 billion) and are projected to double again before 1990 to about $76 billion or about one of every ten dollars spent on health care in the United States (17).

Within LTCFs are three levels of care. Skilled nursing facilities (SNFs) provide 24-hour nursing care and holistic personal needs and are intended to provide some rehabilitative therapeutic goal for each patient. Intermediate care facilities (ICFs) provide more custodial than nursing care

TABLE 62.4   Consultant Pharmacist Qualifications[a]

GUIDELINE 1

The consultant pharmacist seeks the qualifications outlined in these guidelines as a consultant pharmacist.

Interpretation

The consultant pharmacist seeks to meet the following qualifying guidelines to practice in a long-term care facility. Licensure to practice is understood.

Training

The consultant pharmacist should have:

1. Knowledge of the state and federal laws and regulations governing the operations of the long-term care facility in which he/she practices.
2. Knowledge of all state and federal laws and regulations governing the acquisition, disposition, handling, storage, and administration of drugs in the long-term care facility in which he/she practices.
3. Knowledge of the legal responsibilities of the consultant pharmacist to the long-term care facility.
4. Knowledge and proficiency in the evaluation of the long-term care facility's compliance with all state and federal laws and regulations governing the acquisition, disposition, handling, storage, and administration of drugs.
5. Proficiency in assessing the nursing staff's performance in delivery of pharmaceutical services.
6. Proficiency in evaluation and monitoring drug administration systems.
7. Knowledge and proficiency in formulation of policies and procedures for all aspects of pharmaceutical services in the long-term care facility.
8. Knowledge of stability characteristics and storage requirements for drugs and biologicals.
9. Knowledge of the responsibilities of and proficiency in the conduct of committees responsible for governing the development and performance of pharmaceutical services in the long-term care facility.
10. Experience in training the staff of the long-term care facility in the areas of performance of pharmaceutical services, laws and regulations governing the handling, storage, administration, acquisition, and disposition of the drugs in the facility, and the use and effects of drugs and drug products.
11. The ability to effectively communicate with physicians and other health professionals concerning the care and treatment of patients.
12. Appreciation for the essentials of clinical diagnosis and comprehension of the medical management of the patient.
13. Knowledge of the physiology of the aging process and how it affects drug therapy.
14. Knowledge of the social and psychological needs of the aged patient as it relates to drug therapy.
15. Understanding the rational use of drugs, the proper application of drugs to disease states, the principles of pharmacology and pharmacokinetics, mechanisms of action, commercial drug combinations, dosage forms, recommended dosage ranges, factors which influence the physiological availability and biological activity of drugs, the influence of sex, age, and secondary disease states on the course of treatment, the potential interaction of other administered drugs, foods, and diagnostic tests on drug therapy.
16. Understanding the proper interpretation and application of laboratory tests as they relate to the clinical use of drugs.
17. Understanding of the development and application of the parameters necessary for the monitoring of drug therapy.
18. The ability to obtain patient drug histories and perform patient interviews.

[a]Reprinted by permission from *Guidelines for Consultant Pharmacists Practicing in Long-Term Care Facilities.* Arlington, VA, American Society of Consultant Pharmacists, 1981.

TABLE 62.5   Consultant Pharmacist Supervision Guidelines[a]

GUIDELINE 5

The consultant pharmacist supervises the entire spectrum of the pharmaceutical services in the long-term care facility, seeking as a goal the attainment and maintenance of the highest quality pharmaceutical services.

Interpretation

Definition: Pharmaceutical Services

Pharmaceutical services refers to all aspects of the acquisition, handling, storage, and administration of drugs in the long-term care facility, including all systems, methods, documentation, and facilities for: receipt and interpretation of physicians' orders; ordering and receipt of medications (from all sources), both house and individual patient supplies, on a routine and emergency basis; handling of emergency drug supplies; labeling and storage of all drugs, biologicals, and poisonous substances housed and used in the facility; disposition, release, and administration of all drugs, and biologicals used in the facility; parameters for use and administration of drugs and quality control of the service; and all aspects of the pharmacist's consultant service to patients.

Definition: Directing/Supervising

The consultant pharmacist actually directs development of the pharmaceutical services, the policies and procedures, the parameters for drug use, and the quality control standards. Directing being used in the common sense of the word.

The consultant pharmacist, as supervisor, acts as an overseer.

In these capacities the consultant pharmacist interacts directly with all members of the staff involved in development and performance of pharmaceutical services; however, the administrative staff of the facility is responsible to direct and supervise the staff in performance of pharmaceutical services, the correction of problems, and the carrying out of the recommendations and directions of the consultant pharmacist.

Definition: Monitoring

Monitoring involves review, evaluation, problem detection, and problem solving. The term "monitoring" refers to checking and auditing. The consultant pharmacist need not perform the actual checks; however, he/she directly oversees the process and assesses and interprets the findings and prepares and presents reports of findings and recommendations.

Considerations

1. The consultant pharmacist visits the LTC facility at least monthly to perform the above functions.
2. The consultant pharmacist logs all visits to the LTC facility showing time spent and function performed.
3. The consultant pharmacist provides appropriate in-service education for the LTC facility staff.
4. The consultant pharmacist monitors all aspects of the pharmaceutical services on at least quarterly basis and submits a *quarterly report* on the status of the development and performance of the services to the administrative staff and, where established, the committee or governing body responsible for overseeing the services.

Supervision

Supervision of pharmaceutical services includes but is not limited:

1. Directing, supervising, and monitoring the development of all aspects of pharmaceutical services.
2. Directing and supervising the development of all policies and procedures for the services.
3. Overseeing and monitoring the implementation and application of all policies and procedures for the services.
4. Overseeing and monitoring the performance of the services for accuracy, conformance with facility policies and procedures, and compliance with state and federal laws and regulations.
5. Participating in solving problems with the development and performance of the services.
6. Directing, supervising, and monitoring the development, implementation, and application of all parameters for drug use and administration in the facility.
7. Directing, supervising, and monitoring the development, implementation, and application of all necessary quality control standards for the services.
8. Participation in the training of the individual staff members involved in the performance of pharmaceutical services in the areas of orientation, performance of the services, state and federal laws and regulations, and use and effects of drugs and drug products used in the facility.
9. Supervising the dissemination of necessary drug information to the administrative nursing and medical staff of the facility and patients where necessary.
10. Participation in supervising and coordinating the interaction of all disciplines interacting with pharmaceutical services in the facility.
11. Reporting on the status of the development and performance of the services to the administrative staff of the facility, and where established the governing body or committee charged with overseeing the development and performance of pharmaceutic services.
12. Actively participating, where established, on the committee or governing body charged with overseeing the development and performance of pharmaceutical services.

[a]Reprinted by permission from *Guidelines for Consultant Pharmacists Practicing in Long-Term Care Facilities.* Arlington, VA, American Society of Consultant Pharmacists, 1981.

to those persons who can still provide some of these personal needs. A subcategory of the ICF is that intended for the mentally retarded (ICF-MR) patient who is usually at the age range from childhood to early adulthood and needs some help in activities of daily living, nursing, and occupational and rehabilitative therapy.

With the advent of prospective payment mechanisms and diagnosis-related groups, those financing acute hospital care are looking to LTCFs and agencies such as home health and alternative health services as well as congregate housing,

hospice, community physical and mental health centers, and personal care options to lower the overall cost per patient. For example, long-term hospital stays for extended courses of parenteral or enteral nutritional therapy or antimicrobial regimens may be a thing of the past, with the same care available outside of the institutional environment at a much lower cost.

These additional less costly levels of care can provide excellent opportunities for consultant pharmacist activity. Whereas the services of a pharmacist are now required only

TABLE 62.6   Drug Regimen Review Guidelines[a]

GUIDELINE 6

The consultant pharmacist assesses the drug therapy of each patient at least monthly.

Interpretation

1. *Drug Therapy Review*

The consultant pharmacist assesses the drug therapy of each patient in the long-term care facility at least, on a monthly basis. The review is performed primarily at the facility. The consultant makes special provisions to assure that a newly admitted patient's drug therapy is reviewed as soon as possible after admission.

Intent of the Therapeutic Review

The consultant pharmacist applies his/her specialized knowledge and experience in the field of pharmacology and pharmaceutics to review the patient's drug therapy; to assess the appropriateness and rationality of the therapy as prescribed by the patient's physician; to determine that the therapy is optimal and economic; that the therapy, as designed, carries the least possible risk of adverse effects; that the therapy is successful and, where not, that the therapeutic failure is not the result of inappropriate therapy, inappropriate drug administration, or error in administration; and that necessary and appropriate parameters for use and monitoring of the drug therapy are established and being properly applied.

Considerations

The consultant pharmacist considers all drug orders and all other orders related to and/or pertinent to the drug therapy. He/she considers all pertinent patient data, including patient drug and food allergies, diet activities, diagnoses, medical history, physical assessments, current complaints, progress, vital signs, weight records, laboratory and other diagnostic tests, and any other data necessary to thoroughly evaluate the appropriateness and rationality of the drug therapy.

The consultant pharmacist engages, as necessary, in consultation with the nursing staff, patient, the patient's physician, and other disciplines involved with the care of the patient to complete a thorough and effective evaluation of the patient's drug therapy.

Comments/Recommendations and Recommendation

The consultant pharmacist makes comments and recommendations to the attending physician and, where appropriate, the nursing staff regarding necessary deletions, additions, alternatives to the drug regimen, alterations in dosage, time and route of administration, necessity for laboratory, diagnostic, and vital signs tests, and any other comments and recommendations necessary to ensure that the optimal drug therapy is established, is being achieved, and is being properly monitored. The consultant pharmacist documents the performance of the review and documents comments and recommendations.

2. *Drug History Taking*

The consultant pharmacist sees that proper drug history information is obtained on admission of each new patient.

3. *Continuity of Care*

The consultant pharmacist sees that all pertinent drug information becomes part of the patient's medical record.

[a]Reprinted by permission from *Guidelines for Consultant Pharmacists Practicing in Long-Term Care Facilities.* Arlington, VA, American Society of Consultant Pharmacists, 1981.

in LTCFs, there are no barriers to compensation for cost-effective consultant activity in the following areas:

1. *Home health care and other agencies serving long-term care clients.* Intended to be an alternative to either acute or long-term hospitalization, home health care is either institutionally based as an extension of the hospital, LTCF, or as a freestanding agency. On a physician's order, home health care provides a set number of patient visits per month and monthly evaluations from a team usually consisting of a registered nurse, a social worker, various therapists, and a nutritionist. Despite recent difficulties in establishing the overall cost effectiveness of this level of care (without pharmacist consultation) compared to institutionalization, several studies (18,19) have indicated a significant number of patients (one fourth to one third) have drug-related problems that may indicate the need for a legislated or regulatory mandate for the consultant pharmacist similar to that for the LTCF. Other agencies serving long-term care clients include area councils on aging, senior citizen's centers, and community mental health centers (20).

2. *Alternative health services.* Alternative health service is an experimental program in some states where qualified individuals may take a patient (or patients), who may be a candidate for ICF certification, into their home for a fee that is much less than the usual monthly nursing home cost. The individual agrees to supervise activities of daily living, food, laundry, and some medication. It remains to be determined

whether this will become a viable level of care, but the consultant and agencies providing referral and supervision of these patients may well need to be aware of a potential consultation opportunity and the abuse potential of some rest home environments that sparked the scandals in the nursing home industry in the 1960s, lest the cycle repeat itself.

3. *Day care.* Adult day care centers are flourishing, usually as an extension of or associated with area senior citizen's centers or councils on aging. Some states are promulgating specific regulations for their operation. Ideally, an adult day care center should be a licensed facility that provides an organized program of weekday, daytime therapeutic, social, and health activities aimed at rehabilitation to the self-care or personal level of family supervision, or as a further alternative to institutionalization. There appear to be a number of administrative, distributive, and clinical activities that can be efficiently and effectively provided by the consultant pharmacist (21).

4. *Congregate housing.* The high-rise apartment complex that offers a place to reside, a social system, and some administrative supervision of overall personal capability and security is a further opportunity for consultant pharmacist activity. One study has found that most drug-related problems in persons residing in this type of housing occur in those 75 years of age or older (22). Improved compliance in a noncompliant geriatric congregate housing facility pop-

ulation has been shown with weekly consultant clinical pharmacist visits and special reminder packaging of medication (23). It should be recalled that the key factor in drug-related hospital admissions, which account for up to one third of geriatric admissions, is noncompliance (24).

5. *Hospice.* Holistic care of the terminally ill patient should involve the consultant pharmacist in medication monitoring and supervision, especially in pain management.

6. *Community and state physical and mental health centers.* Most states have a public health emphasis in physical and mental health that addresses the needs of the medically indigent patient. Without innovative consultant pharmacist activity, there is little doubt that excessive drug dosages, waste, pilferage, and drug-associated morbidity and mortality occur in this population (24,25).

6. *Personal or self-care.* As the least expensive level of care, the opportunity for personal determination of care-associated expenses depends much more on the individualistic rather than the paternalistic philosophy of health care, the educational level, and the mental capability of patients to learn proper self-care habits, as well as consultant pharmacists' desire to teach patients or their families to take care of themselves. Numerous third-party payers are providing compensation for consultant educational activities with patients and families (26). Whereas these services plus medication monitoring and supervision most logically arise from community pharmacy practice, there remain precious few studies documenting these expanded consultative roles.

CONSULTANT FUNCTIONS

The administrative and distributive functions of the consultant pharmacist may be acquired by trial-and-error field experience. The clinical activities of the consultant pharmacist is the area in which most consultants acknowledge the greatest need for additional training.

Standards for baccalaureate and doctoral clinical training are set by the American Council on Pharmaceutical Education and postdoctoral training by the ASHP, and are usually administered through schools of pharmacy and hospital pharmacy departments. The clinical activities of the consultant pharmacist can be viewed as a continuum of effort from the time the patient enters the LTCFs, agencies, or pharmacy services through periodic evaluations and subsequent care.

Twelve areas of clinical responsibilities are listed below. Few consultants thus far have developed all areas to the point of minimal proficiency. This list, therefore, represents a compilation of clinical activities now being performed that may be a goal for many and minimal proficiency for some consultants.

1. *Drug history.* A complete drug history is essential from several points of view. The first concerns continuity of care, particularly if the LTCF attending physician is not the same practitioner who provided care in the community.

Second, compliance and drug use are extremely important from the standpoint of the patients' subsequent need for drugs in the facility. Furthermore, the starting point of any clinical activity should be a complete knowledge of all prescription and over-the-counter drugs taken by the patient before admission, as well as the use pattern of each drug.

A preadmission or admission survey checklist to be completed by the patient and the family is an invaluable tool.

2. *Problem list.* Developing a complete problem list requires the consultant pharmacist to be thoroughly familiar with the chart, not merely the drug orders. In addition, the physician's history and physical, the nurses' history, assessment, and subsequent nurses' notes, along with social, family, dietary, and drug history all give background information that help establish verified problems for the individual patient, particularly those related to drug therapy. In essence, one cannot establish a rationale for therapy without a knowledge of historical events in the patient's life. The consultant may be the initiator of problem-oriented medical record keeping (POMR) in an LTCF.

3. *Parametric monitoring of the LTCF patient.* Parametric monitoring of the LTCF patient requires the consultant to be thoroughly familiar with pharmacotherapeutics, using knowledge of the anatomy, pathology, and pathophysiology of specific disease states and realistic therapeutic end points or goals of therapy in terms of each patient problem. The two main types of parameters with which the consultant pharmacist is concerned are (1) physical parameters, including the vital signs, symptoms, and complaints offered and observations made by all health care personnel; and (2) laboratory parameters (i.e., which lab test should be done on admission and routinely for each particular drug or groups of drugs a patient is taking).

4. *Patient-oriented regimen review.* The patient-oriented regimen review draws on the first three activities. It is based on knowledge of the patient's prior drug use, verified problems, and parameters of the individual patient's problems to be monitored. The pharmacist reviews the patient's progress toward therapeutic end points to verify the need for continued therapy or to suggest changes that could improve the patient's response and/or prevent problems.

The review of the therapeutic regimen, however, also involves assessing the integrity of the distribution system (i.e., checking for medication errors). The essential documents for a patient-oriented drug review include the pharmacist's dispensing records, records of drugs that have been dispensed to the patient (nurses' Kardex and/or administration records), and the patient's chart, especially orders and progress and nurses' notes.

5. *Communication of clinically significant problems.* Communication of clinically significant problems is perhaps the area of greatest concern for the consultant pharmacist and other health care personnel. Practical methods of communicating anticipated, suspected, or realized problems of individual patients should be stratified in terms of increasing significance as doubtful, potential, possible, probable, and documented problems.

The urgency of a problem may necessitate an immediate phone call to the prescriber. In less urgent situations, written means may be used. Official vs unofficial means of communication are also important.

Problems of documented significance affecting patient care should be placed in the universal progress notes of the patient, preferably in a problem-oriented fashion. In fact, regulation requires notation in the chart that the review has been conducted and whether a problem is found. Documented or probably significant problems should be carefully communicated in terms of unofficial means as simple as a note on the chart, a two-way communication form with a line drawn down the middle for physicians', nurses', and pharmacists' responses, or by keeping a nursing pharmacy log on which all communicants sign off (28).

Nevertheless, records should be kept of all suspected problems to document one's activities. On the other hand, no statement should be put in the chart that one is unwilling to back in court testimony with qualified professional opinions or judgment.

6. *Adverse drug reactions and interactions.* Adverse drug reactions and interactions are a source of primary concern to the consultant in the initial and subsequent assessments of the patient's regimen. Individual adverse reactions should be classified as to (1) side effects, (2) idiosyncratic, and (3) toxic effects, or (4) allergic reactions, listed in the hierarchy form previously mentioned and appropriately noted in the patient's chart and monthly report of the drug regimen review.

7. *Patient care rounds and conferences.* Patient care rounds and conferences are an extremely important activity, in which the consultant's contribution to discussions is invaluable, but in many facilities it is a practical impossibility for the consultant to be present when rounds are to be made unless there is a specified time during which the individual physician would see the majority of patients. There should be a regular schedule of patient care rounds and individual monthly or bimonthly assessments of each patient's problem, with consideration of the consultant's recommendations.

8. *Pharmacokinetic and nutritional consultations.* Pharmacokinetic consultation is extremely important because drugs are in general metabolized more slowly and excreted more slowly in the elderly patient. Knowledge of the drugs for which this is important (e.g., digoxin) is indeed an area of concern about medication errors and assessing the patient's response to therapy.

9. *Patient, family, prescriber, and LTCF personnel education.* It is extremely important to change or modify the situations or address problems raised by the consultant. In-service education and newsletters are methods that generally produce the best results—among patients and families as well—and make the prescriber aware of significant new developments that may benefit the LTCF patient or reinforce the drug knowledge of the LTCF personnel. Education comes at this point in the continuum because it does provide a method for modifying behavior, response, or activities in the areas previously mentioned (numbers 1-9).

10. *Objective drug information retrieval, analysis, and communication.* It is extremely important to review claims made for new drugs or new uses for old drugs, as well as drug comparisons (i.e., is a new drug really better, does it possess significant advantages, does it produce significant side effects that may not have been documented by the manufacturer, does it benefit a particular type of patient?). (See Section III, "Drug Information and Drug Actions.")

11. *Primary care activities of the consultant pharmacist.* Primary care by the consultant pharmacist in LTCFs is the most recent clinical activity of the consultant. The state of California currently has changed its regulations to allow consultant clinical pharmacists with doctoral level training

to provide primary care under physician supervision to SNF patients. The results of this study may provide a basis for further primary care functions for the consultant pharmacist (30).

Administrative Activities

The consultant pharmacist in long-term care is in many ways like a hospital pharmacy director in that he or she must supervise *all* aspects of the comprehensive pharmaceutical services delivered to patients. Previous chapters in this text document most of these activities. For the LTCF or agency there may be some differences that bear emphasis in administration. They are committee functions, in-service education, policy and procedure, and reports of the consultant.

Committee Functions

In examining the committee functions of the consultant pharmacist in LTCFs, one must consider, in particular, practical methods and expectations, committee purpose and responsibilities, along with an assessment of policy and procedure changes.

The three main committees that the consultant should be a part of in LTCFs are the Pharmaceutical Services Committee (PSC), Infection Control Committee (ICC), and Utilization Review Committee (URC). Additional consultant functions that may use a committee format include in-service and patient/family education and patient care.

It should be noted that federal surveyor standards employed by the various state field surveyors will look for documentation of the consultants' activities in each area. In some cases, very specific guidelines have been developed.

In each committee it is essential that:

1. All members understand the purpose and responsibilities of the committee.
2. Goals and objectives are realistic.
3. Adequate resource material is available, especially in patient data, literature references, and other input from the consultant. A motion should be tabled if more documentation is needed to reach an objective opinion.
4. All must recognize resistance to change as being part of human nature. Effective communications as to why change is needed may be helpful.
5. All must recognize that impasses may occur. This indicates the need for more documentation and discussion outside of the formal meeting.
6. Even when new policies and procedures have been established, assessment of the implementation, effectiveness, and total system effects must be an ongoing responsibility of each committee member.
7. Agenda and activities must adequately document committee work.

Pharmaceutical Services Committee (PSC). The PSC should consist of the provider and the consultant pharmacist administrator, one physician (ideally the medical director), and the director of nursing services. It has the responsibility for developing and evaluating written policies and procedures (P&P) concerning drug therapy distribution, administration, accountability control, and use.

The PSC develops and annually updates the pharmacy P&P manual. It further determines the level and types of medication services needed by the patient and how well the staff discharges these services.

Where possible, a formulary system should be developed to minimize drug therapy costs. In addition, the PSC has the overriding final responsibility for the optimal use of the medication modality of treatment in the facility. Some specific areas of concern would be:

1. Minimizing medication or charting errors
2. Anticipating and preventing adverse reactions and interactions
3. Reducing irrational prescribing
4. Simplifying the drug administration procedure

The PSC must meet at least quarterly. The consultant's monthly reports and follow-up should be considered, and persistent communication difficulties remedied by committee (not consultant) letter to the individual prescriber. The consultant does not have to document change; only that an attempt was made to communicate concerning problems. Some problem areas may involve multiple psychotherapeutic drugs, nightly hypnotic drug use, bowel care, vitamin and hematinic use, digoxin use, and diuretic use without a laboratory assessment of serum potassium and creatinine levels. Nursing follow-up should be noted, especially where serious medications errors have occurred.

Infection Control Committee (ICC). The ICC should include representatives of all professional and service staff/departments of the facility (i.e., medical, pharmacy, nursing, administration, dietary, social work, occupational and physical therapy, housekeeping, maintenance).

The committee should develop methods for investigating, controlling, and preventing infections in the facility. In particular, attention has to be paid to handwashing technique (especially between incontinent patients), floor cleaners, antiseptic use, bed-linen changes, catheter care, and prophylactic antimicrobial and topical antibiotic use (especially the aminoglycosides).

The consultant should also monitor staff performance using his or her knowledge of nosocomial infections, bacterial susceptibility, resistance to antibiotics, and antiseptics for given situations.

Utilization Review Committee (URC). All professional staff members of the facility should belong to the URC. Its main objective should be the optimal use of all professional services—sufficiency, level, frequency, appropriateness, and cost effectiveness.

Recognizing inappropriate drug use is the primary function of the consultant on this committee. In a positive way, the consultant should also be able to provide information on less expensive yet efficacious approaches to medicating documented patient problems.

In some facilities, the Patient Care Committee may function as an extension of the URC. The consultant addresses those points of the care plan that pertain to drug therapy—whether therapeutic benefits can be expected, over how long a period a therapeutic trial may be warranted, and the efficacy rating of specific drugs, continuous psychotherapeutic

drug therapy without dose changes, nutritional and vitamin supplements, decubitus treatment, and laxative use.

In-Service Education

In-service education by the consultant pharmacist centers on the following three main areas:

1. A problem-oriented approach that addresses current problems with the drug distribution system, therapeutic effects, adverse reactions, inappropriate drug use, and the need for further assessment by observation and/or laboratory tests
2. Review of specific patient therapeutic problems that could be avoided by better drug monitoring
3. An ongoing review and quizzing on the practical pharmacology of the drugs most commonly used in the facility to ensure that staff members are familiar with the drugs being administered

Patient/family education is important in avoiding drug-related problems. Unauthorized drugs, foods, and salt substitutes can create significant patient problems.

In self-care units or areas studies show that 60% of uninstructed patients make errors in drug use. Patient education can reduce this to a 2-3% error rate via increased patient/family knowledge of therapy (what the drug is for, how to take it, what to expect, etc) (31).

Policy and Procedure in Long-Term Care

The authority for the development of a P&P manual comes from the PSC of the facility. Whereas the pharmacist may provide a draft form of this manual, it is essential that all policies be workable for the nursing and medical staffs. In fact, rules proposed in 1980 as Conditions of Participation would have required this and have tacitly been enforced since this date.

Scope. The pharmacy P&P manual should cover all aspects of life and accurate drug use control and services, from acquisition of the drug through administration and observation of drug effects on the patient.

Guidelines. Since the ultimate assessment of the efficacy of the P&P manual is in the hands of the state surveyor and is influenced by federal and state guidelines, attention should be directed to the most current guidelines, which are found in the *Federal Register*, July 14, 1980, proposed rules changes for SNFs and ICFs.

Regulations Changes. The most important development over the past decade is that the director of nursing assumes co-responsibility for providing and supervising pharmaceutical services. For the director of nursing, this means assurance that drug orders are expeditiously filled, administered, and documented safely and accurately. In addition, there are limits on unaccounted for Schedule II-IV drugs and drug administration error rates. The Drug Enforcement Administration accepts *no* unaccounted for Schedule drugs. Stop orders are also required in the 1980 revised regulations. The final significant change concerns the pharmacist.

In addition to the drug regimen review and report of all SNF faculty patients, all ICF patients should have a similar review conducted by the pharmacist rather than by the nurses. No separate regulations exist for the ICF patient; all are de facto combined despite the Secretary of Health and Human Services Statement that the proposed changes would not be enforced. It has also been suggested that these regimen reviews be integrated into patient care planning activity.

Pertinent P&P Points. The following points should be considered in a comprehensive P&P manual:

1. Purpose of the manual
2. P&P authorization—PSC makeup
3. Pharmacist services agreement (provider and consultant)
4. Patient drug history and drugs brought into facility
5. Patient drug regimen review
6. Drug formulary and product selection
7. Drug ordering and delivery and distribution system
8. Emergency order provisions
9. Drug administration and documentation
10. Stop orders
11. Drug returns, discontinuation and disposal
12. Discharge pass/LOA medications
13. Controlled substances
14. Bedside medications
15. Drug samples
16. Investigational drugs
17. Reports
18. Medication errors
19. Adverse reactions
20. Follow-up on problems

This should not be reviewed as an all-inclusive list of topics to be considered in a pharmacy P&P manual. Several references at the end of this chapter will aid in the formulation of a complete P&P manual (32,33).

Caveat. The P&P manual is a dynamic record of what will be done and how it will be done. Any dynamic system changes constantly, and the manual should be updated and reviewed at least annually by the PSC.

Reports

Reports from consultants are used to document the need for their services, as well as the performance of drug-related functions and responsibilities under contracts between institutions and/or agencies.

For the purposes of this chapter, it is assumed that the provider and the consultant may be one and the same person or two individuals.

Some facilities still encourage pharmacists to participate in a "paper consultant" activity. In the face of ever stronger federal and state guidelines, this is a practice that is certain to decline. More and more, "indicators" are being employed to determine facility and consultant compliance.

Federal regulations now specify that the report must be done at least quarterly. Monthly reports with a quarterly summary that might serve as a working agenda for the quarterly PSC meeting are preferable.

The content of the report will vary with contractual responsibilities and the extent of the facility's needs. In gen-

eral, three areas should be addressed—administrative, distributive, and clinical (or patient oriented).

Administrative. The administrative section deals with problems in overall performance by those concerned in prescribing, dispensing, and administering drugs. Problems in communication are of chief concern, especially where multiple providers and prescribers are employed. Committee functions discussed in a previous section may help rectify some problems. Personal contacts, however, are preferred. Pertinent questions include:

1. Are committees functioning or serving their purpose?
2. Are personal contacts between the consultant, provider(s), prescriber(s), and those administering drugs effective? If so, to what degree? What are the recurring problems?

Verbal or written discussions may be summarized as to content, changes, or comments, and subsequent response or lack of response or change.

Distributive. The distributive section concerns acquiring, ordering, dispensing, administering, and verifying drugs. Pertinent questions that should be addressed include:

1. Is the prescriber seeing the patient and signing orders to make the orders legal?
2. Are drugs and treatments being given as ordered or signed off as being given? Do dispensing refill records indicate the same?
3. Are orders being recopied correctly? Do the orders, pharmacy profile, medication administration record (MAR), and prescription containers (non–unit dose) agree? If medication cards or tickets are used, do they agree with the above?
4. Are missed or extra doses accounted for? Is wastage or spillage being reported?
5. Are any drugs in short supply locally or regionally? Have the orders been filled promptly? Were the orders given to the provider promptly?
6. Are standing or routine orders in use or legal? If so, are stop orders employed?
7. Are prn drugs being used appropriately and signed off in the MAR and the effects noted in nursing notes? If prn drugs are being used several times a day, should they be regularly scheduled to save a special call, as well as the nurse's time?
8. Are stop orders in effect for all drugs? If so, is the physician called at least 24 hours before the stopping order for critical drugs (e.g., anti-infectives, anticoagulants, narcotic analgesics)?
9. Is there a method for determining medication errors—charting, counts, verification of administration?
10. Are incident reports filed for critical medication errors that affect patient care? Does the consultant review these? Can you reduce or prevent their recurrence? How?

Clinical (or Patient-Oriented). The clinical (or patient-oriented) section presents a patient-by-patient summary of clinical and distributive problems, irregularities, or deficiencies noted and/or communicated to those prescribing, dispensing, and administering drugs using the following format:

Chart 1

Patients of Dr. _____

Review for _____ _____ _____
              (Month)   (Year)   (Facility)

Patient Name	Problem/ Recommendation	Response/ Results
1. _____	_____	_____
2. _____	_____	_____
3. _____	_____	_____
4. _____	_____	_____

Drug Distribution Systems in Long-Term Care

The system by which drugs are ordered, filled, dispensed, administered, and recorded should be continually evaluated and revised to meet patient and facility needs, as well as professional and regulatory standards. A drug distribution system is defined as the sum of activities that provide patient medications.

Staff members in long-term care facilities and agencies must be knowledgeable about the drug distribution system (or systems) used for their patients and residents. It is essential that the administrator, the director of nursing, and other members of the nursing staff accept the challenge to educate everyone who administers drugs and treatment under a nursing license.

At the same time, provider/vendor pharmacists—especially consultant pharmacists—need to cooperate in a plan that guarantees a thorough understanding of the drug distribution system. The ultimate goal is to ensure maximum efficiency and a minimum error rate and to cut down on wasted staff time and waste in medications.

System Components

A review of the components of a sound drug distribution system is the first step to understanding it. They include:

1. Ordering the medication
2. Filling the medication order
3. Expeditious delivery of the medication
4. Checking the medication order
5. Entering the order in the MAR
6. Assigning appropriate administration times, schedules, and stop orders
7. Patient's identification and drug administration as appropriate vital signs and patient's condition are evident
8. Verifying drug administration, refusal, omission, or other action
9. Refilling chronic use medications or verifying validity of stop orders
10. Recopying drug orders, the MAR, and the verifying agreement with prior orders

The P&P manual as written by the PSC should state what system is to be employed and how each of these steps is to be accomplished. This manual is a dynamic description of the system. Not only must it be understood by all, it must also be evaluated and changed to meet the needs of the individual facility as conditions dictate. This means that the PSC should examine the P&P manual at least annually to determine just how well the system is meeting the needs of safe drug distribution and the needs of the patient and the facility.

Problem Areas

The following problem areas may make it more difficult for the consultant to supervise the distribution system:

1. Multiple drug providers
2. Incomplete, missing pharmacy dispensing records or failure to supply pharmacy dispensing records to the consultant
3. Incomplete or incorrect MARs and chart orders
4. Turnover of nursing personnel
5. Failure of all personnel to read, comprehend, and adhere to the pharmacy P&P manual
6. Poor compliance with prior consultant recommendations
7. Failure to recognize that a problem exists

The solutions to these problems are obvious but not always easy to accomplish. A single provider who furnishes adequate records, charges that are accurate, and MARs that reflect actual use, in-service training with quizzes on the distribution system, the P&P manual, and problems detected (along with solutions), and motivated pharmacy and nursing professionals who reliably anticipate, prevent, and/or correct problems is taking a long stride toward a solution.

Although the present staff may well understand how the drug distribution system is supposed to work, the problem of constant nursing staff turnover in the LTCF or agency demands a procedure to ensure that new staff comprehend the system.

Types of Systems

Four basic types of drug distribution systems are in use: (1) floor stock, (2) individual prescription, (3) a combination of floor stock and individual prescription, and (4) unit dose in individual doses to doses per administration time for the month.

The first three falsely appear to be the least expensive in terms of total system drug cost. They do, however, share the disadvantage of an increased potential for medication errors, financial losses caused by misappropriation, decomposition, expiration, discards, and increased inventory and an inordinate amount of nursing personnel time in dose preparation (up to 40% of nurses' time). Unit dose is strictly defined (33), a 24-hour supply of unit of use packages of each medication are recorded on a patient profile and the MAR and are accounted for by the nurse and the pharmacist. In long-term care a 3- to 7-day supply of unit dose packaging (solid dose forms only) may be most feasible in current practice.

Whereas the cost of unit of use packaging increases the cost per dose and pharmacy technician personnel are required to set up the cart for the pharmacist's inspection, a unit dose system carries the following advantages:

1. Reduced incidence of medication errors
2. Decrease in overall (total personnel, drugs) cost of medication distribution
3. More efficient use of nursing personnel who could be directed to patient care involvement
4. Improved drug use control
5. More accurate patient billing for drugs
6. Fewer drug discards and/or credits

Although there are a number of variations to this system, a number of packaging systems are not unit dose in the sense that there are separate packages of each dose. There are card systems with doses prepackaged in a 30-day blister pack supply for each daily administration schedule time of the drug. Souffle cup setups of unpackaged doses with medication cards are another inappropriately named system. Pharmacies supplying unit of use packages in larger than 24-hour supplies (typically 2-30 days) may be considered to be offering a modified unit dose system.

LTCFs may employ partial unit dose systems in that only certain dose forms are unit-of-use packaged (e.g., solid oral dose forms). Total unit dose refers to a system in which all oral, peroral, and injectable dose forms come in a ready-to-administer form.

Implementing Unit Dose

Whereas some studies of unit dose provided documentation of the need for and cost effectiveness of such a system, state and private third-party payment groups have in large measure been reluctant to compensate equitably for such a system. At the same time, maximum allowable cost (MAC) ceilings (which supposedly may allow for unit dose packaging cost) on the reimbursable cost per dosage unit have made it at times difficult for the provider pharmacist to dispense a quality drug, much less with unit-of-use packaging.

According to the Title XIX *Medical Assistance Manual* (Section 6-160-30), "Authorized Prescription Pricing Methods, a . . . higher level of [state] reimbursement [could] be offered to pharmacies employing a unit dose system."

The responsibility for working out a payment mechanism rests with the provider, the LTCF, and the third-party payment groups.

12-Point System Checklist

Unit dose in LTCFs can be just as poor as the other three systems if:
1. 24-hour pharmacist or first-dose service is not available from a state or emergency drug kit
2. A long lag time exists between order initiation and drug readiness for patient administration
3. Inaccurate and/or incomplete records are kept
4. Careless cart filling, checking, and replacement occurs
5. Extra doses are supplied to account for waste, pilferage, or unaccounted for medicines
6. Excessive floor stock or bulk liquids are also used
7. Nurses remove the drug(s) from the unit dose package and place in souffle cups before medication rounds
8. Pharmacists do not find out why unadministered doses (other than prns) come back in the cart or exchange cassettes
9. Systems are used in which nurses still use drug tickets or cards to pass medications
10. Systems do not list and document all drugs (regularly scheduled and prn, as well as treatments and fluids) in a place readily visible to the physician, the nurse, and the pharmacist

11. Systems are used in which pharmacy and nursing personnel are not constantly checking each other by relying on their records, knowledge, and experience
12. Systems are used in which nurses borrow medication as starter doses or for supposed or actual missing doses (35)

Medication distribution control is indeed an LTCF team responsibility and part of the consultant's distributive supervisory function.

Medication Errors in Long-Term Care

A medication error is defined in a total system sense as an act of commission or omission pertaining to prescribing, dispensing, or administering drugs. The clinical ramifications of medication errors may range from insignificant to terminal. Unfortunately, health care professionals involved in prescribing, dispensing, and administering drugs make characteristic errors, as do patients, but medication errors are made by both professionals and patients.

Prescriber Errors

It is essential to have a complete and appropriate drug order for the patient. Prescriber errors include:
1. Incorrect or confusing nomenclature (abbreviations, acronyms, symbols). Only standard nomenclature should be used.
2. Inappropriate dose. Lean body weight and renal and hepatic function knowledge must be used. Dose requirements may be 20-50% lower for the elderly patient.
3. Failure to specify strength.
4. Failure to specify exact dose.
5. Incorrect or unspecified route of administration or dosage form. A concise formulary helps to rectify errors 3, 4, and 5. Those dispensing and administering the drug must also clarify incomplete information.
6. Inappropriate delegation of authority. Clear lines of responsibility must be established.
7. Illegible written orders.
8. Confusing oral orders. Clarification is essential (errors 7 and 8).
9. Failure to look at the total problem and the drug list of the patient before prescribing.
10. Failure to periodically assess the need for continued therapy. Other health professionals must contribute to the assessment process in errors 9 and 10, as well as cross check all types of errors.

The literature contains little information on the prescriber's role in creating drug hazards in the institution. Lack of prescriber documentation of history, therapy needs, progress, and outcome have been noted. A basic question has been raised concerning the rationality of preadmission drug therapy. One study found that primary diagnoses were inaccurate in 64% of SNF admissions. It also found that 84% of patients lacked or had inaccurate secondary diagnoses. Misdiagnoses of mental problems were the most common error (31).

Dispensing Errors

Medication errors in dispensing include:

1. Dispensing the wrong drug. The person administering the drug should be familiar with each medication and should never hesitate to question a change in dosage form size, color, or appearance.

2. Dispensing a drug of questionable quality and/or bioavailability. MAC ceilings may make this an increasing problem, but there are reliable manufacturers of generic products.

3. Incorrect or incomplete labeling of the drug, drug container, or the MAR. Regulatory standards by state agencies specify labeling requirements for drugs and the MAR.

4. Incorrect number of doses. It is crucial to account for each dose by comparing dispensing and administration records.

5. Failure to specify or clarify drug scheduling. The pharmacist should schedule drugs, especially oral forms, to maximize absorption, minimize gastrointestinal upset, and prevent the most common interactions between drugs (e.g., antacids with digoxin, iron salts, tetracyclines).

6. Failure to set up an efficient and safe distribution system.

7. Failure to specify stop order times. Specific stop orders and administration should be agreed on by the PSC for all regularly scheduled and prn drugs.

Few studies have been conducted concerning dispensing errors. It is essential that there be constant cross-checking between the nurse and the pharmacist to prevent, reduce, or correct errors in dispensing and administering drugs.

Administration Errors

Among the errors in administration are:

1. Omissions. Failure to give or chart the drug; omissions for which there are no apparent reasons. This can be further broken down into (1) doses given and not charted, (2) doses charted and not given, and (3) doses neither charted nor given. Accounting for each dose dispensed is essential.

2. Wrong dosage. The medicine cup is the greatest source of error with liquids, especially with smaller volumes. Oral dosing syringes enable one to more accurately measure smaller quantities of liquids.

3. Extra or unordered dose(s) given. Careful attention to the reconciliation of doses dispensed and administered should detect these errors.

4. Unordered medication. These errors occur when there is no order for the drug or the wrong patient receives an ordered drug.

5. Wrong dosage form or route of administration. Using a different form (tablet, capsule, suspension, injection) or route (po vs injection primarily).

6. Wrong time. Variously interpreted to be 30 minutes to 2 hours before or after the dose is ordered.

7. Deteriorated or outdated medication. Constant vigilance is mandatory to ensure the quality of each drug dispensed and administered.

Medication errors in administration can be classified as known or unknown. Although 100% reporting of known errors may occur, this is only the tip of the iceberg. Whereas up to one fourth of doses may be given in error with tra-

ditional floor stock and individual prescription systems, this error rate may be reduced to 3-20% of doses with unit dose systems, consultant pharmacist monitoring, and increased nursing supervision of administration (31).

Factors in administration errors include:

1. The number of drugs per patient. A systematic increase in errors has been reported when six or more drugs per patient are ordered.

2. The number of medication passes per patient day. Convenient administration schedules combining drug schedules should be attempted. In addition, many drugs (most anticonvulsants, thiazide, diuretics, some antihypertensives, many psychotropics) can be given once or twice rather than three to four times a day with no drop in therapeutic levels.

3. Poor communication. A nursing-pharmacy log should be kept on each nursing station to facilitate the communication of any events concerning drugs.

4. Lack of established procedure and/or knowledge of same. Policy and procedure concerning drug prescribing, dispensing, and administration should be clearly defined in the P&P manual of the PSC and read by all professionals.

5. Failure to note that a problem has occurred. The consultant pharmacist is responsible by DEA regulation for reconciling doses dispensed and administered for all Schedule II-IV drugs. In addition, each patient MAR sheet should be compared with pharmacy dispensing records to determine possible errors for all drugs.

This chapter has briefly discussed the need and scope of consultant pharmacy practice. For further background reading refer to the References.

REFERENCES

1. Cooper JW: Drug-related problems in geriatric long term care facility patients. *N Engl J Med* (submitted for publication).
2. Cooper JW: Effect of initiation, termination and reinitiation of consultant clinical pharmacist services in a geriatric long term care facility. *Med Care* 23:84-88, 1985.
3. Cheung A, Kayne R: An application of clinical pharmacy services in extended care facilities. *Calif Pharm* 23:22-25, 1975.
4. Thompson J, Floyd R: Cost-analysis of comprehensive consultant pharmacist services in the skilled nursing facility: A progress report *Calif Pharm* 26:22-25, 1978.
5. Strandberg LR, Dawson GW, Mathieson D, Rawlings J, Clark BG: Effect of comprehensive pharmaceutical services on drug use in long term care facilities. *Am J Hosp Pharm* 37:92-94, 1980.
6. Kidder S: The potential cost-benefit of drug monitoring services in skilled nursing facilities. *NARD J* 19:21-22, 1978.
7. *Federal Register,* January 17, 1974, p 228.
8. American Society of Consultant Pharmacists: *ASCP/Special Bulletin July—1980*. HCFA 42 CFR parts 405, 442 and 483), Arlington, VA, ASCP, 1980.
9. American Society of Consultant Pharmacists: *ASCP Special Bulletin— July 1982*, Section 3160FF, Survey procedures for pharmaceutical services in long term care facilities, and Section 3161, Indicators for surveyor assessment of the performance of drug regimen reviews. Arlington, VA, ASCP, 1982.
10. Joint Commission on Accreditation of Hospitals, Chicago.
11. *Medical Assistance Manual.* Title XIX, part 6-160-30.
12. *Guidelines for Consultant Pharmacists Practicing in Long-Term Care Facilities.* Arlington, VA, American Society of Consultant Pharmacists, 1981.
13. Gerson CK (ed): *More than Dispensing.* Washington, DC, American Pharmaceutical Association, 1980.
14. ASHP supplemental standards and learning objectives for residency training on geriatric pharmacy practice. *Am J Hosp Pharm* 39:1972-1974, 1982.

15. Kalman SH, Schlegal JF: Standards of practice for the profession of pharmacy. *Am Pharm* NS19:21-35, 1979.
16. Russell LB: An aging population and the use of medical care. *Med Care* 19:633-643, 1981.
17. Kingston ER, Scheffler RM: Aging: Issues and economic trends for the 1980's. *Inquiry* 18:197-213, 1981.
18. Cooper JW, Griffin DL, Francisco GE, Francis WR: Drug-related problems detected by consultant pharmacist participation in home health care. *Hosp Formul* 20:643-650, 1985.
19. Solomon DK, Baumgartner RP, Weismann AM, et al: Pharmaceutical services to improve drug therapy for home health patients. *Am J Hosp Pharm* 35:535-557, 1978.
20. Jinks MA: Pharmacy-consulting service to agencies serving elderly clients. *Am J Hosp Pharm* 40:1542-1544, 1983.
21. Williams BR: The pharmacist in adult day care centers. *Today's Nurs Home* 5:19,23-25, 1984.
22. Wade WE, Cobb HH, Cooper JW: Drug-related problems in a multiple site ambulatory geriatric population (abstract). Paper presented at the American Society of Hospital Pharmacists' 18th Midyear Clinical Meeting, Atlanta, December 7, 1983.
23. Joyner JL, Hikmat FT, Catania PN: Evaluation of a medication-monitoring service for geriatric patients in a congregate housing facility. *Am J Hosp Pharm* 40:1509-1512, 1983.
24. Frisk PA, Cooper JW, Campbell NA: Community-hospital pharmacist detection of drug-related problems upon admission to small community hospitals. *Am J Hosp Pharm* 34:738-742, 1977.
25. Wade WE, Whaley JA, Cooper JW, Brown RH: Pharmacist involve-
ment in Georgia public health departments preliminary report of two pilot studies. *Ga Pharm J* 3:20-22, 1981.
26. Doyal LE: Cost-effectiveness of the clinical pharmacist in community mental health center. Paper presented to the Department of Pharmacy Practice, College of Pharmacy, University of Georgia, Athens, April 1984.
27. *ASHP Task Force Final Report on Payment for Pharmacy Services.* Bethesda, American Society of Hospital Pharmacists, 1979.
28. Cooper JW: Monitoring drug therapy for the long-term care client. In Pagliaro LA, Pagliaro AM (eds): *Pharmacologic Aspects of Aging.* St. Louis, CV Mosby, 1983.
29. Cooper JW: Nutritional changes in long-term care patients. Paper presented to the Southeastern Society of Hospital Pharmacists, Athens, April 1984.
30. Thompson JF, McGhan WF, Ruffalo JT, et al: Outcome of a trial of clinical pharmacists prescribing drug therapy in a skilled-nursing facility in 1980-82 (University of Southern California Pharmacist Prescribing Project). Cited in *Am J Hosp Pharm* 40:1344, 1983.
31. Cooper JW: Drug therapy in the elderly. Is it all it could be? *Am Pharm* NS18:25-26, 1978.
32. Caruthers KS: *Development and Implementing a Pharmacy Policy and Procedure Manual for Skilled Nursing Facilities.* Sacramento, California Pharmaceutical Association Academy of Long Term Care, 1977.
33. *ASCP Policy and Procedure Manual.* Arlington, VA, ASCP, .
34. ASHP statement on hospital drug control systems. *Am J Hosp Pharm* 31:1198, 1974.
35. Davis N: A poor unit dose system versus a traditional system. *Hosp Formul* 13:478, 1978.

CHAPTER 63

Drug Regimen Review

RALPH KALIES

Quality assurance is not a newly found need of society and the individual, but dates back to at least 2000 BC. A Babylonian inscription reads, "If the doctor shall open an abscess with a blunt knife and shall kill the patient or shall destroy the sight of the eye, his hands shall be cut off." The need for quality assurance still exists in today's society. Indicators of such a need may be the increase in malpractice claims and the requirement of some third-party payment programs to obtain a second opinion before surgery is performed. Quality assurance does not only involve major medical interventions, but should also involve the drug prescription, which is often taken too lightly by our society and the practitioners prescribing such agents. Cheung and Kayne (1) put it this way: "Increased utilization of an even greater number of complex, highly potent and potentially toxic drugs, both prescription and nonprescription, for a full range of medical problems and patient complaints has resulted in an incidence of iatrogenic disease and therapeutic misadventures which is approaching the dimensions of a public health crisis."

Of all hospitalizations in the United States, 3% are related to an adverse response to a medication (5). Cheung and Kayne further stated that 15-30% of hospitalized patients experienced adverse drug reactions that increased the average hospital stay to nearly double when compared to patients who did not suffer adverse drug reactions. Of these, 10% are life threatening (2). The conservative cost estimate for these adverse reactions is about $3 billion per year (1).

THE ELDERLY

The elderly population is probably more at risk for iatrogenic disease than the general population as a whole. The elderly have altered pharmacokinetics (i.e., distribution, metabolism, excretion) of drugs because of decreased hepatic and renal function, alterations in body composition and blood flow, and a decrease in qualitative changes in the protein binding of drugs (3). In general, the efficiency of the individual organs of the body is lessened with age. Other potential complications of concern are the presence of multiple chronic diseases and changes in eating habits. These phenomena may lead to a higher rate of iatrogenic disease. The elderly population (persons over 65 years of age) is approximately 11% of the total U.S. population, but they consume 30% of the health care dollar and account for approximately 25% of the health care dollar spent on drugs (4-6). Greater than 85% of elderly ambulatory patients and approximately 95% of elderly, institutionalized patients receive medication (7,8). This is estimated to increase to 40% of health care dollar spent on drugs (9). By the year 2000, as the elderly population grows, it is projected they will consume 50% of all of the prescribed medications in this country (10). By the year 1995 the percentage of the population over 65 years of age is expected to be 17%, with the fastest growing percentage of that population being those over 85 hears of age.

As a result of multiple medication, pathologic conditions, and altered pharmacokinetics, the elderly are at greater risk of having adverse drug reactions (11,12). Seidl (13) showed the incidence of adverse drug reactions among patients 70-80 years of age was two times the incidence in patients 40-50 years of age. Melmon (14) reported similar findings. Frisk et al (15) found that 30% of patients over 65 years of age admitted to a small community hospital were there for drug-related reasons. Caranasco (16) found that adverse drug reactions may lead to hospitalization. This particular study looked at 6063 consecutive admissions and found that 3% were attributed to adverse drug reactions; 41% of these were patients over 60 years of age. Cluff et al (17) attributed adverse drug reactions to multiple drug therapy, the pharmacokinetic changes of aging, and noncompliance.

Of the elderly population, currently 2-5% are institutionalized. This number is also expected to increase. Nursing home beds in 1954 numbered 172,000; in 1979 they numbered 1.4 million; and today there are approximately 1.5-1.7 million patients in these facilities. It is projected that by the year 2000 there will be 2.8 million nursing home patients, in other words, an approximate doubling in 20 years' time (18,19).

The patients in long-term care facilities have special problems differentiating them from the ambulatory elderly and other institutionalized patients. The typical patient in a long-term care facility usually has 3.1 chronic conditions, and physical impairment is high (1). Prolonged and multiple drug management is common, with 6.1 different drugs being given on the average. Patients are more often in the geriatric group and may react differently to usual drug dosages. The attending physician sees the patient less frequently than hospitalized patients, and many times orders are written before the patient is seen by the physician. The nurse-to-patient ratio is low when compared to the hospitalized patient (1). The therapeutic goal of caring for patients in long-term care facilities also differs because it is a managing role rather than a curing one. This management may become complicated because one third of the elderly in long-term care facilities receive more than eight drugs daily and some receive as many as 12-16 (3). Of hospitalized patients in skilled nursing facilities 23% had the potential of having been drug-induced hospitalizations (20). Even more sobering is that elderly patients institutionalized for more than 6 months have little chance of being discharged to any place other than to a hospital (21).

In the 1960s, health care was becoming part of an interesting philosophy of this society. The philosophy was that health care was a right and that every citizen should have this right to health care. The elderly were no exception. The elderly placed a demand on the health care system and concern rose that elderly patients may not be able to meet the rising health care costs facing them. This brought about government payment (public financing) for health care for the elderly and the indigent. This, along with the increasing elderly population, the increasing ability to treat acute illnesses, the inability to treat chronic illnesses leading to a demand for limited medical and nursing care outside of the hospital, the changing living arrangements of families, and the increasing cost of hospitalization, led to the growth of long-term care facilities. That growth is anticipated to continue. Because public money was funneled into long-term care facilities by the government, there was also a concern for quality assurance.

The Social Security Amendments of 1965, Title 18 and Title 19 (Medicare, Medicaid), were enacted. Medicare was to provide medical coverage for patients over 65 years of age and Medicaid was to provide health care for the indigent. Besides funding for these programs, there was also a provision for utilization review. Even with this mandate, drug utilization review was not taken up in earnest.

In 1974, the regulations were revised not only out of concern for patients' well-being, but also because of the cost resulting from treatment without appropriate quality assurance. The new regulations essentially placed the pharmacist into a new role—performing monthly drug regimen reviews in skilled nursing facilities. Reports of any irregularities were to go to the medical director and the administrator. The new conditions of participation are as follows (22):

The skilled nursing facility provides appropriate methods and procedures for the dispensing and administering of drugs and biologicals. Whether drugs and biologicals are obtained from community or institutional pharmacists or stocked by the facility, the facility is responsible for providing such drugs and biologicals for its patients, insofar as they are covered under the programs, and for ensuring that pharmaceutical services are provided in accordance with accepted professional principles and appropriate Federal, State, and local laws. (See 405.1124 (g), (h), and (i).)

(a) *Standard: Supervision of services.* The pharmaceutical services are under the general supervision of a qualified pharmacist who is responsible to the administrative staff for developing, coordinating, and supervising all pharmaceutical services. The pharmacist (if not a full-time employee) devotes a sufficient number

of hours, based on the needs of the facility, during regularly scheduled visits to carry out these responsibilities. The pharmacist reviews the drug regimen of each patient at least monthly, and reports any irregularities to the medical director and administrator. The pharmacist submits a written report at least quarterly to the pharmaceutical services committee on the status of the facility's pharmaceutical service and staff performance.

After 1974, there were many studies done to show the effectiveness of the pharmacist involved in drug regimen review. As an example, Cheung and Kayne (1) found evidence that clinical pharmacists decreased the incidence of medication errors, decreased the incidence of adverse reactions and drug interactions, decreased the number of inappropriate or unnecessary drugs, and decreased the number of drug-induced complications. They also estimated their activity and activity like theirs could save approximately $80,000 a year per 300 patients.

The main point of this study was that pharmacists could be effective in drug regimen review, but problems still remain in regard to drug regimen review in the long-term care facility. There was a problem with reimbursement for drug regimen review that led to paper compliance. Pharmacists were involved in providing the medications and in reviewing the medications for appropriateness. The pharmacist was paid on a fee-for-service basis for the drugs provided, and as the amount of medication dispensed increased, so did the amount of reimbursement received by the pharmacist. The usual result of a drug regimen review is a decrease in the number of drugs. However, this is not necessarily true. This may give pharmacists a disincentive for engaging in rigorous drug regimen review (22). Discounts for drug services to acquire the prescription business also caused some pharmacist to "throw in" the consulting activities (drug regimen review) free of charge, which in itself may have led to suboptimal drug regimen review (23).

Based on the literature and the professional experience of the author, there is room for improvement in quality and/or efficiency in conducting drug regimen review in long-term care facilities. It is also the author's contention that a more systematic approach, taking into account quality assurance research and selected management theory, may result in improvements.

Even if the quality of drug regimen review was optimal at this point in time, quality assurance must also be cost effective: therefore, it is necessary to search for more efficient ways to conduct drug regimen review without compromising quality. This may include, but is not limited to, reviewing the person doing the review, the methods used, and attempting to semi-routinize the process to optimize the use of required resources and personnel.

DRUG REGIMEN REVIEWS IN LONG-TERM CARE FACILITIES

Drug regimen review has been taking place in long-term care facilities for at least the last decade. Besides the typical problems of quality assurance programs in other health delivery systems, the long-term care facility has additional limitations. These limitations are as follows: The long-term care facility handles patients with chronic illnesses. It is difficult to assign a beginning and an end to a chronic illness;

therefore, it is difficult to relate process with outcome. Medications ordered prn are not used for one specific disease, but may be used for many diseases over an extended time, making it difficult to determine the appropriateness of the process or the outcome. Charts in long-term care facilities are often missing information, especially a specific diagnosis. Without a specific diagnosis, it becomes almost impossible to determine the appropriateness of the drug therapy. There is probably a greater range and combination of disease states and levels of severity within one long-term care institution than in an ambulatory population, making it difficult to set up an appropriate quality assurance program. Finally, there is a low level of structure among medical staff members, who may see patients very infrequently and have little contact with other health care professionals or other members of the facility's medical staff. This alone makes it difficult to have an effective drug utilization review or quality assurance program in a long-term care facility.

The limitations just listed are definitely a concern, but they do not preclude the need society perceives for quality assurance or drug regimen review in these facilities.

Many studies have concerned the need for drug regimen review in long-term care facilities because of drug interactions, unusually high uses of psychotropics and tranquilizers, high costs, and inappropriate drug use (20,23-29).

Many studies have also shown the pharmacist's positive impact when conducting drug regimen reviews in long-term care facilities by decreasing costs and improving the drug therapy (30-41).

There has been a question about the validity of all of the potential drug interactions prevented and all of the potential drug problems curbed (and drug-drug interactions are just that, potential). The potential may not lead to an actual clinical situation requiring additional care or a decreased quality of care. This brings out the point of whether the effectiveness shown by many studies is nothing more than a potential effect.

One might also consider that using the consultant pharmacist to conduct drug regimen review in long-term care facilities may not be necessary continuously. The key here is continuous. Regulations require a monthly drug regimen review, but one particular study indicated two things: (1) that drug regimen review may not have to be as frequent as monthly and (2) if it is not continuous on some basis, drug use problems will reappear. Chrymko and Conrad (42) found that by placing a clinical pharmacist in the facility, the number of medications per patient decreased over a 2-month period. They also found that 12 months after removing pharmaceutical clinical services, the medication use increased to almost the level before the pharmaceutical clinical services were implemented. This study indicated that pharmaceutical clinical services in long-term care facilities should at least be long-term if not continuous each month.

There are other questions that need to be asked concerning the pharmacist's involvement in drug regimen review in long-term care facilities. One concerns the lack of adequate financial support for pharmacy consultants, which led to the paper consultant phenomenon. The paper consultant phenomenon is basically a situation in which the pharmacist consultant does not conduct an adequate drug regimen review; many times no drug regimen review is done other than signing that it was completed (23).

The paper consultant phenomenon may also be related to a lack of pharmacist's time to become involved in drug regimen review. Kidder (23) extensively explains the relationship of kickbacks and/or discounts to the potential decreased level of drug regimen review. He stated: "Thus if a discount is paid in order to gain prescription volume one would want to maintain that volume, not reduce it through the performance of indepth drug regimen review."

The complaints that compensation does not reach the pharmacist for drug utilization review and the paper consulting issue led federal Medicaid program administrators to issue the following reimbursement guideline (43):

Consultant pharmacists often complain that although the facility is reimbursed for the cost of pharmacy consultant service, the nursing home operator does not compensate the pharmacist for his consultant services. In such cases, the consultant pharmacist is also the prime vendor of prescribed drugs in the facility and the operator expects him to furnish consultant services free in exchange for obtaining the prescription business. This is illegal, and both the pharmacist and the facility operator are subject to Federal penalties up to a $10,000 fine or a year in prison or both.

In addition, this conflict of interest concern brought about 1977 Health, Education and Welfare guidelines, which stated that in "those geographical areas where it is possible and feasible," selected criteria used to evaluate drug utilization in a facility should be sought (43). Many thought during this period that consultant pharmacists could not objectively review drugs they had dispensed, which in turn would take money out of their pockets if they were to decrease the number of the medications dispensed through effective drug regimen review.

Other questions that need to be investigated concerning the effectiveness of drug regimen review in long-term care facilities are: How effective from a quality and a cost standpoint are these traditional methods of drug regimen review in long-term care facilities? Can these types of methods continually, without explicit criteria or significant structure to their drug regimen review process, meet both quality and cost-effectiveness standards of quality assurance?

The 1981 *State Operations Manual,* more commonly known as the "indicators," gave some description to drug regimen review. The "indicators" are not regulations, but are tools to be used by state surveyors when attempting to assure that appropriate drug regimen review is being done by the consultant pharmacist. It was a new policy statement, which read as follows:

NEW POLICY—Effective Date: April 1, 1982

Section 3160ff, Survey Procedures For Pharmaceutical Services in Long Term Care Facilities; and Section 3161, Indicators For Surveyor Assessment of the Performance Of Drug Regimen Reviews—The regulations for skilled nursing facilities, intermediate care facilities, and intermediate care facilities for the mentally retarded require either a nurse or a pharmacist, depending on the type of facility, to perform reviews of drug therapy on each patient on a periodic basis. In skilled nursing facilities, a number of studies have demonstrated the cost benefit of these reviews. The cost savings is realized through a reduction in the number of prescription orders utilized by the patients. Although this cost benefit potential exists, it is yet to be fully realized. In July 1980, The General Accounting Office released a report: "Problems Remain in Reviews of Medicaid Financed Drug Therapy in Nursing Homes.'' One of the criticisms in the report was the Department's failure to define what was expected in performing a ''drug regimen review.'' The ''Indicators for Surveyor Assessment of the Performance of Drug Regimen Reviews'' (section 3161) provide the State survey and certification agency with guidance for determining compliance with the requirements and generally define what is expected in the drug regimen review task.

State agency surveyor's assessment of the drug regimen review requirements is difficult because, heretofore, there has been little guidance which would aid the surveyor in making compliance/ noncompliance determinations. The purpose of these ''indicators'' is to achieve a greater degree of uniformity, objectivity, and reliability in surveying. In doing so, we hope to gain greater compliance and realize the potential offers.

Our conclusion that these ''indicators'' are necessary for the proper application of the regulations noted above is based upon continuing review of the enforcement of those regulations around the country over the past several years.

These indicators have been extensively tested by experienced surveyors and have been found to be a valid tool. The indicators have been widely circulated to numerous professional groups, and the response from these groups has been very supportive, with many endorsing them in principle.

The ''indicators'' set of explicit criteria (see Appendix 63.1) can be used by lesser trained individuals to determine whether or not an appropriate drug regimen review is being completed. It is in essence a quality assurance audit of a quality assurance audit that may not have been necessary if the drug regimen review had been more explicitly defined to begin with by the initial project developers. Even though the ''indicators'' set forth explicit criteria that provide an indication as to whether appropriate drug regimen review is being conducted in a long-term care facility, not meeting a criterion as it is indicated does not indicate a poor drug regimen review. Rather it must be taken in context with all of the other indicators to determine implicitly whether or not an appropriate drug regimen review is being provided for the residents of the long-term care facility.

The ''indicators'' may make two statements: (1) quality assurance regarding drug regimen review may be handled by explicit criteria and (2) if explicit criteria can be adequately developed, lesser trained, less expensive persons could use it to assure quality or at least to gather explicit information so a higher trained individual can make an implicit decision.

In summary, drug regimen review in long-term care facilities is perceived as a necessity. It has been suggested that the pharmacist might be the most appropriate person to conduct drug regimen reviews in long-term care facilities. There is also evidence that drug regimen reviews conducted by pharmacists in long-term care facilities have been very effective in decreasing the number of medications, potential drug problems, and the costs of medications.

On the other hand, many questions concerning drug regimen reviews in long-term care facilities remain, such as conflict of interest, kickbacks, discounts, paper compliance, and a lack of structured explicit activities, which spawned the ''indicators'' in 1981. Concerning costs, the question remains regarding whether the most cost effective way of conducting drug regimen reviews has been employed in early methodologies.

As time goes on, the number of drug regimen review problems may decrease, and if the proper internalization of information by other health care professionals has occurred, this may diminish the influence of the consultant pharmacist in these types of drug regimen reviews. Therefore, if the costs or methodologies used by the consultant pharmacist remain the same, the cost-benefit ratio will continually increase, making the process not cost effective and, therefore, providing inadequate quality assurance of the drug regimen.

SOME ATTEMPTED METHODS OF DRUG UTILIZATION REVIEW

Gilroy et al (44) used a computerized base method known as Promis in which all patient information is put into a computer and integrated with algorithms to provide feedback for corrective action in everyday medical practice.

Ishikura and Ishizuka (45) used a real-time computer-based system for checking drug interactions. They thought that by using this system they could advise the prescriber about items requiring clinical tests and treatments to prevent side effects, etc. Out of 169,230 prescriptions checked, 8.8% (14,965) were found to contain possible drug interactions.

Schaffner et al (46) looked at three methods to improve antibiotic prescribing in office practices. They used a mail brochure, a drug educator visit, and a physician visit. They found the mail brochure had no detectable effect and the drug educator had only a modest effect. However, the physician visit produced a strong, attributable reduction in prescribing both drug classes in the study.

Avorn and Soumerai (47) tested three methods. One employed no intervention; the second was an innovative series of printed materials urging appropriate drug use; and the third was a set of printed materials along with a visit from a consultant pharmacist who discussed the drugs in question. They found the consultant pharmacist to be the most effective.

Knapp et al (48) described a system of manual drug use review that used coded cards at the time prescriptions (orders) were processed in neighborhood health care centers. They used this to compile a summary of prescribing practices. These prescribing patterns were then reviewed by a committee. Nursing personnel were responsible for administration of medications, appropriate documentation of drug administration, and documentation and observation of medication effects in the nurses' notes. Brodie et al (39) states that the primary source document for drug utilization review in long-term care facilities is the medication administration record (MAR). Secondary sources are the physician's action (output). This is a cyclic process requiring the modification of criteria as the information dictates.

Brodie et al (39) described a model for drug use in long-term care facilities. The conceptual model for long-term care facilities should be directed to deficiencies in the facility and should be achievable within the constraints of the organizational structure and consist of six utilization review principles. (1) Authority—the person or body conducting drug utilization review should have formal authority. (2) The demographics and operational characteristics of the facility should be compiled. (3) Existing drug use profiles and a mechanism for setting standards and reviewing utilization should be developed. Here Brodie suggests that drug utilization review can take place at the same time each patient's drug regimen is reviewed at least monthly by the pharmacist. (4) There should be standards of appropriateness and review—Brodie further states that standards for drug use (standards of appropriateness) are the core of the program if drug utilization review is to function as a quality assurance mechanism. These criteria or standards should be reviewed by the medical staff, pharmacist, physician, director of nursing, and administrator. Brodie further discusses the need for pharmacists to take the leading role in establishing standards. He suggests that drug utilization review programs could be implemented on a selective basis, reviewing only selected medications because of their expense or likelihood of problems. (5) Remedial programs must be dictated by the deficiencies revealed during the drug utilization review program. Brodie thinks that the details for remedial programs are a matter of local decision, unless directed by the needs of the facility. (6) Evaluation is essential to assure that the program is successful.

Vancura and Marttila (49) described a systematic approach to monitor long-term care patients manually. Medical problem areas are listed along with baselines to alert the pharmacist to potential problems such as sensitivities, renal function, liver function, gastrointestinal absorption, catheters, bowel habits, and ambulatory status. It also has a review grid area as a drug reference monitoring device where the date of the drug review is entered along with the initials of the reviewing pharmacist and findings are described under seven general categories (adverse reactions, interactions, laboratory analysis, vital signs, rationality of drug therapy and subcategories, drug administration, recommendations).

Stewart et al (50) used a five-step method that involved selecting the health problem to be studied, developing criteria for care, measuring specific performance data for comparison with the criteria, establishing the audit committee evaluation process, and designing and implementing educational activities.

Vlasses et al (41) used the method of having the pharmacist go in with a notebook containing past history, chronic diseases, current diseases, current health, laboratory tests, and medications and communication forms listing the date, pharmacist's remarks, date of physician's remarks and/or actions that were developed by the APhA Nursing Home Project to give feedback to the nurses, administrators, and attending physicians concerning the patient's drug regimen. Of the recommendations, 59% were instituted.

Shannon and DeMuth (51) looked at 24 different facilities, ten of which used the federal "indicators" in the review and 14 of which did not. They reported that the mean number of medications used per patient when the "indicators" were applied was not significantly different in their sample, but there was a 5.4 vs 6.6 difference for skilled nursing facilities and 3.4 vs 5.8 difference for intermediate-care facilities. Although not significant, there may be an indication that criteria, such as the "indicators," may be useful in conducting drug regimen reviews.

There have been many suggestions, studies, and demonstrations of the need for quality assurance and one of its subprocesses, drug utilization reviewed. Quality assurance should be judged by two basic measures: outcomes of the process and the cost-benefit ratio of the process. Many of the traditional methods of drug utilization review in long-term care facilities are missing key components of an ideal quality assurance program, with some coming closer to the ideal than others.

The literature and my professional experience lead this author to the following list of characteristics of an ideal quality assurance subprocess of drug utilization review in long-term care facilities:

1. There must be a plan for a dynamic and continuous process.
2. There must be a significant degree of structure in the process. (The more structure the more quality may be assured.)
3. There must be organizational support and commitment for the total process.
4. The drug utilization review process must be viewed as a subprocess of the total quality assurance program.
5. The dynamic process must focus first at rational prescribing and the consequent improvement of health care, and second, it should minimize needless expenditures. (Quality is paramount, with diligence toward cost containment.)
6. The process should be implemented at a local level to increase efficiency and acceptance.
7. The process must be qualitative, not merely quantitative.
8. The main focus of the process must be drug class specific for depth and efficiency with priorities given to drug classes with the most potential problems, highest cost, and greatest use.
9. Medical records, especially the physician order sheet, must be complete and accurate to use as primary source documents for drug utilization review.
10. Problems should be looked at impersonally and in a problem-solving manner.
11. The process for collecting information must be valid and reliable.
12. A protocol process must be used to increase quality and decrease cost.
13. All these affected by the protocol must be involved in its construction and/or approval to decrease any sense of loss of autonomy.
14. The process must be based on explicit standards (criteria) containing the following characteristics:
    a. Criteria must be valid and reliable.
    b. There must be a positive relationship between process criteria and healthy outcome.
    c. Criteria must be determined and/or approved by all of the persons the process touches so the values of all are integrated (a consensus, if possible).
    d. Criteria must be precise for the sake of reliability, yet allow for a degree of discretion (exceptions).
    e. Criteria must generally conform to accepted therapeutic and diagnosis measures.
    f. Criteria must be set at least at a minimal level.
    g. Criteria must be set using normative data.
    h. Criteria must be population specific.
    i. Criteria must at least address the following components of the drug use process:
        (1) Drug indicated
        (2) Drug of choice
        (3) Proper form of drug
        (4) Proper dose
        (5) Drug interactions
        (6) Compliance
        (7) Too little therapy
        (8) Reasonable cost
        (9) Exception to rules
        (10) Drug administration
        (11) Drug effectiveness

(12) Documentation
(13) Dietary considerations
(14) Quality of life
15. Authority must be given to use the information found.
16. Deviation from standards must cause remedial feedback to be initiated.
17. Feedback used must have the following characteristics:
   a. Must be patient specific and targeted
   b. Must have an appropriate combination of education and social control
   c. Must be timely
   d. Must not be unnecessarily alarming
   e. Must keep the total patient in mind (situation, provider, economics, social, and other patient factors)
   f. Must not be repetitive for the same situation
   g. Should not be handwritten
   h. Should be person-to-person if possible or necessary
   i. Must be personally directed
   j. Must be supported by research
   k. Must explain the situation and suggest remediation to correct deviation from criteria
18. Responses to feedback must be obtained for use in the evaluation of the total process and individual standards.
19. Evaluation of the process must be continuous.
20. All of those touched by the process must be involved as much as possible in setting up an interdisciplinary team approach that should include the patient and the payer of care.

DEVELOPMENT OF A NEW SYSTEMATIC APPROACH TO DRUG REGIMEN REVIEW IN A LONG-TERM CARE FACILITY

Systematic approach used by KONSULT is defined by the following steps:
1. Select a drug classification.

2. Prepare and present the in-service program for that drug class with elaboration and specific case examples from the facility. The in-service program should be presented to an interdisciplinary group (i.e., nurses, physicians, administrator, dietitian, pharmacists). It should preferably be oral, but written may be more appropriate in some situations.

3. During the in-service program, allow for a discussion concerning the appropriateness, cost, and practicality of the information contained in the in-service program selected.

4. Obtain a near consensus of the interdisciplinary group on the content of the in-service program criteria.

5. Take a preprepared audit criteria aligned with the specific in-service program and adapt it, as necessary, to comply with the group's agreed on in-service information.

6. Review the drug regimen for the content of selected drug classification agents.

7. Ask the yes or no question dictated by the audit criteria of the patient's chart and care plan.

Example: Is the patient on only one antipsychotic agent? (yes—100%; No—0%)

8. If the answer is "Yes—100%," move to the next criterion.

9. If the answer is "No—0%," write down the corresponding (aligned) code under the patient's name and the wildcard and/or wildline variables, if necessary to specify the drug and/or condition being discussed, for the code. The wildcard and wildline variables should be placed in order of use in parenthesis after the code, i.e., code (wildcard) (wildline). A census list with all past comments and recommendations and a space for new codes to be added is used for data collection. The consultant uses this list (the

---

CONSULTANT'S WORKSHEET

Facility: Test Care Center

Name	Room No.	Attending Physician
Smith, Mabel	101	Daniel R. Smith, M.D.
Hay, Ray		Frank Y. Roberts, M.D.

12/27/83   Kevin G. Dilly, Pharm. D.   MS14

Comment: Tagamet (Cimetidine) may be used in doses of 300 mg four times a day with meals & HS. This therapy is not recommended beyond 4 to 6 weeks, unless pathologic hypersecretory conditions exist clinically. Prophylaxis of recurrent ulcers may be best treated with 300-400 mg at bedtime. Tagamet is a relatively expensive product.

Recommendation: May wish to reevaluate continued Cimetidine or multiple dose Cimetidine therapy unless clinical signs of pathologic hypersecretory conditions exist. May wish to discontinue Cimetidine therapy or use a prophylactic regimen of 300-400 mg HS.

Response: None on file.

This response has been characterized as not currently specified.

New data:

Name	Room No.	Attending Physician
One, Testpatient	100	Daniel R. Smith, M.D.

FIGURE 63.1 Consultant pharmacist worksheet.

PHARMACIST'S CONSULTATION

From: Date: 02/18/84

To: Daniel R. Smith, M.D.
    Gerald K. Alkers, R.N.
    Ms. Jane P. Martin
    Samuel H. Benos, M.D.
    Test Care Center

PATIENT: Smith, Mabel   ROOM: 101

CONSULTING PHARMACIST: Ralph F. Kalles   CONSULT DATE: 10/15/83

SUBJECT: Antipsychotic Consult   AP09

Response requested from: Physician, Dir. of Nursing, Administrator, Medical Director

Comment: Patient has orders for Thorazine and Mellaril (antipsychotic agents). One antipsychotic agent in appropriate dose
                    should be sufficient and more favorable for treatment of psychotic state. Since no antipsychotic agent is superior to
                    any other in treating a psychotic state if dosed properly (only the side effects differ), the use of more than one
                    antipsychotic may be inappropriate.

Recommendation: May wish to use only one antipsychotic agent in adequate dose to accomplish antipsychotic effect.

Response requested
_____

Consultant Pharmacist's Signature:_____
_____

In this area you may enter what is called the "request to the respondent," which may be 240 characters long and individualized for each
facility. This area may be used for disclaimers and/or instructions to the respondent(s).
_____

Attending Physician's comments:

Date:_____ Daniel R. Smith, M.D.:_____

FIGURE 63.2 Pharmacist consultation report.

consultant pharmacist worksheet, Fig. 63.1) to indicate what has been done in the past regarding drug regimen review. This can be used to get a handle on where the consultant pharmacist is with the patient's drug regimen and to prevent the irritating repetition of comments and recommendations. Then move on to the next criterion.

Example: Smith, Mable Room 101 AP09 (Thorazine and Mellaril)

This would appear on the report as follows:

COMMENT: Patient has orders for Thorazine and Mellaril (antipsychotic agents). One antipsychotic agent in an appropriate dose should be sufficient and more favorable for the treatment of psychotic states. Since no antipsychotic agent is superior to any other in treating a psychotic state if dosed properly (only the side effects differ), the use of more than one antipsychotic may be inappropriate.

RECOMMENDATION: May wish to use only one antipsychotic agent in an adequate dose to accomplish an antipsychotic effect.

10. Move on to the next patient until a facility review is completed.

11. The appropriate codes, wildcards, and wildlines are then entered into the KONSULT Drug Regimen Review (KDRR) computerized program for processing into reports (Fig. 63.2).

12. The consultant pharmacist reviews the responses and follows them up when necessary. The response information is entered into the KDRR computerized drug regimen review program for future reference.

13. Repeat the process.

A complete description of the KDRR approach is available on request from the author.

REFERENCES

1. Cheung A, Kayne R: An application of clinical pharmacy services for extended care facilities. *Calif Pharm* 22:6-9, September 1975.
2. Miller JA: Bad reactions for drugged country. Report from Symposium on Drug Allergy, Washington, DC. *Science News* 124:392, December 17, 1983.
3. Lamy PP, Krug BH: Drug therapy review in nursing homes: Proposed standards and guidelines. *Contemp Pharm Prac* 4:125-131, Summer 1981.
4. Fisher CR: Differences by age groups in health care spending. *Health Care Financ Rev* 6:65-68, Spring 1980.
5. *Health in the United States, 1976-1977.* Washington, DC, DHEW Publication No. (HRA)77-1232 (PHS)78-1232. U.S. Department of

Health, Education and Welfare, National Center for Health Statistics, 1978.

6. Gibson RM, Fisher CR: Age differences in health care spending, fiscal year 1977. *Soc Sec Bull* 1(3):42, 1979.

7. Laventurier MF, Talley RB: The incidence of drug-drug interactions in a Medi-Cal population. *Calif Pharm* 10:18, 1977.

8. Law R, Chalmers C: Medicines and the elderly people: A general practice survey. *Br J Med* 1:565, 1976.

9. Young LY, Leach DB, Anderson DA, Rice RT: Decreased medication costs in a skilled nursing facility by clinical pharmacy services. *Contemp Pharm Prac* 4:233-237, Fall 1981.

10. Heinz J: Congressional hearing probes drug misuse in the aged. *J Am Pharm Assoc* NS23:5, September 1983.

11. Hurwitz N: Predisposing factors in adverse reactions to drugs. *Br J Med* 1:536, 1969.

12. Smith JW, Seidl LG, Cluff LE: Studies on the epidemiology of adverse drug reactions. V. Clinical factors influencing susceptibility. *Ann Intern Med* 65:629, 1966.

13. Seidl LG, Thornton GF, Smith JW, Cluff LE: Studies of the epidemiology of adverse drug reactions. *Bull Johns Hopkins Hosp* 119:299, 1966.

14. Melmon KL: Preventable drug reactions—causes and cures. *N Engl J Med* 284:1361-1368, 1971.

15. Frisk PA, Cooper JW, Campbell NA: Community-hospital pharmacist detection of drug-related problems upon patient admission to small hospitals. *Am J Hosp Pharm* 34:738-742, 1977.

16. Caranasco GJ: Drug induced illness leading to hospitalization. *JAMA* 228:713, 1974.

17. Cluff LE, Thorton GF, Seidl LG: Studies on the epidemiology of adverse drug reactions. *JAMA* 188:976, 1964.

18. Webster RT: *Future Projection*. Private interview held during the Sixth Annual Midyear Conference of the American Society of Consultant Pharmacists, Dorado, Puerto Rico, May 1984.

19. Russi G: Can drug therapy be improved in nursing home patients? *Iowa Pharm* 15:21-23, 1981.

20. Leroy AA, Morse ML: *A Study of the Impact of Inappropriate Ambulatory Drug Therapy on Hospitalization*. Contract No. HCFA-500-770011. Washington, DC, Department of Health, Education and Welfare, 1977.

21. Sabin, TD et al: Are nursing home diagnosis and treatment inadequate? *JAMA* 3:248, 321-323, 1982.

22. Kidder SW: *Pharmaceutical Services in Skilled Nursing Facilities—The Intent of the Regulations* (reprint). Washington, DC, American Pharmaceutical Association, 1974.

23. Kidder SW: Saving cost, quality and people: Drug reviews in long term care. *Am Pharm* NS18:18-24, July 1978.

24. Laventurier MF, Talley RB, Hefner DL, Kennard LH: Drug utilization and potential drug-drug interactions. *J Am Pharm Assoc* 16:77-81, February 1976.

25. Requarth CH: Medication usage and interaction in the long-term care elderly. *J Geront Nurs* 5:33-37, March/April 1979.

26. Zawadski RT, Glazer GB, Lurie E: Psychotropic drug use among institutionalized and noninstitutionalized Medicaid aged in California. *J Geront* 33:825-834, 1978.

27. Milleren JW: Some contingencies affecting the utilization of tranquilizers in long term care of the elderly. *J Health Soc Behav* 18:206-211, 1977.

28. Hamilton SF: Therapeutic problems and nursing home patients. *Drug Intell Clin Pharm* 10:703-707, 1976.

29. *Nursing Home Care In The United States: Failure in Public Policy.* Supporting Paper No. 2: Drugs in Nursing Homes: Misuse, High Costs, And Kickbacks, Washington, DC, American Association of Retired Persons, 1975.

30. Aycock EK, Osemene PI, Sear AM: Utilization of prn drugs in long-term care facilities in South Carolina. *J South Carol Med Assoc* 75:631-634, 1979.

31. Berchou RC: Effect of a consultant pharmacist on medication use in an institution for the mentally retarded. *Am J Hosp Pharm* 39:1671-1674, 1982.

32. Tsai AE, Cooper JW, McCall CY: Pharmacist impact on hematopoietic and vitamin therapy in a geriatric long term care facility. *Hosp Formul* 17:225-226, 232-234, 241, 1982.

33. Cooper JW, Francisco GE: Psychotropic usage in long term care facility geriatric patients. *Hosp Formul* 16:407-409, 412-413, 417-419, 1981.

34. Glustien JE: Clinical corner: effects of bran on the use of laxative in a chronic care hospital. *Can J Hosp Pharm* 32:145, 1979.

36. Strandberg LR, Dawson GW, Mathieson D, Rawlings J, Clark BG: Effect of comprehensive pharmaceutical services on drug use in long term care facilities. *Am J Hosp Pharm* 37:92-94, 1980.

36. Williamson DH, Cooper Jr JW, Kotzan JA, Gelbart AO: Consultant pharmacist impact on antihypertensive therapy in a geriatric long-term care facility. *Hosp Formul* 19:123-128, 1984.

37. Wilcher DE, Cooper Jr JW: The consultant pharmacist and analgesic anti-inflammatory drug usage in a geriatric long-term facility. *J Am Geriatr Soc* 29:429-432, 1981.

38. Rawlings JL, Frisk PA: Pharmaceutical services for skilled nursing facilities in compliance with federal regulations. *Am J Hosp Pharm* 32:905-908, 1975.

39. Brodie DC, Lofholm P, Benson RA: Model for drug use review in a skilled nursing facility. *J Amer Pharm Assoc* 17:617-620, 623, 1977.

40. Hood JC, Lemberger M, Stewart RB: Promoting appropriate therapy in a long term care facility. *J Am Pharm Assoc* NS1:32-33, 1975.

41. Vlasses PH, Lucarotti RL, Miller DA, Krigstein DJ: Drug therapy review in a skilled nursing facility: An innovative approach. *J Am Pharm Assoc* 17:92-94, 1977.

42. Chrymko MM, Conrad WF: Effect of removing clinical pharmacy input. *Am J Hosp Pharm* 39:641, 1982.

43. Hays, R: Separation of pharmacy consultants and vendors. *ASCP Update,* January 1978, p 2.

44. Gilroy G, Ellinoy BJ, Nelson GE, Cantrill SV: Integration of pharmacy into the computerized problem-oriented medical information systems (PROMIS)—a demonstration project. *Am J Hosp Pharm* 34:155-162, 1977.

45. Ishikura C, Ishizuka H: Evaluation of a computerized drug interaction checking system. *Int J Biomed Computers* 14:311-319, 1983.

46. Schaffner W, Ray WA, Federspiel CF, Miller WO: Improving antibiotic prescribing in office practice. A controlled trial of three educational methods. *JAMA* 250:1728-1732, 1983.

47. Avorn J, Soumerai SB: Use of a computer-based Medicaid drug data to analyze and correct inappropriate medication use. *J Med Syst* 64:377-386, 1982.

48. Knapp DA, Brandon BM, West S, Leavitt DE: Drug use review—a manual system. *J Am Pharm Assoc* 13:417-420, 433, 1973.

49. Vancura EJ, Marttila JK: Monitoring drug therapy: An applied approach. *Contemp Pharm Prac* 4:238-245, 1981.

50. Stewart JE, Kabat HF, Wertheimer AI: Drug usage review sample studies in long-term care facilities. *Am J Hosp Pharm* 33:138-144, 1976.

51. Shannon RC, De Muth JE: Application of federal indicators in nursing-home drug-regimen review. *Am J Hosp Pharm* 41:912-916, 1984.

Appendix 63.1*   "THE INDICATORS"

SOM Appendix N, Part One: Indicators for Surveyor Assessment of the Performance of Drug Regimen Reviews.—This procedure for judging the quality of drug regimen reviews has been updated to reflect greater experience with their use, and to reflect current advances in drug therapy. Specifically, the following changes have been made:

In an ICF, reviews must be performed by a registered nurse. In an ICF/MR however, they may still be performed by either a R.N. or a pharmacist.

Previous subpart II of Part One, Documentation of Drug Reviews, has been relocated as II, E 1 and renamed "Rules for Applying Apparent Irregularities."

The "indicator" dealing with identifying 5 irregularities per 100 patient months has been replaced with one that identifies excessive numbers of reviews being conducted on the same day, i.e., more than 100 reviews.

Under the "Rules for Applying Apparent Irregularities," insignificant irregularities and previously rejected recommendations on significant irregularities can be documented on an annual rather than monthly basis.

New drugs have been added to almost every drug category.

Minimum doses have been deleted from almost every drug category.

The apical stipulation on pulse rate determinations has been deleted.

Electrolyte determinations have been changed. Only serum potassium determinations are suggested now.

Instead of using a urinary bacterial count to assess drugs used in urinary tract infections, a simple urinalysis is designated.

Emphasis has been placed on the use of brand names. Generic names are included only if they are considered to be in common usage.

Six new apparent irregularities have been added: recorded diagnosis with cardiotonics; routine anticholinergic therapy with antipsychotics; continuous use of antibiotic/steroidal ophthalmics; creatinine determinations with aminoglycosides; patients with known allergies to drugs; and crushing of solid dosage forms.

APPENDIX N
Surveyor Procedures for Pharmaceutical Service Requirements in Long-Term Care Facilities

Part One: Indicators for Surveyor Assessment of the Performance of Drug Regimen Reviews
    I. Proper Use of Indicators
    II. Indicators for Assessing Drug Reviews

APPENDIX N
Surveyor Procedures for Pharmaceutical Service Requirements in Long-Term Care Facilities

PART ONE
Indicators for Surveyor Assessment of the Performance of Drug Regimen Reviews

Skilled Nursing Facilities (SNFs) and Intermediate Care Facilities (ICFs) must perform a review of the patient's drug regimen at least monthly (42 CFR 405.1127(a) and 42 CFR 442.336(a)). In intermediate care facilities for the mentally retarded (ICFs/MR) such reviews must be performed on a regular basis, at least quarterly

---

*Reprinted from State Operations Manual, 1985. Washington, DC, Health Care Financing Administraiton, 1985.

(42 CFR 442.483(c)). These reviews must be performed by a pharmacist in a SNF, a registered nurse in the ICF, and a pharmacist or a registered nurse in an ICF/MR. The information collected from these documents (e.g., drug administration records, physician orders, laboratory reports) is analyzed by the pharmacist or registered nurse reviewer to determine whether there are any potential problems with the patient's drug therapy, and whether such drug therapy is achieving the stated objectives established by the physician for that patient. If there are potential problems, or if stated objectives are apparently not being achieved, then the attending physician must be notified.

I. PROPER USE OF INDICATORS

The word indicator describes what the State agency surveyor discerns as patterns of performance by the pharmacist or registered nurse in their conduct of the required drug regimen reviews. Most of these indicators, taken individually, could not lead to a conclusive finding of compliance or noncompliance with the drug regimen review requirements. However, taken together with the compliance history of the facility, they could represent reasonable evidence whether the pharmacist or registered nurse is adequately performing drug regimen reviews. If there is a high degree of deviation from these indicators, *good* reasons for the deviation must be evident from the patients record. These good reasons may often be learned from the pharmacist or registered nurse, and, for this reason, it is recommended that one of these individuals be present during the survey of the drug regimen review requirement.

When conducting surveys of SNFs participating in the Medicare program, the pharmacy condition of participation must be evaluated by reference to these indicators in order for the survey to be considered valid. Under the Medicaid program, States have the choices of using these indicators or, in the alternative, HCFA will accept other survey criteria developed by the State if the State can establish that its criteria are, at a minimum, equal to these indicators in terms of their reliability and objectivity.

When conducting surveys of SNFs participating in the Medicare program, the pharmacy condition of participation must be evaluated by reference to these indicators in order for the survey to be considered valid. Under the Medicaid program, States have the choices of using these indicators or, in the alternative, HCFA will accept other survey criteria developed by the State if the State can establish that its criteria are, at a minimum, equal to these indicators in terms of their reliability and objectivity.

II. INDICATORS FOR ASSESSING DRUG REGIMEN REVIEWS

A. **Reviews Performed Versus Average Census.**—Compare the number of drug regimen reviews performed to the average census of the facility. If the average census is 100, then the number of reviews that would have been performed *per month* would be about 100. However, this simple indicator cannot be absolute, and tolerances must be allowed. For example, the pharmacist or registered nurse may have reviewed only 50 percent of the patients in a particular month, but the other 50 percent are scheduled for review the day after the survey. If the number of reviews falls significantly short of patient census over a number of months, a noncompliance finding is in order.

In ICFs/MR, reviews need only be performed on a quarterly basis. Thus, this indicator must be modified in the ICF/MR to state that all patients are reviewed quarterly rather than monthly.

B. **Reviews Should Be Performed in the Facility.**—A pharmacist or registered nurse reviewer cannot be *required* to perform reviews in the facility. The regulations do not state where the reviews must be performed. However, in order to perform acceptable reviews, the facility's reviewer must be examining data sources such as the patient's drug administration record, physician orders, nursing notes, and laboratory reports. For all practical purposes these data sources are only located in the facility. Thus, to adequately perform reviews, the pharmacist or registered nurse should be conducting them in the facility.

C. **Average Prescription Utilization.**—In 1974, the average prescription utilization per SNF patient was found to be approximately 6.1. The current average is probably unchanged. As a general rule, one could question the adequacy of drug reviews if the facility's average prescription utilization were above 6 per patient. There are qualifications to this indicator:

1. The 6.1 average is a national average. Regional and State variations can be significantly different. The average in the State the surveyor serves may be more meaningful. The Medicaid Management Information System, if one is available, can be of assistance in supplying this specific information.

2. The nature of the patient population (e.g., a high number of patients with multiple chronic diseases) may be such that a higher utilization is appropriate.

3. The assumption that drug regimen reviews reduce utilization may not always be true. A drug regimen review may result in additional drug utilization.

4. The pharmacist or registered nurse may be performing good reviews and recommending that drugs be discontinued, but the physician may not agree with the recommendations.

5. Analysis by the surveyor of the *trend* in prescription utilization is critical. The pharmacist or registered nurse may be changing attitudes about drug therapy, and a slow improvement may be evolving. Thus, if the average is higher than 6 but the trend is toward reduction, the pharmacist or nurse may be adequately performing drug reviews.

6. In an ICF/MR the drug utilization is usually significantly lower. (Approximately 3 per patient per month.) ICFs' drug utilization is usually comparable to SNFs.

In order to estimate the average prescription utilization, examine a sufficient sample of charts to establish a pattern. It is not necessary to calculate an exact average. In determining the average, include all legend and over-the-counter (OTC) drugs.

Count as one prescription any drug order, including as needed (PRN) orders, if *one* dose has been administered in the last 30 days. If a drug has been ordered but never administered in the last 30 days, do not count it in the average. Combination drugs (e.g., aspirin and codeine) should be counted as one prescription.

D. **Excessive Reviews on the Same Date.**—The ability of a pharmacist or a nurse to review patient records is finite. Question the adequacy of review if more than 100 patients have been reviewed on the same day by the same reviewer.

E. **Apparent Irregularities (Potential Drug Therapy Problems).**—Subsection E.2. list drug therapy circumstances which *may* constitute drug irregularities (potential drug therapy problems). The pharmacist or registered nurse should address these apparent irregularities every time they are encountered. Initially learn five to ten of these apparent irregularities and use them in your surveys, then learn five to ten more, and so forth until all are learned.

1. **Rules for Applying Apparent Irregularities**
   a. The pharmacist or registered nurse conducting reviews is responsible for identifying apparent irregularities and notifying an individual having authority to correct the potential problem.
   b. You are responsible for determining whether such *identification* and *notification* has taken place.

c. Do not go any further than determining if *identification* and *notification* has occurred. *It is not necessary to ascertain the disposition of the recommendation made by the pharmacist or registered nurse reviewer. Inquiry into the specific treatment or outcome could be construed as Federal interference with the practice of medicine, which is prohibited by Section 1801 of the Social Security Act.*

d. A record of drug regimen reviews must be maintained in the facility in order to demonstrate that such reviews have been performed. This record may or may not be a part of the patient's medical record depending on the policy of the facility. In any case, each patient must be identified, and documentation of one of the following circumstances must exist:

   (1) If no potential problems were found by the pharmacist or registered nurse reviewer, he or she must have included a signed and dated statement to this effect in the drug regimen review record.

   (2) If a potential problem was found and the pharmacist or registered nurse reviewer deemed it *not* significant, then he or she must have included a signed and dated statement in the record which describes the situation.

   (3) If a potential problem was found that was considered significant, the pharmacist or registered nurse reviewer must have included a signed and dated statement in the record describing the situation and indicating that they communicated this information to an individual with authority to correct it, usually the attending physician.

   (4) The facility's reviewer need not have documented the identification and notification every month (or quarter in ICFs/MR) even if the apparent irregularity continues, provided:

   • It has been deemed insignificant by the pharmacist or registered nurse reviewer, or

   • It has been deemed significant, but the recommendation has been rejected by the individual having authority to correct it.

Under these circumstance, the facility's reviewer may document that he or she has identified an apparent irregularity and notified a person having authority to correct the potential problem on an *annual* basis. This documentation should appear in whatever record the facility decides to use for documenting drug regimen reviews.

2. **List of Apparent Irregularities.**—These drug therapy circumstances *may* constitute drug irregularities (potential drug therapy problems).

NOTE: Generic names are noted only when they are in common usage and are designated by lower case type.

a. Multiple orders of the same drug for the same patient by the same route of administration (e.g., the same chemical entity by different brand names);

b. Drugs administered in disregard of established stop order policies;

c. As needed (PRN) drug orders administered as directed every day for more than 30 days;

d. Patients receiving three or more laxatives *concurrently*. Sequential use need not be questioned. Example of commonly used laxatives are as follows:

Agoral	Haley's M.O.
Cascara Sagrada	Konsyl
Chronulac	Metamucil
Colace	Milk of magnesia
Dialose	Mineral oil
Docusate sodium	Modane Bulk

Dorbantyl   Mondane Soft
Doxinate   Neoloid
Ducolax   Peri-Colace
Effersyllium   Senokot
Fleet's Enema   Surfak
Glycerin suppositories

e. Use of antipsychotics (see paragraph i for list) or antidepressants (see m for list) for less than three days. (Exception: Compazine used as an antinausant)

f. *Continuous* use of the following hypnotic (sleep induction) drugs for more than 30 days.

	Usual Maximum Single Dosage Age 65 & Over	Usual Maximum Single Dosage
Amytal	150 mg	300 mg
Butisol	100 mg	200 mg
Chloral hydrate	750 mg	1500 mg
Dalmane	15 mg	30 mg
Doriden	500 mg	1000 mg
Halcion	0.25 mg	0.5 mg
Nembutal	100 mg	200 mg
Noctec	750 mg	1500 mg
Noludar	200 mg	400 mg
Placidyl	500 mg	1000 mg
Restoril	15 mg	30 mg
Seconal	100 mg	200 mg

g. Use of two or more hypnotic drugs listed in f at the same time;

h. Hypnotic drugs listed in f administered in excess of the listed maximum doses;

i. Use of two or more of the following antipsychotic drugs at the same time;

	Usual Maximum Daily Antipsychotic Dosage for Ages 65 & Over	Usual Maximum Daily Antipsychotic Dosage
Chlorpromazine	800 mg	1600 mg
Haldol	50 mg	100 mg
Loxitane	125 mg	250 mg
Mellaril	400 mg	800 mg
Moban, Lidone	112 mg	225 mg
Navane	30 mg	60 mg
Proketazine	200 mg	400 mg
Prolixin	20 mg	40 mg
Quide	80 mg	160 mg
Repoise	80 mg	160 mg
Serentil	250 mg	500 mg
Stelazine	40 mg	80 mg
Taractan	800 mg	1600 mg
Thioridazine	400 mg	800 mg
Thorazine	800 mg	1600 mg
Tindal	150 mg	300 mg
Trilafon	32 mg	64 mg
Vesprin	100 mg	200 mg

j. Use of the antipsychotic drugs listed in i in excess of the listed daily dosage maximums;

k. Use of the following anxiolytic drugs when their dosages exceed the following maximums:

	Usual Daily Dosage for Age 65 & Over & Age 12 & Under	Usual Daily Dosage for Age Under 65 & Over 12
Ativan	3 mg/day	6 mg/day
Azene	30 mg/day	60 mg/day
Centrax	30 mg/day	60 mg/day
Chlordiazepoxide	40 mg/day	100 mg/day
Diazepam	20 mg/day	60 mg/day
Equanil	600 mg/day	1600 mg/day
Librium	40 mg/day	100 mg/day
Meprobamate	600 mg/day	1600 mg/day
Miltown	600 mg/day	1600 mg/day
Paxipam	80 mg/day	160 mg/day
Serax	60 mg/day	90 mg/day
Valium	20 mg/day	60 mg/day
Tranxene	30 mg/day	60 mg/day
Xanax	2 mg/day	4 mg/day

l. More than two changes of an antidepressant within a 7-day period. Examples of commonly used antidepressants are as follows:

	Usual Maximum Daily Dosage Age 65 & Over	Usual Maximum Daily Dosage
Adapin	150 mg	300 mg
Amitriptyline	150 mg	300 mg
Asendin	200 mg	400 mg
Aventyl	75 mg	150 mg
Desyrel	300 mg	600 mg
Doxepin	150 mg	300 mg
Elavil	150 mg	300 mg
Imipramine	150 mg	300 mg
Ludiomil	150 mg	300 mg
Norpramin	150 mg	300 mg
Pamelor	75 mg	150 mg
Pertofrane	150 mg	300 mg
Sinequan	150 mg	300 mg
SK pramine	150 mg	300 mg
Surmotil	150 mg	300 mg
Tofranil	150 mg	300 mg
Vivactil	30 mg	60 mg

m. Use of the antidepressants listed in l in excess of the listed daily maximum doses;

n. Patients who repeatedly lose seizure control while taking anticonvulsants (e.g., Dilantin (phenytoin), phenobarbital, Mysoline, Depakene (valproic acid));

o. Patients who are taking thyroid drugs and have not had some assessment of thyroid function (e.g., Free T4 Level, T3 Resin update, Free Thyroxin update). Examples of commonly used thyroid drugs are Synthroid, Cytomel, Thyroid Extract;

p. Patients who are taking the following drugs and have not had a blood pressure recorded at least weekly.

Aldomet   Hylorel
Apresoline   Inderal
Blocadren   Ismelin
Capoten   Lasix
Catapres   Lopressor
Chlorothiazide   Minipress
Corgard   Propranolol
Diuril   Reserpine
Dyazide   Serpasil
Furosemide   Tenormin
Hydralazine   Visken
Hydrochlorothiazide Wytensin
Hydrodiuril   Zaroxolyn
Hygroton

q. Patients who are taking anticoagulant therapy and have not had some assessment of blood clotting function at least every month. The most common blood clotting function test is prothrombin time. Examples of commonly used anticoagulants are Coumadin (warfarin), Dicumarol;

r. Patients who are taking cardioactive drugs (see list below) and have not had a pulse rate recorded daily in the first month of therapy and weekly thereafter, *or* the chart shows a pulse consistently below 60 or above 100.

Blocadren	Procan
Calan	Procardia
Corgard	Pronestyl
Digoxin	Propranolol
Inderal	Quionaglute
Isoptin	Quinidine
Lonoxin	Tenormin
Lopressor	Timoptic
Norpace	Viskin

s. Patients who are taking insulin or oral hypoglycemics and have not had a urine sugar test at least daily *or* a blood sugar test at least every 60 days. Example of commonly used hypoglycemics are: Glucotrol, Diabeta, Micronase, Orinase, Diabinese, Dymelor, Tolinase;

t. Patients who are taking iron preparations, folic acid or vitamin B_{12}, and have not had a red blood cell assessment (e.g., hemoglobin, hematocrit) during the first month of therapy. Examples of commonly used iron preparations are: Feosol (ferrous sulfate), Imferon, Fergon (ferrous gluconate);

u. Use of Mandelamine, Hiprex, Bactrim, Septra, Macrodantin, Furdantin, or Urex in chronic urinary tract infections if a urinalysis has not been performed at least once, 30 days after therapy was initiated;

v. Patients taking Mandelamine or Hiprex who have not had a urine pH determination within 30 days after therapy was initiated, or if therapy is continued when urine pH is continually above 6;

w. Use of nitrofurantoin (Furadantin, Macrodantin) for conditions other than treatment or prophylaxis of urinary tract infections, or blood urea nitrogen or serum creatinine levels are not recorded on the chart;

x. Three or more orders for analgesics used at the same time. Examples of commonly used analgesics are:

Acetaminophen	Indocin
Anaprox	Meclomen
Aspirin	Meperidine
Clinoril	Motrin
Darvocet N	Nalfon
Darvon Compound	Naprosyn
Demerol	Percodan
Dolobid	Rufen
Empirin	Tolectin
Empirin with Codeine	Trilisate
Feldine	Tylenol
Ibruprofen	Tylenol with Codeine

y. Patients taking diuretics who have *not* had a serum potassium level determination within 30 days after initiation of therapy. Examples of commonly used diuretics are:

Acetazolamide	Esidrix
Aladactone	Furosemide
Aldactazide	Hydrochlorothiazide
Bumex	Hydrodiuril
Chlorothiazide	Hygroton
Diamox	Lasix
Diuril	Midamor
Dyazide	Moduretic
Dyrenium	Neptazane
Edecrin	Zaroxolyn
Enduron	

z. Patients taking diuretics (see aa. for list) and cardiotonics, e.g., Lanoxin, who have not had a serum potassium determination within 30 days after initiation of the cardiotonic therapy and every 6 months thereafter;

aa. Patients who are taking Butazolinin, Azolid, or Tandearil continuously and have not had at least one CBC determination 30 days after initiation of therapy;

bb. The use of cardiotonics, e.g., Lanoxin, in the absence of documentation of one of the following diagnoses:

Congestive heart failure
Atrial fibrillation
Paroxysmal supraventricular tachycardia
Atrial flutter

cc. The use of anticholinergic therapy, e.g., Artane, Cogentin, or Kemardin, with antipsychotic drugs (see i for list) in the absence of recorded extrapyramidal side effects, e.g., tremor, drooling, shuffling gait;

dd. The continuous use of antibiotic/steroidal ophthalmic preparation, e.g., Cortisporin ophthalmic, Metimyd ophthalmic, or Ophthocort, for periods exceeding 14 days;

ee. The use of the following aminoglycosides (Garamycin, Nebcin, Amikin, Kantrex, Netromycin) in the absence of a serum creatinine determination when therapy was initiated;

ff. Orders for drugs for which there is a known allergy as documented in the patient's record;

gg. The crushing of solid dosage forms when the likely result will cause patient discomfort (e.g., Ducolax) or undesired blood levels (e.g., Theordur).

CHAPTER 64

The Institutional Pharmacist and Community Relations

DAVID ZILZ

The community pharmacist, through his daily contact with the public in providing pharmaceutical services, has always been readily accessible to the community and in a position to establish rapport and personal relationships with the public. The images created have been both negative and positive, but the images have been established solely dependent on the action of that pharmacist. It has occurred from the direct personal contact between the pharmacist and public in the practice site rather than through organized programs (1,2).

Historically, the pharmacist has been viewed as a health practitioner. His duties and responsibilities in drug compounding, dispensing, and health advisory activities left little confusion in the public's mind as to what role the pharmacists played in fulfilling community needs (8).

However, since the proliferation of industrially prepared products and the diminution of compounding activities, and at the same time expanded retailing of nondrug items in mass merchandising centers with small sections called pharmacies, the public's perceived image of the pharmacist as a health professional has been clouded (4,5). The image has become in many instances primarily that of a businessman and secondarily that of a health practitioner in the community (5,6).

There are exceptions in which highly developed professional pharmacies are exclusively supplying drugs, providing consultations and advisory services, and supplying health care pamphlets on numerous health-related issues and are without doubt thought of as health practitioners. In these settings different expectations of the pharmacist's contribution to the community may be evident (7).

On the other hand, the institutional pharmacist until recently has had very limited visibility in the community. It is well recognized that the historical activities and roles of the institutionally based pharmacist have sheltered, if not totally isolated, him from the view of not only the public but also the institution's staff as well. At best it can be presumed that this isolation has prevented any preconceived expectations of the pharmacist. The evolving capabilities and expanding contributions of the institutional practitioner are, therefore, excellent areas for creating positive com-

munity relationships, and improving the image of the individual pharmacist as well as the profession of pharmacy.

The evolving and expanded concepts of what has become accepted as patient-oriented pharmacy practice has stimulated the pharmacist to accept a different self-image and the role he must play in the community, but more important has become the focus and thrust of a purpose allowing and requiring personal contact by the institutional practitioner. The elements of these patient-centered services must not only be provided to the individual patient, but must be publicized, explained, and reiterated to the community in organized community relations (8,9).

THE HOSPITAL PHARMACIST HAS BECOME VISUAL

The institutional practitioner has become very visual to the public as a result of new services that are increasingly being provided from the hospital setting. Especially in large medical centers that have active ambulatory services, the hospital practitioner is daily coming into contact with patients and thereby creating public impressions by direct professional contact. Practitioners, especially those providing clinical services, have demonstrated a very positive image to the public through their practice contributions. This has been seen in direct evaluative and consultative services to the patients within settings designed to create a positive impression on the individual patients and the public.

Recent developments in the more technologic pharmacy services delivered through the home care programs of the hospital has given institutional practitioners another avenue to demonstrate their competence and contribution to the patient's and public's welfare. Through these services they have been able to demonstrate competence in high-level patient training to assure that patient's can manage the intricacy of high-technology self-administration of drugs in their homes. This has been demonstrated in parenteral nutrition, home IV antibiotic administration, and even the ongoing intra-arterial or IV administration of cancer chemotherapeutic and injectable pain medications. These services have given the institutional practitioner an increased opportunity to relate to the patient on a personal and ongoing basis (10-12).

PHARMACISTS AS PART OF HOSPITAL PUBLIC RELATIONS PROGRAMS

Hospitals have become quite aggressive in establishing community relations programs, primarily by providing community health education programs and services. The very aggressive marketing attitudes of the hospital industry have created an entire new environment within which the hospital and institutional pharmacists must now project their public images. This movement from the historical image of the hospital that was strictly for the purpose of relieving suffering and ill health to one that is in the business of health care delivery has changed the image of the entire health care industry and all those who practice within it (13). For instance, there has seldom if ever been the continuous advertising that is now daily observed in daily newspapers and television commercials. Hospital pharmacy practitioners are now in an environment where they have to identify carefully what they want their image to be. They have to decide whether they want to project the image of inexpensive providers of pharmaceutical products, purveyors of new and complicated drug technologies (14), or ombudsmen of patients concerning themselves about patients' drug information and products needs.

Some of these programs may be considered diagnostic or disease screening services, as exemplified by diabetic screening, hypertension screening, and others, but most have a drug-related therapeutic component that requires the drug knowledge of the pharmacist.

One of the most difficult and costly problems in establishing any community relations program is developing the mechanism or forum through which that program can be delivered. By contributing to a part of a hospital-wide program this obstacle is overcome, thereby allowing the pharmacist to expend his energies on the professional and health components of the program rather than on the organizing and publicity efforts that will be done by other members of the hospital organization.

Examples of comprehensive health programs with pharmacist involvement have been described in the literature (15). For instance, both the diabetic program and hypertension program require a detailed review of all prior medication activities by the patient during the screening process. Further, those patients with these diseases that were previously undiagnosed need significant counseling and training on the appropriate use of the drugs used in treating them (16). Patient education on drug therapy is an invaluable contribution that the pharmacist can make in a hospital-wide public service program.

Hospitals also sponsor health education seminars. An example is a hospital that provided a seminar on diabetes one morning each month. This seminar was presented to parents and patients by an interdisciplinary staff composed of a physician, nurse, dietician, and pharmacist. The patients were interested in this format as a means not only to hear presentations on the disease process and care of the disease, but also to hear discussions and questions raised by other patients with the same disease. More significant, however,

was the opportunity to obtain authoritative and accepted information from an interdisciplinary team. The pharmacist's contribution focused primarily on three areas. First, insulin-related aspects such as mixing, storage, and uses; second, instructions on the appropriate use of diabetic testing agents, items often neglected and misunderstood; and third, a comprehensive discussion of the role of oral hypoglycemia agents in the disease process.

AVAILABILITY OF MASS MEDIA TO HOSPITAL

Most medium and large hospitals have individuals dedicated as public relations officers. Small hospitals may have individuals doubling in that capacity with other activities. They cultivate relationships with members of the press and radio and television stations. Their contact with the mass media allows another excellent potential for presenting information programs to the public. The educational television networks and radio networks are required to make available a certain portion of the broadcast week for public services activities. Educational television especially provides topics of interest in health. Entire program sequences or shows of 30 minutes may be provided at no charge to participants. Both television and radio will often have 1-minute public service "spots" available for items of importance to health. In all cases, it is necessary to have well-thought-out and expertly constructed presentations to be effective and to ensure that the desired image is projected. A poorly presented or developed program will probably not be accepted and, if it should, would create a negative impression, and thus be counterproductive to the objective of establishing respected community relations.

Examples of the pharmacist presenting both lengthy comprehensive programs and short topics can be illustrated by the following programs broadcasted and televised in the author's home city.

All members of the pharmacy departments of each of the hospitals of the community presented a series of five programs each 30 minutes in length on educational television regarding various aspects of pharmaceutical services in hospitals and other drug-related topics. The first program described what hospital pharmacists are, how they are trained, what functions they perform, and how the practice differs from what is routinely seen by the television audience. The programs also described how unit dose systems operate in hospitals to ensure the safety of medications the patient receives, the precautionary measures and other advantages of pharmacy admixture systems, and an elaboration on the principles of incompatibilities and interactions. Other sessions described the working of the poison and drug information center and how they support the needed and requested information on drugs. The final comprehensive session described factors to consider in taking medications in the home, their storage, and appropriate administration and self-monitoring principles.

Spot topics of 1 minute's duration continue to occur on radio with emphasis on compliance, correct use of over-the-counter drugs, and poison prevention topics, which will be discussed in more detail later in the chapter.

Few readers of the general press obtain factual, descriptive stories on the institutional practice of pharmacy. Only once has an article been written that occurred in the Sunday edition of every major syndicated paper nationally. *Parade* magazine in the fall of 1975 provided a comprehensive description of the activities, services, and contributions of institutional practitioners. This article, read by millions of readers, was perhaps the single most significant article relating to the community the contribution of institutional practitioners. Although this is and should be a sought-after level of positive exposure, it is seldom offered to the profession.

PROVIDING HEALTH-RELATED BROCHURES

The pharmacists and the pharmacy department can provide numerous pamphlets for patients. These can also be on topics other than medications and thereby present an image to the community of a practitioner with broader knowledge and interests in health.

The following is a partial list of organizations that provide pamphlets that can be made available in waiting areas or for distribution to patients either in a community practice or an institutional setting: American Cancer Society, American Heart Association, American Kidney Foundation, American Lung Association, American Medical Association, American Nursing Association, American Pharmaceutical Association, American Society of Hospital Pharmacists, National Cancer Institute, National Heart, Lung, and Blood Institute.

Many of the pamphlets are free on request, although there may be a charge for selected items. In addition to brochures that are of general interest to health, there are numerous pharmacy-related brochures designed for patient's use, available on request from the national and state professional pharmacy organizations.

An example of a brochure specifically designed to describe what services the institutional practitioner performs was developed by the American Society of Hospital Pharmacists (ASHP). It was provided to its members for distribution to patients in the hospitals (17).

There have also been publications by professional pharmacy organizations to demonstrate to the public that the profession is capable of and willing to provide unbiased information in a factual, reliable and nonemotional manner. The ASHP published a book, *Consumer Drug Digest,* which was written in lay language and discussed the purpose and action of drugs, side effects, precautions, hints on how patients can monitor their own drug therapy, as well as dosage and storage information (18).

A group of health professionals created an organization, including several national pharmacy organizations, to distribute information on drug-related topics to the public. The title of this group is the National Council on Patient Information and Education (19).

POISON PREVENTION: A SPECIAL CASE

Both community and institutional pharmacists have contributed greatly and successfully to community programs on poison prevention activities (20,21).

The national and local publications feature articles highlighting the extent of the problem, kinds of poisoning, items commonly ingested resulting in poisonings, points on safeguarding the home to prevent accidents from occurring, and, should they occur, methods of emergency treatment.

Institutional practitioners involved with drug and poison information centers have gained considerable publicity. These practitioners have been featured in local articles providing information, ideas, and treatment services available. These programs, done in cooperation with community pharmacists who have provided emetic agents to nearly every home with small children in some communities, have received acclaim from the communities.

The pharmacist is a practitioner who can and should provide the stimulus within both the institution and the community to ensure that a comprehensive publicity program on poison prevention occurs each year.

THE INSTITUTIONAL PHARMACIST AND THE LEGISLATIVE PROCESS

Although pharmacists have been elected to various political offices and have been able, in that capacity, to have a significant impact on public affairs and public policy, this is not a frequent occurrence compared to other professionals such as physicians.

Pharmacists, however, have been active in public affairs through other political processes. Through both national and state professional organizations, the pharmacist can provide significant factual information about complex issues. All of the major pharmacy organizations have councils or committees that concentrate on the health care issues in the legislative and administrative areas of national, state, and local government. Institutional pharmacists should familiarize themselves with the structure and mechanism of these organizations (22) so that they are in a position to assist these groups by providing their expertise on issues related to institutional practice.

In addition to functioning within the pharmacy organizations, contributions can be made in the political process by the individual directly, but not as efficiently as with organized groups. Information on all of the issues in the legislative process is available from political action groups such as the State Taxpayers Alliances that provide information summaries on the status of legislative issues. Pharmacy organizations have presented programs to educate and inform individual pharmacists on methods to provide commentary and influence on these issues (23-26). The ASHP in its *Chapter Officers Manual* has provided a very comprehensive, detailed program on the political process. It is desirable for every institutional practitioner to become familiar with the process through both the pharmacy organizations and those that can be used by an individual in the legislative and law-making team.

OTHER POSSIBILITIES FOR COMMUNITY EXPOSURE

A number of states have well-organized continuing education programs for citizens of those states. One avenue for presenting these programs is through an extension division of a university system. These programs can be telecast or broadcast to the entire state through a "tele-lecture" series, thereby providing accessibility to all sizes of communities, whether distant, or near the university. Stations are strategically located in communities, often in hospitals, and provide drug-related information to many other users of the extension program. Involvement in these programs allows institutional pharmacists to contribute to the drug knowledge via a well-established mechanism and thereby enhance the prestige in the community.

With the increasing interest of the public in more self-reliance in controlling their own health, many professions have been able to provide tests that consumers can take to determine how effectively they are managing. Pharmacists in community practice and institutional practice have concentrated on medications using the same techniques. The Academy of Pharmacy Practice of the American Pharmaceutical Association (APhA) has developed a series of slide/tape programs for presentation by a pharmacist to community groups. These include the *National Medication Awareness Test,* the *Health Check Test,* and the *Self-Medication Awareness Test.* Using technology of this nature allows for sophisticated methods of community exposure and results in a very positive professional image.

Pharmacists' social activities should not be underestimated as a potential means of community relations activities. Local awareness that pharmacists are available and knowledgeable can enhance their prestige and they can provide a valuable service. Although there may be reluctance to describe the practitioner's capabilities and offer them, once they become known the community does not hesitate to rely on this expertise. Although personal conveniences may be disrupted by the community's needs, the personal availability is appreciated.

THE ELDERLY NEED SPECIAL EMPHASIS

It has become clear to anyone who has studied the demographics of the population of the United States that considerable emphasis must be placed on the increasing older population. Pharmacists should be more concerned and pay more attention to this phenomenon than any other health professional, because the elderly use more medication than any other segment of the society. Further, they have more difficulty in managing their medication than other segments of society because many of them are on multiple and complicated drug regimens. As a group they are very concerned about the financial impact drug consumption has on them and the drain it has on their fixed income.

Because of the many drug needs of the elderly, pharmacists should consider concentrating on providing public programs that serve them. In addition, effort directed toward groups such as home health can visiting nurses' associations who work closely with them can also benefit a great deal from the knowledge best provided by a pharmacist (27-29).

INTRAPROFESSIONAL COOPERATION NEEDED

A unified approach and common objectives are keystones to achieving goals in political and public awareness missions. Equally important is the need for cooperation in daily practice between the community and the institutional phar-

macist. An earlier study (30) showed that attempts by one hospital pharmacy to provide at discharge a condensed but comprehensive summary of the major drug activities that occurred on patients whose community pharmacists maintained a patient profile were received with a mixed reaction. Generally, those community practitioners who maintained independent practices or were from small communities were most appreciative and able to use effectively the information by incorporating it into that patient's profile. The information provided consisted of allergic manifestations discovered, changes of therapy on discharge in contrast to medication on admission, quantities of medication that the patient had access to on discharge to assist in assuring that refills were obtained when drugs were critical, and other key information to assist the community pharmacist in the ongoing support of the patient. Some chain stores and others in the study, however, felt the information was of no benefit to them in that mode of their practice.

This type of program information flowing from the hospital to the community, although extremely desirable, is practically nonexistent. It is an example of a program that, in future years, may be seen as common practice.

There are activities, however, where cooperation is occurring on a daily basis. Clinical pharmacy practitioners often call on community pharmacists with patient profiles to unravel drug histories for physicians in hospitals. Networks are established to deter drug abuse problems by prescription forgery methods. Borrowing and loaning drugs during times of emergency or shortages occur routinely between stores and hospitals. In one area, a common formulary was established between the physicians, community practitioner and institutional pharmacists (31). All of these programs occur when the pharmacists in both settings recognize the need to support each others' service to enhance the patients' and communities' health needs.

There is one area that in some locations prevents the development of a cooperative attitude. This basis is financial in nature and relates to the outpatient or dispensing to the hospital's outpatient clinic patient. As with any activity that creates friction, resolution and harmony on all other activities may be achieved by open discussion of the implications and the need for a hospital to implement such services. Often the programs are misunderstood because they are not fully discussed.

PRACTICE SETTING MOST SIGNIFICANT

Although all the activities above are approaches to establish community and public rapport, the most significant are those actions occurring in the individual practice settings of both community and institutional practitioners. Public and patient expectations and impressions are based on the activities and the aura of the practice setting. The more professional and the broader the involvement in health care programs, the greater the expectations of the community of the contribution of the institutional pharmacist to its needs. The specific items, activities, and services to be added and deleted from the practice setting are constantly changing. Pharmacists must be prepared to change to meet these needs if they wish to maintain a positive image of progressive individuals ready to provide for the community's needs.

Sensitivity to community needs and the creativity and boldness to be able to deliver the services needed are the contribution that will allow the institutional pharmacist to establish continued community relations.

REFERENCES

1. Steward JE, Kabat HF, Purahit A: Consumer-pharmacist congruence—understanding consumer wants and needs. *J Am Pharm Assoc* NS17:358-361, 1977.
2. Frank JT: Pharmacy's quest for professional direction. *Drug Intell Clin Pharm* 9:45-46, 1975.
3. Gold BH, Nelson AA: Economic security and professional reality. *J Am Pharm Assoc* NS16:546-550, 1976.
4. Francke DE: Commentaries on the report of the study commission on pharmacy. *Drugs in Health Care* 3(2):68-69, Spring 1976.
5. Norwood GJ, Seibert JJ, Gagnon JP: Attitudes of rural consumers and physicians toward expanded roles of pharmacist. *J Am Pharm Assoc* NS16:551-554, 1976.
6. Yellin AK, Norwood GJ: The public's attitude toward pharmacy. *J Am Pharm Assoc* NS14:61-65, 1974.
7. White EV: A family pharmacist takes a critical look at the report of the study commission on pharmacy. *Drug Intell Clin Pharm* 11:94-101, 1977.
8. Stallman M: How to select a pharmacist: Development, filming and analysis of a television presentation. *J Am Pharm Assoc* NS17:507-509, 1972.
9. American Pharmaceutical Association: Ask Your Pharmacist, a successful newspaper column. *Pharm Weekly* Vol. 16, No. 34, August 20, 1977.
10. Bertino J: Home Antibiotic Therapy. U.S. Pharmacist Hospital Edition. 9:H 13-15, 1984.
11. Swenson JP: Training patients to administer intravenous antibiotics at home. *Am J Hosp Pharm* 38:1480, 1981.
12. Cohen MR: Treatment of severe, chronic pain by continuous parenteral infusion of morphine. *Hosp Pharm* 18:618-624, 1983.
13. Louden T: Opportunities—and competition—in home healthcare are on the rise. *Mod Healthcare* :109-112, December 1983.
14. How will Pharmacy Fare in the 21st Century? *Am Druggist* pp 123-127, May 1984.
15. American Pharmaceutical Association: Pennsylvania pharmacists blitz patients via radio. *Pharm Weekly* Vol. 16, No. 35, August 27, 1977.
16. Gurwick E, Emmanual S: A comprehensive health care program. *J Am Pharm Assoc* NS14:71-79, 1974.
17. *Meet Your Hospital Pharmacist*. Bethesda, American Society of Hospital Pharmacists, 1981.
18. *Consumer Drug Digest*. Bethesda, American Society of Hospital Pharmacists, 1982.
19. NCPIE Campaign, PO Box 1080, Purcellville, Va 22132-0180.
20. Simpson TR Jr, Slmpson TR III: Poison control revisited. *J Am Pharm Assoc* NS16:659-663, 1976.
21. Picchioni A: The oldest new program in poison control. *Am Pharm* NS20:71, February 1980.
22. *American Society of Hospital Pharmacists Chapters Office Manual*, ed 2. Bethesda, ASHP, 1977.
23. Wisconsin Pharmaceutical Association: 77 legislative directory, *WI Pharm* 21:3:80-117, 1977.
24. Henry R, Hammell B: Conference on legislation and political action. *WI Pharm* 18:5:134-138, 1975.
25. Munson ML: Today's politically active pharmacist. *WI Pharm* 18:6:187-191, 1975.
26. Olszewski DA: Fellow pharmacists. *WI Pharm* 21:9:331, 1977.
27. Shimp L, Ascione F, Flynn-Breeden L: Home medication review. *Am Pharm* NS20:266-267, May 1980.
28. Stalpes B: Learning about the elderly, closing the gap. *Am Pharm* NS20:259-263, May 1980.
29. Feinberg M: Reaching the elderly, some new approaches. *Am Pharm* NS20:264-265, May 1980.
30. Zilz AD, Silberg R: Drug profiles follow patients into community/monitoring continued. *Hospitals* 46:68-72, December 1972.
31. Kunin CM, Dierks JW: Physicians-pharmacists voluntary program to improve prescription practice. *N Engl J Med* 280:1442-1446, 1969.

CHAPTER 65

Legal Aspects of Institutional Practice

JOSEPH L. FINK III

Pharmacy is frequently and inextricably intertwined with the law. One will often hear pharmacy referred to as "the most regulated profession." This is true because of the nature of the products and services with which pharmacists deal—they can be of great benefit in speeding health and reducing the impact of various maladies. Yet at the same time they possess the potential to wreak great harm and even death. For this reason society has constructed a complex series of legal requirements to control the distribution and use of drugs, thereby, it is hoped, minimizing the potential for harmful effect.

This chapter deals with the law as it applies to hospital pharmacy practice. Legal principles related to professional practice are discussed, such as those pertaining to pharmaceutical services, standards of professional practice, drug control laws, and professional liability issues.

Specifically excluded from coverage are those laws pertaining to the business aspects of pharmacy practice such as commercial law, the law of sales, laws pertaining to business organizational forms, and tax laws. Likewise, laws dealing with the employment relationship, such as equal employment opportunity laws, minimum wage laws, pension rights, employee safety requirements, employment contracts, and collective bargaining, are not covered.

This discussion of the law as it applies to pharmacy practice in the institutional setting is designed to provide an overview and orientation to the field. It is not to be viewed as an exhaustive discussion of the many and varied legal topics that can arise in the course of professional practice. Appendices 65.4 and 65.5 contain citations for legal materials and references for some articles and books that will assist the interested reader in pursuing additional information on the subjects discussed here.

This chapter is not intended to provide legal advice. Rather, it is designed to assist pharmacists, pharmacy students, and others to identify potential legal entanglements so that further information and counsel can be sought. In some cases it will be necessary to consult an attorney for a legal interpretation of the law on a certain point or application of the law to a given factual situation. Under such circumstances, the attorney serving the institution should be consulted. Some words of caution are appropriate, however, regarding use of the attorney serving the institution. First, although the number of attorneys limiting their practices to health law has increased tremendously in recent years, in many institutions the legal counsel will be provided by a local attorney whose only exposure to pharmacy-related issues is the occasional question from the pharmacy staff at the institution. Thus, in such cases, as with many other situations, how the question is posed to the attorney can be of pivotal importance. The pharmacist should give thorough consideration to the various ways most questions can be phrased because the proper wording of a question can increase the possibilities of receiving the best legal advice. Second, in some situations the legal interests of the institution and the pharmacist may not coincide. In cases where the pharmacist may be to blame for an error, the institution may attempt to isolate itself from the employee pharmacist, laying all of the blame at the feet of the pharmacist. In such cases, pharmacists should secure their own legal counsel to protect their interests and rights and not depend on the institution's attorney.

PHARMACEUTICAL SERVICES

The Pharmacy

The first question that arises in hospital pharmacy is whether any legal requirements must be met before pharmaceutical services may be provided within the institution. Generally state pharmacy laws require a state board of pharmacy license or permit before a pharmacy may be operated. An exception to this general rule in most cases is a pharmacy operated on federal land, such as Veterans Administration and Indian Health Service facilities. Registration with the U.S. Drug Enforcement Administration is required to purchase and dispense controlled substances. The pharmacy as an integral part of the hospital also must meet the requirements of the Joint Commission on Accreditation of Hospitals (JCAH) if accreditation by that organization is sought. Furthermore, many specific technical requirements must be met; these are found in the state pharmacy laws and the U.S. Social Security Administration's Conditions of Participation. These requirements relate to adequate space, equipment, references, and other physical conditions of the pharmacy.

Personnel

In addition to the requirements that concern the operation of a pharmacy within a hospital, there also are legal factors that affect the personnel within the department of pharmaceutical services.

Pharmacists. The most important principle relating to the operation of a pharmacy is that only a pharmacist may practice pharmacy and manage or be in charge of the pharmacy, and to do so he or she must be licensed by the state. Each state imposes its own requirements of education, training, and testing to become licensed as a pharmacist. There may also be additional requirements such as in the case of long-term care facilities seeking federal certification for Medicare or Medicaid, where the conditions of participation require that the pharmacist have ''training or experience in the specialized functions of institutional pharmacy.''

Residents. The foregoing does not mean that other personnel may not be employed in the pharmacy. Pharmacy residents who are enrolled in some specialized, advanced training program generally are already licensed as pharmacists. If they are so licensed, they may provide the same services as a pharmacist.

Pharmacy Interns. Pharmacy interns are generally recognized in state pharmacy laws, but each state may have special requirements for the employment of interns relating to the specific practice experience they must obtain, hours they must work, and reports that must be filed with the board of pharmacy. Some states give interns more leeway than technicians (e.g., in some states an intern may take an oral order for a controlled substance whereas a technician may not).

Supportive Personnel. Other types of supportive personnel may also be used in a hospital pharmacy. Some state boards of pharmacy have specified by regulation what acts may lawfully be performed by supportive personnel, but others have not. Thus, exactly what tasks they may legally perform is sometimes unclear. Certainly, secretaries, clerks, stockboys, and janitors may be employed.

On the other hand, pharmacists are the only individuals permitted to practice pharmacy, and a gray area arises when the tasks being performed by supportive personnel might be interpreted as constituting the practice of pharmacy. The questions arise in connection with the use of technicians who, in some manner, are involved with processing drug orders, drug preparation, and distribution. Answers to specific questions will depend on the interpretation of each state's laws, regulations, and judicial rulings. Nevertheless, it is safe to say that the activities of technicians should be limited to manipulative or mechanical tasks; they should not exercise the discretion or judgment of pharmacists concerning compounding, dispensing, and drug use, and appropriate in-process and technical controls should be used to ensure quality. Their work should be monitored and checked by a pharmacist.

Standards of Professional Practice

Legal Standards. A number of readily identifiable standards have legal significance in the practice of hospital pharmacy. State and federal laws and regulations contain rules that must be followed in practice. Important federal laws and regulations are listed in Appendix 65.1, whereas the primary state laws are identified in Appendix 65.2. Judicial rulings are also important because they contain court interpretations of applicable laws and regulations and principles of constitutional and common law.

Quasi-legal Standards. In addition to these legal standards, certain quasi-legal standards must be consulted in practice, such as those requirements imposed by accrediting agencies such as the JCAH (see Chapter 4). The United States Pharmacopeial Convention publishes drug standards, including those relating to compounding, packaging, and labeling that are enforceable under the Federal Food, Drug and Cosmetic Act (FDCA).

Practice Standards. Professional standards also have a bearing on practice. The American Pharmaceutical Association's Code of Ethics (Appendix 65.3) is a pronouncement by the profession of the ethical standards applicable in pharmacy practice. Likewise, the many statements and guidelines of the American Society of Hospital Pharmacists reflect the level of acceptable current practice. In addition, in a liability suit a pharmacist's performance will be evaluated in light of the performance standards created by his or her peers. More will be said about that in the professional liability section of this chapter.

Areas of Special Interest

In recent years, certain aspects of practice have received heightened interest, from both a legal and a practice point of view. Questions have been raised about the legality of certain practices, whether pharmacists are authorized to provide certain services, what standards apply to these activities, and what new or expanded potential liabilities might attach.

One of the areas of special interest is clinical pharmacy, including patient consultation, taking patient histories, adjusting drug dosages, measuring certain vital signs, and administering medication.

Another area concerns the selection of the drug to be dispensed or administered based on a physician's diagnosis or the selection of the particular brand of drug to be dispensed.

Responsibility for and participation in quality assurance programs is a third area and includes a review of pharmaceutical services and drug use within utilization review programs.

This is not an exhaustive listing of areas of special interest, but it is representative. Unfortunately, not all of the questions related to these practice activities have answers. When a service or practice is questionable, the pharmacist should be sure to maintain subject matter expertise and conduct his affairs with the highest degree of diligence. He or she should not fail to provide the fullest possible scope of service to his patients nor should he or she fail to be innovative in his practice.

DRUG LAWS

Drugs, the stock in trade of pharmacy, are highly regulated commodities under both federal and state laws. Among the most important federal laws that have a direct impact on drugs are the FDCA, the Controlled Substances Act (CSA), the Poison Prevention Packaging Act (PPPA), and alcohol tax laws, which are surveyed in this section.

Food, Drug and Cosmetic Act

The Law. FDCA and applicable regulations are administered by the U.S. Food and Drug Administration (FDA). This law prohibits the introduction of foods, drugs, cosmetics, devices, and diagnostic aids that are adulterated or misbranded into interstate commerce. In general terms, adulteration occurs if a product contains any filthy, putrid, or decomposed substance, if it was processed or held under unsanitary conditions, or if its strength, purity, or quality does not comply with its label. Misbranding results if the labeling is false or misleading or if it does not contain directions for use, precautions, warnings, and other information specified in the FDCA. Drugs are also subject to new drug approvals, investigational new drug (IND) procedures, premarket clearance for safety and effectiveness, good manufacturing practice, manufacturer registration, and a host of other legal requirements.

Use of Investigational Drugs. In terms of hospital pharmacy practice, there are certain areas to watch. Investigational drug use occurs with certain regularity in many hospitals. The pharmacist should be fully aware of the distinction between an investigational use of a drug and its use for the treatment of a disease or condition. (These are distinguished below under "Unapproved Uses.") In the former situation, all of the IND requirements of the FDCA must be met concerning records and reports, informed patient consent, and institutional review procedures, whereas in the latter situations these requirements do not apply.

Unapproved Uses. This legal issue can arise not only with new substances but also with currently marketed products if the prescriber orders a drug to be used in a dosage level or patient population or for a use or by a route of administration not included in the product's FDA approved labeling. The legality of such an order depends on whether the drug is used for treatment or for investigational purposes. The FDCA does not restrict the use for which drugs may be used in treating a patient. If, however, the use is an investigational procedure, evidenced by the record keeping, patient selection, product coding, and other procedures designed to assist in drawing scientific conclusions, then the IND requirements must be followed. Generally speaking, if the objective of drug use is to collect research data, the IND requirements apply, whereas if the objective is to treat without a research component, the requirements do not apply. Obviously, in many cases the distinction will be less than patently clear.

Labeling. Labeling requirements under the FDCA are also important. Dispensing labels must contain (1) the name and address of the dispenser, (2) the serial number of the prescription order, (3) the date of the prescription or its dispensing, (4) the name of the prescriber, (5) the name of the patient, if stated on the prescription, and (6) directions for use and cautionary statements contained in the prescription, if any. Labeling requirements also affect other activities such as prescription price advertisements, the addition of generic names to labels, the name of the actual product manufacturer, and patient package inserts. This area is constantly evolving and should be followed carefully.

Manufacturing. Drug manufacturing requirements as found in the good manufacturing practices (GMP) regula-

tions may have an impact on hospital practice. Basic questions that arise concern the applicability of GMP to centralized IV additive programs, unit dose packaging operations, bulk compounding activities, and the preparation of radiopharmaceuticals. A basic question is whether the drugs are prepared solely for the institution's own use or whether they are distributed to other hospitals or pharmacies. In the latter case, the hospital may be considered a manufacturer, in which case these requirements would apply, as would the requirement to register with the FDA as manufacturer, packer, or distributer.

Controlled Substances Act

The Act. The CSA regulates fewer drugs than the FDCA, but it is no less critical in the practice of pharmacy. In fact, the impact of this area of the law is viewed by some as being more onerous than that of the FDCA. The CSA and regulations promulgated by the enforcement agency, the Drug Enforcement Administration (DEA), contain many specific duties and obligations that must be carried out by pharmacists in their practice. These requirements run from registration before distributing controlled substances to maintaining inventory records, making reports, executing powers of attorney, and special labeling.

Classification of Drugs. Controlled substances are divided into five schedules, depending on their relative potential for abuse, current accepted medical use, safety for use, and relative physical and psychologic dependence.

Schedule I includes certain opiates, opiate derivatives, and hallucinogenic substances such as heroin, LSD, and other drugs that have no currently accepted medical use.

Schedule II includes most of the drugs that were formerly Class A narcotics, such as opium, coca leaves, their various derivatives, synthetic narcotics, and amphetamine, methamphetamine, and other potent stimulants.

Schedule III consists of many of the same narcotics found in Schedule II but in preparations of lesser concentration that may vary by drug and dosage form. Nalorphine is also included. Stimulants not covered elsewhere are included, as well as depressants such as barbiturates and synthetic hypnotics.

Schedule IV includes 11 depressants with a low potential for abuse, such as chloral hydrate, phenobarbital, paraldehyde, meprobamate, and others.

Schedule V is comprised primarily of exempt narcotic cough preparations, camphorated tincture of opium, and diphenoxylate with atropine sulfate. It should be noted that states also have the authority to place controlled substances in the parallel set of schedules that exists under state law. As a result, the possibility exists that more strict control of a given drug product may exist under state law than under federal law. In such cases the more stringent standard prevails.

Registration. All hospitals that wish to purchase and use controlled substances must register annually with the DEA. One registration covers both inpatient and outpatient dispensing. It covers all acts of compounding, dispensing, and administration, and individual employees need not be registered independently. It would not cover manufacturing and distributing to other hospitals; a separate registration would be necessary for that. Separate registration is also needed for each location or principal place of business.

Physicians in private practice must be independently registered to prescribe controlled substances for their hospitalized patients. However, interns or residents employed by the hospital may, under carefully prescribed circumstances, use the hospital's registration to order controlled substances for hospital patients.

Inventories. Physical inventories must be taken of all controlled substances every 2 years after the initial inventory is taken at the start of business. Inventory records must be kept for 2 years. A perpetual inventory is not required, but the inventory must contain a complete and accurate record of all controlled substances. Exact counts of substances in Schedule I or II must be made. If a substance in Schedule III, IV, or V is in a broken package of 1000 units or less, an estimated count or measure may be made.

Records. Records of receipt and disposition of all controlled substances also must be kept for 2 years. This enables the DEA to account for all drugs purchased, dispensed, and still on hand. Records and inventories for substances in Schedule I or II must be maintained separately from all other records whereas those records for substances in Schedules III, IV, and V must be readily retrievable, if they are not separate.

Records of receipt include official order forms or ordinary business records such as invoices or packing slips. The primary record of disposition is the prescription or, in the case of hospitals, the chart order. Prescriptions for Schedule II substances must be filed separately, but those prescriptions for Schedule III, IV, or V drugs may be filed with other prescriptions if stamped in red ink in the lower right-hand corner with the letter "C" no less than 1 inch high. Inpatient charts are generally distilled to yield more manageable records for controlled substances. Certificate of use (proof of use) sheets, medication administration records (MAR), and/or computerized records may be maintained. The computer record or the MAR is the preferred record to use because of the ease of retrieval and detection of diversion.

Official Order Forms. Official order forms are required to purchase substances in Schedule I or II. Only the person whose authorized signature appears in the original registration form may execute an official order form. If the authorized signature is not that of the hospital pharmacist, a power of attorney should be filed with the DEA to allow the pharmacist to execute orders.

Prescribing and Dispensing. Prescriptions under the CSA must be issued for a legitimate medical purpose and not for purposes of detoxification or maintenance of narcotic addicts and must contain the following information: (1) name of the patient, (2) address of the patient, (3) name of the practitioner, (4) address of the practitioner, (5) the DEA registration number of the practitioner, (6) the name, strength, and quantity of medication, and (7) directions for use, if any. Schedule II substances require written prescriptions prepared with ink, indelible pencil, or a typewriter and must be dated and signed manually on that day. Schedule II prescriptions may not be refilled. Oral prescriptions are permissible for substances in Schedules III and IV and may be refilled up to five times within 6 months of issuance. Sched-

ule V drugs or nonlegend drugs in other schedules may be sold without prescription when sold personally by a pharmacist to purchasers at least 18 years of age within specified quantity limits, and a record must be maintained in a bound book.

When dispensing controlled substances, the label must state (1) the date of filling, (2) the pharmacy's name, (3) the pharmacy's address, (4) the serial number of the prescription, (5) the name of the patient, (6) the name of the prescriber, (7) directions for use, and (8) the statement, "Caution: Federal law prohibits transfer of this drug to any person other than the patient for whom it was prescribed," except that this last cautionary statement is not required for Schedule V substances.

Security. All registrants must provide effective controls and procedures to guard against theft and diversion of controlled substances. Controlled substances may be stored in a securely locked, substantially constructed cabinet or dispersed throughout the stock of noncontrolled substances in such a manner as to obstruct the theft or diversion of the controlled substances unless more stringent rules are contained in state law or regulations. Also registrants may not allow any employee access to controlled substances if that employee has had an application for registration denied or has had a registration revoked. When controlled substances are stored at nursing units, they should be kept in a securely locked area, and only authorized personnel should have access to these drugs.

The Poison Prevention Packaging Act

The PPPA provides for special packaging to protect children from serious personal injury or illness that could result, in part, from ingesting medications that are sold for home use. All oral prescription drugs, products containing controlled substances, and aspirin and other salicylates are some of the products requiring special safety packaging if such products are sold or dispensed by the pharmacy for home use by patients of the hospital. The requirements for safety closures do not apply to medications intended for use within the institution. Nor do they apply to certain products that are exempted by regulation.

Pharmacists should be aware that covered products may be dispensed in noncomplying packages if the physician or purchaser requests it. Blanket orders from a physician are invalid; requests for noncomplying packaging must be stated with each prescription. In the case of consumer requests for noncomplying packaging, it is recommended that pharmacists retain a written record of the request.

Alcohol Tax Laws

Under federal tax laws, hospitals and similar institutions may use alcohol, tax free, for medical or scientific purposes. This is true whether the hospital or sanitarium is operated on a profit or nonprofit basis. The regulations contain strict rules for record keeping and monthly reports on such alcohol use. Tax-free alcohol may not be used for beverage purposes or in any food products.

PROFESSIONAL LIABILITY

Criminal Accountability

Various types of liabilities can arise in practicing such a complex and highly regulated profession as pharmacy. Both criminal and civil sanctions can be applied for transgressing legal prohibitions. They can range from civil and administrative penalties to steep fines and long-term imprisonments. Licenses may be suspended or revoked or limitations placed on one's right to practice. In some cases the violation may constitute a misdemeanor and in others it may be a felony. Fines run from $25 for the violation of a pharmacy act to $50,000 for repeated violation of the CSA.

There are many types of laws that, when violated, could result in action against pharmacists, for example:

State pharmacy act requirements of practice

FDCA standards of adulteration and misbranding

CSA requirements for record keeping and labeling

Social Security Act prohibition against kickbacks and false claims

Internal Revenue Code tax payments on income and alcohol

Antitrust prohibitions against fixing prices and unfair competition.

Negligence

Aside from a few unlikely intentional torts that might arise from professional practice, the area of greatest concern to pharmacists is that of negligence, which encompasses malpractice, and product liability, which encompasses breach of warranty (discussed below).

Negligence, or in this case malpractice, is a course of conduct that creates an unreasonable risk by falling below the standard of conduct acceptable by law. It amounts to carelessness, a lack of foresight, or neglect. Certain elements are necessary to maintain a lawsuit for negligence:

1. There must be a legal duty owed to the patient or plaintiff and that duty must be breached.
2. The patient or plaintiff must suffer damages.
3. The breach of the duty must have been the proximate or direct cause of the damages.
4. The defendant (pharmacist) must have no valid defenses to assert.

Breach of Duty. The duty, or standard of care, that pharmacists owe to patients usually flows from the practices of one's professional peers. That is, the level of practice of other pharmacists with similar skills, knowledge, training, and experience will be used to establish a standard by which the performance of a pharmacist being sued is measured. The legal system works by having the jury listen to the testimony of other reputable practitioners of pharmacy describing how they would have handled the transaction in question. The jury then draws a conclusion regarding what a mythical reasonable and prudent pharmacist would or would not have done under the circumstances.

For a number of years, courts ruled that the frame of reference was to be a local one based on the practices of professionals in the same or similar communities. In recent years, however, the courts have been moving away from a local standard and using more of a national standard that reflects the level of practice around the nation.

Pharmacists are held to an extremely stringent standard of care, sometimes referred to as the "highest degree of care" or a "very special degree of responsibility." Some courts will refer to the pharmacist's responsibility or legal duty as requiring "ordinary care" but with reference to that special and peculiar practice of pharmacy and with a degree of vigilance and prudence commensurate with the dangers involved.

Whereas courts and juries will usually look to the practices of professional peers to determine legal duty, in some situations the law will infer a duty from other sources. Some of these sources of legal duty were previously mentioned (e.g., JCAH Standards, Medicare and Medicaid Conditions of Participation, state pharmacy practice acts, statements or standards of professional organizations, etc).

Over the years, negligence on the part of the pharmacist has been found where the wrong drug was dispensed, where the quantity of ingredients was improper, where the wrong route of administration was used, and where a continuous supply of medication was not available, each leading to the patient suffering damages.

Damages. For a negligence suit to be successful, the patient or plaintiff must have suffered legally recognized damages. It should be emphasized that not all damages are sufficient to support a malpractice claim. The damages must at least be sufficient to cross a threshold constituting substantial damages. That is, there must be some amount of damage sufficient to warrant the legal action. Unfortunately, there is no specific dollar amount that indicates where this threshold lies; it must be determined on a case-by-case basis.

Sometimes the issue of whether damages have indeed occurred is complex. For example, in a case where a pharmacist dispensed a sedative rather than the prescribed oral contraceptive, the issue was whether the birth of a child constitutes legally recognized damage, or is such a birth to be viewed as a blessing, as it would be in normal circumstances. In this case, the expense of raising the child was considered to be an unexpected and undesired outcome and the pharmacist was ordered to assist with the cost of rearing the child.

Proximate or Direct Cause. For the patient or plaintiff's malpractice claim to be successful, he or she must establish that the breach of the legal duty was the direct or proximate cuase of the damages suffered. In most cases based on drug use this is the most difficult element of the case to establish given fact that such causal relationships are not easily established.

The law requires that the breach of the duty be shown to have led directly and without interruption to the damages. One case that exemplifies this rule involved a pharmacist who compounded and dispensed some medication using an incorrect vehicle. The pharmacy was determined not to have been negligent because the damages were not directly caused by the incorrect vehicle. In fact, it was found that the medication would have caused the adverse reaction even if the correct vehicle had been used. Hence, the pharmacist's error was not the direct or proximate cause of the injury.

Valid Defenses. Even if the plaintiff is able to establish the previous three elements, he or she may be prevented from prevailing in the suit because the pharmacist has some valid defenses to assert. These defenses will exculpate the defendant pharmacist.

One such defense that can be made is the statute of limitations, a legislatively imposed time limit within which the lawsuit must be commenced. If the plaintiff delays too long in filing the suit, he or she will lose forever the right to bring suit for the damages suffered. In most states the statute of limitations is 1 or 2 years from the time of the discovery of the injury.

Another defense is that the plaintiff in some way contributed to the damages suffered. The traditional rule in this area is that if the plaintiff was negligent and contributed to the injury through negligence, then he or she is totally barred from recovery. However, the modern rule now followed in a majority of states is known as comparative negligence. Under this approach, the jury apportions blame between the plaintiff and the defendant, deciding who was how much at fault. The judgment awarded the plaintiff is then reduced by the percentage of the damages attributed to the plaintiff. This can be viewed as a partial defense in that it reduces the amount the defendant is required to pay.

Breach of Warranties

Negligence as a basis for liability claims requires that someone must have breached a duty, etc. Liability claims can also be based on breach of warranty, which does not require proof of negligence. The law of warranties comes into play because pharmacists, in addition to providing a service, also sell a product. When products are sold, warranties may accompany the sale. Express warranties are statements made at the time of sale that describe the ability of the product to perform (e.g., "this product will cure your cough"). If it does not, the express warranty has been breached. An implied warranty, on the other hand, is one present in the transaction not because of a statement affirmatively made by the seller at the time of the transaction but present in the sale because of the law.

Two primary warranties implied in a transaction by the law are the implied warranty of merchantibility and the implied warranty of fitness for a particular purpose. Merchantibility means the products are acceptable within the trade and of quality suitable for sale. Fitness for a particular purpose means that the goods are appropriate for a particular use for which they were ordered. A typical situation where this would be encountered is where the purchaser describes to the seller the need to which the product will be applied and then relies on the knowledge and expertise of the seller to select a suitable product.

Under these rules, expired medication would not be considered merchantable because the possibility exists that it may be decomposed beyond the point of being acceptable. Likewise, a product that has no value in treating a cough would not be fit for treating a cough. Simple proof of the breach of these warranties can lead to liability.

Professional Liability Insurance

No matter how skilled or how careful a pharmacist is, the possibility of liability arising out of professional practice always exists. The risk of liability is directly proportionate to the number of standards that must be met, and with all the laws, regulations, and standards that apply in pharmacy, the risk is high.

Each practicing pharmacist should have professional liability insurance coverage whether he or she is an owner, supervisor, or employee. Group professional and personal liability insurance are available to pharmacists at reasonable cost from professional pharmacy associations such as the American Society of Hospital Pharmacists. There are two advantages to purchasing professional liability insurance through professional organizations. First, the rates are lower because of group sales. Second, the sponsoring organization will ordinarily have the wording of the policy scrutinized by its attorney to assure that the language provides optimal protection for the insured pharmacist.

CONCLUSION

Although the law affecting pharmacy practice is complex, sufficient time should be devoted to attempting to understand it. By doing so one can minimize liability exposure and assure compliance with legal requirements. In the pharmacy department with multiple staff members, it might be wise to assign one pharmacist the responsibility of keeping up with legal developments affecting pharmacy practice in institutions so that someone on the staff will have detailed knowledge in this area.

Appendix 65.1
CITATIONS TO RELEVANT FEDERAL STATUTES AND REGULATIONS

Statutes

Alcohol Tax Law. 26 U.S.C. §§5214, 5271.

Animal Welfare Act of 1970. 7 U.S.C. §§2131-2155.

Atomic Energy Act of 1954. 42 U.S.C. §§2022-2201.

Controlled Substances Act of 1970, P.L. No. 91-513, 84 Stat. 1236 (codified in scattered sections of 18, 19, 21, 31, 40, 42, and 49 U.S.C.).

Federal Food, Drug and Cosmetic Act. 21 U.S.C. §§301-392.

Health Maintenance Organization Act of 1973. P.L. No. 92-222, 87 Stat. 914 (codified in scattered sections of 12 and 42 U.S.C.).

Narcotic Addict Treatment Act of 1974. P.L. No. 93-281, 88 Stat. 124 (codified in various sections of 21 U.S.C.).

Poison Prevention Packaging Act of 1970. P.L. No. 91-601, 84 Stat. 1670 (codified in 15 U.S.C. §§1471-1476, and scattered sections of 7 and 21 U.S.C.).

Social Security Amendments of 1965 (Medicare and Medicaid). Pub. L. No. 89-97, 79 Stat. 286 (codified in scattered sections of 18, 26, 42 and 45 U.S.C.).

Regulations

Consumer Product Safety Commission (Poison Prevention Packaging Act). 16 C.F.R. §§1700-1704 (1984).

Drug Enforcement Administration. 21 C.F.R. §§1301-1316 (1984).

Food and Drug Administration. 21 C.F.R. §§1-1230 (1984).

Internal Revenue Service (Alcohol Tax Law). 26 C.F.R. §§213.1-213.176 (1984).

Social Security Administration (Medicare); Health Care Financing Administration (Medicaid). Hospitals–20 C.F.R. §405 (1984); Skilled Nursing Facilities–20 C.F.R. §405 (1984); Intermediate Care Facilities–20 C.F.R. §§249-250 (1984); HMOs–42 C.F.R. §110 (1984).

Appendix 65.2
COMMON STATE LAWS AFFECTING PHARMACY*

Hazardous Substances Labeling Act

State Food, Drug and Cosmetic Act

State Pharmacy Act

State Poison Law

Uniform Controlled Substances Act

Uniform Narcotic Drug Act

---

*These are the most commonly encountered titles for state laws affecting pharmacy. Sometimes states use separate or differently titled laws to control foods, drugs, cosmetics, narcotics, stimulants, hazardous substances, etc.

Appendix 65.3
AMERICAN PHARMACEUTICAL ASSOCIATION CODE OF ETHICS*

Preamble

These principles of professional conduct are established to guide pharmacists in relationships with patients, fellow practitioners, other health professionals, and the public.

A Pharmacist should hold the health and safety of pa-

tients to be of first consideration and should render to each patient the full measure of professional ability as an essential health practitioner.

A Pharmacist should never knowingly condone the dispensing, promoting, or distributing of drugs or medical devices, or assist therein, that are not of good quality, that do not meet standards required by law, or that lack therapeutic value for the patient.

A Pharmacist should always strive to perfect and enlarge

---

*Approved by APhA Active and Life members August 1969, amended December 1975, revised July 1981.

professional knowledge. A pharmacist should utilize and make available this knowledge as may be required in accordance with the best professional judgment.

A Pharmacist has the duty to observe the law, to uphold the dignity and honor of the profession, and to accept its ethical principles. A pharmacist should not engage in any activity that will bring discredit to the profession and should expose, without fear or favor, illegal or unethical conduct in the profession.

A Pharmacist should seek at all times only fair and reasonable remuneration for professional services. A pharmacist should never agree to, or participate in, transactions with practitioners of other health professions or any other person under which fees are divided or that may cause financial or other exploitation in connection with the rendering of professional services.

A Pharmacist should respect the confidential and personal nature of professional records; except where the best interest of the patient requires or the law demands, a pharmacist should not disclose such information to anyone without proper patient authorization.

A Pharmacist should not agree to practice under terms or conditions that interfere with or impair the proper exercise of professional judgment and skill, that cause a deterioration of the quality of professional services, or that require consent to unethical conduct.

A Pharmacist should strive to provide information to patients regarding professional services truthfully, accurately, and fully and should avoid misleading patients regarding the nature, cost, or value of these professional services.

A Pharmacist should associate with organizations having for their objective the betterment of the profession of pharmacy and should contribute time and funds to carry on the work of these organizations.

Appendix 65.4
LEGAL ARTICLES IN THE AMERICAN JOURNAL OF HOSPITAL PHARMACY

Volume	Date	Page	Title
25	1968	528	Medication errors and legal implications of drug handling on the patient floor
26	1969	346	Taxability of income of hospital pharmacy residents in ASHP-accredited residency programs
26	1969	404	Legal responsibility of the hospital pharmacist for rational drug therapy
26	1969	537	Regulation on the sale of narcotics through hospitals and related institutions: Monkey on our backs?
27	1970	318	Federal legislation: An examination and prognosis
27	1970	684	Federal legislation: An examination and prognosis: Part II
27	1970	848	State union law: A look at the new Pennsylvania public employee relations act
27	1970	1011	Federal legislation: An examination and prognosis: Part III
28	1971	127	National health insurance: A look at what Congress is prescribing
28	1971	290	Comprehensive drug abuse prevention and control act of 1970
28	1971	707	State narcotic and drug abuse laws: A combination of ingredients
29	1972	168	Some legal considerations in the formation of a group practice
29	1972	774	Some legal considerations in the formation of a group practice: Part II
29	1972	970	The Florida "Institutional Pharmacy" Law
30	1973	168	The new methadone regulations
30	1973	723	PSROs and pharmacy
30	1973	1067	The legal basis for clinical pharmacy
31	1974	86	Some legal aspects of the hospital formulary system
31	1974	402	Health maintenance organization act of 1973
32	1975	212	Implications of certificate of need legislation for institutional pharmacy practice
32	1975	1159	Maximum allowable costs for medications in hospitals
33	1976	475	Current federal legislation
33	1976	572	Portland Retail Druggists Association vs Abbott Laboratories et al, part I
33	1976	648	Portland Retail Druggist Association vs Abbott Laboratories et al, part II
33	1976	814	Legal implications of preparing and dispensing drugs under conditions not in a product's official labeling
33	1976	937	The Federal Drug and Devices Act and the Drug Safety Amendments of 1976
33	1976	1049	Federal health planning, part I: Legislative background
33	1976	1211	Health planning, part II: The National Health Planning and Resources Development Act of 1974
33	1976	1308	Medical devices amendments of 1976
34	1977	90	Antisubstitution law changes and the hospital formulary system
34	1977	541	Effect of NLRB rulings and collective bargaining by hospital pharmacists
35	1978	81	Regulatory aspects of investigational new drugs
		729	Drug Regulation Reform Act
36	1979	85	Pharmacy inspections: Constitutional without a warrant?
36	1979	226	Patient package inserts and the pharmacist's responsibility

Volume	Date	Page	Title
37	1980	537	Implications of the Lannett and Pharmadyne decisions
37	1980	1546	Legal standard of due care for pharmacists in institutional practice
37	1980	1656	Institutional pharmacists' guide to complying with PPI regulations
38	1981	218	Liability of the pharmacist as a therapeutic consultant
38	1981	222	Update on the Lannett and Pharmadyne decisions
38	1981	892	Role of JCAH standards in negligence suits
38	1981	1768	Legality of mandatory continuing professional education
38	1981	1949	Therapeutic substitution and the hospital formulary system
39	1982	1544	Pharmacists as a liability-reducing factor
40	1983	111	"Procompetition" and the continuing struggle to contain health care costs
40	1983	282	Legal implications of preparing and dispensing approved drugs for unlabeled indications
40	1983	439	Pharmacist liability for suicide by drug overdose
40	1983	739	Recent Supreme Court antitrust rulings in health care
41	1984	942	Medicare coverage of hospice care
41	1984	1115	Legal issues associated with the handling of cytotoxic drugs (special feature)
41	1984	2074	Legal aspects of termination of employment
42	1985	352	Legal aspects of outpatient drug transactions in nonprofit hospitals
42	1985	849	Repercussions of The Drug Price Competition and Patent Term Restoration Act of 1984
42	1985	1572	Robinson-Patman update: DeModena v. Kaiser Foundation Health Plan

Appendix 65.5
BOOKS ON PHARMACY LAW

Bonnie RJ, Sonnenreich MR: *Legal Aspects of Drug Dependence.* Cleveland, CRC Press, 1975.

DeMarco CT: *Pharmacy and the Law,* ed 2. Rockville, MD, Aspen Systems, 1984.

Eldridge WB: *Narcotics and the Law,* ed 2. Chicago, University of Chicago Press, 1969.

Fink III JL, Marquardt KW, Simonsmeier LM: *Pharmacy Law Digest.* Media, PA, Harwal Publishing, 1985.

Gibson JT: *Medication Law and Behavior.* New York, John Wiley & Sons, 1976.

Hassan WE: *Law for the Pharmacy Student.* Philadelphia, Lea & Febiger, 1971.

Hickmon LE: *Pharmacy Practice for Trial Lawyers.* Norcross, GA, Harrison Co, 1981.

Merrill RA, Hutt PB: *Food and Drug Law: Cases and Materials.* Mineola, NY, Foundation Press, 1980.

Patterson RM, Robinson RE: *Drugs in Litigation: Damage Awards Involving Prescription and Nonprescription Drugs,* ed 2. Indianapolis, Allen Smith, 1982.

Rheingold PD: *Drug Litigation,* ed 3. New York, Practicing Law Institute, 1981.

Strauss S (ed): *The Pharmacist and the Law.* Baltimore, Williams & Wilkins, 1980.

Uelman GF, Haddox VG: *Cases, Text and Materials on Drug Abuse and the Law.* St Paul, West Publishing, 1974.

Wetherbee H, White BD: *Cases and Materials on Pharmacy Law.* St Paul, West Publishing, 1980.

CHAPTER 66

Professional Relations

MICHAEL L. KLEINBERG

In an editorial in the *American Journal of Hospital Pharmacy,* William Zellmer (1) described the sometimes uneasy relationship between hospital pharmacists and pharmaceutical manufacturers:

The purpose of contemporary pharmacy is the advancement of rational drug therapy. This purpose is incompatible with certain goals of the industry which include the promotion of drug product sales to generate profits and returns on investment. The patient-oriented roles to which pharmacy aspires (e.g., drug product selection, patient education and counseling, drug information services, management of drug therapy for chronic illnesses) require the pharmacist to be an independent practitioner. In order to establish and maintain his credibility, the pharmacist must be free from any hint of alliance with the manufacturers and distributors of drug products.

The methods used by the pharmaceutical company to achieve its objectives are linked closely to the hospital. Most new drug entities are tested and evaluated on hospitalized patients, and the hospital pharmacist may be involved with the drug company to develop and test their product. Mutual questions regarding drug stability, packaging, storage, and pharmacokinetics are answered in research protocols designed by the drug company and the hospital pharmacist. Producing a product that will help the consumer and that can easily be controlled by the hospital will benefit both the pharmaceutical industry and the hospital pharmacist.

In defining a relationship between the hospital pharmacist and the pharmaceutical industry, it is necessary to define the objectives or goals for each. A clear sense as to why each group exists will help foster this interrelationship.

The hospital, for the most part, exists to perform one of four functions. These include delivering patient care; teaching physicians and other health professionals; laboratory and clinical research; and service to the community. An example of a hospital mission statement is shown in Figure 66.1.

Defining the goals of the pharmaceutical industry is equally important. See Figure 66.2 for an example of its goals.

In both examples, the goal of making a profit was not included. This, however, belongs in both statements. The hospital requires the production of revenue for growth and for upgrading services and technology. The hospital is responsible to its owners, be it a private corporation or government owned. The pharmaceutical industry needs a profit to continue its activities and growth and is responsible to its shareholders.

By looking at the goals of both the hospital and the pharmaceutical industry, one can see how the interrelationship can be developed so that both groups may achieve their own individual goals. Examples of this include developing drug distribution systems, innovative drug delivery systems, patient and professional educational services, and clinical and technical research activities. When both groups work together, both benefit. The hospital pharmacist is able to provide innovative distribution and clinical services, and the pharmaceutical industry is able to provide a product that can be used.

MEDICAL SERVICE REPRESENTATIVES

The medical service representative (MSR) is the liaison between the pharmaceutical industry and the hospital. The goals of the MSR are the same as those of his or her company, i.e., to obtain a marketable product and to sell that product. The MSR achieves these goals by interacting with various health professionals in the institution. These include physicians, residents, interns, nurses, and pharmacists.

The typical functions of an MSR are listed in Table 66.1. Obtaining information on available drugs is important to the hospital pharmacist. This information should be concise and accurate. A form may be developed to record this information. Independent clinical studies should be part of the

TABLE 66.1 Functions of the Medical Service Representative

A. Provide current information on available drugs
   1. Dose
   2. Use (new use)
   3. Side effects
   4. Compatibility
   5. Pharmacology
   6. Pharmacokinetics
B. Provide current information and possible solutions on company services or problems
   1. Availability of continuing educational programs
   2. Drug recalls
   3. Return goods
   4. Drug prices
   5. Back orders

MISSION STATEMENT
UCSD MEDICAL CENTER

UCSD Medical Center is the only general acute care institution in San Diego and Imperial Counties that serves as the primary teaching hospital for the University of California, San Diego School of Medicine and is open to all members of the general civilian population. As such, UCSD Medical Center must fulfill simultaneously three principal missions:

• To deliver comprehensive, high quality patient care that is responsive to the needs of the San Diego region as a whole and of the local community.

• To provide an environment appropriate for the education of physicians and allied health professionals.

• To provide an environment that supports and encourages clinical research.

In addition to these primary missions, the Medical Center is committed to working closely with other hospitals, government agencies, health care organizations and community groups to identify community health needs and problems and to contribute toward their resolution. Where appropriate, UCSD Medical Center, in conjunction with the University of California, San Diego School of Medicine, will also seek to provide selected services to patients from Mexico, Central and South America, and the Pacific Basin.

Patient Care
UCSD Medical Center is committed to providing highly specialized services for the treatment of major illnesses and injury to the San Diego region as a whole and primary and secondary services as required to meet local community needs and the educational and research objectives of the University of California, San Diego School of Medicine. All patient care will be rendered in a personal and sensitive manner without regard to race, creed, or national origin. In discharging these responsibilities, UCSD Medical Center will foster the growth and development of the clinically active faculty, other health professionals and staff.

Education
UCSD Medical Center, in concert with the University of California, San Diego School of Medicine, is committed to educating physicians, nurses and other health professionals to meet future health care needs. In order to produce professionals of high competence and integrity with a broad view of health care and its roles in society, UCSD Medical Center will maintain and develop a spectrum of primary, secondary and tertiary services and will endeavor to attract a culturally and economically diverse patient population.

Research
Basic and clinical research is essential to continued advancement in the understanding and treatment of disease and to improvement in the health status of the population. Such research contributes substantially both to the general public well-being and to the educational and patient care missions of the UCSD Medical Center. UCSD Medical Center is therefore committed to providing an environment conducive to clinical investigation.

Community Responsibility
UCSD Medical Center recognizes the crucial importance of social, environmental and economic factors in the health of the community. The Medical Center will take an active role in promoting, assisting, developing and conducting programs leading to improvements in the community health.

FIGURE 66.1

GOALS OF THE PHARMACEUTICAL INDUSTRY

1. To provide pharmaceutical products through research.

2. To promote pharmaceutical products in an ethical manner.

3. To provide to the professional community information on pharmaceutical products.

FIGURE 66.2

UCSD
Medical Center
Department of Pharmacy

PHARMACEUTICAL SALES REPRESENTATIVES COMMITTEE

I. GENERAL INFORMATION

These guidelines have been developed by the Pharmaceutical Sales Representatives Committee to assist and guide all Pharmaceutical Sales Representatives who call upon the University of California Medical Center, San Diego.

A Pharmaceutical Sales Representative (PSR) is defined as the representative of a pharmaceutical company having products/service which are the responsibility of the Department of Pharmacy to evaluate or purchase.

The Committee serves as an ad hoc committee to the Pharmacy and Therapeutics Committee. The names of current members are available through the Director of Pharmacy.

The purpose and function of the Committee are:

(1) Development, implementation, and enforcement of policies and peer review concerning the activities of the Pharmaceutical Sales Representatives in the Hospital.

(2) Maintenance of effective communication between the hospital professional staff and the pharmaceutical industry representatives.

(3) Efficient utilization of health care personnel time through implementation of the PSR guidelines.

The Pharmaceutical Sales Representative Committee is composed of three (3) representatives of pharmaceutical companies and three (3) members of the Department of Pharmacy, a physician-member of the Pharmacy and Therapeutics Committee, and the Director of Pharmacy.

Pharmaceutical company members of the Committee will be selected with consideration of the following criteria:

(a) Representatives who are at the facility on a routine basis.

(b) Representatives whose company's products involve several classes of drugs.

(c) Representatives interested in serving on the Committee should submit their names to the Department of Pharmacy office by October 1st of each year.

(d) Recommendations will be requested from the Medical Service Society.

Terms of Office

(1) Term of office will run from January to December.

(2) Original committee members will hold office until December 1984; thereafter one position will change each year and term of office will run for three years.

(3) If a vacancy should occur in mid-term, the Committee will be responsible for notifying other representatives of the vacancy. Representatives interested in filling this unexpired term will be requested to submit their names. Replacement will then be selected by the Committee.

Policies developed by the PSR Committee are forwarded to the Pharmacy and Therapeutics Committee, and with the approval of that Committee are submitted to the Hospital Executive Committee. Policies will be communicated to the medical center professional staff by means of DIScourse, the Drug Information bulletin.

The Committee will meet six (6) times yearly. Each meeting will be scheduled three weeks before the Pharmacy and Therapeutics Committee meeting. A representative wishing to attend a meeting of the Committee will leave a note with the Department of the Pharmacy Administrative Assistant. The Committee will invite the representative's attendance.

The Committee will maintain two (2) log books. One book will contain all information to representatives from the Committee. The second book will be used for communicating information between representatives and also with the Department of Pharmacy.

The Committee will also issue identifying badges. The badges will be maintained in the Department of Pharmacy office and will be worn by the representatives while in the Hospital. Badges will be signed out when coming to the Hospital for a visit and returned at the end of that visit.

II. PROCEDURES FOR NEWLY ASSIGNED PSRs

A. All newly assigned PSRs shall introduce themselves to the Administrative Assistant in the Pharmacy Office and secure an appointment with the Pharmacist Purchasing Agent.

B. During this initial meeting, the Pharmacy Administrative Assistant will provide the new PSR with:

(1) One (1) copy of the PSR Guidelines; PSR will sign for these guidelines.

(2) One (1) copy of the PSR Guidelines for delivery to the PSR's District Manager.

(3) A list of names, addresses, and telephone numbers of PSRs currently serving on the Committee.

(4) A brief orientation to the PSR Guidelines.

(5) A description of the Drug Information Service, Hospital Purchasing Department, and Pharmacy Purchasing Section and procedures for visiting the Purchasing Section.

C. Following the initial meeting, the PSR shall:

(1) Give the Administrative Assistant three business cards bearing name, current address, and telephone number for inclusion in the PSR log.

(2) Delete the previous PSR's card from the file maintained by the Pharmacy Administrative Assistant.

(3) Request the Pharmacy Administrative Assistant to order you a name tag (a personal in-house authorization badge), payment to be made in advance, and sign in the PSR log. A temporary badge will be issued until your name badge is received.

(4) Make an appointment with the Drug Information Director to assure that appropriate information on the company's product are on file.

FIGURE 66.3

(5) Check the PSR file for messages addressed to the predecessor or the company.

(6) With the PSR Committee List provided, check the PSR log to determine if a PSR on the Committee is in-house to contact for orientation. If a meeting cannot be arranged, the new PSR should contact a PSR on the Committee at home to arrange for orientation at a convenient time for both parties.

(7) Read the PSR guidelines thoroughly before attempting to contact Hospital Personnel and before the orientation by a PSR on the Committee.

(8) Check for PSR announcements in the PSR sign-in area.

III. STANDARD PROCEDURES

A. All PSRs calling on the University of California Medical Center, San Diego, shall come to the Department of Pharmacy office prior to visiting other areas of the Hospital or Clinics. Representatives shall sign the PSR log in which there will be space for noting departments or personnel on whom the representative will call. These entries in the PSR log do not provide authorization for representatives to call on restricted areas. Each time that a PSR signs in at the Pharmacy, s/he shall secure an in-house authorization badge from the file box in the PSR sign-in area. This badge shall be worn visibly at all times in-house. This badge is recognized by Security and will assist the PSR during visits within the Hospital. If the badge is lost, a $5.00 fee will be charged for replacement. A temporary badge may be obtained at the Pharmacy Office until a new badge is secured.

B. PSRs shall first inform the Drug Information Director and the Pharmacist Purchasing Agent of the therapeutic and supply-price aspects, respectively, of new or nonformulary drugs which they wish to discuss in the Hospital. No restrictions will be placed on discussion of such drugs in the hospital unless the Department of Pharmacy determines that the use of the product is detrimental to patient care.

C. PSRs shall provide the Drug Information Director with monograph packets on new drugs their companies release as soon as such information is made available. Information on changes pertaining to currently available drugs (i.e., indications, dosage, routes of administration, formulation, etc.) shall be provided to the Drug Information Director before discussion with hospital personnel. A copy of any material to be distributed in the University of California Medical Center, San Diego, shall be left with the Drug Information Director.

D. Each PSR shall assure current address and telephone number are filed in the Pharmacy Office.

E. On each visit, PSRs shall check in the PSR log for their messages and acknowledge receipt of these messages.

F. On each visit, PSRs shall check in the PSR sign-in area for announcements and minutes of the PSR Committee meetings.

IV. PSR ACTIVITIES WITHIN THE HOSPITAL

A. Only one representative per company shall visit a clinic or patient care area at a time. An exception to this is permitted for a newly hired PSR who may be accompanied by the manager or senior PSR during his/her training period or with approval of the Director of Pharmacy.

B. Operating Suites and Delivery Suites: PSRs may enter these suites by appointment only.

C. Patient Care Areas: PSRs may enter patient care divisions only on the specific invitation of a specific physician, nursing supervisor, or pharmacist. PSRs shall pass through the divisions only when there is not a convenient alternate route to their destination.

D. Respect for Individual Time: Physicians, pharmacists, nurses, and other professionals are busy with patient care responsibilities. Respect should be given to their time and commitments.

V. SAMPLE POLICY

A. Office Use: It is the policy to discourage the use and storage of sample drugs in offices and clinics. The indiscriminate supply of samples can lead to overuse, and may encourage theft or diversion. However, it is recognized that a minimal number of sample drugs may be desirable in specific offices or clinics. The following rules should apply:

(1) No samples will be left in any office or clinic without express permission of the P&T Committee.

(2) Permission for specific samples may be requested only by faculty physicians.

(3) Faculty physicians may request permission to keep samples in their office or clinic by notifying the P&T Committee of their intent, name specific samples to be stored and amounts to be on hand, and storage conditions.
The P&T Committee will notify the faculty physician in writing of their concurrence.

B. Permission to keep specific samples can be given on interim approval by the Chairman of the P&T Committee or Director of Pharmacy. This approval is effective only until the next scheduled P&T meeting. Notification may be made to the Director of Pharmacy.

C. No samples will be left in any hospital nursing unit, non-physician's office, or on the premises—with the exceptions listed above.

D. Personal Use: Requested drugs for physicians' own use shall be delivered directly to the physician. This will generally be by direct mail from the drug company.
This policy also applies to nutritional products.

VI. RULES FOR ENFORCEMENT OF GUIDELINES FOR PSRs

A. Person or persons filing a complaint shall be interviewed by the Review Committee or by the P&T Committee.

B. PSR accused of infraction shall be interviewed by the Review Committee after person filing complaint has been interviewed.

C. Review Committee shall then decide if an infraction has occured and, if so, will determine the severity of the infraction and report their findings to the full Committee for resolution.

D. For minor infractions, a verbal warning will be given followed in writing by a letter. For major or repeated infractions, the penalty will be greater than a warning and a letter will be sent to the PSRs District Manager and/or the home office.

E. Penalties will range from written warning to exclusion of the individual from the hospital. The Committe will recommend to the P&T Committee action to be taken.

FIGURE 66-3, cont'd

UNIVERSITY OF CALIFORNIA MEDICAL CENTER
SAN DIEGO

UNIVERSITY HOSPITAL
225 W. DICKINSON STREET
SAN DIEGO, CALIFORNIA 92103

SUBJECT: RULES FOR PHARMACEUTICAL EXHIBITS

1. Exhibits are held in the Cafeteria Small Dining Rooms, during the hours 7:00 AM to 11:00 AM on the first Wednesday of each month. These exhibits are open to the physicians, pharmacists, nurses, and other members of the hospital professional staff.
   a. All exhibits must be set up no later than 7:15 AM on the exhibit date.
   b. No exhibit shall be dismantled and removed prior to 11:00 AM.
2. Exhibitors may request exhibit space by submitting an application form along with a ten dollar ($10.00) registration fee. Checks should be made payable to the Medical Service Society. (See application procedures attached.)
   a. Exhibitors will check into the Pharmacy Administration office on the exhibit date and pick up a validated display permit and Vendor's Hospital Pass.
3. Exhibits will be kept to a reasonable size; a floor area not to exceed 4' by 5' is desired.
   a. Each exhibitor should be prepared to supply his/her own table, since a sufficient number may not be available.
   b. The exhibitors are responsible for returning the room to its original condition prior to the exhibit.
4. Only materials of an educational nature will be displayed and available.
   a. No drug samples, whether legend or non-legend, will be given out at displays.
   b. Representatives wishing to leave samples for a physician's personal use may leave the requested samples in the Pharmacy Department marked for the physician's attention. Representatives will not be permitted in other areas of the hospital for the express purpose of delivering samples.
5. Due to limited exhibit space, only one representative per exhibit space is permitted.
   a. Training and supervisory visitations are not exceptions to this rule.
   b. Exhibitors may not leave the display unattended.
6. Only those products approved by the Director, Department of Pharmacy may be displayed. Normally, only Formulary Products will be approved for display.
7. University Hospital reserves the right to refuse displays to representatives who have previously violated "Regulations for Pharmaceutical Representatives" or these exhibit rules.
8. Exhibitors will keep a validated display permit in view during their exhibit.

FIGURE 66.4

APPLICATION PROCEDURES FOR PHARMACEUTICAL EXHIBITS

Because a limited amount of exhibit space is available, it is not possible to accommodate all the pharmaceutical representatives who wish to exhibit each month. In order to assign exhibit space in as equitable a manner as possible, the following procedure for accepting applications for exhibits is in effect.

a. Each representative is assigned to one of three groups (see attached list). Any representative whose company has displayed regularly at University Hospital since January 1979 was assigned to a group. Each group has fourteen representatives assigned. Fifteen (15) exhibit spaces are available.
b. The groups will be assigned to a specific month's exhibit on a three (3) month rotation.
   Participation of each company was reviewed in January 1982, and the groups adjusted accordingly.
c. The Alternate Group includes the pharmaceutical representatives who have not exhibited since January 1981, and all nonpharmaceutical representatives.
d. The representatives in groups I, II, and III have priority in submitting applications to exhibit in the specific month assigned.
   1. This priority must be exercised by the last Wednesday of the month preceding the assigned exhibit.
   2. Any exhibit space left vacant one week prior to the exhibit date is open to any representative in the Alternate Group, and any representative in the other two groups.
   3. Applications for vacant exhibit space may be made no sooner than the Wednesday morning preceding the exhibit date (i.e., one week prior to the exhibit).
   4. Applications for vacant exhibit space will be accepted in order of receipt.
e. If a representative does not use scheduled and verified exhibit space, no refund may be granted and the representative's exhibit privileges may be curtailed at the discretion of the Director of Pharmacy.
f. Responsibility for coordinating with other representatives, the room set-up, specific display locations, and refreshments is assigned to one representative, who is selected by exhibitors to represent the group. This representative is given the privilege of displaying each month.

FIGURE 66.5

reference material used by the MSR. The MSR should be aware of any drug recall that the company initiates and should make arrangements to provide help in obtaining other supplies. In addition, during a hospital-wide disaster the MSR should be available to provide needed help. Although functions of individual MSRs may differ, their main goal is to promote the products of their company.

To maximize the usefulness of an MSR in the hospital, it is necessary to develop guidelines to control his or her activities. Without these guidelines, control over the type of information being disseminated, visits to restricted areas of the hospital, improper use of hospital personnel time, and inappropriate drug sampling may become problems. To control the MSR, specific guidelines or standards should be developed by the hospital.

These standards should be in writing and discussed with each MSR by the pharmacist. The pharmacist should keep a log of current MSRs with their telephone numbers and the date that the standards were discussed. The standards should include the following information:

1. Registration and orientation. The hospital should identify those people who fall into the classification of an MSR. These people should be given appropriate orientation to hospital rules and regulations.

2. Identification. It is important for visitors to be identified when they are in the hospital. Proper identification should be displayed at all times.

3. Authorized areas. Various areas of the hospital should be off limits to the MSR. The confidentiality of the patient and the patient's records must be maintained.

4. New drug requests. The mechanism to obtain a new product in the hospital should be outlined to the MSR. If the hospital has a formulary system, this should be explained to the MSR.

5. Samples. Drug samples left in various areas of the hospital may lead to inappropriate use. Control of all drugs within the hospital is the responsibility of the pharmacy department.

6. Exhibits. Displays are one way to disseminate information to the hospital staff. Without proper control, displays may lead to confusion as to which drugs are presently available in the institution.

Examples of written guidelines are given in Figures 66.3-66.6.

THE OHIO STATE UNIVERSITY HOSPITALS

Policy on Detailing by Medical Service Representatives

The Ohio State University Hospitals recognizes that Medical Service Representatives* play an important role as sources of information to staff members and employees of the hospitals in the selection, purchase, use and maintenance of pharmaceuticals and related supplies. However, the representative is a guest of the hospital and, as such, should provide his/her services in accordance with accepted rules of conduct and in a manner which provide the greatest benefit to the hospital and its staff. It is therefore necessary for all representatives to subscribe to the following rules:

1. Representatives shall wear an identification tag with their name and the name of their company while visiting the hospital.

2. Representatives are not permitted on any nursing or other patient care area, Emergency Department, or Ambulatory Clinics except by invitation of a member of the medical staff, the directors of Nursing or Pharmacy or their designee, or other hospital department head.

3. Representatives may detail attending staff members, department heads, and designees only by appointment scheduled in advance.

4. Representatives may not detail medical resident staff except by appointment and permission from the chief of the clinical division to which the resident is assigned.

5. Representatives are not permitted to use the hospital paging system to arrange appointments.

6. Medical, nursing, and other allied students may not be contacted by representatives except by invitation from a faculty member.

7. Drug samples or other drug packages are not allowed to be left on any patient care nursing unit, emergency department, or Ambulatory Clinics. Requests for drug samples by members of the medical staff may be delivered only to the physician's office.

8. Representatives are not permitted to prepare a formulary request form for an attending or resident physician's signature and they may not call on members of the Pharmacy and Therapeutics Committee to review any pending formulary requests.

9. Educational or other materials may be distributed only by U.S. mail. Requested materials may be delivered personally to the physician at his/her request.

10. Representatives are not permitted to attend medical and other educational conferences scheduled in the hospitals and medical school unless specifically invited by a member of the Attending Staff.

11. Representatives should keep the Department of Pharmacy informed of various matters affecting their company's drugs such as FDA recall notices, reformulation changes, price adjustments, new products, and materials to be left for evaluation in the hospitals. Representatives will visit the Pharmacy to provide any updated information relevant to their drug products and to authorize return of outdated products.

12. Representatives are expected to adhere to the hospitals' policies and regulations and to follow accepted professional protocol and conduct. Members of the hospital staff should report infractions of these rules or evidence of misconduct by representatives to the office of the Director of Pharmacy for proper disposition.

*Medical Service Representatives as used herein shall include salesmen, detail men, representatives or other employees or manufacturers, distributors, wholesalers, or suppliers of pharmaceuticals and related supplies.

Approved by the Pharmacy and Therapeutics Committee and the Medical Staff Administrative Committee.

FIGURE 66.6

THE OHIO STATE UNIVERSITY HOSPITAL

RETURN GOODS AUTHORIZATION

The Ohio State University is hereby authorized to return the products listed below for credit, subject to the return policies of the company. Credit should be issued on Ohio State University Purchase Order No. _____. The credit memorandum should be sent to:

The Ohio State University
Auditing Department
1800 Cannon Drive
Columbus, Ohio 43210

Return merchandise should be shipped to:

_____
_____
_____
_____

_____
Company Name

_____
Signature of Representative

Quantity   Item Description, size, N.D.C. number, etc.

FIGURE 66.7

IMPROVING RELATIONSHIPS

The MSR and the pharmacist should discuss problems and exchange ideas. An unusual increase or decrease in drug use may lead to out-of-stock items or to an excessive inventory. The pharmacist should be aware of any new use of a drug so that he or she may plan the inventory accordingly. In addition, if the pharmaceutical company is unable to supply its drug, then the MSR should work with the pharmacist to maintain needed drugs.

Drugs that are no longer used or that are out of date are an added inventory expense for the hospital. The MSR should work with the pharmacist to obtain credit for the items. The pharmacist may want to itemize these drugs (Fig. 66.7) or have the MSR perform this task. Pharmaceutical companies may want to change their product-dating procedures. If drugs were dated to expire only in January or July, the hospital pharmacist would be able to control more effectively returns and outdated items. An exchange of ed-

ucational material would also benefit the pharmacist and the MSR. The pharmaceutical company offers a great deal of educational material relating to its drugs and the diseases the drugs are used for. The pharmacist can use this information in promoting a rational drug therapy.

The pharmacist, in addition, may coordinate and participate in staff development programs. The MSR may increase his or her knowledge by attending these programs.

To improve the relationship between the pharmaceutical industry and the hospital pharmacist, communication should be increased between the two areas. One way to improve this communication is to have a formal orientation program for the MSR. This orientation program may be used to discuss the standards for the MSR at the hospital and, in addition, to provide the MSR with information so that he or she is familiar with the various hospital systems. A thorough understanding of the purchasing system (bids, vendor registration, use of wholesalers), drug delivery system (unit dose, IV admixtures), and formulary system will aid the MSR in providing necessary services to the pharmacist.

Finally, communication between the pharmaceutical industry and the hospital pharmacist must be open and ongoing. The hospital pharmacist must communicate his needs to the industry and the industry must strive to meet these needs. Scientific information regarding the physical nature of a drug (stability, compatibility, pH) and the clinical nature of a drug (pharmacokinetics) must be communicated to the pharmacist. Likewise, the pharmaceutical industry must communicate its needs to the hospital pharmacist and the hospital pharmacist must take time to meet these needs.

REFERENCES

1. Zellmer WA: Report of the study commission on pharmacy: Pharmacy and the pharmaceutical industry. *Am J Hosp Pharm* 33:893, 1976.

ADDITIONAL READING

Industry peer review opens hospital. *Hospitals* 47:66, 1973.
Burkholder D: The role of the pharmaceutical detailman in a large teaching hospital. *Am J Hosp Pharm* 20:275, 1963.
Hassan W: Medical service representation-pharmacist relationship. In *Hospital Pharmacy*. Philadelphia, Lea & Febiger, 1981.
Jeffrey L: Communication between medical service representatives and physicians. *Am J Hosp Pharm* 15:584, 1958.
Katz S, Triboletti M: The pharmaceutical industry's obligation to clinical pharmacists. *Drug Intell Clin Pharm* 11:740, 1977.
Lipman A: Therapeutic substitution. *Hosp Forul* 18:841, 1983.
Lipman A, Mullen H: Quality control of medical service representative activities in the hospital. *Am J Hosp Pharm* 31:167, 1974.
Phillips D, Smith J: Hospital-based training for pharmaceutical manufacturer's representatives. *Am J Hosp Pharm* 40:1661, 1983.
Stolar M: The need to improve hospital investigational drug policies and procedures. *Hosp Formul* 18:79, 1983.
Turco S: What hospital pharmacists expect from a medical service representative. *Hosp Pharm* 9:126, 1974.
Zellmer W: The euphoria factor. *Am J Hosp Pharm* 40:51, 1983.

CHAPTER 67

Disaster Plans

ZACHARY I. HANAN and CARMENCITA TRANQUILINO

Disasters may occur at anytime and can result from natural phenomena such as earthquakes, hurricanes, floods, tornadoes, volcanic eruptions, and tidal waves or from accidental or nuclear disasters. A disaster has been defined as a sudden calamitous event bringing great damage, loss, or destruction (1).

Hospitals have traditionally acknowledged their responsibility to have developed plans for handling mass casualty emergencies in accordance with their responsibility to provide the best possible care and treatment to the communities they serve.

Each type of disaster, whether natural, accidental, or nuclear, requires specific personnel and material resources and facilities different from one another. Therefore, it is necessary for hospitals to consider the potential for specific types of natural or accidental disasters that may have a potential for occurring within their specific geographic area, and to plan accordingly. Although it is beyond the scope of this chapter to delve into the total hospital disaster preparedness necessary to cope with the types of disasters that may occur, the objective is to focus on the specific goals of the department of pharmacy during a disaster, and how to best meet them. It is apparent these goals will be similar for most institutions, but the specific pharmaceutical supplies and manpower necessary to handle them may be dramatically different for a natural disaster vs a mass transit vs a nuclear disaster. It should be noted that additional considerations for a disaster plan for a possible nuclear accident take on a somewhat different complexity. The recent experience of the nuclear accident at Three Mile Island, near Harrisburg, Pennsylvania, illustrates the need for hospitals to consider a disaster plan that encompasses dealing with patients (and vehicles) exposed to nuclear radiation (triage, decontamination) and plans that may necessitate the area-wide evacuation of staff and patients (2).

The JCAH (3) specifies that it is the responsibility of each hospital and its medical staff to help promote, develop, and implement a community-based emergency plan. This plan should be based on each hospital's emergency capabilities, which may range from providing simple first aid to preparing casualties for transfer elsewhere, or to administering comprehensive care.

The 1985 *Accreditation Manual for Hospitals (AMH)*, under Standard V of the "Plant, Technology, and Safety Management" section, defines elements that are integral to a community disaster plan. This plan should address the need for an efficient system of notifying and assigning personnel, a unified medical command, sufficient utilities, food, and medical supplies, and a method for converting specified areas of the hospital into triage, observation, and treatment centers. The plan also should provide for a means of promptly identifying and transporting patients who are immediately dischargeable or transferable, for establishing a centralized public information center, and for developing security measures to control access to the health care facility in an emergency. In addition, a plan should provide for instructions on the use of elevators, alternative communication systems for use when normal communication systems are out or overtaxed, and the use of a special disaster medical record or tag that accompanies disaster victims at all times.

The standard emphasizes that the disaster plan should be developed in conjunction with other emergency facilities and civil authorities in the community to provide an efficient network of transportation and supplies to manage emergencies and to establish an effective chain of command.

To test the effectiveness of its written plan, each facility must conduct at least two drills each year. These rehearsals should be carried out with the participation of such local services as the fire, police, and civil defense departments and other area hospitals. Drills should be realistic and must involve medical, administrative, nursing, and other hospital staffs. Actual patient evacuation during the drills is optional. Each drill must be reviewed and a written report documenting its effectiveness must be developed.

Several basic principles for any plan dealing with a major disaster are (4):

1. It must be simple.
2. It must be capable of taking effect immediately.
3. It must be flexible to allow for variations in the type of disaster.
4. It must be adaptable to nights and weekends when the number of available staff is less than during the normal day staffing.
5. It should follow normal hospital procedure as much as possible to avoid the confusion of a disaster situation, and because only a small number to whom the disaster plan is issued will actually read it.

In consideration of these broad principles, institutions have used a number of options in writing their disaster

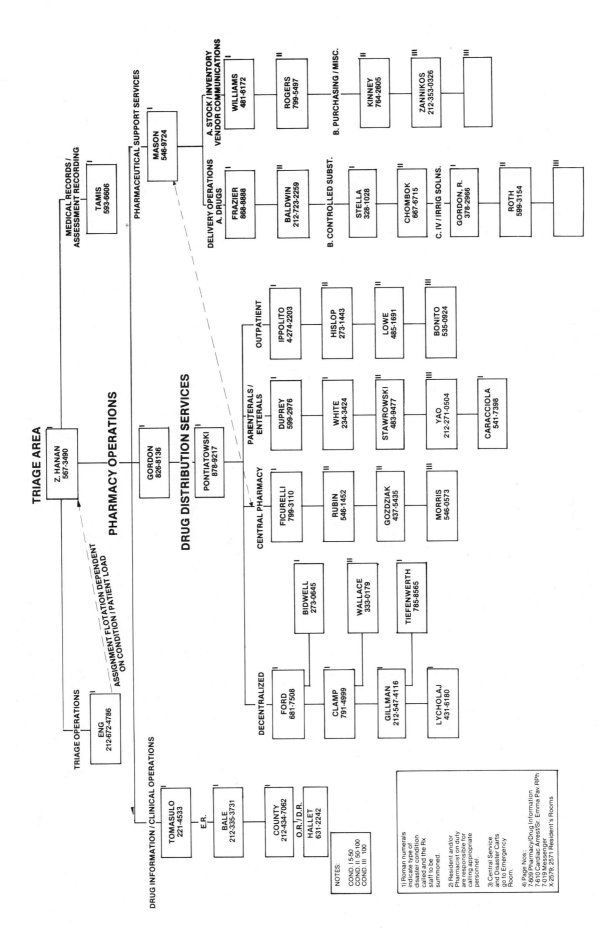

FIGURE 67.1 Department of Pharmacy, Mercy Hospital disaster alert plan.

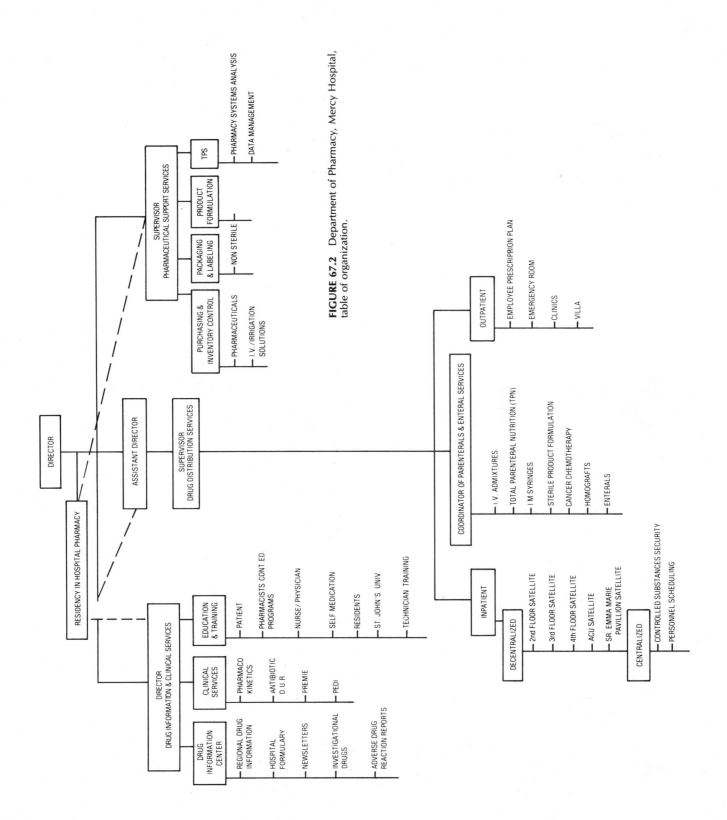

FIGURE 67.2 Department of Pharmacy, Mercy Hospital, table of organization.

manuals in the establishment of procedures for disaster preparedness (5-7). Disaster manuals should be concise and are best expressed as lists, charts, or in a looseleaf form for ease of updating.

Specifically, the disaster goals for a department of pharmacy have been outlined as follows (8,9):

1. To contact and provide sufficient pharmacy personnel to perform the required pharmaceutical services for both disaster victims and the patient needs within the hospital.
2. To establish a method of obtaining and providing an efficient supply of pharmaceuticals meeting the needs of a disaster.

In our institution, the Department of Pharmacy has selected the development of a disaster alert plan (Fig. 67.1) that follows a format similar to that of the department's organizational chart (Fig. 67.2). The disaster alert plan outlines the following:

1. Reference to the possible number of casualties of the disaster (condition I, II, III)
2. Pharmacy personnel and their home telephone numbers
3. The sequence of telephone calls that are to be made by the respective pharmacy personnel on duty when the disaster alert is called
4. Areas of service responsibility once pharmacy personnel arrive within the hospital

DISASTER COMMUNICATIONS AND PERSONNEL ASSIGNMENTS

Disaster communications for the department of pharmacy follow the same basic principles as outlined above for a disaster. The department's disaster plan can be described as follows:

Simple: The disaster chart is simple in that it is similar in format to the department's organization chart. Personnel assignments and responsibilities are, for the most part, almost identical to that of the organizational chart.

Immediate implementation: Pharmacy personnel within the hospital, on notification of a disaster alert, can immediately implement the chain of communication with appropriate off-duty pharmacy personnel.

Flexibility: The type of disaster (and potential number of casualties) can be easily adapted and communicated following the format of the disaster alert plan. Roman numerals adjacent to each of the names of pharmacy personnel indicate the type of disaster condition called (e.g., condition I, 5-50 victims, condition II, 50-100 victims, condition III, over 100 victims). Depending on the type of disaster, the appropriate number of specific pharmacy staff can be summoned.

Adaptable: The disaster alert plan is adaptable to days, nights, and weekends. Depending on when the disaster alert is called, pharmacy personnel may be on duty at the hospital, staffing their respective positions, or if they are off-duty, once they arrive at the hospital they assume their responsibilities as outlined and/or as assigned in the disaster alert plan.

Normal hospital procedure: The disaster alert plan, following the outline of the pharmacy organization chart, allows the pharmacy staff to follow normal hospital procedures and to automatically assume their respective positions. As such, the disaster plan can be easily adapted in the confusion, noise, and tragedy of a disaster situation.

SUPPLY OF PHARMACEUTICALS

The second goal of the pharmacy disaster plan, that of obtaining and providing an efficient supply of pharmaceuticals, can be met with consideration of the following:

A. Emergency room and disaster cart medications
B. Emergency procurement
   1. Pharmaceutic manufacturers
      a. Pharmaceuticals and IV solutions
      b. Drug information
   2. Drug wholesalers
   3. Local community and hospital pharmacies

EMERGENCY ROOM AND DISASTER CART MEDICATIONS

Ambulatory injured patients usually outnumber the more seriously injured in any disaster and the care of ambulatory injured patients will normally be rendered in the emergency department. The principles of triage, the sorting and allocation of treatment to disaster victims according to a system of priorities designed to maximize the number of survivors, are usually devoted to urgent measures in one area of the hospital with the primary objective of stabilizing the patients' conditions before transfering them to specific treatment areas such as a nursing unit or discharge. Treatment in the triage area will be immediate and will normally include, but is not limited to, control of hemorrhage, IV infusion, treating shock, covering large wounds or burns, taking blood for cross-matching administering, analgesics or sedatives, managing patients contaminated by radiation, etc. The provision of pharmaceuticals specifically during triage is limited to very specific drugs necessary for the immediate treatment of trauma, burns, or radiation injuries. An outline of emergency room and disaster cart medications (Table 67.1) by therapeutic class has been established with the approval of the Pharmacy and Therapeutics Committee. Some hospitals have established disaster carts or kits of pharmaceuticals housing only those pharmaceuticals necessary solely for immediate treatment and use in the triage area. The cart or kit may be stored in the emergency room or the pharmacy and can be wheeled or carried to the triage area by the pharmacist(s) assigned to this area as the need arises. The pharmaceuticals included in the emergency room are meant to be comprehensive in scope but limited in terms of numbers of drugs, without unnecessary therapeutic duplication, whereas the asterisked pharmaceuticals are those designed for use on the disaster cart.

Within our institution, the triage area is adjacent to the emergency room, and as the need for additional supplies of pharmaceuticals are necessary they can be obtained from the emergency room stock of medications. In addition, as outlined in the disaster alert plan, through the Division of Pharmaceutical Support Services of the department, the delivery of pharmaceuticals, controlled drugs, and IV and irrigation solutions will be provided as necessary to replenish stocks in both the emergency room and on the disaster cart in the triage area.

TABLE 67.1   Emergency Room and Disaster Cart Medications

4:00	Antihistamines	24:00	Cardiovascular drugs
	Chlorpheniramine	24:04	Cardiac drugs
	Diphenhydramine[a]		Bretylium tosylate
	Promethazine		Digoxin
8:00	Anti-infective agents		Lidocaine HCL
	8:12.02 Aminoglycosides		Procainamide
	Gentamicin		Propranolol
	8:12.04 Antifungal agents		Verapamil
	Amphotericin B	24:08	Hypotensive agents
	Nystatin		Diazoxide
	8:12.06 Cephalosporins		Hydralazine
	Cefazolin		Methyldopa
	Cephalexin		Nitroprusside
	8:12.07 Misc. beta-lactams		Reserpine
	Cefoxitin	24.12	Vasodilating agents
	8:12.16 Penicillins		Isosorbide dinitrate
	Ampicillin		Nitroglycerin
	Oxacillin	28:00	Central nervous system agents
	Penicillin G benzathine		28:08.04 Nonsteroidal anti-inflamatory agents
	Penicillin G potassium		Aspirin
	Penicillin G procaine		Phenylbutazone
	8:12.24 Tetracyclines		28:08.08 Opiate agonists
8:24	Sulfonamides		Codeine sulfate[a]
	Sulfamethoxazole		Fentanyl citrate[a]
	Sulfisoxazole		Meperidine[a]
8:36	Urinary anti-infectives		Morphine sulfate
	Phenazopyridine		Percodan
8:40	Misc. anti-infectives		28:08.12 Opiate partial agonists
	Bactrim		Nalbuphine
12:00	Autonomic drugs		28:08.92 Miscellaneous analgesics
12:04	Cholinergics		Acetaminophen
	Neostigmine[a]	28:10	Opiate antagonists
	12:08.04 Anti-parkinsonians		Naloxone
	Benztropine mesylate	28:12	Anticonvulsants
	12:08.08 Antispasmotics		28:12.04 Barbiturates
	Atropine sulfate[a]		Phenobarbital[a]
	Donnatal		28:12.12 Hydantoins
	Propantheline		Phenytoin
	Scopolamine HBR		28:12.92 Misc. anticonvulsants
12:12	Adrenergic agents		Magnesium sulfate 50%
	Dopamine HCL[a]		28:16.08 Tranquilizers
	Epinephrine[a]		Chlorpromazine
	Isoetharine		Haloperidol
	Isoproterenol		28:16.12 Misc. psychotherapeutic agents
	Metaraminol bitartrate		28:24.04 Barbiturates
	Norepinephrine		Pentobarbital sodium
12:16	Adrenergic blockers		Phenobarbital
	Cafergot		Secobarbital sodium
	Phentolamine		28:24.08 Benzodiazepines
12:20	Muscle relaxants		Chlordiazepoxide
	Methocarbamol		Clorazepate
	Pancuronium bromide		Diazepam[a]
	Succinylcholine[a]		28:24.92 Misc. anxiolytics
16:00	Blood derivatives		Hydroxyzine
	Albumin		Chloral hydrate
20:00	Blood formation and coagulation agents	36:00	Diagnostic agents
	20:12.04 Anticoagulants	36:04	Adrenal insufficiency
	Heparin sodium		Corticotropin
	20:12.08 Antiheparin agents	38:00	Disinfectants
	Protamine sulfate		Chlorhexidine[a]
	20:12.16 Hemostatics		Hydrogen peroxide[a]
	Aminocarproic acid[a]		Isopropyl alcohol[a]
	Gelatin absorbable[a]		Povidone iodine[a]
	Thrombin	40:00	Electrolyte caloric and water balance

[a]Pharmaceuticals that may be considered for a disaster cart or kit, solely for immediate treatment and use in the triage area.

TABLE 67.1, cont'd

40:04	Acidifying agents Ammonium chloride		Cyclopentolate Homatropine HBR Phenylephrine
40:08	Aklalinizing agents Sodium bicarbonate	52:32	Vasoconstrictors Oxymetozoline Phenylephrine
40:10	Ammonia detoxicants Lactulose	52:36	Misc eye, ear, nose, and throat agents Balanced salt solution ophthemic agents Fluorescein sodium[a] Lacri-lube
40:12	Replacement solutions Dext 5% 33S Dext 5% 45S Dext 5% W Dextrose 5% Lact/R[a] Dextrose 5% Ringers[a] Dextrose 5% water[a] Hetastarch[a] Potassium chloride[a] Ringer's injection[a] Ringer's lactate[a] Sodium chloride[a]	56:04	Gastrointestinal drugs Activated charcoal Aluminum hydroxide Mylanta
		56:08	Antidiarrhea agents Kaolin pectin Lomotil Paregoric
40:20	Caloric agents Dextrose[a]	56:10	Antiflatulents Simethicone
40:24	Salt and sugar substitutes	56:12	Cathartics and laxatives Bisacodyl Cascara sagrada Citrate of magnesium Phosphate enema
40:28	Diuretics Ethacrynic acid Furosemide Hydrochlorothiazide Mannitol		
		56:20	Emetics Ipecac
40:36	Irrigating solutions Sodium chloride 0.9%[a] Water for irrigation[a]	56:22	Antiemetics Dimenhydrinate Meclizine Prochlorperazine Trimethobenzamide
40:40	Uricosuric agents Probenicid		
48:00	Antitussives, expectorants, and mucolytics	56:40	Misc. gastrointestinal agents Cimetidine
48:16	Expectorants Guaifenesin Potassium iodine	68:00	Hormones and synthetic substitutes
		68:04	Adrenals Dexamethasone[a] Hydrocortisone sodium[a] Methylprednisolone Triamcinolone
48:24	Mucolytic agents Acetylcysteine 10%		

52:00	Eye, ear, nose and throat agents
	  52:04.04 Antibiotics
	                Chloramphenicol
	                Cortisporin
	                Gentamicin sulfate
	                Neo-Cortef
	                Neodecardron
	                Neosporin
	                Otobiotic
	                Polysporin
	  52:04.06 Antivirals
	                Idoxuridine
	  52:04.08 Sulfonamides
	                Sulfacetamide 10%
		68:16	Estrogens
			Premarin

		68:20	Antidiabetic agents
			  68:20.08 Insulins
			                Insulin lente
			                Insulin NPH
			                Insulin regular
			  68:20.92 Misc. antidiabetic agents
			                Glucagon

		68:28	Pituitary agents Vasopressin

52:08	Anti-inflammatory agents
	Dexamethasone
	Prednisolone
		68:36	Thyroid and antithyroid agents
			  68:36.08 Antithyroid agents
			                Potassium iodide[a]

52:10	Carbonic anhdrase inhibitors Acetazolamide	72:00	Local anesthetic agents Dibucaine HCL Lidocaine HCL[a] Procaine 1%
52:16	Local anesthetics Auralgan		
52:20	Miotics Pilocarpine	76:00	Oxytocics Oxytocin
52:24	Mydriatics Atropine sulfate	80:00	Serums, toxoids, and vaccines
		80:04	Serums

TABLE 67.1 Emergency Room and Disaster Cart Medications—cont'd

	Hepatitis B immune globulin Gamma globulin Tetanus immune globulin		84:06	Anti-inflammatory agents Bethamethasone Triamcinolone
80:08	Toxoids Tetanus toxoid absorbable		86:16	Respiratory muscle relaxants Aminophylline Tedral Theophylline
84:00	Skin and mucous membrane agents		96:00	Pharmaceutical aids Acetone Compound tincture of benzoin Petrolatum white surgical lubricant Talc
	84:04.04	Antibiotics Bacitracin Neosporin Polysporin		
	84:04.08	Antifungals Gentian violet Nystatin		
	84:04.16	Misc anti-infective agents Mafenide acetate[a] Silver sulfadiazine[a]		

EMERGENCY PROCUREMENT

Special considerations should also be given to establishing a mechanism for the emergency procurement of pharmaceuticals that are in short supply or high demand. Local hospital and community pharmacies, drug wholesalers, and pharmaceutical manufacturers should be identified as possible sources of drugs, supplies, and drug information. Lists of emergency phone numbers of pharmaceutical companies (10,11), local hospital and community pharmacies, and drug wholesalers for both sources of supply and assistance in the provision of drug information should be up to date and readily available. The National Clearing House for Poison Control Centers maintains a listing of emergency telephone numbers supplied by manufacturers that also contains a list of pharmaceutical companies (12).

CONCLUSION

Disaster planning in hospitals demands time and effort in anticipation of potential events that may never happen. Although disasters can vary dramatically, there are a number of basic components and predictable elements that merit advance consideration. Following the simple framework established for pharmacy involvement, the goals for providing sufficient pharmacy personnel and providing an efficient supply of pharmaceuticals can be met reasonably and efficiently under the stress of a disaster situation.

REFERENCES

1. *Webster's Ninth New Collegiate Dictionary.* Springfield, MA, Merriam-Webster, 1984.
2. Vinsel DB: Hospitals must plan for nuclear accidents. *Hospitals* 54:113-121, 1980.
3. Affeldt JE: Accreditation issues. *Hosp Med Staff* June 1983, pp 25-26, 1983.
4. Williams DJ: Major disasters—disaster planning in hospitals. *Br J Hosp Med* 308-322, 1979.
5. Ibid.
6. Henze HM, Harrison DC, et al: Disaster planning: Planning a first response. *J Ambulatory Care Mgt* 79-83, 1981.
7. Moore TD: Administrative approach to disaster preparedness in the pharmacy. *Am J Hosp Pharm* 36:1337-1341, 1979.
8. Bradgon RL, Gousse GC, et al: Regional disaster planning for hospital pharmacies. *Am J Hosp Pharm* 39:1913-1915, 1982.
9. Tranquilino C, Hanan ZI: Disaster alert plan for a hospital pharmacy. *Am J Hosp Pharm* 32:1259-1260, 1975.
10. Larson RL: Emergency telephone numbers of pharmaceutical companies. *Hosp Pharm* 18:333-338, 1983.
11. Larson RL: Effective communication in emergency situations. *J Am Pharm Assoc* NS24:58-66.
12. National Clearing House for Poison Control Centers: Emergency phone numbers. *Bulletin* 23:1-11, 1979.

Index